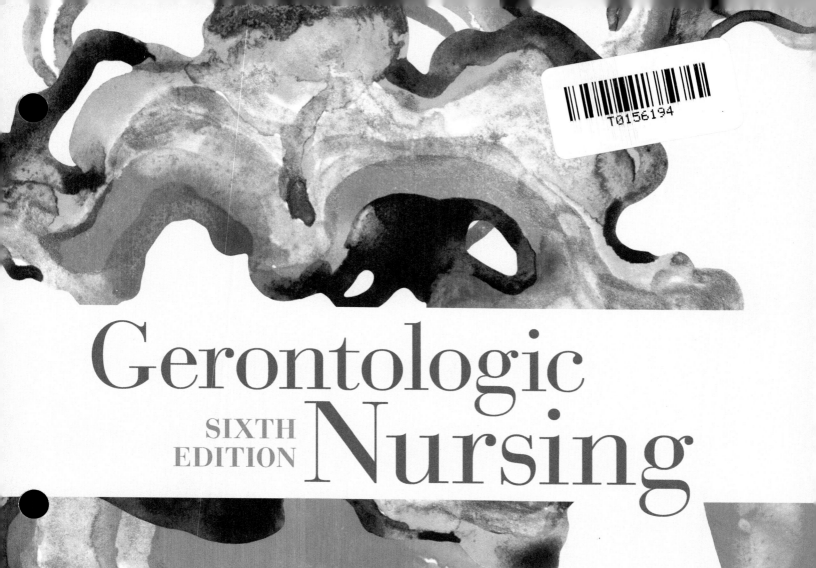

Gerontologic

SIXTH EDITION

Nursing

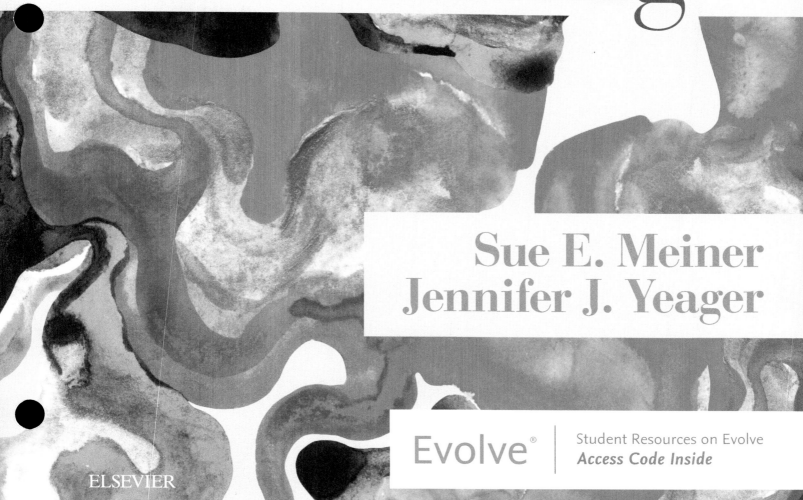

Sue E. Meiner
Jennifer J. Yeager

Evolve® | Student Resources on Evolve
Access Code Inside

ELSEVIER

Evolve®

YOU'VE JUST PURCHASED
MORE THAN A TEXTBOOK!

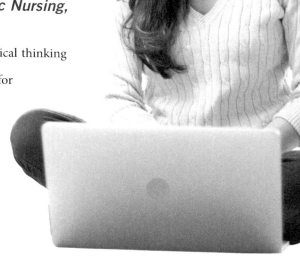

Evolve Student Resources for *Meiner: Gerontologic Nursing,*
6th Edition, **include the following:**

- **Case Studies** designed to apply knowledge and stimulate critical thinking

- 145 **NCLEX-RN® review questions** that cover each chapter for further study.

Activate the complete learning experience that comes with each
NEW textbook purchase by registering with your scratch-off access code at

http://evolve.elsevier.com/Meiner/gerontologic

If you purchased a used book and the scratch-off code at right has
already been revealed, the code may have been used and cannot
be re-used for registration. To purchase a new code to access these
valuable study resources, simply follow the link above.

REGISTER TODAY!

ELSEVIER

Gerontologic Nursing

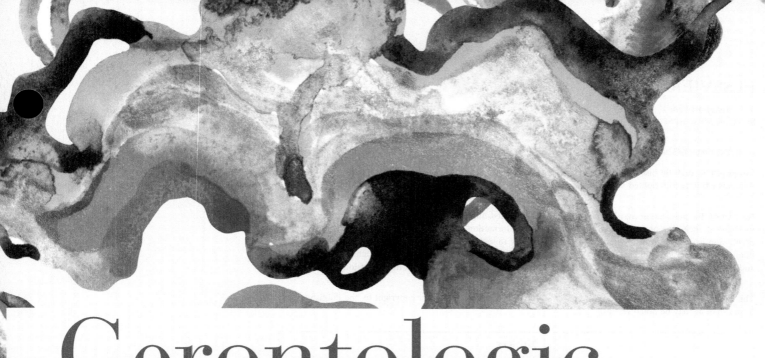

Gerontologic Nursing

SIXTH EDITION

Sue E. Meiner EdD, APRN, BC-GNP

President
Consultant on Health Issues, Inc.
McKinney, Texas
Formerly:
Nurse Practitioner in Private Practice
Las Vegas, Nevada
and
Assistant Professor
University of Nevada, Las Vegas
Las Vegas, Nevada

Jennifer J. Yeager PhD, RN, APRN

Assistant Professor and Director of the Graduate Nursing Program
Tarleton State University
Stephenville, Texas

ELSEVIER

ELSEVIER

3251 Riverport Lane
St. Louis, Missouri 63043

GERONTOLOGIC NURSING, SIXTH EDITION

ISBN: 978-0-323-49811-1

Notices

Library of Congress Control Number: 2018944983

Senior Content Strategist: Sandra Clark
Content Development Manager: Lisa Newton
Content Development Specialist: Laurel Shea
Publishing Services Manager: Deepthi Unni
Project Manager: Janish Ashwin Paul
Design Direction: Amy Buxton

Working together
to grow libraries in
developing countries

www.elsevier.com • www.bookaid.org

Printed in the United States of America
Last digit is the print number: 9 8 7 6 5 4 3 2 1

Special thanks to my husband, Tracy, for his dedicated support and reminders to "chapter, chapter, chapter"; and to my children Jacob and Joshua, thank you for keeping my spirits high. Of course, I wouldn't be me without bringing attention to Xander, my American Staffordshire Terrier, who spent many evenings curled up on my lap while I revised chapters.

Jennifer J. Yeager

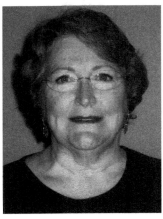

Sue E. Meiner, EdD, APRN, GNP-BC, began her nursing career in 1962 in St. Louis, Missouri. She began as a Licensed Practical Nurse (L.P.N.) prior to the availability of Associate Degree Nursing programs in the Midwest. She graduated from the second class of the Associate in Applied Science degree (A.D.N.) program from St. Louis Community College (Meramec campus). Continuing her education in nursing, she completed a Bachelor of Science in Nursing (B.S.N.) and a Master's of Science in Nursing (M.S.N.) from St. Louis University. Later she received her Doctor of Education (EdD) from Southern Illinois University at Edwardsville, and a Certificate as a Gerontological Nurse Practitioner from the Barnes-Jewish Hospital College of Nursing in St. Louis. Dr. Meiner held certifications as both a Gerontological Clinical Nurse Specialist and a Gerontological Nurse Practitioner from the American Nurses Credentialing Center (A.N.C.C.) of the American Nurses Association (ANA). She took additional courses toward counseling at Lindenwood College, St. Charles, Missouri. She has received numerous awards and has been asked to speak at local, regional, and national conferences and workshops. Dr. Meiner worked as a staff nurse in hospitals in the St. Louis area as well as home health nursing. Over time she worked as a hospital nursing supervisor and interim director of nursing. While her main clinical interest was in medical-surgical nursing, she began to focus on the special care needs of the older adult. She has practiced nursing for over 50 years; however, the last 30 years have been heavily focused in geriatric nursing. She has taught nursing at the L.P.N., A.D.N., B.S.N., and M.S.N. levels of education. She has been the Director of Nursing Programs at the L.P.N. and A.D.N. levels. Before returning to full-time clinical practice in Las Vegas as a Nurse Practitioner, she taught the final course of clinical nursing at the master's level at the University of Nevada, Las Vegas, School of Nursing. Her clinical practice was directed at chronic and tertiary pain management, with a focus on the needs of the older adult. Dr. Meiner has engaged in the support of nursing through advocacy of both nurses and patients and their families by serving part time as a Forensic Nurse. She has been active in legal nurse consulting since 1988 and incorporated her company in the early 2000s. Throughout those 25 years, she provided case reviews and expert witness testimony at depositions and trials across the United States. She authored and edited *Nursing Documentation: Legal Focus across Practice Setting* in 2000, as well as authored, coauthored, or edited multiple textbooks, and has written multiple professional articles on nursing care and issues. During 5 years in the 1980s, she was elected to serve her community of Creve Coeur, Missouri, as a Director of the Fire Protection District. In her free time, Dr. Meiner enjoys national and international travel and spending time with her family.

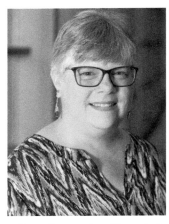

Jennifer J. Yeager, PhD, RN, APRN: I was called to be a nurse during my senior year in high school. I simply woke up one morning knowing that I was supposed to be a nurse; up till the day before, I had planned on becoming an English teacher. I am the only nurse in a large family of teachers.

The Air Force paid my way through nursing school in Portland, Oregon. So, after college, I moved to Texas to be a nurse at Wilford Hall Medical Center in San Antonio. I love the state; when I left the Air Force after six years, I stayed in Texas.

While I was in school in Portland, I looked at my instructors and knew I was supposed to fill their shoes one day. In the back of my mind, I set the goal to earn my doctoral degree before I turned 50 and become a nursing instructor. I met my goal through determination and hard work.

I have taught at Tarleton State University since 2007. Teaching students the art and science of nursing is the most wonderful opportunity imaginable. Although my background has been working with the elderly, I teach a variety of courses.

Reaching my goal meant sacrifice for both my family and me, but it has been worth it. Setting goals and reaching them through hard work, dedication, learning through mistakes but never quitting makes reaching the goal all the sweeter.

CONTRIBUTORS

Joanne Alderman, MSN, APRN-CNS, RN-BC, FNGNA
President, National Gerontological Nursing Association
President, National Organization, AMC-Geneva, Illinois
Physician/APRN Collaborative Community Practice
NICHE Coordinator
Grant Project Leader
CMS/OSDH
Tulsa, Oklahoma

Carol Ann Amann, PhD, MSN, RN-BC, CDP, FNGNA
Assistant Professor
Villa Maria School of Nursing
Gannon University
Erie, Pennsylvania

Linda Anne Bub, MSN, RN, GCNS-BC, FNGNA
Manager Nurse Residency and Onboarding
Aurora Academy
Aurora Health Care
Milwaukee, Wisconsin

Neva L. Crogan, PhD, ARNP, GNP-BC, ACHPN, FAAN
Professor of Nursing
Gonzaga University
Spokane, Washington

Beth Culross, PhD, RN, GCNS-BC, CRRN, FNGNA
Assistant Professor
College of Nursing
University of Nebraska Medical Center
Omaha, Nebraska

Ashley Davis, MSN, RN, PCCN
Instructor
Department of Nursing
Tarleton State University
Stephenville, Texas

Laurie M. Malone, PhD GNP-BC FAANP, FGSA
Professor of Nursing
Community and Family Practiced Nursing
University of North Carolina at Greensboro
Greensboro, North Carolina

Debra L. Sanders, PhD, RN, GCNS-BC
Assistant Professor of Nursing
Bloomsburg University
Bloomsburg, Pennsylvania

Colleen Steinhauser, MSN
Assistant Professor of Nursing
Nebraska Methodist College
Omaha, Nebraska

Mary Winton, PhD
Assistant Professor of Nursing
Tarleton State University
Stephenville, Texas

REVIEWERS

Rita Ferguson, PhD, RN, CHPN, CNE
Clinical Assistant Professor
College of Nursing
The University of Alabama in Huntsville
Huntsville, Alabama

Shelly Hanko, PhD, FNP-BC
Director of MSN Program
College of Nursing
University of Missouri–St. Louis
St. Louis, Missouri

Anna Rachel Olson, DNP, RN, APN, APRN, ANP/GNP-BC
Nurse Practitioner
Banner Health, Western Region
Adjunct Faculty, per diem
University of Northern Colorado
Loveland, Colorado

Janet P. Tracy, PhD, RN, CNE
Professor Emerita
Department of Nursing
William Paterson University
Wayne, New Jersey

Yakima Young-Shields, EdD, MSN, ANP-BC, APRN, ANCC
Assistant Teaching Professor
College of Nursing
University of Missouri–St. Louis
Adult-Geriatric NP Coordinator
Internal Medicine PCP
SSM Health Primary Care
St. Louis, Missouri

PREFACE

The field of gerontologic nursing has blossomed over the past decades as the population of Baby Boomers entered retirement age. The provision of quality health care for older adults is an ever-growing challenge. Issues related to health and illness across the care continuum must be provided within a cost-effective and resource-sparse environment. The largest group of patients in hospitals (outside of obstetric and pediatric units) is older adults. Residents of long-term care facilities and rehabilitation hospitals are predominantly older adults. The specialty of gerontologic nursing is in greater demand more than ever before.

Gerontologic Nursing, sixth edition, has been revised to provide today's students with a solid foundation to meet the future challenges of gerontologic nursing practice. This textbook provides comprehensive, theoretic, and practical information concerning concepts and issues relevant to the care of older adults across the care continuum. The extensive coverage of material provides the student with the information necessary to make sound clinical judgments while emphasizing the concepts, skills, and techniques of gerontologic nursing practice. Psychologic and sociocultural issues and aspects of older adult care are given special emphasis and are integrated throughout the textbook, reflecting the reality of practice with this unique population. Care of both well and sick older adults and their families and caregivers is included.

Intended for use by nursing students in all levels of professional nursing programs, *Gerontologic Nursing* was developed for use in either gerontologic nursing or medical-surgical courses, or within programs that integrate gerontologic content throughout the educational program.

ORGANIZATION

The 29 chapters in *Gerontologic Nursing* are divided into six parts:

Part 1, Introduction to Gerontologic Nursing, includes four chapters that serve as the foundation for the remainder of the textbook. These chapters provide a historical overview of gerontologic nursing and demographics related to aging; theories to guide care of the older adult; practice standards and legal and ethical issues related to care of the older adult across the care continuum; and assessment of the older adult, with a focus on cognition and functional status.

Part 2, Influences on Health and Illness, includes chapters on cultural, family, and socioeconomic and environmental influences. Health promotion and illness/disability prevention are also included.

Part 3, Influences on Quality of Life, details the needs and nursing care of older adults in the areas of nutrition, sleep and activity, safety, issues related to sexuality, pain management, and infection and inflammation.

Part 4, Diagnostic Studies and Pharmacologic Management, focuses on the nurse's role in effectively managing the nursing care of older patients related to drugs and aging, as well as laboratory and diagnostic testing in older adult patients.

Part 5, Nursing Care of Physiologic and Psychologic Disorders, contains chapters detailing nursing management of older adults with diseases or conditions affecting the function of body systems: integumentary, sensory, cardiovascular, respiratory, gastrointestinal, urinary, musculoskeletal, cognitive and neurologic, and endocrine.

Part 6, Health Care Transitions, contains chapters that detail nursing management of older adults as they transition across the care continuum, from wellness, to illness, to end-of-life care.

In organizing the textbook every attempt was made to ensure a logical sequence by grouping related topics. However, it is not necessary to read the text in sequence. A detailed table of contents and an extensive index is included. It is hoped that this approach provides easy access to information of interest.

FORMAT

The sixth edition has been revised and reflects the growth and change of gerontologic nursing practice and the learning needs of today's student. The presentation of content has been designed for ease of use and reference. The textbook's visual appeal has been carefully planned to make it both aesthetically pleasing and easy to read and follow. Clinical examples depict nurses practicing in many different roles in a wide variety of practice settings, reflecting current practice patterns.

All body system chapters include an overview of age-related changes in structure and function. Common problems and conditions within each of the chapters are presented in a format that includes the definition, etiology, pathophysiology, and typical clinical presentation for each. The *Nursing Management* of the problems and conditions is central to each of these chapters and follows the nursing process format of assessment, diagnosis, planning and expected outcomes, intervention, and evaluation. *Nursing Care Plans* for selected problems and conditions begin with a realistic clinical situation and emphasize nursing diagnoses pertinent to the situation, expected outcomes, and nursing interventions, all within an easy-to-reference, two-column format.

FEATURES

Each chapter begins with Learning Objectives to help the student focus on important subject matter, followed by *What Would You Do?* scenarios to stimulate thinking. Patient/Family Teaching boxes are included where appropriate, providing key information on what to teach patients and families to enhance their knowledge and promote active participation in their care. Health Promotion/Illness Prevention boxes are included in the text, which identify activities and interventions that promote a healthy lifestyle and prevent disease and illness. Nutritional Considerations boxes are found throughout the text to stress the importance of nutrition in the care of older adults. Evidence-Based Practice boxes are presented in each chapter to emphasize the application of relevant study findings to current nursing practice and allow students to reflect on how to integrate evidence-based practice into everyday nursing practice. Cultural Awareness boxes are included where applicable to develop the student's cultural sensitivity and promote the delivery of culture-specific care. Home Care boxes are presented at the end of appropriate chapters to provide pragmatic sugges-

tions for care of the homebound patient and family. Finally, each chapter concludes with a brief summary, followed by Key Points that highlight important principles discussed in the chapter. Critical Thinking Exercises at the end of every chapter stimulate students to carefully consider the material learned and apply their knowledge to the situation presented.

As the scope of gerontologic nursing practice continues to expand, so must the knowledge guiding that practice reflect the most current standards and guidelines. Every effort has been made to incorporate the most current standards and guidelines from appropriate agencies into the sixth edition of this text.

Jennifer J. Yeager

ACKNOWLEDGMENTS

Heartfelt thanks must be given to Sue Meiner for placing her trust in me to continue her work on this text. The development of this sixth edition would not have been possible without the combined efforts of many talented professionals who supported me throughout the entire process. Without the tireless work of the contributing authors, who have dedicated their careers to caring for older adults, this edition would not be possible.

A special recognition goes to the editorial and production team at Elsevier. This team of professionals worked extremely hard to assist me in meeting the deadlines. I want to call special attention to Laurel Shea, who kept me on track down to the last second. Her patience is greatly appreciated!

Jennifer J. Yeager

CONTENTS

PART I

Introduction to Gerontologic Nursing

Overview of Gerontologic Nursing

Jennifer J. Yeager, PhD, RN, APRN

ⓔ http://evolve.elsevier.com/Meiner/gerontologic

LEARNING OBJECTIVES

On completion of this chapter, the reader will be able to:

1. Trace the historic development of gerontologic nursing as a specialty.
2. Distinguish the educational preparation, practice roles, and certification requirements of the gerontologic nurse generalist, acute or primary care nurse practitioner, and adult-gerontologic clinical nurse specialist.
3. Discuss the major demographic trends in the United States in relation to the older adult population.
4. Describe the effects of each of the following factors on the health, well-being, and life expectancy of older adults:
   - Gender
   - Marital status
   - Race or ethnicity
   - Living situation
   - Educational status
   - Economic status
   - Functional status
5. Discuss how the aging of society will affect the future of health care delivery.
6. Explore the concept of ageism as it relates to the care of older adults in various settings.
7. Identify the issues influencing gerontologic nursing education.
8. Analyze the issues affecting gerontologic nursing research.

WHAT WOULD YOU DO?

What would you do if you were faced with the following situations?

- You have been a nurse for 6 years; many of your patients are over the age of 65. Your supervisor requests you become certified as a gerontology nurse; upon reflection, you realize this is a wonderful idea. What steps would you take to achieve this goal?
- You discover your 78-year-old patient has been cutting her pills in half. Because of this, her hypertension is uncontrolled. What factors might play into this decision?

FOUNDATIONS OF THE SPECIALTY OF GERONTOLOGIC NURSING

One in seven Americans are over the age of 65. Between 2005 and 2015, there was a 30% growth in the number of adults over 65 years of age. The number of older adults has grown steadily since 1900, and they continue to be the fastest growing segment of the population (Administration on Aging [AOA], 2017). The specialty of gerontologic nursing has grown in recognition since the Baby Boomers began to turn 65 years old in 2011. However, this has not always been the case, and the struggle for recognition can be traced back to the beginning of the 20th century.

Previous author: Sue E. Meiner, EdD, APRN, BC, GNP.

History and Evolution

Burnside (1988) conducted an extensive review of historical materials related to gerontologic nursing. Researching the years between 1900 and 1940, she found 23 writings with a focus on older adults that covered such topics as rural nursing, almshouses, and private duty nursing, as well as early case studies and clinical issues addressing home care for fractured femurs, dementia, and delirium. An anonymous *American Journal of Nursing* editorial in 1925 is thought to be one of the earliest calls for a nursing specialty in older adult care ("Care of the Aged," 1925).

Similarly, Stevens (1994), examined journal articles between 1903 and 1990, looking for those with a focus on nursing care of the older adult, health concerns of the older adult, or other issues facing older adults. Between 1903 and 1950, only one article was published. Between 1960 and 1990, a steady increase in literature with a focus on the older adult was noted.

Professional Origins

In 1966 the American Nurses Association (ANA) established the Division of Geriatric Nursing Practice and defined geriatric nursing as "concerned with the assessment of nursing needs of older people; planning and implementing nursing care to meet those needs; and evaluating the effectiveness of such care." In 1976, the name *The Division of Geriatric Nursing Practice* was changed to *The Division of Gerontologic Nursing Practice* to reflect the nursing roles of providing care to healthy, ill, and frail older persons. The division came to be called *The Council of*

Gerontologic Nursing in 1984 to encompass issues beyond clinical practice. Certification for the Gerontologic Clinical Nurse Specialist (GCNS) was established through the ANA in 1989. In 2013 the differences in acute care and primary care for gerontologic nurse practitioners (GNPs) were identified and separate certification examinations were established by the American Nurses Credentialing Center (American Nurses Credentialing Center [ANCC], 2017).

Standards of Practice

The years 1960 to 1970 were characterized by many "firsts," as the specialty devoted to the care of older adults began its exciting development. Journals, textbooks, workshops and seminars, formal education programs, professional certification, and research with a focus on gerontologic nursing have since evolved. However, the singular event that truly legitimized the specialty occurred in 1969 when a committee appointed by the ANA Division of Geriatric Nursing Practice completed the first *Standards of Practice for Geriatric Nursing*. These standards were widely circulated during the next several years; in 1976 they were revised, and the title was changed to *Standards of Gerontological Nursing Practice*. In 1981 *A Statement on the Scope of Gerontological Nursing Practice* was published. The revised *Scope and Standards of Gerontological Nursing Practice* was published in 1987, 1995, and 2010. The changes to this document reflect the comprehensive concepts and dimensions of practice for the nurse working with older adults. In 2010 the revised *Scope and Standards of Gerontological Nursing Practice* not only reflected the nature and scope of current gerontologic nursing practice but also incorporated the concepts of health promotion, health maintenance, disease prevention, and self-care (ANA, 2017).

In 2017 the ANA revised its statement incorporating the *Nursing: Scope & Standards of Practice* (3rd ed., revised 2015) and the *Code of Ethics for Nurses with Interpretative Statements* (revised 2015) to provide a resource "of the duties that all registered nurses, regardless of role, population, or specialty, are expected to perform competently. Those standards are identified in two categories: a) Standards of Practice that describe a competent level of nursing practice as demonstrated by the nursing process, and b) Standards of Professional Performance that describe a competent level of behavior in the professional role" (ANA, 2017, p. 4). Further information can be found on the ANA website: http://www.nursingworld.org.

Another hallmark in the continued growth of the gerontologic nursing specialty occurred in 1973 when the first gerontologic nurses were certified through the ANA. Certification is an additional credential granted by the ANCC (a subsidiary of the ANA), providing a means of recognizing specialized knowledge and clinical competence (ANCC, 2017). Certification is usually voluntary. In some cases, certification may mean eligibility for third-party reimbursement for nursing services rendered. From the initial certification offering as a generalist in gerontologic nursing, to the first GNP examination offering in 1979, to the GCNS examination first administered in 1989, the gerontologic nursing specialty has continued to grow and attract a high level of interest. The first combined certification for either acute care Adult-Gerontologic Nurse Specialist (AGCNS) or primary care AGCNS examination took place in 2014. Eligibility criteria for the application process to take any one of the four certification examinations can be found in Box 1.1. Because changes are fluid, contact the ANCC credentialing center for up-to-date requirements. Additional information can be retrieved from http://www.nursecredentialing.org/Certification.aspx.

Roles
The Generalist Nurse

The growth of the nursing profession, increasing educational opportunities, demographic changes, and changes in health care delivery systems have all influenced the development of the generalist nurse's role in adult and gerontologic nursing as well as the advanced practice roles. The generalist in gerontologic nursing has completed a basic entry-level educational program and is licensed as a registered nurse (RN). A generalist nurse may practice in a wide variety of settings, including home and the community. The challenge of the gerontologic nurse generalist is to identify older adults' strengths and assist them to maximize their independence. Older adults should participate as much as possible in making decisions about their care. The generalist nurse consults with the advanced practice nurse and other interdisciplinary health care professionals for assistance in meeting the complex care needs of older adults.

The Clinical Nurse Specialist

The AGCNS has the requirement of at least a master's degree in nursing and must be licensed as an RN. The first clinical nurse specialist program was launched in 1966 at Duke University. The gerontologic master's program typically focuses on the advanced knowledge and skills required to care for younger through older adults in a wide variety of settings, and the graduate is prepared to assume a leadership role in the delivery of that care. AGCNSs have an expert understanding of the dynamics, pathophysiology, and psychosocial aspects of aging. They use advanced diagnostic and assessment skills and nursing interventions to manage and improve patient care (ANCC, 2017). The AGCNS functions as a clinician, educator, consultant, administrator, or researcher to plan care or improve the quality of nursing care for adults and their families. Specialists provide comprehensive care based on theory and research. Today, AGCNSs may be found practicing in acute care hospitals, long-term care or home care settings, or independent practices.

The Nurse Practitioner

The Adult Gerontologic Acute Care or Primary Care Nurse Practitioner (AGACNP/AGPCNP) may be educationally prepared in various ways but must hold a license as an RN. In the early 1970s the first AGNPs were prepared primarily through continuing education programs. Another early group of AGNPs received their training and clinical supervision from physicians. Only since the late 1980s has master's level education with a focus on primary care been available. As a provider of primary care and a case manager, the AGNP conducts health assessments; identifies nursing diagnoses; and plans, implements, and evaluates nursing care for adult and older patients.

BOX 1.1   American Nurses Credentialing Center Eligibility Requirements for Certification in Gerontologic Nursing

Gerontological Nurse (Registered Nurse—Board Certified [RN-BC])

The nurse must meet all the following requirements before application for examination:

1. Currently hold an active registered nurse (RN) license in the United States or its territories or the professional, legally recognized equivalent in another country.
2. Have practiced the equivalent of 2 years, full time, as an RN.
3. Have completed clinical practice of at least 2000 hours in gerontologic nursing within the past 3 years.
4. Have had 30 contact hours of continuing education applicable to gerontologic nursing within the past 3 years.

Adult-Gerontology Acute Care Nurse Practitioner (AGACNP–BC)

The nurse must meet all the following requirements:

1. Currently hold an active RN license in the United States or its territories or the professional, legally recognized equivalent in another country.
2. Hold a master's, postgraduate, or doctorate degree from an adult-gerontology acute care nurse practitioner program accredited by the Commission on Collegiate Nursing Education (CCNE) or the Accreditation Commission for Education in Nursing (ACEN).
3. A minimum of 500 faculty-supervised clinical hours must be included in the adult-gerontology acute care nurse practitioner role and population.
4. Three separate, comprehensive graduate-level courses in the following:
   a. Advanced physiology/pathophysiology, including general principles that apply across the life span
   b. Advanced health assessment, which includes assessment of all human systems, advanced assessment techniques, concepts, and approaches
   c. Advanced pharmacology, which includes pharmacodynamics, pharmacokinetics, and pharmacotherapeutics of all broad categories of agents

Adult-Gerontology Primary Care Nurse Practitioner (AGPCNP–BC)

The nurse must meet all the following requirements:

1. Currently hold an active RN license in the United States or its territories or the professional, legally recognized equivalent in another country.
2. Hold a master's, postgraduate, or doctorate degree from an adult-gerontology primary care nurse practitioner program accredited by the CCNE or the ACEN.

3. A minimum of 500 hours of faculty-supervised clinical hours must be included in the adult-gerontology primary care nurse practitioner role and population.
4. Three separate, comprehensive graduate-level courses in the following:
   a. Advanced physiology/pathophysiology, including general principles that apply across the life span
   b. Advanced health assessment, which includes assessment of all human systems, advanced assessment techniques, concepts, and approaches
   c. Advanced pharmacology, which includes pharmacodynamics, pharmacokinetics, and pharmacotherapeutics
5. Content in:
   a. Health promotion and/or maintenance
   b. Differential diagnosis and disease management, including the use and prescription of pharmacologic and nonpharmacologic interventions

Adult-Gerontology Clinical Nurse Specialist (AGCNS–BC)

The nurse must meet all the following requirements:

1. Currently hold an active RN license in the United States or its territories or the professional, legally recognized equivalent in another country.
2. Hold a master's, postgraduate, or doctorate degree from an adult-gerontology clinical nurse specialist program accredited by the CCNE or the ACEN.
3. A minimum of 500 hours of faculty-supervised clinical hours must be included in the adult-gerontology clinical nurse specialist role and population. The adult-gerontology clinical nurse specialist program must include content across the health continuum from wellness through acute care.
4. Three separate, comprehensive graduate-level courses in the following:
   a. Advanced physiology/pathophysiology, including general principles that apply across the life span
   b. Advanced health assessment, which includes assessment of all human systems, advanced assessment techniques, concepts, and approaches
   c. Advanced pharmacology, which includes pharmacodynamics, pharmacokinetics, and pharmacotherapeutics of all broad categories of agents
5. Content in:
   a. Health promotion and/or maintenance
   b. Differential diagnosis and disease management, including the use and prescription of pharmacologic and nonpharmacologic interventions

More details on these certifications can be found online at http://nursecredentialing.org/Certification.

Modified from ANCC Certification Center. (2017). Retrieved from http://www.nursecredentialing.org/Certification. Accessed on November 6, 2017. To keep abreast of the changing scope, standards, and education requirements, the eligibility criteria are reviewed annually and are subject to change. When applying to take a certification examination, request a current catalog from ANCC; compliance with the current eligibility criteria is required. Applications can be downloaded from the Internet.

The AGNP has knowledge and skills to detect and manage limited acute and chronic stable conditions; coordination and collaboration with other health care providers is a related essential function. The acute care or primary care AGNP's activities include interventions for health promotion, maintenance, and restoration. AGNPs provide acute or primary ambulatory care in an independent practice or in a collaborative practice with a physician; they also practice in settings across the continuum of care, including the acute care hospital, subacute care center, ambulatory care setting, and long-term care setting. Health maintenance organizations (HMOs) are now including acute care or primary care AGNPs on their provider panels. Certification can elevate the status of the nurse practicing with older adults in any setting. More important, it enables the nurse to ensure the delivery of quality care to older adult patients. In most states in the United States, AGNPs hold prescriptive authority for most drugs. Each state has determined the type and extent of prescriptive authority permitted.

Terminology

Any discussion of older adult nursing is complicated by the wide variety of terms used interchangeably to describe the specialty. Some terms are used because of personal preference or because they suggest a certain perspective. Still others are avoided because of the negative inferences they evoke. As described in the preceding overview of the evolution of the specialty, the terminology has changed over the years. The following are the most commonly used terms and definitions:

- *Geriatrics*—from the Greek *geras,* meaning "old age," geriatrics is the branch of medicine that deals with the diseases and problems of old age. Viewed by many nurses as having limited application to nursing because of its medical and disease orientation, the term *geriatrics* is generally not used when describing the nursing care of older adults.
- *Gerontology*—from the Greek *geron,* meaning "old man," gerontology is the scientific study of the process of aging and the problems of older adults; it includes biologic, sociologic, psychological, and economic aspects.
- *Gerontologic nursing*—this specialty of nursing involves assessing the health and functional status of older adults, planning and implementing health care and services to meet identified needs, and evaluating the effectiveness of such care. *Gerontologic nursing* is the term most often used by nurses specializing in this field.
- *Gerontic nursing*—this term was developed by Gunter and Estes in 1979 and is meant to be more inclusive than *geriatric* or *gerontologic nursing* because it is not limited to diseases or scientific principles. Gerontic nursing connotes the nursing of older persons—the art and practice of nurturing, caring, and comforting. This term has not gained wide acceptance, but some view it as a more appropriate description of the specialty.

These terms and their usage spark a great deal of interest and controversy among nurses practicing with older adults. As the specialty continues to grow and develop, it is likely that the terminology will too.

DEMOGRAPHIC PROFILE OF THE OLDER POPULATION

Nursing care of the older adult has come a long way from its beginning in almshouses and nursing homes. Nurses today find themselves caring for older adults in a wide variety of settings, including, but not limited to, emergency departments, medical-surgical and critical care units in hospitals, outpatient clinics and surgical centers, home care agencies, hospices, and rehabilitation and long-term care centers. Nurses in any of these settings need only count the number of adults 65 or older to understand firsthand what demographers have termed the *graying of America*. Although this trend has already attracted the attention of the health care marketplace, it promises to become an even greater influence on health care organizations. It is clearly a trend that promises to shape the future practice of nursing in profound and dramatic ways.

Demography is the science dealing with the distribution, density, and vital statistics of human populations. What follows is a review of basic demographic facts about older adults. Keep in mind while reading that the rates and intensity of aging are highly variable and individual. It occurs gradually and in no predictable sequence.

Before examining the statistics surrounding aging in America, it is important to understand how society arrived at the age of 65 as the beginning of older adulthood. Many ascribe this definition of retirement age to Germany, the first nation to adopt an insurance program for older adults in 1889, under the direction of Chancellor Otto Von Bismark, who stated, "...those who are disabled from work by age and invalidity have a well-grounded claim to care from the state" (Social Security History, n.d., para. 1). However, the decision to adopt 65 as the age of retirement in the United States was based on actuarial studies and evaluation of state old-age pension systems already in place at the time. Within the existing systems, retirement age varied between 65 and 70. Studies "showed that using age 65 produced a manageable system that could easily be made self-sustaining with only modest levels of payroll taxation" (Age 65 Retirement, n.d., para. 3).

When the American Social Security program was established in 1935, it was believed that age 65 would be a reasonable age for allocating benefits and services. Today, with so many older persons living productive, highly functional lives well beyond age 65, this age has become an inappropriate one for determining whether a person is old. However, demographic information and other forms of data are still reported using age 65 as the defining standard for *old*. Consequently, it is not uncommon to see older persons classified as *young-old, middle-old,* or *old-old.*

Although grouping older persons is useful in some circumstances, nurses are cautioned against thinking all persons older than age 65 as similar. In fact, older persons are far from a homogeneous group. Landmarks for human growth and development are well established for infancy through middle age, but few landmarks have been discretely defined for older adulthood. In fact, most developmental landmarks described for later life categorize all older persons in the older-than-65 group. One could argue, from a developmental perspective, that great differences exist among 65-, 75-, 85-, and 95-year-olds as they do among 2-, 3-, 4-, and 5-year-olds; yet, no definitive landmarks for older adult development have been established. Consequently, nurses are urged to view each older patient as one would any patient—a being with a richly diverse and unique array of internal and external variables that ultimately influence how the person thinks and acts. Understanding how the variables interact with and affect older adults enables the nurse to provide individualized care. Additionally, nurses are encouraged to use each patient as his or her own standard, comparing the patient's previous pattern of health and function with current status.

The Older Population

For several decades, the American Association of Retired Persons (AARP) has maintained a yearly update of the key indicators of well-being of older adults in America. The AARP is a nonprofit, nonpartisan membership organization for people age 50 or older. The AARP is dedicated to enhancing the quality of life for all Americans as they age. The association acknowledges that its members receive a wide range of unique benefits, special products, and services (AARP, n.d.). Additional information can be found at their website: https://www.aarp.org.

The federal government maintains aging statistics available to the public. These publications include an annual chart book with the name of the year. Information can be found at https://www.acl.gov/aging-and-disability-in-america/data-and-research/profile-older-americans. This is now a part of public census and reporting data.

The rapid growth of the older adult population segment is not just an American issue. According to the United Nations Population Fund (UNFPA, 2012), the rapid aging of the world population "is an unprecedented phenomenon that is affecting nearly all countries of the world" (p. 20). It is a result of falling fertility rates, reduced infant and child mortality, improved sanitation, advances in vaccination, and increasing survival at older ages. In developed countries, life expectancy is 78 years; in developing countries, life expectancy is 68 years. Life expectancy is expected to continue to increase. By 2050, those born in developed countries are expected to live an average of 83 years; those in developing countries are expected to live an average of 74 years (UNFPA, 2012).

Highlights of the Profile of Older Americans

As stated previously, people are living longer. The population aged 85 and older increased to 6.3 million in 2015 and are expected to reach 14.6 million by 2040. Adults 65 and older numbered 47.8 million, which is an increase of 30% since 2005. One in every seven Americans is an older adult. This accounts for 14.9% of the population of the United States (AOA, 2017). See Fig. 1.1 for population trends of persons 65 years or older through 2060.

Gender and Marital Status

Women live longer than men for a variety of reasons, including reduced maternal mortality, decreased death rates from accidents, and increased death rates in men from all chronic diseases except diabetes. The protective effects of estrogen, versus that of testosterone, are also hypothesized to play a role in female longevity (Robson, 2015; Williams, 2017). Older adults reaching age 65 have an average life expectancy of an additional 19.4 years (20.6 years for women and 18 years for men). Older women continue to outnumber older men—in 2015 there were 26.7 million older women compared with 21.1 million older men. Older men are much more likely to be married than older women—70% of men versus 45% of women. In 2016 34% of women older than age 65 were widows (AOA, 2017). Nearly half (46%) of older women over the age of 75 live alone. Marital status is an important determinant of health and well-being because it influences income, mobility, housing, intimacy, and social interaction.

The differences between the proportions of older women and older men is expected to continue to increase as the size of the age group older than 85 increases, and it is a group in which women represent the majority. This demographic fact has important health care and policy implications because most older women are likely to be poor, live alone, and have a greater degree of functional impairment and chronic disease. The resulting increased reliance on social, financial, and health-related resources, coupled with emerging health care reforms, points to an uncertain future for older women. Because of these considerations, many gerontologists view aging as significantly a woman's problem. The nursing profession, and gerontologic nurses in particular, must assume a prominent role in the political arena and advocate for an agenda that addresses this important issue.

Race and Ethnicity

"By 2044, more than half of all Americans are projected to belong to a minority group" (Colby & Ortman, 2015, p.1). Statistics from 2015 indicate that 22% of persons 65 or older were

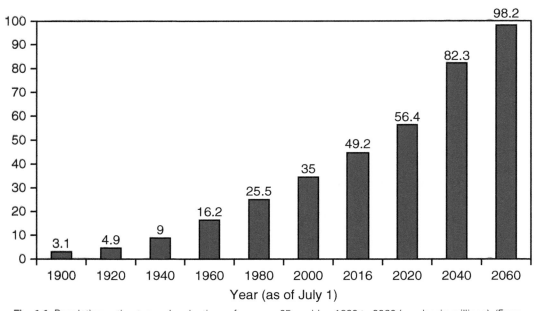

Fig. 1.1 Population estimates and projections of persons 65 or older: 1900 to 2060 (number in millions). (From Administration on Aging. [2018]. *2017 profile of older Americans.* Washington, DC: Administration for Community Living, U.S. Department of Health and Human Services.)

minorities: 9% were African Americans (not Hispanic), 4% were Asian or Pacific Islander (non-Hispanic), and fewer than 1% were American Indian or Native Hawaiian. In addition, 0.7% of persons older than 65 identified themselves as being of two or more races. Persons of Hispanic origin (of any race) were 8% of the older population (AOA, 2017).

People of Hispanic origin may be of any race, but their origins are in the Spanish-speaking countries of Central or South America. The census counts them by racial groups, usually as white, black, or other. The higher proportion of older whites is expected to remain stable and continue into the mid-twenty-first century, at which time the nonwhite segment of the population is expected to increase at a higher rate. Hispanics will continue to be one of the fastest-growing segments, and the numbers of African Americans, Native Americans, Native Alaskans, Asians, and Pacific Islanders will also increase. The nursing profession must consider the effect of such changing demographic characteristics, as the health status of diverse populations presents unique nursing care challenges.

Living Arrangements

Living arrangements differ according to the needs and preferences of each person. Most older adults prefer to live in their own homes and communities (referred to as *aging in place*). The older adult's home may be a single-family home (68%), an apartment (19%) or duplex-type home (6%), a manufactured or mobile home (6%), or RV (0.1%; Johnson & Appold, 2017). The arrangements might include living alone, with family members, or with an unrelated individual. For those living independently, additional in-home care may be required; assisted-living communities, continuing care retirement communities, group homes, and the controlled environments of long-term care are also options. A person's overall degree of health and well-being greatly influences the selection of housing as they age. Ideally, housing should be selected to promote functional independence, but the need for safety and social interaction must also be considered.

Statistics show that approximately 3.1% of all adults older than 65 are institutionalized in long-term care facilities or nursing homes. About 29% of noninstitutionalized older adults, or 13.6 million persons, live alone, according to recent figures. Women comprise most of this group; they number 9.3 million compared with 4.3 million men. Of women older than 75, nearly half live alone (AOA, 2017).

As people age, they are more vulnerable to multiple losses and frailty. Frail older adults need more intensive care across all health care settings. Despite the growth of life-extending therapies and the continuous development of highly sophisticated treatment measures, the current health care delivery system is still not equipped to effectively manage the needs of this segment of the population.

Older adults have unique responses to the factors that influence their health status. Advancing age is associated with more physical frailty because of the increased incidence of chronic disease, greater vulnerability to illness and injury, diminished physical functioning, and the increased likelihood of developing cognitive impairment. Additionally, psychological, social, environmental, and financial factors play a significant role in the level of frailty. Nevertheless, not *all* older adults are frail. The expectation of wellness, even in the presence of chronic illness and significant impairment, must be incorporated into the consciousness *and* practice of nurses who interact with this population. (See Fig. 1.2 for living arrangements of persons age 65 and older.)

In 2015 the median value of homes owned by older persons was $150,000; the median year of construction for these homes was 1969. About 78% percent of homeowners had paid off their homes. However, much of an older adult's income went to housing costs: 36% for homeowners and 78% for renters (AOA, 2017).

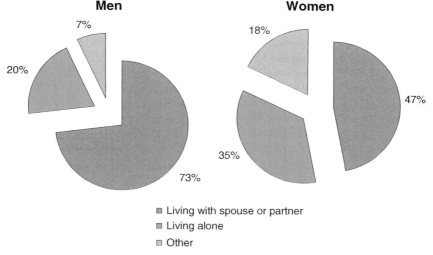

Men

7%
20%
73%

Women

18%
47%
35%

- Living with spouse or partner
- Living alone
- Other

Fig. 1.2 Living arrangements of persons 65 or older: 2016. (From Administration on Aging. [2017]. *A profile of older Americans: 2016*. Washington, DC: Administration for Community Living, U.S. Department of Health and Human Services.)

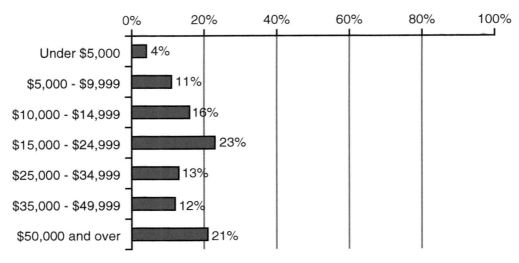

$22,887 median for 45.9 million persons 65+ reporting income

Fig. 1.3 Percentage distribution by income for individuals 65 or older. (From Administration on Aging. [2017]. *A profile of older Americans: 2016.* Washington, DC: Administration for Community Living, U.S. Department of Health and Human Services.)

Geographic Distribution

Older adults, as a group, are less likely to change residences compared with other age groups. This has been an important factor in the growth of the population 65 or older living in metropolitan and nonmetropolitan areas. However, various factors may influence the decision to move. Functional and health status may require older persons to move to be near caregivers. Dwindling financial resources may necessitate a move to a more economical location; conversely, economic stability or affluence may afford the opportunity to move to a retirement community or a location with a temperate climate and recreational offerings.

Education

The educational level of the older adult population has been steadily increasing. Between 1970 and 2016, the percentage of older adults who had completed high school increased from 28% to 85%. In 2016 about 28% had earned their bachelor's degree or higher (AOA, 2017).

Educational levels are significantly different between whites and nonwhites. In 2016 90% of whites had completed high school, whereas only 80% of Asians, 77% of African Americans, 71% of American Indian and Alaska Natives, and 54% of Hispanics had achieved the same level of education (AOA, 2017).

Low levels of education may impair the older adult's ability to live a healthy lifestyle, access service and benefit programs, recognize health problems and seek appropriate care, and follow recommendations for care. The literacy level of older adult patients also affects patient educational processes; thus it is an important consideration in discharge planning, health promotion, and illness/disability prevention.

Income and Poverty

The median income of older adults in 2015 was $31,372 for older men and $18,250 for older women. For all older persons reporting income in 2015, 15% reported less than $10,000 and

46% reported $25,000 or more (Fig. 1.3). The major source of income for older individuals and couples in 2014 was Social Security (reported by 84% of older persons), a plan originally developed to be a supplemental source of income in old age. Other income sources in order of rank were income from assets (reported by 62%), earnings (reported by 29%), private pensions (reported by 37%), and government employee pensions (reported by 16%; AOA, 2017).

Family households headed by persons 65 or older had a median income of $57,360 in 2015. Nonwhites continued to have substantially lower incomes than their white counterparts. African Americans had a median income of $43,855 and Hispanics $42334, whereas whites had a median income of $60,266. About 5% of all family households headed by an older adult had annual median incomes of less than $15,000; 72% had incomes of $35,000 or more (Fig. 1.4).

More than 4.2 million older adults were living below the poverty level in 2015. Another 2.4 million older persons were classified as near-poor, with incomes between the poverty level and 125% of the level (AOA, 2017).

Gender and race are significant indicators of poverty. Older women had a poverty rate higher than older men in 2017 (10.3% versus 7%). Only 6.6% of older whites were poor in 2015 compared with 18.4% of older African Americans, 11.8% of Asians, and 17.5% of older Hispanics (AOA, 2017).

The most important factors in the relationship between income and health are the lifestyle changes imposed by reduced or dwindling financial resources. Persons unable to meet their basic needs typically reduce the amount spent on health care or avoid spending any health-related dollars.

Employment

About 8.8 million older adults (18.9%) were classified as labor force participants (employed or actively seeking employment) in 2015, of which 23.4% were men and 15.3% were women.

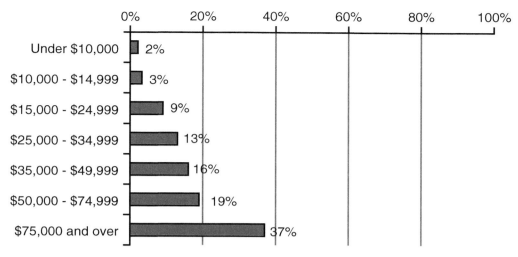

$57,360 median for 16.6 million family households 65+

Fig. 1.4 Percentage distribution by income in households headed by persons 65 or older. (From Administration on Aging. [2017]. *A profile of older Americans: 2016.* Washington, DC: Administration for Community Living, U.S. Department of Health and Human Services.)

The labor force participation of older men decreased from a high of 63.1% in 1900 to a low of 15.8% in 1985. The numbers remained constant from 1985 until 2002, at which time it began increasing; it has steadily increased ever since. The number of older women in the labor force rose only slightly from 1900 (8.3%) to 1956, at which time the rate was 10.9%. A slight decrease occurred in 1985 (7.3%); labor force participation of older women has been increasing since 2000 (9.7%) to the current level (AOA, 2017).

Following the financial crisis in 2008, many older men and women have continued to work past the expected retirement age of 66 (for those born before 1960). Part-time work has increased past the point at which Social Security payments are received. As the age for full Social Security payments rises to 67 years or older (for those born after 1960), this trend is expected to continue (Span, 2016). The cost of living in the United States has increased, job growth has slowed, and the amount of debt incurred by everyone has increased. The U.S. economic growth outlook in 2018 is expected to continue to be slow (Conerly, 2016).

HEALTH STATUS OF OLDER ADULTS

Old age is not synonymous with disease. Although selected portions of this text addresses disease and disability in old age by emphasizing the provision of age-appropriate nursing care of persons with various conditions, the implication is not that disease is a normal, expected outcome of aging. Clearly, risks of health problems and disability increase with age, but older adults are not necessarily incapacitated by these problems. They may have multiple, complex health problems resulting in sickness and institutionalization, but nurses should not consider this the norm for older adults.

Because of the high concentration of morbidity and frequent use of health services by certain high-risk groups of older adults,

delivery systems are now forced to manage resources more effectively. Strategies to maximize health and prevent disease in older adults are incorporated into health insurance plans. Incentives have prompted the development of innovative programs and services lines that improve outcomes and lower costs for healthy and chronically ill older adults. These proactive developments hold promise for the future care of older adults and provide opportunities to redefine gerontologic nursing practice. The notion of incorporating an expectation of wellness, even when treating those who have chronic disease and functional impairment, is one that is reshaping the care of older adults. Nurses must remember that older adults with disease, disability, or both can be considered healthy and well to some degree on the health–illness continuum. In fact, older adults already tend to view their personal health positively despite the presence of chronic illness, disease, and impairment.

Self-Assessed Health and Chronic Disease

Noninstitutionalized older adults over the age of 75 routinely assessed (39%) their own health as good or excellent. Most older adults have one or more chronic conditions. In 2015 the most common conditions for noninstitutionalized older adults over the age of 75 were arthritis and hypertension. In 2016 70% of those over age 65 received their influenza vaccine and 68% reported receiving the pneumococcal vaccine. About 30% of adults over age 65 are obese. Nearly half of those between ages 65 and 74 report physical activity; it drops to 29% of those 75 years of age and older. Only 9% of older adults report smoking; 8% report heavy drinking. Less than 3% report some form of psychological distress (AOA, 2017).

Overall cause of death has not changed in recent years. According to Nichols (2017), nearly 75% of all deaths stem from the following 10 causes: heart disease, cancer (lung), chronic respiratory disease (COPD), accidents, stroke, Alzheimer's disease, diabetes, influenza/pneumonia, kidney disease, and suicide.

Functional Status

The degree of functional ability is of greater concern to older adults and nurses than the incidence and prevalence of chronic disease. *Functional ability* is defined as the capacity to carry out the basic self-care activities that ensure overall health and well-being. Functional ability is classified in many measurement tools by activities of daily living (ADLs), such as bathing, dressing, eating, transferring, and toileting (Katz, Ford, Moskowitz, Jackson, & Jaffe, 1963), and instrumental ADLs, which include home-management activities such as shopping, cooking, housekeeping, laundry, and handling money (Lawton & Brody, 1969). These measurement tools were identified more than 45 years ago, but they remain the most used and effective measurement tools available.

The use of such measurement tools or scales to determine the effect of chronic disease and normal aging on physical, psychological, and social function provides objective information about a person's overall degree of health. Assessment of the effect of chronic disease and age-related decreases in functional status enables nurses to determine needs, plan interventions, and evaluate outcomes.

Chronic disease and disability may impair physical and emotional health, self-care ability, and independence. Interventions to improve the health and functional status of older adults and prevent complications of chronic disease and disability may avert the onset of physical frailty and cognitive impairment, two conditions that increase the likelihood of institutionalization.

Health Care Expenditure and Use

Through Medicare, the federal government funds most of health care in the United States for persons aged 65 or older. The Medicare insurance program is for people age 65 or older, younger than 65 with certain disabilities, and any age with end-stage renal disease (ESRD: permanent kidney failure requiring dialysis or a kidney transplantation). The different parts of Medicare include Part A (hospital insurance), Part B (medical insurance), Part C (Medicare advantage plans such as HMOs or preferred provider organizations [PPOs]), and Part D (Medicare prescription drug coverage) (Centers for Medicare and Medicaid Services [CMS], 2017). Some basics of these types of coverage include Part A services such as blood transfusions, home health services, hospice care, hospital stays as an inpatient, and residency in a skilled nursing facility (CMS, 2017).

The Affordable Care Act (ACA) of 2010 improved the cost of prescription drugs for more than 10.7 million Medicare beneficiaries, and saved them more than $20.8 billion since it was enacted. The ACA facilitated these savings by bridging the Medicare Part D "donut hole" (Box 1.2). From 2013 through 2020 Medicare beneficiaries pay reduced costs for generic and brand-name medications (in 2016, beneficiaries in the "donut hole" received a 55% discount on brand-name drugs and a 42% discount on generic drugs). By 2020, the coverage gap will be closed, that is, there will be no more "donut hole," and recipients will pay only 25% of the costs of medications until the yearly out-of-pocket spending limit is reached (National Committee to Preserve Medicare & Social Security, n.d.; Jaffe, 2017). For more information on the many benefits or services, go to https://www.medicare.gov or call 1-800-633-4227.

Implications for Health Care Delivery

Although the future direction of health care is uncertain, based on the demographic profile, it can confidently be surmised that nurses in a wide variety of settings and roles will be challenged to provide care to an increasingly divergent, complex group of older persons. An urgent need exists for gerontologic nurses to (1) create roles that meet the needs of older adults across the continuum of care; (2) develop models of care delivery directed at all levels of prevention, with special emphasis on primary prevention and health promotion services in community-based settings; and (3) assume positions of leadership and influence not only in institutions and settings where care is currently provided to older adults but also in the political arena. The overriding fact to remember is that most of the problems experienced by older adults fall within the scope of *nursing* practice.

The following descriptions of select settings of care are given as an overview and are not intended to be inclusive. Rather, they represent the settings where much of the care is provided to older adults.

Acute Care Setting

The time when the hospital was the hub of the health care delivery system has clearly passed. Political climate, market forces, technological advances, and economics are a few of the major external forces that have brought about the significant changes seen in recent years in this traditional care setting. Although the shift is away from the acute care setting toward a wide array of community-based alternatives, a segment of the older adult population will continue to need care in a hospital setting. Acute conditions such as stroke, hip fracture, congestive heart failure, and infections are common in older adults and are still treated in the hospital, as are critical health problems requiring medical and surgical treatments. However, few acute care hospitals adequately manage the care of their older adult patients in terms of preventing functional decline and promoting independence, which is why the hospital setting continues to be one of the most dangerous for older persons.

Subacute care units are aimed at the high-risk hospitalized older population. Such units typically provide intensive physical and functional interventions to bridge the gap between hospital and home. These units may be in freestanding facilities, hospital-based, or they may be part of a traditional nursing or rehabilitation facility that has upgraded the physical unit as well as the staff providing the care. The units provide such treatments as chemotherapy, wound care, intravenous therapy, and ventilator care.

BOX 1.2   Medicare Part D "Donut Hole"

Before the Affordable Care Act changes to Part D, prescription drug coverage, a "donut hole" in coverage existed. This was the result of the Medicare recipient paying the first $310 toward medications and then paying 25% of the cost of the prescriptions until reaching $2800 of costs. Once this limit was attained, no benefits were applied toward the cost of prescriptions until $4550 was spent. Then the recipient was only responsible for about 5% of the cost of the remainder of medications for that fiscal year.

Because they may be caring for frail, high-risk, older adults, nurses in the acute care workforce of today need to recognize that they should quickly acquire the necessary knowledge and skills for delivering timely, age-appropriate care—knowledge that includes (1) an understanding of normal aging and abnormal aging; (2) strong assessment skills to detect subtle changes that indicate impending, serious problems; (3) excellent communication skills when interacting with well older adults, but also those with delirium, dementia, and depression; (4) a keen understanding of rehabilitation principles as they apply to the maintenance and promotion of functional ability in older adults; and (5) sensitivity and patience so that older adults are treated with dignity and respect. It is imperative for acute care nurses to incorporate this knowledge and these skills into their daily practice with older adult patients because hospitalized older adults in the future will likely be even frailer than they are today.

Nursing Facilities

As discussed, the emphasis on reducing costs in the hospital setting through more rapid discharge has led to shifting more acutely ill residents to nursing facilities, which are traditionally referred to as *nursing homes* or *long-term care facilities*. Unfortunately, some of these facilities do not have an adequate number of qualified, professional nursing staff members to provide the complex care these residents require, or the staff does not have up-to-date knowledge and skills. In addition, the nursing staff mix may not be sufficient to meet the needs of this more acutely ill population. Finally, the physical environment and systems for delivering care in the traditional nursing facility may not be the most appropriate for meeting the needs of this acutely ill, more unstable population.

The population of adults older than 85, whose members have decreased functional abilities, is increasing in size and represents the group typically found in nursing facilities. Their care needs, coupled with those of the more acutely ill residents who are increasingly being placed in nursing facilities, have already placed great demands on many of these institutions. In the immediate future, these forces promise to continue putting pressure on nursing facilities. Economics, particularly as driven by health care reform, will determine the future of these institutions.

As the role of the advanced practice nurse continues to progress, opportunities for implementing various models of service delivery to nursing facility residents are growing. For example, AGACNPs are serving as case managers and coordinators of care in this setting. AGPCNPs are providing primary care services to nursing facility residents, demonstrating delivery of high-quality health care. AGCNSs are providing staff education and training and serving as consultants to the nursing staff in assessing and planning nursing care for residents with complex health conditions. Significant gains have been made in the quality of nursing facility resident care because of economic and legislative reforms that have allowed nurses to practice in these innovative ways. Although the momentum is growing, advanced practice nurses are challenged to continue to serve as leaders in promoting continued reform and advocating higher standards of care.

Home Care

The desire and preference of most older persons to stay in their own homes for as long as possible is a major driving force influencing the need for increased home care services. Additional factors are the recent economic, governmental, and technological developments that have led to sicker patients being discharged from the hospital after shorter stays, with needs for high-tech care and complex equipment (The Joint Commission, 2011).

Older home care patients have multiple, complex problems. In addition to possessing the knowledge and skills previously noted, home care nurses must be self-directed and capable of functioning with a multidisciplinary team widely dispersed throughout the community. Keen clinical judgment is essential because the home care nurse is often called on to make decisions about whether patients should be referred to a physician. In addition to physical and psychosocial assessments, the home care nurse is responsible for determining older patients' functional status. Assessment of home safety and family dynamics, knowledge and use of community resources, knowledge of the older adult's acute and chronic conditions, and lifestyle implications are the responsibility of the home care nurse. Excellent coordination and collaboration skills are necessary because the home care nurse is the primary resource for older patients; home care nurses call in other resources as warranted. Finally, a genuine respect for the older adult's wishes, preferences, and rights to live at home is vital.

Nurses caring for homebound older adults need to become involved in conducting community assessments that focus specifically on the aged population. The data obtained from this type of assessment may be used to plan age-specific programs and services aimed at all levels of prevention (i.e., refinement of health screening, health promotion, and health maintenance activities). Linking these activities to existing community-based programs and organizations already used by older persons is a logical place to begin.

With rapidly increasing health care costs, the Independence at Home Act, a part of the ACA, is a demonstration project that provides primary care teams to deliver care to high-risk patients at home. The focus of the project is to "improve the overall quality of care and quality of life for patients served, while lowering health care costs by forestalling the need for care in institutional settings" ("Independence at Home," 2017, para. 1). Six quality outcomes are monitored in the project:

- Follow-up within 48 hours of an acute change in condition (hospitalization, emergency department visit, or hospital discharge)
- Medication reconciliation in the home 48 hours after hospital discharge or emergency department visit
- Documentation of patient preferences
- Hospital readmission within 30 days of discharge
- Hospital admission for a problem that could have been addressed in ambulatory care setting
- Emergency department visit for a problem that could have been addressed in ambulatory care setting

Year 2 results of the demonstration project showed a $746 savings per beneficiary ("Independence at Home," 2017).

Continuum of Care

The shift from acute care, hospital-based organizations to fully integrated health systems has resulted in a highly competitive and intricate system of care. HMOs, PPOs, provider service organizations (PSOs), and independent practice associations (IPAs) are just a few of the current health systems. More health care is being delivered on an ambulatory basis. With this shift to community-based care, greater emphasis is being placed on health promotion and disease prevention, so that the goals of maximum health and independence can be achieved. Gerontologic nurses must advocate for *all* older persons along the continuum of care, promoting interventions that result in their highest level of wellness, functionality, and independence.

Continuing efforts to restructure the health care system for the older adult population must consider the wide range of care needed by this group. Any health care system that evolves for this population must integrate programs of care that allow for ease of movement along the continuum. As eloquently stated by Ebersole and Hess (1990), "Fragmented or superficial care is particularly dangerous to the elderly. Their functions become more and more interdependent as they age. A small disturbance is like a pebble in a still lake. The ripples extend outward in all directions." The future of health care for older adults remains in flux. Older adults and their caregivers are anxiously awaiting the new choices that will be presented in hopes of more effectively meeting the needs of a growing and demographically changing population.

EFFECT OF AN AGING POPULATION ON GERONTOLOGIC NURSING

Given the demographic projections presented previously in this chapter and the development of gerontologic nursing as a specialty, the current challenge is to participate in the development of an appropriate health care delivery framework for older adults that considers their unique needs. Now is the time for all gerontologic nurses to create a new vision for education, practice, and research.

Ageism

Ageism is a term coined by Butler in 1969 to describe the deep and profound prejudice in American society against older adults. In a society that highly values youth and vitality, it is no surprise that ageism exists. Butler compares ageism to bigotry: "Ageism can be seen as a process of systematic stereotyping of and discrimination against people because they are old, just as racism and sexism accomplishes this with skin color and gender. I see ageism manifested in a wide range of phenomena, on both individual and institution levels—stereotypes and myths, outright disdain and dislike, simple subtle avoidance of contact, and discriminatory practices in housing, employment, and services of all kinds" (Butler, 1989; Butler, 2005 as stated in Achenbaum, 2015).

Butler (1993) also discusses the development of a "new ageism" in recent years caused by forces such as the economic gains of older adults, their increasing vigor and productivity, and their growing political influence. He added that for these and even more subtle reasons, the older population is considered a threat by many who fear their ever-increasing numbers will only further drain financial resources, slow economic growth, and create intergenerational conflict. Some of the suggestions Butler proposes to fight this "new ageism" include building coalitions among advocates of all age groups; recognizing that older persons themselves are an economic market and developing ways to capitalize on it; investing in biomedical, behavioral, and social research to eliminate many of the costly chronic conditions of old age and strengthen social networks; and fostering the development of a healthy philosophy on aging. A sense of hope, pride, confidence, security, and integrity can greatly enhance the quality of life for older adults. Persons of *all* ages are stakeholders in developing strategies and solutions to this end. Only then will we be able to eliminate the negative attitudes and discriminatory practices that harm us all.

Unfortunately, the nursing profession is not immune to ageism. Because generally negative attitudes about older people are held by society at large—and nurses are members of society—it follows that some nurses may have ageist views. Studies have found such attitudes among nursing recruits, which is a finding that has significant implications for practice, education, and research.

Nursing Education

The need for adequately prepared nurses to care for the growing population of older adults continues to intensify. Gerontologic nursing content must be an intricate component throughout the nursing curricula in all nursing educational programs.

The pioneering work of Gunter and Estes (1979) defined an educational program specific to five levels of nursing: (1) nursing assistants/technicians, (2) licensed practical/vocational nurses, (3) RNs, (4) nurses with graduate education at the master's degree level, and (5) nurses with graduate education at the doctoral level. Although no reports in the nursing literature describe the use of this framework for curriculum development, this work has been an invaluable reference for nurse educators and in-service education staff members in various settings because it is the first attempt to provide a conceptual framework, delineation, and definition for the specialty. Since the first publication of this work, the published literature has cited some agreement among nurse educators as to what constitutes essential gerontologic content in the baccalaureate program.

Through the Community College–Nursing Home Partnership Project has offered ideas about essential gerontologic nursing content in the associate degree program (Waters, 1991). However, despite the many recommendations that have been made, unanimous agreement as to what constituted *core* gerontologic nursing content at any level of nursing education was not published until 1996, with an updated text in 2002. The second edition of the *National Gerontological Nursing Association Core Curriculum for Gerontological Nursing* (Luggen & Meiner, 2002) set the tone for the guideline of essentials in gerontologic education. These texts were developed in conjunction with the National Gerontological Nursing

Association (NGNA) and were originally conceived as a tool to prepare candidates for the ANCC Certification Examination for the Gerontologic Nurse. Gerontologic nursing educational programs in colleges, universities, and nursing schools would do well to use current texts as a content outline for development of their programs.

In 2008 the AACN published *The Essentials of Baccalaureate Education for Professional Nursing Practice.* It addressed the inclusion of geriatric nursing content and clinical experience. This document was updated in 2010, with additional information from the Hartford Institute for Geriatric Nursing, as *Recommended Baccalaureate Competencies and Curricular Guidelines for the Nursing Care of Older Adults.* These works have encouraged nursing educational programs at all levels to add geriatric nursing content with clinical experiences to enhance nurses' responsibilities, knowledge, and skills to the practice of nursing.

EVIDENCE-BASED PRACTICE

Dedicated Education Unit—Long-Term Care

Background
The shortage of nurses prepared to provide safe and effective care for older adults in long-term care (LTC) nursing facilities is becoming worse and may threaten the ability of health care reform in improving elder care and reducing costs. LTC nursing is perceived negatively by nursing students. Faculty at a baccalaureate nursing program in the northwestern United States set out to determine whether implementation of the Portland Model Dedicated Education Unit (DEU) in an LTC facility would improve the quality and rigor of the LTC clinical experience and improve student and staff satisfaction with the LTC clinical experience.

Sample/Setting
Three-hundred and thirteen student participants enrolled in the first adult health course in the baccalaureate nursing program and direct entry master's program were randomized to have their first medical/surgical clinical experience in either an acute care DEU or DEU-LTC.

Methods
In this quasiexperimental, mixed methods study, rigor was measured through formative and summative simulations, course grades, and standardized examinations. Satisfaction was evaluated using focus groups held at the LTC facility, guided by opening questions, and allowed to progress naturally. The focus groups were held with students and LTC staff.

Findings
No significant differences were found between students attending clinical at the acute care DEU and the DEU-LTC on any measure of rigor. Focus group discussions revealed students enjoyed their clinical at the DEU-LTC, even though they did not get to have much experience with intravenous drugs and calling physicians. The tradeoff was they were able to administer drugs to patients with dementia, perform wound care, and hang tube feedings.

Implications
The DEU-LTC was an effective clinical teaching environment that provided positive clinical experiences for students and professional development opportunities for the LTC facility staff.

From O'Lynn, C. (2013). Comparison between the Portland model dedicated education unit in acute care and long-term care settings in meeting medical-surgical nursing course outcomes: A pilot study. *Geriatric Nursing, 34,* 187–193.

In terms of program evaluation and outcomes, these documents assist in meeting the challenges set forth by evolutions in health care, nursing curricula, instructional strategies, and clinical practice models that respond to major trends in health care. Nurse educators must develop clinical practice sites for students, outside the comfort of the institutional setting, that reflect the emerging trends of community-based care with a focus on health promotion, disease prevention, and the preservation of functional abilities. Nurse faculty members with formal preparation in the field of gerontologic nursing are imperative if students are to be adequately prepared to meet the needs of the older adult population.

Assuring nursing students that they will be sufficiently prepared to practice in the future—a future that will undeniably include the care of older adults in a wide variety of settings—necessitates answering many questions concerning nursing education. The primary issue is not whether to include gerontologic nursing content but the extent of its inclusion. Until a sufficient number of nurse faculty members are prepared in the specialty, this question will remain unanswered, and students will continue to be inadequately prepared for the future of nursing.

Nursing Practice

Gerontologic nursing practice continues to evolve as new issues concerning the health care delivery system in general and the health of older adults in particular demand attention. The continuing movement of health care away from acute care hospitals, economics as a driving force in health care delivery, the changes in managed care, the expanding role of the RN, and the use of unlicensed assistive personnel (UAPs) has implications for the future of gerontologic nursing.

Today's older adult health care consumers are more knowledgeable and discerning and thus better informed as they become more active decision makers about their health and well-being. Because they have greater financial resources than they had in the past, older adult consumers are able to exercise more options in all aspects of their daily lives.

As care continues to shift from hospitals to ambulatory or community-based sites, older adults are demanding more programs and services aimed at (1) health maintenance and promotion and (2) disease and disability prevention. Gerontologic nurses play an integral role in effecting these changes in the various emerging practice arenas. They practice in clinics, the home care environment, and older adult living communities that range from independent homes to rehabilitation centers. Parish nurses in all 50 states provide a wide range of services to older adults living in their service areas; this type of nursing practice is likely to continue to expand. Gerontologic nurses work as case managers in various practice sites, including hospitals and community-based ambulatory settings. As health care systems adjust to meet the needs of the growing population of older adults, so will the opportunities for gerontologic nursing practice.

Advanced practice gerontologic nurses are practicing independently in some states; others work with a collaborating physician in primary care, urgent care, and long-term care facilities.

Gerontologic nurses must continue to educate older persons about their care options and lobby for legislation at the state and federal levels for expansion of reimbursement opportunities for advanced practice nurses who care for older adults.

Considering the increasing number of older adults requiring functional assistance to remain at home, in semiindependent living settings, or in other alternative settings, gerontologic nurses need to be vigilant as care functions normally performed by RNs are transferred to UAPs. It is unclear whether UAPs are a viable solution for providing safe, high-quality, cost-effective care to older adult patients in any setting. However, with appropriate education and training, it may be possible to use UAPs in select situations. For this to be successful, nurses need to take a greater role in the education of UAPs within an appropriate practice framework and ensure that they meet established competency criteria.

Additional skills required by nurses to support aging of older adults includes the ability to teach families and other caregivers about safe and effective caregiving techniques as well as the services and resources available in the community. Because many of these older patients have varying degrees of functional impairment, nurses must have a comprehensive knowledge of functional assessment, as well as intervention and management strategies from a rehabilitative perspective. Gerontologic nurses need lifestyle counseling skills because the emphasis on health promotion and disease prevention continues to grow, and older adults assume more responsibility for their health. Most gerontologic nurses have had little experience with education and counseling related to preretirement planning, but such skills are invaluable when assisting older adults through life transitions.

Despite change and advancements in the delivery of health care services, the traditional medical model continues to endure in the acute care setting and long-term care. Future models of care must consider the effect of many intervening factors on the health status of older adults. Psychological, social, environmental, and economic needs must be given equal consideration to presenting physical needs. The ability to comprehensively assess these areas requires the nurse to possess refined and highly discriminating assessment skills. This will become increasingly more important as nurses take on more responsibility for the care and treatment of older adults across all settings. Equally important will be the development of coordination and collaboration skills, communication and human relations skills, and the ability to influence others, because future practice models and sites will likely reflect a true team approach to older adult care.

Nursing Research

The evolution of gerontologic nursing research can be seen in the publications and organizations that regularly review and disseminate evidence-based practice findings. The *Journal of Gerontological Nursing* has been in publication since the mid-1970s. The peer-reviewed journal publishes articles on the practice of gerontologic nursing across the continuum of care in a variety of health care settings. *Geriatric Nursing,* the official journal of the American Assisted Living Nurses Association, the National Gerontological Nursing Association, and the Gerontological Advanced Practice Nurses Association, began publication in 1980. This journal addresses current issues related to pharmacotherapy, advance directives, staff development and management, legal issues, patient and caregiver education, infection control, and many other relevant topics. *Research in Gerontological Nursing* began bimonthly publication in 2008; this journal focuses on interdisciplinary gerontologic nursing research relevant to educators, clinicians, and policymakers involved in the care of older adults across all health care settings.

The leading gerontologic nursing research questions for the future should be framed within larger issues such as patient-centered outcomes, health promotion and maintenance, prevention of disease and disability, and early detection of disease and illness—all within traditional and alternative health care delivery systems. Knowledge built through research is imperative for the development of a safe and sound knowledge base that guides clinical practice as well as for the promotion of the specialty.

The incredible growth in research on aging has largely been the result of the birth of Medicare and Medicaid in 1965. Although private funding is available for gerontologic research, it is difficult to find. Information regarding federal funding for specific research areas may require significant investigation. The National Institute on Aging provides information related to research funding (https://www.nia.nih.gov/research) as does https://www.grants.gov. Smaller research grants are available through nursing organizations such as Sigma Theta Tau International and the American Nurses Foundation.

Evidence-Based Practice

In 2011 the Committee on the Robert Wood Johnson Foundation Initiative on the Future of Nursing at the Institute of Medicine published *The Future of Nursing: Leading Change, Advancing Health.* The report summary states we have:

> … the opportunity to transform its health care system to provide seamless, affordable, quality care that is accessible to all, patient centered, and evidence based and leads to improved health outcomes. Achieving this transformation will require remodeling many aspects of the health care system. This is especially true for the nursing profession, the largest segment of the health care workforce. This report offers recommendations that collectively serve as a blueprint to (1) ensure that nurses can practice to the full extent of their education and training, (2) improve nursing education, (3) provide opportunities for nurses to assume leadership positions and to serve as full partners in health care redesign and improvement efforts, and (4) improve data collection for workforce planning and policy making. (Institute of Medicine, 2011, p. 1)

Nursing research and evidence-based practice play an integral role in meeting the Future of Nursing recommendations. The Iowa Model of Evidence-Based Practice to Promote Quality Care (Fig. 1.5) provides a multistep process to facilitate evaluation and implementation of evidence in practice. From selecting an appropriate clinical question, forming a team, implementing and evaluating practice changes, to dissemination of results, the model is a guide to quality improvement (Iowa Model Collaborative, 2017).

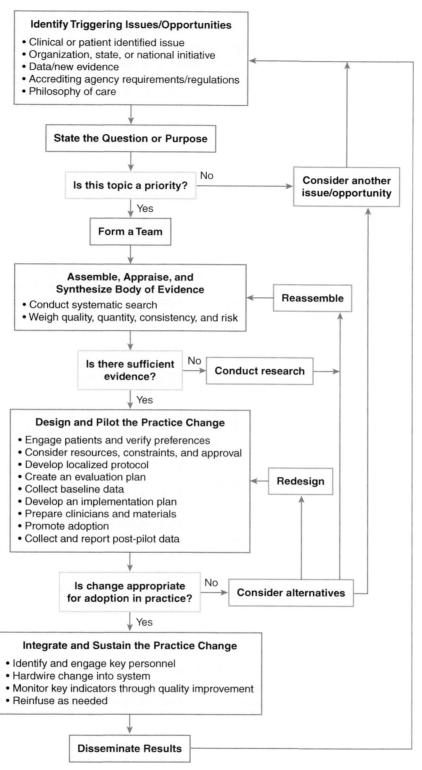

Fig. 1.5 The Iowa Model Revised: Evidence-based Practice to Promote Excellence in Health Care. (Redrawn from Iowa Model Collaborative. [2017]. Iowa Model of Evidence-Based Practice: Revisions and Validation. *Worldviews on Evidence-Based Nursing, 14*[3], 175–182.)

SUMMARY

Nursing care of older adults is recognized as a legitimate specialty. The important groundwork that has been laid serves as the basis from which the specialty will forge into the future. Gerontologic nurses at all levels of educational preparation and in all settings of care must venture into that future with creativity, pride, and determination as they meet their professional responsibility to provide quality care to older adults everywhere. Now is the time to seize the opportunity to advance gerontologic nursing education, practice, and research for the benefit of the older adult population—a population that continues to grow.

KEY POINTS

- The growth of the nursing profession, increasing educational opportunities, demographic changes, and changes in health care delivery systems have all influenced the development of gerontologic nursing roles.
- *Age 65 or older* is widely accepted and used for reporting demographic statistics about older persons; however, turning 65 does not automatically mean a person is "old."
- Nurses are cautioned against thinking of all older adults as alike, even though most demographic data places all adults over 65 into a single reporting group.
- Adults 65 or older currently represent about 14.9% of the total population of the United States
- The most rapid and dramatic growth for the older adult population in the United States to date is occurring now as the baby boomers reach 65 years old.
- About 3.1% of persons older than 65 live in long-term care facilities, but the percentage increases dramatically with advancing age.
- Gender and race are significant indicators of poverty; older women have a poverty rate significantly higher than older men, and a higher percentage of aging African Americans and Hispanics are poor, compared with the percentage of whites.
- Estimates indicate that most adults over 65 have one or more chronic health conditions.
- Three leading causes of death among older adults are cardiovascular diseases, cancer, and COPD.
- Ageism is prejudice against the old just because they are old.
- Nurses in a variety of settings and roles provide age-appropriate and age-specific care based on a comprehensive and scientific knowledge base.
- Gerontologic nursing content should be included in all nursing education programs.
- Evidence-based practice has the potential to improve care for the older adult.

CRITICAL-THINKING EXERCISES

1. Care of the older person today is considerably different from what it was in 1960. Cite examples of how and why the care of older adults is different today than it was in the past.
2. When reporting for work, you note that you have been assigned to two 74-year-old women for the evening. Is it safe to assume that the care of these two women will be similar because they are the same age? Why or why not? How would their care be enhanced or be compromised if they were treated similarly?
3. As a student, you are often assigned to care for older adults. At what point in your education do you feel information related to the care of the older adult should be included? In early classes, later in the program, or throughout your nursing program? Support your position.

REFERENCES

Achenbaum, W. A. (2015). A history of ageism since 1969. [Blog]. Retrieved November 6, 2017 from http://www.asaging.org/blog/history-ageism-1969.

Administration on Aging. (2017). *A profile of older Americans: 2017.* Washington, DC: Administration for Community Living, U. S. Department of Health and Human Services.

Age 65 Retirement. (n.d.). Retrieved November 6, 2017 from https://www.ssa.gov/history/age65.html.

American Association of Retired Persons. (n.d.). *AARP member benefits guide.* Lakewood, CA: Author.

American Nurses Association. (2017). Website. Accessed November 6, 2017 http://www.nursingworld.org/.

American Nurses Credentialing Center. (2017). Website. Accessed November 6, 2017 http://www.nursecredentialing.org/Certification.aspx.

Burnside, I. M. (1988). *Nursing and the aged: A self-care approach* (3rd ed.). New York: McGraw-Hill.

Butler, R. N. (1993). Dispelling ageism: The cross-cutting intervention. *Generations, 17*(2), 75.

Care of the Aged. (1925). *The American Journal of Nursing, 25*(5), 394.

Centers for Medicare and Medicaid Services. (2017). *Medicare & You.* Washington, DC: Author.

Colby, S. L., & Ortman, J. M. (2015). Projections of the size and composition of the US population: 2014 to 2060. In *P25-1143.* Retrieved from census.gov.

Conerly, B. (2016). US economic forecast 2017-2018: Mild rebound. Retrieved from https://www.forbes.com/sites/billconerly/2016/09/16/u-s-economic-forecast-2017-2018-mild-rebound/#18087c05337f.

Ebersole, P., & Hess, P. (1990). *Toward healthy aging: Human needs and nursing response* (3rd ed.). St Louis: Mosby.

Gunter, L., & Estes, C. (1979). *Education for gerontic nursing.* New York: Springer.

Institute of Medicine. (2011). *The future of nursing: Leading change, advancing health.* Washington, DC: National Academies Press.

Collaborative, Iowa Model. (2017). Iowa Model of Evidence-Based Practice: Revisions and validation. *Worldviews on Evidence-Based Nursing, 14*(3), 175–182.

Jaffe, I. (2017). Obamacare repeal could threaten provisions that help older adults. Retrieved from http://www.npr.org/sections/health-shots/2017/01/28/511994587/obamacare-repeal-could-threaten-provisions-that-help-older-adults.

Johnson Jr., J. H., & Appold, S. J. (2017). US older adults: Demographics, living arrangements, and barriers to aging in place. [uisc05301701]. Kenan Institute of Private Enterprise. Retrieved from www.kenaninstitute.unc.edu.

Katz, S., Ford, A. B., Moskowitz, R. W., Jackson, B. A., & Jaffe, M. W. (1963). Studies of illness in the aged. The index of ADL: a standardized measure of biological and psychosocial function. *JAMA: The Journal of the American Medical Association, 185,* 94.

Lawton, M. P., & Brody, E. M. (1969). Assessment of older people: Self-maintaining and instrumental activities of daily living. *Gerontologist, 9,* 179.

Luggen, A. S., & Meiner, S. E. (2002). *NGNA core curriculum for gerontological nursing* (2nd ed.). St. Louis: Mosby.

National Committee to Preserve Medicare & Social Security. (n.d.). How the Affordable Care Act helps seniors. Retrieved November 6, 2017 from http://www.ncpssm.org/publicpolicy/medicare/documents/articleid/216/how-the-affordable-care-act-helps-seniorsover.

Nichols, H. (2017). The top 10 leading causes of death in the United States. Retrieved November 6, 2017 from https://www.medicalnewstoday.com/articles/282929.php.

Robson, D. (2015). *Why do women live longer than men?* Retrieved November 6, 2017 from http://www.bbc.com/future/story/20151001-why-women-live-longer-than-men.

Social Security History. (n.d.). Retrieved May 1, 2018 from https://www.ssa.gov/history/ottob.html.

Span, P. (2016). Of retirement age, but remaining in the work force. Retrieved from https://www.nytimes.com/2016/08/02/health/retirement-working-longer.html.

Stevens, J. (1994). A history of nursing the elderly. *Australian Nursing Journal, 1*(8), 23–25.

The Joint Commission. (2011). Home – the best place for health care. Retrieved from www.jointcommission.org.

United Nations Population Fund. (2012). *Aging in the twenty-first century: A celebration and a challenge.* New York, NY: Author.

Waters, V. (Ed.), (1991). *Teaching gerontology: The curriculum imperative.* New York: National League for Nursing Press.

Williams, M.E. (2017). *Why do women live longer than men?* [Blog]. Retrieved November 6, 2017 from https://www.psychologytoday.com/blog/the-art-and-science-aging-well/201702/why-do-women-live-longer-men.

Theories Related to Care of the Older Adult

Jennifer J. Yeager, PhD, RN, APRN

ⓔ http://evolve.elsevier.com/Meiner/gerontologic

LEARNING OBJECTIVES

On completion of this chapter, the reader will be able to:

1. Define aging from biologic, sociologic, and psychological frameworks.
2. Apply nursing theory to the care of older adults.
3. Discuss the rationale for using an eclectic approach in the development of aging theories.
4. Develop nursing interventions based on the psychosocial issues and biologic changes associated with older adulthood.
5. Discuss several nursing implications for each of the major biologic, sociologic, and psychological theories of aging.
6. Describe the evolution of the Roy Adaptation Model to fit a middle-range nursing theory of successful aging.

WHAT WOULD YOU DO?

What would you do if you were faced with the following situations?
* After your morning report, you are prioritizing care for your five older adult patients. Which theory(ies) could aid in this process?
* You are caring for a 92-year-old hospice patient. His care could be best guided by what theory?

Theories of aging have been debated since the time of the ancient Greeks. In the twelfth century, thoughts were centered on predetermination and an unalterable plan for life and death. The philosopher Maimonides thought that precautions and careful living might prolong life. In the late 1400s, Leonardo da Vinci attempted to explain aging as physiologic changes while studying the structure of the human body. Studies were few until the late 1900s when world populations began to have increasing numbers of older adults. Scholars have sought to embrace a theory that can explain the entire aging phenomenon. However, many scholars have concluded that no one definition or theory explains all aspects of aging; rather, scientists have found that several theories may be combined to explain various aspects of the complex phenomenon we call aging.

Theories function to help make sense of a phenomenon; they provide a sense of order and give a perspective from which to view the facts. Theories provide a springboard for discussion and research. Some theories are presented in this chapter because of their historical value; for the most part, they have been abandoned because of a lack of empiric evidence. Other theories are the result of ongoing advances made in biotechnology and, as such, provide glimpses into our future.

Human aging is influenced by a composite of biologic, psychological, sociologic, functional, and spiritual factors. Aging may be viewed as a continuum of events that occur from conception to death (Ignatavicius, Workman, & Rebar, 2018). Biologic, sociologic, and psychological theories of aging attempt to explain and explore the various dimensions of aging. No single gerontologic nursing theory has been accepted by this specialty, which requires nurses to use an eclectic approach from other disciplines as the basis of clinical decision making (Comfort, 1970) (Box 2.1).

By incorporating a holistic approach to the care of older adults, nurses can view this ever-increasing portion of the population more comprehensively. Interactions between gerontologic nurses and older adults are not limited to specific diseases or physiologic processes, absolute developmental tasks, or psychosocial changes. Nurses can synthesize various aspects of the different aging theories and visualize older adults interfacing with their total environment, including physical, mental/emotional, social, and spiritual aspects. Therefore an eclectic approach provides an excellent foundation as nurses plan high-quality care for older adults.

Theories of aging attempt to explain this phenomenon of aging as it occurs over the life span. Several basic assumptions and concepts have been accepted over the years to guide research and clinical practice related to aging (Hornsby, 2010). Human aging is viewed as a total process that begins at conception. Because individuals have unique genetic, social, psychological, and economic factors intertwined in their lives, the course of aging varies from individual to individual.

Previous author: Sue E. Meiner, EdD, APRN, BC, GNP.

BOX 2.1   **Theories of Aging**

Biologic
Concerned with answering basic questions regarding physiologic processes that occur in all living organisms over time (Hayflick, 1996).

Sociologic
Focused on the roles and relationships within which individuals engage in later life (Hogstel, 1995).

Psychological
Influenced by both biology and sociology; addresses how a person responds to the tasks of his or her age.

Nursing
Helps to describe and explain phenomena; predicts and prescribes nursing interventions for the range of different situations encountered in the profession of nursing (Garcia & Maya, 2015).

Moral/Spiritual
Examines how an individual seeks to explain and validate his or her existence (Edelman & Mandle, 2003).

Senescence, defined as a change in the behavior of an organism with age, leading to a decreased power of survival and adjustment, also occurs. The recognition of the universal truths is what we attempt to discover through the theories of aging.

BIOLOGIC THEORIES OF AGING

Biologic theories are concerned with answering basic questions regarding the physiologic processes that occur in all living organisms as they chronologically age. These age-related changes occur independent of any external or pathologic influence. The primary question being addressed relates to the factors that trigger the actual aging process in organisms. These theories generally view aging as occurring at molecular, cellular, and even systemic levels. In addition, biologic theories are not meant to be exclusionary. Theories may be combined to explain phenomena (Hayflick, 1996, 2007).

The foci of biologic theories include explanations of the following: (1) deleterious effects leading to decreasing function of the organism, (2) gradually occurring age-related changes that progress over time, and (3) intrinsic changes that may affect all members of a species because of chronologic age. The decreasing function of an organism may lead to a complete failure of either an organ or an entire system (Hayflick, 1996, 2004, 2007). In addition, according to these theories, all organs in any one organism do not age at the same rate, and any single organ does not necessarily age at the same rate in different individuals of the same species (Warner, 2004).

Mitochondrial Free Radical Theory

Free radicals are byproducts of fundamental metabolic activities within the body. Free radical production may increase because of environmental pollutants such as ozone, pesticides, and radiation. Normally, they are neutralized by enzymatic activity or natural antioxidants. However, if they are not neutralized, they may attach themselves to other molecules. These highly reactive free radicals react with the molecules in cell membranes, in particular, cell membranes of unsaturated lipids such as mitochondria, lysosomes, and nuclear membranes. This action monopolizes the receptor sites on the membrane, thereby inhibiting the interaction with other substances that normally use this site; this chemical reaction is called *lipid peroxidation.* Therefore the mitochondria, for example, can no longer function as efficiently, and their cell membranes may become damaged, which results in increased permeability. If excessive fluid is either lost or gained, the internal homeostasis is disrupted, and cell death may result.

Other deleterious results are related to free radical molecules in the body. Although these molecules do not contain DNA themselves, they may cause mutations in the DNA–RNA transcription, thereby producing mutations of the original protein. In nervous and muscle tissue, to which free radicals have a high affinity, a substance called *lipofuscin* has been found and is thought to be indicative of chronologic age. Strong support for this theory has continued over the past 35+ years (Jang & Van Remmen, 2009).

Lipofuscin, a lipid- and protein-enriched pigmented material, has been found to accumulate in older adults' tissues and is commonly referred to as "age spots." As the lipofuscin's presence increases, healthy tissue is slowly deprived of oxygen and its nutrient supply. Further degeneration of surrounding tissue eventually leads to actual death of the tissue. The body does have naturally occurring antioxidants, or protective mechanisms. Vitamins C and E are two of these substances that can inhibit the functioning of the free radicals or possibly decrease their production in the body.

Harman (1956) was the first to suggest that the administration of chemicals terminating the propagation of free radicals would extend the life span or delay the aging process. Animal research demonstrated that administration of antioxidants did increase the average length of life, possibly because of the delayed appearance of diseases that may have eventually killed the animals studied. It appears that the administration of antioxidants postpones the appearance of diseases such as cardiovascular disease and cancer, two of the most common causes of death. Antioxidants also appear to influence the decline of the immune system and degenerative neurologic diseases, both of which affect morbidity and mortality (Hayflick, 1996; Weinert & Timiras, 2003; Yu, 1993, 1998).

Cross-Linkage Theory

The cross-linkage theory of aging hypothesizes that with age, some proteins become increasingly cross-linked or enmeshed and may impede metabolic processes by obstructing the passage of nutrients and wastes between the intracellular and extracellular compartments. According to this theory, normally separated molecular structures are bound together through chemical reactions.

This primarily involves collagen, which is a relatively inert long-chain macromolecule produced by fibroblasts. As new fibers are created, they become enmeshed with old fibers and form an actual chemical cross-link. The result of this cross-linkage process is an increase in the density of the collagen molecule but a decrease in its capacity to both transport nutrients to the cells and remove waste products from the cells. Eventually, this results in a decrease in the structure's function. An example of this would be the changes associated with aging skin. The skin of a baby is soft and pliable, whereas aging skin loses much of its suppleness and elasticity. This aging process is like the process of tanning leather, which purposefully creates cross-links (Bjorkstein, 1976; Hayflick, 1996, 2004).

Cross-linkage agents have been found in unsaturated fats; in polyvalent metal ions such as aluminum, zinc, and magnesium; and in association with excessive radiation exposure. Many of the medications ingested by the older population (such as antacids and coagulants) contain aluminum, as does baking powder, a common cooking ingredient. Some research supports a combination of exercise and dietary restrictions in helping to inhibit the cross-linkage process as well as the use of vitamin C prophylactically as an antioxidant agent (Bjorkstein, 1976).

One researcher, Cerani, has shown that blood glucose reacts with bodily proteins to form cross-links. He has found that the crystallin of the lens of the eye, membranes of the kidney, and blood vessels are especially susceptible to cross-linking under the conditions of increased glucose. Cerani suggests increased levels of blood glucose cause increased amounts of cross-linking, which accelerate lens, kidney, and blood vessel diseases (Schneider, 1992). This research was more recently updated by Eyetsemitan, who identified the stiffening of blood vessels with an increase in thickness caused by the cross-linking of protein and glucose. The products of this effect are identified as AGEs, or *advanced glycation end-products* (Eyetsemitan, 2007).

Cross-linkage theory proposes that as a person ages and the immune system becomes less efficient, the body's defense mechanism cannot remove the cross-linking agent before it becomes securely established. Cross-linkage has been proposed as a primary cause of arteriosclerosis, decrease in the efficiency of the immune system, and the loss of elasticity often seen in older adult skin.

Hayflick Limit Theory

One of the first proposed biologic theories is based on a study completed in 1961 by Hayflick and Moorehead. This study included an experiment on fetal fibroblastic cells and their reproductive capabilities. The results of this landmark study changed the way scientists viewed the biologic aging process.

Hayflick and Moorehead's study showed that functional changes do occur within cells and are responsible for the aging of the cells and the organism. The study further supported the hypothesis that a cumulative effect of improper functioning of cells and eventual loss of cells in organs and tissues are therefore responsible for the aging phenomenon. This study contradicted earlier studies by Carrel and Ebeling, in which chick embryo cells were kept alive indefinitely in a laboratory; the conclusion from this 1912 experiment was that cells do not wear out but continue to function normally forever. An interesting aspect of the 1961 study was that freezing was found to halt the biologic cellular clock (Hayflick & Moorehead, 1961).

This 1961 study found that unlimited cell division did not occur; the immortality of individual cells was found to be more an abnormal occurrence than a normal one. Therefore this study seemed to support the Hayflick Limit Theory. Life expectancy was generally seen as preprogrammed within a species-specific range; this biologic clock for humans was estimated at 110 to 120 years (Gerhard & Cristofalo, 1992; Hayflick, 1996). Based on the conclusions of this experiment, the Hayflick Limit Theory is sometimes called the "Biologic Clock Theory," "Cellular Aging Theory," or "Genetic Theory."

Immunologic Theory

The immune system is a network of specialized cells, tissues, and organs that provide the body with protection against invading organisms. Its primary role is to differentiate self from nonself, thereby protecting the organism from attack by pathogens. It has been found that as a person ages, the immune system functions less effectively. The term *immunosenescence* has been given to this age-related decrease in function.

Essential components of the immune system are T lymphocytes, which are responsible for cell-mediated immunity, and B lymphocytes, the antibodies responsible for humoral immunity. Both T and B lymphocytes may respond to an invasion of an organism, although one may provide more protection than the other in certain situations. The changes that occur with aging are most apparent in T lymphocytes, although changes also occur in the functioning capabilities of B lymphocytes. Accompanying these changes is a decrease in the body's defense against foreign pathogens; this manifests as an increased incidence of infectious diseases and an increase in the production of autoantibodies, which lead to a propensity to develop autoimmune-related diseases (De la Fuente, 2008; Hayflick, 1996; Weinert & Timiras, 2003) (Box 2.2).

The changes in the immune system cannot be explained by an exact cause-and-effect relationship, but they do seem to increase with advancing age. These changes include a decrease in humoral immune response, often predisposing older adults to (1) decreased resistance to a tumor cell challenge and the development of cancer, (2) decreased ability to initiate the immune process and mobilize the body's defenses against aggressively attacking pathogens, and (3) heightened production of autoantigens, often leading to an increase in autoimmune-related diseases.

Immunodeficient conditions such as human immunodeficiency virus (HIV) infection and immune suppression in organ

---

BOX 2.2   Changes in Cell-Mediated Immune Function Secondary to Aging

- *Increase in autoantibodies because of altered immune system regulation:* This predisposes an individual to autoimmune diseases such as systemic lupus erythematosus and rheumatoid arthritis.
- *Low rate of T-lymphocyte proliferation in response to a stimulus:* This causes older adults to respond more slowly to allergic stimulants.
- *Reduced response to foreign materials, resulting in an increased number of infections:* This is a result of a decrease in cytotoxic or killer T cells.
- *Generalized T-lymphocyte dysfunctions, which reduce the response to certain viral antigens, allografts, and tumor cells:* This results in an increased incidence of cancer in older adults.

transplant recipients have demonstrated a relationship between immunocompetence and cancer development. HIV infection has been associated with several forms of cancer such as Kaposi sarcoma. Recipients of organ transplants are 80 times more likely to develop cancer compared with the rest of the population (Black & Hawks, 2005).

Implications for Nursing

When interacting with the older population, caregivers must relate the key concepts of the biologic theories to the care provided. Although these theories do not provide *the answer*, they certainly can explain some of the changes seen in the aging individual. Aging and disease do not necessarily go hand in hand, and the nurse caring for older adults needs to have a clear understanding of the difference between age-related changes and those that may be pathologic. Nurses must remember that scientists are still in the process of discovering what "normal" aging is.

Among biologic theories of aging, two concepts have gained wide acceptance: (1) The limited replicative capacity of certain cells causes overexpression of damaged genes and oxidative damage to cells; and (2) free radicals may cause damage to cells over time. Based on these concepts, gerontologic nurses can promote the health of older adult patients in many ways. Helping with smoking cessation would be one example of health promotion. Cigarette smoking causes increased cell turnover in the oral cavity, bronchial tree, and alveoli. Smoking also introduces carcinogens into the body, which may result in an increased rate of cell damage that can lead to cancer. Using the same principles, nurses can develop a health promotional activity for education regarding sun exposure. Excessive

exposure to ultraviolet light is another example of a substance causing rapid turnover of cells, which may lead to mutations and ultimately malignancies. To reduce free radical damage, nurses can also advise patients to ingest a varied, nutritious diet using the food pyramid as a guide and suggest supplementation with antioxidants such as vitamins C and E (Goldstein, 1993). Physical activity continues to play an important role in the lives of older adults. Daily routines need to incorporate opportunities that capitalize on existing abilities, strengthen muscles, and prevent further atrophy of muscles from disuse. Encouraging older adults to participate in activities may prove a challenge to nurses interacting with these patients (Carter, 2003).

Performing activities of daily living (ADLs) requires the functional use of extremities. Daily exercises that enhance upper arm strength and hand dexterity contribute to older adults' ability to successfully perform dressing and grooming activities. Even chair-based activities such as deep breathing increase the oxygen flow to the brain, thereby promoting clear mental cognition, minimizing dizziness, and increasing stamina with activity.

Encouraging older adults to participate in daily walking, even on a limited basis, facilitates peripheral circulation and promotes the development of collateral circulation. Walking also helps with weight control, which often becomes a problem in older adults. Additional benefits of walking include (1) replacement of fat with muscle tissue, (2) prevention of muscle atrophy, and (3) a generalized increase in the person's sense of well-being.

The health care delivery system is beginning to focus on disease prevention and health promotion, and older adults must be included in this focus. Stereotypical views that older adults

EVIDENCE-BASED PRACTICE

Relationship Between Health Literacy and Health-Promotion Activities in Older Adults

Background
Health literacy is limited in a large portion of older adults. Limited health literacy has been shown to be a strong predictor of poor health outcomes. Limited health literacy is also associated with low use of preventive health services and poor adherence to therapeutic regimens.

Sample/Setting
There were 707 random and purposefully selected respondents who participated in the Health and Retirement Study sponsored by the National Institute on Aging. Respondents were predominantly white (92%), female (57%), and married (81%). Most (95%) had completed high school; nearly 45% had completed college.

Methods
Secondary analysis of cross-sectional data was used to determine health literacy, perceived control over health, perceived health care discrimination, and perceived social standing. Health literacy was measured using the Test of Functional Health Literacy, which determined whether participants could read and understand two written passages. Perceived control was measured using a single item asking, "How would you rate the amount of control you have these days over your health" ("0" = no control; "10" = very much control). Social standing was measured using the MacArthur Scale of Subjective Social Status, where respondents marked a rung on a ladder where they believed they stood in society. Health care discrimination was measured by asking, "In day-to-day life, how often has any of

the following things happened to you" (You receive poorer service or treatment than other people from doctors or hospitals [almost every day, at least once a week, a few times a month, a few times a year, less than once a year, never]). Additionally, eight specific health behaviors were measured: flu immunization, cholesterol testing, mammography, breast self-examination, prostate examination, current tobacco use, and moderate and vigorous physical activity.

Findings
Significant differences were found between participants with adequate and inadequate self-reported health literacy in perceived control over health and in perceived social standing. Significant associations were found between self-reported health literacy and mammography, moderate physical activity, and tobacco use. Participants with adequate self-reported health literacy were more likely to report having a mammogram within the past 2 years, more likely to perform moderate physical activity, and less likely to use tobacco.

Implications
Results of this study provide evidence of the relationship between health literacy and health promotion activities and control over health. With this information in mind, nurses should use appropriate screening tools to identify older adults at risk for poorer health outcomes related to health literacy and intervene to improve health promotion activities and control of health.

From Fernandez, D. M., Larson, J. L., & Zikmund-Fisher, B. J. (2016). Associations between health literacy and preventive health behaviors among older adults: Findings from the health and retirement study. *BMC Public Health, 16,* 596. doi: 10.1186/s12889-016-3267-7.

are "too old to learn new things" must be replaced by factual knowledge about the cognitive abilities of older adults. It is necessary for patient teaching to stress the concept that certain conditions or diseases are not inevitable just because of advancing years. A high level of wellness is needed to help minimize the potential damage caused by disease in later years. Although aging brings with it a decrease in the normal functioning of the immune system, older adults should not suffer needlessly from infections or disease. Encouraging preventive measures such as annual influenza vaccination or a one-time inoculation with the pneumococcal vaccine is essential to providing a high-quality life experience for the older population.

Other applications of biologic theories include the recognition that stress, both physical and psychological, has an effect on the aging process. In planning interventions, nurses should pay attention to the various stress factors in an older person's life. Activities to minimize stress and promote healthy coping mechanisms must be included in the patient-teaching plan for older adults.

Teaching the basic techniques of relaxation, guided imagery, visualization, distraction, and music therapy facilitate a sense of control over potential stress-producing situations. Additional options, including heat or cold application, therapeutic touch, and massage therapy, could be explored. Being aware of individual cultural preferences and sharing these with other health care professionals will further promote positive interactions with older adults in all settings.

SOCIOLOGIC THEORIES OF AGING

Sociologic theories focus on changing roles and relationships (Box 2.3). In some respects, sociologic theories relate to various social adaptations in the lives of older adults. One of the easiest ways to view the sociologic theories is within the context of the societal values at the time in which they were developed.

BOX 2.3 Sociologic Theories of Aging

Activity Theory
Individuals need to remain active to age successfully. Activity is necessary to maintain life satisfaction and a positive self-concept (Havighurst, Neugarten, & Tobin,1963).

Continuity Theory
Individuals will respond to aging in the same way they have responded to previous life events. The same habits, commitments, preferences, and other personality characteristics developed during adulthood are maintained in older adulthood (Havighurst, Neugarten, & Tobin, 1963).

Age Stratification Theory
Society consists of groups of cohorts that age collectively. The people and roles in these cohorts change and influence each other, as does society at large. Therefore a high degree of interdependence exists between older adults and society (Riley, 1985).

Person–Environment Fit Theory
Everyone has personal competencies that assist the person in dealing with the environment. These competencies may change with aging, thus affecting the older person's ability to interrelate with the environment (Lawton, 1982).

The early research was carried out largely on institutionalized and ill older persons, which skewed the collected information. Contemporary research is being conducted in a variety of more naturalistic environments, reflecting more accurately the diversity of the aging population.

During the 1960s, sociologists focused on the losses of old age and the way individuals adjusted to these losses in the context of their roles and reference groups. A decade later, society began to have a broader view of aging as reflected in the aging theories proposed during this period. These theories focused on more global, societal, and structural factors that influenced the lives of aging persons. The 1980s and 1990s brought other changes into focus, as sociologists began to explore interrelationships, especially those between older adults and the physical, political, environmental, and even socioeconomic milieu in which they lived.

Activity Theory

Havighurst first proposed the idea that aging successfully is related to staying active. It was not until 10 years later that the phrase "activity theory" was coined by Havighurst and his associates (Havighurst, Neugarten, & Tobin, 1963).

This theory sees activity as necessary to maintain a person's life satisfaction and positive self-concept. By remaining active, the older person stays engaged and gains satisfaction with aging. This theory is based on three assumptions: (1) It is better to be active than inactive; (2) it is better to be happy than unhappy; and (3) an older individual is the best judge of his or her own success in achieving the first two assumptions (Havighurst, 1972). Within the context of this theory, activity may be viewed broadly as physical or intellectual. Therefore even with illness or advancing age, the older person can remain "active" and achieve a sense of life satisfaction (Havighurst et al., 1963).

Continuity Theory

The continuity theory proposes that how a person has been throughout life is how that person will *continue* to be through the remainder of life (Havighurst et al., 1963). Old age is not viewed as a terminal or final part of life separated from the rest of a person's life. According to this theory, the latter part of life is a continuation of the earlier part and therefore an integral component of the entire life cycle. When viewed from this perspective, the theory is a developmental theory. Simply stated, the theory proposes that, as people age, they try to maintain or continue previous habits, preferences, commitments, values, beliefs, and the factors that have contributed to their personalities (Havighurst et al., 1963).

Age Stratification Theory

Beginning in the 1970s, theorists on aging began to focus more broadly on societal and structural factors that influenced how the older population was being viewed. The age stratification theory is only one example of a theory addressing societal values. The key societal issue addressed in this theory is the concept of interdependence between the aging person and society at large (Riley, Johnson, & Foner, 1972).

This theory views the aging person as an individual element of society and also as a member, with peers, interacting in a social process. The theory attempts to explain the interdependence between older adults and society, and how they constantly influence each other in a variety of ways.

Riley (1985) identifies the five major concepts of this theory: (1) Each individual progresses through society in groups of cohorts that are collectively aging socially, biologically, and psychologically; (2) new cohorts are continually born, and each of them experiences their own unique sense of history; (3) society itself can be divided into various strata, according to the parameters of age and roles; (4) not only are people and roles within every stratum continuously changing but so is society at large; and (5) the interaction between individual aging people and the entire society is not stagnant but remains dynamic.

Person–Environment Fit Theory

Another aging theory relates to the individual's personal competence within the environment in which they interact. This theory, proposed by Lawton (1982), examines the concept of interrelationships among the competencies of a group of persons, older adults, and their society or environment.

All people, including older persons, have certain personal competencies that help mold and shape them throughout life. Lawton (1982) identified these personal competencies as including ego strength, motor skills, individual biologic health, and cognitive and sensory–perceptual capacities. All these help people deal with the environment in which they live.

As a person ages, changes or even decreases may occur in some of these personal competencies. These changes influence the individual's abilities to interrelate with the environment. If a person develops one or more chronic diseases such as rheumatoid arthritis or cardiovascular disease, then competencies may be impaired, and the level of interrelatedness may be limited.

The theory further proposes that, as a person ages, the environment becomes more threatening, and he or she may feel incompetent dealing with it. In a society constantly making rapid technologic advances, this theory helps explain why an older person might feel inadequate and may retreat from society.

Implications for Nursing

It is important to remember that all older adults cannot be grouped collectively as just *one* segment of the population. Many differences exist within the aged population. The young-old (ages 65 to 74), the middle-old (ages 75 to 84), the old-old (more than 85), and the elite-old (more than 100 years old) are four distinct cohort groups, and the individuals within each of these cohort groups have their own history. Variation exists among even the same cohort group based on culture, life experiences, gender, and health and family status. Nurses need to be aware that whatever similarities exist among the individuals of a cohort group, they are still individuals. Older adults are not a homogeneous sociologic group, and care needs to be taken not to treat them as if they were.

Older adults respond to current experiences based on their past life encounters, beliefs, and expectations. If their "typical" reaction to stress, challenges, or fear is to disengage from interactions, then current situations often produce the same responses. Because older adults are individuals, their responses must be respected. However, it is within the nurse's scope of practice to identify maladaptive responses and intervene to protect the integrity of the person.

Withdrawal in older adults may be a manifestation of a deeper problem such as depression. Using assessment skills and specific tools, nurses can further investigate and plan appropriate interventions to help resolve a potentially adverse situation. Older adults may refuse to engage in an activity because of fear of failure or frustration at not being able to perform the activity. Planning realistic activities for particular patient groups is crucial to successful group interaction. The successful completion of a group activity provides an opportunity for increasing an older person's self-confidence, whereas frustration over an impossible task further promotes feelings of inadequacy and uselessness.

By examining the past and being aware of significant events or even beliefs about health and illness, the health care provider can develop a deeper understanding of *why* these older adults act the way they do or believe in certain things. The health care provider can also gain insight into how a group of older adults responds to illness and views healthy aging. This knowledge and insight can certainly assist in planning not only activities but also meaningful patient teaching.

Another application of the sociologic theories relates to helping individuals adapt to various limitations and securing appropriate living arrangements. After the passage of the 1990 Americans with Disabilities Act, most buildings are now easily accessible to those with special needs. These special needs may include doorways wide enough for wheelchairs, ramps in addition to stairs, handrails in hallways, and working elevators. Although these changes assist younger members of society with limited physical capabilities, they also benefit older adults. In addition, older adults might consider the installation of medical alert devices, preprogrammed or large-numbered phones, and even special security systems.

Helping older adults adjust to limitations while accentuating positive attributes may enable them to remain independent and may perpetuate a high quality of life during later years. These adaptations may encourage older adults to remain in the community, perhaps even in the family home, instead of being prematurely institutionalized. Older adults continue to feel valued and viewed as active members of society when allowed to maintain a sense of control over their living environment.

In some cities in the United States, multigenerational communities are developing, fostering a sharing of different cultures as well as generations. Schools are promoting "adopt a grandparent" programs, day care centers are combining services for children and older adults, and older volunteers visit hospitalized children or make telephone calls to "latchkey" children after school. These are examples of the practical application of sociologic aging theories. Older adults are continuing to be active, engaging or disengaging as they wish, and remaining valued members of society.

PSYCHOLOGICAL THEORIES OF AGING

The basic assumption of the psychological theories of aging is that development does not end when a person reaches adulthood but remains a dynamic process throughout the life span (Box 2.4). As a person passes from middle life to later life, his or her roles, abilities, perspectives, and belief systems enter a stage of transition. The nurse, by providing holistic care, seeks to employ strategies to enhance patients' quality of life (Hogstel, 1995). The psychological theories of aging are much broader in scope than the earlier theories because they are influenced by both biology and sociology. Therefore psychological aging cannot readily be separated from biologic and sociologic influences.

BOX 2.4 Psychological Theories of Aging

Maslow's Hierarchy of Human Needs
Human motivation is viewed as a hierarchy of needs critical to the growth and development of all people. Individuals are viewed as active participants in life, striving for self-actualization (Carson & Arnold, 1996).

Jung's Theory of Individualism
Development is viewed as occurring throughout adulthood, with self-realization as the goal of personality development. As individuals age, they can transform into a more spiritual being.

Erikson's Eight Stages of Life
All people experience eight psychosocial stages during a lifetime. Each stage represents a crisis, where the goal is to integrate physical maturation and psychosocial demands. At each stage, the person can resolve the crisis. Successful mastery prepares an individual for continued development. Individuals always have within themselves an opportunity to rework a previous psychosocial stage into a more successful outcome (Carson & Arnold, 1996).

Selective Optimization With Compensation
Physical capacity diminishes with age. An individual who ages successfully compensates for these deficits through selection, optimization, and compensation (Schroots, 1996).

As people age, various adaptive changes help them cope with or accept some of the biologic changes. Some of the adaptive mechanisms include memory, learning capacity, feelings, intellectual functioning, and motivations to perform or not perform activities (Birren & Cunningham, 1985). Psychological aging, therefore, includes not only behavioral changes but also developmental aspects related to the lives of older adults. How does behavior change in relation to advancing age? Are these behavioral changes consistent in pattern from one individual to another? Theorists are searching for answers to questions such as these.

Maslow's Hierarchy of Human Needs

According to this theory, everyone has an innate internal hierarchy of needs that motivate all human behaviors (Maslow, 1954). These human needs have different orders of priority. When people achieve fulfillment of their elemental needs, they strive to meet the needs on the next level, continuing until the highest order of needs is reached. These human needs are often depicted as a pyramid, with the most elemental needs at the base (Fig. 2.1).

The initial human needs each person must meet relate to physiologic needs—the needs for basic survival. Initially, a starving person worries about obtaining food to survive. Once this need is met, the next concern is about safety and security. These needs must be met, at least to some extent, before the person becomes concerned with the needs for love, acceptance, and a feeling of belonging. According to Maslow (1968), as each succeeding layer of needs is addressed, the individual is motivated to look to the needs at the next higher step.

Maslow's fully developed, self-actualized person displays high levels of all the following characteristics: perception of reality; acceptance of self, others, and nature; spontaneity; problem-solving ability; self-direction; detachment and the desire for privacy; freshness of peak experiences; identification with other human beings; satisfying and changing relationships with other people; a democratic character structure; creativity;

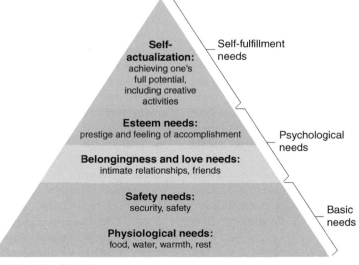

Fig. 2.1 Maslow's hierarchy of needs.

and a sense of values (Maslow, 1968). Maslow's ideal self-actualized person is probably only attained by about 1% of the population (Thomas & Chess, 1977). Nevertheless, the person developing in a healthy way is always moving toward more self-fulfilling levels.

Jung's Theory of Individualism

The Swiss psychologist Carl Jung (1960) proposed a theory of personality development throughout life: childhood, youth and young adulthood, middle age, and old age. An individual's personality is composed of the ego, the personal unconsciousness, and the collective unconsciousness. According to this theory, a person's personality is visualized as oriented either toward the external world (extroversion) or toward subjective, inner experiences (introversion). A balance between these two forces, which are present in every individual, is essential for mental health.

Applying his theory to individuals as they progress through life, Jung proposed that it is at the onset of middle age that the person begins to question values, beliefs, and possible dreams left unrealized. The phrase *midlife crisis,* popularized by this theory, refers to a period of emotional, and sometimes behavioral, turmoil that heralds the onset of middle age. This period may last for several years, with the exact time and duration varying from person to person.

During this period, the individual often searches for answers about reaching goals, questioning whether a part of his or her personality or "true self" has been neglected and whether time is running out for the completion of these quests. This may be the first time the individual becomes aware of the effects of the aging process and the fact that the first part of the adult life is over. This realization does not necessarily signal a time of trauma. For many people, it is just another "rite of passage."

As the person ages chronologically, the personality often begins to change from being outwardly focused, concerned about establishing oneself in society, to becoming more inward, as the individual begins to search for answers from within. Successful aging, according to Jung's theory, is when a person looks inward and values himself or herself for more than just current physical limitations or losses. The individual accepts past accomplishments and limitations (Jung, 1960).

Eight Stages of Life

In 1959, Erikson (1993) proposed a theory of psychological development that reflects cultural and societal influences. The major focus of development in this theory is on an individual's ego structure, or sense of self, especially in response to the ways in which society shapes its development. In each of the eight stages identified by Erikson, a "crisis" occurs that affects the development of the person's ego. The way a person masters any particular stage influences future success or lack of success in mastering the next stage of development.

When considering older adults, one must focus attention on the developmental tasks of both middle adulthood and older adulthood. The task of middle adulthood is resolving the conflict between generativity and stagnation. During older adulthood, the developmental task needing resolution is balancing the

TABLE 2.1   Summary of Erikson's Theory
Middle and Older Adulthood

Stages and Ages	Characteristics of Stages	Theory Addendum
Generativity vs. Self-Absorption or Stagnation		
40–65 years old; middle adulthood Mode: nurturing Virtue: care	Mature adults are concerned with establishing and guiding the next generation. Adults look beyond the self and express concern for the future of the world in general.	Self-absorbed adults will be preoccupied with their personal well-being and material gains. Preoccupation with self leads to stagnation of life.
Ego Integrity vs. Despair		
65 years to death; older adulthood Mode: acceptance Virtue: wisdom	Older adults can look back with a sense of satisfaction and acceptance of life and death.	Unsuccessful resolution of this crisis may result in a sense of despair, in which individuals view life as a series of misfortunes, disappointments, and failures.

Modified from Potter, P. A., & Perry, A. G. (2004). *Fundamentals of nursing* (5th ed.). St. Louis, MO: Mosby.

search for integrity and wholeness with a sense of despair (Table 2.1) (Potter & Perry, 2004).

In 1968, Peck expanded Erikson's original theory regarding the eighth stage of older adulthood. Erikson had grouped all individuals together into "old age" beginning at age 65, not anticipating that a person could live another 30 to 40 years beyond this milestone. Because people were living longer, an obvious need arose to identify additional stages for older adults. Peck (1968) expanded the eighth stage, ego integrity versus despair, into three stages: (1) ego differentiation versus work role preoccupation, (2) body transcendence versus body preoccupation, and (3) ego transcendence versus ego preoccupation (Ignatavicius et al., 2018).

During the stage of ego differentiation versus work role preoccupation, the task for older adults is to achieve identity and feelings of worth from sources other than the work role. The onset of retirement and termination of the work role may reduce feelings of self-worth. In contrast, a person with a well-differentiated ego, who is defined by many dimensions, can find other roles to replace the work role as the major defining source for self-esteem.

The second stage, body transcendence versus body preoccupation, refers to the older person's view of the physical changes that occur because of the aging process. The task is to adjust or transcend the declines that may occur to maintain feelings of well-being. This task can be successfully resolved by focusing on the satisfaction obtained from interpersonal interactions and psychosocial activities.

The third and final task, ego transcendence versus ego preoccupation, involves acceptance of the individual's eventual death without dwelling on the prospect of it. Remaining actively involved with a future that extends beyond a person's mortality is the adjustment that must be made to achieve ego transcendence.

Selective Optimization With Compensation

Baltes (1987) has conducted a series of studies on the psychological processes of development and aging from a life span perspective and formulated a psychological model of successful aging. This theory's central focus is that individuals develop certain strategies to manage the losses of function that occur over time. This general process of adaptation consists of three interacting elements: (1) *selection,* which refers to an increasing restriction on one's life to fewer domains of functioning because of an age-related loss; (2) *optimization,* which reflects the view that people engage in behaviors to enrich their lives; and (3) *compensation,* which results from restrictions caused by aging, requiring older adults to compensate for any losses by developing suitable, alternative adaptations (Schroots, 1996).

The lifelong process of selective optimization with compensation allows people to age successfully. Schroots (1996) cited the famous pianist Arthur Rubinstein to illustrate an application of these elements. Rubinstein stated that, as he grew older, he first reduced his repertoire and played a smaller number of pieces (selection); second, he practiced these more often (optimization); and third, he slowed down his playing right before fast movements, producing a contrast that enhanced the impression of speed in the fast movements (compensation). These concepts of selection, optimization, and compensation can be applied to any aspect of older adulthood to demonstrate successful coping with declining functions.

Implications for Nursing

Integrating the psychological aging theories into nursing practice becomes increasingly important as the U.S. population continues to age. Present and future generations can learn from the past. Older adults should be encouraged to engage in a "life review" process; this may be accomplished using a variety of techniques such as reminiscence, oral histories, and storytelling. Looking back over one's life's accomplishments or failures is crucial in assisting older adults to accomplish developmental tasks (as in ego integrity), to promote positive self-esteem, and to acknowledge that one "did not live in vain."

As nurses apply the psychological theories to the care of older adults in any setting, they help dispel many of the myths about old age. An older person talking about retirement, worrying about physical living space, and even planning funeral arrangements are all part of the developmental tasks appropriate for this age group. Instead of trying to change the topic or telling the person not to be so "morbid," the nurse must understand that, in each stage of life, specific developmental tasks need to be achieved. Instead of hampering their achievement, the nurse should facilitate them.

Nurses also need to keep in mind that intellectual functioning remains intact in most older adults. A younger person can gain much by observing older persons, listening to how they have coped with life experiences, and discussing his or her plans with them.

As other humanistic psychologists did, Maslow focused on the human potential, which sets an effective and positive foundation for nurse–patient interactions. Maslow's theory also sets priorities for the nurse in relationship to patient needs.

Employing Maslow's theory, the nurse recognizes that essential needs such as food, water, oxygen, elimination, and rest must be met before self-actualization needs. The nurse recognizes, for example, that patient education will be more successful if patients are well rested (Carson & Arnold, 1996).

In planning activities for older adults, nurses need to remember that all individuals enjoy feeling needed and respected, and being considered contributing members of society. Perhaps activities such as recording oral history, creating a mural, or reviewing a person's lifetime through pictures could be included. Not only would such activities demonstrate that the individual is valued, but they would also serve to pass on information from one generation to the next; this is an important task that is often overlooked.

Programs promoting interaction between older adults and young children might prove beneficial to all concerned. For some older adults, caring for small children represented a happy time in their lives. Rocking, cuddling, and playing with children might bring back feelings of being valued and needed. The touching aspects of this activity are also important in relieving stress; many older adults no longer experience any type of meaningful physical contact with others, yet all individuals need this type of contact.

As eyesight and manual dexterity diminish, many older adults enjoy the opportunity to cook or to work in a garden. Often, the feel of dirt between the fingers is relaxing and brings back memories of growing beautiful flowers and prize vegetables in the past. For the older woman, preparing a meal may be an activity she has not been able to do for several years, and with assistance, she may find baking cookies a pleasant activity filled with memories of holidays and loved ones, or prizes at the county fair. Older men may also enjoy cooking and should not be left out of this activity. Preparing muffins for a morning snack would be an activity in which everyone could participate.

NURSING THEORIES

Theory of Successful Aging

One midrange nursing theory related to aging was derived from Sr. Calista Roy's Adaptation Model. In this theory, successful aging is defined as "an individual's perception of a favorable outcome in adapting to the cumulative physiologic and functional alterations associated with the passage of time, while experiencing spiritual connectedness, and a sense of meaning and purpose in life" (Flood, 2005, p. 36). With the conceptual definition of successful aging in mind, Flood (2005) integrated concepts from Roy's Adaptation Model (RAM) with those of Lars Tornstams' 1989 Sociological Theory of Gerotranscendence in the development of the Theory of Successful Aging. The theory identifies three coping mechanisms (adaptation of functional performance mechanisms, intrapsychic factors, and spirituality) that describe the older adult's response to their environment. This response provides feedback within these identified mechanisms, promoting gerotranscendence. In this theory, gerotranscendence is defined as "a coping process that occurs when there is a major shift in the person's worldview, where a person examines one's place within the world and in

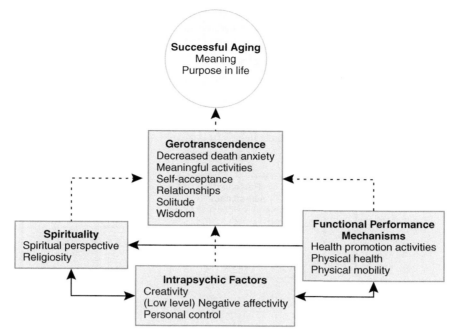

Fig. 2.2 Theory of Successful Aging. (Courtesy of Dr. Meredith Troutman-Jordan.)

relation to others ... includ[ing] decreased death anxiety, engagement in meaningful activities, changes in relationships, self-acceptance and wisdom" (Flood, 2005, p. 38). In turn, the feedback loop centered on the three coping mechanisms, and gerotranscendence facilitates successful aging (Fig. 2.2). The Theory of Successful Aging guides the gerontologic nurse in the provision of mental, physical, and spiritual nursing interventions aimed at promoting positive coping and successful aging (Flood, 2005).

Health Promotion Model

The Health Promotion Model (HPM), revised by Nola Pender in 1996, identifies health as a dynamic state directed at improving the person's overall sense of well-being. In this model, health is not viewed as simply the absence of disease. Health is multidimensional in nature and influenced by the person's environment. The three components comprising health are (1) the unique characteristics and experiences of the person that affect subsequent actions; (2) the person's behavior and cognitive affect, which provide motivation and can be modified through nursing interventions; and (3) behavioral outcomes which should result in optimum health and functional ability, and improved quality of life (Fig. 2.3) (Current Nursing, 2011). Gerontologic nurses can effectively use this model to guide health teaching and improve adherence to health promotion and disease prevention guidelines.

Comfort Theory

Comfort theory is a midrange nursing theory developed by Katharine Kolcaba during the 1990s. In this theory, comfort is defined as "the immediate experience of being strengthened through having the needs for relief, ease, and transcendence met in four contexts of experience (physical, psychospiritual,

social, and environmental)" (as quoted in Kolcaba & DiMarco, 2005, p. 188). Comfort is composed of three components: (1) *relief* occurs when specific comfort needs are met; (2) *ease* is the absence of discomfort; and (3) *transcendence* occurs when a patient can rise above their discomfort when it cannot be completely relieved. The theory recognizes the importance of patient involvement in identifying their needs. Comfort is the holistic outcome of nursing interventions (Fig. 2.4) (Kolcaba & DiMarco, 2005). Comfort theory has direct application for gerontologic nurses who practice in medical/surgical environments, as well as those in hospice and palliative care.

MORAL AND SPIRITUAL DEVELOPMENT

Human beings seek to explain and validate their existence in the world. For many individuals, this occurs through their development as moral and spiritual thinkers. Kolberg has postulated a theory of moral development based on interviews with young persons. He recognized distinct sequential stages of moral thinking. Although he did not study older adults, parallels could be drawn between his highest stage of moral development, Universal Ethical Principles, and Maslow's highest level of Self-Transcendent Needs. In each instance, only a small segment of the population reaches this highest level of development, where their personal needs are sublimated for the greater good of society (Edelman & Mandle, 2003; Levin & Chatters, 1998; Mehta, 1997).

It is important for the nurse to acknowledge the spiritual dimension of a person and support spiritual expression and growth (Hogstel, 1995). *Spirituality* no longer merely denotes religious affiliation; it synthesizes a person's contemplative experience. Illness, a life crisis, or even the recognition

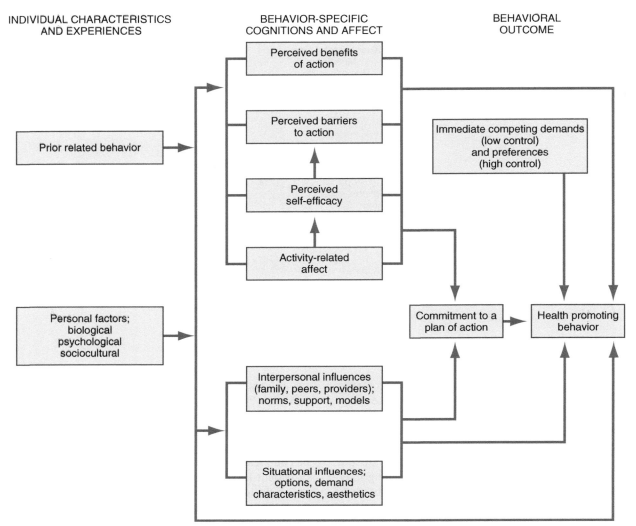

INDIVIDUAL CHARACTERISTICS
AND EXPERIENCES

BEHAVIOR-SPECIFIC
COGNITIONS AND AFFECT

BEHAVIORAL
OUTCOME

Fig. 2.3 Health Promotion Model. (From Pender, N. J., Murdaugh, C.L., & Parsons, M. A. [2006]. *Health promotion in nursing practice* [5th ed.]. Upper Saddle River, NJ: Prentice-Hall Health, Inc. Reprinted by permission of Pearson Education, Inc., New York.)

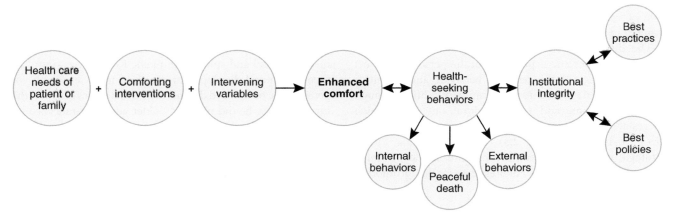

Fig. 2.4 Theory of Comfort. Redrawn from Krinsky, R., Murillo, I., & Johnson, J. [2014]. A practical application of Katharine Kolcaba's comfort theory to cardiac patients. *Applied Nursing Research, 27*[2], 148.)

that one's days on Earth are limited may cause a person to contemplate spirituality. The nurse can assist patients in finding meaning in their life crises. Research has begun to explore the relationship between patient-centered outcomes and spirituality. A correlation between successful outcomes and spirituality has been demonstrated in some of this research. Regardless of outcomes, nurses need to address spirituality as a component in holistic care (Phipps et al., 2003).

SUMMARY

When interacting with older adults, the nurse often plays a key role as the coordinator of the health care team. Nurses have the background to incorporate information from a variety of sources when planning care for older adults. By using an eclectic approach to the aging theories, the nurse will have a broad background from which to draw specific details to provide clarity, explanations, or additional insight to a given situation.

Biologic theories help the nurse understand how the physical body may change with advancing years and what factors may increase older adults' vulnerability to stress or disease. The nurse will also be able to develop health promotional strategies on behalf of older patients. Understanding the sociologic theories broadens the nurse's view of older adults and their interactions with society. The psychological theories provide an understanding of the values and beliefs an older person may possess. These theories enable a nurse to understand the phases of the life span and the developmental tasks faced by older adults. Nursing theories help to describe and explain phenomena and to predict and prescribe nursing interventions for the range of different situations nurses encounter when providing care for older adults. By integrating the various components of these theories, nurses can plan high-quality care for this population. As the U.S. population continues to age, nurses with the capability to understand and apply the theories of aging from several disciplines will be the leaders of gerontologic nursing. These nurses will contribute to increasingly holistic care and an improved quality of life for older adults.

KEY POINTS

- No one theory explains the biologic, sociologic, or psychological aging processes.
- An eclectic approach incorporating concepts from biology, sociology, and psychology was used in developing aging theories.
- The biologic theories address what factors trigger the aging process in organisms.
- A change in the efficiency of immune processes may predispose individuals to disease with advancing age.
- The biologic theories alone *do not* provide a comprehensive explanation of the aging process.
- Reminiscence is supported by the sociologic theories and assists older adults in appreciating memories.
- Everyone is unique. Older adults are not a homogeneous population.
- The activity theory remains popular because it reflects current societal beliefs about aging.
- As a person ages, various adaptive changes occur that may assist the person in coping with or accepting some of the biologic changes.
- Human development is a process that occurs over the life span.
- The Theory of Successful Aging was derived from Sr. Calista Roy's Adaptation Model.

CRITICAL-THINKING EXERCISES

1. Discuss how sociologic theories of aging may be influenced by changing societal values (e.g., advanced technology or a community health care focus) in the next decade.
2. A 64-year-old woman believes that heart disease and poor circulation are inevitable consequences of growing older and is resistant to altering her ADLs and dietary regimen. How would you respond?
3. Think of various programs and institutions in your community that care for older persons. Identify two, and discuss the sociologic aging theories represented in each example.
4. A 77-year-old man frequently talks about how he wishes he were as strong and energetic as he was when he was younger. His family consistently changes the topic or criticizes him for being so grim. How would you intervene in this situation?
5. What health promotion strategies would you recommend facilitating for successful aging?
6. Imagine yourself at age 70. Describe your appearance, your health issues, and your lifestyle.

REFERENCES

Alvarado, A. M., & Salazar, A. M. (2015). Adaptation to chronic benign pain in elderly adults. *Invest Educ Enferm*, 33(1), 138–147.

Baltes, P. B. (1987). *Lifespan development and behavior.* (Vol. 7). Hillsdale, NJ: Lawrence Erlbaum.

Birren, J. E., & Cunningham, W. R. (1985). Research on the psychology of aging. In J. E. Birren & K. W. Scheie (Eds.), *Handbook of the psychology of aging.* New York: Van Nostrand Reinhold.

Bjorkstein, J. (1976). The cross-linkage theory of aging: Clinical implications. *Comprehensive Therapy, 11,* 65.

Black, J. M., & Hawks, J. H. (2005). *Medical-surgical nursing: Clinical management for positive outcomes.* Philadelphia: WB Saunders.

Carson, V. B., & Arnold, E. N. (1996). *Mental health nursing, the nurse–patient journey.* Philadelphia: WB Saunders.

Carter, K. F. (2003). Behaviors of older men in the community: Correlates producing active composure. *Journal of Gerontological Nursing, 29*(10), 37.

Comfort, A. (1970). Biological theories of aging. *Human Development, 13,* 127.

Current Nursing. (2011). Health Promotion Model. Retrieved February 18, 2018 from http://currentnursing.com/nursing_theory/health_promotion_model.html.

De la Fuente, M. (2008). Role of neuroimmunomodulation in aging. *Neuroimmunomodulation, 15*, 213.

Edelman, C. L., & Mandle, C. L. (2003). *Health promotion throughout the lifespan* (5th ed.). St Louis: Mosby.

Erikson, E. (1993). *Childhood and society* (35th ed.). New York: WW Norton.

Eyetsemitan, F. E. (2007). Perception of aging in different cultures. In M. Robinson, W. Novelli, C. Pearson, & L. Norris (Eds.), *Global health and global aging* (p. 58). San Francisio: Wiley.

Flood, M. (2005). Mid-range nursing theory of successful aging. *The Journal of Theory Construction & Testing, 9*(2), 35.

Gerhard, G., & Cristofalo, V. (1992). The limits of biogerontology. *Generations, 16*(4), 55.

Goldstein, S. (1993). The biology of aging: Looking to defuse the time bomb. *Geriatrics, 48*(9), 76.

Harman, D. (1956). Aging: A theory based on free radical and radiation chemistry. *Journal of Gerontology, 11*, 298.

Havighurst, R. J. (1972). *Developmental tasks and education* (3rd ed.). New York: David McKay.

Havighurst, R. J., Neugarten, B. L., & Tobin, S. S. (1963). Disengagement, personality and life satisfaction in the later years. In P. Hansen (Ed.), *Age with a future*. Copenhagen: Munksgaard.

Hayflick, L. (1996). *How and why we age*. New York: Ballantine Books.

Hayflick, L. (2004). The not-so-close relationship between biological aging and age-associated pathologies in humans. *Journal of Gerontology, 59A*, B547.

Hayflick, L. (2007). Biological aging is no longer an unsolved problem. *Annals of the New York Academy of Sciences, 1100*, 1.

Hayflick, L., & Moorehead, P. S. (1961). The serial cultivation of human diploid cell strains. *Experimental Cell Research, 25*, 585.

Hogstel, M. O. (1995). *Geropsychiatric nursing* (2nd ed.). St Louis: Mosby.

Hornsby, P. J. (2010). Senescence and life span. *Pflugers Archiv: European Journal of Physiology, 459*, 291.

Ignatavicius, D. D., Workman, M. L., & Rebar, C. (2018). *Medical-surgical nursing: Concepts for interprofessional collaborative care* (9th ed.). St. Louis: Elsevier.

Jang, Y., & Van Remmen, H. (2009). The mitochondrial theory of aging: Insight from transgenic and knockout mouse models. *Experimental Gerontology, 44*, 256.

Jung, C. (1960). The stages of life. In 8. *Collected works: The structure and dynamics of the psyche*. New York: Pantheon Books.

Kolcaba, K., & DiMarco, M. A. (2005). Comfort Theory and Its Application to Pediatric Nursing. *Pediatric Nursing, 31*(3), 187–194.

Lawton, M. P. (1982). Competence, environmental press, and the adaptation of older people. In M. P. Lawton, P. G. Windley, & T. O. Byerts (Eds.), *Aging and the environment: Theoretical approaches*. New York: Springer.

Levin, J. S., & Chatters, L. M. (1998). Religion, health, and psychological well-being in older adults: Findings from three national surveys. *Journal of Aging and Health, 10*(4), 504.

Maslow, A. (1954). *Motivation and personality*. New York: Harper & Row.

Maslow, A. (1968). *Toward a psychology of being* (2nd ed.). Princeton, NJ: Van Nostrand Reinhold.

Mehta, K. K. (1997). The impact of religious beliefs and practices on aging: A cross-cultural comparison. *Journal of Aging Studies, 11*(2), 101.

Peck, R. (1968). Psychological development in the second half of life. In B. Neugarten (Ed.), *Middle age and aging*. Chicago: University of Chicago Press.

Phipps, W. J., Monahan, F. D., Sands, J. K., et al. (2003). *Medical-surgical nursing: Health and illness perspectives* (7th ed.). St Louis: Mosby.

Potter, P. A., & Perry, A. G. (2004). *Fundamentals of nursing* (5th ed.). St Louis: Mosby.

Riley, M. W. (1985). Age strata in social systems. In R. H. Binstock & E. Shanas (Eds.), *Handbook of aging and social sciences*. New York: Van Nostrand Reinhold.

Riley, M. W., Johnson, M., & Foner, A. (1972). In *Aging and society: a sociology of age stratification: Vol. 3*. New York: Russell Sage Foundation.

Schneider, E. (1992). Biological theories of aging. *Generations, 16*(4), 7.

Schroots, E. (1996). Theoretical developments in the psychology of aging. *Gerontologist, 36*(6), 742.

Thomas, A., & Chess, S. (1977). *Temperament and development*. New York: Brunner/Masel.

Warner, H. R. (2004). Current status of efforts to measure and modulate the biological rate of aging. *Journal of Gerontology, 59A*(7), 692.

Weinert, B. T., & Timiras, P. S. (2003). Theories of aging. *Journal of Applied Physiology, 95*, 1706.

Yu, B. P. (1993). *Free radicals in aging*. Boca Raton, Fla: CRC Press.

Yu, B. P. (1998). *Methods in aging research*. Boca Raton, Fla: CRC Press.

3

Legal and Ethical Issues

Carol Ann Amann, PhD, RN-BC, CDP, FNGNA

ⓔ http://evolve.elsevier.com/Meiner/gerontologic

LEARNING OBJECTIVES

On completion of this chapter, the reader will be able to:

1. Discuss how professional standards are used to measure the degree to which the legal duties of patients' nursing care are met.
2. State the sources and definitions of laws such as statutes, regulations, and case law, as well as the levels at which the laws were made such as federal, state, and local laws.
3. Explore why older adults are considered a vulnerable population, why this is legally significant, and the legal implications of such a designation.
4. Discuss the reasons behind the sweeping nursing facility reform legislation known as the Omnibus Budget Reconciliation Act (OBRA) of 1987 and understand its continuing significance and effect for residents and caregivers in nursing facilities.
5. Identify the OBRA's three major parts and describe the key areas addressed in each.
6. State the rationale behind the Affordable Care Act and cite who the Act was developed to benefit.
7. Discuss the legal history of the doctrine of autonomy and self-determination and cite major laws that have influenced contemporary thought and practice.
8. Identify the three broad categories of elder abuse, define seven types of abuse, and discuss the responsibility of the nurse in responding to suspected abuse of older adults.
9. Name and state the purpose tools known as "advance directives" and Physician Orders for Life-Sustaining Treatment (POLST).
10. Explain the requirements of the four major provisions of the Patient Self-Determination Act (PSDA) and the nurse's responsibility with respect to advance directives.
11. Describe the values history and how it can help patients and health care professionals in preparing for end-of-life decisions.
12. Identify at least three ethical issues nurses may face in caring for older adults in the areas of care of the terminally ill, organ donation, and self-determination.
13. State the function and role, as well as the recommended membership composition, of an institutional ethics committee.
14. Relate at least three major reasons why the skillful practice of professional nursing can improve the quality of life for older adults in health care settings.
15. Discuss social media policies and their effect on patients and professional practice.

WHAT WOULD YOU DO?

What would you do if you were faced with the following situations?

- You are viewing social media at home when you notice one of your coworker's posts complaining about an elderly patient on your unit. The post reveals that the patient has Alzheimer's disease and is "crazy" and states, "I can't wait until she is transferred out of here and back to Comfort Care Homes. After this shift, you will find me at the bar, line them up, I will need it." Additionally, the coworker's full name, occupation, and employer is listed on their "about me" page. What would you do regarding this posting?

- An elderly patient arrives in the emergency department with their caregiver present. On assessment, you note multiple stages of ecchymosis on their upper arms. The patient is vague about the nature of their injury and states, "Oh, I fell and hurt my arms." The caregiver interjects that the patient is "clumsy and does not follow directions." You suspect there is more to the patient's story and would like to investigate this further. What will you do?

- A patient and their family ask you what the difference is between a living will (advance directive) and a Physician Orders for Life-Sustaining Treatment (POLST) form. How will you best explain this to them?

How the health needs of older adults will be met is an ongoing concern not only for physical care but also to provide for legal and ethical standards to be applied within the care setting. The unique characteristics and needs of older

adults pose significant questions of legal and ethical significance. Older adults depend upon and expect the health care system to deliver the care that optimizes their health status and promotes care to reach their highest level of functioning. Their quality of life often depends on the type and quality of nursing care they receive. This chapter focuses on legal

Previous author: Sue E. Meiner, EdD, APRN, BC, GNP.

concerns of nurses who care for older adults and the ethical issues that may be encountered.

PROFESSIONAL STANDARDS: THEIR ORIGIN AND LEGAL SIGNIFICANCE

Health care providers have a general obligation to live up to accepted, prudent, or customary standards of care, which may be determined on a regional or national basis. Nurses are responsible for providing care to their level of education, inclusive of the degree, skill, and diligence measured and recognized by applicable standards of care. The duty of care and nurse advocacy roles increase as patients' physical and mental conditions and ability for self-care decline.

Nursing standards of practice are measured according to the expected level of professional practice of those in similar roles and clinical fields. For example, the standards of practice of a gerontologic nurse practicing at the generalist level would be measured against the practice of other nurse generalists practicing in gerontology. The advanced practice gerontologic nurse, who holds a minimum of a master's degree in an applicable field, would be expected to conform to standards established for similarly situated advanced practice nurses.

A standard of care is a guideline for nursing practice and establishes an expectation for the nurse to provide safe, effective, and appropriate care. It is used to evaluate whether care administered to patients meets the appropriate level of skill and diligence that can reasonably be expected, given the nurse's level of skill, education, and experience. Standards may originate from many sources. Both state and federal statutes may help establish standards, although conformity with a state's minimum standards does not necessarily prove that due care was provided. Conformity with local, state, and federal standards or comparison with similar facilities (benchmarking) may be considered evidence of proper care (Agency for Healthcare Research and Quality [AHRQ], 2013). Some jurisdictions in the United States call this the *community standard of care.* Note that the community standard of care can be more restrictive within organizations but cannot be lower or hold fewer expectations than the federal standard.

The published standards of professional organizations, representing the opinion of experts in the field, are important in establishing the proper standard of care. The *Scope and Standards of Gerontological Nursing Practice,* originally published in 1994 by the American Nurses Association (ANA), is one example. Nurses who care for older patients should be familiar with these standards. In 2010 the *Scope and Standards of Practice: Nursing* was updated and has not been revised since then. Refer to http://www.nursingworld.org for additional information.

Most health care facilities, at some point, seek accreditation status. This means that they voluntarily undergo a detailed survey by an organization with the skill and expertise to evaluate their services. One of the best-known accreditation organizations is The Joint Commission (TJC), previously known as the Joint Commission on Accreditation of Healthcare Organizations (JCAHO). Because it is a well-known and long-existing organization, the standards established and used by the TJC to review health care facilities are often referred to in court cases to ascertain the appropriate standard of care. Thus the standards set by TJC are often considered the "industry standard" even for facilities that are not accredited (Weden, 2016).

Federal and state statutes require nursing facilities to have written health care and safety policies, and these have been used successfully to establish a standard of care in court cases. Bylaws and internal rules and policies also help establish the standard of care in an organization, although, depending on the circumstances, their importance may vary. In any event, it is important for nurses to be aware of their organization's policies; failure to follow "your own rules" clearly poses a liability risk—both to the nurse and the organization.

OVERVIEW OF RELEVANT LAWS

Sources of Law

Statutes are laws created by legislation and are enacted at the federal and state levels. Common laws are principles and rules of action and derive authority from judgments and decrees of the court; they are also known as *case law* (Syam, 2014). Regulations are rules of action and conduct developed to explain and interpret statutes and to prescribe methods for carrying out statutory mandates. Regulations are also promulgated at the federal and state levels.

Health Insurance Portability and Accountability Act of 1996 (HIPAA)

Recent changes in federal law provide additional protection to individuals and their family members when they need to buy, change, or continue their health insurance. These important laws affect the health benefits of millions of working Americans and their families. It is important that nurses understand these regulations, as well as laws in their respective states, to help them make more informed choices for themselves or to inform their patients of the options available. The Health Insurance Portability and Accountability Act of 1996 (HIPAA) may:

1. Increase a person's ability to get health care coverage when the person begins a new job;
2. Lower the chance of losing existing health coverage, whether the coverage is through a job or through individual health insurance;
3. Help maintain continuous health coverage when a change of job occurs; and
4. Help purchase health insurance coverage individually if the coverage is lost under an employer's group health plan and no other health coverage is available (Health and Human Services, 2017).

Among the specific protections of HIPAA, it:

1. Limits the use of preexisting condition exclusions;
2. Prohibits group health plans from discriminating by denying coverage or charging extra for coverage based on the person's or a family member's past or present poor health;
3. Guarantees certain small employers and individuals who lost job-related coverage the right to purchase health insurance; and

4. Guarantees, in most cases, that employers or individuals who purchase health insurance can renew the coverage regardless of any health conditions of individuals covered under the insurance policy (Health and Human Services, 2017).

Several misunderstandings exist about what HIPAA provides. Note the following:

1. HIPAA does *not* require employers to offer or pay for health coverage for employees or family coverage for spouses and dependents.
2. HIPAA does *not* guarantee health coverage for all workers.
3. HIPAA does *not* control the amount an insurer may charge for coverage.
4. HIPAA does *not* require group health plans to offer specific benefits.
5. HIPAA does *not* permit people to keep the same health coverage they had in their old job when they move to a new job.
6. HIPAA does *not* eliminate all use of preexisting condition exclusions.
7. HIPAA does *not* replace the state as the primary regulator of health insurance (Health and Human Services, 2017).

ELDER ABUSE AND PROTECTIVE SERVICES

It has already been noted that the incidence of illness and disability increases with age. With aging, the older adult's health status often leads to changes in living arrangements both in homes and institutions. Often, a crisis or a sudden change emerges that leaves the older adult unable to continue in his or her own residence or perform self-care. These changes affect not only older adults but also often their family and others who must see to their care and living needs. Without enacting appropriate interventions and resources, this can lead to neglect, deliberate abuse, or exploitation of older adults.

In addition, as older adults' abilities to manage their personal affairs are compromised, the necessity of turning the management of certain activities over to others may also open the door to mistreatment. The legal recognition of this vulnerability is reflected in laws enacted specifically to protect older adults. Unfortunately, mistreatment is not defined in the same manner across each state. However, it is known that it occurs recurrently, episodically, and not usually as an isolated incident. (Factora, 2017).

The need to protect older adults from abuse is a subject of growing public policy interest. Elder abuse, including neglect and exploitation, is reported to be experienced by 1 out of every 10 people, ages 60 and older (Centers for Disease Control, 2017). However, given the potential for hiding incidents of elder abuse in domestic settings as a "family secret" or out of fear, the incidents of elder abuse are likely grossly underreported. Cultural differences have also led to poor identification of the reaction to abuse.

Elder abuse is defined by state laws, which vary from state to state. However, three basic categories of elder abuse exist: (1) domestic elder abuse, (2) institutional elder abuse, and (3) self-neglect or self-abuse (U.S. Legal, 2016). *Domestic elder abuse* refers to forms of maltreatment by someone who has a special relationship with the older adult, for example, a family member or caregiver. *Institutional abuse* refers to abuse that occurs in residential institutions such as nursing facilities, usually committed by someone who is a paid caregiver such as a nursing facility staff member. Self-neglect is usually related to a diminished physical or mental decline. It is identified by a failure or refusal to provide oneself with adequate shelter, food, water, hygiene, safety, clothing, or health care. Within the three broad categories as noted, there are several recognized types of elder abuse.

An analysis of existing definitions inclusive of elder abuse, neglect, and exploitation was conducted by the National Center of Elder Abuse (NCEA). Seven types of elder abuse were identified (NCEA, n.d.):

1. Physical abuse—use of physical force that may result in bodily injury, physical pain, or impairment
2. Sexual abuse—nonconsensual sexual contact of any kind with an older adult
3. Emotional abuse—infliction of anguish, pain, or distress through verbal or nonverbal acts
4. Financial and material exploitation—illegal or improper use of an older adult's funds, property, or assets
5. Neglect—the refusal or failure of a person to fulfill any part of his or her obligations or duties to an older adult
6. Abandonment—the desertion of an older adult by an individual who has physical custody of the older adult or by a person who has assumed responsibility for providing care to the older adult
7. Self-neglect—behaviors of an older adult that threaten the older adult's health or safety

Elder abuse generally occurs as the result of many complex factors. Abuse or the potential for abuse may be a result of caregiver stress. The physical and emotional demands of caring for a physically or mentally impaired person can be great, and the caregiver may not be prepared to undertake the responsibility. Supportive resources may also be lacking. Unpaid caregivers, be they family or a significant other, often report anxiety symptoms and depression (Kudra, Lees, & Morrell-Scott, 2017). Additionally, caregivers with less social support and poor coping mechanisms are at a higher risk of experiencing depression and anxiety disorders, which can lead to burnout and abuse in some situations.

Nurses must be alert to recognize signs and symptoms of abuse and caregiver stress. Signs of physical abuse may be visible, for example, bruises, wounds, or fractures. They may also be less apparent, for example, an older adult's report of being hit or mistreated or a sudden change in behavior. Sexual abuse may be detectable by the presence of signs such as bruises in the genital area or unexplained vaginal bleeding/discharge. Other forms of abuse such as the taking of pornographic photographs may be more difficult to detect. Signs of neglect, self or caregiver related, may include unsanitary living conditions or the older adult being malnourished or dehydrated. In addition, the nurse should be alert to signs of financial or material exploitation, for example, the unexplained disappearance of funds or valuable possessions.

Because signs and symptoms of elder abuse in its many forms may be difficult to detect, the nurse must be educated in this regard and be alert to the actions of others such as nursing attendants involved in the care of older adults. It has been well documented that health care professionals, from all levels, lack adequate education and training with respect to the unique health care needs of older adults (White et al., 2015). As the number of elderly requiring care increases, it is paramount that ongoing education inclusive of stress management, abuse identification, and abuse prevention be included as required elements in ongoing training and education.

The term *adult protective services* refers to the range of laws and regulations enacted to deal with abusive situations. The laws and regulations are typically administered by an agency within the state, for example, the Department of Social Services and individual state's Department of Health, which receives and investigates complaints. Specific responses to safeguard abused or at-risk older adults may include protective orders and legal involvement to shield older adults from abusive persons; elder abuse statutes that outlaw harmful acts victimizing older adults; and interventions to protect older residents of nursing facilities from abuse inclusive of psychological, physical, and social needs of abused older adults (Du Mont, Kosa, Macdonald, Elliot, & Yaffe, 2015).

Elder abuse laws levy criminal penalties against those who commit harmful acts against older adults. Many states' laws enhance the penalties for criminal offenses against older persons, for example, some violent or property-related offenses outlaw any acts that victimize older adults (e.g., see Connecticut General Statutes Annals §46a-15). These laws typically apply to the abuse of older adults in the community. States may also levy penalties for acts of elder abuse committed by those responsible for the care of older adults in nursing facilities or other institutions. These laws are in addition to those already in effect to protect the rights of patients in facilities governed by federal regulation. Most states have mandatory reporting requirements for nurses, other health care workers, and facility employees who have a reasonable suspicion of elder abuse.

The definition of what constitutes elder abuse under these statutes varies. For example, emotional abuse may be in the form of acts such as "ridiculing or demeaning ... or making derogatory remarks to a ... resident"[1]; "any nonaccidental infliction of physical injury, sexual abuse, or mental injury"[2]; and "unauthorized use of physical or chemical restraint, medication, or isolation."[3] For the purposes of these types of statutes, some states define the term *older adults* as those 60 years or older. It is important for nurses to know the legal requirements relating to the abuse of older adults for the state in which they practice.

Most states designate certain professionals, such as nurses or other caregivers, as "mandated reporters." This means that the mandated reporter is *required* by law to report suspected cases of abuse, neglect, or exploitation. Failure to report as required under this law may result in imposition of civil penalties, criminal penalties, or both.

A report of suspected abuse may be required on a "reasonable suspicion." This implies that actual knowledge or certainty is not necessary. Most states provide immunity from civil liability for anyone reporting older adult abuse based on reasonable suspicion and in good faith, even if it is later shown that the reporter was mistaken. However, it is interesting to note that the majority of elder abuse reports are in fact substantiated after investigation (Oregon State Bar, 2015).

In most care settings, nurses are mandated reporters. To be responsive to this legal obligation and because of the great variation among the states, nurses should determine the specific reporting requirements of their jurisdictions, including where reports and complaints are received and in what form they must be made.

Nurses must be aware of their responsibility to respect and to preserve the autonomy and individual rights of older adults. All people, including older adults, have the right to decide what is to be done to them, as well as the right to exercise maximum control of their personal environments and living conditions. The nurse's responsibility in this regard emanates from both legal and professional standards.

The fact of ongoing legislative responses to the identification and preservation of these rights underscores this point. The nurse as a trusted health professional is often closest to older patients and therefore may be in the best position to communicate and understand their wishes. This presents both an unequaled opportunity and a legally recognizable and indisputable responsibility to advocate on their behalf. Thus the need to be legally informed and professionally conscientious in practice is greater than ever.

Medicare and Medicaid

The federal government, under the Social Security Act, has the primary responsibility for providing medical services to certain older adults, those with disabilities, or certain other classified American citizens. The government fulfills this obligation through the Medicare and Medicaid programs. These programs were enacted as part of the Social Security Amendments of 1965 (P.L. No. 89–97, July 30, 1965).[4] Several amendments have been added over the years, and the continuation or proposed modifications of amendments is ongoing.

The U.S. Department of Health and Human Services (DHHS) promulgated regulations for the Medicare and Medicaid programs until July 1, 2001. At that time, the Health Care Financing Administration (HCFA) became the Centers for Medicare and Medicaid Services (CMS). The restructured agency aims to increase emphasis on responsiveness to the beneficiaries and providers, and quality improvement is one of the goals (Fig. 3.1).

Two levels of care are generally associated with nursing facilities: skilled and intermediate. *Skilled* nursing facilities (SNFs) provide technical and complex care and offer a higher level of care provided by professional staff. Medicare pays for skilled care in a long-term care facility only on a case-by-case basis for a limited period of time. Coverage includes nursing, physical

---

[1]Delaware Title 16 § §1132 and 1135.

[2]Illinois Chapter 111½¶ 4161-176.

[3]California Welfare and Institutions § §15600–15637.

[4]42 U.S.C. §3001 (1965).

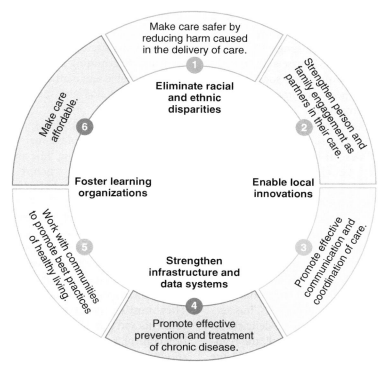

Fig. 3.1 Centers for Medicare and Medicaid Services Quality Strategy goals. (Redrawn from Healthcare and technology. [2015]. Is fee-for-service dead? Retrieved from http://www.myhealthtechblog.com/2015/04/fee-for-service.html)

therapy, occupational therapy, and speech therapy. Medicaid pays for both intermediate and skilled care for indigent persons. *Intermediate* care is considered custodial in nature and is supervised by professional nurses.

The Omnibus Budget Reconciliation Act of 1987 (OBRA), a landmark piece of legislation enacted October 1990, refers to SNFs only in relation to Medicare facilities and has merged the distinctions *skilled* and *intermediate* into the single term *nursing facility* for Medicaid purposes. For survey purposes, a single set of survey requirements is used. Survey and certification procedures and the process by which the CMS evaluates and determines whether a provider is compliant with the Medicare and Medicaid requirements can be found through the Health Standards and Quality Bureau housed within the CMS.

NURSING FACILITY REFORM

As of 2014, the number of nursing facilities in the United States was 15,600 with 1.7 million licensed beds and more than 1.4 million older adults in residence (Centers for Disease Control, 2016).

The OBRA applies to all Medicare- and Medicaid-certified nursing facilities, including (1) beds in acute care hospitals certified to be used as long-term nursing care beds at times when they are not needed for acute care purposes (so-called swing beds) and (2) beds in acute care hospitals certified as separate units for Medicare-approved services (so-called distinct part units). The OBRA is the most sweeping reform affecting Medicare and Medicaid nursing facilities since the programs began.

Evidence that the health and safety of nursing facility residents have improved as a result of these stringent regulations and sweeping reforms is quite evident. Such improvements, among other things, include reduction in the overuse of antipsychotic drugs, inappropriate use of restraints, and inappropriate use of indwelling urinary catheters. Since 2001, the CMS has increased the number of penalties levied on poor-quality nursing facilities (CMS, 2017).

However, the CMS has also identified areas requiring greater regulatory oversight. Nursing facility surveys are too predictable and are rarely conducted on weekends or during evening hours. Some states rarely cite nursing facilities for substandard care, which is an indication that their inspections may be inadequate. Nursing facility residents continue to suffer from pressure ulcers and skin breakdown, malnutrition and dehydration, and various forms of abuse (Levinson, 2013). For these reasons, new enforcement tools are being added to the regulatory oversight of the nations' nursing facilities. Some of these additional measures are discussed in the following section.

OBRA's Three Major Parts

The OBRA provisions are divided into three parts: (1) provision of service requirements for nursing facilities, (2) survey and certification processes, and (3) enforcement mechanisms and sanctions.

The provision of service requirements for nursing facilities includes resident assessments, preadmission and annual screening of residents, maintenance and public posting of minimal nurse staffing levels, required and approved nurse aide training programs and competency levels, and professional social worker services in facilities with 120 or more beds. The important focus is on specifying and ensuring resident rights.

The survey and certification process was substantially revised with the enactment of the OBRA. New survey methods have been established to evaluate facilities. In brief, each facility is subject to a standard annual survey. Any change in facility management or ownership is further evaluated by a "special" survey. If any survey suggests that care may be substandard, the facility may be subject to a more detailed "extended" survey. States are also evaluated for the effectiveness of their survey process through a "validation" survey. Furthermore, federal authorities may make an independent and binding determination of a facility's compliance through a "special compliance" survey.

A new range of enforcement mechanisms and sanctions have been brought forth since the enactment of the OBRA. Thus several corrective measures may be applied to repair deficiencies based on the severity of the risk to residents. Overall, the regulations focus on the quality of life of nursing facility residents and emphasize their individual rights. As a direct result from the OBRA, a new regulatory environment was created to empower residents and provide them with a greater voice regarding quality of life issues.

Provision of Service Requirements

Quality of Care. Nursing facility residents must be assessed to detect medical problems, evaluation of their capacity to perform daily life functions, and identification of significant impairments in their functional capacity. In Medicare- and Medicaid-certified long-term care facilities, physicians evaluate residents at the time of admission, then reassessment must be completed by a health care provider at 30 days and 90 days, with any change in condition, and at 1-year intervals. A state-specified instrument must be used to conduct the initial or intake assessment, which is based on a uniform data set, referred to as the *minimum data set* (MDS), established by the DHHS.

This assessment is used to develop an initial baseline plan of care for each resident and must be accomplished with in the first 48 hours of admission (CMS, 2017). The plan must quantify expected levels of functioning and must be reviewed quarterly. MDS assessment categories include resident background, daily pattern of activity, cognition, physical functioning, psychosocial status, pharmacologic use, health problems, and specific body systems (CMS, 2017).

A similar uniform approach to the assessment of adult home care patients, known as the *outcome and assessment information set* (OASIS-C), is used across the country. The goal of this tool is to provide a set of essential data items necessary for measuring patient outcomes that have utility for such purposes as outcome monitoring, clinical assessment, and care planning. As of January 1, 2015, the CMS (2015) issued new rules relating to home health agencies that include the required collection of OASIS-C data.

The assessment and planning of care for nursing facility residents is a significant role for the professional nurse. As can be seen from this discussion of nursing facility reform, it is a central point for determining the care and services that residents will need. Careful assessment and planning require the professional nurse to be skilled and knowledgeable in carrying out these functions.

The advent of the OBRA and nursing facility reform has ushered in increased professional accountability. It has increased the demands on nursing time and performance, forced nursing facilities to change the structure of their operation, and resulted in a different image of what nursing facilities are and how they care for their residents.

Medicare SNFs and Medicaid nursing facilities must have licensed nursing services available around the clock, 7 days a week. A registered nurse (RN) must be on duty a minimum of 8 hours a day, 7 days a week.

Nursing assistants must be trained according to regulatory specifications and pass state-approved competency evaluations. They must receive classroom training before any contact with residents and training in areas such as interpersonal skills, infection control, safety procedures, and resident rights. Regulations specific to curriculum and training requirements are developed at the individual state level to govern the profession. Many but not all states require ongoing continuing education in topics such as elder care or working with cognitively impaired residents, for example (Freeman, 2017).

Resident Rights. A primary thrust of the OBRA's nursing facility reform provision is to protect and promote the rights of residents to enhance their quality of life. Thus the legislation contains numerous requirements to ensure the preservation of a resident's rights.[5] Disclosure obligations on nursing facilities to apprise residents of their rights have been required by the OBRA; residents are to be notified, both orally and in writing, of their rights and responsibilities and of all rules governing resident conduct. Notification and disclosure must take place before or up to the time of admission and must be updated and reviewed during the residents' stay. Box 3.1 provides an example of statements from the OBRA's resident bill of rights, as adapted from the Code of Federal Regulations (CFR). Most facilities have developed a contract for new residents (or a family member or other responsible person) to sign at the time of admission. This is usually called the *admission agreement.* This agreement sets forth the rights, obligations, and expectations of each party. It is an effective way to inform residents of a facility's rules, regulations, and philosophy of care. This is a practical way to meet the OBRA's notification and disclosure requirements.

As with any agreement, it can only be a valid contract if the parties entering into the agreement can understand its provisions. If a resident is not capable of doing this, then a family member or other responsible person may sign on the resident's behalf. The laws of the particular state should be explored to determine who is permitted to contract on behalf of the resident.

Transfer or discharge of residents is permissible by the facility per the OBRA regulations in the following situations: (1) if

---

[5]OBRA '87 at § 4211(a), 42 U.S.C.A. § 139r(c) (West Supp 1989).

BOX 3.1 Resident Bill of Rights

A facility must protect and must promote the exercise of rights for all residents. The following are some of those rights:

1. The right to select a personal attending physician and to receive complete information about one's care and treatment, including access to all records pertaining to the resident
2. Freedom from physical or mental abuse, corporal punishment, involuntary seclusion, and any unwarranted physical or chemical restraints
3. Privacy regarding accommodations, medical treatment, mail and telephone communication, visits, and meetings of family and resident groups
4. Confidentiality regarding personal and clinical records
5. Residing in a facility and receiving services with reasonable accommodation of individual needs and preferences
6. Protesting one's treatment or care without discrimination or reprisal, including the refusal to participate in experimental research
7. Participation in resident and family groups
8. Participation in social, religious, and community activities
9. The right to examine the federal or state authorities' surveys of a nursing facility

Modified from 42 CFR § 483.10.

the facility cannot meet the residents' needs, (2) if their stay is no longer required for their medical condition, (3) if they fail to pay for their care as agreed to, or (4) if the facility ceases to operate. These provisions provide a 30-day notice and are designed to establish the basic right of a resident to remain in a facility and not be transferred involuntarily unless one of these conditions exists; they also ensure that a resident has been given proper notice with the opportunity to appeal the decision. This was, in part, a response to situations in which older residents of nursing facilities were "ousted" without notice and perhaps without regard to the detrimental effects (both physical and emotional) of being uprooted from familiar surroundings.

The requirement for a bill of rights for residents is a new requirement. Many states have had such provisions in their facility licensure statutes for many years. Medicare and Medicaid regulations have also included resident rights requirements for some time. The OBRA strengthened and enhanced the importance of these requirements by enforcing them as part of the facility survey process. Although the specific contents of resident's rights laws vary considerably from state to state, both the state and federal contents have some similarities. Both are concerned with physician selection, medical decision making, privacy, dignity, the ability to pursue grievances, discharge and transfer rights, and access to visitors and services (Medicare.gov, n.d.).

Unnecessary Drug Use and Chemical and Physical Restraints. The OBRA regulations require nursing facility residents be free of unnecessary drugs of all types; chemical restraints, commonly thought of as psychotropic drugs; and physical restraints. Chemical restraints are inclusive of drugs used to limit or inhibit specific behaviors or movements, such as antipsychotics, benzodiazepines, other anxiolytic and sedative drugs, and hypnotics. The drug use guidelines are based on the principles that certain problems can be handled with nonpharmacologic methods and interventions should be utilized and ruled out as correcting the issue before drug therapy is initiated. Furthermore, when used, drugs must either maintain or demonstrate improvement of a resident's functional status.

Guidelines, as noted by the OBRA, detail doses but do not set maximum dosage limitations. Dosage detailing draws attention to the ongoing need for a comprehensive assessment and review of appropriate drug/dosage use to be completed for each resident. Surveyors review the duration of drug therapy regimens and look for documentation of indications for the use of the drug therapy. Nurses should also carefully document observed effects of drug therapy. This is an area in which the nurse should exercise their skill, knowledge, critical thinking, and leadership by working with others on the resident's care team to ensure that the resident is not overmedicated or unnecessarily medicated. For example, the nurse may work with the interdisciplinary care team to plan nondrug interventions.

The nurse, as an advocate for the practice and resident, is in a position to inform the health care provider about the OBRA's guidelines regarding drug use. This may not only be new information for the provider, but it may also provide a sound explanation that can be used when speaking with a resident's family who may request drug interventions. In fact, the nurse is in the best position to work with residents and their families to provide information, give instruction on alternative nonpharmacologic interventions, and reinforce best practice about this important approach to care.

Drug toxicities have been underestimated, and at times drugs have been used to meet the desires of nurses or other facility staff for "environmental control," for example, to settle residents down for sleep. The need to manage the environment may pose a genuine dilemma for nurses because certain resident behaviors such as yelling or wandering into other residents' rooms may be disruptive. Such behaviors may cause family members to pressure nurses to calm down such residents or take other steps to stop the bothersome behavior. Nursing facility residents may be challenging despite the nursing staff's intent to provide appropriate levels of care inclusive of a behavioral assessment to identify the cause. However, drug therapy should not be used for convenience or environmental control but rather for resident-specific interventions to address the issue.

The OBRA's guidelines require that antipsychotic drugs be used at the minimum dose necessary. This minimization must be ensured through careful monitoring and documentation by the staff to identify why a behavioral problem may exist and whether the antipsychotic treatment is effecting a positive change in the target symptom. Residents receiving an antipsychotic drug must have an indication for the use of the drug based on one of the following conditions:

1. Schizophrenia
2. Schizoid-affective disorder
3. Delusional disorder
4. Acute psychosis
5. Mania with psychotic mood
6. Brief reactive psychosis
7. Atypical psychosis
8. Tourette syndrome
9. Huntington chorea

10. Short-term symptomatic treatment of nausea, vomiting, hiccups, or itching
11. Dementia associated with psychotic or violent features that represent a danger to the patients or others

Reasons for the use of antipsychotic drugs must be documented in the physician's orders and in the resident care plan. They should not be used for behaviors such as restlessness, insomnia, yelling or screaming, and wandering, or because of the staff's inability to manage the resident.

The OBRA mandates a 25% reduction in dose trial, unless the drug has been tried previously and has resulted in decompensation of the resident or if the resident has one of the 11 conditions listed earlier. A "reduction in dose trial" consists of a reduction in the dose of the drug coupled with observations to note the return of symptoms or any adverse side effects. The dose is gradually increased until the optimal effectiveness in treatment response and the minimum necessary dose are achieved.

The provider's order must include the following specific information: (1) the reasons for the use of antipsychotic drugs, including medical indications; (2) the target behaviors that the drug therapy is intended to treat; (3) the goals of therapy; and (4) common side effects. These notations must also be entered in the resident's care plan. The observations and charting made by the nurse must also address these specific points.

Physical restraints are appliances that inhibit free physical movement, for example, limb restraints, vests, jackets, and waist belts. Wheelchairs, geriatric chairs, and side rails may, in some circumstances, also be forms of physical restraint (DHHS, 2014). This type of restraint may be used only when specific medical indications exist and when a provider has written a specific order for their use. The order must include the type of restraint, the condition or specific behavior for which it is to be applied, and a specified time or duration for its use. Orders for a restraint must be reevaluated and, if use is to be continued, periodically reassessed.

Documentation of the behavior or condition that led to the order for a restraint, both chemical and physical; interventions utilized before restraints; and ongoing monitoring of the resident's condition must be undertaken. When physical restraints are used, the resident must be observed and the restraints released at regular intervals. Records documenting these activities must be kept.

Reductions in the use of physical restraints and almost universal use of CMS's resident assessment system are indications that nursing facility reform is working. Recent reports indicate that antipsychotic drug use is down, resulting in economic benefits and improving the quality of life for nursing facility residents (California Advocates for Nursing Home Reform [CANHR], 2016). Nurses have been successful in employing interventions directed toward avoiding the use of chemical or physical restraints. Some of these interventions are companionship; increased patient supervision; meeting physical needs such as toileting, exercise, or hunger; modifying staff attitudes; 1:1 safety sitters; and distraction and other psychosocial approaches. Nurses are in a unique position to positively affect the quality of life of institutionalized older adults. Nurses should continue to educate others about behavior management techniques to decrease the incidence of chemical and physical restraint usage.

A facility is not absolved from regulatory liability by the mere presence of a provider's written order for restraints of any kind. The nursing staff as directed by the Nurse Practice Act and the ANA *Code of Ethics for Nurses* is professionally responsible for challenging all questionable orders. For example, statement three and its interpretation in the *Code of Ethics for Nurses* identify the nurses' responsibility to "safeguard the patient," and to challenge any "questionable practice in the provision of health care" (ANA, 2015). Nurses should participate in the development of problem-solving procedures established to provide constructive and effective ways to resolve disputes involving patient care issues. Such procedures generally provide an avenue of communication that may be used to resolve questions or disagreements that arise between health care professionals. When a question or issue does arise, the nurse must institute the dispute resolution procedure promptly.

Urinary Incontinence. Urinary incontinence is commonly noted in SNFs. In fact, more than half of nursing facility residents are incontinent. Left untreated, this condition may lead to other physical problems such as infections and skin breakdown. Because this is a prevalent condition and one that has implications for the quality and enjoyment of life, it may be expected to remain a major area of regulatory scrutiny. Under the OBRA, nursing facilities are required to include incontinence in the comprehensive assessment of a resident's functions and to provide the necessary treatment inclusive of bladder retraining, prompted voiding, pelvic floor exercises, etc. (Kow, Carr, & Whytock, 2013). Furthermore, surveyors of the state Division of Aging focus on this problem by evaluating its occurrence in the nursing facilities they survey and assessing the extent to which residents are involved in bladder training programs.

Nurses should be familiar with guidelines and procedures for management of incontinence, for example, the Agency for Health Care Policy and Research Guidelines. Charting should be specific to reflect the presence and extent of the problem of incontinence, and it should note the treatment plan that has been established and the effects of the treatment. From the OBRA perspective, behavioral approaches are preferable to more intense mechanical or chemical therapies.

Facility Survey and Certification

The CMS is determined to see that every nursing facility implements and complies with the letter and spirit of the OBRA's requirements. This determination is enforced through a process of surveying facilities that certifies a facility's compliance with the OBRA's laws and regulations. The enactment of the OBRA created a new survey process. In general, the standard survey is conducted to review the quality of care by evaluation of criteria such as medical, nursing, and rehabilitative care; dietary services; infection control; and the physical environment.

Written care plans and resident assessments are evaluated for their adequacy and accuracy, and the surveyors look for compliance with residents' rights. The OBRA's long-term care survey processes have a renewed emphasis on the outcome of resident care rather than mere paper compliance with regulatory requirements.

By contractual arrangement with the DHHS, state survey agencies are authorized to certify the compliance of facilities.

States are also required to educate facility staff regarding the survey process and are further authorized to investigate complaints of all types. Based on reports of persistent problems in nursing facilities that spearheaded government involvement, the CMS strives to strengthen federal oversight of nursing facility quality and safety standards. These steps include increasing the frequency of inspections for repeat offenders or facilities with serious violations. In addition, contrary to past practices, more inspections are carried out on weekends and evenings. This approach serves to target states with weak inspections systems and compliance. In doing so, there is assurance that state surveyors are enforcing the policies of the CMS to sanction nursing facilities with serious violations.

Surveys are conducted by a multidisciplinary survey team of professionals, including at least one RN. Survey participants include facility personnel, residents and their families, and the state's long-term care public advocate that investigates complaints, known as an ombudsman. Surveyors interview residents and ask them about facility policies and procedures. They observe staff in the performance of their duties, and staff may be asked to complete forms required by the survey team.

Enforcement Mechanisms and Sanctions

The DHHS and the states may apply sanctions or penalties against a facility for failure to meet requirements and standards. Such sanctions include civil monetary penalties, appointment of a temporary manager to run a facility while deficiencies are remedied, or even closure of a facility or transfer of residents to another facility (or both). In addition, the CMS and some State Department of Health offices publish individual nursing facility survey results and violation records on the Internet to increase accountability and flag repeated offenders for families and the public.

If sanctions are applied, they must be appropriate to the facility deficiency. This often depends on whether an immediate threat to the health and safety of residents exists. Sanctions may also be increased if there are repeated or uncorrected deficiencies. Deficiencies are analyzed based on the scope of the deficiency—that is, whether it constitutes a pattern of activity or whether it is an isolated or sporadic occurrence—and the severity of the deficiency—that is, the extent to which it presents a threat to the safety and welfare of residents. To assist in analysis, the scope and severity factors are laid out in a gridlike fashion, and sanctions are applied based on the result of this analysis.

It is important for the nurse to understand that officials, authorized by the state or federal agencies that oversee the operation of nursing facilities (or any licensed health care institution or setting), may enter and review activities within an organization at any time. They are not required to announce the visit in advance; OBRA's regulations specifically prohibit this for the annual standard survey, and nurses must respond to their questions and requests for information and records once proper identification is shown.

The Director of Nursing (DON) of the organization has a significant role in the survey process. If requested to do so by the surveyor, the director may participate in rounds or other activities of the surveyor; the director is also present at a closing conference in which the overall results of the survey are discussed.

Often, the surveyors follow up the visit by telephone, or they may return for additional visits to a facility if further information is needed. A written report of the survey is ultimately sent to the facility; if deficiencies or violations are present, the DON and other members of the nursing staff may participate in formulating a plan of correction to submit to the regulatory officials.

During an inspection, a surveyor may find information suggesting that the practice of a licensed nurse may have been improper or may not have met the proper standard of care. For example, a nurse may have a high incidence of medication errors or may not have taken proper action when a patient or resident experienced a change in condition. In such cases, the surveyor may forward the record showing the relevant findings to the appropriate state agency or board for review of the nurse's practice, requesting a determination of whether the nurse may have violated their state's nurse practice act. The board may find no basis for further action and not proceed, or it may require a hearing or other measure that could lead to disciplinary action. Disciplinary action could range from a reprimand, to required educational remediation, to suspension or revocation of the nurse's license. This again underscores the need for nurses to be diligent, current, conscientious, and accountable in their professional practice.

Proposed Legislative Changes

The federal government, although recognizing improvements in the care of nursing facility residents, has also been alarmed by reports of persistent serious problems. Ongoing changes and a commitment to improved health care to address issues are goals of the CMS.

Congress has taken some steps to ensure a safe environment for nursing facility residents. For example, the OBRA requires all states to establish and maintain a registry of nurse aides who are unfit to provide care because of abusive or criminal histories. In addition, states currently require nursing facilities to do criminal background checks on new job applicants, inclusive of student nurses training in the extended care facilities.

Affordable Care Act

The Affordable Care Act (ACA) was passed by Congress on March 21, 2010, and signed into law on March 23, 2010, by former President Barack Obama. The ACA represents the largest change in the United States Health Care System since 1965 when Medicare and Medicaid were enacted and initiated. The main goal of the ACA is to reduce the number of Americans who do not have health insurance and to further reduce the overall costs of health care in the United States (eHealth, 2016).

Legislative changes to the ACA in 2017 repealed the individual mandate, eliminated cost-sharing reductions, increased state Medicaid waivers and the expansion of Association Health Plans (AHPs) (Beaton, 2018). The overall impact of these changes to the ACA is yet to be determined.

All Americans will be able to obtain health insurance regardless of their community rating, preexisting medical conditions, or age. Everyone within the same age group and location must be charged the same premium. Failure to secure coverage may lead to penalties assessed by a health insurance tax.

AUTONOMY AND SELF-DETERMINATION

The right to self-determination has its basis in the doctrine of informed consent. *Informed consent* is the process by which competent individuals are provided with information that enables them to make a reasonable decision about any treatment or intervention to be performed on them. A great deal of legal analysis has been applied to the question, "What is enough information for a person to make a reasonable decision?" It is generally accepted that for consent to be valid and legally sufficient, a standard of disclosure must be met that includes the diagnosis, the nature and purpose of the treatment, the risks of the treatment, the probability of success of the treatment, available treatment alternatives, and the consequences of not receiving the treatment.

Informed consent has developed from strong judicial deference toward individual autonomy, reflecting a belief that individuals have a right to be free from nonconsensual interference with their persons, and the basic moral principle that it is wrong to force others to act against their will (DHHS, 2016). The judicial system's strong deference toward individual autonomy in the medical context was articulated long ago by Justice Benjamin Cardozo: Every human being of adult years and sound mind has a right to determine what shall be done with his own body.[6]

The right to self-determination has a long-standing basis in common or case law and has roots under the right of liberty guaranteed by the U.S. Constitution. These common law rights, to a significant extent, have been codified, acted on by legislatures, and enacted into statutory law. The codification of these legal rights should serve to make the legal tools of self-determination more readily available to the citizenry.

Nurses should be careful, however, on those occasions in which the opposite effect occurs. Rather than making mechanisms for the exercise of consent more available, the codification of these rights sometimes results in a view that the absence of a legal, written tool or directive such as a living will (LW) or a signed consent form means that a patient's decision has not been made. However, there may be other sources of information that express a person's wishes, and caregivers should not presume that the absence of a written document is the same as a lack of consent. Rather, nurses must remember that the right to decide what shall be done for and to oneself is a fundamental right. Legal tools should be used to assist, not detract, from that basic human right. The nurse's role as advocate has a high degree of importance in this regard.

The right to self-determination covers all decisions about one's care and treatment, including the removal of life support or life-sustaining treatments and life-prolonging or life-saving measures. These issues are particularly relevant to older adults. Although individuals of all ages are concerned with these matters and young persons do die, incapacity and infirmity are more common in old age. Therefore more frequent discussion of the need to preserve the right to self-determination occurs among older adults.

The doctrine and standards of informed consent are intended to apply to the decision-making capability of one who is competent to make such a decision. In this context, the term *competent* refers to the ability to understand the proposed treatment or procedure and thereby make an informed decision. When a person is not competent, a surrogate may make the decision. This is known as "substituted" judgment.

Do Not Resuscitate Orders

A "do not resuscitate" (DNR) order is a specific order from a health care provider, entered on the patient/resident's order sheet or by using computerized physician order entry (CPOE) systems. Code status or DNR orders have been used for many years. The order instructs health care providers not to use or order specific methods of life-saving therapy, referred to as *cardiopulmonary resuscitation* (CPR). This generally includes measures and therapies used to restore cardiac function or to support ventilation in the event of a cardiac or respiratory arrest[7] and to handle emergencies caused by sudden loss of oxygen supply to the brain because of lung or cardiac failure. In some states, consent to CPR is presumed unless a DNR order has been issued.[8] Competent individuals may choose to forego any treatment or care, even if the choice will result in death.

For a person to choose to accept or reject medical care, that person must be determined to be competent. The reluctance of courts to articulate a standard for competence has resulted in very few reported opinions that state any formal opinion of competency. Rather, courts prefer to involve physicians, often psychiatrists, and other caregivers in testifying about the mental state of a person, and the courts base the determination of competency on that information.

The capacity to make decisions is applicable only to the decision being made at the time. Even if a person has appointed an agent to manage his or her affairs, this does not necessarily mean that the person is incompetent in any total sense. "It is ethically inappropriate to assign blanket 'incapacity to decide' to the [older adult] patient based on isolated areas of irrationality."[9]

In a court determination of competency, the nurse may be called on to testify and will be asked to offer information relative to their assessment of the client's behavior or verbalizations that may give evidence of the person's state of mind. The medical record is extremely important in this type of proceeding, and the nurse will want to use it to back up any testimony given; this is yet another reason as to why documentation is so vitally important.

Older adults are more often faced with issues concerning the right to self-determination, and in such matters, patients' statements and other indications of their wishes, as well as their state of mind, are critical. Nurses should keep these points in mind when they are responsible for the care of older adults, and they

---

[6]*Schloendorf v. Society of New York Hospital*, 211 N.Y. 125, 129 (1914).

[7]McKinney's consolidated laws of New York annotated, Public Health Law § 2961(4).

[8]McKinney's consolidated laws of New York annotated, Public Health Law § 2962(1) (McKinney, 1993).

[9]Lieberson AD, *Advance medical directives*, vol. 1, September 1997, Sec 30.3, p 453.

should make certain that records and notations, assessments, and other ongoing observations are carefully, objectively, and accurately documented. If a time comes when a nurse needs to refer to records to testify in a court proceeding, the information provided will be used to help determine how an individual's basic rights are being addressed. A nurse can be secure in knowing that everything morally, ethically, and legally has been done to see that the resident's rights are respected.

Guidelines for DNR Policies in Nursing Facilities

Nurses often raise questions and are faced with dilemmas about DNR policies because of inconsistency or uncertainty in either the existing policy or the application of procedures. Because the nurse may be the only health care professional present in the nursing facility at any given time, it is imperative for the nurse to request that the facility have a detailed and specific policy to provide the necessary guidance.

If a facility does develop a DNR policy, the following guidelines should be considered. Whatever policies are adopted should be well communicated to the staff and should be adhered to scrupulously. The policy should indicate:

- That a facility must have competently trained staff available 24 hours a day to provide CPR (Consumer Voice, n.d.).
- Whether CPR will be performed unless a DNR order exists.
- The conditions under which the facility will issue DNR orders. These factors should be in compliance with applicable state law; thus it is necessary to examine the DNR provisions of the jurisdiction. Considerations include required health care provider consultations regarding medical conditions and documented discussions with the patient and family members.
- That competency is established, again with proper documentation or medical consultation, as may be indicated by applicable state law.
- The origin of consent for the order: by the patient, while competent; by an advance medical directive (AMD); or by a substitute or surrogate decision maker.
- Provision for renewal of DNR orders at appropriate intervals with ongoing documentation of the condition to note changes.

Advance Medical Directives

AMDs are documents that permit people to set forth in writing their wishes and preferences regarding health care. These legal documents are used to indicate the patient/resident's health care decisions if the time should come when they are unable to speak for themselves. Some AMDs also permit people to designate someone to convey their wishes in the event they are rendered unable to do so. The AMD is helpful to professionals because it provides information and guidance based on the person's wishes of their treatment decisions.

Many issues pose problems to the professional in honoring advance directives. First, an advance directive is not operative until the patient is no longer capable of decision making (Mayo Clinic, 2017). Therefore the first decision must be whether a patient is capable of making a decision or whether the advance directive must be followed. At times, the patient may be awake and responsive but not clear in his or her ability

to think or communicate. However, if a determination of incapacity is made, then an advance directive may be looked to, as it would speak when the person cannot.

Sometimes, the policy of the provider or the judgment of the treating physician may not be in accord with the patient's wishes. In such cases, it is necessary to advise the patient of this. For example, if a nursing facility does not offer CPR and the patient desires that option, then the facility must advise the patient and offer the option of transfer. In the same way, a physician who does not agree with or cannot carry out the patient's wishes must advise the patient of this and must then transfer the care of the patient to another physician as soon as it is practical to do so.

The right to self-determination is well grounded in the common law and is interpreted in the U.S. Constitution under the right of liberty. The statutory developments and codification of these principles promote communication and make it easier for individuals to exercise their right to autonomy.

Physician Orders for Life-Sustaining Treatment (POLST)

Physician Orders for Life-Sustaining Treatment, or more commonly known as POLST, is a process of communicating health care wishes during a medical crisis or decline in health (National POLST Paradigm, Fundamental Policy Principles, 2017). This tool is seeing more frequent use and allows the patient to communicate with their physician to set forth medical orders to be followed. The POLST form is not meant to replace traditional end-of-life care communication tools such as advance directives or "no code" or DNR statuses. Rather, it augments these tools to provide a comprehensive set of patient preferences for care, more so than simply a DNR. Table 3.1 compares POLST with advance directives.

As a portable medical order, the POLST form is an ongoing order set that reflects the patient's current preferences for care (National POLST paradigm, 2017). As such, this form needs to be reviewed with the patient to assure their needs regarding end-of-life care are met. Although POLST forms may have slight variations from state to state, they are all inclusive of the following three sections: (1) cardiopulmonary resuscitation (CPR), (2) medical interventions, and (3) artificially administered nutrition (Fig. 3.2).

Legal Tools

Living Wills or Designation of Health Care Agents

LWs are intended to provide written expressions of a patient's wishes regarding the use of medical treatments in the event of a terminal illness or condition. Health care agent designations entail appointing a trusted person to express the patient's wishes regarding the withholding or withdrawal of life support when the patient is cognitively stable and aware of their decisions.

Allowing for variations among states, LWs are generally not effective until (1) the attending physician has the document and the patient has been determined to be incompetent, (2) the physician has determined the patient has a terminal condition or a condition such that any therapy provided would only prolong dying, and (3) the physician has written the appropriate orders in the medical record (Mayo Clinic, 2017). The LW is not the

TABLE 3.1   Comparing Physician Orders for Life-Sustaining Treatment (POLST) and Advance Directives

	POLST Paradigm Form	Advance Directives
Type of Document	Medical order	Legal document
Who Completes	Health care professional	Individual
Appoints a Surrogate	Seriously ill, frail, individuals with a life expectancy of less than 1 year	All competent adults
What Is Communicated	Specific medical orders for treatment wishes	General wishes about treatment, may help guide treatment after a medical emergency
Can Emergency Medical Services (EMS) Use?	Yes	No
Ease in Locating	Easy to find Patient has original Copy is placed in medical record	Copy is provided to health care professionals for placement in medical record

From National POLST Paradigm. (n.d.). *POLST &. advance directives.* Retrieved from http://polst.org/wp-content/uploads/2018/01/2018.01_POLST-vs-AD-Chart.pdf

Fig. 3.2 Components of a Physician Orders for Life-Sustaining Treatment (POLST) form. Section A applies only when the patient is unresponsive, has no pulse, and is not breathing; this section does not apply to any other medical circumstance. Section B gives medical orders when CPR is not required, but the patient still has a medical emergency and cannot communicate. Section C is where orders are given about artificial nutrition (and in some states artificial hydration) for when the patient cannot eat. (From National POLST Paradigm. [2017]. *POLST paradigm form elements.* Retrieved from http://oregonpolst.org/form-details)

same instrument as a DNR. The DNR is a medical directive, not a personal directive (Florida State University, n.d.).

States differ in the type of written instruments used for these purposes. For example, New York does not have an LW statute as such but does have a health care proxy provision, which combines the elements of the LW and the designation of a health care agent. As you enter practice, it is wise to understand your state's practice.

General Provisions in Living Wills

Any competent adult may execute LWs. Most statutes contain specific language excluding euthanasia and declaring that

withholding care in compliance with the document does not constitute suicide.

Most statutes require that the patient's signature be witnessed. The witness usually does not have to attest to the patient's mental competence; however, many forms require that the witness indicate that the principal "appeared" to be of sound mind.

In general, it is also prohibited for an owner or employee of a facility in which a patient resides to serve as a witness to a signature, unless the owner is a relative. In some states, a person who has an interest in the patient's estate may not serve as a witness or be designated as the health care agent.

Pain and comfort measures may not be withheld. The patient has the right to revoke or change their LW at any time if they remain cognizant and aware of the changes and possible repercussions.

Durable or General Power of Attorney: Differences and Indications

The durable power of attorney for health care (DPAHC) is a legal instrument by which a person may designate someone else to make health care decisions at a time in the future when he or she may be rendered incompetent. This is called a *springing power,* which comes into effect in the future on occurrence of a specific event—in this case, the incompetence of the patient.

The person delegating the power of attorney for health care is called the *principal,* whereas the person to whom the power is granted is known as the *agent.* A DPAHC is different from a general power of attorney in that a general power of attorney would become invalid upon determination of the incompetence of the principal; thus the DPAHC allows the designation of a legally enforceable surrogate decision maker. The role of the designated surrogate in this situation is to make the decisions that most closely align with the patient's wishes, desires, and values.

The DPAHC has an advantage over the LW in that the designated agent may assess the current situation, ask questions, and gather information to assist in determining the probable wishes of the patient. The LW, however, speaks for the patient who cannot speak for himself or herself.

All states now have laws providing for types of LW documents, DPAHCs, or both. Because specifics of the laws vary from state to state, it is important for the nurse to be knowledgeable of the laws in the state in which he or she practices. Furthermore, the nurse needs to keep abreast of changes within the laws. Depending on a nurse's work environment, resources for this information may be the facility administration, risk management staff, legal counsel, or another appropriate source.

Decision Diagram

The decision diagram assists the patient to understand the thought process that should be followed when trying to analyze end-of-life decision-making situations (Box 3.2). If patients are competent, then they can make their own decisions. While competent, a person may prepare for potential future incompetence by executing an AMD and by discussing personal wishes with health care professionals and family members so that they fully understand that person's specific preferences for future care and treatment.

When the time comes for an AMD to be used, a verification of incompetence will be made. This is normally accomplished through medical judgment and family discussion. Laws of any jurisdiction should be evaluated to see what documentation and procedures are required.

Once a person is deemed incompetent, substituted decision-making alternatives must be chosen. If a person has not executed an AMD, other people are looked to for their knowledge about the patient's wishes. If all agree about the patient's medical condition, then the statutory order of priority for surrogates can be looked to for designation of the decision maker. If an AMD has been executed and an agreement exists among health care professionals and family, then the wishes may be carried out according to the AMD.

Where lack of agreement or confusion is present, it may be necessary to seek a court-ordered conservator or, in some

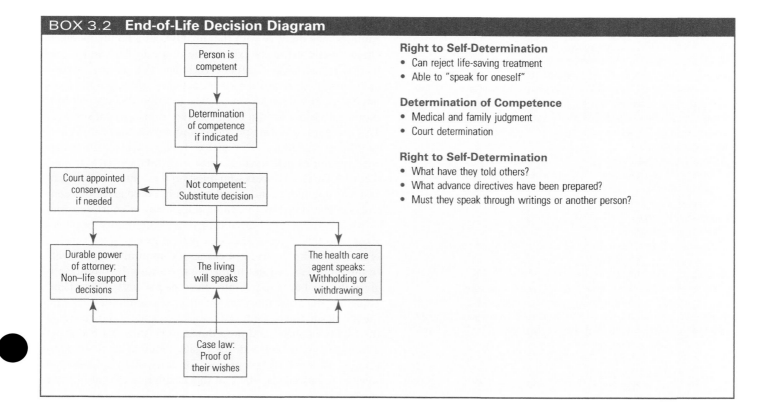

BOX 3.2   End-of-Life Decision Diagram

Person is competent

Determination of competence if indicated

Not competent: Substitute decision

Court appointed conservator if needed

Durable power of attorney: Non–life support decisions

The living will speaks

The health care agent speaks: Withholding or withdrawing

Case law: Proof of their wishes

Right to Self-Determination
- Can reject life-saving treatment
- Able to "speak for oneself"

Determination of Competence
- Medical and family judgment
- Court determination

Right to Self-Determination
- What have they told others?
- What advance directives have been prepared?
- Must they speak through writings or another person?

jurisdictions, a guardian. This person then acts as the surrogate and decides according to the patient's wishes as can best be determined by available information. They also make decisions in the best interests of the patient. This refers to a conservator (guardian) of the person, as opposed to a conservator (guardian) of property, who deals with matters related to an individual's property and belongings. The court-appointed conservator/guardian has priority over other decision makers. This person may be a spouse, parent, or other family member. It may also be any person the court determines may best serve the interests of the patient. For a paradigm of end-of-life decision making, see Box 3.2.

An example of a typical LW document is presented in Box 3.3, and an example of a document concerning appointment of a health care agent is presented in Box 3.4. States usually provide forms for these purposes but may not require that the specific form be used. Rather, most simply require that the executed

---

BOX 3.3   Living Will

Connecticut General Statutes § 19A-575. Form of Document

Any person 18 years of age or older may execute a document which shall contain directions as to specific life support systems which such person chooses to have administered. Such document shall be signed and dated by the maker with at least two witnesses and may be substantially in the following form:

Document Concerning Withholding or Withdrawal of Life Support Systems

If the time comes when I am incapacitated to the point where I can no longer actively take part in decisions for my own life, and am unable to direct my physician as to my own medical care, I wish this statement to stand as a testament of my wishes.

"I .... (NAME) request that, if my condition is deemed terminal or if it is determined that I will be permanently unconscious, I be allowed to die and not be kept alive through life support systems. By terminal condition, I mean that I have an incurable or irreversible medical condition which, without the administration of life support systems, will, in the opinion of my attending physician, result in death within a relatively short time. By permanently unconscious I mean that I am in a permanent coma or persistent vegetative state that is an irreversible condition in which I am at no time aware of myself or the environment and show no behavioral response to the environment. The life support systems that I do not want included, but are not limited to:

Artificial respiration

Cardiopulmonary resuscitation

Artificial means of providing nutrition and hydration (Cross out any initial life support systems you want administered.)

I do not intend any direct taking of my life, but only that my dying not be unreasonably prolonged.

Other specific requests:

This request is made, after careful reflection, while I am of sound mind.

.... (Signature)

.... (Date)

This document was signed in our presence, by the above-named

.... (NAME) who appeared to be 18 years of age or older, of sound mind, and able to understand the nature and consequences of health care decisions at the time the document was signed.

.... (Witness)

.... (Address)

.... (Witness)

.... (Address)

BOX 3.4   Health Care Agent

Connecticut Health Care Agent (C.G.S. § 19A-577)

(a) Any person 18 years of age or older may execute a document that may, but need not, be in substantially the following form:

Document Concerning the Appointment of Health Care Agent

I appoint.................... (NAME) to be my health care agent. If my attending physician determines that I am unable to understand and appreciate the nature and consequences of health care decisions and to reach and communicate an informed decision regarding treatment, my health care agent is authorized to:

1) convey to my physician my wishes concerning the withholding or removal of life support systems.

2) take whatever actions are necessary to ensure that my wishes are given effect.

If this person is unwilling or unable to serve as my health care agent, I appoint.................... (NAME) to be my alternative health care agent.

This request is made, after careful reflection, while I am of sound mind.

.... (Signature)

.... (Date)

This document was signed in our presence, by the above-named

.... (NAME) who appeared to be 18 years of age or older, of sound mind, and able to understand the nature and consequences of health care decisions at the time the document was signed.

.... (Witness)

.... (Address)

.... (Witness)

.... (Address)

---

documents be in substantially the same form. In any event, the laws of the jurisdiction should be reviewed to see if a specific form or document is required.

Conflicts Between Directives and Family Desires

Families may disagree with the directives of a family member. Often, family members express the desire to have more care than is requested by a patient. Although the law consistently upholds the expressed desires of patients, often families continue to exert influence over medical decisions, even when they support decisions known to be contrary to the patient's wishes. This can put health care providers and nurses in confusing and conflicting situations. Designated health care agents either appointed or by patient choice may also find themselves in conflict with family members who question the control of the agent and may not understand why the agent has been given this control. Yet it is our duty to uphold the patient or court decision.

Most AMD statutes specifically provide immunity for physicians who follow the wishes of a patient as expressed therein. Nurses should note, in most cases, this immunity applies only to the physician and not to the nurse because the physician is given the legal duty to put into effect the patient's wishes. Consequently, the nurse must rely on effective communication with the physician, the patient, and the family, and on the quality of the facility's policies and procedures, to be sure that his or her actions are consistent with the legally required steps. In addition, an effective ethical process for discussion and problem solving, discussed elsewhere in this chapter, is critical in these situations.

THE PATIENT SELF-DETERMINATION ACT

The Patient Self-Determination Act[10] (PSDA) came into effect on December 1, 1991. The intent of this law is to ensure that patients are given information about the extent to which their rights are protected under state law. The PSDA itself does not create any new substantive legal right for individuals regarding their decision making. Rather, its focus is on education and communication.

The PSDA requires hospitals, nursing facilities, and other health care providers who receive federal funds such as Medicare or Medicaid to give patients written information explaining their legal options for refusing or accepting treatment should they become incapacitated.

Background: The Cruzan Case

On January 11, 1983, Nancy Cruzan, a healthy 25-year-old woman, was seriously injured in an automobile accident; she became comatose and remained in a persistent vegetative state. Seven years later, the U.S. Supreme Court considered whether her life support could be withdrawn. Her parents, who had also been designated her coguardians by a judgment of the court, sought a court order to withdraw the artificial feeding and hydration equipment after it became apparent that she had virtually no chance of regaining her cognitive facilities.[11]

In June 1990, in a 5-to-4 decision, the Court held that because there was no clear and convincing evidence of Nancy's desire to have life-sustaining treatment withdrawn under such circumstances, her parents did not have the authority to carry out such a request. The Court affirmed that the Missouri Supreme Court was within its rights to request more evidence to indicate what Nancy's decision would be if she were able to make that decision herself. It was in this decision that the Court permitted the state of Missouri (and thus made it constitutionally permissible) to require "clear and convincing proof" as the standard needed to determine a person's wishes regarding the withdrawal of life support.

Most states have not adopted this rigorous standard of proof for such decisions. In most jurisdictions, family members, those close to the individual, or other surrogate decision makers may make decisions for a patient who has not left specific oral or written instructions (American Bar Association, 2017).

Clear and Convincing Proof

It is difficult, if not impossible, to come up with a precise meaning of "clear and convincing proof." Although this standard is not applied in most states, a discussion is presented here to provide insight into the Cruzan case, to help understand the significance of the Court's decision to initiate AMD legislation nationwide and to enact the PSDA, and to provide some clarification for understanding a lesser standard of proof.

The clear and convincing standard is an intermediate standard of evidence, higher than a "preponderance of the evidence" but below "certainty beyond a reasonable doubt." An AMD may help meet this standard. However, in the absence of an AMD, the evidence required to meet this standard is somewhat cloudy. Documents such as an LW would be accorded more weight than oral statements.

Westchester County Medical Center on Behalf of O'Connor[12] described the clear and convincing standard as "a firm and settled commitment… under circumstances like those presented"; it must be "more than immediate reactions to the unsettling experience of seeing or hearing another's unnecessarily prolonged death."[13]

The Cruzan decision must be examined for the areas of clarification it provides. Although it does not declare a "right to die" as such, it does provide much stimulus for the development of state legislation to clarify the existing rights to self-determination. In addition, it also served as the catalyst for the enactment of the PSDA: A competent person has a constitutionally protected right under the Fourteenth Amendment to refuse medical treatment, even life-saving nutrition and hydration; an incompetent or incapacitated person may have that right exercised by a surrogate.[14]

In her concurring opinion, U.S. Supreme Court Justice Sandra Day O'Connor made the following points (the interpretation is the author's analysis of points taken from the concurring opinion of O'Connor): Artificial provision of nutrition and hydration involves intrusion and restraint and invokes the same due process concerns as any other medical treatment. One does not by incompetence lose one's due process liberty interests. The U.S. Constitution may require the states to implement the decision of a client's duly appointed surrogate.[15]

The Four Significant Provisions of the PSDA

The PSDA has four significant provisions:
1. It requires hospitals, SNFs, home health agencies, hospice programs, and health maintenance organizations (HMOs) that participate in Medicare and Medicaid programs to maintain written policies and procedures guaranteeing that every adult receiving medical care is given written information regarding his or her involvement in treatment decisions. This information must include (1) individual rights under state law, either statutory or case law; and (2) written policies of the provider or organization regarding the protection of such rights. When state advance directive laws change, facilities must update their materials accordingly but no later than 90 days after the changes in state laws.
   - The information must be provided by hospitals at the time of admission, nursing facilities at the time of admission as a resident, hospice programs at the time of the initial

---

[10]42 U.S.C. §§ 1395 and 1396 (1990), as amended, 60 FR 33262, June 27, 1995.

[11]*Cruzan v Director, Missouri Department of Health* (1990, US), 111 L Ed 2d 224, 234, 110 S Ct 2841.

[12]72 NY2d 517, 534 NYS2d 886, 531 NE2d 607 (1988).

[13]72 NY2d 517, 534 NYS2d 886, 531 NE2d 607 (1988) at 903.

[14]*Cruzan v. Director, Missouri Department of Health*, 111 L Ed 2d 224, 110 S Ct 2841 (1990).

[15]Modified from *Cruzan v. Director, Missouri Department of Health* [1990, US] 111 L Ed 2d 224, 247–251, 110 S Ct 2841.

receipt of hospice care, HMOs at the time of enrollment, and home health agencies in advance of the individual coming under the agencies' care.

- The PSDA further requires distribution of written information that describes each facility's policy for protecting the rights of patients. *Each patient's medical record must document whether the patient has executed an AMD.*
- The PSDA also provides protection against discrimination or refusal to provide care based on whether an individual has executed an AMD.
- A facility may engage a contractor to perform services required by the PSDA, but it retains the legal obligations for compliance with the law.
- If a patient or resident is incapacitated at the time of admission, the required information may be furnished to the family member or responsible party, but the patient or resident must be provided with the material when he or she is no longer incapacitated.

2. The provider must provide for education of staff and community on issues concerning AMDs but is not required to provide the public with the same material it provides patients.
3. States are required to develop a written description of the law concerning AMDs in their respective jurisdictions and to distribute the material to providers who provide it to patients according to the requirements of the PSDA.
4. The secretary of the DHHS was also required to develop and implement a national campaign to inform the public of the option to execute AMDs and of the patient's right to participate in and direct his or her health care decisions.

Nurses' Responsibilities

Nurses should know the laws of the state in which they practice. The nurse has a responsibility to facilitate discussions and direct patients regarding informed decision making, including but not limited to advance directives to the appropriate source. As such, many organizations have included the following questions in their nursing admission assessment:

- Do you have basic information about AMDs, including LWs and durable power of attorney?
- Do you wish to initiate an AMD?
- If you have already prepared an AMD, can you provide it now?
- Have you discussed your end-of-life choices with your family or designated surrogate and health care team workers?

Problems and Ethical Dilemmas Associated With Implementation of the PSDA

Although public and medical professionals overwhelmingly support AMDs, patients have historically been reluctant to complete them. Even distribution of forms and information has failed to increase the participation rate.

Other research indicates that care of dying patients may not be keeping pace with national guidelines or legal decisions upholding patients' rights to accept or refuse treatment. Physicians may be reluctant to discuss AMDs with their patients. The major barriers to this communication process are lack of knowledge about AMDs and the belief that AMDs are not necessary for young healthy patients. Other studies have found that patients' personal desires do not always get attention, and physicians try to avoid discussion of grim subjects (Taylor, Gustin, & Wells-DiGregorio, n.d.).

Questions arise about the effectiveness of AMDs in situations where, for example, the person is away from home, a person changes his or her mind, or an unanticipated event occurs. Some approaches have been recommended regarding these issues. For example, some states have included in the language of LW provisions that a validly executed LW from another jurisdiction will be honored. However, if any uncertainty exists, it is probably wise to have people from the other state execute a new document as soon as possible.

AMD provisions appropriately allow people to change their minds at any time and by any means. Nurses need to be alert to any indications from a patient of their intent to do so. Because of the person's medical condition, subtle signs such as a gesture or a nod of the head may be easily overlooked.

The protocols established by facilities to comply with the PSDA may turn the "tangible indicators of extremely important and personal decisions into just another piece of paper" (LaPuma, Orrentlicher, & Moss, 1991).

Many have questioned whether the time of admission to a hospital or a nursing facility is the best time to discuss AMDs when patients may be fearful, uncomfortable, in pain, and anxious. Health professionals' concern lies in that the patients' emotional states may affect their level of understanding and competence. It is important for the nurse to facilitate this discussion, however, using the professional skills and understanding necessary to comply with the PSDA.

Conflicts between medical judgment and patient choices are bound to become more common. It will be necessary to take steps to ensure that the directives of patients are accorded appropriate compliance and that the judgment of health care professionals is respected.

As discussed previously, both the PSDA and the OBRA require that a facility or a physician who is unable to comply with the patient's wishes notify the patient when it is appropriate to be transferred to another facility or to the care of another physician. This ensures that the patient's wishes are respected and preserves the integrity of the medical practitioner and provider. The medical record should reflect only the facts of such a situation. It is neither necessary nor appropriate to "make a case" in the record as to which party was right or wrong. It is appropriate only to show that proper procedures were followed and that all relevant matters were fully explained.

Many unanswered questions in the PSDA still remain and will have to be sorted out over time. For example, how is the matter handled with those who are illiterate? What should the nurse do if patients refuse to produce their AMDs? In the case of surrogate decision makers, what about the response of a designated agent who is then called on to decide about the removal of life support? If and when the time comes, will the person be able to carry out the principal's wishes? Will the instructions left by the patient be clear enough to ensure that those wishes are carried out? To address these issues, one must rely on their experience and knowledge, and follow organizational and legal policies regarding AMDs and PSDA.

The responsibility to make these truly profound decisions may arise at times of great personal difficulty and may, in fact, be more demanding than the agent ever thought possible. A realistic approach to these points at the time such instruments are executed will help resolve such dilemmas. The nurse should be alert for opportunities to gain information from both patients and their families or health agents to gauge their level of understanding. The nurse's role in clarifying matters and in explaining information may help alleviate the emotional dilemma associated with carrying out end-of-life decisions.

VALUES HISTORY

Directives such as LWs, DPAHCs, and for some states POLSTs are easing some of the difficult situations faced by health care professionals and families when making decisions about treatment to prolong life. However, criticism of such documents is that they hold a degree of ambiguity and, as such, may not offer insight into the person's own values or underlying beliefs regarding such directives (Saha et al., 2016).

A values history may help add this dimension to decision making regarding AMDs. The values history is an instrument that asks questions related to quality versus length of life and tries to determine what values a person sees as important to maintain during terminal care. The instrument asks people to specify their wishes regarding several types of medical situations. It presents the types of treatment that may be available in each situation and describes the persons with whom these matters have been discussed in the past and who should be involved in the actual decision making.

As a practical matter, its use may be limited by the time required for discussion with the physician or by the physician's discomfort or reluctance to directly address the issues. However, this should not serve as a reason to abandon this potentially useful tool.

The values history has important implications for the nurse. The values history is really more than a document with questions and answers. It is a process of reflection. These reflections add information gained over a lifetime. The close interpersonal relationships that nurses develop with patients and families and their high degree of communication skills speak to the critical role they can play in this process. As life-and-death situations become more complex and begin to demand factual knowledge of the patient's wishes, the values history may help preserve the autonomy of the individual.

The values history may encourage extended conversation between individuals and their physicians and other health care professionals. This type of instrument may increase autonomy by providing a better basis for representing the patient's desires when they can no longer express their wishes. A copy of the values history developed at the University of New Mexico is included in Appendix A.

NURSES' ETHICAL CODE AND END-OF-LIFE CARE

Ethics relate to the moral actions, behavior, and character of an individual. Nurses occupy one of the most trusted positions in society, and conforming to a code of ethics gives evidence of acceptance of that responsibility and trust. A code of ethical conduct offers general principles to guide and to evaluate nursing actions (ANA, 2015). The role of the health care professional is to advocate, promote and improve patient autonomy, maintain or improve health status, and do no harm (ANA, n.d.).

The nurse–patient relationship is built on trust, and nurses' understanding of the key ethical principles is the basis of a trusting relationship. The key ethical principles should serve as a framework for nursing decision making and application of professional judgment. These key ethical principles are autonomy or self-determination, beneficence (doing good), nonmaleficence (avoiding evil), justice (allocation of resources), and veracity (truthfulness) (ANA, n.d.). Issues related to ageism, ethnicity, sexual orientation, gender, physical or mental disability, and race are critical areas of difference that may affect the provider–patient relationship (Ouchida & Lachs, 2015). These factors must be acknowledged and addressed if the moral and ethical principles of the provider–patient relationship are to be respected.

The *Scope and Standards of Gerontological Nursing Practice,* Professional Performance Standard V, states that a gerontologic nurse's practice is guided by the Code for Nurses, established by the ANA as the guide for ethical decision making in the practice of nursing (ANA, 2015). The code explains the values and ideals that serve as a framework for nurses' ethical decision making and conduct. A violation of the ethical code may not be a violation of law. The state's nursing association may act against a nurse who has committed a violation of the ethical code. More important, the ethical code serves to regulate professional practice from within the profession and ensure ethical conduct in the professional setting. Maintaining mutual respect among practitioners in the field is arguably one of the best ways to bring respect to the profession and to oneself.

Ethical directives guide and direct the nurse caring for dying patients. Care of the terminally ill and dying should be done with professional and ethical deliberation.

Ethical Dilemmas and Considerations
Euthanasia, Suicide, and Assisted Suicide

The issue of physician-assisted suicide has become a front-burner national debate. Calls to legalize physician-assisted suicide have increased, and public support and interest in the subject has grown in recent years (Sulmasy, Mueller, & Snyder, 2017). Personal and professional views on this issue are at best controversial. However, grass roots efforts to change and shape public policy on this issue will continue. The American Medical Association (AMA) and the American College of Physicians (ACP) have maintained their opposition to physician-assisted suicide, stating "The ACP does not support the legalization of physician-assisted suicide, the practice of which raises ethical, clinical, and other concerns" (Sulmasy, Mueller, & Snyder, 2017, para 14).

However, many citizens, some physicians, and some other health care professionals believe that doctors should be allowed to help severely ill persons take their own lives. In most states, assisted suicide is considered an illegal act. However, an act of affirmative euthanasia (actual administration of the instrumentality that causes death) constitutes an illegal criminal offense in all 50 states.

Additionally, the *Code of Ethics for Nurses* prohibits nurses from participating in assisted suicide. The ANA's position statement holds that "The nursing profession's opposition to nurse participation in euthanasia does not negate the obligation of the nurse to provide compassionate, ethically justified end-of-life care which includes the promotion of comfort and the alleviation of suffering, adequate pain control, and at times, foregoing life-sustaining treatments" (ANA, 2013).

On November 8, 1994, Oregon voters approved ballot Measure 16, otherwise known as Oregon's Death with Dignity Act. Despite legal challenges, Oregon voters reaffirmed the measure in 1997. Under the Oregon law, physicians may prescribe life-ending medications for patients to self-administer to anyone considered mentally competent, a resident of Oregon, and diagnosed as having less than 6 months to live (Oregon Health Authority, 2014). The patient may take the lethal dose only after a 15-day waiting period. The law does not specify what medications may be used.

Precise information on the incidence of "assisted dying" type activities across the United States is not available. If such acts occur, they may be handled with subtlety and thus may be unlikely to be recognized as affirmative euthanasia. Actions such as failure to take steps to prevent a suicide, deliberate administration of a medication in a dosage that will suppress respiration and cause death, or administering heavy doses of pain medications needed to comfort a terminally ill patient may be intentional or inadvertent acts of assisting suicide or euthanasia. The nurse may be in the middle of a conflict between the therapeutic necessity of treatment and the likely outcomes. Unlike an act of affirmative euthanasia where the nurse's actions are clear, in situations where there are competing interests (therapeutic necessity and likely outcomes), the nurse must rely on patients' needs and his or her own professional judgment. The nurse should not hesitate to request assistance from the institutional ethics committee to help cope with such dilemmas.

What about the person who, although not terminally ill or in a persistent vegetative state, is in her 80s and wishes to stop eating or drinking with the intent of causing her own death? In a 1987 case,[16] the New York Supreme Court denied the petition of a nursing facility administrator to authorize forced feeding. Although physicians disagreed regarding the resident's competence, the court decided that she was competent and had the right to determine what was to be done with her body. It found that refraining from force-feeding is not abetting suicide.

In these challenging times, the nurse may be confronted by unanswered questions, ambiguity, and decisional conflicts in their employment setting. Nurses must hone their ethical and analytical skills to deal effectively with these situations and look to the learning tools and information available to them.

Reference has already been made to the Code for Nurses (ANA, 2015), which has established the ethical framework for nursing practice. In addition, nurses should look to their patient's statements, either written or verbal. Nurses should be alert to their own visceral reaction—that is, does the situation "feel right"?—and identify the issues that cause concern. By answering these questions and proceeding in a cautious and deliberate manner, nurses can usually determine the proper action.

EVIDENCE-BASED PRACTICE
Depression and Spousal Self-Euthanasia

Background

This article provides the first qualitative account of spousal self-euthanasia in older people, a previously unexplored phenomenon. The researchers investigate the lived experience of a Dutch elderly couple who strongly wished—and chose—to die together at a self-directed moment, despite not suffering from a life-threatening disease or severe depression. The anticipatory fear of further deterioration, further losing control, and not being able to control time and manner of death in the future compelled the couple to make this ultimate decision.

Sample/Setting

This research focused on the experience of one elderly couple (aged over 70 years) by presenting two personal accounts from an insider perspective. Interviews inclusive of personal accounts from an insider perspective regarding an elderly couple aged over 70 years were conducted.

Methods

A case study through family interviews was completed regarding two married older adults who committed simultaneous suicide through a "lived experience." A thematic existential phenomenological method was utilized to report data.

Findings

After self-directed spousal self-euthanasia, the respondent confirmed that both (husband and wife) feared separation, dependency, and physical decline more than death. "They wanted to abandon life in all serenity."

Implications

The article outlines practical implications nurses and health care providers working in gerontology should be aware of regarding consequences of the effects of depression and the relationship between self-euthanasia and depression in elderly people. The authors felt that encouraging people to discuss the emotional tensions about the different concerns and sense of time is the most appropriate intervention to understand the desire to end one's life.

From van Wijngaarden, E., Leget, C., & Goossensen, A. (2016). Till death do us part: The lived experience of an elderly couple who chose to end their lives by spousal self-euthanasia. *The Gerontologist, 56*(6), 1062–1071.

Experimentation and Research

As previously discussed, nursing facility residents are accorded specific rights with respect to their treatments. The patient or resident bill of rights entitles them to choose a primary physician and terminate their relationship if so desired. Furthermore, they have the right to be informed about their medical conditions and proposed plans of treatment. Nursing facility

---

[16]*In re Application of Brooks*, NY Sup CT, Albany County, June 10, 1987.

residents, or any patients, may refuse to participate in experimental research,[17] and they may refuse to be examined, observed, or treated by students or other staff without jeopardizing their access to care.[18]

The goals of research are different from the goals of care. Research seeks to acquire knowledge with no intended benefit to the subjects because much of clinical research is conducted to determine effective treatments or potential benefits of new drugs and medical devices. This is a complex and controversial subject. Key points to consider in such issues are the goals and value of the research, conflicts between institutional interests and researchers, and the medical interests of the individual.

DHHS regulations may permit waiving the right to informed consent under the following specific circumstances: the research poses only a minimum risk; no adverse effects on the rights and welfare of the subjects will occur; the research cannot be carried out effectively without the waiver; and, whenever possible, the participants will be provided with pertinent information during or after participation.

Only a full review of the research, including legal analysis, determines whether a waiver of informed consent can be justified. It may be that the right to informed consent cannot be waived even when the research poses minimum risk.

An appropriate institutional review board (IRB) should examine research involving humans. All aspects of the proposed study must be evaluated to ensure that the research is justified and of benefit and that the individual rights of all persons, including those of volunteer participants, are not sacrificed. Nurses, as a professional group closely involved with the clinical aspects of human research, should be represented on the review board.

Both state and federal regulatory provisions govern human research investigations. The diligent efforts of the research review board consider not only these laws and regulations but also their application to the benefits of the proposed research. A nurse involved in any aspect of human research should ask to see the details of the proposed study and the deliberations and decision of the institutional review board. It is not improper for a nurse to ask to attend a meeting of the review board if the nurse is involved in carrying out any aspect of the research or has any information of importance to the board's deliberations. Furthermore, the nurse should report to the board any time issues arise with respect to the research if it appears that individual rights are in question.

Organ Donation

Technologic and medical advances have facilitated the successful transplantation of vital organs, and such procedures have become routine at many medical centers. However, this success has exacerbated the ethical questions involving the allocation of scarce donor organs. In 2014 the *Washington Post* noted "About 30 Americans a day either die on the waiting list or are removed

from it because they have become too ill to receive a transplant" (Humphreys, 2014, para 2). From this statistic, questions arise such as: Which individuals should have priority for receiving donated organs? Should relatives, for example, be permitted to donate kidneys? What about the risks of such procedures to the donors? What about the psychological issues and family dynamics? Should donors be compensated, or should recipients pay for their organs? What about animal organ transplants?

Recognizing that the number of recipients waiting is more than that of available donors, the federal government has taken steps to promote organ donation. Hospitals in the United States are now required to report *all* deaths to the local organ procurement organization (OPO) or Organ Procurement and Transplantation Networks (OPTN). This would permit the nation's OPOs, which collect organs and coordinate donations daily, to determine whether a person is a suitable donor while following specific guidelines set forth based on the organ and potential recipient (Organ Procurement and Transplantation Network, n. d.) The DHHS believes that this measure, which is now a condition for participating in the Medicare program, will save lives by substantially increasing organ donations in the United States.

Standards of informed consent must be adhered to with respect to both donors and recipients. In Pennsylvania and West Virginia, for example, the Center for Organ Recovery and Education (CORE) notes: "If the patient is a registered donor, the family is notified that CORE will proceed with organ—and, if applicable, tissue—recovery. If the individual is not registered, the family is asked to give their authorization for organ and/or tissue recovery. If the family authorizes donation, the legal next-of-kin signs a donor consent form" (CORE, 2017, para 2).

In dealing with the ethical issues faced in these situations, the answers are not clear cut and may depend on individual values. However, when it is necessary to sort out conflicts or report anything believed to be illegal or unethical, the nurse should consider obtaining guidance from an institutional ethics committee or other ethical resource.

Ethics Committees

Institutional biomedical ethics committees play a pivotal role in dealing with sensitive conflicts about treatment decisions. Ethics committees act as the primary organizational mechanism for studying, educating about, and providing advice on value conflicts and dilemmas faced in health care (Geppert & Shelton, 2016). Ethics committees serve in a voluntary capacity in a consultative role and do not act as a decision-making body (University of Kansas Medical Center, 2017). Their primary objective is to carefully evaluate differing positions to achieve a consensus that is ethically and legally acceptable to all parties. Ethics committees do not have any legal authority. Their main purpose is to create a forum where patients, patient representatives, and providers can express and consider different points of view.

Two-thirds of general hospitals with more than 200 beds have panels of ethics committees. Their presence in nursing facilities is not as common. Membership on ethics committees should be diverse to help maintain a balanced view among professionals, laypersons, and special interest groups. If constructed in this manner, the committee will offer a variety of perspectives to those

---

[17]For example, see Annotated Code of Maryland, 1957, § 19-344(f); and Vermont Statutes Annotated, Title 18 § 1852(a)(10) and Title 33 § 3781 (3), as redesignated by Act 219, L. 1990, effective July 1, 1990.

[18]For example, see 1990 edition, General Laws of Massachusetts, supplemented by the 1991 Supplement, Chapter 111: 70E9h.

seeking guidance. The nurse's role as a member of an ethics committee is crucial. Representation should include administrative and staff nurses, as well as nurses practicing in specialty areas.

Ethics committees' primary purposes are to (1) provide education and help guide policy making regarding ethical issues, (2) facilitate the resolution of ethical dilemmas, and (3) take an activist role in involving all interested parties in promoting the best care for patients (Geppert & Shelton, 2016; University of Kansas Medical Center, 2017).

Issues and topics that might be discussed by an ethics committee include but are not limited to euthanasia; patient competency and decision-making capacities; guardianship issues; DNR orders and policies; patient refusal of treatment; starting, continuing, or stopping treatment; informed consent; use of feeding tubes; use of restraints; and the list goes on. Basically, anything that composes an ethical dilemma can be brought before the committee.

An organization considering the establishment of an ethics committee should be prepared to make the necessary commitment of time and resources. A committee should be visible and available, and should publish clear notice of means to obtain access.

Social Media

Social media has taken the world by storm and will continue to do so. Rarely can you go anywhere without connectivity to the world around us. Sadly, this type of media raises ethical issues as well within the health care environment. According to Ventola (2014), by using social media, health care providers have "tools to share information, to debate health care policy and practice issues, to promote health behaviors, to engage with the public, and to educate and interact with patients, caregivers, students, and colleagues" (para. 5). However, there are risks to using social media, inclusive of: poor quality information, posting of unprofessional content that can damage professional image, and breaches of patient privacy whether intentional or accidental, to name a few. Nursing boards have disciplined nurses for violations involving online disclosure of patients' personal health information and imposed sanctions ranging from letters of concern to license suspensions (Ventola, 2014).

"In 2009, a U.S. District Court upheld the expulsion of a nursing student for violating the school's honor code by making obscene remarks about the race, sex, and religion of patients under her care. The court concluded that the school's honor code and confidentiality agreement signed by each nursing student governed the standards of acceptable behavior, dismissing the student's claim that her right to freedom of speech had been violated. A similar ruling was made in a case in which a student posted pictures of herself as a drunken pirate on social media" (Ventola, 2014).

The ANA in concert with the National Council of State Boards of Nursing (NCSBN) in 2011 developed principles for social networking for nurses and nursing students to set forth expectations of professional nurses in this digital age (Box 3.5).

🏠 HOME CARE

- Remember that home care agencies' standards are based on the *Scope and Standards of Gerontological Nursing Practice,* originally published by the American Nurses Association (1995) and revised in 2010.
- Assess for older adult abuse and notify the proper authorities (e.g., local older adult protective services or ombudsman program).
- On initial assessment, inform homebound older adults and their caregivers of home care patient rights. Have them sign a copy that documents that they have been informed of their rights.
- Inform caregivers and homebound older adults of their right to self-determination. Document that homebound older adults, caregivers, or both have been informed by obtaining signatures. AMDs must be part of a clinical assessment.
- Obtain a copy of homebound older adults' AMDs, and keep them on file in their charts. Send copies to the physicians to file.
- Remember that the physician must sign a DNR order within 48 hours as specified by Medicare regulations.
- To help caregivers and homebound older adults make decisions about treatment used to prolong life, consider using a values history. The values history is an instrument that asks questions related to quality versus length of life and the values that persons see as being important to maintain during terminal care.

BOX 3.5   ANA's Principles for Social Networking

1. Nurses must not transmit or place online individually identifiable patient information.
2. Nurses must observe ethically prescribed professional patient–nurse boundaries.
3. Nurses should understand that patients, colleagues, institutions, and employers may view postings.
4. Nurses should take advantage of privacy settings and seek to separate personal and professional information online.
5. Nurses should bring content that could harm a patient's privacy, rights, or welfare to the attention of appropriate authorities.
6. Nurses should participate in developing institutional policies governing online conduct.

Six Tips to Avoid Problems

1. Remember that standards of professionalism are the same online as in any other circumstance.
2. Do not share or post information or photos gained through the nurse–patient relationship.
3. Maintain professional boundaries in the use of electronic media. Online contact with patients blur this boundary.
4. Do not make disparaging remarks about patients, employers, or coworkers, even if they are not identified.
5. Do not take photos or videos of patients on personal devices, including cell phones.
6. Promptly report a breach of confidentiality or privacy.

From American Nurses Association. (n.d.). *6 Tips for Nurses Using Social Media.* Retrieved from https://www.nursingworld.org/~4af5ec/globalassets/docs/ana/ethics/6_tips_for_nurses_using_social_media_card_web.pdf. Data from American Nurses Association. (2011). *Principles for social networking and the nurse.* Silver Spring, MD: Author; National Council of State Boards of Nursing. (2011). *White Paper: A nurses's guide to the use of social media.* Chicago, IL: Author.

SUMMARY

This chapter presented the legal and ethical issues associated with the nursing care of older adults. Professional standards of practice were identified as the legal measure against which nursing practice is judged, and sources of such standards were identified. Laws applicable to older adults generally were presented, and because older adults who reside in nursing facilities are particularly vulnerable, nursing facility regulations were comprehensively covered, including issues involving quality of life and rights of residents.

Issues associated with autonomy and self-determination were described, including physician-assisted suicide, DNR orders, POLST, AMDs, end-of-life decision making, and organ donation. Ethical considerations were discussed, including issues associated with euthanasia and human research. Nurses have a significant role in assisting to meet the health care needs of older adults, whose unique characteristics, vulnerabilities, and needs present great and varied challenges. The older person's quality of life is affected to a great extent by the quality of nursing care he or she receives.

KEY POINTS

- The nurse's duty to patients is to provide care according to a measurable standard. When patients' physical and mental conditions and their ability to care for themselves decline, the duty of care increases.
- Older adults, particularly infirm older adults, are considered a vulnerable population; therefore their treatment in licensed health care institutions and other settings (including the home) is carefully regulated.
- Evidence provided to the U.S. Congress in 1983 suggested widespread abuse of residents in nursing facilities and resulted in the enactment of the OBRA, the most sweeping reform affecting Medicare and Medicaid nursing facilities since those programs began. Results of the reforms have been mixed, and reports of continuing problems affecting quality of care for older adults persist, causing Congress to consider closer regulation and more stringent enforcement.
- The OBRA focuses on the quality of life of residents in nursing facilities and assurances of the preservation of their human rights and due process interests. The regulations address virtually every element of life in a nursing facility. The OBRA's regulations are enforced through a survey process that focuses on the outcomes of residential care and include sanctions designed to force compliance, analyzed according to the scope and severity of violations.
- A strong judicial deference toward individual autonomy ensures that every human has the right to determine what shall be done with his or her own body. These rights are guaranteed in the U.S. Constitution and have been additionally interpreted in case law and state laws.
- Legal tools and instruments such as AMDs, DNR, POLST orders, designation of health care agents, and durable powers of attorney help people plan for future decision making so that their wishes can be carried out even when they are no longer able to speak for themselves. The presence of these instruments may add to the information available about an individual's wishes, but care should be taken to avoid equating the instruments themselves with the existence of these fundamental human rights.
- The right to self-determination was given even more emphasis with the passage of the PSDA. This law requires health care providers to inform and educate patients about their rights as they exist under the laws of each state.
- Physician-assisted suicide and issues surrounding the care of terminally ill older persons are subjects of national interest and debate, as well as judicial and legislative interest, and the role and obligation of the nurse in such matters must be carefully monitored.
- The technologic and medical advancements that help people live longer also contribute to the complicated ethical dilemmas that exist in the care of older adults. Ethics committees help in these matters by responding to the need for the education of and communication between caregivers and patients.
- It is preferable to resolve patient care dilemmas at the bedside rather than in the courtroom. The courts prefer that patients, their families, and health care professionals handle such matters. With careful guidance and discussion, this can often be achieved.

CRITICAL-THINKING EXERCISES

1. An 85-year-old man has been able to care for himself with minimum assistance until recently. Should he and his family decide that it is time for him to move to a long-term care facility? How will his rights as an individual be protected, because he will be giving up his independence? Explain.
2. A 95-year-old man resides in a long-term care facility. He has signed an advance medical directive (AMD) in case he becomes seriously ill. A 73-year-old woman is being treated in the hospital for a recent cerebral vascular accident that has left her severely incapacitated. Her family has requested a do not resuscitate (DNR) order. How do these two instruments differ? In what ways do they protect each person's rights?
3. You are the nurse in charge of a wing of a nursing facility. During rounds one evening, an older, sometimes confused resident tells you that a nurse aide "pushed her around" during dinner that evening. What issues are presented, and what actions should you take?

REFERENCES

Abuse Intervention: n.d. A Delphi Consensus Survey. *PLoS ONE. 10* (12): e0140760. doi:10.1371/journal.pone.0140760.

Agency for Healthcare Research and Quality [AHRQ]. (2013). Module 7: Measuring and benchmarking clinical performance. Retrieved from https://www.ahrq.gov/professionals/prevention-chronic-care/improve/system/pfhandbook/mod7.html.

American Bar Association. (2017). When you can't make the decision: Living wills, powers of attorney and other disability issues. Retrieved from https://www.americanbar.org/content/dam/aba/migrated/publiced/practical/books/wills/chapter_12.authcheckdam.pdf.

American Nurses Association. (n.d.). Short definitions of ethical principles and theories: Familiar words, what do they mean? Retrieved from http://www.nursingworld.org/MainMenuCategories/EthicsStandards/Resources/Ethics-Definitions.pdf.

American Nurses Association. (2015). *Code of ethics for nurses with interpretive statements.* Silver Spring, MD: American Nurses Association/nursebooks.org.

American Nurses Association [ANA]. (2013). Euthanasia, assisted suicide, and aid in dying. Retrieved from http://www.nursingworld.org/euthanasiaanddying.

American Nurses Association. (2011). *Principles for social networking and the nurse.* Silver Spring, MD: Author.

Beaton, T. (2018). Affordable Care Act changes may breing a rock 2018 for payers. Retrieved May 1, 2018 from https://healthpayerintelligence.com/news/affordable-care-act-changes-may-bring-a-rocky-2018-for-payers.

California Advocates for Nursing Home Reform [CANHR]. (2016). Restraint-free care. Retrieved from http://www.canhr.org/factsheets/nh_fs/html/fs_RestraintFreeCare.htm.

Centers for Disease Control. (2017). Elder abuse prevention. Retrieved from https://www.cdc.gov/features/elderabuse/index.html.

Centers for Disease Control. (2016). *National Center for Health Statistics. Nursing Home Care.* Retrieved from https://www.cdc.gov/nchs/fastats/nursing-home-care.htm.

Center for Medicare and Medicaid Services [CMS]. (2017). Nursing home enforcement - frequently asked questions. Retrieved from https://www.cms.gov/Medicare/Provider-Enrollment-and-Certification/SurveyCertificationEnforcement/Downloads/NH-Enforcement-FAQ.pdf.

Center for Medicare and Medicaid Services [CMS]. (2017). 2017 RAI user's manual provider updates. Retrieved from https://downloads.cms.gov/files/MDS-RAI-Users-Manual-Provider-Updates.pdf.

Center for Medicare and Medicaid Services [CMS]. (2015). OASIS-C1 Data sets. Retrieved from https://www.cms.gov/Medicare/Quality-Initiatives-Patient-Assessment-Instruments/HomeHealthQualityInits/OASIS-C1-DataSets.html.

Center for Organ Recovery and Education [CORE]. (2017). Donor designation and family consent. Retrieved from https://www.core.org/for-professionals/donor-designation-and-family-consent/.

Consumer Voice. (n.d.) Federal law and regulations on nurse staffing issues. Retrieved from http://theconsumervoice.org/uploads/files/issues/Federal-Law-Regulations-Final.pdf.

Du Mont, J., Kosa, D., Macdonald, S., Elliot, S., & Yaffe, M. (2015). Determining possible professionals and respective roles and responsibilities for a model comprehensive elder. *PLoS ONE, 10*(12), e0140760.

eHealth. (2016). History and timeline of the affordable care act (ACA). Retrieved from https://resources.ehealthinsurance.com/affordable-care-act/history-timeline-affordable-care-act-aca.

Factora, R. (2017). Elder abuse: How to recognize the signs, what to do. Retrieved from https://health.clevelandclinic.org/2017/07/elder-abuse-how-to-recognize-the-signs-what-to-do/.

Florida State University. (n.d.). What is the difference between POLST and a living will? Retrieved from http://www.med.fsu.edu/userFiles/file/POLST%20article%20by%20Dr_%20Dan%20Doty.pdf.

Freeman, J. (2017). State continuing education requirements for nurses' aides. Retrieved from http://classroom.synonym.com/state-education-requirements-nurses-aides-6883206.html.

Geppert, C., & Shelton, W. (2016). Health care ethics committees as mediators of social values and the culture of medicine. *AMA Journal of Ethics., 18*(5), 534–539. https://doi.org/10.1001/journalofethics.2016.18.05.msoc1-1605.

Health and Human Services. (2017). The HIPAA privacy rule. Retrieved from https://www.hhs.gov/hipaa/for-professionals/privacy/laws-regulations/combined-regulation-text/index.html.

Healthcare and technology. (2015). Is fee-for-service dead? Retrieved from http://www.lawtechtv.com/.a/6a00d8341e18e853ef01b8d1091a45970c-pi.

Humphreys, K. (2014). An organ shortage kills 30 Americans every day. Is it time to pay donors? *Washington Post.* Retrieved from https://www.washingtonpost.com/news/wonk/wp/2014/10/20/an-organ-shortage-kills-30-americans-every-day-is-it-time-to-pay-donors/?utm_term=.bd9b39380dbc.

Kow, J., Carr, M., & Whytock, S. (2013). Diagnosis and management of urinary incontinence in residential care. *BCMJ., 55*(2), 96–100.

Kudra, A., Lees, C., & Morrell-Scott, N. (2017). Measuring carer burden in informal carers of patients with long-term conditions. *British Journal of Community., 22*(5), 230–236.

LaPuma, J., Orrentlicher, D., & Moss, R. J. (1991). Advance directives on admission: Clinical implications and analysis of the Patient Self-Determination Act. *JAMA, 266,* 402.

Levinson, D. (2013). *Skilled nursing facilities often fail to meet care planning and discharge planning requirements.* Department of Health and Human Services: Office of the Inspector General. Retrieved from https://oig.hhs.gov/oei/reports/oei-02-09-00201.pdf.

Mayo Clinic. (2017). Living wills and advance directives for medical decisions. Retrieved from http://www.mayoclinic.org/healthy-lifestyle/consumer-health/in-depth/living-wills/art-20046303.

Medicare.gov. (n.d.). Rights & protections in a nursing home. Retrieved from https://www.medicare.gov/what-medicare-covers/part-a/rights-in-nursing-home.html.

National Center on Elder Abuse [NCEA]. (n.d.). Types of abuse. Retrieved from https://ncea.acl.gov/faq/abusetypes.html.

National Council of State Boards of Nursing. (2011). *White Paper: A nurses' guide to the use of social media.* Chicago, IL: Author.

National POLST Paradigm. (2017). *Appropriate POLST paradigm form use policy.* Retrieved from http://polst.org/wp-content/uploads/2017/05/2017.05.18-Appropriate-POLST-Paradigm-Form-Use-Policy.pdf.

National POLST Paradigm. (2017). *Fundamental policy principles.* Retrieved from http://polst.org/wp-content/uploads/2017/04/2017.02.10-National-POLST-Paradigm-Fundamental-Policy-Priniciples.pdf.

National POLST Paradigm. (2017). *POLST vs. advance directives.* Retrieved from http://polst.org/wp-content/uploads/2017/03/2017.03.27-POLST-vs.-ADs.pdf.

National POLST Paradigm. (2017). *POLST paradigm form elements.* Retrieved from http://polst.org/about/polst-form-elements/.

Oregon Health Authority. (2014). Oregon's death with dignity act—2013. Retrieved from http://www.oregon.gov/oha/ph/ProviderPartnerResources/EvaluationResearch/DeathwithDignityAct/Documents/year16.pdf.

Oregon State Bar. (2015). Oregon elder abuse reporting requirements. Retrieved from http://www.osbar.org/cle/library/2015/EAR115_Handbook.pdf.

Organ Procurement and Transplantation Network. (n.d.). How organ allocation works. Health Resources and Service Administration [HRSA], U.S. Department of Health & Human Services [DHHS]. Retrieved from https://optn.transplant.hrsa.gov/learn/about-transplantation/how-organ-allocation-works/.

Ouchida, K. M., & Lachs, M. S, (2015). Not for doctors only: Ageism in healthcare. *Generations: Journal of the American Society on Aging.* Retrieved from http://asaging.org/blog/not-doctors-only-ageism-healthcare.

Saha, D., Moreno, C., Csete, M., Kury Perez, E., Cubeddu, L. Farcy, D., Henry, S.,…Goldszer, R. (2016). *Outcomes of patients who have do not resuscitate status prior to being admitted to an intensive care unit.* Hindawi Publishing Corporation: Scientifica https://doi.org/10.1155/2016/1513946.

Sulmasy, S., Mueller, P., & Snyder, L. (2017). Ethics and the legalization of physician-assisted suicide: An American College of Physician's position paper. *Annals of Internal Medicine.* Retrieved from http://annals.org/aim/article/2654458/ethics-legalization-physician-assisted-suicide-american-college-physicians-position-paper.

Syam, P. (2014). *What is the difference between common law and civil law?.* Washington University Law. Retrieved from https://onlinelaw.wustl.edu/blog/common-law-vs-civil-law/.

Taylor, R. M., Gustin, J. L., & Wells-DiGregorio, S. M. (n.d.). Improving do-not-resuscitate discussions: A framework for physicians. *The Journal of Supportive Oncology, 8,* 42–44. Retrieved from https://osuwmcdigital.osu.edu/sitetool/sites/palliativepublic/documents/rotatorreading/DNR_How_to_Do_It.pdf.

University of Kansas Medical Center. (2017). Hospital ethics committee. Retrieved from http://www.kumc.edu/school-of-medicine/history-and-philosophy-of-medicine/ethics/hospital-ethics-committee.html.

University of New Mexico. (n.d.). Values history. Center for Health and Law Ethics, Institute of Public Law, University of New Mexico, Albuquerque. Retrieved from http://hscethics.unm.edu/common/pdf/values-history.pdf.

U.S. Department of Health and Human Services [DHHS] (2016). A guide to informed consent - information sheet. Retrieved from https://www.fda.gov/RegulatoryInformation/Guidances/ucm126431.htm.

U.S. Department of Health and Human Services [DHHS]. (2014). CMS/CDRH letter regarding physical restraint definition. Retrieved from https://www.fda.gov/MedicalDevices/ProductsandMedicalProcedures/GeneralHospitalDevicesandSupplies/HospitalBeds/ucm123678.htm.

U. S. Legal. (2016). *Types of elder abuse.* Retrieved from https://elderlaw.uslegal.com/types-of-elder-abuse/.

van Wijngaarden, E., Leget, C., & Goossensen, A. (2016). Till death do us part: The lived experience of an elderly couple who chose to end their lives by spousal self-euthanasia. *The Gerontologist., 56*(6), 1062–1071.

Ventola, C. L. (2014). Social media and health care professionals: benefits, risks, and best practices. *Pharmacy & Therapeutics [P&T]., 39*(7), 491–499. 520. Retrieved from https://www.ncbi.nlm.nih.gov/pmc/articles/PMC4103576/.

Weden, M. L. (2016). *Why do hospitals get accredited by The Joint Commission? In Intermedix.* Retrieved from http://healthcare.intermedix.com/blog/why-do-hospitals-get-accredited-by-the-joint-commission.

White, J., Duncan, D., Burr, D., Nicholson, T., Bonaguro, J., & Abrahamson, K. (2015). Substance abuse policies in long-term care facilities: A survey with implications for education of long-term care providers. *Educational Gerontology., 41,* 519–526.

4

Assessment of the Older Adult

Jennifer J. Yeager, PhD, RN, APRN

http://evolve.elsevier.com/Meiner/gerontologic

Previous author: Sue E. Meiner, EdD, APRN, BC, GNP.

LEARNING OBJECTIVES

On completion of this chapter, the reader will be able to:

1. Explain the interrelationship between the physical and psychosocial aspects of aging as it affects the assessment process.
2. Describe how the atypical presentation of illness in older adults affects the assessment process.
3. Compare the clinical presentation of delirium and dementia.
4. Describe the assessment modifications that may be necessary when assessing older adults.
5. Describe strategies to ensure collection of relevant and comprehensive health histories for older adults.
6. Identify the basic components of a health history for older adults.
7. List the principles to observe when conducting physical examinations of older adults.
8. Explain the rationale for assessing functional status in older adults.
9. Describe the elements of a functional assessment.
10. Describe the basic components of cognitive assessment.
11. Explain the rationale for assessing social function in older adults.
12. Conduct a comprehensive health assessment on an older adult patient.

WHAT WOULD YOU DO?

What would you do if you were faced with the following situations?

- Your 99-year-old patient is recovering from open reduction and internal fixation, right femur. The femur was fractured during a fall at home. Since surgery yesterday morning, your patient has been oriented to person only. When you bring her breakfast into the room this morning, she pushes the tray away, holds out her hand, and with a big smile says, "Look, look, he finally proposed. Evel Knievel asked me to marry him." What is going on with your patient? How would you determine this?
- Your 82-year-old patient has been diagnosed with leukemia and is undergoing chemotherapy. On his home health intake at 3 p.m., you note he is frail, sitting on the sofa with his head on his chest. He is unshaven and wearing pajamas. His feet are bare on the carpeted floor. What additional assessments should you complete to ensure optimal outcomes from your nursing interventions?

The nursing process is a problem-solving process that provides the organizational framework for the provision of nursing care. Assessment, the crucial foundation on which the remaining steps of the process are built, includes the collection and analysis of data and results in a nursing diagnosis. A nursing-focused assessment is crucial in determining nursing diagnoses amenable to nursing intervention. Unless the approach to assessment maintains a *nursing* focus, the sequential steps of the nursing process—diagnosis, planning, implementation, and evaluation—cannot be carried out.

A nursing focus evolves from an awareness and understanding of the definition of nursing. This is defined by the American Nurses Association (ANA, 2015):

> *Nursing is the protection, promotion, and optimization of health and abilities, prevention of illness and injury, facilitation of healing, alleviation of suffering through the diagnosis and treatment of human response, and advocacy in the care of individuals, families, groups, communities, and populations. (p. 1)*

Furthermore, the ANA (2015) identifies tenets that characterize the practice of nursing across all settings:

1. Caring and health are central to the practice of the registered nurse.
2. Nursing practice is individualized.
3. Registered nurses use the nursing process to plan and provide individualized care for health care consumers.
4. Nurses coordinate care by establishing partnerships.
5. A strong link exists between the professional work environment and the registered nurse's ability to provide quality health care and achieve optimal outcomes. (pp. 8–9)

Tenet number three establishes the nursing process as the foundation of nursing care. As stated previously, assessment provides the basis for all components of the nursing process.

During assessment, the nurse collects subjective and objective data about the patient and his or her environment that assist the nurse in determining a response to health and illness. A comprehensive, *nursing-focused* assessment of these responses establishes a database about a patient's ability to meet the full range of "physical, functional, psychosocial, emotional, cognitive, sexual, cultural, age-related, environmental, spiritual/transpersonal, and economic needs" (ANA, 2015, p. 53). Patient responses that reveal an inability to satisfactorily meet these needs indicate a need for nursing care.

Nursing-focused assessment of older adults occurs across all settings: hospitals, homes, long-term care facilities, senior centers, congregate living units, hospice facilities, and independent or group nursing practices. The setting dictates the way data collection and analysis should be managed to best serve patients. Although the setting may vary, the purpose of nursing-focused assessment of older adults remains that of determining the older person's ability to meet any health- and illness-related needs. Specifically, the purpose of older adult assessment is to identify patient strengths and limitations so that effective and appropriate interventions can be delivered to support, promote, and restore optimal function, and prevent disability and dependence.

Gerontologic nurses recognize that assessing the older adult involves the application of a broad range of skills and abilities, as well as consideration of many complex and varied issues. Nursing-focused assessment based on a sound, scientific gerontologic knowledge base, coupled with repeated practice to acquire the *art* of assessment, is essential for the nurse to recognize responses that reflect unmet needs. Many frameworks and tools are available to guide the nurse in assessing older adults. Regardless of the framework or tool used, the nurse should collect the data while observing the following key principles: (1) the use of an individual, person-centered approach; (2) a view of patients as participants in health monitoring and treatment; and (3) an emphasis on patients' functional ability.

SPECIAL CONSIDERATIONS AFFECTING ASSESSMENT

Nursing assessment of older adults is a complex and challenging process that must take into account the following points to ensure a patient-centered approach. The first is the interrelationship between physical and psychosocial aspects of aging. Next is an assessment of the nature of disease and disability and their effects on functional status. The third is to tailor the nursing assessment to the individual older adult.

Interrelationship Between Physical and Psychosocial Aspects of Aging

The health of people of all ages is subject to the influence of multiple physical and psychosocial factors within the environment. The balance achieved within that environment of many factors greatly influences a person's health status. Factors such as reduced ability to respond to stress, increased frequency and multiplicity of loss, and physical changes associated with normal aging may combine to place older adults at high risk for loss of functional ability. Consider the following case, which illustrates how the interaction of select physical and psychosocial factors may seriously compromise function.

Mrs. M, age 83, arrived in the emergency room after being found in her home by a neighbor. The neighbor had become concerned because he noticed Mrs. M had not picked up her newspapers for the past 3 days. She was found in her bed, weak and lethargic. She stated that she had the flu for the past week, so she was unable to eat or drink much because of the associated nausea and vomiting. Except for her mild hypertension, which is medically managed with an antihypertensive agent, she had enjoyed relatively good health before this acute illness. She was admitted to the hospital with pneumonia. Because of the emergent nature of the admission, Mrs. M does not have any personal belongings with her, including her hearing aid, glasses, and dentures. She develops congestive heart failure after treatment of her dehydration with intravenous fluids. She becomes confused and agitated, and haloperidol is administered to her. Her impaired mobility, resulting from the chemical restraint, has caused urinary and fecal incontinence, and she has developed a stage 2 pressure injury on her coccyx. She needs to be fed because of confusion and eats very little. She sleeps at intervals throughout the day and night, and when she is awake, she is usually crying.

Table 4.1 depicts the serious outcomes related to the interplay of physical and psychosocial factors in this case. Undue emphasis should not be placed on individual weaknesses; the gerontologic nurse should identify the patient's strengths and abilities, and build the plan of care on these. However, in a situation such as that of Mrs. M, the nurse should be aware of the potential for the consequences identified in Table 4.1. In older adults, the cause of one problem is often best understood in light of associated problems. Careful consideration must be given to the interrelationships among physical, psychosocial, and environmental aspects of every patient situation.

Nature of Disease and Disability, and Their Effects on Functional Status

Aging does not necessarily result in disease and disability. Although the prevalence of chronic disease increases with age, older adults remain functionally independent. However, what cannot be ignored is that chronic disease increases older adults' vulnerability to functional decline. Comprehensive assessment of physical and psychosocial function, as well as environmental issues, is important because it can provide valuable clues to a disease's effect on functional status. Self-reported vague signs and symptoms such as lethargy, incontinence, decreased appetite, and weight loss may be indicators of functional impairment. Ignoring older adults' vague symptomatology exposes them to an increased risk of physical

TABLE 4.1   **Effect of Selected Variables on Functional Status**

Variable	Effect
Visual and auditory loss	Apathy Confusion, disorientation Dependency, loss of control
Multiple strange and unfamiliar environments	Confusion, agitation Dependency, loss of control Sleep disturbance Relocation stress
Acute medical illness	Mobility impairment Dependency, loss of control Sleep disturbance Pressure injury Inadequate food intake
Altered pharmacokinetics and pharmacodynamics	Persistent confusion Drug toxicity Potential for further mobility impairment, loss of function, and altered patterns of bowel and bladder elimination Loss of appetite, which, in turn, affects wound healing, bowel function, and energy level; dehydration Sleep disturbance (oversedation)

Adapted from Lueckenotte, A. G. (1998). *Pocket guide to gerontologic assessment* (3rd ed.). St. Louis, MO: Mosby.

frailty. Physical frailty, or impairment of physical abilities needed to live independently, is a major contributor to the need for long-term care. Therefore it is essential to thoroughly investigate reports of nonspecific signs and symptoms to determine whether underlying conditions may be contributing to the older person's frailty.

Declining organ and system function and diminishing physiologic reserve with advancing age are well documented in the literature. Such normal changes of aging may make the body more susceptible to disease and disability, the risk of which increases with advancing age. It may be difficult for the nurse to differentiate normal age-related findings from indicators of disease or disability. In fact, it is not uncommon for nurses and older adults alike to mistakenly attribute vague signs and symptoms to normal aging changes or just "growing old." However, it is essential for the nurse to determine what is "normal" versus what may be an indicator of disease or disability so that treatable conditions are not disregarded.

Age-Related Changes

Declining physiologic function and increased prevalence of disease are a result of a reduction in the body's ability to respond to stress in all of its forms. Typical physiologic changes include decreased renal and hepatic blood flow and mass, decreased lean body mass and muscle mass, along with decreased total body water and increased adipose tissue, all leading to a potential for altered pharmacokinetic and

pharmacodynamic responses to drugs. With age, the immune system has a decreased ability to respond to invading microorganisms secondary to decreased T-cell and B-cell function. Additionally, as individuals age, they are more susceptible to cancer due to an increase in damage to cellular DNA and a decreased ability to repair this damage. Baroreceptors have a reduced response to physiologic changes increasing the risk of syncope in older adults. The incidence of diabetes increases secondary to increased insulin resistance and glucose intolerance.

The important point is that older adults have less ability than younger adults to manage issues such as acute illness, blood loss, the high-technology environment of the hospital, or other issues. It is important for nurses to assess older adults for the presence of physical, psychosocial, and environmental stressors and their physical and cognitive manifestations.

Atypical Presentation of Illness

Determining older adults' physical and psychosocial health status is not easy, secondary to altered presentation of illness. Vague signs and symptoms of illness, coupled with altered parameters for laboratory values and drug dosages, make diagnosis and treatment difficult in older adults. With advanced age, the body does not respond as vigorously to illness or disease because of diminished physiologic reserve. The diminished reserve poses no particular problems for older people as they carry out their daily routines; however, in times of physical and emotional stress, older people will not always exhibit the expected or classic signs and symptoms. The characteristic presentation of illness in older adults is more commonly one of blunted or atypical signs and symptoms.

The signs and symptoms exhibited by the older adult often differ from the "classic" examples provided in pathophysiology textbooks. For example, in the case of pneumonia, older adults may exhibit a dry cough instead of the classic productive cough. Also, the presenting signs and symptoms may be unrelated to the actual problem, for example, the confusion accompanying a urinary tract infection. Finally, the expected signs and symptoms may not be present at all, as in the case of a myocardial infarction that occurs without chest pain (Table 4.2). All these atypical presentations challenge the nurse to conduct careful and thorough assessments and analyses of symptoms to ensure appropriate treatment.

The nurse should assume heterogeneity rather than homogeneity when caring for older people. It is crucial to respect the uniqueness of each person's life experiences, strengths, cultural practices, values, and beliefs, and to preserve the individuality created by those experiences. The older person's experiences represent a rich and vast background that the nurse can use to develop an individualized plan of care. The nurse can compare the older adult's own previous patterns of physical and psychosocial health and function with the current status, using the individual as the standard.

Cognitive Assessment

As can be seen in Box 4.1, delirium is one of the most common, atypical presentations of illness in older adults, representing a

TABLE 4.2   Atypical Presentation of Illness in Older Adults

Problem	Classic Presentation in Young Patients	Presentation in Older Adult Patients
Urinary tract infection	Dysuria, frequency, urgency, nocturia	Dysuria, frequency, and urgency often *absent;* nocturia *sometimes* present. Incontinence, delirium, falls, dizziness, confusion, fatigue, weakness, and anorexia are other signs.
Myocardial infarction	Severe substernal chest pain, diaphoresis, nausea, dyspnea	Sometimes *no* chest pain; or atypical pain location such as in jaw, neck, shoulder, epigastric area. Dyspnea may or may not be present. Other signs are tachypnea, arrhythmia, hypotension, restlessness, syncope, confusion, and fatigue/weakness. A fall may be a prodrome.
Pneumonia	Cough productive of purulent sputum, chills and fever, pleuritic chest pain, elevated white blood cell (WBC) count	Cough may be mild and nonproductive, or absent; chills and fever and/or elevated white blood cells also may be absent. Tachypnea, slight cyanosis, delirium, anorexia, nausea and vomiting, confusion, malaise and tachycardia may be present.
Heart failure	Increased dyspnea (orthopnea, paroxysmal nocturnal dyspnea), fatigue, weight gain, pedal edema, nocturia, bibasilar crackles	Anorexia, confusion, agitation, weakness, restlessness, delirium, cyanosis, and falls may be present. Cough, may not report dyspnea.
Hyperthyroidism	Heat intolerance, fast pace, exophthalmos, increased pulse, hyperreflexia, tremor	Subtle symptoms, lethargy, weakness, depression, atrial fibrillation, tachycardia, weight loss, fatigue, palpitations, tremor, and heart failure.
Hypothyroidism	Weakness, fatigue, cold intolerance, lethargy, skin dryness and scaling, constipation	Often presents without overt symptoms; cognitive dysfunction, fatigue, anorexia, and arthralgias may be present. Delirium, dementia, depression/lethargy, constipation, weight loss, and muscle weakness/unsteady gait are common.
Depression	Dysphoric mood and thoughts, withdrawal, crying, weight loss, constipation, insomnia	Any of classic symptoms *may or may not* be present. Memory and concentration problems, cognitive and behavioral changes, increased dependency, anxiety, and increased sleep. Muscle aches, abdominal pain or tightness, flatulence, nausea and vomiting, dry mouth, and headaches. Be alert for congestive heart failure, diabetes, cancer, infectious diseases, and anemia. Cardiovascular agents, anxiolytics, amphetamines, narcotics, and hormones may also play a role.

Modified from Besdine, R. W. (2016). *Unusual presentation of illness in the elderly.* Retrieved February 19, 2018, from http://www.merckmanuals.com/professional/geriatrics/approach-to-the-geriatric-patient/unusual-presentations-of-illness-in-the-elderly; and Henderson, M. L. (1986). Altered presentations. *American Journal of Nursing, 15,* 1104.

EVIDENCE-BASED PRACTICE

Recognition of Atypical Presentation of Illness in Older Adults

Background

Prompt recognition of acute myocardial infarction (AMI) symptoms and initiation of lifesaving measures in the emergency department (ED) is necessary to save lives. Symptom recognition is challenging in older adults who arrive at the ED with atypical symptoms.

Sample and Setting

Cardiac units at three regional hospitals in Hong Kong participated in this study. Consecutive samples were recruited, consisting of patients over 18 years of age with confirmed diagnosis of AMI. The developmental cohort consisted of 300 participants; the validation cohort consisted of 97 participants.

Methods

This was a risk-prediction model development study, designed to develop and validate a risk scoring system to predict atypical symptom presentation among AMI patients.

Findings

There were 24.3% of patients in the development cohort and 24.7% of patients in the validation cohort who presented with atypical symptoms. Five predictors made statistically significant contribution to atypical AMI presentation: age ≥ 75; female; diagnosis of diabetes; previous AMI; and no history of hyperlipidemia.

Implications

Timely recognition of AMI and initiation of lifesaving treatment is crucial to decreasing morbidity and mortality. Identification of predictors of atypical presentation has the potential to improve recognition of atypical presentation of AMI for triage nurses in the ED.

From Li, P. W. C., & Yu, D. S. F. (2017). Recognition of atypical symptoms of acute myocardial infarction: Development and validation of a risk scoring system. *Journal of Cardiovascular Nursing, 32*(2), 99-106. doi: 10.1097/JCN.0000000000000321.

BOX 4.1   Physiologic, Psychological, and Environmental Causes of Delirium in Hospitalized Older Adults

Physiologic

A. Primary cerebral disease
   1. Nonstructural factors
   2. Structural factors
      a. Vascular insufficiency—transient ischemic attacks, cerebrovascular accidents, thrombosis
      b. Central nervous system infection—acute and chronic meningitis, neurosyphilis, brain abscess
      c. Trauma—subdural hematoma, concussion, contusion, intracranial hemorrhage
      d. Tumors—primary and metastatic
      e. Normal pressure hydrocephalus
B. Extracranial disease
   1. Cardiovascular abnormalities
   2. Pulmonary abnormalities
   3. Systemic infective processes—acute and chronic
   4. Metabolic disturbances
   5. Drug intoxications—therapeutic and substance use disorder
   6. Endocrine disturbance
   7. Nutritional deficiencies
   8. Physiologic stress—pain, surgery
   9. Alterations in temperature regulation—hypothermia and hyperthermia
   10. Unknown physiologic abnormality—sometimes defined as pseudodelirium
       a. Decreased cardiac output state—myocardial infarction, arrhythmias, congestive heart failure, cardiogenic shock
       b. Alterations in peripheral vascular resistance—increased and decreased states
       c. Vascular occlusion—disseminated intravascular coagulopathy, emboli
       d. Inadequate gas exchange states—pulmonary disease, alveolar hypoventilation
       e. Infection—pneumonias
       f. Viral
       g. Bacterial—endocarditis, pyelonephritis, cystitis, mycosis
       h. Electrolyte abnormalities—hypercalcemia, hyponatremia and hypernatremia, hypokalemia and hyperkalemia, hypochloremia and hyperchloremia, hyperphosphatemia
       i. Acidosis and alkalosis
       j. Hypoglycemia and hyperglycemia
       k. Acute and chronic renal failure
       l. Volume depletion—hemorrhage, inadequate fluid intake, diuretics
       m. Hepatic failure
       n. Porphyria
       o. Misuse of prescribed drugs
       p. Side effects of therapeutic drugs
       q. Drug–drug interactions
       r. Improper use of over-the-counter drugs
       s. Ingestion of heavy metals and industrial poisons
       t. Hypothyroidism and hyperthyroidism
       u. Diabetes mellitus
       v. Hypopituitarism
       w. Hypoparathyroidism and hyperparathyroidism
       x. B vitamins
       y. Vitamin C
       z. Protein

Psychological
   1. Severe emotional stress—postoperative states, relocation, hospitalization
   2. Depression
   3. Anxiety
   4. Pain—acute and chronic
   5. Fatigue
   6. Grief
   7. Sensory-perceptual deficits—noise, alteration in function of senses
   8. Mania
   9. Paranoia
   10. Situational disturbances

Environmental
   1. Unfamiliar environment creating a lack of meaning in the environment
   2. Sensory deprivation or environmental monotony creating a lack of meaning in the environment
   3. Sensory overload
   4. Immobilization—therapeutic, physical, pharmacologic
   5. Sleep deprivation
   6. Lack of temporospatial reference points

Modified from Foreman, M. D. (1986). Acute confusional states in hospitalized elderly: A research dilemma. *Nursing Research, 35*(1), 34.

wide variety of potential problems. The nurse, as an advocate for older adults, may need to remind other team members that a sudden change in cognitive function is often the result of illness, not aging. Knowing older adults' baseline mental status is essential to avoid overlooking a serious illness manifesting itself with delirium. Box 4.1 outlines the multivariate causes of delirium that the nurse must consider during assessment.

One of the more challenging aspects of assessment of an older adult is distinguishing reversible delirium from irreversible cognitive changes such as those seen in dementia and related disorders. In contrast to the characteristics of delirium noted previously, dementia is a global, sustained deterioration of cognitive function in an alert patient. Other diagnostic features of dementia include evidence of significant cognitive decline over time along with deficits in learning and memory, language, executive function, attention, perceptual and motor skills, and social interactions (UpToDate, 2018). Table 4.3 depicts the distinguishing features of delirium and dementia. Keep in mind that delirium predominantly affects attention and is typically reversible; dementia predominantly affects memory and is irreversible.

Assessment may be complex because of the multiple associated characteristics of delirium and dementia. In fact, it is not uncommon for delirium to be superimposed on dementia. In this case, the symptoms of a new illness may be accentuated or masked, thus confounding assessment. Therefore the nurse must have a clear understanding of the differences between delirium and dementia, and must recognize

TABLE 4.3   Differentiating Delirium and Dementia

Clinical Feature	Delirium	Dementia
Onset	Sudden, with a definite beginning point	Slow and gradual, with an uncertain beginning point
Duration	Days to weeks, although it may be longer	Usually permanent
Cause	Almost always another condition (e.g., infection, dehydration, use or withdrawal of certain drugs)	Usually a chronic brain disorder (e.g., Alzheimer's disease, Lewy body dementia, vascular dementia)
Course	Usually reversible	Slowly progressive
Effect at night	Almost always worse	Often worse
Attention	Greatly impaired	Unimpaired until dementia has become severe
Level of consciousness	Variably impaired	Unimpaired until dementia has become severe
Orientation	Varies	Impaired
Use of language	Slow, often incoherent, and inappropriate	Sometimes difficulty finding the right word
Memory	Varies	Lost, especially for recent events

From the Merck Manual, edited by Robert Porter. Copyright 2014 by Merck Sharp & Dohme Corp., a subsidiary of Merck & Co, Inc, Kenilworth, NJ. Available at http://www.msdmanuals.com/professional. Accessed February 19, 2018.

that only subtle evidence may be present to indicate the existence of a problem. Also, it may not be possible or desirable to complete the total assessment during the first encounter with the patient. In conducting the initial assessment of the course of the presenting symptoms, the nurse should remember that families and friends of the patient may be valuable sources of data regarding the onset, duration, and associated symptoms.

Tailoring the Nursing Assessment to the Older Person

The health assessment may be collected in a variety of physical settings, including the hospital, home, office, day care center, and long-term care facility. Any of these settings may be adapted to be conducive to the free exchange of information between the nurse and an older adult. The overall atmosphere established by the nurse should be one that conveys trust, caring, and confidentiality. The following general suggestions related to preparation of the environment and consideration of individual patient needs foster the collection of meaningful data.

🌐 CULTURAL AWARENESS

Cultural Assessment

Culturally sensitive assessment is necessary to achieve quality care outcomes. At a minimum, the following questions should be included as part of every geriatric assessment:

* What is your ethnicity?
* What is your preferred language?
* Do you know that interpreter services are available free of charge? Do you want to choose one of the available interpreter services (online, telephone, in person)?
* How much education did you complete (none, <7th grade, ≥7th grade)?

From American Geriatrics Society Ethnogeriatrics Committee. (2016). Achieving high-quality multicultural geriatric care. *Journal of the American Geriatrics Society, 64,* 255-260. doi: 10.1111/jgs.13924.

Environmental modifications made during the assessment should consider sensory and musculoskeletal changes in the older adult. The following points should be considered in preparation of the environment:

* Provide adequate space, particularly if the patient uses a mobility aid.
* Minimize noise and distraction such as those generated by a television, radio, intercom, or other nearby activity.
* Set a comfortable, sufficiently warm temperature and ensure no drafts are present.
* Use diffuse lighting with increased illumination; avoid directional or localized light.
* Avoid glossy or highly polished surfaces, including floors, walls, ceilings, and furnishings.
* Place the patient in a comfortable seating position that facilitates information exchange.
* Ensure the older adult's proximity to a bathroom.
* Keep water or other preferred fluids available.
* Provide a place to hang or store garments and belongings.
* Maintain absolute privacy.
* Plan the assessment, considering the older adult's energy level, pace, and adaptability. More than one session may be necessary to complete the assessment.
* Be patient, relaxed, and unhurried.
* Allow the patient plenty of time to respond to questions and directions.
* Maximize the use of silence to allow the patient time to collect thoughts before responding.
* Be alert to signs of increasing fatigue such as sighing, grimacing, irritability, leaning against objects for support, dropping of the head and shoulders, and progressive slowing.
* Conduct the assessment during the patient's peak energy time.

Regardless of the degree of disability and decline an older adult patient may exhibit, they have assets and capabilities that allow functioning within the limitations imposed by chronic disease. During the assessment, the nurse must provide an environment that gives the older adult the opportunity to demonstrate those abilities. Failure to do so could result in inaccurate conclusions about the older adult's functional ability, which may lead to inappropriate care and treatment:

- Assess more than once and at different times of the day.
- Measure performance under the most favorable of conditions.
- Take advantage of natural opportunities that would elicit assets and capabilities; collect data during bathing, grooming, and mealtime.
- Ensure that assistive sensory devices (glasses, hearing aid) and mobility devices (walker, cane, prosthesis) are in place and functioning correctly.
- Interview family, friends, and significant others involved in the patient's care to validate assessment data.
- Use body language, touch, eye contact, and speech to promote the patient's maximum degree of participation.
- Be aware of the patient's emotional state and concerns; fear, anxiety, and boredom may lead to inaccurate assessment conclusions regarding functional ability.

THE HEALTH HISTORY

The nursing health history—the first phase of a comprehensive, nursing-focused health assessment—provides a subjective account of the older adult's current and past health status. The interview forms the basis of a therapeutic nurse–patient relationship in which the patient's well-being is the mutual concern. Establishing this relationship with the older adult is essential for gathering useful, significant data. The data obtained from the health history alerts the nurse to focus on key areas of the physical examination that require further investigation. By talking with the nurse about health concerns, the older adult increases their awareness of health, and topics for health teaching can be identified. Finally, the process of recounting a patient's history in a purposeful, systematic way may have the therapeutic effect of serving as a life review.

Although many formats exist for the nursing health history, all have similar basic components. The nursing health history for the older adult should include assessment of functional, cognitive, affective, and social well-being. Specific tools for the collection of these data are addressed later in this chapter.

The physical, psychosocial, cultural, and functional aspects of the older adult patient require adaptations in interviewing styles and techniques. Making adaptations that reflect a genuine sensitivity toward the older adult and a sound, theoretic knowledge base of aging enhances the interview process.

The Interviewer

The interviewer's ability to elicit meaningful data from the patient depends on the interviewer's attitudes and stereotypes about aging and older people. The nurse must be aware of these factors because they affect nurse–patient communication during the assessment (see Cultural Awareness box).

⊕ CULTURAL AWARENESS

Cultural Considerations and the Interviewer

Health care personnel must be mindful of the different approaches to health care each culture prefers. Research indicates that persons who consider themselves without prejudice tend to express overt prejudice. Self-awareness can help overcome this issue and facilitate compassionate, culturally appropriate care (American Geriatrics Society [AGS] Ethnogeriatrics Committee, 2016).

- Be respectful of, interested in, and understanding of other cultures without being judgmental.
- Avoid stereotyping by race, gender, age, ethnicity, religion, sexual orientation, socioeconomic status, and other social categories.
- Know the traditional health-related beliefs and practices prevalent among members of a patient's cultural group and encourage patients to discuss their cultural beliefs and practices.
- Learn about the traditional or folk illnesses and folk remedies common to patients' cultural groups.
- Try to understand patient perceptions of appropriate wellness and illness behaviors and expectations of health care providers in times of health and illness.
- Study the cultural expressions and manifestations of caring and noncaring behaviors expected by patients.
- Avoid stereotypical associations with violence, poverty, crime, low level of education, nonadherent behaviors, and nonadherence to time-regimented schedules, and avoid any other stereotypes that may adversely affect nurse–patient relationships.
- Be aware that patients who have lived in the United States for many years may have become increasingly westernized and have fewer remaining practices of their birth culture.
- Learn to value the richness of cultural diversity as an asset rather than a hindrance to communication and effective intervention.

Attitude is a feeling, value, or belief about something that determines behavior. If the nurse has an attitude that characterizes older adults as less healthy and alert, and more dependent, then the interview structure will reflect this attitude. For example, if the nurse believes that dependence in self-care normally accompanies advanced age, the patient will not be questioned about strengths and abilities. The resulting inaccurate functional assessment will do little to promote patient independence. Myths and stereotypes about older adults also may affect the nurse's questioning. For example, believing that older adults do not participate in sexual relationships may result in the nurse's failure to interview the patient about sexual health matters. The nurse's own anxiety and fear of personal aging, as well as a lack of knowledge about older people, contribute to commonly held negative attitudes, myths, and stereotypes about older people. Gerontologic nurses have a responsibility to themselves and to their older adult patients to improve their understanding of the aging process and aging people.

To ensure a successful interview, the nurse should explain the reason for the interview to the patient and give a brief overview of the format to be followed. This alleviates anxiety and uncertainty, and the patient can then focus on telling the story. Another strategy that can be employed in some settings is to give the patient selected portions of the interview form to complete *before* meeting with the nurse. This allows patients sufficient time to recall their life histories, thus facilitating the collection of important health-related data.

Older people have lengthy and often complicated histories. A goal-directed interviewing process helps the patient share the pertinent information, but the tendency to reminisce may make it difficult for the patient to stay focused on the topic. *Guided reminiscence,* however, can elicit valuable data and can promote a supportive therapeutic relationship. Using such a technique helps the nurse balance the need to collect the required information with the patient's need to relate what is personally important. For example, the patient may relate a story about a social outing that seems irrelevant but may reveal important information about available resources and support systems. The interplay of the previously noted factors may necessitate more than one encounter with the patient to complete the data collection. Setting a time limit in advance helps the patient focus on the interview and aids with the problem of diminished time perception. Keeping an easy-to-read clock within view of the patient may be helpful.

Because of the need to structure the interview, nurses tend to exhibit controlling behavior with patients. To promote patient comfort and sharing of data, the nurse should work with the patient to establish the organization of the interview. The patient should feel that the nurse is a caring person who treats others with respect. Self-esteem is enhanced if the patient feels included in the decision-making process.

At the beginning of the interview, the nurse and patient need to determine the most effective and comfortable distance and position for the session. The ability to see and hear is critical to the communication process with an older adult, and adaptations to account for any disability must include consideration of personal space requirements.

The appropriate use of touch during the interview may reduce the anxiety associated with the initial encounter. The importance and comfort of touch is highly individual, but older persons need and appreciate it. Touch should always convey respect, caring, and sensitivity. Nurses should not be surprised if an older person reciprocates because of an unmet need for intimacy.

Finally, the nurse does not have to obtain the entire history in the traditional manner of a seated, face-to-face interview. In fact, this technique may be inappropriate with the older adult, depending on the situation. The nurse should not overlook the natural opportunities available in the setting for gathering information. Interviewing the patient at mealtime, or even while participating in a game, hobby, or other social activity, often provides more meaningful data about a variety of areas.

The Patient

Several factors influence the patient's ability to participate meaningfully in the interview. The nurse must be aware of these factors because they affect the older adult's ability to communicate all the information necessary for determining appropriate, comprehensive interventions. Sensory–perceptual deficits, anxiety, reduced energy level, pain, multiple and interrelated health problems, and the tendency to reminisce are the major patient factors requiring special consideration while the nurse elicits the health history. Table 4.4 contains recommendations for managing these factors.

TABLE 4.4 Patient Factors Affecting History Taking and Recommendations

Factor	Recommendations
Visual deficit	Position self in full view of patient. Provide diffused, bright light; avoid glare. Ensure patient's glasses are worn, in good working order, and clean. Face patient when speaking; do not cover mouth.
Hearing deficit	Speak directly to patient in clear, low tones at a moderate rate; do not cover mouth. Articulate consonants with special care. Repeat if patient does not understand question initially, and then restate. Speak toward patient's "good" ear. Reduce background noises. Ensure patient's hearing aid is worn, turned on, and working properly.
Anxiety	Give patient sufficient time to respond to questions. Establish rapport and trust by acknowledging expressed concerns. Determine mutual expectations of interview. Use open-ended questions that indicate an interest in learning about the patient. Explain why information is needed. Use a conversational style. Allow for some degree of life review. Offer a cup of coffee, tea, or soup. Address the patient by name often.
Reduced energy level	Position comfortably to promote alertness. Allow for more than one assessment encounter; vary the meeting times. Be alert to subtle signs of fatigue, inability to concentrate, reduced attention span, restlessness, or posture. Be patient; establish a slow pace for the interview.
Pain	Position patient comfortably to reduce pain. Ask patient about degree of pain; intervene before interview or reschedule. Comfort and communicate through touch. Use distraction techniques. Provide a relaxed, "warm" environment.
Multiple and interrelated health problems	Be alert to subjective and objective cues about body systems and emotional and cognitive function. Give patient opportunity to prioritize physical and psychosocial health concerns. Be supportive and reassuring about deficits created by multiple diseases. Complete full analysis on all reported symptoms. Be alert to reporting of new or changing symptoms. Allow for more than one interview time. Compare and validate data with old records, family, friends, or confidants.
Tendency to reminisce	Structure reminiscence to gather necessary data. Express interest and concern for issues raised by reminiscing. Put memories into chronologic perspective to appreciate the significance and span of patient's life.

From Lueckenotte, A. G. (1998). *Pocket guide to gerontologic assessment* (3rd ed.). St. Louis, MO: Mosby.

Electronic Health Records

With the advent of electronic health records (EHR), patients and providers have voiced concerns that the connection they have with each other has been undermined and become impersonal. To alleviate some issues related to their use, if possible, keep the keyboard or monitor in a position that lets you face the older adult. Patients have noted that eye contact with their health care provider is an important component of communication. Input as much data into the EHR before talking to the older adult, then alternate talking and inputting data to maintain eye contact and personal connection with the older adult. On a positive note, patients like use of the EHR as it reduced repetition of information; additionally, when health care providers shared the information in the EHR with the patient, they felt it facilitated communication and made them feel a part of the health care planning process (Rose, Richter, & Kapustin, 2014).

The Health History Format

Box 4.2 provides a brief overview of components of the health history. When possible, refer to old records to obtain information that will lessen the time required of both the patient and the interviewer.

Patient Profile or Biographic Data

This profile is basic, factual data about the older adult. In this section, it is often useful to comment on the reliability of the information source. For example, if the patient's cognitive ability prevents giving accurate information, secondary sources such as family, friends, or other medical records should be consulted. Knowledge of the source of the data alerts the reader or user to the context within which he or she must consider the information. Take time to clarify advance directives such as the existence of a living will, powers of attorney for health care and finances, and code status.

Family Profile

This information about immediate family members gives a quick overview of who may be living in the patient's home or who may represent important support systems for the patient. These data also establish a basis for a later description of family health history.

Occupational Profile

Information about work history and experiences may alert the nurse to possible health risks or exposures, lifestyle or social patterns, activity level, and intellectual performance. Retirement concerns may also be identified. Obtaining the patient's perception of the adequacy of income for meeting daily living needs may have implications for designing nursing interventions. Financial resources and health have an interdependent relationship.

Living Environment Profile

Any nursing interventions for the patient must be planned with consideration of the living environment. The degree of function, safety and security, and feelings of well-being are a few of the areas affected by a patient's living environment.

Recreation or Leisure Profile

Identifying what the patient does to relax and have fun, and how the patient uses free time may provide clues to some of the patient's social and emotional dimensions.

Resources or Support Systems Used

Obtaining information about the various health care providers and agencies used by the patient may alert the nurse to patterns of use of health care and related services, perceptions of such resources, and attitudes about the importance of health maintenance and promotion. The importance of religion in all its

---

BOX 4.2 **Basic Components of a Nursing Health History**

Patient Profile/Biographic Data: Address and telephone number; date and place of birth, age; gender; race; religion; marital status; education; name, address, and telephone number of nearest contact person; advance directives

Family Profile: Family members' names and addresses, year and cause of death of deceased spouse and children

Occupational Profile: Current work or retirement status, previous jobs, source(s) of income and perceived adequacy for needs

Living Environment Profile: Type of dwelling; number of rooms, levels, and people residing; degree of privacy; name, address, and telephone number of nearest neighbor

Recreation/Leisure Profile: Hobbies or interests, organization memberships, vacations or travel

Resources/Support Systems Used: Names of physician(s), hospital, clinics, and other community services used

Description of Typical Day: Type and amount of time spent in each activity

Present Health Status: Description of perception of health in past 1 year and 5 years, health screenings, chief complaint and full symptom analysis, prescribed and self-prescribed drugs, immunizations, allergies, eating and nutritional patterns

Past Health Status: Previous illnesses throughout life, traumatic injuries, hospitalizations, operations, obstetric history

Family History: Health status of immediate and living relatives, causes of death of immediate relatives, survey for risk of specific diseases and disorders

Review of Systems: Head-to-toe review of all body systems and review of health promotion habits for same

---

⊕ CULTURAL AWARENESS

Health Literacy

Health literacy is "the degree to which individuals have the capacity to obtain, process, and understand basic health information and services needed to make appropriate health decisions" (AGS Ethnogeriatrics Committee, 2016, p. 257). Nearly 60% of older adults have limited health literacy; this number rises when the older adult has less than a high school education and is a minority. Limited health literacy has been associated with an increased risk of mortality, poor understanding of prescribed drugs on discharge, and failure to use preventive health services. Universal adoption of the "teach-back" technique and keeping printed and oral education at the 6th grade reading level or lower (in the preferred language of the older adult) has been shown to compensate for limited health literacy (AGS Ethnogeriatrics Committee, 2016).

dimensions, including participation in church-related activities, is an important area to assess. Frequently, the church "family" is a significant source of support for the older adult.

Description of a Typical Day

Identifying the activities of a patient during a full 24-hour period provides data about practices that either support or hinder healthy living. Analysis of the usual activities carried out by the patient may explain symptoms described later in the Review of Systems section. Clues about the patient's relationships, lifestyle practices, and spiritual dimensions may also be uncovered.

Present Health Status

The patient's perception of health in both the past year and the past 5 years, coupled with information about health habits, reveals much about his or her physical integrity. Based on how the patient responds, the nurse may be able to ascertain whether the patient needs health maintenance, promotion, or restoration.

The chief complaint, stated in the patient's own words, enables the nurse to specifically identify why the patient is seeking health care. It is best to ask about this using a term other than *chief complaint,* because patients may take offense at that choice of words. If a symptom is the reason, usually its duration is also included. A complete and careful symptom analysis may be carried out for the chief complaint by collecting information on the factors identified in Table 4.5. When the patient does not display specific symptomatology but instead has broader health

TABLE 4.5 Symptom Analysis Factors

Dimensions of a Symptom	Questions to Ask
1. Location	Where do you feel it? Does it move around? Does it radiate? Show me where it hurts.
2. Quality or character	What does it feel like?
3. Quantity or severity	On a scale of 1–10, with 10 being the worst pain you could have, how would you rate the discomfort you have now? How does this interfere with your usual activities? How bad is it?"
4. Timing	When did you first notice it? How long does it last? How often does it happen?"
5. Setting	Does this occur in a particular place or under certain circumstances? Is it associated with any specific activity?
6. Aggravating or alleviating factors	What makes it better? What makes it worse?
7. Associated symptoms	Have you noticed other changes that occur with this symptom?

From Barkauskas, V. H., et al. (1998). *Health and physical assessment* (2nd ed.). St. Louis, MO: Mosby.

concerns, the nurse should identify those concerns to begin establishing potential nursing interventions.

Information about the patient's knowledge and understanding of his or her current health state, including treatments and management strategies, helps the nurse focus on possible areas of health teaching and reinforcement, identify a patient's access to and use of resources, discover coping styles and strategies, and determine health behavior patterns. Data about the patient's perception of functional ability regarding perceived health problems and medical diagnoses provide valuable insight into the individual's overall sense of physical, social, emotional, and cognitive well-being.

Drugs

Assessment of the older adult's current drugs is usually accomplished by having the patient bring in *all* prescription and over-the-counter drugs, as well as regularly and occasionally used home remedies. The nurse should also inquire about the patient's use of herbal and other related products and ask how each drug is taken—by the oral, topical, inhaled, or other route. Obtaining the drugs in this manner allows the nurse to examine drug labels, which may show the use of multiple physicians and pharmacies. Also, this helps the nurse determine the patient's pattern of drug taking (including adherence), his or her knowledge of drugs, the expiration dates of drugs, and the potential risk for drug interactions.

Immunization and Health Screening Status

The older adult's immunization status for specific diseases and illnesses is particularly important because of the degree of risk for this age group. More attention is increasingly paid to the immunization status of the older adult population, primarily because of inappropriate use and underuse of vaccines in the past, especially the influenza and pneumococcal vaccines. Tetanus and diphtheria toxoids (Td) boosters are recommended at 10-year intervals for those who have been previously immunized as adults or children. Adults over the age of 60 should receive the herpes zoster immunization whether they remember having had chicken pox or not. Older adults should still participate in health screenings for the most recent recommendations. Tuberculosis, a disease that was once well controlled, is now resurfacing in this country. Older adults who may have had a tubercular lesion at a young age may experience a reactivation because of age-related immune system changes, chronic illness, and poor nutrition. Frail and institutionalized older adults are particularly vulnerable and should be screened for exposure or active disease through an annual purified protein derivative (PPD) test.

Allergies

Determining the older adult's drug, food, and other contact and environmental allergies is essential for planning nursing interventions. It is particularly important to note the patient's reaction to the allergen and the usual treatment.

Nutrition

A 24-hour diet recall is a useful screening tool that provides information about the intake of daily requirements, including

⊕ CULTURAL AWARENESS

Cultural Assessment of Nutritional Needs

- What is the meaning of food and eating to the patient?
- What does the patient eat during:
  - A typical day?
  - Special events such as secular or religious holidays? (e.g., Muslims fast during the month of Ramadan; Catholics may not eat meat on Fridays during Lent.)
- How does the patient define food? (For some, food may mean survival; for others, food is a reflection of status; food can be pleasure or mean community.)
- What is the timing and sequencing of meals?
- With whom does the patient usually eat? (e.g., alone, with others of the same gender, with spouse)
- What does the patient believe constitutes a "healthy" versus "unhealthy" diet?
- From what sources (e.g., ethnic grocery store, home garden, restaurant) does the patient obtain food items? Who usually does the grocery shopping?
- How are foods prepared? (e.g., type of preparation; cooking oil used; length of time food is cooked; amount and type of seasoning added before, during, and after preparation)
- Has the patient chosen a nutritional practice such as vegetarianism or abstinence from alcoholic beverages?
- Do religious beliefs and practices influence the patient's diet or eating habits (e.g., amount, type, preparations, or designation of acceptable food items or combinations)? Ask the patient to explain the religious calendar and guidelines that govern these dietary practices, including exemptions for older adults and the sick.

the intake of "empty" calories, the adherence to prescribed dietary therapies, and the practice of unusual or "fad" diets. The nurse should also assess the time meals and snacks are eaten. If a 24-hour recall cannot be obtained or the information gleaned raises more questions, having the patient keep a food diary for a select period may be indicated. The diets of older adults may be nutritionally inadequate because of advanced age, multiple chronic illnesses, lack of financial resources, mobility impairments, dental health problems, and loneliness. The diet recall and diary provide nutritional assessment data that reflect the patient's overall health and well-being.

Previous Health Status

Because a person's present health status may depend on past health conditions, it is essential to gather data about common childhood illnesses, serious or chronic illnesses, trauma, hospitalizations, operations, and obstetric history. The patient's history of measles, mumps, rubella, chickenpox, diphtheria, pertussis, tetanus, rheumatic fever, and poliomyelitis should be obtained to identify potential risk factors for future health problems.

An older adult patient may not know what diseases are considered serious or may not fully appreciate why it is important to ask about the history of certain diseases. In such cases, the nurse should ask the patient specifically about the history of certain diseases. It is also important to note the dates of onset or occurrence and the treatment measures prescribed for each disease.

For the older adult the history of traumatic injuries should be completely described, and the date, time, place, circumstances surrounding the incidents, and effect of the incidents on the patient's overall function should be noted. Based on the information gathered about previous hospitalizations, operations, and obstetric history, additional data may be needed to gain a complete picture of the older adult's health status. The patient may need to be guided through this process because of forgetfulness or because of a lengthy, complicated personal history.

Family History

Collecting a family health history provides valuable information about inherited diseases and familial tendencies, whether environmental or genetic, for the purposes of identifying risk and determining the need for preventive services. In surveying the health of blood relatives, the nurse should note the degree of overall health, the presence of disease or illness, and age (if deceased, the cause of death). By collecting these data, the nurse may also be able to identify the existence and degree of family support systems. Data are usually recorded in a family tree format.

Review of Systems

The review is generally a head-to-toe screening to ascertain the presence or absence of key symptoms within each of the body systems. It is important to question the patient in lay terminology and, if a positive response is elicited, conduct a complete symptom analysis to clarify the course of the symptomatology (see Table 4.5). To reduce confusion and ensure the collection of accurate data, the nurse should ask the patient for only one piece of information at a time. Information obtained here alerts the nurse about what to focus on during the physical examination.

Approach to Physical Assessment

The objective information acquired in the physical assessment adds to the subjective database already gathered. Together, these components serve as the basis for establishing nursing diagnoses and planning, developing interventions, and evaluating nursing care.

Physical assessment is typically performed after the health history. The approach should be a systematic and deliberate one that allows the nurse to (1) determine patient strengths and capabilities, as well as disabilities and limitations; (2) verify and gain objective support for subjective findings; and (3) gather objective data not previously known.

No single right way exists to put together the parts of the physical assessment, but a head-to-toe approach is generally the most efficient. The sequence used to conduct the physical assessment within this approach is a highly individual one, depending on the older adult patient. In all cases, however, a side-to-side comparison of findings is made using the patient as the control. To increase mastery in conducting an integrated and comprehensive physical assessment, the nurse should develop a method of organization and use it consistently.

Ultimately, the practice setting and patient condition together determine the type and method of examination to be performed. For example, an older adult admitted to an acute care hospital with a medical diagnosis of heart failure initially requires respiratory and cardiovascular system assessments to plan appropriate interventions for improving activity tolerance. In the home care setting, assessment of the patient's musculoskeletal system is a priority for determining the potential for fall-related injuries and the ability to perform basic self-care tasks. The frail, immobile patient in a long-term care setting requires an initial skin assessment to determine the risk for pressure injury development and preventive measures required. Regular examination of the skin thereafter is necessary to assess the effectiveness of the preventive measures instituted.

In all situations, complete physical assessments are important and should eventually be carried out, but the patient and setting dictate priorities. Consider the subjective patient data already obtained in terms of the urgency of the situation, the acute or chronic nature of the problem, the extent of the problem in terms of body systems affected, and the interrelatedness of physical and psychosocial factors in determining where to begin.

SPICES is an efficient acronym to help gather information necessary to identify patient problems in six common areas identified as increasing mortality risk, leading to increased cost and longer hospitalizations in older adults. Positive findings in these areas guide the nurse to implement preventive and therapeutic interventions. The acronym SPICES stands for:

Sleep disorders: Ask the patient how well they usually sleep.

Problems with eating or feeding: Ask the patient why they do not feel like eating.

Incontinence (of bowel or bladder): Ask the patient if they usually make it to the bathroom on time.

Confusion: Assessed through observation and use of appropriate assessment tools.

Evidence of falls: Ask the patient how often they have fallen. Obtain additional data from secondary sources (e.g., family, caregivers, or long-term care facility).

Skin breakdown: Assess for risk factors using appropriate assessment tools.

When using this tool, alterations in any area should lead to additional assessment in the area indicated (Fulmer, 2007).

General Guidelines

Regardless of the approach and sequence used, the following principles should be considered during the physical assessment of an older adult:

- Recognize that the older adult may have no previous experience with a nurse conducting a physical assessment; each step should be explained, and the patient reassured. The examiner needs to project warmth, sincerity, and interest to allay any anxiety or fear.
- Be alert to the older patient's energy level. If the situation warrants it, complete the most important parts of the assessment first, and complete the other parts of the assessment at another time. Generally, it should take approximately 30 to 45 minutes to conduct the head-to-toe assessment.

- Respect the patient's modesty. Allow privacy for changing into a gown; if assistance is needed, assist in such a way as to not expose the patient's body or cause embarrassment.
- Keep the patient comfortably draped. Do not unnecessarily expose a body part; expose only the part to be examined.
- Sequence the assessment to keep position changes to a minimum. Patients with limited range of motion and strength may require assistance. Be prepared to use alternative positions if the patient is unable to assume the usual position for assessment of a body part.
- Develop an efficient sequence for assessment that minimizes both nurse and patient movement. Variations that may be necessary will not be disruptive if the sequence is consistently followed. Working from one side of the patient, generally the right side, promotes efficiency.
- Make sure the patient is comfortable. Offer a blanket for added warmth or a pillow or alternative position for comfort.
- Explain each step in simple terms. Give clear, concise directions and instructions for performing required movements.
- Warn of any discomfort that might occur. Be gentle.
- Probe painful areas last.
- For reassurance, share findings with the patient when possible. Encourage the patient to ask questions.
- Take advantage of "teachable moments" that may occur while conducting the assessment (e.g., breast self-examination).
- Develop a standard format on which to note selected findings. Not all data need to be recorded, but the goal is to reduce the potential for forgetting certain data, particularly measurements.

Equipment and Skills

Because the older adult patient may become easily fatigued during the physical assessment, the nurse should ensure proper function and readiness of all equipment before the assessment begins to avoid unnecessary delays. Place the equipment within easy reach and in the order in which it will be used. The traditional techniques of inspection, palpation, percussion, and auscultation are used with older adults, with age-specific variations for some areas.

ADDITIONAL ASSESSMENT MEASURES

The use of standardized tools and measures of functional status are important adjuncts to traditional assessment, as they enable health care providers to objectively determine the older person's ability to function independently in spite of disease, altered cognition, and other disability. These assessments include determination of the patient's ability to perform activities of daily living (ADLs) and instrumental activities of daily living (IADLs), as well as the patient's cognitive, affective, and social levels of function. Obtaining these additional data provides a more comprehensive view of the effect of all the interrelated variables on the older adult's total functioning.

Functional Status Assessment

Functional status is considered a significant component of an older adult's quality of life. Assessing functional status has long been viewed as an essential piece of the overall clinical evaluation of an older person. Functional status assessment is a measurement of the older adult's ability to perform basic self-care tasks, or ADLs, and tasks that require more complex activities for independent living, or IADLs (Kane & Kane, 1981). Determination of the degree of functional independence in these areas helps identify a patient's abilities and limitations, leading to appropriate interventions.

The patient's situation determines the location and time when any of the scales or tools should be administered, as well as the number of times the patient may need to be tested to ensure accurate results. Many tools are available, but the nurse should use only those that are valid, reliable, and relevant to the practice setting. A description of the tools appropriate for use with older adults in most settings is given in the following sections.

The Katz Index of ADLs (Katz et al., 1963) (Fig. 4.1) is a tool widely used to determine the results of treatment and the prognosis in older and chronically ill people. The index ranks adequacy of performance in six functions: bathing, dressing, toileting, transferring, continence, and feeding. A dichotomous rating of independence or dependence is made for each of the functions. One point is given for each dependent item. Only people who can perform the function without any help at all are rated as independent; the actual evaluation form merely shows the rater how a dependent item is determined. The order of items reflects the natural progression in loss and restoration of function, based on studies conducted by Katz and his colleagues (Kane & Kane, 1981). The Katz Index is a useful tool for the nurse because it describes the patient's functional level at a specific point in time and objectively measures the effects of the treatment intended to restore function. The tool takes only about 5 minutes to administer and may be used in most settings.

Older adults in most health care settings benefit from functional status assessment, but those in acute care settings are

Katz Index of Independence in Activities of Daily Living

ACTIVITIES POINTS (1 OR 0)	INDEPENDENCE: (1 POINT) **NO** supervision, direction or personal assistance	DEPENDENCE: (0 POINTS) **WITH** supervision, direction, personal assistance or total care
BATHING POINTS:_____	**(1 POINT)** Bathes self completely or needs help in bathing only a single part of the body such as the back, genital area or disabled extremity.	**(0 POINTS)** Needs help with bathing more than one part of the body, getting in or out of the tub or shower. Requires total bathing.
DRESSING POINTS:_____	**(1 POINT)** Gets clothes from closets and drawers and puts on clothes and outer garments complete with fasteners. May have help tying shoes.	**(0 POINTS)** Needs help with dressing self or needs to be completely dressed.
TOILETING POINTS:_____	**(1 POINT)** Goes to toilet, gets on and off, arranges clothes, cleans genital area without help.	**(0 POINTS)** Needs help transferring to the toilet, cleaning self or uses bedpan or commode.
TRANSFERRING POINTS:_____	**(1 POINT)** Moves in and out of bed or chair unassisted. Mechanical transferring aides are acceptable.	**(0 POINTS)** Needs help in moving from bed to chair or requires a complete transfer.
CONTINENCE POINTS:_____	**(1 POINT)** Exercises complete self control over urination and defecation.	**(0 POINTS)** Is partially or totally incontinent of bowel or bladder.
FEEDING POINTS:_____	**(1 POINT)** Gets food from plate into mouth without help. Preparation of food may be done by another person.	**(0 POINTS)** Needs partial or total help with feeding or requires parenteral feeding.

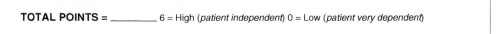

TOTAL POINTS = _____ 6 = High (*patient independent*) 0 = Low (*patient very dependent*)

Fig. 4.1 Katz Index of Independence in Activities of Daily Living. (Adapted from Katz, S., Down, T. D., Cash, H. R., & Grotz, R. C. [1970]. Progress in the development of the index of ADL. *The Gerontologist, 10*[1], 20-30. Copyright © The Gerontological Society of America.)

particularly in need of such an assessment because of their advanced age, level of acuity, comorbidity, and risk for iatrogenic conditions such as urinary incontinence, falls, delirium, and polypharmacy. The hospitalization experience for older adults may cause loss of function and self-care ability because of the many extrinsic risk factors associated with this setting, including aggressive treatment interventions, bed rest, lack of exercise, insufficient nutritional intake, and iatrogenic infection. Box 4.3 provides a clinical practice protocol to guide acute care nurses in the functional assessment process for older adults (Kresevic & Mezey, 1997). Nurses in this setting are in a key position to assess the older adult's function and implement interventions aimed at preventing decline. Specialized care units known as *acute care for elders* (ACE) units have been developed in hospitals around the country to better address these issues. Research has demonstrated this age-specific, comprehensive approach reduces morbidity and mortality associated with hospitalizing older adults (Gorman, 2016).

Nurses practicing in all settings should begin incorporating valid and reliable tools into routine assessments to determine a patient's baseline functional ability. However, the nurse should remember the following points:

- The environment in which the tool is administered will affect scores.
- The patient's affective and cognitive state will affect performance.
- The result represents but one piece of the total assessment.

Cognitive and Affective Assessment

The purpose of a mental status assessment in the older adult is to determine the patient's level of cognitive function (which implies all those processes associated with mentation or intellectual function). This assessment is usually integrated into the interview and physical examination, and testing is conducted in a natural, nonthreatening manner with consideration of ethnicity. Table 4.6 identifies typical areas assessed in a mental status assessment.

The multiple physiologic, psychological, and environmental causes of cognitive impairment in older adults, coupled with the view that mental impairment is a normal, age-related process, often lead to incomplete assessment of this problem. Standardized examinations test a variety of cognitive functions, aiding the identification of deficits that affect overall functional ability. Formal, systematic testing of mental status helps the nurse determine which behaviors are impaired and warrant intervention.

The Montreal Cognitive Assessment (MoCA) (Fig. 4.2) was developed as a quick screening tool for mild cognitive impairment and Alzheimer's dementia. It assesses attention, concentration, executive functions, memory, language, visuoconstructional skills, conceptual thinking, calculations, and orientation. The tool has extensive testing in multiple languages in older adults over 85 years of age covering a wide range of disorders affecting cognition. The total possible score is 30 points, with a score of 26 or more considered normal. To compensate for a limited educational background, older adults with only 4 to 9 years of

education should have 2 points added to the total score; for those with only 10 to 12 years of education, 1 point should be added to the total score. A modified version of the tool is available for use in older adults with visual impairment (Doerflinger, 2012).

The Mini-Cog is an instrument that combines a simple test of memory with a clock drawing test. It was created by researchers at the University of Washington led by Soo Borson. The Mini-Cog is both quick and easy to use, and has been found to be as effective as longer, more time-consuming instruments in accurately identifying cognitive impairment (Borson et al., 2003). It is relatively uninfluenced by education level or language.

Affective status measurement tools are used to differentiate serious depression that affects many domains of function from the low mood common to many people. Depression is common in older adults and is often associated with confusion and disorientation, so older people with depression are often mistakenly labeled as having dementia. It is important to note here that depressed people usually respond to items on mental status examinations by saying, "I don't know," which leads to poor performance. Because mental status examinations are not able to distinguish between dementia and depression, a response of "I don't know" should be interpreted as a sign that further affective assessment is warranted.

The Geriatric Depression Scale: Short Form (GDS; Fig. 4.3), a valid and reliable tool, is derived from the original 30-question scale. It is a convenient instrument designed specifically for use with older people to screen for depression (Yesavage & Brink, 1983). Of the 15 items on the short form GDS, 10 indicate depression when answered positively; the remaining 5 (questions 1, 5, 7, 11, and 13) indicate depression when answered negatively. A score of 0 to 4 is considered normal; a score greater than or equal to 5 indicates depression (Greenberg, 2007).

The instruments described here for assessing cognitive and affective status are valuable screening tools that the nurse may use to supplement other assessments. They may also be used to monitor a patient's condition over time. The results of any mental or affective status examination should never be accepted as conclusive; they are subject to change based on further workup or after treatment interventions have been implemented.

Social Assessment

Several legitimate reasons exist for the need for health care providers to screen for social function in older people, despite the diverse concepts of what constitutes social function (Kane & Kane, 1981). First, social function is correlated with physical and mental function. Alterations in activity patterns may negatively affect physical and mental health, and vice versa. Second, an individual's social well-being may positively affect his or her ability to cope with physical impairments and the ability to remain independent. Third, a satisfactory level of social function is a significant outcome in and of itself. The quality of life an older person experiences is closely linked to social function dimensions such as self-esteem, life satisfaction, socioeconomic status, and physical health and functional status.

BOX 4.3   Nursing Standard of Practice Protocol: Assessment of Function in Acute Care

The following nursing care protocol has been designed to assist bedside nurses in monitoring function in older patients, preventing decline, and maintaining the function of older adults during acute hospitalization.

Objective: The goal of nursing care is to maximize the physical functioning and prevent or minimize declines in ADL function.

I. Background

A. The functional status of individuals describes the capacity to safely perform ADLs. Functional status is a sensitive indicator of health or illness in older adults and therefore a critical nursing assessment.

B. Some functional decline may be prevented or ameliorated with prompt and aggressive nursing intervention (e.g., ambulation, enhanced communication, adaptive equipment).

C. Some functional decline may occur progressively and is not reversible. This decline often accompanies chronic and terminal disease states such as Parkinson disease and dementia.

D. Functional status is influenced by physiologic aging changes, acute and chronic illness, and adaptation. Functional decline is often the initial symptom of acute illness such as infections (pneumonia, urinary tract infection). These declines are usually reversible.

E. Functional status is contingent on cognition and sensory capacity, including vision and hearing.

F. Risk factors for functional decline include injuries, acute illness, drug side effects, depression, malnutrition, and decreased mobility (including the use of physical restraints).

G. Additional complications of functional decline include loss of independence, loss of socialization, and increased risk for long-term institutionalization and depression.

H. Recovery of function can also be a measure of return to health such as in those individuals recovering from exacerbations of cardiovascular disease.

II. Assessment Parameters

A. A comprehensive functional assessment of older adults includes independent performance of basic ADLs, social activities, or IADLs; the assistance needed to *accomplish* these tasks; and the sensory ability, cognition, and capacity to ambulate.

  1. Basic ADLs
    a. Bathing
    b. Dressing
    c. Grooming
    d. Eating
    e. Continence
    f. Transferring

  2. IADLs
    a. Meal preparation
    b. Shopping
    c. Drug administration
    d. Housework
    e. Transportation
    f. Accounting

B. Older adult patients view their health in terms of how well they can function rather than in terms of disease alone.

C. The clinician should document functional status and recent or progressive declines in function.

D. Function should be assessed over time to validate capacity, decline, or progress.

E. Standard instruments selected to assess function should be efficient to administer and easy to interpret and provide useful, practical information for clinicians.

F. Multidisciplinary team conferences should be scheduled.

III. Care Strategies

A. Strategies to maximize function

  1. Maintain individual's daily routine. Help the patient to maintain physical, cognitive, and social functions through physical activity and socialization: encourage ambulation; allow flexible visitation, including pets; and encourage reading the newspaper.

  2. Educate older adults and caregivers on the value of independent functioning and the consequences of functional decline.
    a. Physiologic and psychological value of independent functioning
    b. Reversible functional decline associated with acute illness
    c. Strategies to prevent functional decline—exercise, nutrition, and socialization
    d. Sources of assistance to manage decline

  3. Encourage activity, including routine exercise, range of motion exercises, and ambulation to maintain activity, flexibility, and function.

  4. Minimize bed rest.

  5. Explore alternatives to physical restraint use.

  6. Judiciously use psychoactive drugs in geriatric dosages.

  7. Design environments with handrails, wide doorways, raised toilet seats, shower seats, enhanced lighting, low beds, and chairs.

  8. Help individuals regain baseline function after acute illnesses by the use of exercise, physical therapy consultation, and increasing nutrition.

  9. Obtain assessment for physical and occupational therapies needed to help regain function.

B. Strategies to help individuals cope with functional decline

  1. Help older adults and family determine realistic functional capacity with interdisciplinary consultation.

  2. Provide caregiver education and support for families of individuals when decline cannot be ameliorated in spite of nursing and rehabilitative efforts.

  3. Carefully document all intervention strategies and patient responses.

  4. Provide information to caregivers on causes of functional decline related to the patient's disorder.

  5. Provide education to address safety care needs for falls, injuries, and common complications. Alternative care settings may be required to ensure safety.

  6. Provide sufficient protein and calories to ensure adequate intake and prevent further decline.

  7. Provide caregiver support and community services such as home care, nursing, and physical and occupational therapy services to manage functional decline.

IV. Expected Outcomes

A. Patients can

  1. Maintain a safe level of ADLs and ambulation.

  2. Make necessary adaptations to maintain safety and independence, including assistive devices and environmental adaptations.

B. Provider can demonstrate

  1. Increased assessment, identification, and management of patients susceptible to or experiencing functional decline.

  2. Ongoing documentation of capacity, interventions, goals, and outcomes.

  3. Competence in preventive and restorative strategies for function.

Continued

BOX 4.3   Nursing Standard of Practice Protocol: Assessment of Function in Acute Care—cont'd

C. Institution can demonstrate
   1. Decrease in incidence and prevalence of functional decline in all care settings.
   2. Decrease in morbidity and mortality rates associated with functional decline.
   3. Decreased use of physical restraints.
   4. Decreased incidence of delirium.
   5. Increase in prevalence of patients who leave hospital with baseline functional status.
   6. Decreased readmission rate.
   7. Increased use of rehabilitative services (occupational and physical therapy).
   8. Support of institutional policies and programs that promote function.
      a. Caregiver educational efforts
      b. Walking programs
      c. Continence programs
      d. Self-feeding initiatives
      e. Elder group activities

ADL, Activities of daily living; *IADL,* instrumental activities of daily living.
Modified from Kresevic, D. M., & Mezey, M. (1997). Assessment of function: Critically important to acute care of elders. *Geriatric Nursing, 18*(5), 216.

TABLE 4.6   Mental Status Assessment

Examination Component	Area to Assess
General appearance	Observe physical appearance, coordination of movements, grooming and hygiene, facial expression, and posture as measures of mental function.
Alertness	Note level of consciousness (alert, lethargic, obtunded, stuporous, or comatose).
Mood or affect	Note verbal and nonverbal behaviors for appropriateness, degree, and range of affect.
Speech	Evaluate comprehension of and ability to use the spoken language; note volume, pace, amount, and degree of spontaneity.
Orientation	Note awareness of person, place, and time.
Attention and concentration	Note ability to attend to or concentrate on stimuli.
Judgment	Note ability to evaluate a situation and determine appropriate reaction or response.
Memory	Note ability to accurately register, retain, and recall data or events (may need to verify with collateral sources).
Perception	Note presence or absence of delusions or visual and auditory hallucinations.
Thought content and processes	Observe for organized, coherent thoughts; note ability to relate history in a clear, sequential, and logical manner.

The relationship the older adult has with family plays a central role in the overall level of health and well-being. The assessment of this aspect of the patient's social system may yield vital information about an important part of the total support network. Contrary to popular belief, families provide substantial help to their older members. Consequently, the level of family involvement and support cannot be disregarded when collecting data.

Support for people outside the family plays an increasingly significant role in the lives of many older persons today. Faith-based community support, especially in the form of the parish nurse program, is evolving as a meaningful source of help for older persons who have no family or who have family in distant geographic locations. The nurse must regard these "nontraditional" sources of social support as legitimate when assessing the older adult's social system.

One of the components of the Older Adults Resources and Services (OARS) Multidimensional Functional Assessment Questionnaire, developed at Duke University, is the Social Resource Scale (Duke University Center for the Study of Aging and Human Development, 1988) (Fig. 4.4). The questions extract data about family structure, patterns of friendship and visiting, availability of a confidant, satisfaction with the degree of social interaction, and availability of a helper in the event of illness or disability. Different questions (noted in italics in Fig. 4.4) are used for patients residing in institutions. The interviewer rates the patient using a six-point scale ranging from "excellent social resources" to "totally socially impaired" based on the responses to the questions.

For all the additional assessment measures discussed previously, the nurse should bear in mind that these are meant to augment the traditional health assessment, not replace it. Care needs to be taken to ensure the tools are used appropriately regarding purpose, setting, timing, and safety. Doing so leads to a more accurate appraisal on which to base nursing diagnostic statements and to plan suitable and effective interventions.

LABORATORY DATA

The last component of a comprehensive assessment is evaluation of laboratory tests. The results of laboratory tests validate history and physical examination findings and identify potential health problems not pointed out by the patient or the nurse. Data are considered in relation to established norms based on age and gender.

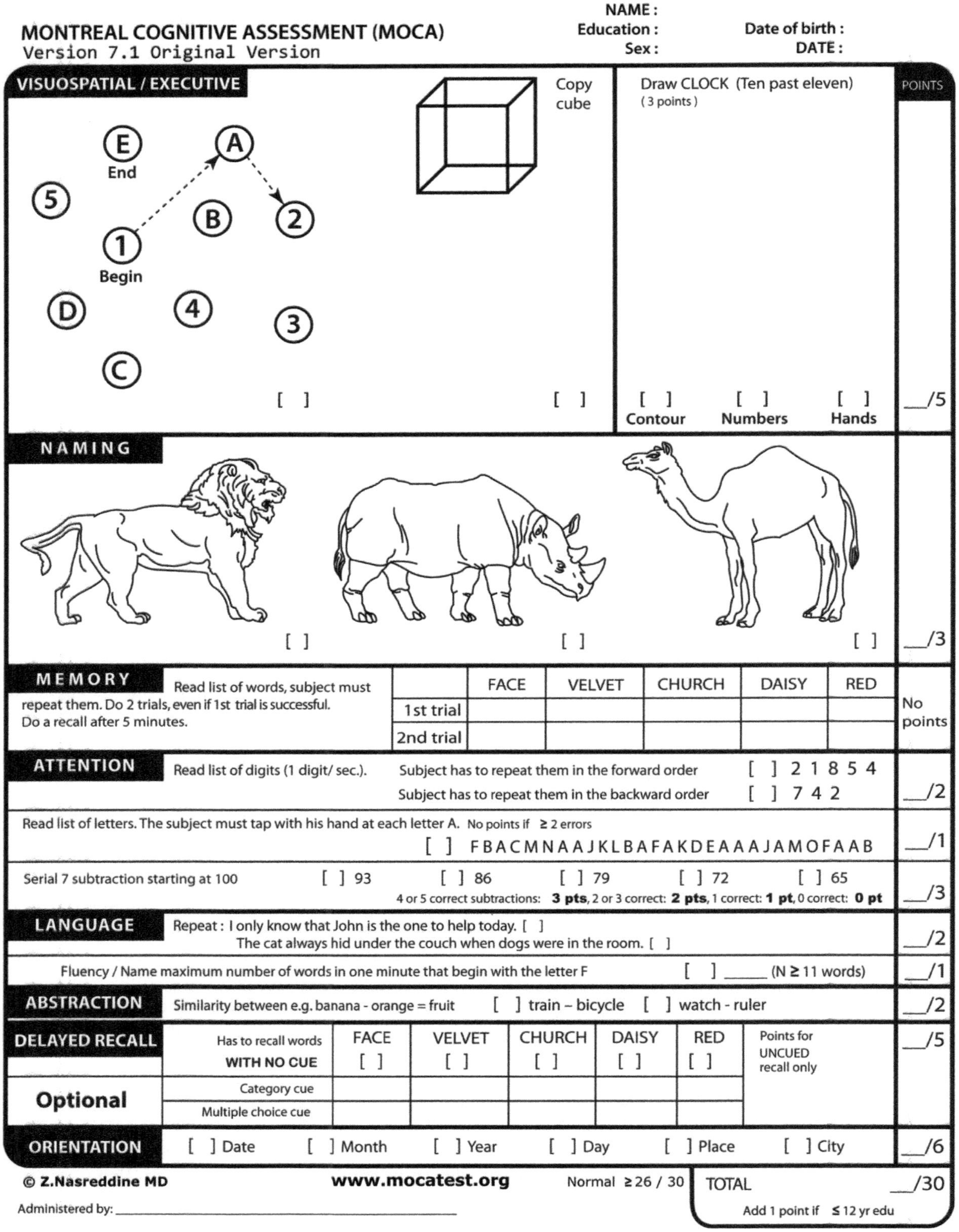

MONTREAL COGNITIVE ASSESSMENT (MOCA)
Version 7.1 Original Version

NAME :
Education :   Date of birth :
Sex :   DATE :

VISUOSPATIAL / EXECUTIVE		POINTS

Copy cube

Draw CLOCK (Ten past eleven)
(3 points)

[ ]   [ ]   [ ]   [ ]   [ ]   __/5
                              Contour   Numbers   Hands

NAMING

[ ]   [ ]   [ ]   __/3

MEMORY	Read list of words, subject must repeat them. Do 2 trials, even if 1st trial is successful. Do a recall after 5 minutes.		FACE	VELVET	CHURCH	DAISY	RED	No points
		1st trial						
		2nd trial						

ATTENTION	Read list of digits (1 digit/ sec.).	Subject has to repeat them in the forward order	[ ] 2 1 8 5 4	
		Subject has to repeat them in the backward order	[ ] 7 4 2	__/2

Read list of letters. The subject must tap with his hand at each letter A. No points if ≥ 2 errors
[ ] F B A C M N A A J K L B A F A K D E A A A J A M O F A A B   __/1

Serial 7 subtraction starting at 100   [ ] 93   [ ] 86   [ ] 79   [ ] 72   [ ] 65
4 or 5 correct subtractions: **3 pts**, 2 or 3 correct: **2 pts**, 1 correct: **1 pt**, 0 correct: **0 pt**   __/3

LANGUAGE	Repeat : I only know that John is the one to help today. [ ] The cat always hid under the couch when dogs were in the room. [ ]	__/2

Fluency / Name maximum number of words in one minute that begin with the letter F   [ ] _____ (N ≥ 11 words)   __/1

ABSTRACTION	Similarity between e.g. banana - orange = fruit [ ] train – bicycle [ ] watch - ruler	__/2

DELAYED RECALL	Has to recall words WITH NO CUE	FACE [ ]	VELVET [ ]	CHURCH [ ]	DAISY [ ]	RED [ ]	Points for UNCUED recall only	__/5
Optional	Category cue							
	Multiple choice cue							

ORIENTATION	[ ] Date [ ] Month [ ] Year [ ] Day [ ] Place [ ] City	__/6

© Z.Nasreddine MD   **www.mocatest.org**   Normal ≥ 26 / 30   TOTAL   __/30

Administered by: _____   Add 1 point if ≤ 12 yr edu

Fig. 4.2 Montreal Cognitive Assessment. (Copyright © Dr. Ziad S. Nasreddine, MD, FRCP. The Montreal Cognitive Assessment [MoCA©]. McGill University and Sherbrooke University Canada. Reproduced with permission.)

Geriatric Depression Scale: Short Form

Choose the best answer for how you have felt over the past week:

1. Are you basically satisfied with your life? YES / **NO**

2. Have you dropped many of your activities and interests? **YES**/NO

3. Do you feel that your life is empty? **YES**/NO

4. Do you often get bored? **YES**/NO

5. Are you in good spirits most of the time? YES / **NO**

6. Are you afraid that something bad is going to happen to you? **YES**/NO

7. Do you feel happy most of the time? YES / **NO**

8. Do you often feel helpless? **YES**/NO

9. Do you prefer to stay at home, rather than going out and doing new things? **YES**/NO

10. Do you feel you have more problems with memory than most? **YES**/NO

11. Do you think it is wonderful to be alive now? YES / **NO**

12. Do you feel pretty worthless the way you are now? **YES**/NO

13. Do you feel full of energy? YES / **NO**

14. Do you feel that your situation is hopeless? **YES**/NO

15. Do you think that most people are better off than you are? **YES**/NO

Answers in **bold** indicate depression. Score 1 point for each bolded answer.

A score >5 points is suggestive of depression.
A score ≥10 points is almost always indicative of depression.
A score >5 points should warrant a follow-up comprehensive assessment.

Fig. 4.3 Geriatric Depression Scale: Short Form. (Adapted from Aging Clinical Research Center. [n.d.] *Geriatric depression scale.* Retrieved from https://web.stanford.edu/~yesavage/GDS.html.)

SUMMARY

This chapter presented the components of a comprehensive nursing-focused assessment for an older adult, including special considerations to ensure an age-specific approach, as well as pragmatic modifications for conducting the assessment with this unique age group. Components of the health history and physical assessment were discussed, and consideration was given to additional functional status assessment measures that can be used with older adults. Compiling an accurate and thorough assessment of an older adult patient, which serves as the foundation for the remaining steps of the nursing process, involves the blending of many skills and is an art not easily mastered.

KEY POINTS

- The less vigorous response to illness and disease in older adults because of diminished physiologic reserve, coupled with the diminished stress response, causes an atypical presentation of and response to illness and disease.
- Cognitive change is one of the most common manifestations of illness in old age.
- Delirium in the older adult requires a complete workup to identify the cause so that appropriate interventions can be developed to reverse it.

- Conducting a health assessment with an older adult requires modification of the environment, consideration of the patient's energy level and adaptability, and the observance of the opportunity for demonstrating assets and capabilities.
- Sensory-perceptual deficits, anxiety, reduced energy level, pain, multiple and interrelated health problems, and the tendency to reminisce are the major factors requiring special consideration by the nurse while conducting the health history with the older adult.

Now I'd like to ask you some questions about your family and friends.

Are you single, married, widowed, divorced, or separated?

1 Single	3 Widowed	5 Separated
2 Married	4 Divorced	___ Not answered

If "2" ask following:

Does your spouse live here also?*

1 yes   0 no

___ Not answered

Who lives with you?

(Check "Yes" or "No" for each of the following.)

Yes	No	
___	___	No one
___	___	Husband or wife
___	___	Children
___	___	Grandchildren
___	___	Parents
___	___	Grandparents
___	___	Brothers and sisters
___	___	Other relatives (does not include in-laws covered in the above categories)
___	___	Friends
___	___	Nonrelated paid help (includes free room)
___	___	Others (specify)_____

In the past year about how often did you leave here to visit your family and/or friends for weekends or holidays or to go on shopping trips or outings?*

1 Once a week or more

2 One to three times a month

3 Less than once a month or only on holidays

4 Never

___ Not answered

How many people do you know well enough to visit with in their homes?

3 Five or more

2 Three to four

1 One to two

0 None

___ Not answered

About how many times did you talk to someone—friends, relatives, or others—on the telephone in the past week (either you called them or they called you)? (If subject has no phone, question still applies.)

3 Once a day or more

2 Twice

1 Once

0 Not at all

___ Not answered

How many times during the past week did you spend some time with someone who does not live with you, that is, you went to see them, or they came to visit you, or you went out to do things together?

3 Once a day or more

2 Two to six

1 Once

0 Not at all

___ Not answered

How many times in the past week did you visit with someone, either with people who live here or people who visited you here?*

3 Once a day or more

2 Two to six

1 Once

0 Not at all

___ Not answered

Do you have someone you can trust and confide in?

1 Yes

0 No

___ Not answered

Do you find yourself feeling lonely quite often, sometimes, or almost never?

0 Quite often

1 Sometimes

2 Almost never

___ Not answered

Do you see your relatives and friends as often as you want to, or not?

1 As often as wants to

0 Not as often as wants to

___ Not answered

Is there someone (outside this place) who would give you any help at all if you were sick or disabled (e.g., your husband/wife, a member of your family, or a friend)?

1 Yes

0 No one willing and able to help

___ Not answered

If "yes," ask A and B.

A. Is there someone (outside this place) who would take care of you as long as needed, or only for a short time, or only someone who would help you now and then (e.g., taking you to the doctor, or fixing lunch occasionally)?

3 Someone who would take care of subject indefinitely (as long as needed)

2 Someone who would take care of subject for a short time (a few weeks to six months)

1 Someone who would help subject now and then (taking him to the doctor or fixing lunch, etc.)

___ Not answered

B. Who is this person?

Name _____

Relationship _____

RATING SCALE

Rate the current social resources of the person being evaluated along the 6-point scale presented below. Circle the one number

Fig. 4.4 OARS Social Resources Scale, modified for community and institutional use. *Indicates questions that are intended for residents of institutions. (Reprinted from the OARS Multidimensional Functional Assessment Questionnaire. [1988]. With permission of the Center for the Study of Aging and Human Development, Duke University Medical Center, Durham, NC.)

(Continued)

that best describes the person's present circumstances.

1. *Excellent Social Resources:* Social relationships are very satisfying and extensive; at least one person would take care of him (her) indefinitely.

2. *Good Social Resources:* Social relationships are fairly satisfying and adequate and at least one person would take care of him (her) indefinitely, or social relationships are very satisfying and extensive, and only short-term help is available.

3. *Mildly Socially Impaired:* Social relationships are unsatisfactory, of poor quality, few; but at least one person would take care of him (her) indefinitely, or social relationships are fairly satisfactory and adequate, and only short-term help is available.

4. *Moderately Socially Impaired:* Social relationships are unsatisfactory, of poor quality, few; and only short-term care is available, or social relationships are at least adequate or satisfactory, but help would only be available now and then.

5. *Severely Socially Impaired:* Social relationships are unsatisfactory, of poor quality, few; and help would be available only now and then, or social relationships are at least satisfactory or adequate, but help is not available even now and then.

6. *Totally Socially Impaired:* Social relationships are unsatisfactory, of poor quality, few; and help is not available even now and then.

Fig. 4.4, cont'd

- An older adult's physical health alone does not provide a reliable measure of functional ability; assessment of physical, cognitive, affective, and social function provides a comprehensive view of the older adult's total degree of function.
- The purpose of a nursing-focused assessment of the older adult is to identify patient strengths and limitations so that effective and appropriate interventions can be delivered to promote optimum function and to prevent disability and dependence.
- An older adult's reduced ability to respond to stress and the physical changes associated with normal aging combine to place the older adult at high risk of loss of functional ability.
- A comprehensive assessment of an older adult's report of nonspecific signs and symptoms is essential for determining the presence of underlying conditions that may lead to a functional decline.
- To compensate for the lack of definitive standards for what constitutes "normal" in older adults, the nurse may compare the older patient's own previous patterns of physical and psychosocial health and function with the patient's status.

CRITICAL-THINKING EXERCISES

1. You are interviewing a 79-year-old man who was just admitted to the hospital. He states that he is hard of hearing; you note that he is restless and apprehensive. How would you revise your history-taking interview based on these initial observations?

2. Three individuals, 65, 81, and 95 years of age, have blood pressure readings of 152/88, 168/90, and 170/92 mm Hg, respectively. The nurse infers that all older people are hypertensive. Analyze the nurse's conclusion. Is faulty logic being used in this situation? What assumption(s) did the nurse make regarding older people in general?

REFERENCES

American Geriatrics Society Ethnogeriatrics Committee. (2016). Achieving high-quality multicultural geriatric care. *Journal of the American Geriatrics Society, 64,* 255–260. https://doi.org/10.1111/jgs.13924.

American Nurses Association. (2015). *Nursing: Scope and standards of practice* (3rd ed.). Silver Spring, MD: Author.

Barkauskas, V. H., et al. (1998). *Health and physical assessment* (2nd ed.). St. Louis: Mosby.

Besdine, R.W. (2016). Unusual presentation of illness in the elderly. Retrieved February 19, 2018 from http://www.merckmanuals.com/professional/geriatrics/approach-to-the-geriatric-patient/unusual-presentations-of-illness-in-the-elderly.

Borson, S., et al. (2003). The Mini-Cog as a screen for dementia: Validation in a population-based sample. *Journal of the American Geriatrics Society, 51*(10), 1451.

Doerflinger, D.M.C. (2012). Mental status assessment in older adults: Montreal Cognitive Assessment. Retrieved February 19, 2018, from https://consultgeri.org/try-this/general-assessment/issue-3.2.pdf.

Duke University Center for the Study of Aging and Human Development. (1988). *OARS multidimensional functional assessment: Questionnaire.* Durham, NC: Duke University.

Foreman, M.D. (1986). Acute confusional states in hospitalized elderly: A research dilemma. *Nursing Research, 35*(1), 34.

Fulmer, T. (2007). Fulmer SPICES. *American Journal of Nursing, 107* (10), 40–48.

Gorman, A. (2016). *Hospital units tailored to older patients can help prevent decline.* Retrieved from https://www.npr.org/sections/health-shots/2016/08/09/486608559/hospital-units-tailored-to-older-patients-can-help-prevent-decline.

Greenberg, S. A. (2007). The Geriatric Depression Scale: Short Form. *American Journal of Nursing, 107*(10), 60–69.

Huang, J. (2016). *Overview of delirium and dementia.* Retrieved February 19, 2018 from http://www.merckmanuals.com/professional/neurologic-disorders/delirium-and-dementia/overview-of-delirium-and-dementia.

Kane, R. A., & Kane, R. L. (1981). *Assessing the elderly: A practical guide to measurement.* Lexington, MA: Lexington Books.

Katz, S., Ford, A. B., & Moskowitz, R. W. (1963). Studies of illness in the aged: The index of ADL—A standardized measure of biological and psychosocial function. *JAMA, 185*, 914.

Kresevic, D. M., & Mezey, M. (1997). Assessment of function: Critically important to acute care of elders. *Geriatric Nursing, 18*(5), 216.

Lueckenotte, A. G. (1998). *Pocket guide to gerontologic assessment.* (3rd ed.). St. Louis: Mosby.

Rose, D., Richter, L. T., & Kapustin, J. (2014). Patient experiences with electronic medical records: Lessons learned. *Journal of the American Association of Nurse Practitioners, 26*(12), 674–680. https://doi.org/10.1002/2327-6924.12170.

UpToDate. (2018). DSM-IV and DSM-5 criteria for dementia. Retrieved February 19, 2018. https://www.uptodate.com/contents/image?imageKey=NEURO%2F91276.

Yesavage, J. A., & Brink, T. L. (1983). Development and validation of a geriatric depression screening scale: A preliminary report. *Journal of Psychiatric Research, 17*, 37.

WEBSITES

ConsultGeri, a clinical website of The Hartford Institute for Geriatric Nursing. https://consultgeri.org.

Montreal Cognitive Assessment (MoCA). http://www.mocatest.org/splash/.

The Registered Nurses' Association of Ontario (RNAO). http://rnao.ca/.

PART II

Influences on Health and Illness

5

Cultural Influences

Carol Ann Amann, PhD, RN-BC, CDP, FNGNA

ⓔ http://evolve.elsevier.com/Meiner/gerontologic

LEARNING OBJECTIVES

On completion of this chapter, the learner will:

1. Discuss the major demographic trends in the United States in relation to the various older adult ethnic populations.
2. Analyze the nursing implications of ethnic demographic changes.
3. Differentiate between *culture, ethnicity,* and *race.*
4. Identify potential barriers to care for the ethnic older person.
5. Discuss cultural variations in beliefs about health, illness, and treatment.
6. Describe how differences in cultural patterns may result in a potential conflict between a gerontologic nurse and an older person or his or her family members.
7. Identify methods to improve the quality of interactions between the nurse and the older adult as it relates to culture, relationships, and behavior.
8. Apply linguistically appropriate techniques in communicating with an ethnic older person.
9. Discuss ways in which planning and implementation of nursing interventions can be adapted to older adults' ethnicity.

WHAT WOULD YOU DO?

What would you do if you were faced with the following situations?

- You are caring for an elderly person who has limited comprehension of the English language. To provide the person with the highest level of care, what will need to be added to the plan of care to ensure there is appropriate communication?
- You are the nurse caring for patients of diverse ethnicities. After looking inward of yourself, your beliefs, and potential biases, how will you best change your perceptions of a culture different from your own? How will you integrate culture into care?
- You are interviewing an elderly Hispanic patient recently admitted to your facility with abdominal pain. There is no medical interpreter present. The daughter states, "Don't worry, I know all about her medical history and I will interpret for her." What would you do?

DIVERSITY OF THE OLDER ADULT POPULATION IN THE UNITED STATES

The population of the United States is becoming more racially and ethnically diverse. A significant shift in the percentage of persons who identify with ethnic groups other than those classified as white and of Northern European descent have increased. It is projected that, by 2044, persons from groups that have long been counted as statistical minorities will assume membership in what has been called the *emerging majority* (Ortman, Velkoff, & Hogan, 2014).

Previous author: Ramesh C. Upadhyaya, RN, CRRN, MSN, MBA, PhD(c).

Although older adults of color will still be outnumbered by their white counterparts for years to come, tremendous growth is anticipated. Projections by the United States Census Bureau note that, by 2044, the composition of racial and ethnic identity as we experience today will shift. Whites will comprise 49.7% of the population compared with 25% for Hispanics, 12.7% for blacks, 7.9% for Asians, and 3.7% for multiracial persons (Frey, 2014). By 2030 into 2060, the number of older Hispanics is expected to be the largest of any other group described as a minority (Tables 5.1 and 5.2).

It must be noted that the figures and projections we have today are drawn from the U.S. Census Bureau in which persons of color are often underrepresented and those who are in the United States illegally are not included at all. In reality, the numbers of ethnic older adults in the United States may be or may become substantially higher (Table 5.3).

Furthermore, within the broad census categories, considerable diversity exists. A person who identifies himself or herself as a Native American or Alaskan Native is a member of one of more than 500 tribal groups and may prefer to be referred to as a member of a specific tribe such as the Cherokee Nation, for example. Although commonalities exist, each tribe has unique cultural features and practices. Similarly, older adults who consider themselves Asian/Pacific Islanders may be from one of more than a dozen countries from the Pacific Rim and speak at least one of the thousand or more languages or dialects.

Adding to the diversity in the United States is the influx of immigrants. The immigrant population has grown at a faster rate than that of native-born citizens. Although access to the

TABLE 5.1 Population by Race and Hispanic Origin: 2014 and 2060

Race and Hispanic Origin[a] Total Population	2014		2060		CHANGE, 2014-2060	
	Number 318,748	Percent 100.0	Number 416,795	Percent 100.0	Number 98,047	Percent 30.8
One Race	310,753	97.5	390,772	93.8	80,020	25.8
White	246,940	77.5	285,314	68.5	38,374	15.5
Non-Hispanic White	198,103	62.2	181,930	43.6	−16,174	−8.2
Black or African American	42,039	13.2	59,693	14.3	17,654	42.0
American Indian and Alaska Native	3,957	1.2	5,607	1.3	1,650	41.7
Asian	17,083	5.4	38,965	9.3	21,882	128.1
Native Hawaiian and Other Pacific Islander	734	0.2	1,194	0.3	460	62.6
Two or More Races	7,995	2.5	26,022	6.2	18,027	225.5
Race Alone or in Combination[b]						
White	254,009	79.7	309,567	74.3	55,558	21.9
Black or African American	45,562	14.3	74,530	17.9	28,968	63.6
American Indian and Alaska Native	6,528	2.0	10,169	2.4	3,640	55.8
Asian	19,983	6.3	48,575	11.7	28,592	143.1
Native Hawaiian and Other Pacific Islander	1,458	0.5	2,929	0.7	1,470	100.8
Hispanic or Latino Origin						
Hispanic	55,410	17.4	119,044	28.6	63,635	114.8
Not Hispanic	263,338	82.6	297,750	71.4	34,412	13.1

[a]Hispanic origin is considered an ethnicity, not a race. Hispanics may be of any race. Responses of "Some Other Race" from the 2010 Census are modified. For more information, see www.census.gov/popest/data/historical/files/MRSF-01-US1.pdf.
[b]"In combination" means in combination with one or more other races. The sum of the five race groups adds to more than the total population, and 100%, because individuals may report more than one race.
From Colby, S. L., & Ortman, J. M. (2015). *Projections of the size and composition of the U.S. population: 2014 to 2060: Population estimates and projections.* Retrieved from https://www.census.gov/content/dam/Census/library/publications/2015/demo/p25-1143.pdf. Data from U.S. Census Bureau, 2014 National Projections.

TABLE 5.2 The Population Continues to Be More Diverse

Nationally, all race and ethnic groups grew between July 1, 2015, and July 1, 2016. Throughout the release references to race groups indicate people who would be included in that group alone or in combination with any other race group, unless otherwise noted (United States Census, 2017).

Hispanic population	Grew by 2.0% to 57.5 million.
Asian population	Grew by 3.0% to 21.4 million.
Native Hawaiian and Other Pacific Islander population	Grew by 2.1% to 1.5 million.
American Indian and Alaska Native population	Grew by 1.4% to 6.7 million.
Black or African American population	Grew by 1.2% to 46.8 million.
White population	Grew by 0.5% to 256.0 million.
Those who identified as being of two or more races	Grew by 3.0% to 8.5 million.
Non-Hispanic white alone population	Grew by 5,000 people, remaining at 198.0 million.

From U.S. Census Bureau. (2017). *The nation's older population is still growing, census bureau reports.* Retrieved from https://www.census. gov/newsroom/press-releases/2017/cb17-100.html.

United States is tenuous related to global politics, older adults are frequently emigrating from their country of origin to the United States to reunite with their adult children; they may live in their adult children's households, where they assist with homemaking and care for younger children in the family, and are cared for in return. As this influx continues, senior communities and heath care facilities will need to advance their cultural competence to support older adults in all settings with activities, meal planning, and programs reflective of their diverse participants. To accomplish this task, long-term strategies to strengthen policies and programs that enhance the health and well-being of diverse older people need to be undertaken (Espinoza, 2017).

Certain communities and regions in the United States are decidedly more diverse than others. Today and in the future, nurses may provide care to older adults from multiple ethnic groups in a single day. It is likely that many of these older adults will not speak the same language as the nurse. As such, appropriate arrangements for interpretive services and interventions must be undertaken to provide culturally appropriate care.

TABLE 5.3   Cultural Diversity in the United States

The Hispanic Population (All Races)	Among states, California had the largest Hispanic total population (15.3 million) in 2016, whereas Texas had the largest numeric increase in the Hispanic population (233,100). New Mexico had the highest Hispanic share of its total population at 48.5%. • Among counties, Los Angeles County, Calif., had the largest Hispanic population (4.9 million) in 2016, whereas Harris County, Texas, had the largest numeric increase (39,600). Starr County, Texas, had the highest Hispanic share of the population (96.3%).
The White Population	Among states, California had the largest white population on July 1, 2016 (29.9 million). Texas had the largest numeric increase since 2015 (281,200). Maine had the highest percentage of its population in this group (96.5%). • Among counties, Los Angeles County, Calif., had the largest white population in 2016 (7.5 million). Maricopa County, Ariz., had the largest numeric increase from last year (59,100). McPherson County, Neb., was the county with the highest white percentage of the population (99.6%).
The Black or African American Population	New York had the largest black or African American population of any state or equivalent in 2016 (3.8 million). Texas had the largest numeric increase (91,900). The District of Columbia had the highest percentage of its total population being black or African American (49.4%). • Among counties, Cook County, Ill. (Chicago), had the largest black or African American population in 2016 (1.3 million). Harris County, Texas, had the largest numeric increase since 2015 (16,400). Claiborne County, Miss., was the county with the highest black or African American percentage of the population in the nation (86.3%).
The Asian Population	California had the largest Asian population of any state (6.6 million), and the largest numeric increase (152,400). Hawaii had the highest percentage for this group (57.0%). • Among counties, Los Angeles County, Calif., had the largest Asian population of any county (1.7 million), as well as the largest numeric increase (22,400). Honolulu County, Hawaii, had the highest percentage in the nation for this group (61.3%).
The American Indian and Alaska Native Population	California had the largest American Indian and Alaska Native population of any state in 2016 (1.1 million), while Texas had the largest numeric increase since July 1, 2015 (10,800). Alaska had the highest percentage (19.9%) of the American Indian and Alaska Native population. • Among counties, Los Angeles County, Calif., had the largest American Indian and Alaska Native population of any county in 2016 (233,200), and Maricopa County, Ariz., held the greatest increase from the previous year (4,100). Kusilvak Census Area, Alaska, had the highest share for this group (91.8%).
The Native Hawaiian and Other Pacific Islander Population	Hawaii had the largest Native Hawaiian and Other Pacific Islander population of any state in 2016 (381,000). Since 2015, this group increased the most in California (4,900). Hawaii had the highest percentage of its population in this group in 2016 (26.7%). • Among counties, Honolulu County, Hawaii, had the largest Native Hawaiian and Other Pacific Islander population (245,600) in 2016, and Clark County, Nev., had the largest increase during the last year (1,500).
The Population of Two or More Races	Among states, more people who identified as being of two or more races lived in California (1.5 million) than in any other state, with an increase of 32,900 from 2015. Hawaii had the highest percentage for this group (23.7%). • Among counties, Los Angeles County, Calif., had the largest population of two or more races in 2016 (305,000). Maricopa County, Ariz., had the highest numeric increase since 2015 (5,300). Hawaii County, Hawaii, had the highest share for this group (30.1%).
The Non-Hispanic White Alone Population	Among states, California had the largest non-Hispanic white alone population on July 1, 2016 (14.8 million). Florida had the largest numeric increase since 2015 (114,200). Maine had the highest percentage of its population in this group (93.5%). • Among counties, Los Angeles County, Calif., had the largest non-Hispanic white alone population in 2016 (2.7 million). Maricopa County, Ariz., had the largest numeric increase from last year (24,700). Keya Paha County, Neb., was the county with the highest share of its total population in this group (98.0%).

From U.S. Census Bureau. (2017). *The nation's older population is still growing, census bureau reports.* Retrieved from https://www.census.gov/newsroom/press-releases/2017/cb17-100.html.

CULTURALLY SENSITIVE GERONTOLOGIC NURSING CARE

The diversity of values, beliefs, languages, and historical life experiences of older adults today challenge nurses to gain new awareness, knowledge, and skills to provide culturally and linguistically appropriate care. When language becomes a barrier to care, working with professional medical interpreters may be helpful. To give the most sensitive care, it is necessary to step outside of cultural bias and accept that other cultures have different ways of perceiving the world that are as valid as one's own. Increasing awareness, knowledge, and skills are the tools needed to begin to overcome the barriers to culturally compassionate care to reduce health disparities (see Evidence-Based Practice box).

EVIDENCE-BASED PRACTICE

Discriminatory Practices Within Vulnerable Cultures

Background
Perceived discrimination while seeking heath care services is commonly associated with poor physical and mental health outcomes. This study examined self-reported discrimination from a subset of the Asian American population: Asian Indians, the third largest Asian American subgroup in the United States (Misra & Hunte, 2016).

Sample/Setting
The sample consisted of 1824 Asian Indian adults in six states across the United States.

Methods
A cross-sectional survey was utilized to identify perceptions of discrimination in health care services provided.

Findings
Asian Indians who reported poor self-rated health were approximately twice as likely to perceived discrimination when seeking care compared with those in good or excellent health status. Asian Indians who lived for more than 10 years in the United States and had chronic illnesses were more likely to perceive discrimination when seeking health care.

Implications
The gerontologic nurse should be aware of discriminatory practices in caring for patients with varied cultures. The study authors noted that the perception of interpersonal discrimination when seeking heath care services affects future heath care utilization. This may exacerbate the overall health burden of those who have chronic health conditions. As a result, management of chronic disease states may be hindered leading to decreased quality of life. Developing an understanding of various cultures and caring for patients in a nonbiased manner by eliminating discriminatory practices will improve patient outcomes.

From Misra, R., & Hunte, H. (2016). Perceived discrimination and health outcomes among Asian Indians in the United States. *BMC Health Services Research,16,* 567. DOI 10.1186/s12913-016-1821-8.

Awareness

Providing culturally appropriate care begins with an introspective look at our own beliefs and attitudes inclusive of those commonly seen in the community at large and in the community of health care. Awareness of one's thoughts and feelings about others who are culturally different from oneself is necessary. These thoughts and feelings may be hidden from you but may be evident to others. To be aware of these thoughts and feelings about others, you can begin to share or write down personal memories of those first experiences of cultural differences. A good starting point to begin the process of discovery is to conduct a cultural self-assessment such as the one found in the Cultural Awareness box on self-assessment.

Awareness is also enhanced through the acquisition of new knowledge about cultures and the common barriers to high-quality health care too often faced by persons from ethnically distinct groups.

CULTURAL AWARENESS

Self-assessment

1. What are my personal beliefs about older adults from different cultures?
2. What experiences have influenced my values, biases, ideas, and attitudes toward older adults from different cultures?
3. What are my values as they relate to health, illness, and health-related practices?
4. How do my values and attitudes affect my clinical judgments?
5. How do my values influence my thinking and behaving?
6. What are my personal habits and typical communication patterns when interacting with others? How would these be perceived by older adults of different cultures?

Knowledge

Increased knowledge is a prerequisite for culturally appropriate care given to all persons, regardless of race or ethnicity. Developing cross-cultural knowledge is essential for the delivery of sensitive care. Frustration and conflict among older adult patients, nurses, and other health care providers can be lessened or avoided. Courses in anthropology (political, economic, and cultural), world religions, intercultural communication, scientific health and folk care systems, cross-cultural nutrition, and languages are relevant. Such information helps students, practitioners, and health care institutions become more culturally sensitive to the diversity of their present and potential patient populations. It will allow the nurse to improve patient health outcomes and, in doing so, reduce persistent health disparities (Purnell, 2012).

Cultural Concepts

Several key terms and concepts are discussed here to clarify those that are often used incorrectly or interchangeably in any discussion related to culture and ethnicity.

Culture is a universal phenomenon. It is the shared and learned beliefs, expectations, and behaviors of a group of people. Style of dress, food preferences, language, and social systems are expressions of culture. Cultures may share similarities, but no two are exactly alike. Cultural knowledge is transmitted from one member to another through the process called *enculturation*. It provides individuals with a sense of security and a blueprint for interacting within the family, community, and country. Culture allows members of the group to predict each other's behavior and respond appropriately, including during one's own aging and that of community members. Culture is universal and adaptive, and it exists at the microlevel of the individual or family and at the macrolevel in terms of a region, country, or a specific group (see Boxes 5.1 through 5.4).

Cultural beliefs about what is right and wrong are known as *values*. Values provide a standard from which judgments are made, are learned early in childhood, and are expressed throughout the life span. An example of this is the importance of filial responsibility in many cultures outside those of Northern European origins. This is the expectation that the needs of older adults will be met by their children.

BOX 5.1 Anglo American (European American) Culture (Mainly U.S. Middle and Upper Classes)

Cultural Values

- Individualism—focus on a self-reliant person
- Independence and freedom
- Competition and achievement
- Materialism (items and money)
- Technologic dependence
- Instantaneous actions
- Youth and beauty
- Equal rights to both sexes
- Leisure time
- Reliance on scientific facts and numbers
- Less respect for authority and older adults
- Generosity in time of crisis

Culture Care Meanings and Action Modes

- Alleviating stress:
  - Physical means
  - Emotional means
- Personalized acts:
  - Doing special things
  - Giving individual attention
- Self-reliance (individualism) by:
  - Reliance on self
  - Reliance on self (self-care)
  - Becoming as independent as possible
  - Reliance on technology
- Health instruction:
  - Explaining how "to do" this care for self
  - Giving the "medical" facts

From Leininger, M (Ed.). (1991). *Culture care diversity and universality: A theory of nursing.* Sudbury, MA: National League for Nursing, Jones and Bartlett.

BOX 5.2 Appalachian Culture

Cultural Values

- Keeping ties with kin from the "hollows"
- Personalized religion
- Folk practices as "the best ways of life"
- Guarding against "strangers"
- Being frugal; often using home remedies
- Staying near home for protection
- Mother as decision maker
- Community interdependency

Culture Care Meanings and Action Modes

- Knowing and trusting "true friends"
- Being kind to others
- Being watchful of strangers or outsiders
- Doing for others; less for self
- Keeping with kin and local folks
- Using home remedies "first and last"
- Taking help from kin as needed (primary care)
- Helping people stay away from the hospital—"the place where people die"

From Leininger, M (Ed.). (1991). *Culture care diversity and universality: A theory of nursing.* Sudbury, MA: National League for Nursing, Jones and Bartlett.

BOX 5.3 Black Culture

Cultural Values

- Extended family networks
- Religion (many are Baptists)
- Interdependence with blacks
- Daily survival
- Technology (e.g., radio, car)
- Folk (soul) foods
- Folk healing modes
- Music and physical activities

Culture Care Meanings and Action Modes

- Concern for "my brothers and sisters"
- Being involved
- Providing a presence (physical)
- Family support and "get-togethers"
- Touching appropriately
- Reliance on folk home remedies
- Reliance on Jesus to "save us" with prayers and songs

From Leininger, M (Ed.). (1991). *Culture care diversity and universality: A theory of nursing.* Sudbury, MA: National League for Nursing, Jones and Bartlett.

BOX 5.4 Arab American Muslim Culture

Culture Care Meanings and Action Modes

- Providing family care and support—a responsibility
- Offering respect and private time for religious beliefs and prayers (five times each day)
- Respecting and protecting cultural differences in gender roles
- Knowing cultural taboos and norms (e.g., no pork, alcohol, or smoking)
- Recognizing honor and obligation
- Helping others to "save face" and preserve cultural values
- Obligation and responsibility to visit the sick
- Following the teachings of the Koran
- Helping children and elderly when they are ill

From Leininger, M (Ed.). (1991). *Culture care diversity and universality: A theory of nursing.* Sudbury, MA: National League for Nursing, Jones and Bartlett.

Acculturation is a process that occurs when a member of one cultural group adopts the values, beliefs, expectations, and behaviors of another group, usually in an attempt to become recognized as a member of the new group. Issues surrounding acculturation are particularly relevant for ethnic older persons. Many emigrate to join their children's families who have established themselves in a new homeland. They may live in ethnically homogeneous neighborhoods such as "Little Italy," "Little Havana," "Chinatown," or other such locations. They may have little interest or need to adopt the mainstream culture of the new country and may retain practices and expectations of the "old country." Their children, on the other hand, may live in two cultures, that of their parents and that of the community, including their workplaces. This phenomenon has produced a considerable amount of intergenerational conflict.

Race is the outward expression of specific genetically influenced, hereditary traits such as skin color and eye color, facial structures, hair texture, and body shape and proportions. Many older adults would have married members of their same ethnic or racial group, but this is becoming less common among younger persons. This, too, may serve as a source of familial conflict as traditions and expectations clash.

Ethnicity is defined as a social differentiation of people based on group membership, shared history, and common characteristics. For example, the term *Hispanic* or *Latino* is often applied to persons who speak the Spanish language and practice the Catholic religion. However, those who identify themselves as Latino may have been born in any number of countries and be of any race.

Ethnic identity refers to an individual's identification with a group of persons who share similar beliefs and values. Ethnic identity cannot be assumed by appearance, language, or other outward features. The author once asked an older black woman, "May I assume you identify yourself as an African American?" To which she replied, "Well, no—I have always thought of myself as just an American and don't think in terms of 'African American.'"

Gerontologic nursing care is provided to all persons in all settings without regard to personal characteristics (see Home Care box).

🏠 HOME CARE

1. Ascertain whether the older adult was born in America or came to the United States as a child, young adult, or later in life. This may affect his or her level of knowledge of Western medicine and care, as well as his or her eligibility for benefits and services. Adapt communication styles as needed to reduce the potential for conflict. Refer to the appropriate agency or social worker for assistance, if necessary.
2. Assess the caregiver's and patient's concepts and perceptions of health and illness.
3. Communicate with persons with different linguistic or cultural patterns (e.g., eye contact) in a way in which information may be clear and understandable.
4. Assess the home environment for evidence of cultural values, and determine views on health and illness concepts. Ask the patient if there are any cultural practices they prefer or currently use. Incorporate these data into the care plan to meet the cultural needs of the individual and family.

However, evidence of racial and ethnic disparities in health care and health outcomes exists across the range of illness and services and all age groups (Agency for Healthcare Research and Quality [AHRQ], 2013). Socioeconomic factors account for some of these differences but so do racism and ageism in the health care encounter. Significant for older adults, alarming differences are seen in the rate of angioplasty, use of pain medication, timing of mammography, and mortality associated with prostate cancer, to name only a few (AHRQ, 2015; Chatterjee, He, & Keating, 2013; Davis, Buchanan, & Green, 2013).

Gerontologic nurses who provide culturally sensitive care can contribute to the reduction of health disparities through awareness of, sensitivity to, and knowledge of both overt and covert barriers to caring (Neese, 2017). Among these barriers are ethnocentrism and racism. Both are triggers to cultural conflict in the nursing situation. In gerontologic nursing, the barriers are reinforced by ageism.

Ethnocentrism is the belief that one's own ethnic group, race, or nation of origin is superior to that of another's. In nursing, we have our own unique culture with the expectation that patients adapt to our methods of care provision. Nurses and the health care system expect patients to be on time for appointments and follow instructions, among other requirements. If we care for older adults in an institutional setting, we expect they will agree to the frequency of prescribed bathing, eating (and timing of this), and sleep and rest cycles. The more an individual accepts the institution's culture, the more content he or she will appear to be. The individual most likely will be identified as "compliant" or a "good patient." Such a nursing home resident will eat the meals provided even if the food does not look like or taste like what he or she has always eaten. A non–English-speaking resident will cooperate with the staff, with or without the help of an interpreter. Those who resist may be considered "noncompliant," "combative," or "a difficult patient." However, some of the emerging models of care such as the Green House Model and the Eden Alternatives in nursing facilities are attempting to reverse this care trend and create homelike environments (Amann & LeBlanc, 2013).

Racism is having negative beliefs, attitudes, or behavior toward a person or group of persons based solely on skin color. Racism results in hostile attitudes of prejudice and the differential treatment and behavior of discrimination, and is directed at a specific ethnic or minority group. It has also been found to be a factor in reduced health outcomes in persons from those groups considered "minorities." The same description may be applied to discrimination based on age. The following example illustrates racism:

> A gerontologic nurse responded to a call from an older patient's room. For some unknown reason, the patient, repeatedly and without comment, dropped his watch on the floor while talking to the nurse. She calmly picked it up, handed it back to him, and continued talking. During one of the droppings, an aide walked in the room, picked up the watch, and attempted to hand it back to him. The patient immediately started yelling and cursing at the aide for attempting to steal his watch. When telling this story, the nurse thought the whole situation odd but not too remarkable. It was not until she learned about subtle racism in health care settings that she recognized the patient's harmful, racist behavior: He was white and so was she, but the aide was black.

Cultural conflict is the anxiety experienced when people interact with individuals who have beliefs, values, customs, languages, and ways of life different than their own. Consider this example:

> An immigrant Korean nurse was instructed to walk with an 80-year-old black patient. The patient complained that he was tired and wanted to remain in bed. The nurse did not insist. The European American nurse manager reprimanded the immigrant Korean nurse for not walking with the patient as ordered. The immigrant Korean nurse commented to another Korean nurse, "These Americans do not respect their elders; they talk to them as if they were children."

Older adults are revered by the Korean culture. Cultural conflicts may occur when caregivers apply their own cultural norms to others without understanding the rationale for the action.

Beliefs About Health and Illness

Beliefs about health, disease causation, and appropriate treatment are grounded in culture. The significance attached to illness symptoms and the expectation of outcomes are influenced by past experiences. Knowledge about a person's beliefs about health and illness is especially important in gerontologic nursing because elders have had a lifetime of experience with illness of self, family, and others within their ethnic and cultural groups (Spector, 2017). Beliefs about health, illness, and treatment can be loosely divided into three theoretical categories: magico-religious, balance and harmony, and biomedical.

In the *magico-religious theory*, health, illness, and effectiveness of treatment are believed to be caused by the actions of a higher power (e.g., God, gods, or supernatural forces or agents). Health is viewed as a blessing or reward from a higher source and illness as a punishment for breaching rules, breaking a taboo, or displeasing the source of power. Beliefs that illness and disease causation originate from the wrath of God are prevalent among members of the Holiness, Pentecostal, and Fundamental Baptist churches.

Examples of magical causes of illness are voodoo, especially among persons from the Caribbean; root work among southern black Americans; hexing among Mexican Americans; and Gaba among Filipino Americans. For other religious beliefs of different groups, see Box 5.5.

Treatments may involve religious practices such as praying, meditating, fasting, wearing amulets, burning candles, and

---

BOX 5.5   Religious Beliefs of 23 Different Groups That Can Affect Nursing Care

Adventist (Seventh Day Adventist; Church of God)
- May believe in divine healing and practice anointing with oil; use of prayer
- May desire communion or baptism when ill
- Believe in human choice and God's sovereignty
- May oppose hypnosis as therapy

Baptist (27 Groups)
- Laying on of hands (some groups)
- May resist some therapies such as abortion
- Believe God functions through physician
- May believe in predestination; may respond passively to care

Black Muslim
- Faith healing unacceptable
- Always maintain personal habits of cleanliness

Buddhist Churches of America
- Believe illness to be a trial to aid development of soul; illness because of karmic causes
- May be reluctant to have surgery or certain treatments on holy days
- Believe cleanliness to be of great importance
- Family may request Buddhist priest for counseling

Church of Christ Scientist (Christian Science)
- Deny the existence of health crisis; see sickness and sin as errors of the mind that can be altered by prayer
- Oppose human intervention with drugs or other therapies; however, accept legally required immunizations
- Many believe that disease is a human mental concept that can be dispelled by "spiritual truth" to the extent that they refuse all medical treatment

Church of Jesus Christ of Latter Day Saints (Mormon)
- Devout adherents believe in divine healing through anointment with oil, laying on of hands by certain church members holding the priesthood, and prayers
- Medical therapy not prohibited; members have free will to choose treatments

Eastern Orthodox (in Turkey, Egypt, Syria, Romania, Bulgaria, Cyprus, Albania, and Other Countries)
- Believe in anointing of the sick
- No conflict with medical science

Episcopal (Anglican)
- May believe in spiritual healing
- Rite for anointing sick available but not mandatory

Friends (Quakers)
- No special rites or restrictions

Greek Orthodox
- Each health crisis handled by ordained priest; deacon may also serve in some cases
- Holy Communion administered in hospital
- May desire Sacrament of the Holy Unction performed by priest

Hindu
- Illness or injury believed to represent sins committed in previous life
- Accept most modern medical practices

Islam (Muslim/Moslem)
- Faith healing not acceptable unless patient's psychological condition is deteriorating; performed for morale
- Ritual washing after prayer; prayer takes place five times daily (on rising, midday, afternoon, early evening, and before bed); during prayer, face Mecca and kneel on prayer rug

Jehovah's Witness
- Generally, absolutely opposed to transfusions of whole blood, packed red blood cells, platelets, and fresh or frozen plasma, including banking of own blood; individuals may sometimes be persuaded in emergencies
- May be opposed to use of albumin, globulin, factor replacement (hemophilia), and vaccines
- Not opposed to non–blood plasma expanders

Judaism (Orthodox and Conservative)
- May resist surgical or medical procedures on Sabbath unless emergent, which extends from sundown Friday until sundown Saturday
- Seriously ill and pregnant women are exempt from fasting
- May follow Kosher diet; however, illness is grounds for violating dietary laws (e.g., patient with congestive heart failure does not have to use kosher meats, which are high in sodium)
- May refuse autopsies to be performed on loved ones

Continued

BOX 5.5 Religious Beliefs of 23 Different Groups That Can Affect Nursing Care—cont'd

Lutheran
- Church or pastor notified of hospitalization (with patient permission or by their designee)
- Communion may be given before or after surgery or similar crisis

Mennonite (Similar to Amish)
- No illness rituals
- Deep concern for dignity and self-determination of individual; would conflict with shock treatment or medical treatment affecting personality or will

Methodist
- Communion may be requested before surgery or similar crisis

Nazarene
- Church official administers communion and laying on of hands
- Believe in divine healing but without excluding medical treatment

Pentecostal (Assembly of God, Four-Square)
- No restrictions regarding medical care
- Deliverance from sickness provided for by atonement; may pray for divine intervention in health matters and seek God in prayer for themselves and others when ill

Orthodox Presbyterian
- Communion administered when appropriate and convenient
- Blood transfusion accepted when advisable
- Pastor or elder should be called for ill person
- Believe science should be used for relief of suffering

Roman Catholic
- Encourage anointing of sick, although older members of the church may see this as equivalent to "extreme unction," or "last rites"; may require careful explanation if reluctance is associated with fear of imminent death
- Traditional church teaching does not approve of contraceptives or abortion

Russian Orthodox
- Cross necklace is important and should be removed only when necessary and replaced as soon as possible
- Believe in divine healing but without excluding medical treatment

Unitarian Universalist
- Most believe in general goodness of fellow humans and appreciate expression of that goodness through visits from clergy and fellow parishioners during times of illness

Adapted from Leininger, M. & McFarland, M. (2002). *Transcultural nursing: Concepts, theories and practice* (3rd ed.). New York: McGraw-Hill; Purnell, L. (2012). *Transcultural health care: A culturally competent approach* (4th ed.). New York: FA Davis; Spector, R. (2012). *Cultural diversity in health and illness* (8th ed.). Upper Saddle River, NJ: Prentice-Hall.

establishing family altars. Any or all of these practices may be incorporated into the care of the patient. Such practices may be used both curatively and preventively.

Significant conflict with nurses may result when a patient refuses biomedical treatments because accepting treatment is viewed as a sign of disrespect for God or their source of power, and as challenging God's will. Although this belief is more common in certain groups, many nurses have engaged in magico-religious healing practices such as joining the patient in prayer. Other practices such as "laying on of hands," or Reiki, are also becoming more widely accepted.

Others view health as a sign of *balance*—of the right amount of exercise, food, sleep, evacuation, interpersonal relationships, or geophysical and metaphysical forces in the universe, for example, chi. Disturbances in balance are believed to result in disharmony and subsequent illness. Appropriate interventions, therefore, are methods that restore balance, for example, following a strict American Dietetic Association diet, following a diet in which the sodium intake does not upset the fluid balance, or balancing sleep with activity. Historical manifestations of philosophies of balance are the "yin and yang" of ancient China and the "hot and cold theory" common throughout the world.

The yin and yang theory is an ancient Chinese theory that has been used for the past 5000 years. It is common throughout Asia. Many Chinese and other Asian groups apply it in their lives along with practices of Western medicine. The theory posits that all organisms and things in the universe consist of yin or yang energy forces. The seat of the energy forces is within the autonomic nervous system. Health is a state of perfect balance between yin and yang. When a person is in balance, he or she experiences a feeling of inner and outer peace. Illness represents an imbalance of yin and yang. Balance may be restored by herbs, acupuncture, acupressure, or massage to specific points on the body called meridian points.

According to the *hot and cold theory*, illness may be classified as either "hot" or "cold." The treatments (including food) provided must be balanced with the illness to be effective. Hot foods and treatments are needed for "cold" illnesses, and cold foods and treatments are needed for "hot" illnesses. The culturally caring nurse would ask older adults whether they have a belief about the hotness or coldness of a condition and what accommodations are needed.

Another theoretical perspective on health, illness, and treatment is called the *biomedical* or *Western* perspective. The body is viewed as a functioning machine. A part may fall into disrepair and need adjustment or become susceptible to infection. Health is a state of optimal functioning as well as the absence of disease-causing microorganisms such as bacteria or viruses. When microorganisms enter the body, they overpower its natural resistance. Treatment is directed at repair or removal of the damaged part or administration of drugs to kill or retard the growth of the causative organism. The biomedical perspective is the one most prevalent in what are called "Western cultures."

In most cultures, older adults are likely to treat themselves informally for familiar or chronic conditions they have successfully treated in the past, based on one or several of the beliefs just described. When self-treatment fails, a person may consult with another known to be knowledgeable or experienced with the problem, for example, a community healer. Only when this fails do most people seek professional help within a formal health care system. This is especially true of older adults who were born in a non-Western country other than the one in which they reside. Older immigrants may be accustomed to brewing certain herbs, grasses, plants, and leaves to make herbal teas, drinks, solutions, poultices, decoctions, and medicines to prevent and treat illness. Many of the same drugs prescribed by physicians are prepared by older adult immigrants at less expense than buying the drug at the pharmacy. These products may be available in ethnic neighborhood grocery stores or botánicas. Others grow their own treatments in potted plants and backyard herb and vegetable gardens (Spector, 2017).

Transcending Cultural Concepts

As with health beliefs, various concepts may transcend cultures. These beliefs may have a significant influence in the method in which the patient seeks out and/or receives health care. As older adults acquire more and more chronic diseases, these concepts may become more important in the effort to provide the highest quality and culturally sensitive care.

Time Orientation

Time orientation refers to one's primary focus—toward the past, present, or future. The focus of a person who is future-oriented is consistent with the biomedical practices of Western medicine. Holders of a *future orientation* accept that what we do now affects our future health. This means that a problem noted today can "wait" until an office appointment with a health care provider tomorrow—that the problem will still be there and the delay will not necessarily affect the outcome. This also means that health screenings will help detect a problem today for potentially better health in the days, weeks, or years ahead. As the nurse caring for the patient, the concept of health prevention may be worth pursuing.

Quite different from individuals with a future perspective, *persons oriented to the present* perceive a new health problem requires immediate attention. The outcome is noted as occurring in the present, not the future. Preventive actions are not consistent with this approach. This may be a partial explanation of the use of emergency departments when same-day appointments are not available from one's own heath care provider. This difficulty with same-day access may partially explain the new industry known as "retail health clinics."

Persons *oriented to the past* perceive present health and health problems as the result of past actions, from a past life, earlier in this life, or from events and circumstances related to one's ancestors. Illness may also be viewed as a punishment for past deeds. For example, dishonoring ancestors by failing to perform certain rituals may result in illness. An older adult used to maintaining traditional customs may refuse preventive services while receiving care in a future-oriented system or may resist present orientations seen in nursing facilities.

Conflicts between the future-oriented, Westernized world of the nurse and persons with past or present orientations are not hard to imagine. Patients are likely to be labeled as noncompliant for failure to keep appointments or for failure to participate in preventive measures such as immunizations or even a turn and positioning schedule to avoid pressure ulcers.

The nurse should listen closely to the older adult to find out which orientation he or she values most, then figure out ways to work with it within their plan of care rather than to continue to expect the patient to conform. In this way, we reach beyond our ethnocentrism to improve the quality of the care we provide and improve patient-centered outcomes.

Individualist and Collectivist Orientations

From the individualist orientation of white "mainstream" Americans and Northern Europeans, autonomy and individual responsibility are paramount. Identity and self-esteem are bound to the self rather than to a group. Decisions on health care practices and treatment should be made autonomously. This cultural value was placed into law through the passing of the Patient Self-Determination Act (PSDA) of 1990 in the United States (American Bar Association, n.d.). The PSDA formalized the concept that the individual, without the help of family or friends, makes all decisions about his or her health care. The Health Insurance Portability and Accountability Act (HIPAA) further codified the role of the individual as the ultimate "owner" of health information (U.S. Department of Health & Human Services, 2017). Others may have access to this private information only with the express permission of the owner.

This approach is in sharp contrast to that held by most or all persons from non-Western cultures, including Native Americans and persons from Mediterranean Europe. Those from a collectivist perspective derive their identity from affiliation with and participation in a social group such as a family or clan. The needs of the group are more important than those of the individual, and decisions are made with consideration on the overall effect it may have on the group. Health care decisions may be made by a group such as tribal elders or by a group leader such as the oldest son. This means that neither the PSDA nor the HIPAA are appropriate. For example, in some Latino culture groups, it is inappropriate to inform an older adult of his or her diagnosis or prognosis. Instead, it is expected that this information be conveyed to the oldest male in the family, for example, the husband or the son. To do otherwise shows disrespect of the older adult and thus the family.

When a nurse who values individuality provides care for one who has a collectivist perspective, the potential for cultural conflict exists, as illustrated by the following scenario:

An older Filipino woman is seen in her home by a public health nurse and is found to have a blood pressure of 210/100 mm Hg and a blood glucose level of 380 milligrams per deciliter (mg/dL). The nurse insists on arranging immediate transportation to an acute care facility. The older Filipino woman insists that she must wait until her only child returns home from work to decide her disposition and treatment. She is concerned about the family's welfare and wants to ensure that income is not lost by her child leaving work early. The family also jointly decides if they can afford a heath care provider visit and a possible hospitalization because the patient does not have health insurance. The nurse's main concern is the health of the woman, and the woman's concern is her family. The nurse is operating from the value that dictates that an individual be independent and responsible for personal health care decisions.

Context

A final perspective is that of *context.* In the 1970s, E.T. Hall described the interactional patterns of high context (universalism) and low context (particularism). This theory has stood the test of time and is very useful when relating to another person cross-culturally; the theory refers to the characteristics of relationships and behaviors toward others (Liu, 2016). When a person from a high-context culture interacts with the nurse, a more personal relationship is expected. For example, the nurse is expected to ask about family members and should appear friendly and genuinely interested in the person first and concerned with what might be called *nursing tasks* second. Body language is more important than spoken words because it is there that the true meaning of the communication is considered to reside.

In stark contrast are those whose relationships and behaviors are of low context such as those from the culture of health care drawn from primarily English and German roots. Low-context health care encounters are task-oriented and only secondarily concerned about the relationship between the nurse and the older adult. Individual identity is not as important: Ms. Gomez is not the 82-year-old recent immigrant from Mexico, mother of seven, and grandmother of 30 but is the "fractured hip in 203." For the person from a low-context culture, small talk may be considered a waste of time; a direct approach is expected, with the literal message, "Just tell me what is wrong with me!" Negligible attention is given to nonverbal communication, and verbal communication is kept to only what is necessary.

Most cultures across the globe are high-context cultures. The culturally sensitive nurse is skilled enough to assess the patterns of those cared for and can move between contexts in the provision of caring.

SKILLS

The most important skills are those associated with sensitive intercultural communication. The linguistically competent gerontologic nurse will be able to appropriately use the conventions of the handshake, silence, and eye contact. He or she will also have developed fundamental skills related to working with interpreters.

Handshake

In the United States, the customary greeting in the business world consists of smiling, extending the hand, and grasping the other person's hand. The quality of the handshake is open to varied interpretation. A firm handshake in European American culture is considered a sign of good character and strength. A weak handshake may be viewed negatively. Traditional Native American older adults may interpret a vigorous handshake as a sign of aggression. They may offer a hand, but it is more of a passing of the hand with light touch, which could be misinterpreted as a sign of not being welcome or of weakness.

In some situations, any type of handshake may be inappropriate. For example, older Russian immigrants may interpret a handshake as insolent and frivolous. Physical contact, inclusive of handshakes, between members of the opposite sex is strongly discouraged with older adults from the Middle East and those from a traditional Muslim background (Walton, Akram, & Hossain, 2014).

The effective nurse is careful to follow correct etiquette with his or her patients, whenever possible. The best way to know the appropriate response is to follow the lead of the patient; waiting for the patient to extend a hand or asking permission for any physical contact are also good safe rules to follow.

Eye Contact

In the European American culture, direct eye contact is a sign of honesty and trustworthiness. Nursing students are taught to establish and maintain eye contact when interacting with patients. However, this was not the expected behavior for many older adults in their youth, when avoiding direct eye contact was interpreted as a sign of deference. This pattern continues to be the norm in other countries. Traditional Native American older adults may avoid eye contact with the nurse. They may move their eyes slowly from the floor to the ceiling and around the room. This behavior may lead the nurse to erroneous conclusions but may also cause the nurse to reflect the apparent appropriate behavior with this patient.

In many Asian cultures, looking one directly in the eyes implies equality. Older adults may avoid eye contact with physicians and nurses because health care professionals are viewed as authority figures. Direct eye contact is considered disrespectful in most Asian cultures.

Gender issues are also present in maintaining eye contact. In Middle Eastern Muslim cultures, direct eye contact between the sexes, like touch, may be forbidden except between husband and wife. It is interpreted as a sexual invitation. Nurses may want to avoid direct eye contact with patients and physicians of the opposite gender from a Middle Eastern culture if this is what is observed.

Interpreters

The gerontologic nurse can increase the linguistic competence of care through the appropriate use of interpreters. *Interpretation* is the processing of oral language in a manner that preserves the meaning and tone of the original language without adding or deleting anything. The interpreter's job is to work with two different linguistic codes in a way that will produce equivalent messages (United States Department of Labor, 2015). The interpreter informs the older person what the nurse has said and the nurse what the older person has said, without altering meaning or adding opinion.

An important distinction exists between the terms "interpreter" and "translator." An interpreter decodes the spoken word, whereas a translator decodes the written word. The translator must further decode meaning and therefore may use different words when translating a written document from what the interpreter uses. Although advancements have been made, downloaded translation applications are not recommended for translating full documents at this time.

An interpreter is needed any time the nurse and the patient speak different languages, when the patient has limited English proficiency, or when cultural tradition prevents the patient from speaking directly to the nurse. In 2016 an amendment was made to the Affordable Care Act (ACA) further providing provisions on medical interpreters. According to this amendment, a "qualified interpreter" is defined as an interpreter who "via a remote interpreting service or an on-site appearance":

1. Adheres to generally accepted interpreter ethics principles, including client confidentiality;
2. Has demonstrated proficiency in speaking and understanding both spoken English and at least one other spoken language; and
3. Is able to interpret effectively, accurately, and impartially, both receptively and expressly, to and from such language(s) and English, using any necessary specialized vocabulary and phraseology (Hunt, 2016, paras 6–7).

For issues of complex decision making, it is necessary to have an interpreter present, for example, determining an older person's wishes regarding consent, patient teaching, and decisions on life-prolonging measures.

It is ideal to engage persons trained in medical interpretation who are of the same sex and social status of the older person. The interpreter should be a mature individual so that potential problems of age differentials are avoided. When working with an interpreter, the nurse first introduces herself or himself and the interpreter to the patient, and sets down guidelines for the interview. Sentences should be short, employ the active voice, and avoid metaphors and other idioms because they may be impossible to translate from one language to another. Before the session, the nurse asks the interpreter to say exactly what is being said and directs all the conversation to the patient (Minnesota Department of Human Services Online, 2017).

CULTURAL COMPETENCE FRAMEWORKS

Many nursing frameworks are available to assist in providing culturally competent care. The website of the Transcultural Nursing Society (https://www.tcns.org/theoriesandmodels/) provides information regarding multiple theories and models related to cultural care.

Leininger

A popular theory that has stood the test of time is Leininger's Theory of Cultural Care Diversity and Universality. This unique theory has been recommended for use with the older adult population; it was designed primarily to assist nurses in discovering ways to provide culturally appropriate care to people who have different cultural perspectives than those of the professional nurse (Leininger & McFarland, 2002).

Leininger's theory uses worldview, social structure, language, ethnohistory, environmental context, folk systems, and professional systems as the framework for looking at the influences on cultural care and well-being. The components of cultural and social structure dimensions are technologic, religious, philosophic, kinship, social, political, legal, economic, and educational factors, as well as cultural values and ways of life.

Leininger theorizes three modes of action for the professional nurse to provide culturally congruent care: (1) cultural care preservation or maintenance, (2) cultural care accommodation or negotiation, and (3) cultural care repatterning or restructuring. Leininger defines the three modes of nurse decisions and actions as follows:

1. *Cultural care preservation* or *maintenance* refers to those assistive, supportive, facilitative, or enabling professional actions and decisions that help people of a particular culture to retain and to maintain their well-being, to recover from illness, or face handicaps or death.
2. *Cultural care accommodation* or *negotiation* refers to those assistive, supportive, facilitative, or enabling professional actions and decisions that help people of a designated culture adapt to or negotiate with others for a beneficial or satisfying health outcome.
3. *Cultural care repatterning* or *restructuring* refers to those assistive, supportive, facilitative, or enabling professional actions and decisions that help patients reorder, change, or greatly modify their ways of life for new, different, and beneficial health care patterns while respecting their cultural values and beliefs, and still providing beneficial or healthier ways of life than existed before the changes were established (Leininger, 1991).

This theory may be used with individuals, families, groups, communities, and institutions in diverse health care delivery systems. Leininger developed the Sunrise Model (Fig. 5.1) to depict the components of the theory and the interrelationship of its components (Leininger & McFarland, 2002). This model may be used as a visual and cognitive map to guide the nurse in teasing out essential data from all the dimensions of the influencers to gain clues for providing culturally sensitive care.

The Explanatory Model

Kleinman, Eisenberg, and Good (1978) presented an alternative far-reaching proposition. They suggested that to provide culturally sensitive and competent care, the gerontologic nurse should explore the meaning of the health problem from the patient's perspective. This was a radical approach at the time, but one that is becoming more relevant as global diversity continues to grow. See Box 5.6 for an explanation and assessment approach that the gerontologic nurse might use in coming to know the older adult from a culture different from that of the nurse.

The LEARN Model

The LEARN Model (Berlin & Folkes, 1992) uses the same approach as the Explanatory Model. This model is a useful tool to guide the nurse with older adult interactions of any ethnicity in the clinical setting. The premise of the tool is that the nurse will increase his or her cultural sensitivity, become instrumental in providing more culturally competent care, and consequently contribute to the reduction of health disparities. The model consists of the following steps:

L   Listen carefully to what the older person is saying. Attend not just to the words but to the nonverbal communication and the meaning behind the stories. Listen to the person's perception of the situation, desired goals, and ideas for treatment.

E   Explain your perception of the situation and the problem(s).

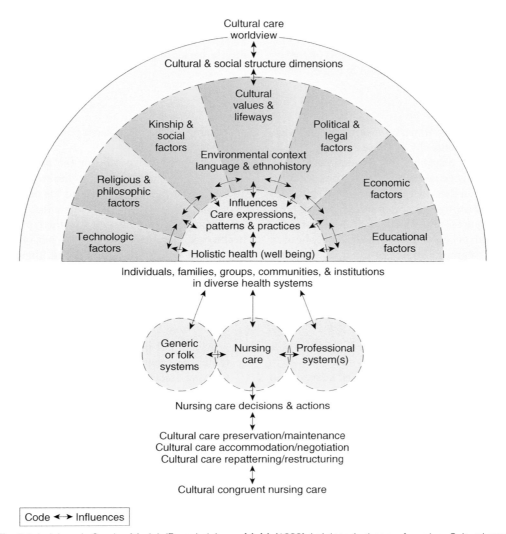

Cultural care worldview

Cultural & social structure dimensions

Cultural values & lifeways

Kinship & social factors

Political & legal factors

Environmental context language & ethnohistory

Religious & philosophic factors

Economic factors

Influences
Care expressions, patterns & practices

Technologic factors

Educational factors

Holistic health (well being)

Individuals, families, groups, communities, & institutions in diverse health systems

Generic or folk systems — Nursing care — Professional system(s)

Nursing care decisions & actions

Cultural care preservation/maintenance
Cultural care accommodation/negotiation
Cultural care repatterning/restructuring

Cultural congruent nursing care

Code ←→ Influences

Fig. 5.1 Leininger's Sunrise Model. (From Leininger, M. M. [1988]. Leininger's theory of nursing: Cultural care diversity and universality. *Nursing Science Quarterly, 1*[4], 152–160.)

BOX 5.6 Kleinman's Theory of Explanatory Models

Kleinman proposed that instead of simply asking patients, "Where does it hurt?" we need to focus on encouraging the patient to respond to questioning as "Why," "When," "How," and "What Next" (Kandula, 2013). To elicit data, begin with finding a common term for the problem or illness: "What do you call your illness or problem?" "What name does your illness(es) have?" (Kleinman's 8 Questions, n.d.) Then follow the cultural care questions as noted here to elicit information:

1. What do you think caused this problem?
2. Why do you think this problem started and when did it start?
3. What do you think this problem does inside your body? How does it work?
4. How severe is this problem? Will it have a short or long course?
5. What kind of treatment do you think you should receive?
6. What are the most important results you hope to receive from this treatment?
7. What are the chief problems this illness has caused?
8. What do you fear most about the illness/problem?

Kleinman's 8 Questions. (n.d.). Retrieved May 1, 2018 from http://www.nursingassets.umn.edu/effectiveinterculturalcommunications/content/modules/strategies/kleinman.html

---

A Acknowledge and discuss both the similarities and the differences between your perceptions and goals and those of the older person.

R Recommend a plan of action that takes both perspectives into account.

N Negotiate a plan that is mutually acceptable.

The ETHNIC Model

The mnemonic ETHNIC is another simple and useful tool to guide health care professionals to elicit culturally competent information from older adults (Levin, Like, & Gottlieb, 2000):

E Explanation (How do you explain your illness?)

T Treatment (What treatment have you tried?)

H Healers (Have you sought any advice from folk healers?)

N Negotiate (mutually acceptable options)

I Intervention (agree on)

C Collaboration (with patient, family, and healers)

Nursing skills required to work across cultures include the application of new knowledge. Leininger's Sunrise Model

(Leininger, 1991; Leininger & McFarland, 2002) provides a complex framework for a comprehensive assessment of the culture and the person. However, the Explanatory Model offered by Kleinman et al. (1978), LEARN Model (Berlin & Folkes, 1992), and ETHNIC Model (Levin, Like, & Gottlieb, 2000) may be more useful in the day-to-day interactions with persons from diverse backgrounds.

SUMMARY

Gerontologic nurses develop awareness, sensitivity, knowledge, and skills in the delivery of culturally sensitive and linguistically competent care to a steadily diversifying older adult population. Conducting a self-assessment enables nurses to become aware of their strengths and weaknesses in their knowledge and skills needed in cross-cultural caring and communication. The positive stereotypical information provided in this chapter, for example, common health beliefs or death practices, may be used as a starting point for communication. For example, the nurse might ask, "It is my understanding that remaining active in the church is important to many in the black community. Is this important to you? If so, how is your stroke affecting this aspect of your life?"

Culturally sensitive care for the patient or resident begins with an understanding of the health care practices, values, and beliefs of the older adult and his or her family. Members of distinct ethnic and racial groups across the globe are suffering from compromised outcomes in their pursuit and receipt of health care. Gerontologic nurses are in a unique position to take the lead in providing culturally and linguistically appropriate care. In doing so, they can contribute to the national agenda to reduce health disparities and improve patient outcomes.

KEY POINTS

- The current older adult population in the United States is becoming more culturally diverse.
- Culture is a universal phenomenon that is learned and transmitted from one generation to another, providing the blueprint for a person's beliefs, behaviors, attitudes, and values.
- Culture affects all dimensions of health and well-being, so the nurse must consider patients' cultures when planning, delivering, and evaluating nursing care.
- Ethnocentrism, discrimination, and racism contribute to health disparities.
- Providing culturally appropriate care requires awareness, new knowledge, and new skills.
- The nurse should be knowledgeable about the predominant health practices of the cultural groups for which care is provided, but he or she should still individualize the care rather than generalize about all patients in any given group.
- Cultural assessment tools and instruments need to be free from bias and previously tested on the ethnic group for whom they are intended.
- Nurses caring for older adults from diverse ethnic and cultural backgrounds should be aware that nurse–patient relationships may be based on different orientations to communication than the typical Western mode.
- Nurses should conduct a cultural self-assessment to determine how they are influenced by their own cultures and how their cultures affect their interactions with people of different cultures.
- Nursing interventions should be adapted to meet the cultural needs of older adult patients.

CRITICAL-THINKING EXERCISES

1. In what ways do you value diversity in the world around you? How do you incorporate this in your patient care?
2. What are the limitations of using only race or ethnicity in identifying older patients?
3. Interview two or more older patients from the same ethnic group and compare/contrast their cultural adaptation.
4. What knowledge must the nurse possess to avoid stereotyping or generalizing about older patients?
5. How would you respond to a colleague who just made a racist remark or joke?
6. How would you recognize cultural conflict? How would you respond to it?
7. What are the nurse's responsibilities when discussing the use of cultural preferences related to practice, medicine, and nutrition with older diverse patients?
8. Discuss ethical conflicts that may arise among older patients whose values and beliefs are different from your own.
9. What specific cultural nursing skills are needed in caring for older patients from another ethnic group?
10. In what ways can you expand on your cultural awareness?

REFERENCES

Agency for Healthcare Research and Quality [AHRQ]. (2015). *National Healthcare Quality and Disparities Report.* Retrieved from https://www.ahrq.gov/sites/default/files/wysiwyg/research/findings/nhqrdr/nhqdr14/2014nhqdr-intro.pdf.

Agency for Healthcare Research and Quality [AHRQ]. (2013). *Program brief: Minority health: Recent findings.* AHRQ Pub. No. 12(13)-P005-EF. Retrieved from https://www.ahrq.gov/sites/default/files/wysiwyg/research/findings/factsheets/minority/minorfind/minorfind.pdf.

Amann, C. A., & LeBlanc, R. (2013). Chapter 32: Caring across the continuum. In Mauk (Ed.), *Gerontological nursing: Competencies for care* (3rd ed.). Jones and Bartlett: Sudbury, Massachusetts.

American Bar Association (ABA). (2014). *Patient self-determination act.* Retrieved from www.americanbar.org/groups/public_education/resources/law_issues_for_consumers/patient_self_determination_act.html.

Berlin, E., & Folkes, W. (1992). A teaching framework for cross-cultural health care: Application in family practice. *The Western Journal of Medicine, 39,* 934.

Chatterjee, N. A., He, Y., & Keating, N. L. (2013). Racial differences in breast cancer stage at diagnosis in the mammography era. *American Journal of Public Health, 103*(1), 170–176.

Colby, S. L., & Ortman, J. M. (2015). *Projections of the size and composition of the U.S. population: 2014 to 2060: Population estimates and projections.* Retrieved from https://www.census.gov/content/dam/Census/library/publications/2015/demo/p25-1143.pdf.

Davis, J. L., Buchanan, K. L., & Green, L. (2013). Racial/ethnic differences in cancer prevention beliefs: Applying the health belief model framework. *American Journal of Health Promotion, 27*(6), 384–389.

Espinoza, R. (n.d.) Meeting the needs of elders of color and LGBT elders. Grant makers in aging 2017. Retrieved from https://www.giaging.org/issues/diverse-elders/.

Frey, W. H. (2014). *New projections point to a majority minority nation in 2044.* Retrieved from https://www.brookings.edu/blog/the-avenue/2014/12/12/new-projections-point-to-a-majority-minority-nation-in-2044/.

Gurman, T., & Moran, A. (2008). Predictors of appropriate use of interpreters: Identifying professional development training needs for labor and delivery clinical staff serving Spanish-speaking patient. *Journal of Health Care for the Poor and Underserved, 19*(4), 1303.

Hadziabdic, E., Heikkila, K., Albin, B., & Hjelm, K. (2011). Problems and consequences in the use of professional interpreters: Qualitative analysis of incidents from primary healthcare. *Nursing Inquiry, 18,* 253–261.

Hunt, D. (2016). *New 2016 ACA rules significantly affect the law of language access.* Retrieved from https://www.cmelearning.com/new-2016-aca-rules-significantly-affect-the-law-of-language-access/.

Kandula, N. (2013). *The Patient Explanatory Mode.* Retrieved from https://news.northwestern.edu/stories/2013/06/opinion-health-blog-kandula-/.

Kleinman, A., Eisenberg, L., & Good, B. (1978). Culture, illness and care: Clinical lessons from anthropological and cross-cultural research. *Annals of Internal Medicine, 88,* 251.

Kleinman's 8 Questions. (n.d.) University of Minnesota. Retrieved from http://www.nursingassets.umn.edu/effectiveintercultural communications/content/modules/strategies/kleinman.html.

Leininger, M. (1991). The theory of culture care diversity and universality. In M. Leininger (Ed.), *Culture care diversity and universality: A theory of nursing.* Sudbury, MA: National League for Nursing, Jones and Bartlett.

Leininger, M., & McFarland, M. (2002). *Transcultural nursing: Concepts, theories and practice* (3rd ed.). New York: McGraw-Hill.

Levin, S. J., Like, R. C., & Gottlieb, J. E. (2000). ETHNIC: a framework for culturally competent clinical practice. In: Appendix: Useful clinical interviewing mnemonics. *Patient Care, 34*(9), 188–189.

Liu, M. (2016). Verbal communication styles and culture. In *Oxford Research Encyclopedia of Communication.* Oxford, UK: Oxford University Press. https://doi.org/10.1093/acrefore/9780190228613.013.162.

Minnesota Department of Human Services Online. (2017). *Tips for working with interpreters.* Retrieved from http://www.dhs.state.mn.us/main/idcplg?IdcService=GET_DYNAMIC_CONVERSION&RevisionSelectionMethod=LatestReleased&dDocName=id_051607.

Misra, R., & Hunte, H. (2016). Perceived discrimination and health outcomes among Asian Indians in the United States. *BMC Health Services Research, 16,* 567. https://doi.org/10.1186/s12913-016-1821-8.

Neese, B. (2017). *A guide to culturally competent nursing care.* Retrieved from http://blog.div ersitynursing.com/blog/a-guide-to-culturally-competent-nursing-care.

Ortman, J., Velkoff, V., & Hogan, H. (2014). *An aging nation: The older population in the United States, Current Population Reports, P25-1140.* Washington, DC: U.S. Census Bureau. Retrieved from https://www.census.gov/prod/2014pubs/p25-1140.pdf.

Purnell, L. (2012). *Transcultural health care: A culturally competent approach* (4th ed.). New York: FA Davis.

Spector, R. (2017). *Cultural diversity in health and illness* (9th ed.). Upper Saddle River, NJ: Prentice-Hall.

Transcultural Nursing Society. (2017). Retrieved from http://www.tcns.org/Theories.html.

United States Census Bureau. (2017). *The nation's older population is still growing, census bureau reports.* Retrieved from https://www.census.gov/newsroom/press-releases/2017/cb17-100.html.

United States Department of Health & Human Services [DHHS]. (2017). Your health information, your rights. Retrieved from https://www.healthit.gov/sites/default/files/YourHealthInformationYourRights_Infographic-Web.pdf.

United States Department of Labor. (2015). *Interpreters and translators.* Retrieved from https://www.bls.gov/ooh/media-and-communication/interpreters-and-translators.htm.

Walton, L. M., Akram, F., RDMS, BS, & Hossain, F., BBA. (2014). Health beliefs of Muslim women and implications for health care providers: Exploratory study on the health beliefs of Muslim women. *Online Journal of Health Ethics, 10*(2). Retrieved from http://aquila.usm.edu/ojhe/vol10/iss2/5/.

6

Family Influences

Jennifer J. Yeager, PhD, RN, APRN

e http://evolve.elsevier.com/Meiner/gerontologic

LEARNING OBJECTIVES

On completion of this chapter, the reader will be able to:

1. Gain an understanding of the role of families in the lives of older adults.
2. Identify demographic and social trends that affect families of older adults.
3. Understand common dilemmas and decisions older adults and their families face.
4. Develop approaches that can be suggested to families faced with specific aging-related concerns.
5. Identify common stresses that family caregivers experience.
6. Identify interventions to support families.
7. Plan strategies for working more effectively one-on-one with families of older adult patients.

WHAT WOULD YOU DO?

What would you do if you were faced with the following situations?

- You have been married 45 years. Your husband recently had a severe stroke and cannot communicate. He managed the family finances and made all the family decisions. You do not know anything about your financial affairs. What would you do?
- Your parents, in their late 70s, are mentally competent, but their physical condition means they cannot manage alone in their home. They require all kinds of help and reject any other living situation or paying outsiders for services. What do you do?
- Your father is dying. You promised that no heroic measures would be taken to prolong his life; he did not want to die "with tubes hooked up to my body." Your brother demands the physician use all possible measures to keep your father alive. What do you do?
- Your father's reactions and eyesight are poor. You do not want your children with him when he is driving. He always takes the grandchildren to get ice cream and will be hurt if you say the children cannot ride with him. How do you approach this situation?

ROLE AND FUNCTION OF FAMILIES

Families play a significant role in the lives of most older persons. When family is not involved, it generally is because the older person has no living relatives nearby or there have been long-standing relationship problems; 85% of senior citizens will need in-home assistance at some point in their lives. About 78% of in-home care is provided by unpaid family members and friends, and about 79% of people who need long-term care remain at home (Society of Certified Senior Advisors [CSA], 2013). This means that most care for older adults is provided in the home environment. Community services generally are used only after

a family's resources have been depleted. However, several demographic and social trends have affected families' abilities to provide support. These trends include the following:

- **Increasing aging population.** Since 1900, the percentage of Americans 65+ has more than tripled (from 4.1% in 1900 to 19.9% in 2015), and the number has increased more than 15 times (from 3.1 million to 47.8 million). The older population itself is increasingly older. In 2015, the 65- to 74-year age group (27.6 million) was more than 12 times larger than in 1900; the 75- to 84-year group (13.9 million) was more than 17 times larger; and the 85+ group (6.3 million) was 51 times larger. About 3.5 million persons celebrated their 65th birthdays in 2015. Census estimates showed an annual net increase between 2014 and 2015 of 1.6 million in the number of persons 65 and over. Between 1980 and 2015, the centenarian population experienced a larger percentage increase than did the total population. Persons age 100 or older numbered 76,974 in 2015 (0.2% of the total 65+ population). This is more than double the 1980 figure of 32,194 (Administration of Aging [AOA], 2017).
- **Living arrangements.** In 2016, 59% of noninstitutionalized persons age 65 and older lived with their spouses or partner. About 29% lived alone. In 2015, approximately 1 million grandparents age 60 and over provided the basic needs for one or more grandchildren under age 18 living with them. Approximately 3.1% of the 65+ group lived in an institutional setting such as a nursing home or assisted living. This percentage increases with age (1% for 65–74 years to 9% for 85 and older) (AOA, 2017).
- **Disability and activity.** The AOA measures disability based on limitations in activities of daily living (ADLs) and instrumental activities of daily living (IADLs). ADLs include activities such as bathing, dressing, eating, and ambulation.

Previous author: Elizabeth C. Mueth, MLS, AHIP.

IADLs include preparing meals, shopping, managing money, using the telephone, housework, and taking medication. According to data collected in 2013, 30% of noninstitutionalized Medicare beneficiaries reported difficulty performing one or more ADLs, and 12% reported difficulty with one or more IADLs (AOA, 2017).

- **Decrease in birth rate.** Birth rates have hit an historic low; there were 1,818 births per 1000 women in 2016. Although there has been a decline in birth rates, and the U.S. birthrate is "below replacement level" (replacement level is 2,100 births per 1,000 women), the overall population has grown as a result of immigration (Bakalor, 2017; Kaplan, 2017). The U.S. birthrate has implications for family caregiving for aging parents.

- **Increase in employment of women.** Roughly 66% of family caregivers are women. In 2016, women comprised 56.8% of the workforce, with 42% having a college degree. Although great strides have been made in equal pay, in 2016 women working full-time only earned 82% of what men earned (compared with 62% in 1979) (Bureau of Labor Statistics [BLS], 2017). Approximately 15% of older adult women work full time (5.6% of the workforce) (AOA, 2017). Employment status throughout a woman's life has implications not only for family caregiving but for financial security in later years.

- **M**obility of families.** Families today may live not only in different cities from those of their older relatives but also in different states, regions, or countries. In fact, according to 2010 U.S. Census Bureau data (U.S. Census Bureau, 2012), 13% of the U.S. population has migrated since the last census. Geographic distance makes it more difficult to directly provide the ongoing assistance an older family member may need.

- **Increase in blended families.** Divorce rates for younger adults have been declining since the 1970s. There are 6.9 marriages per 1,000 population; 3.2 divorces per 1,000 population (Centers for Disease Control and Prevention [CDC], 2017). However, divorce among those 50 and over is increasing. In 2015, for every 1,000 married adults over 50, 10 marriages ended in divorce; this is double from 1990. Nearly half of these divorces occurred in second marriages or higher; more than a third occurred in couples married at least 30 years (Stepler, 2017). Divorce and remarriage may increase the complexity of family relationships and decision making and may affect helping patterns. Difficulties may arise from family conflicts, the different perspectives of birth children and stepchildren, and the logistics of caring for two persons who do not live together. However, in some situations, remarriage increases the pool of family members available to provide care.

- **Older adults providing and receiving support.** Many older adults receive financial help from adult children, but many give support (money, child care, shelter) to their adult children and grandchildren.

- **The state of the senior housing industry.** About 95% of Americans age 65 or older have incorporated elements for aging into their homes. The most common are main-level bathrooms and bedrooms. The aging-in-place model remains strong, as 90% of the 65+ age group plans to stay in their current homes if possible. Assisted living is becoming more popular, as adult children need more support in caring for their aging parents. Although 90% of institutionalized seniors still reside in nursing homes, the rapidly increasing number of alternatives has caused the number of nursing homes to decrease. The number of older adults living in continuing-care retirement communities (CCRCs) nearly doubled from 1997 to 2007, although occupancy rates have begun to decline with the decline in the housing market (CSA, 2013).

- **Caregiver workplace issues.** Caring for older adult family members is becoming the new normal for American families. Employers lose close to $25 billion annually from employees missing work to care for loved ones. Often, employers interpret this as a lack of commitment to career. Family responsibilities discrimination (FRD) is becoming a public policy issue. No law exists to protect caregivers as a group (Krooks, 2013). The Family Medical Leave Act (FMLA) allows eligible employees up to 12 weeks of unpaid leave to care for a parent, spouse, or child, but caregiving for an older adult parent may take up to 20 hours per week for as many as 5 years. Another limitation of the law is that family members with a different relationship (grandchild, niece, etc.) to the older adult are not protected by the law. Also, less than half of American employees are considered "eligible" under the law (Yang & Grimm, 2013).

For more on the family views of various cultures regarding older adults, see the Cultural Awareness box.

🌐 CULTURAL AWARENESS
Modern Attitudes Toward Older Adults

Despite widely held beliefs that Eastern and Latin American cultures hold their older adults in higher regard than the West, North and Fiske have found this does not necessarily hold true in the twenty-first century. Factors such as industrialism, economics, aging rate of the population, and decreasing birth rates have affected attitudes toward older adults; "attitudes toward older adults derive from modern cultural realities" (p. 1009).

Intergenerational care common in Latin America does not translate to positive views or dispelled stereotypes. In their meta-analysis, North and Fiske determined that, although Latin American cultures believed wisdom comes with age, older adults were also perceived as less attractive, having decreased ability to care for themselves, and not being able to learn new tasks. In Asian countries with high percentages of their population comprised of older adults, resentment, societal perceptions of burden, and conflict over resources have resulted in increased rates of abuse and abandonment. South Korea, Taiwan, and China have the highest rates of suicide among their older adult populations.

Nurses caring for older adults must keep this information in mind and not hold preconceived cultural assumptions regarding the value of older adults in any given group. Each older adult and their family situation must be assessed and interventions planned collaboratively based on individualized needs.

From North, M. S., & Fiske, S. T. (2015). Modern attitudes toward older adults in the aging world: A cross-cultural meta-analysis. *Psychological Bulletin, 141*(5), 993-1021. doi: 10.1037/a0039469

COMMON LATE-LIFE FAMILY ISSUES AND DECISIONS

When changes occur in an older person's functioning, family members are often involved in making decisions about the person's living situation, arranging for social services, health care, and caregiving. They also can facilitate, obstruct, or prohibit the older family member's access to care and services.

Some of the most common issues and difficult decisions families face include changes in living arrangements, nursing facility placement, financial and legal concerns, end-of-life health care decisions, vehicle driving issues, and family caregiving.

Changes in Living Arrangements

Many families face the question, "What should we do?" when an older family member begins to have problems living alone. Common scenarios heard from families include the following (Schmall, 1994):

- "Dad is so unsteady on his feet. He's already fallen twice this month. I'm scared he'll fall again and really injure himself the next time. He refuses help, and he won't move. I don't know what to do."
- "Mom had a stroke, and the doctor says she can't return home. It looks like she will have to live with us or go to a nursing facility. We have never gotten along, but she'll be very angry if we place her in a nursing facility."
- "Grandmother has become increasingly depressed and isolated in her home. She doesn't cook, and she hardly eats. She has outlived most of her friends. Wouldn't she be better off living in a group setting where meals, activities, and social contact are provided?"

Family members are often emotionally torn between allowing a person to be as independent as possible and creating a more secure environment. They may wonder whether they should force a change, particularly if they believe the person's choice is not in their best interest. The family may be focused on the advantages of a group living situation (e.g., good nutrition, socialization, and security). However, an older person may view a move as a loss of independence or as being "one step closer to the grave."

The nurse plays an important role in the following:

- Providing an objective assessment of an older person's functional ability
- Exploring ways to maintain an older relative in their home and the advantages and disadvantages of other living arrangement options
- Helping families understand the older person's perspective of the meaning of home and the significance of accepting help or moving to a new environment

It can be particularly frustrating when a family knows an older relative has difficulty functioning independently yet refuses to accept help in the home. However, as long as the older person has the mental capacity to make decisions, they cannot be forced to accept help. To deal successfully with resistance, a family first must understand the reasons underlying the resistance. Encourage family members to ask themselves these questions:

- Is my family member concerned about the effect of costs on their or my personal financial resources?
- Does my relative think they do not need any help?
- Does my family member view agency assistance as "welfare" or "charity"?
- Is my family member concerned about having a stranger in the house?

- Does my relative believe that the tasks I want to hire someone to do are ones that they can do or that "family should do," or do they feel that it would not be done to their standards?
- Does my family member view acceptance of outside help as a loss of control and independence?
- Are the requirements of community agencies—financial disclosure, application process, interviews—overwhelming to my family member?

Depending on the answers to these questions, it may be helpful to share one or more of the following suggestions with the family (Schmall, Cleland, & Sturdevant, 1999):

- **Deal with your relative's perceptions and feelings.** For example, if your older mother thinks she does not have any problems, be objective and specific in describing your observations. Indicate that you know it must be hard to experience change. If your father views government-supported services as "welfare," emphasize that he has paid for the service through taxes.
- **Approach your family member in a way that prevents him or her from feeling helpless.** Many people, regardless of age, find it difficult to ask for or accept help. Try to present the need for assistance in a positive way, emphasizing how it will enable the person to live more independently. Generally, emphasizing the ways in which a person is dependent only increases resistance.
- **Suggest only one change or service at a time.** If possible, begin with a small change. Most people need time to think about and accept changes. Introducing ideas slowly rather than pushing for immediate action increases the chances of acceptance.
- **Suggest a trial period.** Some people are more willing to try a service when they initially see it as a short-term arrangement rather than a long-term commitment. Some families have found that giving a service as a gift works.
- **Focus on your needs.** If an older person persists in asserting, "I'm okay. I don't need help," it may be helpful to focus on the family's needs rather than the older person's needs. For example, saying, "I would feel better if . . ." or "I care about you and I worry about . . ." or "Will you consider trying this for me so I will worry less?" sometimes makes it easier for a person to try a service.
- **Consider who has "listening leverage."** Sometimes an older person's willingness to listen to a concern, consider a service, or think about moving from their home is strongly influenced by who initiates the discussion. For example, an adult child may not be the best person to raise a particular issue with an older parent. An older person may "hear" the information better when it is shared by a certain family member, a close friend, or a doctor (Box 6.1) (Hartford Institute for Geriatric Nursing, 2014).

Deciding About a Care Facility

Until about 25 years ago, only two options were available to older adults who could no longer live alone: move in with their children or move into a long-term care facility. In the mid-1980s, a new option was born: assisted living. Many older people needed help with things such as housekeeping, meals, laundry, or transportation, but otherwise they were able to function on

BOX 6.1 Hartford Institute for Geriatric Nursing at New York University

Mission

"To ensure older adults achieve optimal health and quality of life."

Vision

"Older adults will experience a quality of life that reflects wellness and optimal function, characterized by engagement in their health care and health-related behaviors. Anyone involved in older adult care understands the unique needs of that population and has access to the resources they need to decrease the incidence and mitigate the impact of chronic disease and social determinants of health."

Values

- Interprofessional practice
- Care coordination
- Chronic disease management
- Quality care
- Better patient outcomes
- Population health
- Cost effective health care
- Person/family engagement

The resources link provides a connection to ConsultGeri.org:

- The General Assessment Try This:® Series
- Specialty Practice Series
- Dementia Series
- Quality Improvement Series

Additional programs and resources can be found here: https://consultgeri.org/

From Hartford Institute for Geriatric Nursing. (2014). Retrieved from https://hign.org/.

their own. Baby boomers latched onto this concept, and the industry has grown exponentially. Perhaps the fastest-growing care facility option is the continuing-care retirement community (CCRC), which often look a lot more like four-star resorts than long-term care facilities. Amenities may include restaurants, pools, fitness centers, and spas. The attraction of CCRCs is health care for life. This type of community typically allows residents to live independently as long as they can and gives them access to increased care, in the same location, when they need it. Today, more than 2000 CCRCs exist nationwide. The biggest drawback to CCRCs is the cost; although some facilities charge monthly fees, others require a lump sum buy-in, the cost ranging from $250,000 to $1 million (Wasik, 2016).

The decision to move an older family member into any type of care facility is difficult for most families. It is often a decision filled with guilt, sadness, anxiety, doubt, and anger—even when the older person makes the decision. The difficulty of the decision is reflected in these comments:

- "It was easier to bury my first husband than to place my second husband in a nursing home."
- "My parents have lived together in the same house for more than 50 years. Even though they know that they need more help and have agreed that they need to move where they can get more help, they are having a very difficult time coming to grips with the necessity to downsize into a retirement apartment."

Dealing with the family's feelings about placement is as important as stressing the need for long-term care. Many families view facilities negatively because of what they have seen in the media concerning neglect, abuse, and abandonment. Cultural considerations may also affect feelings about placement.

A common feeling that families express when faced with care facility placement is guilt. Guilt may come from several sources, including (1) pressures and comments from others ("I would never place my mother in a care facility," or "If you really loved me, you would take care of me"); (2) family tradition and values ("My family has always believed in taking care of its own—and that means you provide care to family members at home"); (3) the meaning of nursing facility placement ("I'm abandoning my husband," "I should be able to take care of my mother. She took care of me when I needed care," or "You do not put someone you love in a nursing facility"); and (4) promises ("I promised Mother I would always take care of Dad," or "When I married, I promised 'till death do us part'").

It may help to talk with family members about the potential benefits of a care facility. For many people, it is not easy walking into a care facility for the first time. It is helpful to prepare families about what to expect and to give guidelines for evaluating facilities, moving an older family member into a care facility, and helping an older family member adjust to the changes.

For more information, see Questions to Consider When Moving from Independent Living to a Supervised Living Facility (Boxes 6.2 and 6.3) and Internet Resources (Table 6.1).

Financial and Legal Concerns

Major financial issues some families face include paying for long-term care, helping an older person who has problems managing money, knowing about and accessing resources for the older family member whose income is not sufficient, and planning for and talking about potential incapacity.

One of the most important things a nurse can do is to become knowledgeable about the community resources that can help families faced with financial and legal concerns, eligibility requirements for programs, program access issues, and options

BOX 6.2 Should I Move My Parents Into My Home?

Take the time to consider the following 10 questions when deciding whether to have someone live with you:

- What kind of care will your parent need?
- How much assistance and supervision can you provide?
- How well do you get along?
- Is your home parent-friendly, and if not, can you make it so?
- Will your parent contribute financially?
- How do your spouse and children feel about the move-in?
- Will your parent be able to live by the rules of your house?
- Will you and your family be able to adjust to the lifestyle changes involved in having a parent in the house?
- Do you have the time to take this on?
- Will your parent have a social network available?

From Naman, M. (2018). *10 Factors To Consider Before Moving Elderly Parents In*. Retrieved from https://www.caring.com/articles/moving-in-aging-relative-or-parent.

BOX 6.3   Questions to Consider When Moving From Independent Living to a Supervised Living Facility

1. Is the move permanent or temporary?
2. Does the patient view the facility as a safety net or dumping ground?
3. Who is in control of the patient's finances?
4. What are the personal space needs of the patient?
5. Will these needs be met in the facility?
6. Does the patient understand the diagnosis and prognosis of the illness that is precipitating the placement?
7. What has the patient's living situation been (did the patient live alone or with others)?
8. Does the patient have long-term friends and associates in reasonable proximity to the facility to allow visiting?
9. Does the patient have a pet or pets whose care must be arranged, or does the facility allow pets?

From Baldwin, K. & Shaul, M. (2001). When your patient can no longer live independently: A guide to supporting the patient and family. *Journal of Gerontological Nursing, 27*(11), 10.

TABLE 6.1   Internet Resources for Caregivers

Organization	URL	Resources
Administration on Aging (AOA)	https://www.acl.gov/about-acl/administration-aging	Promotes the well-being of older individuals by providing services and programs designed to help them live independently in their homes and communities.
American Association of Retired Persons (AARP)	http://www.aarp.org	An excellent site with many topics and links of interest to older persons and their families.
American Health Care Association (AHCA)	http://www.ahcancal.org	Represents the long-term care community to the nation at large; serve as a force for change, providing information, education, and administrative tools that enhance quality at every level.
Centers for Medicare and Medicaid Services (CMS)	http://www.cms.gov	Clearing house for information related to Medicare, Medicaid and other recourses empower patients to work with their doctors and make health care decisions that are best for them
Aging Life Care Association	https://www.aginglifecare.org/	A holistic, client-centered approach to caring for older adults or others facing ongoing health challenges.
National Family Caregivers Association	http://www.caregiveraction.org	A nonprofit organization providing education, peer support, and resources to family caregivers across the country free of charge.

for older persons who need assistance in managing their finances. If a family and their older relative have not already discussed potential financial concerns, encourage them to do so.

Many families do not discuss finances before a crisis—and then it is often too late. Sometimes adult children hesitate to discuss financial concerns for fear of appearing overly interested in inheritance. This is the last subject that parents want to talk about with their children, but it is also the most important. Children should convey that they do not want to know how much their parents have—or might leave in their will; rather, they want to make sure that a current and complete plan exists. When a person has been diagnosed with Alzheimer's disease or a related disorder, it is critical that the family make financial and legal plans while the older person is able to participate. At this point it would be appropriate to execute a general durable power of attorney, which appoints someone to act as agent for legal, financial, and sometimes health matters when the person is no longer able to do so. Once the person becomes incapacitated, if plans have not been made, the options are fewer, more complex, and more intrusive. A family may need to seek a conservatorship, which requires court action (Levy, 2013).

Older persons with limited mobility, diminished vision, or loss of hand dexterity may need only minimum assistance with finances (e.g., help with reading fine print, balancing a checkbook, preparing checks for signature, or dealing with Medicare or other benefit programs). Others who are homebound because of poor health but who still are able to direct their finances may need someone to implement their directives. In such situations, a family's objective should be to assist, not to take away control. The goal is to choose the least intrusive intervention that will enable the older person to remain as independent as possible.

End-of-Life Health Care Decisions

The use of life-sustaining procedures is another difficult decision, especially when family members are uncertain about the older person's wishes or they disagree about "what Mom (or Dad) would want." The main interests of patients nearing the end of life are pain and symptom control, financial and health decision planning, funeral arrangements, being at peace with God, maintaining dignity and cleanliness, and saying goodbye (Auer, 2008).

It is important for the nurse to realize that life's final developmental stage ultimately ends in death. Thus end-of-life decisions are common for most patients and their families. Often, this process does not begin until after the patient has lost the ability to participate in the decision. Some patients and families may need repeated reminders to handle these decisions. Goal setting is a useful tool to help them along. In addition, caregivers could mention that they have completed some of the same planning for themselves (Auer, 2008) (Table 6.2).

A useful tool to help with end-of-life planning is "Five Wishes," an easy-to-use legal document written in everyday language. It is "America's most popular living will." "Five Wishes" meets the legal requirements for a living will in all but eight states. The wishes are (Aging with Dignity, 2013):

TABLE 6.2 Common End-of-Life Documents

Type of Document	Definition	Signature
Do-Not-Resuscitate (DNR) Order	Executed by a competent person indicating that if heartbeat and breathing cease, no attempts to restore them should be made.	Physician, Nurse Practitioner, or patient (state law dependent)
Out of Hospital DNR or Physician Orders for Life-Sustaining Treatment (POLST)	This gives the EMS providers permission not to perform CPR. Without an out-of-hospital DNR order or POLST, emergency crews must perform CPR.	Patient signature and signature of physician and two witnesses (state law dependent)
Health Care Proxy or Medical Power of Attorney	Designates a surrogate decision maker for health care matters that takes effect on one's incompetency. Decisions must be made following the person's relevant instructions or in his or her best interests.	Patient or witnesses (state law dependent)
Living Will	Directs that extraordinary measures not be used to artificially prolong life if recovery cannot reasonably be expected. These measures may be specified.	Patient or witnesses (state law dependent)
Advance Health Directive	Explains person's wishes about treatment in the case of incompetency or inability to communicate. Often used in conjunction with a Health Care Proxy or Power of Attorney.	Patient or witnesses (state law dependent)

1. The person I want to make health care decisions for me when I cannot
2. The kind of medical treatment I want or do not want
3. How comfortable I want to be
4. How I want people to treat me
5. What I want my loved ones to know

End-of-life caregiving by health care professionals differs greatly from that provided by family members. For health care professionals, usually, a wealth of experience is available to draw from and support from colleagues to share in the burdens. Families generally do not have the same life experiences to draw from in these situations. In a study by Phillips and Reed (2009), eight themes were identified to form the core characteristics of end-of-life caregiving:

1. **It is unpredictable.** Each crisis could be the last or just the next in a series of crises.
2. **It is intense.** It is constant and engulfing. A feeling of overwhelming responsibility exists and cannot be shared.
3. **It is complex.** Complex treatment regimens must be balanced with complex interpersonal relationships with the patient and other family members.
4. **It is frightening.** Situations such as falls, bleeding, behavior problems, or medication reactions frighten many caregivers.
5. **It is anguishing.** Watching the suffering of a beloved family member causes many caregivers severe angst.
6. **It is profoundly moving.** Many precious moments have spiritual or sacred overtones.
7. **It is affirming.** Bonding with the older patient is a moving experience.
8. **It involves dissolving familiar social boundaries.** Caregivers and older adults share intimacies such as toileting, changing diapers, or catheter care, which would otherwise not be shared.

The Issue of Driving

Driving is a critical issue for seniors—and for this country. Older drivers are more likely to get into multiple-vehicle accidents than younger drivers, including teenagers. Older adults are also more likely to get traffic citations for failing to yield, turning improperly, and running red lights and stop signs, which are indications of decreased driving ability. Car accidents are more dangerous for seniors than for younger people. A person 65 or older involved in a car accident is more likely to be seriously hurt, more likely to require hospitalization, and more likely to die than younger people involved in the same crash. In particular, fatal crash rates rise sharply after a driver has reached the age of 70 (Help Guides, 2013).

Safe driving is an important issue for our country's older adults. Everyone ages differently, so some people are perfectly capable of continuing to drive in their 70s, 80s, and beyond. Many older adults, however, are at higher risk for road accidents. A few of the factors that contribute to increased risk are as follows:

- Loss of hearing acuity
- Loss of visual acuity
- Limited mobility and increased reaction time
- Medications
- Dementia or mental impairment

Driving symbolizes autonomy, control, competence, self-reliance, freedom, and belonging to the mainstream of society, so older persons alter their driving when their abilities decline. They may drive only during daylight hours, avoid heavy traffic times, and limit the geographic area in which they drive or limit driving to less complicated roadways. Some couples begin driving in tandem, with the passenger acting as copilot. Sometimes, after the death of a spouse, family members notice that "for the first time, Dad is having problems with driving." What they may not realize is that Dad had problems with driving before his wife died, but she had served as his eyes and ears when he was behind the wheel.

Families face a difficult time when an older relative shows signs of unsafe driving. They may be both worried about safety and reluctant to raise concerns with their family member or to take action. The issue is even more complicated when the older person is cognitively impaired and does not perceive his or her deterioration and potential driving risk. Studies show that persons with Alzheimer's disease are likely to rate themselves as highly capable of driving when they are not.

Sometimes, a family member may rationalize that "Mom only drives short distances in the neighborhood" or may think, "I just can't ask Dad not to drive. The car is too important to him." Some families are continually faced with a cognitively impaired person who cannot remember from day to day that he or she cannot drive and insists on driving. The following tips are offered for talking to a loved one about driving (Help Guides, 2013):

1. Be respectful but do not back down if you have a legitimate concern.
2. Give specific examples. Instead of "You are not a safe driver," try "You have a harder time turning your head than you used to."
3. Find strength in numbers. If more than one person has noticed, it becomes more believable.
4. Help find alternatives. Offer rides or set up an account with a senior transit or taxi company.
5. Understand the difficulty of the transition. If it is safe to do so, try "weaning" the senior from driving. Start with only driving in daylight or only to familiar places. Perhaps set up transportation to specific appointments to get them used to the idea.

Families may need assistance in assessing a person's driving ability and how to best carry out a recommendation that their relative should limit or discontinue driving. Health care professionals play a critical role in discussing the issue of driving with older persons. Some older persons view health care professionals as being more objective than the family and thus are more willing to listen to their advice and recommendations. Many participants in focus groups indicated that family advice alone would not influence their decision to quit driving. A written prescription from a physician or other health care professional that simply states "no driving" may remind the cognitively impaired person and divert blame from the family. Families also may need information about how to make a car inoperable for the cognitively impaired person.

If family members will be addressing the issue of driving with an older relative, the nurse could suggest they first check some of the resources in Table 6.3.

Family Caregiving

Family caregiving is primarily provided by the adult children of the older person. Often, the varying levels of participation among siblings may cause stress within the family. It is important for the nurse to recognize the types and levels of family caregiving (Willyard, Miller, Shoemaker, & Addison, 2008):

TABLE 6.3   Online Resources for Older Adults Who Drive

Program	URL	Features
American Association of Retired Persons (AARP) Driver Safety	https://www.aarp.org/auto/driver-safety/	AARP Driver Safety courses designed for older drivers; helps them hone their skills and avoid accidents and traffic violations. Features information on classes and on senior driving in general, including FAQs, driving IQ test, and close call test.
Senior Driving from American Automobile Association (AAA)	http://seniordriving.aaa.com	Features videos, pictures, and text presentations to help seniors learn to drive more safely. Topics include exercising for driving safety, adjusting your car for driving safety, handling common and difficult driving situations, and handling emergencies.
National Highway Traffic Safety Administration: Older Drivers	https://www.nhtsa.gov/road-safety/older-drivers	Offers material to help older adults understand how aging can affect driving and what can be done to continue driving safely.
Clinician's Guide to Assessing and Counseling Older Drivers	https://geriatricscareonline.org/ProductAbstract/clinicians-guide-to-assessing-and-counseling-older-drivers-3rd-edition/B022	Guide includes checklists for vision and motor skills to assist the interprofessional team in evaluating the ability of older adults to operate a motor vehicle safely.
Centers for Disease Control and Prevention: Older Adult Drivers	https://www.cdc.gov/motorvehiclesafety/older_adult_drivers/index.html	Provides information and resources related to older adult driver safety.

Routine Care—regular assistance incorporated into the daily routine of the caregiver

Back-up Care—assistance with routine activities provided only at the request of the main caregiver

Circumscribed Care—participation provided on a regular basis within boundaries set by the caregiver (i.e., taking Mom to get her hair and nails done every Saturday)

Sporadic Care—irregular participation at the caregiver's convenience

Dissociation—potential caregiver does not participate at all in care

Providing care to frail, dependent older adults is becoming increasingly common because of the rapidly aging population. Although many caregivers are spouses, 52% of all parental caregiving is still provided by daughters or daughters-in-law (Wang, Yea-Ing, & Yang, 2010). In addition, the type of care provided for parents by women is different from that provided by men. Just as the age-old concepts of "women's work" and "men's work" imply, a division of labor exists in family caregiving. Women are most likely to handle the more time-consuming and stressful tasks such as housework, hygiene, medications, and meals. Men are more likely to handle matters such as home maintenance, yard work, transportation, and finances (Willyard et al., 2008).

Caregiving may evolve gradually as a family member becomes frail and needs more assistance, or it may begin suddenly as the result of a stroke or accident. A family may adjust better to the demands of caregiving when a relative's need for support gradually increases rather than when the person's functional ability declines rapidly.

A family member with a dementing illness such as Alzheimer's disease will require increasing levels of support and assistance as the disease progresses. The need may progress to where help is required 24 hours a day. Caregivers of patients with dementia often exhibit symptoms of tiredness and depression because of the high levels of stress (Clark & Diamond, 2010).

Losing the person that family members have always known is one of the most difficult aspects of coping with a progressive, dementing illness. As one woman said, "I've already watched the death of my husband. Now I'm watching the death of the disease." Another stated, "The personality that was my husband's is no longer present. I feel as though I am tending the shell of who he was—that is, his body. That is all that remains."

More and more families are faced with long-distance caregiving. They may find themselves driving or flying back and forth to repeated crises, spending long weekends "getting things in order," or "constantly checking on Mom and Dad." Such long-distance managing not only takes time and money but may also be emotionally and physically exhausting. Trying to connect with and coordinate services from a distance may be frustrating, especially if older persons cancel the arrangements made by their families.

Care managers, many of whom are nurses, may be particularly helpful to long-distance caregivers. A care manager can evaluate an older person's situation and needs, establish an interface with health care providers and arrange for needed services, monitor the older person's status and compliance with treatment plans, provide on-the-spot crisis management, and keep the family informed about progress and changes in the older person's condition and situation. Care management services are offered by local Area Agencies on Aging (AAAs), hospitals, and private agencies and practitioners. AAAs can connect families with publicly funded care management services.

Placing the family member in a long-term care facility may merely change the kind of stress felt by the caregiver rather than alleviate it. The caregiver may feel a sense of failure—even when placement is the best decision. Stress also may result from difficult visits, travel to and from the care facility, worry about the quality of the care, family conflicts regarding placement, and the cost of the care. Some family members continue to do tasks in care facilities that they performed when providing care at home (e.g., providing assistance with eating, walking, and personal care).

EVIDENCE-BASED PRACTICE

Aging in Place

Background

Increasing numbers of persons living with dementia has posed significant challenges for policy makers and services. The shift to aging-in-place has brought into focus the toll placed on unpaid carers, who are usually family members.

Sample or Setting

This was a case study of a 53-year-old woman caring for her 80-year-old mother with dementia. She has two adult children: a 27-year-old daughter who has a 1-year-old child, and her 22-year-old son who lives at home while attending university. She works full-time.

Methods

Qualitative analysis of in-depth interview.

Findings

The overarching theme, Negotiating the Interstices, was derived from the following subthemes:

Negotiating self – carer revises own story of who she is and what is important.

Negotiating others – new tasks taken on by carer, seeking information, completing paperwork, care-related discussion, and planning about care arrangements; and negotiation with formal care services, including respite when it is available.

Negotiating work – Supportive workplaces are important for the success of aging-in-place

Implications

It is important for nurses to advocate for improved policies that affect aging-in-place:

High quality, accessible and affordable care services

Flexible work time without penalty and compensation for caregiving

Money to access support services

These changes are necessary for aging-in-place to succeed long term and facilitate the positive intersection of individualization and care.

From Vreugdenhil, A. (2014). Ageing-in-place: Frontline experiences in intergenerational family carers of people with dementia. *Health Sociology Review, 23*(1), 43-52.

Challenges and Opportunities of Caregiving

Few families are prepared to cope with the physical, financial, and emotional costs of caregiving. Most children have not anticipated the possible need to provide care to their aging parents. Caregivers may become frustrated and exhausted because of unrealistic expectations or lack of knowledge and time. When caregiving is combined with other family responsibilities, the caregiver may feel that he or she does not have sufficient time in the day to complete all the tasks (Hendriksson & Arestedt, 2013).

The two types of patients in American nursing homes are as follows (Eskildsen & Price, 2009):

Long-term care—patients needing help for coping with ADLs, incontinence, and dementia. This care is not reimbursed by Medicare. These patients pay out of pocket for their stay until they become impoverished enough to qualify for Medicaid.

Subacute (or postacute) care—patients released from the hospital who are undergoing rehabilitation after stroke, joint replacement, or wound care. This care is reimbursed by Medicare; however, the number of days that will be covered is limited.

The cost of caregiving may place a burden on the finances of many families. It is generally less expensive to provide care at home. LongTermCare.gov estimates some average costs for long-term care in the United States for 2016:

- $225 per day or $6844 per month for a semiprivate room in a nursing home
- $253 per day or $7698 per month for a private room in a nursing home
- $119 per day or $3628 per month for care in an assisted living facility (one-bedroom unit)
- $20.50 per hour for a home health aide
- $20 per hour for homemaker services
- $68 per day for adult day care center

As part of their study of the Aging-In-Place model, Marek et al. (2010) determined that remaining at home with the use of a Nurse Care Coordinator, the costs to Medicare and Medicaid in Missouri were lower for those who remained at home.

If the caregiver is employed, work relationships may be compromised. The caregiver may be interrupted often at work or may need to miss work completely. Caregiving activities may be viewed as "lack of career commitment" (Krooks, 2013) (see Evidence-Based Practice box). Adult day care is one alternative available to the working caregiver; however, programs are limited in number, availability, and hours, and are often costly.

Chronic stress is another challenge to family caregivers. The family's normal routine may be disrupted. If the family providing care is from another locality, the time commitment of coordinating services and care providers may disrupt the family routine. Many families expect the daughter (either the oldest or the one living closest) to be the caregiver, regardless of her other commitments to her household or employer.

Many adult caregivers express frustration regarding the inequality of the contributions by their siblings. The siblings providing most of the care may resent those who are perceived to do less, whereas those who do less may feel guilt or frustration that their suggestions or offers of help are rejected.

Caregiving may also be regarded as a beneficial opportunity. Close-knit families may view the caregiving situation as demonstrating love and commitment. Frail older persons in this situation are reportedly less depressed and more satisfied with their care. Bonds between grandparents and grandchildren may be strengthened, along with other family relationships. Depending on the situation, the younger family may move in with their older relative and as a result may receive room and board, childcare, or financial assistance while they help out with the household chores.

Long-Distance Versus Nearby Family

Conflict may arise between family members who live near an older person and those who live at a distance because of their different perspectives (National Institute on Aging,

2013). To the family member who lives at a distance and sees the older person for only a few days at a time, the care needs may not seem as great as they do to the family member who has daily responsibility. In addition, the person may "perk up" in response to a visit by a rarely seen family member and may not display the symptoms and difficult behavior that he or she exhibited before the visit. Some older persons "dump" on one family member and show a cheerful side to another. Others take out feelings of frustration and loss on those providing day-to-day support and talk in glowing terms about sons and daughters who live at a distance.

Family members who are unable to visit regularly sometimes are shocked at the deterioration in their older relative. They may become upset because they have not been told "just how bad Mom or Dad is." However, they may have only two points of reference: the last time they saw their older relative (which may have been several months or a year earlier) and now. On the other hand, when changes have occurred gradually, family members who have regular contact with the person often are not aware of the degree of change because they have adjusted gradually.

Family conflict may occur because of these different experiences. The nurse often can help family members understand the reasons for different perceptions. It also may be helpful to remind distant family members not to let apparent differences in behavior between what they see and what the local caregiver has said discredit the caregiver. They also need to know that local caregivers often have to compromise with the older person and accept imperfect solutions to problems.

INTERVENTIONS TO SUPPORT FAMILY CAREGIVERS

Education

Many caregivers are unprepared for their new role, which may prove detrimental to both the caregiver and the patient. It is important that health care professionals ask the family what they *want* to know, as well as providing them with information they *need* to know (Box 6.4). The TRAC Study in the United Kingdom (Forster et al., 2011) evaluated a structured, competency-based training program for caregivers of patients who had suffered a stroke. The preliminary results of the study found that both physical and psychological outcomes for both caregivers and patients were improved. The program appears to be cost effective compared with additional health care costs incurred by those who did not participate in the program.

One advantage of education—whether provided one-on-one or in group settings—over other intervention strategies is its non-intrusive nature. Many people who would not attend a support group or seek counseling may attend a program labeled "education." An educational program also may be a springboard for a person to seek other intervention programs. As one woman said,

I avoided going to a support group because I didn't want to air my "dirty laundry." It was not until after I attended an educational program that I realized my concerns and fears were not abnormal. It was then I felt more comfortable talking to others and joining the support group.

BOX 6.4 Managing Stress

10 Symptoms of Caregiver Stress

Denial	*I know Mom is going to get better.*
Anger	*If he asks me that one more time, I'll scream.*
Social withdrawal	*I don't care about getting together with the neighbors any more.*
Anxiety	*What happens when he needs more care than I can provide?*
Depression	*I don't care anymore.*
Exhaustion	*I'm too tired for this.*
Sleeplessness	*What if she wanders out of the house or falls and hurts herself?*
Irritability	*Leave me alone!*
Lack of concentration	*I was so busy that I forgot we had an appointment.*
Health problems	*I can't remember the last time I felt good.*

10 Ways to Manage Stress

1. Understand what is happening as soon as possible
2. Know what community resources are available.
3. Become an educated caregiver.
4. Get help from family, friends, and community resources.
5. Take care of yourself (diet, exercise, plenty of sleep).
6. Manage your level of stress through relaxation techniques, or talk to your doctor.
7. Accept changes as they occur, and be prepared for changing needs.
8. Make legal and financial plans.
9. Give yourself credit, not guilt.
10. Visit your doctor regularly.

From Alzheimer's Association. (2013a). Take care of yourself. Retrieved from http://www.alz.org.

Most caregivers do not have the opportunity for extensive education or training before assuming their role. Often, education programs from rehabilitation services or brochures and booklets from other sources do not adequately prepare the caregiver for the many varied issues they will face at home (Elliott & Pezent, 2008). Although a caregiver's needs for information are diverse, they fall into six general categories (Schmall, 1994):

1. **Understanding the family member's medical condition.** Caregivers need information about the progression, signs, symptoms, and outcomes of medical conditions; common medical treatments; a condition's effect on an older adult's functional abilities; and implications for the caregiver and family. It is important to dispel any myths, misinformation, and unrealistic expectations. For example, when caregivers do not understand behavior caused by a dementia, they often view the person's behavior as intentional.

2. **Improving coping skills.** Coping skills may include stress management, social network-building skills, behavioral management skills, problem-solving skills, and the ability to perform specific tasks of caregiving—such as managing incontinence, feeding a person with swallowing difficulties, or meeting an older adult's emotional needs.

3. **Dealing with family issues.** Family issues often involve getting support from other family members, identifying how

much and what type of help family members can give, and dealing with conflicting feelings toward family members who do not help. Decisions about older adult care and caregiving generally affect not only caregivers and care receivers but also other family members. Anger and family dissension may occur when caregivers do not attend to the thoughts and feelings of family members.

4. **Communicating effectively with older persons.** Family members often need to know how to effectively communicate their concerns to older persons who are competent as well as how to communicate with those who are unable to understand or communicate. Communicating effectively with cognitively impaired persons often requires learning communication skills contrary to those learned over a lifetime; yet using appropriate techniques may reduce stress for everyone. The benefits of such information are reflected in the following adult son's comments:

The hardest thing about dealing with Alzheimer's disease is learning to relate in new ways and accepting my Dad as he is today. What a difference it made for me when I learned in the caregiver class to "step into my Dad's world," rather than keep asking him questions about things he simply could not remember. Our times together are now much more enjoyable for the both of us.

5. **Using community services.** Many caregivers need information about the range of community services, the types of help that are available, how to access services, and care facility options.

6. **Long-term planning.** This includes making legal and financial plans, and considering changes in the current caregiving situation, including possible nursing facility placement.

Two major goals of caregiver education should be to (1) empower caregivers and (2) increase caregiver confidence and competence (Elliott & Pezent, 2008). Feeling powerless may have a significant effect on a caregiver's physical and emotional health. Although the factors that affect feelings of powerlessness are complex and vary from person to person, it is helpful if health care professionals use approaches that do the following (Schmall, 1994):

- **Help caregivers set realistic goals and expectations.** Failing to achieve goals reinforces feelings of powerlessness. Achieving goals increases morale. A caregiver whose goal is to "make Mother happy" is less likely to experience "success" than a caregiver whose goal is to plan one enjoyable activity each week with her mother.
- **Provide caregivers with needed skills.** Being able to do the tasks that need to be done, get needed support, or access community resources enhances feelings of being in control.
- **Enhance caregivers' decision-making skills.** This includes sharing information about options and their potential consequences for older persons, caregivers, and other family members.
- **Help caregivers solve problems.** The ability to solve problems in managing care reduces feelings of powerlessness and stress.

One of the goals of education should be to provide caregivers with the confidence that they need to do a task or take an action. This means it is critical to give caregivers an opportunity to practice skills in a learning environment that is nonthreatening and psychologically safe. Skill building is enhanced when caregivers have the opportunity to practice skills in an educational setting and receive feedback, apply skills in the home environment, and then return to discuss how well the techniques worked, the problems that were encountered, and what they might do differently the next time in applying the skills.

It is important to discuss the barriers caregivers may confront in the real world and ways to overcome these barriers. For example, professionals often talk about the importance of caregivers setting limits, but they do not always prepare caregivers for the possible consequences of doing so. For instance, an older person's manipulative behavior may worsen for a time after a caregiver begins setting limits, particularly if in the past such behavior generally resulted in the older person getting what he or she wanted.

Family members also need to know that at times they may have to step back and wait until a crisis occurs before they can act (e.g., when a mentally intact older family member refuses to go to a physician or refuses to stop drinking despite attempts at intervention). In such situations, however, family members often feel they have failed. They may need help to recognize that "failures" are the result of a challenging situation and not their performance.

Sharing printed information (e.g., handouts the nurse has prepared, pamphlets, articles) and programs is another important way to provide education. Adults also learn independently. Workbooks can provide caregivers with a step-by-step guide for taking action.

Educational materials should be easy to read, with bullet points, definitions of difficult terms, illustrations, and enough white space to keep them from being intimidating. People will not read something that looks like it will be complicated or difficult to understand. Materials should be written in plain language designed to flow, and the materials should avoid medical jargon (Make written material, 2009).

Print materials provided to caregivers, when shared with other family members, may help create a common base of information and understanding (Schmall, 1994). Sometimes other family members "listen" more readily to information in a handout developed by a professional than to the same information shared verbally by caregivers. Printed materials are beneficial for another reason. It is difficult for people who are anxious or in crisis to hear and remember everything that is said. Written information gives them a reference for later use.

Another resource for families is the Internet. Many health and caregiving organizations offer a variety of helpful information through their websites. See Table 6.1 for more information. If families do not have access to the Internet, encourage them to ask the local library for help in locating appropriate websites.

Respite Programs

Respite programs are one of the few services designed specifically to benefit the caregiver. The programs allow caregivers planned time away from their caregiving role. Researchers agree that respite care could potentially improve the well-being of the caregiver as well as possibly delay the institutionalization of the older person in their care. The two basic premises to respite care are (1) shared responsibility for caregiving and (2) caregiver support (Alzheimer's Association, 2013b).

The nurse can help the caregiver understand that it is normal to need a break, and that seeking respite care will not label them as a failure. According to the Alzheimer's Association, respite services also benefit the patient. Caregivers need time to spend with family and friends, run errands, get a haircut, or see a doctor while still having the comfort of knowing that their loved one is well cared for. Benefits to the patient may include interactions with others in a similar situation; safe, supportive environment; and activities that will match their needs and abilities (Alzheimer's Association, 2013a).

Respite services may be provided in home or out of home and for a few hours, a day, overnight, a weekend, or longer. In-home respite care can include companion sitter programs or the temporary use of homemaker or home health services. Out-of-home respite services include adult day programs or short stays in adult foster care homes, long-term care facilities, or hospitals.

Respite services often are underused by caregivers. Barriers to access and use of services include the following (Schmall & Nay, 1993):

- **Lack of awareness.** Often, families are not aware of the availability of respite services or of program eligibility, or they are not familiar with the provider agency.
- **Apprehension.** With in-home respite services, caregivers may be apprehensive about leaving a family member with a "stranger" or nonprofessional.
- **Caregiver attitudes.** Some caregivers think, "I can care (or should be able to care) for my family member myself" or "No one can care for my family member like I can." Others feel guilty and selfish for leaving ill family members in the care of someone else so that they can meet their own needs.
- **Timing.** Caregivers often view respite services as "a last resort." They seek help much too late—when they are in crisis or a family member is severely debilitated and requires care beyond what a program can provide.
- **Finances.** The cost of respite care, or the anticipation of future expenses, is another reason some caregivers may be unwilling to use or delay using such programs. Others are unwilling to pay for a program they view as a "babysitting service."
- **Care receiver resistance.** Negative reactions by care receivers such as resentment toward someone coming into the house or a caregiver's leaving may keep caregivers from using respite programs.
- **Energy required to use the program.** The time and energy required to prepare and transport care receivers may limit use of adult day programs.
- **Program inflexibility and bureaucracy.** Program inflexibility may contribute to caregivers' low usage of respite care.

These are issues the nurse may need to address when working with a caregiver who hesitates or refuses to use a respite program. It is important to first identify the reasons a caregiver is reluctant to use a program and then work with the caregiver to reduce or eliminate the identified barriers.

In general, female caregivers appear to have more difficulty using respite and adult day programs. Because they have been socialized as nurturers and caregivers, women may buy into the view that "caregiving is women's work" and may believe caregiving is something they *should* do. As a result, they may be more reluctant to let go of the caregiver role and to accept outside help. Men, on the other hand, may feel less secure in the caregiver role and may perceive that they lack the necessary skills to take care of someone else. Thus they tend to be more willing to use services.

The nurse should help caregivers recognize that caregiving is a job. Just as employees benefit from regular breaks and vacations, caregivers benefit from a "break" in the job. The nurse should emphasize that the need for respite care begins with the onset of caregiving.

The message a nurse conveys about respite to caregivers may be important. Although respite programs are designed primarily to benefit the caregiver, some caregivers are reluctant to take advantage of services for themselves. Resistance to respite and day care programs may decrease if the nurse emphasizes how a program can benefit care receivers by keeping the caregiver fresh and relaxed.

It is generally assumed that respite is inherently beneficial to caregivers. However, different uses of respite time may lead to different outcomes (Lund et al., 2009). Caregivers who use respite time primarily for discretionary activities such as socializing, rest, and exercise experience more favorable outcomes than caregivers who spend the time primarily in obligatory activities such as doing housework, performing other domestic chores, or providing care to another person. As a nurse, it may be worthwhile to discuss with caregivers how they plan to use respite time and encourage caregivers to engage in discretionary activities that they enjoy.

Even when formal respite services are not available, the nurse plays a vital role in encouraging caregivers to take breaks in caregiving and helping them identify and overcome barriers to obtaining respite. Members of a caregiver's informal support system may be able to provide respite when formal services are unavailable or inaccessible. Some caregivers need help to reach out and ask for assistance, particularly if they view asking for help as a sign of weakness, helplessness, inadequacy, or failure. A written "prescription for respite" by a health care provider for certain hours of respite per week or month may provide the authority a caregiver needs to begin taking breaks from the demands of caregiving.

Support Groups

In many communities, caregiver support groups have developed. Some support groups are oriented to specific diseases such as cancer, Parkinson's disease, lung disease, stroke, or Alzheimer's disease and related dementia. Others are for family caregivers in general.

A support group may be a place where caregivers get advice, gain knowledge about their older relatives' medical conditions

and problems, share experiences and feelings, develop new coping strategies, and learn about community resources and care alternatives. A support group may help normalize a caregiver's experience. Discovering that they are not alone may provide much-needed emotional relief to some caregivers. For the isolated caregiver deprived of intimacy and support from the care receiver, a support group also may provide an acceptable outlet for socializing. Although many caregivers benefit from support groups, they are not for everyone.

Research on support group effectiveness has yielded several broad themes (Golden & Lund, 2009):

Balance—support group members learn to balance their own needs against those of their relatives

Sameness—caregivers realize that others face the same issues

Individuality—group members realize that, although some issues are the same, each person's circumstances may be unique

Family Meetings

Although one family member is generally responsible for caregiving, other family members are important in providing support. However, each family member may have a different idea about what the problem is or how to handle it. For example, one brother might not want a parent's resources—his potential inheritance—spent for in-home care; he may prefer that the family provide the needed care. Another brother may believe "Mom's money is there to spend on her" and prefer to purchase services. Beliefs about what is best often differ, creating family dissension. One person may be adamant that the older person should be kept at home at all costs; another may think a care facility is the best setting. Intense conflicts may result.

Unless differences are discussed and resolved, disagreements among family members usually magnify. A family meeting should be held as early as possible after the need for caregiving arises. Everyone who is concerned or who may be affected by decisions should be involved, including the older person (if possible) for whom plans are being made. Calling distant family members to get their input and keeping them informed may help them feel involved in the decision making. A family member should not be excluded because of distance, personality, family history, or limited resources. It is just as important to invite the difficult, argumentative family member or the one who seldom visits as it is to involve those who are supportive. Such involvement ensures greater success and support for any developed plans and may help prevent later undermining of decisions.

Sometimes, families find it helpful to hold a two-step meeting. The first meeting is held without the older person to discuss ideas and feelings, raise concerns, and identify needed information. The purpose is not to make the decision or to "gang up" on the older person. A second meeting is then held in which the older person is actively involved in identifying and evaluating options and making decisions.

A family meeting is not always easy. It is most difficult for family members who have never discussed emotion-laden concerns, who hold differing values and outlooks in regard to the situation, or who have a history of poor relationships and conflict. A family in conflict may become angry and get sidetracked from current issues and the decisions that need to be made. Old resentments and conflicts that have been dormant since childhood can reemerge with regard to relationships, family roles, expectations, the authority to make decisions, and even inheritance. A family meeting often is even more important in these situations.

If family conflicts or hidden resentments prevent rational discussion, it often helps to have a health care professional skilled in working with older adults and their families facilitate the family meeting. The professional, whether a nurse, social worker, member of the clergy, or counselor, should be well versed in aging-related issues and family dynamics and have group facilitation skills. The mere presence of an "outsider" often keeps the atmosphere calm and the discussion focused and objective. An objective third party also can help move the family past emotions to common interests and can handle many difficult situations. Some practitioners and agencies offer family consultation services that include facilitation of family meetings.

A family meeting is more likely to be successful if the following are considered (Schmall & Stiehl, 1998):

- Hold the family meeting in a neutral setting. However, a family meeting in the older person's home may help give him or her a greater sense of control, especially if the person is feeling a loss of control over his or her life.
- Create a feeling of support and confidentiality.
- Acknowledge that everyone has a different relationship with each other and that current life circumstances vary. These factors need to be respected and considered as decisions are discussed and made.
- Have each family member address the problem from his or her perspective. This increases commitment to the process and contributes to defining "the problem" and reaching agreement on and possible solutions.
- Give everyone the opportunity to express feelings, voice preferences, and offer suggestions without being criticized.
- Keep the family meeting focused on current concerns rather than on other issues, past conflicts, personalities, or resentments.
- Focus on the positive things family members do, or are willing and able to do, and encourage everyone to be honest about their limitations. Sharing information about other responsibilities may help others understand the reasons support might be limited.
- Prepare a written plan about decisions made, what each person will do, and when he or she will do it. A written plan may prevent later disagreements.

WORKING WITH FAMILIES OF OLDER ADULTS: CONSIDERATIONS AND STRATEGIES

Identifying Who the Patient Is and Who the Family Is

Critical questions to ask when working with older adults include the following: Who is the patient? Is it just the older person? Should the older person's family also be considered the "patient"?

Although the older person is generally identified as the patient, it is also appropriate to consider the family as the patient. Family members are often intimately involved in the decisions to be made, affected by potential decisions, or actively involved in caregiving for the older person. If only the needs of the older person are considered and not the needs and situation of the family, the care plan may have less chance for success, particularly if family members will be responsible for carrying it out.

Another significant question to ask is, "Who is family, as defined by the older person?" Many older persons are connected to others by love and friendship, and function as a family to each other. These relationships often extend into caregiving. The following are examples of such "families" (Schmall, 1994):

- Red, who divorced in his early 70s, never had children. His only blood relatives were his nieces, nephews, and older adult sisters, all of whom lived hundreds of miles away. During the past 12 years of his life, nearly all support was provided by a person Red referred to as "my adopted granddaughter." When medical crises occurred and care arrangements were needed, Red looked to his "granddaughter" to make the necessary arrangements.
- Florence's son divorced his first wife, Jane, and remarried. The divorce, however, did not end the relationship between Florence and Jane. Florence continued to view Jane as "the daughter I never had," not as her "ex-daughter-in-law." When Florence became frail, she did not turn to her sons or the current daughters-in-law for help; she turned to Jane for both day-to-day assistance and emotional support.
- Elizabeth and Mary had lived together as a couple for 30 years when Elizabeth was diagnosed with cancer. Although Elizabeth's "blood relatives" were supportive during the downhill course of the disease, Mary was the primary caregiver, the person Elizabeth consulted when she faced medical decisions, and the one who made decisions when Elizabeth was no longer able to do so.

In created but not legally recognized families, it may be important to help individuals take steps—such as completing an advance medical directive (AMD), power of attorney for health care, or durable power of attorney for financial decisions—to ensure that the relationships continue into caregiving, especially if one person loses the capacity to make decisions. As Mary stated, "Elizabeth's giving me power of attorney for health care ensured that our relationship could continue as it had been for 30 years. We knew another couple who were in a similar situation, and the [blood] relatives stepped in and took over control, disregarding the relationship Jim and Bill had for 20 years."

In the health care setting, it may be important to reevaluate the definition of family. If "blood relatives only allowed in intensive care" and other rules are followed, some older persons may be deprived of their most significant sources of support.

Other important questions for the nurse to ask are, "Who is the decision maker?" and "Who owns the care plan?" The nurse's primary role is to empower older persons and their families. This means giving the information, guidelines, options, and skills that will enable them to make the best decisions possible and to better manage a medical condition or their situation. However, it is easy to become frustrated and angry—and eventually experience burnout—if older persons or families choose a course of action that the nurse feels is not the best. Remember, nurses have not failed when an older person or family selects an option different from the nurse's recommendation. Depending on the situation, the primary responsibility for implementation lies with the older person or the family.

Assessing the Family

When an older person's life situation or physical or mental status changes, no easy answers exist. What may be the best answer for one older person and his or her family may be inappropriate for another family whose situation seems the same.

Each older person and family system is different. It may be just as important to understand the family's history, current life circumstances, and needs as it is to know about an older person's needs and level of functioning. A family's willingness to provide care, for example, says nothing about their actual ability to do so. Sometimes, the care an older person needs exceeds that which an individual or family can provide, and the caregiver becomes the "hidden patient." As one adult daughter stated, "My father was the person with Alzheimer's disease, but his illness also killed my mother." Failing to evaluate the ability of family members to provide caregiving is a disservice to older patients.

Information from a family assessment may result in more effective older adult care planning and decision making. Another benefit of assessing how well a caregiver is doing is that it validates a person's caregiving efforts and sends a message that the nurse is concerned about the caregiver's well-being as well as the older adult's health.

Depending on the family, the older adult, and the decisions to be made, the following may be among the important factors to consider in conducting a family assessment.

Past Relationships

Lifetime relationships may influence the family's ability to plan, to make decisions together, and to provide support. Remember, every adult child has a different history with an aging parent, even if they shared the same family events. Families with a history of alcoholism, poor relationships, or abusive behavior cannot always be expected to provide the assistance an older person needs.

Consider the degree of emotional intensity—the closeness, affection, and openness—in the relationships among family members. Parental or spousal disability sometimes threatens a person's identity or the level of emotional relationship that has been established. For example, some married couples, parents, and children have been emotionally distant for many years. Some spouses have shared the same household but have lived separate lives. Some adult children have maintained emotional distance from a parent by living and working at a geographic distance. People in these situations may be reluctant to enter the care system or may have more difficulty with caregiving. It may be unrealistic to expect such family members to meet the emotional needs of the older person; they

may feel more comfortable with meeting a person's instrumental needs, that is, doing tasks.

Family Dynamics

Family dynamics are the ways family members interact with one another, including their communication patterns, family alliances, and symbiotic relationships. What are family members' views about how decisions should be made? How do they view the older adult's role in decisions about his or her life? To what degree are family members paternalistic, that is, to what degree do they expect the older person to submit to their decisions or a health care professional's recommendation?

Roles

It is useful to know whether individual family members have distinctive roles. If so, what role or roles does each person have? What expectations are held by the person fulfilling the role and by other family members? Do any of the roles generate conflict for the people who bear them? For example, family members may have always assumed that if a parent needed care, a particular daughter would provide the care because she is the oldest, lives the closest, is a nurse, or has always taken care of everyone who needed help. The daughter also may have viewed caregiving as her role. However, this "assigned" role may or may not be realistic given the daughter's current life situation or the parent's needs. Sometimes, an older person or a family member may not make a decision until the "decision maker" in the family is consulted. The importance of considering who plays which roles is exemplified by this daughter's comments:

I lived in the same town as my Dad, so when he needed help, I was the one who provided it daily. Dad expected me to help because I was his daughter. But when it came to making decisions, my opinions never counted with him. His son's opinions, however, mattered, and he would listen to them. I think his basic view throughout his life was "women are there to serve men" and "men are, by far, more knowledgeable than women." It didn't matter that I had a college education, and my brother didn't.

Knowing who does what for the older person makes for more effective planning. Old family roles may also come to the foreground when brothers and sisters are brought together to address the care needs of a parent. One daughter stated:

I lived in the same community as my parents, so when they became ill, I did everything that needed to be done and arranged for support services. Both of my sisters lived hundreds of miles away. Although I am a competent businesswoman, it seemed that when both of my sisters, who are older, came home, I immediately became the "baby of the family" again.

The roles of family members vary. Examples of potential roles include the "prime mover," the person who gets things done in the family; the "scapegoat," the person who becomes the focus of attention when problems arise; the "decision maker," a role that may vary depending on whether the decision to be made regards finances, living arrangements, or health care; the "peacemaker," the person who always tries to create peace when family dissension arises; the "pot-stirrer," the person who seems to keep things "stirred up" in the family; the "black sheep"; the "burden bearer"; the "favorite child"; the "model child"; and the "escapee," the person who disappears when there are tough decisions to be made or work to be done.

It may be helpful to identify how family roles, especially those of the older person, are affected because of the older adult's increased frailty. What are the perceptions of family members regarding the role of the older person? Do any adult children perceive that their role is now to "parent their parent"?

Sometimes people talk about "role reversal." Although a family member may take on "parent-like" responsibilities, in the emotional sense a parent is still a parent and a spouse is still a spouse, no matter how dependent a person has become. Decades of adult experiences cannot be repressed. If family members think of an older family member as a child, they are more likely to treat that person as they would treat a child and, in return, get childish behavior.

Consider the older adult's view of his or her role with respect to the rest of the family. For example, does the older person believe he or she is still a contributing family member, or does he or she feel a loss of role? Does the person think he or she is entitled to care from family members, for example, "just because I am your parent?" Paulette tells her story:

> I could see Dad deteriorating. When Dad could no longer live alone at home, he refused to consider anyone but "his daughter helping him." When the time came that Dad had to move from his home, he said to me adamantly, "Your mother took care of her mother and my father until they died," implying that I also should do the same with him. To Dad, "taking care of" meant he would live in our home. He felt that this is "what daughters are supposed to do."

Loyalties and Obligations

This refers to interpersonal allegiances. Family members often struggle with two questions: (1) What should be my primary priority: Meeting the needs of my aging family member? My spouse and children? My career?; and (2) How much do I owe to whom? Caregivers who have not been able to deal with these questions may find themselves stressed by trying to do too much. They may feel guilty because they feel they are not doing enough.

Sometimes, family members, in looking at older adult care issues, also weigh how much various family members "owe" to the person who needs assistance. Is any particular family member viewed as being more obligated or more indebted to providing care because of how much the older person has given him or her in the past? In other words, which family members are viewed as "creditors" and which as "debtors," and to whom do they owe? For example:

> Ann did not feel obligated to provide hands-on care to her mother. She thought, "Mother never did anything to help me. All I got from her was criticism—about everything!" On the other hand, Louise (Ann's younger sister) said,

> "Mother has always been there for me. I don't know what I would have done after my divorce if Mom hadn't opened her doors to me and my three children for those 2 years." Ann also believed Louise "owed" their mother more than she did.

It is important to be aware that levels of stress tend to be higher for the person who provides caregiving only out of a sense of obligation.

Dependence and Independence

Some families accept and adjust more easily than other families to the increased dependence of a family member. Answers to the following questions can help determine how well family members are dealing with or will deal with increased frailty in an older family member:

- What are the attitudes and expectations of family members, including the older person, about dependency?
- Has the family experienced a shift in who is dependent? If so, what is the response of individual family members to this shift?
- Are any family members threatened by the increased dependence of the older person?
- Is the older person giving family members mixed messages about how independent or dependent he or she is?
- Do family members perceive the dependency needs of the person realistically? Is anyone denying, minimizing, or exaggerating the dependence? Is anyone overprotecting or forcing dependency?

Providing caregiving to a family member may be more difficult if the caregiver has been the dependent person in the relationship. The care receiver also may resent the caregiver exercising more control.

Caregiver Stress

It is critical to assess the nature and extent of caregiver stress. The Modified Caregiver Strain Index (MCSI) is a 13-item tool that can be used to quickly screen for caregiver strain (Fig. 6.1). In addition to identifying actual stressors—which may or may not be a direct result of caregiving—the nurse must assess their significance to the caregiver. Other useful areas to assess are a caregiver's style of coping; the caregiver's support system; the caregiver's evaluation of the adequacy of his or her support system; the care needs of the older person, including behavioral and emotional problems, and the caregiver's perception of those care needs; and financial resources.

Just as an older adult's situation can change and require reassessment, so can a family's situation and a caregiver's ability to provide care. The following factors should be considered:

- Change in the older adult's condition
- Change in family structure (marriage, divorce, birth, death)
- Change in employment status of the caregiver

Encouraging Families to Plan in Advance of Need

Families tend not to discuss age-related issues until faced with a crisis (Hebert et al., 2009). As a result, many adult children are often unaware of parental preferences, views about care arrangements, or the existence and location of important documents.

Modified Caregiver Strain Index

Directions: Here is a list of things that other caregivers have found to be difficult. Please put a checkmark in the columns that apply to you. We have included some examples that are common caregiver experiences to help you think about each item. Your situation may be slightly different, but the item could still apply.

	Yes, On a Regular Basis = 2	Yes, Sometimes = 1	No = 0
My sleep is disturbed (For example: the person I care for is in and out of bed or wanders around at night)	_____	_____	_____
Caregiving is inconvenient (For example: helping takes so much time or it's a long drive over to help)	_____	_____	_____
Caregiving is a physical strain (For example: lifting in or out of a chair; effort or concentration is required)	_____	_____	_____
Caregiving is confining (For example: helping restricts free time or I cannot go visiting)	_____	_____	_____
There have been family adjustments (For example: helping has disrupted my routine; there is no privacy)	_____	_____	_____
There have been changes in personal plans (For example: I had to turn down a job; I could not go on vacation)	_____	_____	_____
There have been other demands on my time (For example: other family members need me)	_____	_____	_____
There have been emotional adjustments (For example: severe arguments about caregiving)	_____	_____	_____
Some behavior is upsetting (For example: incontinence; the person cared for has trouble remembering things; or the person I care for accuses people of taking things)	_____	_____	_____
It is upsetting to find the person I care for has changed so much from his/her former self (For example: he/she is a different person than he/she used to be)	_____	_____	_____
There have been work adjustments (For example: I have to take time off for caregiving duties)	_____	_____	_____
Caregiving is a financial strain	_____	_____	_____
I feel completely overwhelmed (For example: I worry about the person I care for; I have concerns about how I will manage)	_____	_____	_____

[Sum responses for "Yes, on a regular basis" (2 pts each) and "yes, sometimes" (1 pt each)]

Total Score =

Fig. 6.1 Modified Caregiver Strain Index. (From Thornton, M., & Travis, S. S. [2003]. Analysis of the reliability of the Modified Caregiver Strain Index. *The Journal of Gerontology, Series B, Psychological Sciences and Social Sciences, 58*[2], S129. Copyright © The Gerontological Society of America. Reproduced by permission of the publisher.)

Planning requires anticipating negative situations—dependency, disability, incapacity, and death—and exploring actions to be taken. Discussing such subjects may be uncomfortable for all family members. For some people, talking about potential incapacity and inability to manage finances is more difficult than talking about death.

A critical time for discussion is when a family member shows signs of deterioration or has been diagnosed with a degenerative disease such as Alzheimer's disease. Waiting for a situation to worsen reduces the options. Although planning does not prevent all problems, it does prepare families to act more effectively if a crisis occurs. Planning may also do the following:

- Help avoid crisis decision making and make decisions easier in difficult times
- Reduce emotional and financial upheaval later
- Ensure that the older person's lifestyle, personal philosophies, and choices are known should a time come when the person is unable to participate in making decisions
- Decrease the possibility that the family will have to take more intrusive, restrictive actions such as petitioning the court for guardianship or conservatorship if their older family member becomes incapacitated
- Reduce disagreements and misunderstandings among family members

Families may find the following suggestions helpful in opening up discussion with a reluctant older family member (Schmall et al., 1999).

Looking for Natural Opportunities to Talk

A natural opportunity might be a life event such as when a friend or another family member experiences a health crisis, is diagnosed with Alzheimer's disease, or moves into a care facility; a situation reported in the media, for example, a person dying without a will; or when the older person is recovering from an illness. If a parent says, "When I die . . .," family members should listen and encourage the expression of feelings. Too often, families discourage discussion by saying things like, "Don't be so morbid," "You'll probably outlive all of us," or "We have lots of time to talk about such things."

Talking About "What Ifs"

A family member might say, "If a time came when you could no longer make decisions about your own health care, who would you want to make decisions for you?" or "If you could no longer care for yourself at home, even with the help of community services, what would you want to happen?"

Sharing Personal Preferences and Plans in the Event of One's Own Illness or Death

It is important for adult children to remember that incapacity is not always a function of getting older. Some parents are more open to discussion when their adult children also have planned for future possibilities, for example, prepared a will, an AMD, or a durable power of attorney.

Expressing Good Intentions and a Willingness to Listen

The objective is to set the right tone for discussion. A loving, caring approach moves a discussion farther than an "I know what's best for you" attitude. A paternalistic approach is likely to create resistance.

An appropriate role for the nurse is to educate older patients about the benefits of planning and the importance of making plans while their capacities are intact. A positive approach is to emphasize that making plans gives people greater control and provides greater assurance that their preferences will be known and honored.

Helping Family Members Communicate Their Concerns Honestly and Positively

Open, honest communication helps build and maintain relationships, but such communication is not easy if family communication has been about "game playing." Adult sons or daughters may say only what they think a parent wants to hear or what they think will not upset a parent. However, this tends to create mistrust and wastes energy as family members "walk on eggshells" around each other.

Family members often express concerns using "you" messages, that is, telling the person what to do or not to do. An example of such a message is, "Mother, you are no longer safe living in your home. It's time for you to move into a retirement facility." The worst "you" message is a threat: "If you don't … then I will …" "You" messages sound dictatorial, create defensiveness and resistance, and close off communication.

An older person is more likely to listen to family members who express their concern about an issue rather than family members who talk as if it is the older person who has the problem. The nurse can suggest they use "I" messages. With a good "I" message, a person states his or her feeling, describes the specific behavior or situation of concern, and gives a concrete reason for the concern. "I" messages are specific rather than general and focus attention on problems, not personalities. An example of an "I" message is, "Mom, because of your recent fall, I'm concerned about your safety living in this house. I'm afraid you might fall again, and the next time, you might not be found for several hours or longer. Can we talk about my concern?"

The words "I am concerned about . . ." sound quite different to a person from "You should . . . ." When done correctly, "I" messages come across as "speaking from the heart." "I" messages also communicate that the person bringing up the issue or concern recognizes that what is being said is his or her belief; this leaves room for other perceptions. It also is more difficult for another person to argue with an "I" message because the speaker merely shared his or her feelings.

Adequately expressing one's concerns to an older family member is only one part of effective communication. Family members also may need help to listen actively and to empathize, that is, to understand the feelings and emotional needs of the older person. Sometimes, when family members think an older person needs to make a change, for example, move to a group-living situation or give up driving, they focus only on the change as being "for the best" and fail to acknowledge the older person's losses and feelings. The older person may experience a wide range of feelings: fear, anger, grief, helplessness, frustration, and relief. It is easier for many older persons to talk openly about their situations, concerns, and feelings if the family member listens, acknowledges, and accepts these feelings.

It is helpful if family members try to imagine how a situation looks and feels from the perspective of the older person. The nurse should encourage adult children to ask themselves, "How would I feel if I were in Dad's shoes?" Older persons who sense empathy and understanding are more willing to listen to concerns expressed by family members.

Additional communication techniques to help caregivers communicate more effectively can be found in *Taking Care of You: Powerful Tools for Caregiving* (http://www.powerful toolsforcaregivers.org/caregiver-classes/).

Involving the Older Person in Decision Making

Too often, the older person, especially if he or she is frail, is excluded from decisions being made about his or her own life. Family members may fail to tell the person about the decisions under consideration or what is happening. A person who is excluded from decision making is more likely to become angry, demanding, helpless, or withdrawn. Plans also are more likely to backfire.

Involvement in decision making provides greater assurance that a person will accept and adapt to a change, even if the change is not the person's preferred choice. A person who is railroaded into a new situation usually adjusts poorly. Change produces anxiety, but not being involved in decisions about a potential change creates even more anxiety and an atmosphere of distrust. Even a person who cannot actively participate in making or carrying out decisions should still be informed about alternatives and plans that are being made.

Only in a few extreme cases, as when people are afflicted with advanced Alzheimer's disease or suffering from a massive stroke, are they unable to make decisions. It is critical for a family to understand that an older family member with memory impairment may be unable to remember discussions or agreements made. However, the person often feels a sense of being involved in what is happening. One son stated:

Talking to a parent about a potential move is good advice, even if it does not always work out. I talked to my mother many times concerning her condition (in response to her own concerns), and we agreed on the appropriate plan. She could not remember even 30 minutes later.

Health care providers need to avoid taking a paternalistic approach, that is, communicating primarily with the family about an older person's condition, care plans, and the decisions to be made even though the older person is present and capable of participating in and making decisions.

Families usually must take greater control in making and carrying out decisions regarding older relatives with Alzheimer's disease or other dementia. It is unrealistic to expect the person with the disease to be able to do so. However, the older person may express anger, hostility, and rejection toward family members. A nurse should prepare family members for such reactions and help them understand that these feelings really are the result of the "pain of the situation." One person wrote about her difficult situation:

My grandmother and I had always been close. As a result of a series of small strokes, changes occurred, which included her driving down streets in the wrong lanes. We tried talking with my grandmother about

her unsafe driving but to no avail. Finally, I had to remove her car from the premises. We talked with her about the reasons she could no longer drive and made plans for meeting her transportation needs. For weeks, my grandmother was angry and accused me of stealing her car. Of course, it hurt, but I also realized that it probably felt to my grandmother as though her car had been stolen, and because of the disease process (and her lifelong personality), it was unrealistic for me to expect her to fully comprehend the true situation.

Validating Feelings

Families experience many emotions when faced with difficult decisions and caregiving. These emotions may include grief, frustration, anger, resentment, embarrassment, or guilt. At times, caregivers may wish that care receivers would die. The increasing frailty of an older family member may become a daily reminder of that person's mortality—and a caregiver's own mortality.

Family members may also need to adjust their perception of the ill person, and this may be emotionally painful. It may not be easy to accept that "my husband is no longer the strong and powerful man he once was," or "my mother who crocheted beautifully now no longer recognizes what to do with a crochet hook." It is particularly painful when the person with Alzheimer's disease or related disorder no longer recognizes a family member. In *The Loss of Self*, Eisdorfer and Cohen (1987) discuss the importance of caregivers "setting emotional distance," that is, creating some detachment by viewing the family member as a person with a disease over which neither the person nor the caregiver has any control, while at the same time maintaining a closeness to the person.

Because feelings, beliefs, and attitudes influence behavior, it is important to address the belief systems and feelings of family members. When feelings are not dealt with, decisions are more likely to be made based on guilt, promises, and "should's and should not's" rather than on the circumstances and what is best for everyone.

Feelings are validated by bringing them up for discussion and acknowledging their commonality. A nurse should emphasize that feelings are neither good nor bad; it is how family members act on their feelings that makes a difference.

Addressing Feelings of Guilt

It is important to deal with feelings of guilt family members may have. Guilt reduces objectivity and the ability to make decisions that are best for everyone. In addition, decisions made on the basis of guilt are likely to create feelings of resentment. For example, family members who feel guilty about moving a relative into a care facility are more likely to be critical of staff, overprotective of their older relative, or reluctant to visit.

Feelings of guilt generally result from the feeling that one has broken a "rule." Most guilt "rules" are black-and-white, inflexible, and impossible to conform to completely. Examples of rules include the following:

- "A good daughter provides care to an ailing parent."
- "You should always keep a promise."
- "I vowed we would be together for better or for worse."
- "A son does not tell his father what to do."
- "A loving person would never put a family member in a nursing facility."

Telling people they have no reason to feel guilty generally does not lessen the feelings of guilt. It is more desirable to help people (1) identify and examine the rules causing the guilt feelings; (2) evaluate the effect of that rule (a critical question to ask is, "Does the rule work to the detriment of anyone—yourself, the person receiving care, or other family members?"); and (3) rewrite the rule, often with qualifiers, to make it more realistic and appropriate to the current situation.

If a promise is the source of guilt feelings, explore the conditions under which the promise was made and the current situation with the person. Usually, the conditions are quite different. Comparing "what was" with "what is" often helps a family member look more objectively at the current situation.

Emphasizing Goodness of Intent of Actions

Sometimes, a family member may say, "I wish I had known this information earlier. I would have done things differently." In most cases, families are trying to make good decisions and do what is best. Actions are generally based on good intentions. For example, after a workshop, one woman wrote:

A year ago, we moved Mother from Texas to Oregon. She had lived in the small Texan community all of her life, and, of course, everyone knew Mom. I now realize why the move has been so difficult for Mom and that she probably would have been less lonely living in Texas, even though it would have meant moving her into a care facility. I came to the workshop feeling guilty, and I could have left the workshop feeling an even heavier load of guilt except that [the nurse] emphasized the goodness of intent behind actions. For me, this was to give Mom the help she needed, to keep Mom out of a nursing facility and in a home environment, and to add the "pleasure of family" to her life.

In working with families, it is important to start with the premise that most families are doing their best. Then a nurse can help them discuss and reinforce the "goodness of intent" underlying their actions when the actual action taken may turn out not to be the best choice.

Recognizing the Nurse's Role as Permission Giver

Because health care professionals are often looked to as "experts," their messages may carry a lot of power and authority with families. The following are 10 important messages that may be helpful for nurses to share, as appropriate, with family caregivers (Ostwald, 2009; Petch & Shamian, 2008):

1. **Take care of yourself.** Providing care to an older family member at the expense of the caregiver's own health or relationships with spouse or children does not benefit anyone, including the person who needs care. Although a caregiver may be unable to mitigate the effect of an illness on the older person, it is critical that the caregiver does not allow a family member's illness to destroy him or her or other family members.

2. **Maintain contact with friends and involvement in outside activities.** This is critical to caregiver well-being. Studies show that caregivers who sacrifice themselves in the care of others and remove pleasurable events from their lives may become emotionally exhausted, depressed, and physically ill. Caregivers should ask, "What happens if my family member enters a care facility or dies? Will I have been so wrapped up in caregiving that I will be 'used up' and without a life separate from caregiving?"

3. **Caregiving to adults is more stressful than child-rearing.** With a baby, a person looks forward to the child's increasing independence. However, with older adult caregiving, the prognosis generally involves decline and increasing dependence, not recovery. In addition, it is generally difficult to predict how long caregiving will be needed.

4. **It is all right not to love (or like) the older person who needs care.** Not all older family members have been lovable or likable. It is important for caregivers to take into consideration personalities and past relationships as they consider their level of involvement in caregiving.

5. **Asking for help is a sign of strength.** Asking for help is not a sign of weakness, inadequacy, or failure. Knowing the limits and reaching out for assistance before a caregiver is beyond them is characteristic of a strong individual and family. It also helps ensure high-quality care for the care receiver.

6. **Caregivers have a right to set limits and to say no.** Trying to do it all or to do it alone only makes caregivers physically and emotionally exhausted.

7. **Begin taking regular breaks early in caregiving—it is not selfish.** Breaks from the demands of caregiving are a must. They are as important to health as diet, rest, and exercise. Respite benefits the care receiver as well as the caregiver; caregivers are likely to be more loving and less exhausted. Caregivers should ask, "If my health deteriorates or I die, what will happen to my family member?" If caregivers wait until they are "burnt out," these breaks will not be enough.

8. **Make caregiving decisions based on the needs of everyone involved.** Decisions should not be made based only on the needs and desires of the older person.

9. **Moving a family member into a care facility can be the most loving step to take.** It does not mean an end to a caring relationship. Being a manager and coordinator of a family member's care is just as important as providing hands-on care. When a caregiver is no longer devoting time to meeting the person's physical and safety needs, he or she will be better able to meet the person's emotional and social needs. Having these needs met adds immensely to a person's quality of life.

10. **Caregivers should focus on what they have done well—and forgive themselves.** Too often, caregivers focus only on what they have not done or have done poorly. They should remind themselves of the many things they have

done well. They should ask, "What are my personal strengths? How have I made a difference for my family member? What have I done that I feel good about?" Not everything will be as caregivers would like. At times, caregivers will wish they had done things differently. They are only human. If they make a mistake, they should admit it, learn from it, and then go on. Although family members and friends may have given these messages, many caregivers do not take such messages to heart until they hear them from a health care professional.

Recommending a Decision-Making Model to Families

Many times, families find it helpful to have a model to follow as they make decisions or solve problems. One six-step model details the importance of gathering information, formulating options, evaluating options, creating a plan, implementing a plan, and reassessing (Schmall et al., 1999).

Step 1. Gathering Information

The goal is for the family to make an informed decision; therefore the first step is for them to clearly identify the issue and to gather pertinent information. Families are often so concerned about making a decision or handling a difficult situation that questions that could provide a better base for decision making go unasked and unanswered. A professional assessment of the older person's health and level of function also may be needed.

Step 2. Formulating Options

Once the issue has been identified, the nurse should help the family see all possible options for resolving it. This involves considering the resources of the older person, the family, and the community.

This should be the brainstorming portion of decision making. By generating a variety of possible options, families increase the chances of a successful outcome. In addition, keeping the decision separate from the possible options or solutions tends to take pressure away from people defending positions.

Step 3. Evaluating Options

After all options have been identified, the next step is for the family to assess the advantages and limitations of each option. It is helpful to first identify criteria or standards by which potential options will be evaluated. These may include financial constraints and personal preferences.

Agreeing on the criteria makes it easier to identify the best options. A good guideline to follow is: "Be easy on people; be

tough on issues." Keeping the focus on the issue, not the positions people take, increases effective decision making. Nurses can help families identify potential consequences of various options.

It is critical that family members be open and honest about their abilities to fulfill any responsibilities associated with an identified alternative. Honest communication helps prevent unrealistic expectations and keeps people from feeling overwhelmed or burdened.

Step 4. Creating a Plan

Sometimes, this is the most difficult aspect of decision making, especially if a single best choice does not seem to exist. However, identifying and evaluating all possible alternatives helps families avoid unsatisfactory decisions that may be regretted later. Also, families sometimes think that a good choice simply does not exist and that they must select "the best of the worst." It is important for the professional to recognize that a plan developed by one family may be quite different from a plan developed by another family whose "problem" appears to be the same.

Some families find that writing down the plan and indicating who has agreed to do which tasks by when help reduce disagreements. A written plan also may be useful later when the plan is reevaluated.

Step 5. Implementing the Plan

The fifth step in decision making is to put the plan into action. As with any decision, a plan should not be considered "final and forever" because situations do change. If possible, it may be helpful to establish a trial period, approaching the decision from the perspective of "This seems like the best decision for now. Let's give it a try for 1 month, and then evaluate the situation and how well our plan is working." This may be difficult to do, especially if the family wants closure to a difficult situation. However, flexibility is a key to high-quality decision making.

Step 6. Reassessing

It is important that the family makes plans for assessing the outcomes of the decision by asking, "How well is the plan working?" and then adjusting the plan as necessary.

Decision making is seldom easy. It is influenced by many factors such as the specific decision being faced, the personalities of family members, the quality of family relationships and communication, whether the older person is mentally intact and capable of full participation in making the decision, whether decisions are being made in advance of need or at a time of crisis, and whether family members are living nearby or at a great distance. However, a model for decision making may provide families with a method for approaching decisions.

▮ SUMMARY

Providing high-quality care to older adults requires recognizing the family's role and assessing and responding to the needs of family members, particularly the caregivers. Family members should be considered a part of the care team, not outsiders. The nurse should invite families to share the knowledge they

have gained through caregiving, particularly when placing an older relative in a care setting.

It is also important to be nonjudgmental and to remember that each family has its own history and values. Nurses need to be aware of their own values regarding what constitutes a family and their feelings about family behavior and relationships. It is important that nurses not allow personal values to prevent them from working effectively with families whose values or relationships with each other may be different. Nurses should not label such families as "dysfunctional." It is necessary to identify the strengths within each family and to build on those strengths while recognizing the family's limitations in providing support and caregiving.

KEY POINTS

- Families are significant in the lives of older persons and provide 80% of the support to older adults.
- Common dilemmas and decisions families face in later life involve changes in living arrangements, nursing facility placement, financial and legal issues, end-of-life medical treatments, the safety of an older family member's driving, and caregiving.
- Moving an older family member to a nursing facility is a difficult decision for most families.
- When working with older adults, it is as important to address the family's needs as to focus on the older person's needs. If only the older person's needs are considered, a care plan is less likely to be successful, particularly if the family is responsible for implementing it.
- Caregiving tends to be more stressful if the care receiver has a dementing illness, behavioral problem, or emotional disturbance than if a care receiver is only physically disabled.
- The meaning a caregiver ascribes to a stressor is a stronger predictor of its effect than the actual stressor.
- Family caregivers often experience restriction of personal activities and social life, emotional strain, competing demands, role conflict, and financial stress. They may need to adjust their expectations in regard to their ill family member, themselves as caregivers, and their stage of life.
- Caregiving for frail older adults differs from providing care to children.
- Education—whether provided one-on-one or in a group setting—should be designed to empower caregivers and to increase their confidence and competence in problem solving, decision making, and applying skills.
- Respite is most effective when a caregiver begins to use it early to prevent physical and emotional exhaustion rather than later to treat it.

- The family meeting is one strategy for a family to use to decide how to share caregiving responsibilities and to reach a consensus about problems, needs, and decisions.
- *Family* is more than relationships determined by blood and marital ties.
- Factors to consider in conducting a family assessment include a history of relationships, family dynamics, family roles, the effect of increased dependence of an older person on all family members, the family's ability to provide the needed care, and the nature and degree of caregiver stress.
- Strategies and considerations for nurses working with families of older adults include the following:
  - Identifying who the patient is and who the family is
  - Assessing the family as well as the older person
  - Encouraging families to plan in advance of need
  - Helping families communicate their concerns to older relatives honestly and in positive ways
  - Involving the older person in decisions to be made about his or her life
  - Validating the feelings and experiences of family members
  - Addressing feelings of guilt
  - Emphasizing the goodness of intent of actions
  - Recognizing the nurse's role as "permission giver"
  - Recommending a decision-making model
  - The nurse should try to "step into the shoes" of family members. Nurses who look at the situation from the perspective of a family member can increase their understanding of "where a person is coming from" and thus can improve their insight and sensitivity.

CRITICAL-THINKING EXERCISES

1. Think about your own family relationships. What individual and family values might influence your care of an older adult and his or her family members? How might your current perceptions change over the next decade?
2. An 83-year-old woman is recovering from pneumonia. She has Alzheimer's disease and has become increasingly hostile and unmanageable in the home setting. Her 65-year-old daughter is distraught about the idea of placing her mother in a long-term care facility but feels she is not able to care for her. What is your role as nurse in this situation?

REFERENCES

Administration on Aging. (2017). *A profile of older Americans: 2016.* Retrieved from https://www.acl.gov/aging-and-disability-in-america/data-and-research/profile-older-americans.

Aging with Dignity. (2013). *Five wishes.* Retrieved September 5, 2013 from http://www.agingwithdignity.org/catalog/product_info.php?products_id=28.

Alzheimer's Association. (2013a). *Take care of yourself.* Retrieved September 3, 2013 from www.alz.org.

Alzheimer's Association. (2013b). Respite care. Retrieved September 6, 2013, from http://www.alz.org/care/alzheimers-dementia-caregiver-respite.asp.

Auer, P. (2008). Primary care end-of-life planning for older adults with chronic illness. *The Journal for Nurse Practitioners, 4*(3), 185.

Bakalor, N. (2017). *U.S. fertility rate reaches record low.* Retrieved from https://www.nytimes.com/2017/07/03/health/united-states-fertility-rate.html.

Bureau of Labor Statistics. (2017). *Women in the labor force: A databook.* Retrieved February 28, 2018 from https://www.bls.gov/opub/reports/womens-databook/2017/home.htm.

Centers for Disease Control and Prevention. (2017). *Marriage and divorce.* Retrieved February 26, 2018 from https://www.cdc.gov/nchs/fastats/marriage-divorce.htm.

Clark, M., & Diamond, P. (2010). Depression in family caregivers of elders: A theoretical model of caregiver burden, sociotrophy, and autonomy. *Research in Nursing & Health, 33,* 20.

Eisdorfer, C., & Cohen, D. (1987). *The loss of self.* New York: Penguin.

Elliott, T., & Pezent, G. (2008). Family caregivers of older persons in rehabilitation. *NeuroRehabilitation, 23*(5), 439.

Eskildsen, M., & Price, T. (2009). Nursing home care in the U.S.A. *Geriatrics & Gerontology International, 9,* 1.

Forster, A., et al. (2011). A cluster randomized controlled trial of a structured training programme for caregivers of inpatients after stroke (TRACS). *International Journal of Stroke, 7*(1), 94.

Golden, M., & Lund, D. (2009). Identifying themes regarding the benefits and limitations of caregiver support group conversations. *Journal of Gerontological Social Work, 52*(2), 154.

Hartford Institute for Geriatric Nursing. (2014). Retrieved September 10, 2013, from http://www.hartfordign.com.

Hebert, R., Schulz, R., Copeland, V. C., & Arnold, R. M. (2009). Pilot testing of a question prompt sheet to encourage family caregivers of cancer patients and physicians to discuss end-of-life issues. *The American Journal of Hospice & Palliative Care, 26*(1), 24.

Help Guides. (2013). *Older driver safety.* Retrieved September 5, 2013 from http://www.helpguide.org/elder/senior_citizen_driving.htm.

Hendricksson, A., & Arestedt, K. (2013). Exploring factors and caregiver outcomes associated with feelings of preparedness for caregiving in family caregivers in palliative care: A correlational, cross-sectional study. *Palliative Medicine, 27*(7), 639.

Kaplan, K. (2017). *Americans keep having fewer babies as U.S. birthrates hit some record lows.* Retrieved from http://www.latimes.com/science/sciencenow/la-sci-sn-us-birth-rate-20170630-htmlstory.html.

Krooks, B. (2013). Elder care emerging as workplace issue. *Westchester County Business Journal, 49*(25), 15.

Levy, D. (2013). *U.S. Department of State: Legal & financial issues in caregiving for older adults.* Retrieved September 5, 2013 from http://www.state.gov/m/dghr/flo/142266.htm.

Lund, D., Utz, R., Caserta, M., & Wright, S. (2009). Examining what caregivers do during respite time to make respite more effective. *Journal of Applied Gerontology, 28*(1), 109.

Make written material easy to read, understandable. (2009). *Hospital Home Health, 26*(1), 9.

Marek, K., Adams, S., Stetzer, F., Popejoy, L., & Rantz, M. (2010). The relationship of community-based nurse care coordination to costs in the Medicare and Medicaid programs. *Research in Nursing & Health, 33,* 235.

National Institute on Aging. (2013). *So far away: Twenty questions for long distance caregivers.* Retrieved September 6, 2013, from http://www.nia.nih.gov/health/publication/so-far-away-twenty-questions-andanswers-about-long-distance-caregiving-o.

Ostwald, S. (2009). Who is caring for the caregiver? Promoting spousal caregiver's health. *Family & Community Health, 32*(1S), S5.

Petch, T., & Shamian, J. (2008). Tapestry of care: Who provides care in the home? *Healthcare Quarterly, 11*(4), 79.

Phillips, L., & Reed, P. (2009). Into the abyss of someone else's dying: The voice of the end-of-life caregiver. *Clinical Nursing Research, 18*(1), 80.

Schmall, V. (1993). In T. Nay (Ed.), *Helping your older family member handle finances.* Corvallis: Oregon State University Extension Service.

Schmall, V. (1994). Family caregiving: A training and education perspective. In M. H. Cantor (Ed.), *Family caregiving: An agenda for the future.* San Francisco: American Society on Aging.

Schmall, V., Cleland, M., & Sturdevant, M. (1999). *Taking care of you: Powerful tools for caregiving* (1st ed.). Portland, OR: Legacy Health Systems.

Schmall, V., & Stiehl, R. (1998). *Coping with caregiving: How to manage stress when caring for elderly relatives, Pacific Northwest Extension Publication, PNW 315.* Corvallis: Oregon State University Extension Service.

Society of Certified Senior Advisors (CSA). (2013). *State of the senior housing industry (white paper).* Retrieved September 5, 2013 from www.csa.us.

Stepler, R. (2017). *Led by Baby Boomers, divorce rates climb for America's 50 + population.* Retrieved February 26, 2018 from http://www.pewresearch.org/fact-tank/2017/03/09/led-by-baby-boomers-divorce-rates-climb-for-americas-50-population/.

U.S. Census Bureau. (2012). *Current population survey 1948–2012.* Retrieved September 3, 2013 from http://www.census.gov/hhes/migration/data/cps/historical/Figure%20A-1.1.png.

Wang, Y., Yea-Ing, L., Chen, M., & Yang, P. (2010). Reconciling work and family caregiving among adult-child family caregivers of older people with dementia: Effects on role strain and depressive symptoms. *Journal of Advanced Nursing, 67*(4), 829.

Wasik, J. F. (2016). *The Everything-in-One Promise of a Continuing Care Community.* Retrieved from https://www.nytimes.com/2016/02/27/your-money/the-everything-in-one-promise-of-a-continuing-care-community.html.

Willyard, J., Miller, K., Shoemaker, M., & Addison, P. (2008). Making sense of sibling responsibility for family caregiving. *Qualitative Health Research, 8*(12), 1673.

Yang, Y., & Grimm, G. (2013). Caring for elder parents: A comparative evaluation of family leave laws. *Journal of Law, Medicine, and Ethics, 41*(2), 501.

7

Socioeconomic and Environmental Influences

Colleen Steinhauser, MSN, RN-BC, FNGNA

(e) http://evolve.elsevier.com/Meiner/gerontologic

LEARNING OBJECTIVES

On completion of this chapter, the reader will be able to:

1. Identify the major socioeconomic and environmental factors that influence the health of older adults.
2. Explain the importance of age cohorts in understanding older adults.
3. Describe the economic factors that influence the lives of older persons.
4. Identify components of the Medicare health insurance programs.
5. Discuss the influence of support systems on the health and well-being of older adults.
6. Distinguish among a conservator, guardian, and durable power of attorney.
7. Discuss environmental factors that affect the safety and security of older adults.
8. Compare and contrast the housing options available for older adults.
9. Compare the influences of income, education, and health status on quality of life.
10. Relate strategies for protecting older persons in the community from criminal victimization.
11. Assess the ability of older adults to be their own advocate.

WHAT WOULD YOU DO?

What would you do if you were faced with the following situations?

- You are the medical surgical nurse on an inpatient unit. An older adult is 2 days postsurgery and set to be discharged. You determine that your patient was homeless before their admission through the emergency department and has no place to go. What options for discharge will your patient have? What can you, as a nurse, do to help your patient after discharge?
- You are a nurse at an internal medicine clinic. You are working with a patient who is 85 years old and lives alone. He has a diagnosis of coronary heart disease and hypertension. He is interested in making some health changes. Based on where he falls in a cohort, what interventions and suggestions would you have for him to make health changes?
- With the advancement of technology to monitor health and assist at home, what are some of the benefits and challenges that this new technology can bring to the older adult population?

Each person is a unique design of genetic inheritance, life experiences, education, and environment. Social status, economic conditions, and environment influence our health and response to illness. Socioeconomic factors such as income, level of education, present health status, and availability of support systems all affect the way older adults perceive the health care system. Benefits and entitlements may influence the availability of high-quality health care. A small number of older adults may not be competent to manage their own health care; they need the protection of a conservator or guardian.

Environmental factors such as geographic area, housing, perceived criminal victimization, and community resources make a difference in older adults' abilities to obtain the type and quality of health care that is appropriate. One of the strongest and most consistent predictors of illness and death is socioeconomic status (Sowa et al., 2016). The environment also influences safety and well-being. Therefore it is imperative that health care professionals understand the socioeconomic and environmental status of older adults. Although, in some cases, illness may lead to poverty, more often poverty causes poor health by its connection with inadequate nutrition, substandard housing, exposure to environmental hazards, unhealthy lifestyles, and decreased access to and use of health care services.

The United States spends more per capita on health care than any other country, and the rate at which spending is increasing. Much of this spending is on health care that controls or reduces the effect of chronic diseases and conditions affecting an increasingly older population; notable examples are prescription drugs and cardiac disease. Adults over the age of 65 average twice as many physician visits than persons younger than 65 (O'Hara & Caswell, 2013).

Older adult health care consumers often depend on the health care professional for advocacy. To be an effective advocate, the nurse must understand the factors that shape the older consumer's perceptions of environment, socioeconomic status, and access to health care.

Previous author: Jennifer J. Yeager, PhD, RN.

SOCIOECONOMIC FACTORS

Age Cohorts

Persons who share the experience of an event or time in history are grouped together in what is called a *cohort*. Strauss and Howe (1992) were the first to name them: the *G.I. Generation,* commonly called the "Greatest Generation," born 1900 to 1924; the *Silent Generation*, born 1925 to 1945; and the *Baby Boomers,* born 1946 to 1964. They share certain experiences at similar stages of physical, psychological, and social development that influence the way they perceive the world. Therefore they develop attitudes and values that are similar (Richardson, 1996). By understanding cohorts, the nurse develops a greater understanding of older adults' value systems. For example, persons who reached maturity during the Great Depression of the 1930s learned the value of having a job and working hard to keep it. Generally, persons in this cohort have been loyal workers. They feel better if they are "doing their jobs." The nurse might increase adherence with a treatment regimen by referring to the need for adherence as an older adult's "job."

Cohort classifications include age, historical events, and geographic area of residence. Today's older Americans have shared many momentous experiences. World War II and the Korean War made impressions on everyone who lived through those events but especially on those who were young at the time. Values and the pace of life, which vary between communities and regions of the country, influence the perceptions of the residents of each region.

The age cohort that reached young adulthood in the post-World War II and Korean War era benefited from a very productive time in American history. The late 1940s, 1950s, and 1960s were times of rapidly increasing earnings and heavy spending. Strong unions negotiated for better pension plans and medical benefits. This cohort became accustomed to contacting professionals for services, thereby becoming more conscious of preventive health care compared with previous generations. This group has become aware of wellness techniques and self-care strategies that improve health. Members of this cohort usually have at least a high school education and often have some form of higher education. Many pursued further educational opportunities. As a group, however, they experience a less cohesive family life. Many have moved from their home communities and have experienced divorce, remarriage, or other circumstances that complicate family support (Johnson, 1992).

The age cohort that matured just before and during World War II was strongly influenced by the war. Those who served in the armed forces were shaped by their direct involvement, while most of those at home worked in the defense industry; experienced rationing of food, clothing, and fuel; and waited for the men and women in the service to come home. Life revolved around the war. Movies and music featured war themes, and rationing was a reminder that all resources were needed primarily for the war effort. Signs and billboards urged people to sign up or to purchase war bonds. Windows of houses displayed stars to honor family members who were serving or who had died in the war; resurgence in popularity of this symbol began with Operation Desert Storm in 1991 and continues today in the homes of families whose loved ones serve in the War in Afghanistan.

The workforce was expanded to include more women, many of whom continued to work after the war. In 1940, 12 million women were working; by 1945, 19 million women were working (Wapner, Demick, & Redondo, 1990). Men and women serving in the armed forces became accustomed to regular physical and dental checkups, and they extended these practices to their families after the war. Veterans took advantage of the G.I. Bill to pursue a college education, which would have been unobtainable otherwise. With the help of veterans' benefits, they purchased houses for little or no money as down payment. Having experienced the trauma of war, this group developed an appetite for the good things in life and willingly paid for them.

Today, the oldest Americans are strongly influenced by having lived through the Great Depression of the 1930s. At the time, today's oldest-old (95 years or older) were struggling to keep families together, and today's younger older adults were attempting to find work and start families. The struggles of those times have shaped the lives of Americans older than 80 years.

Persons of this era are generally frugal and often do not spend money, even if they have it. The oldest-old believe they will outlive their money because they remember what it was like to have nothing. In addition, this age cohort did not have the experience of receiving regular health care. Visits to the doctor or dentist occurred only when necessary, and home remedies were used as the first line of defense. Education often ended with the eighth grade so that children could help support the family. A college education was rare.

During this era, families were close and supportive. However, the family was a closed unit, and personal matters remained within the family. Unhappy family situations, mental illness, family finances, and abusive situations were not usually discussed outside the family. Gender roles were well defined.

Many of today's conveniences, including antibiotics, were not available during the 1930s. The technology now used in health care settings, ranging from electronic thermometers to computed tomography (CT) and positron emission tomography (PET) scanners, represents a true technologic explosion to persons who have witnessed its development. Today's older adult cohort has survived many significant changes. Among those changes is the family living arrangement of grandparents aged 65 or older having the primary responsibility for their grandchildren who live with them; more than 2.7 million children in the United States live with their grandparents (Ellis & Simmons, 2014).

Income Sources

Older adults report income from five sources: (1) Social Security (84%), (2) assets (62%), (3) retirement funds (37%), (4) government pensions (16%), and (5) wages (29%). The median income in 2015 was $31,372 for men and $18,250 for women. In 2015, 8.8% of older adults lived below the poverty level (Administration on Aging [AOA], 2016). Social Security is a benefit package for retired individuals, survivors of participants, and those with disabilities. Funds for Social Security are derived from payroll taxes, and benefits are earned by accumulating credits based on annual income.

Retirement age to begin receiving Social Security retirement benefits is 62 years old but at a reduced percentage (Social Security Administration, n.d.). Those born before 1938 are eligible for full Social Security benefits at age 65. However, beginning in 2003, the age at which full benefits are payable began increasing in gradual steps from 65 to 67 (Table 7.1). For those who wish to delay retirement, the benefit increases by a certain

TABLE 7.1   Age to Receive Full Social Security Benefits

If you start getting benefits at age[a]	Wage earner, the retirement benefit you will receive is reduced to	Spouse, the retirement benefit you will receive is reduced to
62	70.0%	32.5%
62 + 1 month	70.4	32.7
62 + 2 months	70.8	32.9
62 + 3 months	71.3	33.1
62 + 4 months	71.7	33.3
62 + 5 months	72.1	33.5
62 + 6 months	72.5	33.8
62 + 7 months	72.9	34.0
62 + 8 months	73.3	34.2
62 + 9 months	73.8	34.4
62 + 10 months	74.2	34.6
62 + 11 months	74.6	34.8
63	75.0	35.0
63 + 1 month	75.4	35.2
63 + 2 months	75.8	35.4
63 + 3 months	76.3	35.6
63 + 4 months	76.7	35.8
63 + 5 months	77.1	36.0
63 + 6 months	77.5	36.3
63 + 7 months	77.9	36.5
63 + 8 months	78.3	36.7
63 + 9 months	78.8	36.9
63 + 10 months	79.2	37.1
63 + 11 months	79.6	37.3
64	80.0	37.5
64 + 1 month	80.6	37.8
64 + 2 months	81.1	38.2
64 + 3 months	81.7	38.5
64 + 4 months	82.2	38.9
64 + 5 months	82.8	39.2
64 + 6 months	83.3	39.6
64 + 7 months	83.9	39.9
64 + 8 months	84.4	40.3
64 + 9 months	85.0	40.6

TABLE 7.1   Age to Receive Full Social Security Benefits—cont'd

If you start getting benefits at age	Wage earner, the retirement benefit you will receive is reduced to	Spouse, the retirement benefit you will receive is reduced to
64 + 10 months	85.6	41.0
64 + 11 months	86.1	41.3
65	86.7	41.7
65 + 1 month	87.2	42.0
65 + 2 months	87.8	42.4
65 + 3 months	88.3	42.7
65 + 4 months	88.9	43.1
65 + 5 months	89.4	43.4
65 + 6 months	90.0	43.8
65 + 7 months	90.6	44.1
65 + 8 months	91.1	44.4
65 + 9 months	91.7	44.8
65 + 10 months	92.2	45.1
65 + 11 months	92.8	45.5
66	93.3	45.8
66 + 1 month	93.9	46.2
66 + 2 months	94.4	46.5
66 + 3 months	95.0	46.9
66 + 4 months	95.6	47.2
66 + 5 months	96.1	47.6
66 + 6 months	96.7	47.9
66 + 7 months	97.2	48.3
66 + 8 months	97.8	48.6
66 + 9 months	98.3	49.0
66 + 10 months	98.9	49.3
66 + 11 months	99.4	49.7
67	100.0	50.0

[a]If your birthday is on the 1st of the month, then the Social Security Administration figures the benefit as if your birthday were the previous month.
From Social Security Online. (n.d.). *Retirement Age: If you were born in 1960 or later*. Retrieved from https://www.ssa.gov/planners/retire/1960.html.

percentage depending on the year of birth. Widows and widowers are eligible for Social Security under their spouse's benefits beginning at age 60. Surviving spouses with no work experience receive about two-thirds of the overall income earned before the death of their spouses. Very poor older adults depend on another federal government program. Supplemental Security Income (SSI) pays monthly checks to persons who are aged, disabled, or sight impaired, and who have few assets and minimal income. This program is also regulated by the Social Security Administration, but the money to provide benefits is from income tax sources rather than Social Security payroll taxes. Eligibility depends on income and assets. Additional information is obtainable through the Social Security website at http://www.socialsecurity.gov.

Ages 55 to 64

Those in the preretirement age cohort of 55 to 64 are generally in their peak earning years. Most are married, but few have children younger than 18 still residing in the family home. The heavy expenses of child rearing are over, and homeowners have completely or nearly paid for their homes. This age cohort tends to have increased disposable income yet is acutely aware of impending retirement; thus priorities change, and spending begins to decrease.

The recession beginning December 2007 changed the economic picture of this age cohort. Many older adults lost 25% of their private retirement account value. In 2017 the jobless rate for this age group was between 3.1% and 3.5%. Older adults who lose their jobs have a harder time finding gainful employment (an average of 35.5 weeks). Despite the jobless rate, 53% of older adults 55 and over remain employed full time. The increase in the number of older adults in the labor force began with changes to retirement savings beginning in the 1990s when the burden of retirement funding shifted from the employer to the worker. Although older adult workers took financial losses in their retirement portfolios, this had a negligible effect on the number of adults over the age of 55 entering the labor force (American Association of Retired Persons [AARP], 2014; Ghilarducci, 2015; Bureau of Labor Statistics, 2017).

Persons in this age group are generally healthy and have resources to maintain housing. The average annual income of families ages 55 to 64 is more than $ 49,608 (Josephson, 2017). Because of higher earnings, they have contributed more to Social Security than older age groups. Many held jobs with disability benefits, which now may be contributing to income. Those who served in the armed forces may be eligible for veterans' benefits.

Ages 65 to 74

Retirement ordinarily causes income to decrease, most recently by more than 40%. The median income before taxes for households ages 65 and older is a little more than $22,887 (AOA, 2016). Although spending continues to decrease in this age group, especially for such items as clothing, electronics, furniture, and appliances, expenses related to medical care and prescription drugs increase. Additionally, persons in this age group face funeral expenses.

Today, this age group includes many veterans from the Vietnam War. Veterans' benefits are important to this age group because of the increased risk of chronic disease and other acute health problems. Eligibility for veterans' benefits is based on military service, service-related disability, and income. Benefits are considered on an individual basis (U.S. Department of Veterans Affairs, 2016b) (Box 7.1).

Ages 75 to 84

After age 75, women outnumber men in American society. Many persons in this age group live alone, which affects their average household income. Although this age group has reached retirement age, they are projected to have more than a 6% growth rate from 2014 to 2024, more than any other age group (Projections of the Labor Force, 2015). As health problems increase with age, so do expenses for prescriptions and assistive devices such as eyeglasses, hearing aids, and dentures. The

---

BOX 7.1 Veterans' Benefits

Benefits for eligible veterans include the following:
- Disability compensation
- Pension
- Education and training
- Home loan guaranties
- Life insurance
- Burial benefits
- Health care benefits
- Special Monthly Compensation
- Caregiver Program and Services
- Long Term Care Services

From: U. S. Department of Veterans Affairs. (2016). *Federal benefits for veteran, dependents and survivors.* Washington, DC: Office of Public Affairs. Retrieved September 19, 2017 from https://www.va.gov/opa/publications/benefits_book/2016_Federal_Benefits_for_Veterans.pdf.

---

quality of housing deteriorates as houses age and less money is available for maintenance. Decreased strength and endurance reduce the ability to perform household chores.

Ages 85 and Older

This group is the fastest-growing segment of our population (Table 7.2), with more than 6.3 million persons 85 years and over in 2015. By 2040 those the number of Americans over 85 years old is expected to be 14.6 million. Although medical and social advances have prolonged the life span of Americans, this age cohort is at risk for increased chronic disease, resulting in decreased ability to perform activities of daily living (ADLs) and increased expenses for assistance, assistive devices, and medication (AOA, 2016; Ortman, Velkoff, & Hogan, 2014).

This group has the lowest average annual income level of all older Americans; nearly 10% live in poverty (Federal Interagency Forum on Aging-Related Statistics, 2016). Social Security is the primary source of income for this age group, although investments and pensions provide a significant source of additional income. Members of this age group may receive assistance from family, but the amount is small and often sporadic. Few receive wages, salary, or self-employment income.

The 85 or older group is more likely to need assistance with ADLs. They are also more likely to need institutional and home care (Federal Interagency Forum, 2016). Dependence on medication and assistive devices increases.

If persons in this age group live independently, their housing is likely to be old and in need of repairs and maintenance (Federal Interagency Forum, 2016). Adaptations to compensate

---

TABLE 7.2 Projections and Distributions of the Population Aged 65 and Over by Age Group in the United States

Age	2012	2030	2050
65 years and over	43,145	72,774	83,739
65–84 years	37,258	63,829	65,760
85 years and over	5,887	8,946	17,978

Adapted from Ortman, J. M., Velkoff, V. A., Hogan, H. [2014]. *An aging nation: The older population in the United States: Population estimates and projections,* [P25-1140] U. S. Census Bureau.

for decreasing abilities help older adults remain in their homes, but these changes may be costly. Some older adults choose to move in with family or to facilities offering assistance; 3% of persons aged 75 to 84 and 10% of persons 85 and older live in long-term care settings (AOA, 2016).

The nation's political climate and financial stability affect the sources of income for older adults at any time. Decreased interest earnings, for example, affect those with money market investments or certificates of deposit; stock market fluctuations affect the value of stock portfolios and mutual funds; and the political climate affects the type and amount of taxes paid. Since reaching a low point in December 2011, home values have steadily risen (a 6.2% increase) in home values, increasing home equity that can be part of many older adults' portfolio of investments for their retirement years (Boss, 2016).

Poverty

The following information looks at poverty at various times over the past 20 to 30 years. Updates to all statistics take place periodically and can be found by checking with the U.S. Census Bureau at http://www.census.gov/ or with the AOA at http://www.aoa.gov/.

In 2015 8.8% of those age 65 or older were classified as poor, with income at or below the poverty level ($11,400 for family of one; $15,500 for family of two). Nearly 18.4% of African Americans over 65 are poor compared with 6.6% of older Caucasians, 17.5% of older Hispanics, and 11.8% of older Asians. The poverty rate for older women is 10.3%, whereas the rate for older men is 7%. Hispanic women over the age of 65 who live alone have the highest rate of poverty (40.7%) (AOA, 2016).

Low income may affect the quality of life for older adults. For example, basics such as housing and diet may be inadequate. A worn-out wardrobe and lack of transportation may cause the older adult to avoid social contact, leading to isolation. Older adults may delay seeking medical help or may not follow through with the prescribed treatment or medications because of limited income. Eyeglasses, hearing aids, and dental work may become unaffordable luxuries. Identifying an older patient's income level enables the nurse to direct the patient to agencies and services available to those with limited resources (Fig. 7.1A and 7.1B).

Education

Education has been shown to have a strong relationship with health risk factors. The level of education influences earning ability, information absorption, problem-solving ability, value systems, and lifestyle behaviors. A more educated person often has greater access to wellness programs and preventive health options (Zimmerman, Woolf, & Haley, 2015)

The educational level of the older population has increased steadily between 1970 and 2012, reflecting increased mandatory education and better educational opportunities in the last 40 years. The percentage of individuals who completed high school varies by race and ethnic origin; however, 85% of older adults have completed high school, and 28% have earned a bachelor's degree or higher (AOA, 2016).

Many older adults continue their education in their later years. Some complete high school or take college courses. The Servicemen's Readjustment Act of 1944 (known as the *G.I. Bill*)

fostered this trend. This bill offers, in part, tuition assistance and defrayment of living expenses. It has been used by the Vietnam War–era veterans more than any previous generation. Revision of this bill, known as the *Montgomery G.I. Bill,* extended benefits to military veterans through 2008; in 2008, Congress extended benefits to ensure those serving in the military following the September 11, 2001, terrorist attacks could further their education. Other older adults take advantage of continuing education programs such as Road Scholar (for more information, go to http://www.roadscholar.org/) to explore subjects of interest. Seeking educational opportunities in later life has many benefits for older adults. Lifelong learning promotes intellectual growth, increases self-esteem, and enhances socialization. Older adults have an opportunity to stimulate creativity and to remain alert and involved with the world.

Erikson's seventh stage of development stresses how important generativity versus stagnation is to the individual's sense of achievement and fulfillment in life (Cox, 1986). Education provides an opportunity to avoid stagnation and isolation and adds to the enjoyment of later life. Teaching older adults with disabilities may be a challenge for nurses when the teaching is a part of health education. See the Patient/Family Teaching box for suggestions related to the learning environment of those with memory, vision, or adherence issues.

Patient Teaching Strategies

Older adults often have short-term memory deficits or limited vision or hearing abilities that affect teaching. To improve comprehension and adherence, consider the following suggestions:

- Find out what they want to know.
- Provide a comfortable environment with adequate lighting and minimal distractions. Turn off the TV/radio.
- Repeat important information at least three times.
- Present information in several forms: written material, discussion, video and audiotape, and photos and pictures.
- With written material, use large print and clear black letters on a contrasting background.
- Speak at a moderate pace and volume with a low tone of voice. Check for understanding by asking the patient to explain in his or her own words.
- Use appropriate gestures to enhance understanding and face the person.
- Check back later to assess understanding.

Health Status

The health status of older adults influences their socioeconomic status. Eighty percent of older adults have at least one chronic health condition; 50% have two. The most common chronic health problems leading to death in 2015 were heart disease, cancer, chronic obstructive pulmonary disease (COPD, accounting for 50% of deaths), followed by stroke, Alzheimer's disease, and diabetes (Centers for Disease Control and Prevention [CDC], 2016). Many add obesity to this list as well. The influence health problems exert often depends on the older person's perception of the problem. Among noninstitutionalized persons, 44% of those 65 and older consider their health to be excellent or very good (AOA, 2015). Some approach health problems with an attitude of acceptance, whereas others find that chronic problems require considerable energy, and they

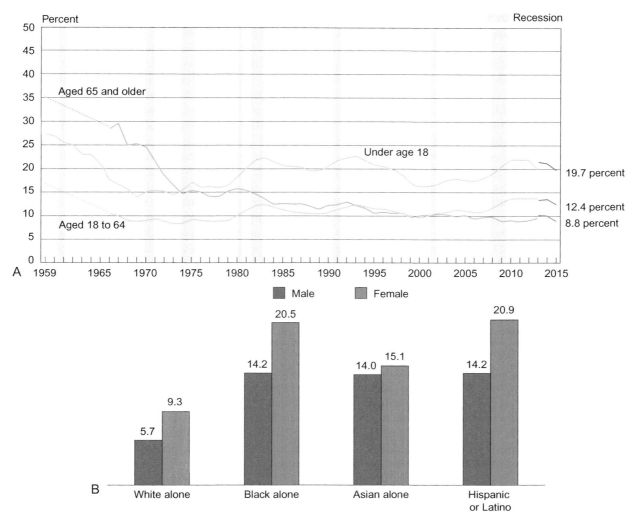

Fig. 7.1 A, Poverty rates by age: United States, 1959 to 2015. **B,** Low-income population by age, race, and Hispanic origin: United States, 2006. *Notes:* Data shown are the percentage of persons with family income below the poverty level. Percent of poverty level is based on family income and family size and composition using U.S. Census Bureau poverty thresholds. Persons of Hispanic origin may be of any race. Black and Asian races include persons of Hispanic and non-Hispanic origin. (**A,** From Proctor, B. D., Semega, J. L., & Kollar, M. A. [2015]. *Income and poverty in the United States: 2015.* Retrieved from https://www.census.gov/content/dam/Census/library/publications/2016/demo/p60-256.pdf. **B,** From West, S.A., Cole, S., Goodkind D., He, W. [2014]. *65 + in the United States: 2010 Special studies current population reports.* U. S. Government Printing Office. Retrieved from https://www.census.gov/content/dam/Census/library/publications/2014/demo/p23-212.pdf.)

spend extensive time and resources finding ways to cope or adapt (Burke & Flaherty, 1993).

Functional status is affected by chronic conditions. The CDC (2016) reports that functional status is important because it serves as an indicator of an older adult's ability to remain independent in the community. Functional ability is measured by the individual's ability to perform ADLs and instrumental activities of daily living (IADLs). ADLs include six personal care activities: (1) eating, (2) toileting, (3) bathing, (4) transferring, (5) dressing, and (6) continence. A quarter of persons with at least one chronic disease experience a decrease in the ability to perform one or more ADLs. The term *IADLs* refers to the following home-management activities: preparing meals, shopping, managing money, using the telephone, doing light housework, doing laundry, using transportation, and taking medications appropriately. Data

concerning the ability to perform ADLs and IADLs were gathered through the National Health Interview Survey. Nurses work with older adults to prolong independence by encouraging self-management of chronic conditions. *Self-management* is defined as learning and practicing the skills necessary to carry on an active and emotionally satisfying life in the face of a chronic condition (Schulman-Green et al., 2012). Education and support help older adults make informed choices, practice positive health behaviors, and take responsibility for the care of a chronic condition.

The amount of money available for food, shelter, clothing, and recreation may be greatly affected by the cost of medication, health care equipment, glasses, hearing aids, dental care, medical care, home care assistance, and nursing facility care, some of which may not be covered by insurance programs. In addition, the insurance premiums themselves may cause financial distress. Restricted finances may affect an older adult's safety, nutritional status, and social opportunities, which may result in an altered quality of life.

By making older adults aware of programs such as equipment loan programs, as well as optical, auditory, and dental assistance programs, the nurse can help them receive services necessary to maintain their health status, thus maximizing their quality of life in spite of restricted finances.

An integrated health care delivery system built on capitated benefits through Medicare and Medicaid funding is called the *Program of All-inclusive Care for the Elderly (PACE)*. The program is a state option under Medicare with additional funding from Medicaid; eligible participants receive primary, acute, and long-term care services in the community. States certify the eligibility of frail individuals who are older than 55 and require the level of care provided at nursing facilities. Full financial responsibility is assumed by the providers of care regardless of the duration of care, amount of services used, or the scope of services provided (Centers for Medicare & Medicaid Services [CMS], 2017).

Insurance Coverage

Older Americans should review their insurance coverage often to determine whether the coverage they have is necessary, appropriate, and adequate. Residential insurance purchased several years ago may be inadequate today. For example, home insurance should cover at least 80% of the replacement cost; however, many older adult homeowners are insured for the assessed value of the home at the time of purchase. Content and liability coverage may also be inadequate. Older homeowners may be unaware that policies are outdated, or they may not be able to afford the premiums an update would require. Insurance checkups reveal inadequacies. Older adults may wish to investigate several insurance companies to find the best coverage for the least cost.

Many older adults have automobiles that have reached maximum depreciation. These automobile owners may still be carrying full coverage when all they need is liability insurance. They may also be able to save money by investigating senior discounts, choosing higher deductibles, and comparing premiums from several companies. Completion of a defensive driving course such as the AARP Driver Safety Program (offered both online and in person; see http://www.aarpdriversafety.org/) may help older adults qualify for lower insurance rates (AARP, n.d.).

Life insurance is valuable when providing for dependents. In old age, the primary reason for life insurance is to cover burial expenses. Term life insurance accomplishes this purpose. Many older adults can substantially reduce life insurance coverage. Proceeds from those policies and premium payments that are no longer due may be redirected for greater benefit.

Health insurance is a necessity for older adults because medical problems—and therefore medical expenses—increase with age. As persons age, they visit the doctor more often (O'Hara & Caswell, 2013). Older adults spend more time in the hospital—double that of those younger than 65 years old (AOA, 2016).

Medicare is a federal health insurance program for persons older than 65, or persons of any age who are disabled or who have chronic kidney disease. Medicare has several parts to provide multiple benefits to older adults.

Part A, the hospital insurance, helps pay for inpatient hospital care and some follow-up care such as a skilled nursing facility, home health services, and hospice care. A person is eligible for Medicare Hospital Insurance if he or she is age 65 or older and (1) is eligible for any type of monthly Social Security benefit or railroad retirement system benefit or (2) is retired from or the spouse of a person who was employed in a Medicare-covered position. It costs nothing for those who contributed to Medicare taxes while they were working. If the person is not eligible for premium-free Part A, a monthly premium may be paid, as long as the person meets citizenship or residency requirements and is age 65 or older or disabled. The 2017 premium amount for people who buy Part A is $413 each month. There are also required deductibles to meet each year and some coinsurance costs ("Medicare 2017 costs at a glance," n.d.).

Part A, the hospital insurance, helps pay for the following:
- Home health care (including durable medical equipment)
- Hospice care
- Hospital inpatient stay
- Mental health inpatient stays
- Skilled nursing facility stay

Part B is medical insurance coverage. Most Medicare recipients pay a premium deducted from monthly Social Security income. In addition, they pay an annual deductible and 20% of the Medicare-approved amount. The 2017 premium amount for Part B starts at $134 or more each month, based on income, with a $183 deductible per year ("Medicare 2017 costs at a glance," n.d.).

Part B, the medical insurance, helps pay for the following:
- Home health services (including durable medical equipment)
- Medical and other services (including inpatient doctor services and outpatient therapies)
- Outpatient mental health services and partial hospitalization for mental health services
- Outpatient hospital services

Medicare Part D refers to the prescription drug program that began in 2004. Eligibility requires that the person have Medicare. Each October through December, eligible persons can use the Medicare website to choose a new plan based on their current medications to find one with the lowest monthly premiums, copays, and deductibles. Older adults who have Medicaid are still eligible; however, they must sign up for a Medicare Prescription Drug Plan to receive their medications. These individuals do not have a copay. Medicare Part D is available regardless of income level. Older adults with limited income may qualify for Extra Help. Refer to http://www.medicare.gov for more information on the Extra Help program (Drug coverage [Part D], n.d.).

Medicare Part A covers medically necessary skilled nursing care for a limited period; custodial care is not covered. In 2016 average daily cost for 1 day in a nursing facility was $225 for a semiprivate room (American Eldercare Research Organization, 2016). In the case of most of the older adults, savings and other assets are exhausted after 6 months or less of nursing facility care. Therefore some persons purchase long-term care insurance. Premiums depend on age at time of purchase and the extent of benefits chosen by the purchaser.

Medicare rules and benefits change often. Medicare Advantage plans ("Medicare Advantage Plans," n.d.) were introduced as a result of the Balanced Budget Act of 1997; until the Medicare Prescription Drug, Improvement, and Modernization Act of 2003, these were known as Medicare + Choice programs, or Medicare Part C. These programs provide comprehensive care through a variety of health care delivery models, including Health Maintenance Organizations, Preferred Provider Organizations, Private Fee-for-Service Plans, Special Needs Plans, and Medicare Medical Savings Account Plans (Balanced Budget Act of 1997; The Official U.S. Government Site for Medicare, n.d.).

Many older adults do not understand how Medicare works and are often confused by the paperwork, billing, and notices they receive regarding claims. They are encouraged to contact the Social Security Administration or the insurance departments of their local medical facilities if they have questions.

Those older adults who are still working may continue to be covered by their employers' health insurance plans. A retiree is sometimes covered by a former employer's health plan or their spouse's employer health plan. If covered by an employer-sponsored insurance policy and enrolled in Medicare, the employer's insurance becomes "primary" and the Medicare insurance is "secondary." Some older adults choose to purchase supplemental insurance to cover copays and deductibles, often referred to as *Medigap policy*. The supplemental insurance is then secondary to Medicare, which is primary. This is very important to know if hospitalization or outpatient surgery centers are to be used.

Medicaid is a federal- and state-funded, state-managed program for low-income individuals and their families. For eligible older adults residing in nursing facilities, it covers health-related care and other services not available in the community because of their mental or physical conditions. Each state has different coverage and requirements; however, general, up-to-date information can be obtained at http://www.medicaid.gov/Medicaid/ltss/index.html.

The Official U.S. Government Site for Medicare (please see https://www.medicare.gov/) provides information to explain Medicare. Insurance trade associations such as the Health Insurance Association of America (HIAA), the Insurance Information Institute (III), and the American Council of Life Insurance (ACLI) publish a variety of free educational materials to help people understand insurance.

Support Systems

Throughout life, people make new acquaintances, develop friendships, and form family circles. People identify with schools, churches or synagogues, clubs, neighborhoods, and towns. These are the places and people they turn to when they need advice or help, want to celebrate, or are grieving. With age, a person loses some of these support systems. Family and friends move away or die, and organizations and neighborhoods change. Changing work roles and financial status may require changes in the groups with whom a person associates. To cope with losses of family members and friends and a decline in health and independence, individuals need a large social network.

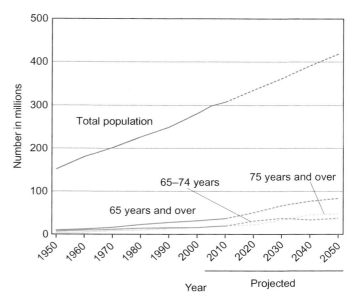

Fig. 7.2 Total population and older population: United States, 1950 to 2050. (From National Center for Health Statistics. [2009]. *United States, 2008 with chartbook,* Hyattsville, MD: National Center for Health Statistics Health.)

A study by Fuller-Iglesias (2015) found that older adults with a larger social network reported an increase in well-being and reduced caregiver burden that might be experienced. Marital status affects older persons in several ways. A married person is likely to live in a household with more income compared with an older adult who lives alone. Nutritional status is likely to be better for the married person than for the person living alone. Men benefit most from marriage. They do not cultivate the close friendships that women do outside the marriage, so the spouse is a vital friend and supporter (see Fig. 7.2 for information on population numbers from 1950 to 2050).

Traditionally, men have not engaged in cooking, cleaning house, mending clothes, and doing the laundry and thus miss these services when they lose their spouses. Also, older women outnumber older men, so many men marry again. In 2015 about 74% of men ages 65 to 74 were living with their spouses; 59% of those older than 85 were living with their spouses. For women, these numbers are much lower. Among women 65 to 74, 58% were married; the number dropped to 17% among those over 85 (Federal Interagency Forum, 2016).

Children continue to provide support to their older parents. About one-half of older adults in the United States live within 18 miles of a child, although this number varies depending on marital status and employment (Bui & Miller, 2015). Many visit at least weekly with children, and most talk on the phone at least once a week with a child. Female children are more likely to assist with hands-on care, whereas male children are more likely to provide business and financial support (Miller & Montgomery, 1990; Federal Interagency Forum, 2016). Although many families are separated by miles, children are concerned about their parents and attempt to arrange needed services for them. Area Agencies on Aging (AAAs), local social service organizations, and private care managers are some resources available.

Many older adults develop family-like relationships with younger neighbors or fellow church members. These relationships provide both emotional and practical support. Research is now considering the effect of older adults who have no family or close friends (*unbefriended elders*) for health care decision making (Pope, 2013; Weiss et al., 2012).

The financial status of older adults may affect their support systems. Older adults tend to feel an obligation to return favors. If someone does something for them, they want to be able to reciprocate. If they are financially unable to do this, they might withdraw so as not to place themselves in an embarrassing position. In addition, the inability to afford suitable clothing or to maintain clean clothing may cause them to withdraw or cause others to avoid them.

The emotional status of older adults may also affect support systems. It may be difficult for friends and family of depressed or negative older persons to maintain contact with them because of the exhibited behaviors of these older adults. A complete health history and physical examination should be conducted to rule out physical causes of emotional problems. Peer counseling, support groups, or professional assistance from mental health professionals, clergy, or a community nursing service may help them express feelings and concerns. Close friends may be able to help the person find the positive aspects of life. Spirituality and religious practice provide positive support for older adults. Participation in religious community events helps eliminate feelings of isolation and diminishes depression. Many older adults use song, prayer, or meditation to express feelings. For many, faith is an effective coping mechanism and provides hope and support through illness and loss (Brennan et al. 2012, Harris et al. 2013).

Benefits

In addition to Social Security, Supplemental Security Income, Medicare, and Medicaid, a variety of other benefits are available to older Americans, and these affect their socioeconomic status. Entitlement programs require the beneficiary meet certain guidelines of income or disability, whereas all older Americans may enjoy other benefits such as senior discounts.

Subsidized housing is available in almost every community in the nation. Most programs are supervised by the U.S. Department of Housing and Urban Development (https://portal.hud.gov/hudportal/HUD), but one major program is under the authority of the Farmers Home Administration of the U.S. Department of Agriculture. Once a person establishes eligibility, he or she may find suitable housing in existing rental buildings or public housing developments. The housing authority then contracts with the building owner for rent payments on the unit, or the renter pays a portion of the rent and the housing authority pays the rest. Eligibility standards differ for each program. An individual's income, assets, and expenses are all considered in determining eligibility.

Another entitlement program available to older adults is Supplemental Nutrition Assistance Program (SNAP). SNAP programs are usually administered by a state's Department of Health and Human Services. Eligibility and the amount of assistance a family may receive are based on family size, available income, and other resources. Nutritious meals are available at senior centers and meal sites throughout the country. A small donation is requested for each meal. If older adults are homebound, home-delivered meals are available in many communities.

Energy assistance is also available. This program is administered differently in each community. Information on the program can be obtained at the local senior center or utility company. Again, income requirements must be met.

In 2015, veterans older than age 65 numbered 20 million in the United States (U.S. Department of Veterans Affairs, 2016). Many of these veterans are eligible for veterans' benefits. The benefit used most often is access to Veterans Affairs (VA) health care. As the population has aged, the large number of veterans from World War II has put a strain on VA health care facilities. As a result, the VA has tightened the rules, making it more difficult to qualify for care. Veterans who require health care because of a war-related injury or disease are given priority. Those needing long-term care are now being referred back to their communities for that care until an opening is available in a VA health care facility. The influx of thousands of veterans of the Middle East wars has reopened the need for acute, subacute, and rehabilitation services for veterans. With the large numbers of amputees with a loss of one or multiple limbs, this group of veterans will become another large group needing senior care in the future (Fig. 7.3).

Area Agencies on Aging

Local AAAs provide several services for older adults. AAAs were created in 1973 as an amendment to the Older Americans Act. The purpose of the agencies is to plan and implement social service programs at the local level. Benefits available through these agencies include the following:
- Nutrition services through group meal sites and home-delivered meals
- Recreational opportunities
- Chore service
- Legal assistance
- Transportation
- Information and referral

It is not the purpose of the AAAs to duplicate the services of other agencies. In fact, these agencies try to encourage community-based services. However, if a service is not available, the AAA attempts to provide it.

Conservators and Guardians

When older adults are unable to handle their own financial affairs, a conservator may be appointed. This does not necessarily indicate that older persons are incompetent. For example, if a person is visually impaired, he or she may voluntarily select a conservator. However, if an older person is incompetent, the court selects the conservator. In either case, the conservator is legally appointed and court supervised.

A guardian may be appointed to handle decisions not related to financial matters. The guardian makes decisions about housing, health care, and other similar matters. This may be the same person as the conservator or a different person.

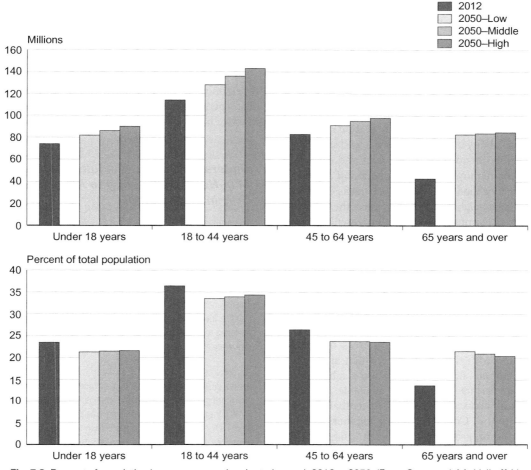

Fig. 7.3 Percent of population by age group and projected growth 2012 to 2050. (From Ortman, J. M., Velkoff, V. A., Hogan, H. [2014]. *An aging nation: The older population in the United States: Population estimates and projections,* [P25-1140] U. S. Census Bureau. Retrieved from https://www.census.gov/prod/2014pubs/p25-1140. pdf. Data from U. S. Census Bureau, 2012 Population Estimates and 2012 National Projections.)

A guardian or conservator may affect a person's socioeconomic status. By handling his or her assets wisely, a conservator may help an older person remain at least financially independent for longer than he or she could have otherwise. By supervising housing and health matters, the knowledgeable guardian may assist the older person in functioning at the highest possible level (Box 7.2).

ENVIRONMENTAL INFLUENCES

Environment contributes to a person's perception of life. Although the environment might not be noticeable unless it is uncomfortable, it does significantly affect emotional and physical health and well-being. *Environment* may be described as hot or cold, dark or light, hard or soft, and safe or dangerous. Environmental factors such as adequate shelter, safety, and comfort contribute to a person's ability to function well. These factors take on added importance to older adults with decreased functional abilities. Geographic location, transportation, housing, and safety issues as they relate to the environment of the older person are discussed in the following sections.

BOX 7.2   Definitions

Conservator—manages an older person's financial resources. An annual report must be filed with the court detailing how the funds were spent on the person's behalf.

Guardianship—is a legal relationship between an appointed person and the disabled individual. Based on state law the guardian can make legal, financial, and health care decisions. The guardian must file an annual report with the court on the individual's condition.

Durable power of attorney—is a document by which one person (the principal) gives legal authority to another (the agent or attorney-in-fact) to act on behalf of the principal. It is called *durable* because it continues to be effective even after the principal has lost capacity as a result of illness or injury. The two types of durable power of attorney are:

- **Durable power of attorney for financial matters**—this authority to handle financial affairs may be as broad or limited as the parties agree upon.

- **Durable power of attorney for health care decisions**—the agent or attorney-in-fact is not required to report actions on behalf of the principal to the court.

From Elder Law Answers. (2017). Guardianship and conservatorship. Elderlaw net. Inc. Retrieved 9/25/17 from www.elderlawanswers.com/guardianship-and-conservatorship-12096.

Geographic Location of Residence

Geographic factors influence individuals differently. Climate is important to older adults because they are susceptible to temperature extremes. Those who live in cold climates need adequate heat and clothing; those in temperate areas need cooling systems during warm seasons. Because older adults are concerned about accidental injuries, weather extremes such as snow and ice may contribute to isolation.

Whether a person lives in an urban or rural location may affect access to services, availability of support systems, and safety perceptions. Urban neighborhoods tend to be older and subject to change because of suburban migration. The notion of a friendly and convenient neighborhood in larger urban areas is rapidly declining. Such changing neighborhoods may affect the socialization of older adults because of the foreign and frightening atmosphere created. Most older Americans have lived in the same geographic area for more than 30 years and do not plan to move.

Older adults residing in rural areas have different problems. Geographic isolation may result in long distances between social contacts and services, and inadequate availability of transportation. However, the social supports obtained through churches, friends, and neighbors are often strong and reliable. Although a larger percentage of older adults in rural areas own their own homes compared with those in metropolitan areas, they occupy a disproportionate share of the nation's substandard housing. Also, fewer formal services are available for older adults living in rural areas (Jaffe, 2015; Rosenthal & Fox, 2000; Ziller, Lenardson, & Coburn, 2012). Neighbors helping neighbors, local clubs or groups, and church congregations often support older adults living in rural areas. However, some individuals enjoy being left alone and away from others and do not want outside involvement. Each community should set standards for being available if needed while permitting personal privacy for the older adults in their area.

Transportation

For many older adults, an automobile is a symbol of independence. In 2015, 47.8 million older adults still had their drivers' licenses (U.S. Department of Transportation, n.d.). In some areas, an automobile is necessary for transportation to shopping areas, medical facilities, and social centers. An older adult's self-assessment, along with care partner and clinician involvement, may determine when an older adult should stop driving. Driving is a form of independence and hard to "give up." Normal physical aging changes and effects of chronic health conditions may require adaptations (day time only driving; limited driving locations; Occupational Therapy consults for adapted devices). Resources are available from the CDC at https://www.cdc.gov/features/olderdrivers/index.html to help start the conversation on when to stop driving (U.S. Department of Transportation, n.d.). One challenge for older adults who do not drive is the availability of public transportation. In a report by AARP (n.d.) in 2015, depending on the size of the metropolitan city, 55% to 62% of older adults had poor access to public transit with 40% of rural older adults having no access to public transportation. Low-cost transportation is an objective of the Older Americans Act and is the responsibility of the AOA. Each AAA is charged with ensuring that transportation is available in its area. Obstacles preventing public transportation use include cost, scheduling, distance from home, availability in rural areas, lack of awareness of the service, and reluctance of some older adults to use public transportation.

Housing

A person's home is a true reflection of the individual, and for the older person, it signifies independence (see Evidence-Based Practice box).

EVIDENCE-BASED PRACTICE

Understanding Older Adults' Need and Acceptance of In-Home Monitoring to Allow Them to Safely Stay in Their Homes

Sample/Setting

Researchers looked at 37 older adults with early dementia and caregiver pairs. Caregivers included spouse, children, and a paid caregiver. Four pairs attended a focus group and 17 pairs participated in focused interviews and questionnaires.

Method

Researchers gathered qualitative and quantitative data using focus groups, interviewing, and questionnaires. In-home monitoring equipment that included motion sensors, contact sensors, smart light bulbs, and a remote control were installed in the older adult's home as part of the research.

Findings

Using descriptive statistics, it was found that less than half believed the monitoring system produced no change in their security (64% older adults, 87% caregivers). Live-in caregiving was provided by 81% of the respondents, and 19% reported providing more than 100 hours of care per week. In the interview portion, deductive analysis was used to develop the following themes: feeling cared for, feeling cared about, and suggestions for change. Feeling cared for had two subthemes: *a sense of control and order,* where the caregivers reported reassurance, and *a sense of being controlled,* which resonated more with the older adult reporting it felt intrusive, threatening, and insulting. Feeling cared about had three subthemes: *a sense of amusement,* where the older adults and caregivers used the monitoring equipment for entertainment with grandchildren or their pets; *a safe place in the home* was seen as reassuring to have the computer and monitoring equipment in the home setting; and the dominate subtheme of *no replacement for caregiver love,* where both sides reported how technology can never replace human interaction and interventions in emergencies. With suggestions for change, there were four subthemes. The first, *do not use a monitoring system on me,* was expressed by a small number of older adults who did not want "robots" working with them. The second, *do not abolish but embellish the system and make it simple,* reported the need to make it user friendly and adaptable to the older adults' needs. Some reported some errors in reporting data. The third subtheme, *do not standardize but customize,* provides more detail in the need to fit the system to the needs of the older adult and caregiver. For the last subtheme, *do not just monitor but prevent and act,* caregivers want the ability to prevent issues from occurring.

Implications

As the population of older adults rises, the number of older adults living in their homes with outside and live-in caregivers will only increase. Use of electronic monitoring equipment to monitor safety, medication reminders, and location devices will become more common. Understanding the older adult and caregiver needs can help them utilize the technology currently available and prompt more research and development of future needs.

From Epstein, I., Aligato, A., Krimmel, T., & Mihailidis, A. (2016) Older adults' and caregivers' perspectives on in-home monitoring technology. *Journal of Gerontological Nursing, 42*(6), 43-50.

After World War II, home ownership was encouraged by offers of insured mortgages and reductions in property taxes and mortgage interest to stimulate the postwar economy. Therefore home ownership was a goal many in the older generation sought to achieve (Burke & Flaherty, 1993). A person's house is often his or her major asset and, in fact, may be the only asset. The older person may have been born and raised there and then raised his or her own children. More often, a young married couple would have bought the house, raised the family in that same house, then continued to live there as a couple or after the death of the spouse.

The availability of features that support older adults' abilities to function in their homes is often a concern. Most homes occupied by older adults were designed for younger, more active individuals. Many older Americans have made modifications in their houses to adapt the environment to specific needs, but many others have yet to do this. For those who wish to remain in their homes but need funds for maintenance and repairs or even extra income, home equity conversion, also known as *reverse mortgage,* might be an alternative. In a reverse mortgage, the homeowner arranges for regular payments from a bank in exchange for the future transfer of the property to the bank.

Older adults who rent face the problem of locating affordable rental property. Once it is located, increases in rental cost may outpace older adults' fixed income. The tenant–property manager relationship may change as property management changes hands. Building structure and appliances may be inadequate to support independent functioning in many rental properties.

In urban areas, some older adults live in single-room-occupancy (SRO) hotels. SRO hotels offer single, sparsely furnished rooms with limited cooking facilities and communal bathrooms. Tenants are traditionally single persons with limited incomes, mental illness, or substance abuse problems. Typically, they have few contacts with other tenants and no family to provide support. An increasing incidence of chronic disease and disability may keep individuals from leaving their rooms and may further restrict the person's living environment. This may affect tenants' physical and mental health by isolating them and preventing access to services.

Safety may be a problem in all these living arrangements. Aging furnaces and appliances; worn linoleum or carpeting; poor lighting; unprotected stairs; lack of smoke alarms and assistive grab bars; and aging, sagging, or broken furniture all pose hazards for older adults. For those who decide to give up their houses, several options are available (Fig. 7.4). Independent housing options may include mobile homes, condominiums, and cooperatives. Increasingly, older adults are sharing houses. They may move in with family into a single room, an accessory apartment, or a portable housing unit on the family property. Others may team up with a group of older adults to buy or rent a house. Typically, in this situation, each person has a private room, and the living, dining, and kitchen areas are shared. Chores are also shared, and in some instances a housekeeper or manager for the house is hired. Some older adults take in boarders to help with expenses and household chores. The boarder is often a younger person who can do the "heavy" housework.

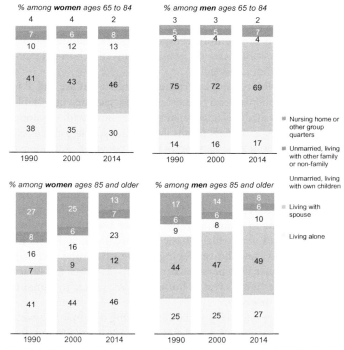

Fig. 7.4 Living situation by age and sex. (From Stepler, R. [2016]. Smaller share of women ages 65 and older are living alone. Pew Research Center, Washington, DC. Retrieved December 29, 2017, from http://www.pewsocialtrends.org/2016/02/18/smaller-share-of-women-ages-65-and-older-are-living-alone/.)

Home matching programs are gaining in popularity. These agencies locate and match persons who can share a home. Through interviews and screenings conducted by the agency, applicants are able to locate a compatible housemate. With home sharing, common areas of the house such as the kitchen and living room are always available for use. However, personal spaces such as bedrooms and bathrooms are private. Home sharing is not for everyone. Agreements need to be in writing regarding expectations from both renter and owner before entering into the arrangement (DiCarlo & Prosper, n.d.).

A growing number of older adults are living a mobile life. These are usually the young-old who live in warmer climates in the winter and cooler climates in the summer. They may own a home in one area and rent in another, or they may use a recreational vehicle as a second home. The real nomads are those who travel all year from place to place in recreational vehicles. As these older adults age and begin to have health problems, they often return to their home communities where long-established support systems of family and friends are available.

Retirement communities appeal to some. In a survey of older Americans, 25% of respondents lived in retirement housing (West, Cole, Goodkind, & He, 2014). These communities may have facilities for independent persons only, or they may include a variety of housing alternatives for those with various levels of dependency. Separate housing units for independent residents, congregate apartment units for those who need meals or housekeeping help, and nursing facilities for those who need more care may be found in a continuing care community.

Residents may move from one level to another as their needs change. Most such communities require a substantial entrance fee in addition to monthly charges. Benefits include activity programs and assistance with housekeeping and chores. Transportation is often included.

For those who require increasing assistance but are still able to function independently, assisted living facilities are viable options. These facilities have separate living units with common dining facilities and social rooms. Meals, transportation, housekeeping, and some laundry services are provided. Most have activity programs and encourage residents to socialize. Staff are present around the clock should a resident need help.

Board and care homes (also known as *sheltered housing, personal care homes, residential care facilities,* and *domiciliary care*) provide a home to a small number of older adults (usually four to six). Services vary widely. Basic rent usually includes room, board, laundry, and housekeeping. Some offer other services such as assistance with personal care for an additional fee. Board and care homes try to create a homelike atmosphere by remaining small and friendly.

Nursing care facilities are another housing option for persons no longer able to function independently. Residents of nursing care facilities depend on assistance with ADLs for survival. The resident occupies a single room or shares a room with one or more persons. The facility is staffed 24 hours a day with nursing professionals and trained personnel who provide needed assistance. The services on the premises generally include meals, personal laundry services, and a hair salon. Activity programming is provided to meet the needs of individual residents. Rehabilitation services are available as required by the residents.

In any assistive facility, it should be noted that residents are renting their room or part of their room, and to them, it is home. It should be arranged as residents wish and furnished with as many personal possessions as possible to provide a sense of historical continuity, belonging, identity, and comfort (Johnson, 1996). Staff should treat residents in a courteous and respectful manner. For example, a person would not go to a friend's house and turn on the television or rearrange the furniture without permission. By recognizing the importance of personal space, staff members reaffirm older adults' rights and enhance their sense of dignity.

When older persons change environments, stress caused by relocation is a possibility. Moving to any new setting is often associated with loss. Older persons may move because of loss of the spouse, health, home, or functional independence. Depression, withdrawal, confusion, increased dependency, lowered life satisfaction, and increased health problems may result from a move, especially if older adults are not prepared or the move is abrupt. If older persons make the decision to move after careful consideration over time, if they are familiar with the new environment, and if they can take cherished possessions with them, the move is made with minimum stress. Preadmission and ongoing assessments of residents and their spouses and family help ease the adjustment (Johansson, Ruzin, Graneheim & Lindgren, 2014). When the move is precipitous with little or no input from the older adults, it may have negative effects on health and may possibly increase the risk of death (Jusela,

Struble, Gallagher, Redman, & Ziemba, 2017; Sullivan & Williams 2017).

A segment of the older population is homeless. Data about homelessness are difficult to quantify because of the nature of the problem. Older adults in the homeless population are defined as those older than 50 because they tend to look and act 10 to 20 years older (DeMallie, North, & Smith, 1997). It is estimated that there were 44,000 homeless older adults in 2010. In 2015, 40% of adults 65 and older were at risk for being homeless with incomes below 200% of the poverty rate (Goldberg, Lang, & Barrington, 2016). In 2008 27% of the individuals residing in shelters were over the age of 50 (National Health Care for the Homeless Council, 2013). Women are increasing in numbers among the homeless older adult communities. Some have some source of income (Social Security Insurance [SSI]), but it is usually insufficient to obtain adequate housing. However, a significant number of homeless are between the ages of 50 and 62; they are not old enough for Medicare. Approximately 30% of homeless older adults have mental illness or dementia. Many may also suffer from chronic illnesses or visual and hearing problems. This population is seen to age 20 to 30 years more than their chronologic age. Impaired judgment may lead to financial mismanagement, eviction, or exploitation of property by others, leading to a loss of residence. Locating a new residence is difficult because of limited income, mental and physical health problems, and a lack of information about affordable housing. Often the only option is placement in long-term care settings that accept Medicaid (Goldberg, Lang, & Barrington, 2016).

Homeless older adults tend to have higher emergency department (ED) usage and require interventions that can connect them with needed services. Medical and mental assessments, emergency shelter, and long-term supervision may be required (National Health Care for the Homeless Council, 2013). Programs are being developed to offer Permanent Supportive Housing to persons older than 50 who are experiencing homelessness that involve case management and personal care services (Brown et al., 2013).

Whatever the housing status of the older person, it must be remembered that each person has a right to determine where to live unless he or she is proven incompetent for self-care. Nurses, as health care professionals, must respect that right and work with the person to maintain as much independence and dignity as possible.

The AARP provides many books on housing options, adaptations, and safety. Many are free or available at minimum cost. The federal government also provides materials on housing options through the Consumer Information Center.

Criminal Victimization

Elder victimization frequently goes unreported. Often, the perpetrator of the crime is someone known to the older adult: an acquaintance, family member, or friend (Box 7.3). Although older adults experience the lowest rates of victimization (3.6 victims per 1000 population, compared with 49.9 per 1000 population of 12- to 24-year-olds from 2003–2013), older adults appear to be particularly susceptible to crimes motivated by

BOX 7.3 Types of Crimes Committed Against Older Adults

The types of crimes most often committed against older adults include the following:

Financial/Material exploitation: illegal or improper use of funds, property, or assets

Sexual abuse or assault: sexual contact without consent

Murder/Homicide: taking of another person's life

Internet crime: illegal activity committed through the Internet (cybercrime)

Identity theft: stealing another's identity or personal data

Emotional/Psychological abuse: verbal or nonverbal means of inflicting pain and suffering

Physical abuse: physical force resulting in injury

Neglect: intentional or unintentional failure to fulfill obligations

Abandonment: desertion

From Morgan, R.E., Mason, B. J. (2014). *Crimes against the elderly, 2003-2013.* U.S. Annapolis Junction, MD: Bureau of Justice Statistics Clearinghouse. Retrieved from https://www.bjs.gov/content/pub/pdf/cae0313.pdf.

BOX 7.4 Older Adult Crime Victims

- 5% of older adults were victims of identity theft.
- Victimization rates are higher among older men than among older women. However, the rates of personal larceny with contact such as purse snatching are higher among older women.
- The rates of victimization are higher among older adults ages 65 to 74 than among those ages 75 or older.
- Older blacks are more likely than older whites to be victims of crime. However, rates of personal larceny that do not involve contact between the victim and offender are greater among whites.
- Older adults with the lowest incomes experience higher violence than those with higher family incomes. The highest rates of personal theft or household crime are seen among older adults with the highest family income.
- The highest rates of victimization for all types of crime are seen among older persons who are either separated or divorced (from among all marital statuses).
- Rates of victimization for all types of crime are highest among older residents in urban cities compared with suburban or rural older adults.
- Older renters are more likely than owners to experience both violence and personal theft. However, older homeowners are more likely than renters to be victims of household crime.

From Morgan, R.E., Mason, B. J. (2014). *Crimes against the elderly, 2003-2013.* U.S. Annapolis Junction, MD: Bureau of Justice Statistics Clearinghouse.

economic gain. Older adults are more likely to be injured in a violent crime. When injured, almost half the older victims receive medical care in a hospital (Morgan & Mason, 2014) (Box 7.4).

Whatever the actual risk, it is the perception of risk by older adults that affects their lifestyles (Policastro, Gainey, & Payne, 2015). Declining health and limited finances contribute to feelings of vulnerability. As a result, older persons may withdraw behind locked doors, becoming isolated. They may rarely leave home and may even refuse to permit services within the home. Such self-imposed social isolation has a negative effect on older adults' overall health and well-being.

Ross, Grossmann, and Schryer (2014) found no compelling evidence to support that older adults are more at risk than younger and middle age adults to be victims of consumer fraud. This calls into question a stereotype that older adults are often victims of fraud and scams. Just 5% of older adults are victims of identity theft, less than approximately 7.8% of adults aged 25 to 64 (Morgan & Mason, 2014). Just how often they are victimized is not known because older adults may not realize what has happened or may be too embarrassed to admit to victimization. After accounting for women being a higher proportion of the older population, they are abused at a higher rate than men. The nation's oldest-old (85 years or older) are abused and neglected at two to three times their proportion of the older adult population (Box 7.5).

In nearly 90% of elder abuse and neglect cases with a known perpetrator, it is a family member such as an adult child or a spouse (Acierno et al., 2010; National Center on Elder Abuse, 1998).

Older adults become victims for several reasons (Box 7.6). They are perceived as vulnerable. The ageist views of society

BOX 7.5 Consumer Frauds Perpetrated Most Against Older Adults

- **Health and medical frauds**—quackery or merchandising of drugs, health aids, or insurance
- **Mail order frauds**—merchandising through the mail that includes false or misleading information about the product
- **Income creation and investment frauds**—get-rich-quick schemes such as pyramid selling, work-at-home scams, the sale of fraudulent franchises, and real estate investment opportunities
- **Social psychological frauds**—merchandising of products and services that exploit fears by promising solutions to problems and loneliness
- **Con games**—schemes such as "pigeon drop," vacation lure, bank swindle, or oil well investment; usually perpetrated by professional con operators
- **Telemarketing scams**—sweepstakes or contests that require payment in advance to enter or claim a prize, with payment usually by credit card; merchandising that pressures people to buy without being sent written information about the products or services that are being sold

BOX 7.6 Reasons Older Adults Are Victims of Fraud

1. Older adults are often lonely and isolated. They are more likely to be at home and therefore available to both door-to-door and phone scams. They welcome con artists who are willing to spend time visiting.
2. Older adults have fewer resources to turn to for advice. They may be reluctant to "bother" friends, family, or professionals.
3. Older adults may be more susceptible to con artists who are polite, who appear knowledgeable, or who represent authority.
4. Older adults often have concerns about maintaining a comfortable lifestyle on a fixed income, affording good medical and long-term care, and providing for spouse and children.
5. Chronic illness leads many older adults to consider medical remedies offered by health fraud promoters.
6. Many older adults believe it is impolite to hang up on a caller or turn someone away at the door.

often portray older adults as weak and gullible; older adults may even see themselves this way.

Older adults are highly visible. Appearance advertises age. Predictability of daily routines and movements make older adults more vulnerable to criminals. They tend to rely on public transportation, and if they live in undesirable urban areas, they are vulnerable when walking to and from public transportation.

The level of dependency is an indicator for victimization. The more dependent an individual is or appears to be, the greater the risk of victimization. Some older adults have a diminished sense of sight or hearing. They may be unable to see well enough to recognize danger in the immediate area. They may not hear well enough to understand what is being said and may not ask for clarification. Loss of physical strength reduces the ability to fight back. With loss of cognitive ability, older adults are less able to reason rationally and are therefore vulnerable to fraud and abuse.

Older adults who have been victimized are likely to be confused, disoriented, fearful, or angry. When trying to assist older adult victims, the nurse should give the impression of nonhostile authority. Firm direction should be tempered with empathy. It is important to listen carefully to victims. This conveys an attitude of empathy and respect and helps the victims sort out the facts. The nurse must remain calm and reassure them that help will be provided throughout this crisis.

The nurse may need to allow time for victims to regain composure. One way to accomplish this is to distract them by asking for demographic information. Inquire about address, phone number, family, and other support systems to help calm them.

Follow-up procedures such as referral to a social service agency or victim support group or a phone call to let a victim know how the case is progressing help victims know that the professional cares. However, precautions must be taken to avoid encouraging excessive dependency.

Community resources for crime victims vary from one area to another. In some communities, victim and witness assistance programs may offer short-term immediate help. Support groups may help victims work through feelings of anger and fear. Volunteer action programs, such as a neighborhood watch, and prevention help older adults feel safer. The AAA is a good resource for information about assistance programs for older persons. Local law enforcement agencies and the Better Business Bureau are also available for help.

Every state has older adult abuse laws that include methods for reporting suspected abuse. Most state laws define abuse and provide a system of investigation. Many states maintain a registry of reports on suspected abuse. Some states mandate professionals working with older adults to report suspected abuse. In other states, reporting is voluntary. The local department of social services or AAA may provide information on reporting requirements.

It is important for older adults to have control over their environment and a voice in the community. Older adults who take responsibility for their own environment feel in control, and those who would victimize older adults recognize that attitude.

ADVOCACY

Older adults as a group are good advocates for their own special needs and interests. They write to legislators, consumer protection groups, government agencies, and other groups that control issues affecting older adults. By advocating for themselves, older adults are taking charge of their environment, their resources, their mental and physical health, and the future of all older adults. Older adults know from experience that they can make a difference.

Some older adults, however, are not able to plead their case. For example, older women were not taught to be assertive and stand up for themselves. The physically or mentally disabled, the undereducated, minority groups, those who do not speak the local language, and the financially disadvantaged all need assistance to take advantage of services and programs that may benefit them.

Advocacy is basic to professional nursing because it seeks to protect the human rights of patients within the health care system (Segesten & Fagring, 1996). Advocacy is an ongoing process as opposed to a single isolated event. As a moral concept, advocacy requires the nurse to speak up for the patient's rights and choices, to help the patient clarify his or her decision, and to protect the patient's privacy and autonomy in decision making (Potter, Perry, Stockhert, & Hall, 2017). The nurse is often the best person to initiate and provide that assistance. The nurse is trained to listen and assess, is aware of aging physiology and psychology, is familiar with community resources, and is motivated to serve older adults. The nurse may be the one member of the formal support group with the most complete information about older adults.

By listening to and consulting with older adults, the nurse develops an understanding of the values and perceptions that guide older adults' thoughts and feelings about life. The nurse forms partnerships with older adults to defend and promote their rights.

The nurse advocate determines what older adults want and then helps find ways to satisfy those desires. If staying at home is important to an older adult, the nurse can assist in enabling the person to stay home. By involving older persons in planning from the start, the nurse establishes partnerships that strengthen older adults' self-esteem, promote dignity, and enhance satisfaction with life.

Within the hospital or nursing facility, the nurse can advocate for older adults by clearly documenting their concerns and problems and any nursing care approaches. The nurse is in a key position to advocate for older adults by bringing problems to the attention of the physician, social services department, or administrator, as appropriate. In cases in which patient competency is questioned, it may be appropriate for the nurse to encourage the patient to obtain legal counsel or to insist on comprehensive evaluations by a qualified geriatric specialist to determine the cause of symptoms.

Whatever the setting, the nurse's advocacy for older adults is important to ensure older adults continue to control their lives. There are many organizations in the United States that advocate for older adults (see Appendix B). Local and regional organizations, including state departments also advocate for older adults of aging and the local AAA.

HOME CARE

Socioeconomic Influences

- Assess older adults' outside sources of income. Many supplemental policies cover excess costs that Medicare does not cover, thus ensuring more equipment and supplies for older adults.
- The goal of home care is to restore older adults' independence by teaching self-management of chronic conditions.
- Use social workers to identify community resources for financial assistance for homebound older adults.
- Arrange for meals to be delivered to homebound older adults, if necessary.
- Contact the Area Agency on Aging for referral to employment and legal services and social opportunities for older adults.

Environmental Influences

- Many meal delivery services provide food that has been prepared and frozen. Assess the functional ability and environment of older adults to ensure they can prepare the food that has been delivered (e.g., make certain they have a stove or microwave and electricity).
- Use a social worker to identify community resources for housing options for homebound older adults with multiple problems.
- Refer to the Area Agency on Aging for resources for home repair and transportation.
- Assess for signs of older adult abuse that may be manifested by consumer frauds. Report any suspicion of consumer fraud.
- Reduce potential for consumer fraud by decreasing social isolation in homebound older adults.

SUMMARY

Older adults' perceptions of the health care system in its entirety are influenced by experience. The nurse needs knowledge about the major historical events that have influenced the perceptions of today's older adults to understand their response to health care issues.

Socioeconomic issues, including income sources, prosperity or poverty, educational level, health status, and formal and informal support systems, affect the ability of older adults to comprehend and comply with health care regimens.

Older adults and their families may not be aware of community resources. The nurse should be aware of housing options, nutrition programs, transportation opportunities, respite programs, and legal assistance programs available in the community.

By understanding the eligibility requirements for benefits and entitlements, the nurse can assist older adults in receiving optimum services. By understanding the necessity for and the availability of conservatorship or guardianship, the nurse can help older adults and their families cope with diminishing abilities.

The sensitive nurse understands the concerns of older adults and supports and reassures them. The nurse can also encourage the older adults' informal support systems of friends and family. Often, the nurse can coordinate the formal and informal support systems for the maximum positive effect on the health and well-being of older adults.

Advocates for older persons, whether the older adults themselves or professionals in the field of aging, can help make socioeconomic and environmental factors a positive influence on older adults.

To provide maximum benefits to aging health care consumers, the nurse must understand the factors that influence health perception. To successfully work with older adults, the nurse must understand not only where they are but also where they have been.

KEY POINTS

- Socioeconomic factors such as income level, income sources, insurance coverage, benefits and entitlements, and educational level influence older adults' perceptions of their health and approach to health care.
- Environmental factors such as geographic location, housing, transportation, and perception of safety influence the availability of services, as well as older adults' knowledge and use of those services.
- The strength of the formal and informal support systems, including community services, medical care, spiritual resources, and family and friends, may affect the maintenance of independence for older adults.
- Experience has a strong influence on shaping value systems, coping skills, and perceptions. It is important to understand the events that occurred early in older adults' lives to understand their values and perceptions.
- Education has a strong positive influence on economic well-being and health status. Education prepares persons to make positive decisions that contribute to a higher perceived quality of life.

- Medicare is a federal program that provides health insurance for older adults. It consists of two parts: Part A is hospital insurance that helps pay for inpatient care and some follow-up care, and Part B is medical insurance that helps pay for physician services and some outpatient services.
- Medicaid is a state-administered program that uses federal funds to provide some medical expenses not covered by Medicare. Each state has different coverage and requirements. Medicaid is designed for persons with very low incomes and minimal assets.
- Older adults who are no longer able to handle their affairs or make decisions about their lives may benefit from a conservator, guardian, or durable power of attorney. A conservator manages financial resources, a guardian makes personal decisions, and a durable power of attorney is a document that names an agent to act on behalf of a person for a specific function, such as in making financial or health care decisions.
- The condition of homes and furnishings, the composition of neighborhoods, and the availability and type of

transportation affect the security and safety of older adults. Aging and outdated homes and appliances, worn furniture, and unreliable transportation may lead to accidents and injury. Deteriorating neighborhoods with changing populations may foster feelings of insecurity in older adults.

- Most communities in America have a variety of housing options to meet the needs of older adults, including single family residences, apartments, congregate housing, shared housing, retirement communities, assisted living facilities, and nursing facilities. Each option provides a different level of service to help older adults maintain maximum independence.

- Perceived victimization in older adults may result in increased suspicion and eventual withdrawal and isolation, which may have negative effects on health and well-being.
- A strong support system helps protect older adults from criminal victimization. Professional service providers, friends, and family may monitor older adults' environments and offer guidance when necessary. Community programs such as neighborhood watch programs and educational programs on victimization help older adults actively participate in crime prevention.
- Through advocacy, nurses can protect the dignity of older adults and improve their quality of life.

CRITICAL-THINKING EXERCISES

1. A 69-year-old chronically ill woman has few financial resources, no formal education, and only one child who can assist her. Her son is married, has four children, and a job that barely manages to support him and his family. Speculate how the woman's situation may affect her perception of her health care. In what ways can the nurse intervene to assist her?

2. A 78-year-old man is a retired banker whose wife died several years ago. He is able to perform all ADLs but needs help with meal preparation and transportation. He lives in a deteriorating neighborhood and no longer feels safe. He does not want to live with family members or completely give up his independence. What housing options would be appropriate for him? What advantages would such housing options offer over living alone?

REFERENCES

Acierno, R., Hernandez, M. A., Amstadter, A. B., Resnick, H. S., Steve, K., Muzzy, W., & Kilpatrick, D. G. (2010). Prevalence and correlates of emotional, physical, sexual, and financial abuse and potential neglect in the United States: The National Elder Mistreatment Study. *American Journal of Public Health, 100*(2), 292–297.

Administration on Aging. (2016). *A profile of older Americans: 2016.* Retrieved December 11, 2017 from https://www.giaging.org/documents/A_Profile_of_Older_Americans__2016.pdf.

American Association of Retired Persons (n.d.) Waiting for a ride: Transit access and America's aging population Retrieved on September 22, 2017 from http://www.aarp.org/content/dam/aarp/livable-communities/learn/transportation/waiting-for-a-ride-transit-access-and-americas-aging-population-aarp.pdf.

American Association of Retired Persons. (n.d.). *Driver safety program.* from, https://www.aarpdriversafety.org/?intcmp=dsp_hp_cw_saferdriving-.

American Association of Retired Persons. (2014). *Staying ahead of the curve 2013: The AARP work and career study.* Washington, DC: The Association.

American Eldercare Research Organization. (2016). *How to pay for nursing home care.* https://www.payingforseniorcare.com/longtermcare/paying-for-nursing-homes.html.

Balanced Budget Act of 1997, Pub. Law No. 105–33, § 1851(a), 1997.

Bekey, M. (1991). Dial S-W-I-N-D-L-E. *Mod Maturity, 34*(2), 31.

Boss, J. (2016). *What to expect for the 2017 housing market.* U. S. News & World Report Acessed September 26, 2017 from https://realestate.usnews.com/real-estate/articles/what-to-expect-for-the-2017-housing-market.

Brennan, P. L., Holland, J. M., Schutte, K. K., & Moos, R. H. (2012). Coping trajectories in later life: A 20-year predictive study. *Aging and Mental Health, 16*(3), 305–316.

Brown, R. T., Thomas, M. L., Cutler, D. F., & Hinderlie, M. (2013). Meeting the housing and care needs of older homeless adults: A permanent supportive housing program targeting homeless elders. *Seniors Housing and Care Journal, 21*(1), 126–135.

Bureau of Labor Statistics. (2017). *Labor force statistics from current population survey.* United States Department of Labor. Retrieved on December 30, 2017 from https://www.bls.gov/web/empsit/cpseea10.htm.

Bui, Q., & Miller, C. C. (2015). The typical American lives only 18 miles from mom. *The New York Times.* Retrieved December 11, 2017 from https://www.nytimes.com/interactive/2015/12/24/upshot/24up-family.html.

Burke, M., & Flaherty, M. J. (1993). Coping strategies and health status of elderly arthritic women. *Journal of Advanced Nursing, 18,* 7.

Centers for Disease Control and Prevention. (2016). *The state of aging & health in America 2013.* Atlanta, GA, Retrieved from https://www.cdc.gov/aging/pdf/state-aging-health-in-america-2013.pdf.

Cox, H. (1986). *Later life.* Englewood Cliffs, NJ: Prentice Hall.

DeMallie, D. A., North, C. S., & Smith, E. M. (1997). Psychiatric disorders among the homeless: A comparison of older and younger groups. *Gerontologist, 37*(1), 61.

DiCarlo, A. S., Prosper, V. (n.d.) *Match-up home sharing program.* Livable New York Resource Manual. Retrieved on December 30, 2017 from https://www.cdc.gov/features/olderdrivers/index.html.

Drug coverage (Part D). (n.d.). Retrieved September 19, 2017, from https://www.medicare.gov/part-d/.

Elder Law Anwers. (2017). *Guardianship and conservatorship.* Elderlaw net. Inc. Retrieved September 25, 2017 from www.elderlawanswers.com/guardianship-and-conservatorship-12096.

Ellis, J. R., & Simmons, T. (2014). *Coresident grandparents and their grandchildren: 2012 population characteristics.* (U.S. Department of

Commerce P20-576). Retrieved from United States Census Bureau website https://www.census.gov/content/dam/Census/library/publications/2014/demo/p20-576.pdf.

Epstein, I., Aligato, A., Krimmel, T., & Mihailidis, A. (2016). Older adults' and caregivers' perspective on in-home monitoring technology. *Journal of Gerontological Nursing., 42*(6), 43–50.

Fattah, E., & Sacco, V. (1989). *Crime and victimization of the elderly.* New York: Springer-Verlag.

Federal Interagency Forum on Aging-Related Statistics. (2016). *Older Americans 2016: Key indicators of well-being.* Retrieved on December 30, 2017 from Administration on Aging website https://agingstats.gov/docs/LatestReport/Older-Americans-2016-Key-Indicators-of-WellBeing.pdf.

Fuller-Iglesias, H. R. (2015). Social ties and psychological well-being in late life: the mediation role of relationship satisfaction. *Aging and Mental Health, 19*(12), 1103–1112. https://doi.org/10.1080/13607863.2014.1003285.

Ghilarducci, T. (2015). The Recession hurt American's retirement accounts more than anybody knew. *The Atlantic.* Retrieved December 30, 2017 from https://www.theatlantic.com/business/archive/2015/10/the-recession-hurt-americans-retirement-accounts-more-than-everyone-thought/410791/.

Goldburg, J., Lang, K., & Barrington, V. (2016). *How to prevent and end homelessness among older adults.* Justice in Aging. Retrieved September 19, 2017 from http://www.justiceinaging.org/wp-content/uploads/2016/04/Homelessness-Older-Adults.pdf.

Harris, G. M., Allen, R. S., Dunn, L., & Parmelee, P. (2013). "Trouble won't last always": Religious coping and meaning in the stress process. *Qualitative Health Research., 23*(6), 773–781. https://doi.org/10.1177/1049732313482590.

Jaffe, S. (2015). Aging in rural America. *Health Affairs, 34*(1), 7–10.

Johansson, A., Ruzin, H. O., Graneheim, U. H., & Lindgren, B. (2014). Remaining connected despite separation—Former family caregivers' experiences of aspects that facilitate and hinder the process of relinquishing the care of a person with dementia to a nursing home. *Aging and Mental Health., 18*(8), 1029–1036. https://doi.org/10.1080/13607863.2014.908456.

Johnson, C. (1992). Divorced and reconstituted families: Effects on the older generation. *Generations, 17*(3), 17.

Johnson, R. (1996). The meaning of relocation among elderly religious sisters. *Western Journal of Nursing Research, 18*(2), 172.

Josephson, A. (2017). *The average salary for Americans at every age. In Business Insider.* Retrieved December 11, 2017 from http://www.businessinsider.com/the-average-salary-for-americans-at-every-age-2017-4.

Jusela C., Struble L., Gallagher N. A., Redman R. W., Ziemba R. A. (2017). Communication Between Acute Care Hospitals and Skilled Nursing Facilities During Care Transitions: A Retrospective Chart Review. Journal of Gerontological Nursing, 43*(3)*:19–28. https://doi.org/10.3928/00989134-20161109-03.

Medicare 2017 costs at a glance. (n.d.). Retrieved September 19, 2017, from https://www.medicare.gov/your-medicare-costs/costs-at-a-glance/costs-at-glance.html.

Medicare Advantage Plans. (n.d.). Retrieved September 19, 2017, from https://www.medicare.gov/sign-up-change-plans/medicare-health-plans/medicare-advantage-plans/medicare-advantage-plans.html.

Miller, B., & Montgomery, A. (1990). Family caregivers and limitations in social activities. *Research on Aging, 12*(1), 72.

Morgan, R. E., & Mason, B. J. (2014). *Crimes against the elderly, 2003-2013 U.S.* Annapolis Junction, MD: Bureau of Justice Statistics Clearinghouse.

Mullin, E. (2013, February 26). How to pay for nursing home costs. *U.S. News & World Report.* Retrieved from http://health.usnews.com/health-news/best-nursing-homes/articles/2013/02/26/how-to-pay-for-nursing-home-costs.

National Center on Elder Abuse. (1998). *National elder abuse incident study.* U.S. Department of Health and Human Services-Administration on Aging. from http://www.ojp.usdoj.gov/ovc/assist/nvaa2000/academy/chapter14.htm.

National Coalition for the Homeless. (2012). http://www.nationalhomeless.org/factsheets/elderly.html.

National Health Care for the Homeless Council. (2013). Aging and Housing Instability: Homelessness among Older and Elderly Adults. *In Focus: A Quarterly Research Review of the National HCH Council.* Retrieved on December 30, 2017 from http://www.nhchc.org/wp-content/uploads/2011/09/infocus_september2013.pdf.

The Official U.S. Government Site for Medicare. (2017). *Nursing homes: Program of All-Inclusive Care for the Elderly (PACE).* Retrieved September 19, 2017, from https://www.medicare.gov/your-medicare-costs/help-paying-costs/pace/pace.html.

The Official U.S. Government Site for Medicare. (n.d.). *How do Medicare Advantage Plans work?* Retrieved September 19, 2017, from http://www.medicare.gov/sign-up-change-plans/medicare-health-plans/medicare-advantage-plans/how-medicare-advantage-plans-work.html.

O'Hara, B., & Caswell, K. (2013). *Health status, health insurance, and medical services utilization: 2010.* [Report]. Retrieved from United States Census Bureau website http://www.census.gov/prod/2012pubs/p70-133.pdf.

Ortman, J. M., Velkoff, V. A., & Hogan, H. (2014). *An aging nation: The older population in the united states, Population estimates and projections* [P25-1140]. U. S. Census Bureau.

Potter, P. A., Perry, A. G., Stockert, P. A., & Hall, A. M. (2017). *Fundamentals of nursing* (9th ed.). St. Louis: Elsevier.

Policastro, C., Gainey, R., & Payne, B. K. (2015). Conceptualizing crimes against older persons: elder abuse, domestic violence, white-collar offending, or just regular 'old' from crime. *Journal of Crime and Justice, 38*(1), 27–41. https://doi.org/10.1080/0735648X.2013.767533.

Pollak, R. A. (2010). *Most Americans live surprisingly close to their mothers.* Retrieved from http://news.wustl.edu/news/Pages/20720.aspx.

Proctor, B. D., Smega, J. L., & Kollar, M. A. (2016). *Income and poverty in the United States: 2015.* (U. S. Department of Commerce P60-256). Retrieved on December 29, 2017 from https://www.census.gov/content/dam/Census/library/publications/2016/demo/p60-256.pdf.

Projections of the labor force, 2014–24. (2015). *Career Outlook.* U.S. Bureau of Labor Statistics.

Pope, T. M. (2013). Making medical decisions for patients without surrogates. *New England Journal of Medicine, 369,* 1976–1978.

Richardson, J. (1996). The cohort factor—As important as diversity. *Aging Today.*

Rosenthal, T. C., & Fox, C. (2000). Access to health care for the rural elderly. *Journal American Medical Association, 284*(16), 2034–2036.

Ross, M., Grossmann, I., & Schryer, E. (2014). Contrary to psychological and popular opinion, there is no compelling evidence that older adults are disproportionately victimized by consumer fraud. *Perspectives on Psychological Science, 9,* 427–442.

Segesten, K., & Fagring, A. (1996). Patient advocacy—An essential part of quality nursing care. *International Nursing Review, 43* (5), 142.

Schulman-Green, D., Jaser, S., Martin, F., Alonzo, A., Grey, M., McKorkle, R, . . . Whittemore, R. (2012). Process of self-management in chronic illness. *Journal of nursing scholarship, 44*(2), 136–144. https://doi.org/10.1111/j.1547-5069.2012.01444.x.

Semega, F. L., Fontenot, D. R., & Kollar, M. A. (2017). *Income, poverty, and health insurance coverage in the United States: 2016.* (U.S. Department of Commerce P60-259). Retrieved from United States Census Bureau website https://www.census.gov/library/publications/2017/demo/p60-259.html.

Social Security Administration (n.d.) *Full Retirement Age: If you were born in 1960 or later,* Retrieved December 10, 2017, from https://www.ssa.gov/planners/retire/1960.html.

Sowa, A., Tobiasz-Adamdzyk, B., Topor-Mady, R., Poscia, A., & Ignazio la Milia, D. (2016). Predictors of healthy aging: Public health policy targets. *BMC Health Services Research, 16*(Suppl 5), 441–453. https://doi.org/10.1186/s12913-016-1520-5.

Strauss, W., & Howe, N. (1992). *Generations: The history of America's future, 1584 to 2069.* New York: William Morrow and Company.

Stepler, R. (2016). *Smaller share of women ages 65 and older are living alone.* Pew Research Center Accessed December 29, 2017 at http://www.pewsocialtrends.org/2016/02/18/smaller-share-of-women-ages-65-and-older-are-living-alone/.

Sullivan G.J., Williams C. (2017). Older Adult Transitions into Long-Term Care: A Meta-Synthesis. Journal of Gerontological Nursing, 43*(3),* 41–49. https://doi.org/10.3928/00989134-20161109-07.

U. S. Department of Transportation (n.d.) *Older drivers.* Retrieved September 22, 2017, from https://www.nhtsa.gov/road-safety/older-drivers.

U. S. Department of Veterans Affairs. (2016a) Veteran population projections 2017-2037. Retrieved on December 29, 2017 from https://www.va.gov/vetdata/docs/Demographics/New_Vetpop_Model/Vetpop_Infographic_Final31.pdf.

U. S. Department of Veterans Affairs. (2016b). *Federal benefits for veteran, dependents and survivors* [2016]. Washington, DC: Office of Public Affairs. Retrieved September 19, 2017 from Veterans Affairs website https://www.va.gov/opa/publications/benefits_book/2016_Federal_Benefits_for_Veterans.pdf.

Wapner, S., Demick, J., & Redondo, I. P. (1990). Cherished possessions and adaptations of older people to nursing homes. *International Journal of Aging and Human Development, 31*(3), 219.

Weiss, B. D., Berman, E. A., Howe, C. L., & Fleming, R. B. (2012). Medical decision-making for older adults without family. *Journal of American Geriatric Society, 60*(11), 2144–2150.

West, S. A., Cole, S., Goodkind, D., & He, W. (2014). *65+ in the United States: 2010 Special studies current population reports.* U. S. Government Printing Office.

Ziller, E. C., Lenardson, J. D., & Coburn, A. F. (2012). Health care access and use among the rural uninsured. *Journal of Healthcare for the Poor and Underserved., 23,* 1327–1345.

Zimmerman, E. B., Woolf, S. H., & Haley, A. (2015). *Understanding the relationship between education and health: A review of evidence and examination of community perspectives. Agency for Healthcare Research and Quality.* Rockville, MD. Retrieved December 11, 2017 from https://www.ahrq.gov/professionals/education/curriculum-tools/population-health/zimmerman.html.

8

Health Promotion and Illness/Disability Prevention

Ashley N. Davis, MSN, RN, PCCN

ⓔ http://evolve.elsevier.com/Meiner/gerontologic

LEARNING OBJECTIVES

On completion of this chapter, the reader will be able to:

1. Define health promotion, health protection, and disease prevention.
2. Identify models of health promotion and wellness.
3. Describe health care provider barriers to health promotion activities.
4. Describe patient barriers to health promotion activities.
5. Describe primary, secondary, tertiary, and quaternary prevention.
6. Plan strategies for nursing's role in health promotion and public policy.
7. Develop approaches to support the empowerment of older adults.

WHAT WOULD YOU DO?

What would you do if you were faced with the following scenarios?

• You are caring for an older adult male in the telemetry unit with a history of hypertension, chronic heart failure, chronic obstructive pulmonary disease, and smoker of 30 pack-years, who was admitted for shortness of breath and unstable hypertension. While performing a medication review, you realize that he is on multiple medications to control blood pressure, including metoprolol, lisinopril, and clonidine. When you ask him about his medication adherence at home, he states, "Sometimes I skip doses of my medication because I have trouble affording them all." What interventions can you do to help your patient?

• You are caring for an older adult female in the medical/surgical unit the day she received the news that there is a possibility her cancer, which has been in remission for 15 years, could be present again. The internist explained to her that he would like to order a CT, MRI, and multiple laboratory tests. Your patient refuses the tests, stating, "I have lived a long and happy life. Even if the cancer is back, I don't plan on wasting my time and energy on treatments. I would rather live each day to the fullest." The internist is adamant that your patient should follow through with the testing because the diagnosis has not yet been confirmed, thus a prognosis cannot be formed. What would you do?

ESSENTIALS OF HEALTH PROMOTION FOR AGING ADULTS

As baby boomers continue to age, it is inevitable that the United States will soon encounter the largest population of older adults thus far. This number will only continue to grow as new advancements in medications and technology are developed. According to the Centers for Disease Control

and Prevention (CDC, 2016), the life expectancy of men is 76.3 years, whereas the life expectancy of women is 81.2 years. Due to this increased life expectancy, the older adult will have more time to benefit from health promotion and disease prevention services that are often underutilized. The increased life expectancy also means that the cost of health care will continue to rise. The only way to offset the rising costs of health care is to utilize health promotion and disease prevention services so that the older adult can minimize or limit the effects of disease. Educating the older adult regarding these services is key to decreasing premature mortality and functional disability, increasing quality of life, and reducing hospital visits and health care spending.

Health promotion and disease prevention activities include primary prevention, or the prevention of disease before it occurs, and secondary prevention, or the detection and treatment of disease at an early stage. Weight management, exercising, managing hypertension, smoking cessation, managing alcohol use, increasing nutrients, and decreasing sun exposure can prevent cardiovascular disease, cerebrovascular accidents, cancer, diabetes, dementia, and falls (Troutman-Jordan & Heath, 2017). These measures, along with age-appropriate screenings, yearly health checkups, and vaccinations, are examples of how the older adult can maintain health and quality of life, and avoid or delay the onset or progression of potential disease (CDC, 2017a). However, ineffective health maintenance is high. Of individuals age 51 years and older, only 12.4% eat enough fruit and 10.9% eat enough vegetables, more than one-third of older adults are obese, one-third of older adults age 75 and older do not engage in physical activity, 8.4% of older adults smoke, and 8% are considered to be heavy drinkers (CDC, 2017b). Under the new American Heart Association (2017) hypertension guidelines, 7.2% of older adults ages 65

Previous authors: Sue E. Meiner, EdD, APRN, BC, GNP, and Dr. Jean Benzel-Lindley, PhD, RN.

to 74, and 3.8% ages 75 and older will require hypertension medication.

The Healthy People 2020 preventive objectives for older adults include increasing the number of older adults who utilize preventive services, increasing the number of older adults who engage in physical activity, and reducing the number of older adults who have moderate to severe functional disabilities (U.S. Department of Health and Human Services, 2014). To attain these goals, the nurse must first understand why the older adult does not adhere to therapeutic regimens or seek out preventive services. Recent findings suggest that affording and maintaining prescriptions; lack of transportation; lack of access to primary and specialty care; poor social infrastructure and coordination of services; limited assisted living and in-home care; and cultural, language, and other economic barriers may be the most prevalent factors for nonadherence (Averill, 2012). Other factors that influence health behaviors in older adults may include cognitive impairment, social support, sensory changes, environment, past experiences, competing priorities, and health literacy. Table 8.1 discusses these factors in greater detail.

Terminology

Health promotion is the science and art of helping people change their lifestyle to move toward a state of optimal health, with *optimal health* being a complete and holistic type of health, or health that focuses on mind, body, and spirit. The promotion of health provides the pathway or process to achieve this balance. Box 8.1 lists areas of health promotion that are the most relevant to older adults. A distinction should be made between health promotion and disease prevention. Health promotion addresses individual responsibility, whereas preventive services are fulfilled by health care providers. Disease prevention focuses

---

BOX 8.1 Areas of Health Promotion Most Relevant to Older Adults

- Increasing physical activity
- Smoking reduction/cessation
- Medication safety
- Spiritual health
- Cardiac health: heart healthy diet, exercise, and preventive medication use
- Psychological/Emotional/Mental health
- Environmental health
- Nutrition
- Social health
- Weight maintenance
- Driving safety

TABLE 8.1 Factors That Influence Health Behaviors in Older Adults

Factor	Description
Affording and maintaining prescriptions	The inability to afford or obtain medications can result in missed doses, cutting pills in half, or replacing them with alternative therapies. The older adult may have to choose between buying their medications, or buying other necessities, such as food.
Transportation gaps	Older adults may be unable to travel long distances to seek care services due to physical limitations or lack of access to transportation.
Care access	Access to care may be limited due to a lack of primary and specialty providers in the area, providers who do not speak their native language, and providers who do not establish meaningful relationships with them.
Poor social infrastructure and coordination of services	The lack of qualified case workers and services provided in long-term care settings can place the older adult at risk for ineffective health maintenance.
Limited assisted living and in-home care	Older adults who need extra assistance to maintain health may not be able to attain these services due to lack of facilities, home health companies, and staffing.
Cultural, language, health literacy, and other economic barriers	Avoidance of seeking preventive care can occur if the older adult's primary language is not English, or if they fear their culture and cultural practices are not completely understood by health care providers. Avoidance can also occur if the older adult is unable to fully comprehend their plan of care due to health care illiteracy. Most older adults rely solely on Social Security for retirement. This is not enough to sustain them, and they may have difficulty paying for services, along with having inadequate health insurance.
Cognitive impairment	As cognitive ability declines, the older adult may forget to take medications or to attend appointments. Cognitive impairments may exclude the patient from driving to obtain services. They often will not understand the effect this has on their future health.
Social support	Social support can encourage good health maintenance behaviors and can help increase access to healthy options.
Sensory changes	The ability to hear and see decreases with age. This can hinder the older adult from driving to receive preventive services and can affect their ability to engage in conversation with health care providers and engage in health maintenance behaviors.
Environment	Rural versus urban areas can determine how accessible health care is. Some living spaces do not facilitate exercise or other physical activities.
Negative past experiences	Negative past experiences with health care providers and staff can hinder the older adult from continuing to seek care.
Competing priorities	The older adult may have multiple other responsibilities that keep them busy and nonadherent to seeking preventive services or engaging in health maintenance behaviors.

Data from Averill, J. B. (2012). Priorities for action in a rural older adults study. *Family Community Health, 35*(4), 358-37; and Fernandez, D., Larson, J., & Zikmund-Fisher, B. (2016). Associations between health literacy and preventive health behaviors among older adults: Findings from the health and retirement study. *BMC Public Health, 16*, 596.

on protecting as many people as possible from the harmful consequences of a threat to health.

Primary prevention is the act of seeking out services and education to prevent disease. Primary prevention measures include activities that help prevent a given health care problem. Examples include immunization against diseases, receiving health-protecting education and counseling, promotion of the use of automobile passenger restraints, home safety, and fall prevention programs. Because successful primary prevention helps avoid the suffering, cost, and burden associated with injury or disease, it is typically considered the most cost-effective form of health care.

Secondary prevention is the act of detecting early disease and seeking care before the disease progresses or symptoms become apparent. Examples of secondary prevention activities include screening tests for cancer and findings of other diseases. If disease is detected early, interventions can be performed to maintain functional ability and increase the chance of survival and wellness.

Tertiary prevention is defined as activities that involve the care of established disease; attempts are made to restore the person to their highest function, minimize the negative effects of disease, and prevent disease-related complications.

Quaternary prevention involves limiting disability caused by chronic symptoms while encouraging efforts to maintain functional ability or reduce any loss of function through adaptation. Quaternary prevention also includes actions to protect from unnecessary medical treatment. The nurse, along with the older adult, should take into consideration comorbidities, present health status, prognosis, and the older adult's desire to continue treatment. Treatment for terminal disease can diminish quality of life instead of prolonging years of life and being beneficial.

MODELS OF HEALTH PROMOTION

This section provides an overview of three models of health promotion. The models selected represent current focus areas of health promotion programs and focus on behavioral aspects of health promotion.

The first is the Transtheoretical Model. This model focuses on an individual progressing through six stages of behavioral changes, including precontemplation (not ready to take action within the next 6 months), contemplation (getting ready to take action within 6 months), preparation (ready to take action immediately), action, maintenance, and termination. The amount of time an individual takes to complete each stage is variable (Prochaska, & Velicer, 1997).

The second is the Health Belief Model. This model was created to help determine certain behaviors that attributed to and prevented participation in preventive measures. This model tries to compare how a person perceives the value of attaining a health goal or service, and how likely a specific action will help to attain that goal. The three key elements include modifying factors such as demographics, sociopsychologic variables (social class, peer pressure), structural barriers (knowledge about the disease, prior experience with the disease), and cues to action (guidance, media advertisements, individual perceptions

(susceptibility, the impact of illness, perceived threat), and the likelihood of action (perceived benefits versus barriers) (Galloway, 2003).

The third and final model is Nola Pender's Health Promotion Model. This model presumes the participant will take an active role in developing and deciding the context in which health behaviors will be modified. The model focuses on achieving a high level of well-being, eventually resulting in self-actualization. Key elements include: (1) perceived health and control of health, (2) perceived personal decision making (self-efficacy, and (3) benefits and barriers to behaviors that promote health (Dehdari, Rahimi, Aryaeian & Gohari, 2014; Galloway, 2003).

The use of a model in the study, research, or practice of nursing provides a framework and guide for implementing interventions in many areas, not only gerontology.

BARRIERS TO HEALTH PROMOTION AND DISEASE PREVENTION

As a vulnerable population, older adults face many barriers to health promotion and disease prevention. The older adult population has often been neglected from receiving health promotion and disease prevention as it was believed that they would not benefit from these services, and they would not change their lifestyle (Golinowska, Groot, Baji, & Pavlova, 2016). Many factors that place the older adult at risk for having ineffective health maintenance are also considered barriers. There are barriers to health promotion from the older adult's perspective and the health care professional's perspective. Both will be addressed here.

Health Care Professionals' Barriers to Health Promotion

Previously it was thought that, due to age, the older adult would not have much more time to benefit from health promotion services; thus health promotion was not a priority of health care providers and was limited to activities that could produce immediate effects. Health care providers did not see the older adult making these drastic changes to their lives. Current research in this area is lacking at the time of this publication. However, one barrier can be due to the fact that because the older adult typically has a wide range of multiple comorbidities, it may be difficult for health care providers to create more individualized health promotion programs for multiple older adults (Golinowska, Groot, Baji, & Pavlova, 2016).

Older Adults' Barriers to Health Promotion

Patient barriers unrelated to health beliefs include lack of transportation, financial limitations, lack of insurance coverage, lack of availability, language barriers, and health illiteracy. Transportation is not readily available to many urban and rural older adults, or it is cost prohibitive. In addition, older adults incur the cost of many preventive services because Medicare does not cover them all (Table 8.2). This may be hard on the fixed, limited income of many older adults. Providers in their area may be scarce, especially for older adults living in rural communities. Older adults might also face a barrier when attempting to

TABLE 8.2   Secondary Prevention

Medicare Reimbursement

Screening/ Preventive Procedure	Medicare Guidelines for Reimbursement
Pneumococcal infection vaccination	The initial vaccine and the second vaccine 1 year later, then every 5 years.
Influenza vaccination	For all older adults annually.
Hepatitis B vaccination	Older adults at a medium or high risk of contracting hepatitis B: once per lifetime.
Mammography	Women older than 40 years are covered for one screening every 12 months.
Papanicolaou test and pelvic examination	Pap test and screening pelvic examination (including clinical breast examination) are covered at 2-year intervals. Annual examinations are covered for women identified as high risk.
Colorectal screening	Annual fecal occult blood test for those older than 50 years. Flexible sigmoidoscopy every 4 years for those older than 50 who are higher risk. For those not high risk, every 10 years. Colonoscopy every 2 years for those at high risk. For those not high risk, every 10 years. Screening barium enemas every 2 years for those older than 50 years and are high risk. For those not high risk, every 4 years.
Osteoporosis	Bone density scans every 2 years for those who meet one or more criteria.
Diabetes screening	Up to twice a year for those at high risk.
Glaucoma screening	Annually for those at high risk (20% and copayment required).
Smoking cessation counseling	Up to 8 face-to-face visits per year.
Physical examination	Within the first 12 months of joining Medicare, then every 12 months.

Data from Medicare.gov. Your medicare coverage. Retrieved May 4, 2018, from https://www.medicare.gov/coverage/preventive-and-screening-services.html.

seek out a provider who is sensitive and understanding of their own language, ethnicity, and culture. Health illiteracy can also place the older adult at risk for medication misunderstandings and nonadherence. All of these barriers could result in delays in receiving care, the inability to receive preventive services, and increased hospitalizations and cost (U.S. Department of Health and Human Services, 2014).

As technology advances, telehealth is coming to the forefront. Telehealth can include videoconference, telephone calls, and other forms of technology for the older adult to communicate with health care providers. Telehealth benefits those who face barriers to accessing traditional means of health care and can be cost effective. However, there are barriers and disadvantages to telehealth, including legal barriers regarding care across state lines, educating the older adult population on the use of telehealth methods, issues with telecommunications connections in rural areas, lack of technological skills/devices and reliability of devices, and attitudes regarding less hands-on care and less ability to assess the patient and home environment (Kelly et al., 2016). One study found that telehealth helps to lower mortality and emergency admission rates among the general population (Steventon et al., 2012). Telehealth should be utilized as a complementary service, along with traditional face-to-face care for the older adult to fully benefit from this service. A current review of the literature suggests that, although telehealth does not correlate with reduced expenditure, an increase in social inclusion and medication adherence has been found (Husebo & Storm, 2014)

Other factors that can affect health promotion are related to ethnicity, culture, and language. Although current research is lacking in this area, nurses need to be aware of the differences in the older adult population in the areas we serve to provide individualized nursing care.

HEALTH PROTECTION

The Healthy People initiative, created by the U.S. Department of Health and Human Services (2014), provides our country with guidelines and objectives for how to achieve a set of new goals every 10 years to obtain optimal health for the entire population. The underlying premise of *Healthy People* is that the health of the individual is almost inseparable from the health of the larger community, and the health of every community in every state determines the overall health status of the country. The overarching goals are to attain high-quality, long lives that are free of preventable disease, disability, and injury; eliminate disparities; create social and physical environments that promote health; and optimize quality of life across the entire life span. At the time of this publication, new guidelines and objectives for *Healthy People 2030* have not been developed.

DISEASE PREVENTION

Primary Preventive Measures

Primary preventive measures refer to some specific action taken to optimize the health of an individual by helping him or her become more resistant to disease or to ensure that the environment will be less harmful. Overall guidelines for Medicare coverage of primary prevention are reviewed in Tables 8.2 and 8.3. Providing ongoing education to the older adult population about the importance of these measures, and that Medicare pays for them, may increase the likelihood of being utilized.

Yearly well visits with a primary care provider are recommended for assessment of the older adult, as well as screening and counseling opportunities. Not only are well visits important to the overall health of the older adult, so too are routine dental visits. Too often dental visits are not prioritized due to lack of access to care, cost, and discomfort associated with examinations. However, poor dental hygiene can lead to dental caries, pain, infection, gum disease, tooth loss, decrease in nutritional intake, cardiovascular disease, and cancer. Due to barriers that

TABLE 8.3   United States Preventive Services Task Force Guidelines for Primary and Secondary Health Promotion Activities for Older Adults

Health Promotion Activity	Recommendation	Supportive Evidence
Mammography	Annually starting at age 50 and continue every 2 years until age 74.	Based on randomized trials. Supportive evidence does not correlate with recommendation as higher stage tumors are reduced with annual screening.
Cervical smear test	Screening is not recommended after age 65 if not high risk, and the previous 3 consecutive screenings were negative within the last 10 years, with the most recent being within the last 5 years.	Based on randomized trials and evidence that harm outweighs benefit.
Colorectal cancer screening	Screening is recommended from age 50-75. After age 75, screening should be based on the individual and prior screening history. Fecal occult screening is recommended yearly, whereas a colonoscopy is recommended every 10 years.	Based on randomized trials. Supportive evidence does not correlate with recommendation as evidence supports fecal occult screening every 2 years. Colonoscopy benefits appear to outweigh the risks.
Prostate examination	Evidence is insufficient to support screening with prostate-specific antigen (PSA) testing in men older than 70 years of age. Men 55-69 years of age should be evaluated on an individual basis.	Based on insufficient evidence to support the benefits of screening. The risks appear to outweigh the benefits.
Osteoporosis screening	Screening is recommended for women age 65 and older. Evidence is insufficient in evaluating men for osteoporosis.	No current evidence evaluates the risks versus benefits.

Data from US Preventive Services Task Force. (2018). USPSTF A and B Recommendations. Retrieved May 2, 2018 from https://www.uspreventiveservicestaskforce.org/Page/Name/uspstf-a-and-b-recommendations/.

prevent the older adult from seeking dental care, a culture change is needed to educate and train primary care providers to perform basic oral examinations, provide education, use dental sealants and fluoride varnish, and make dental referrals when needed (Bussenius, Reznik, & Moore, 2017).

Immunizations are strongly recommended for older adults, especially for those older adults considered to be high risk due to multiple comorbidities and suppressed immune systems, and those who are institutionalized. The recommended immunizations include an annual high-dose influenza vaccination by October of each year and a tetanus vaccination (Td or Tdap) every 10 years. In 2016 only 66.7% and 67.6% of older adult men and women received the influenza vaccine, respectively. These statistics closely correlate to those who received the pneumococcal vaccine. All older adults should receive a vaccination against pneumococcal infection starting at age 65. Ideally, the older adult should first be given an initial dose of PCV13, followed by a dose of PPSV23 a year later. The CDC recommends that all older adults who are considered to be high risk receive a dose of PPSV23 every 5 years (CDC, 2016). Taking into account that the majority of the older adult population is considered to be high risk, it is prudent to educate all older adults about receiving the pneumococcal vaccine every 5 years. The shingles vaccine is recommended once for everyone over the age of 60, whether they have or have not previously had chickenpox or shingles. However, older adults with suppressed immune systems should not receive it due to the live virus within the vaccine (CDC, 2016).

Smoking cessation increases life expectancy, reduces the risk of developing or further complicating heart and lung disease, reduces the risk of cerebrovascular accident and erectile dysfunction, reduces respiratory symptoms, and reduces risk of cancer. These benefits can significantly increase the quality of life of the older adult. Immediate benefits to quitting smoking include a reduction in heart rate and blood pressure and decreased carbon monoxide levels in the blood (World Health Organization [WHO], 2018). There have been recent debates regarding whether or not alcohol or wine consumption has cardiovascular benefits. One study found that increasing alcohol intake in older adults results in cardiotoxic effects (Goncalves et al., 2015). Recent findings also suggest that light alcohol consumption can correlate with a higher level of episodic memory (Downer et al., 2015). Wine can benefit the heart due to the antioxidants found in the grape skin, causing an increase in HDL cholesterol (American Heart Association, 2015). Alcohol use can result in increased accidents such as falls and motor vehicle accidents, can lead to increased suicide rates, can further complicate other medical conditions, and can affect medications. Due to the risks versus benefits of drinking alcohol, it would be safer for the older adult to increase their HDL through eating more antioxidant-rich fruits and vegetables and exercising.

Polypharmacy occurs when the older adult is prescribed or takes multiple medications concurrently that have the possibility of interacting with one another, or when the older adult is taking medications that are not necessary to their conditions. This occurs when care is sought out from multiple providers who do not collaborate in the care of the older adult. Polypharmacy can result in increased hospitalizations and health care spending due to adverse drug events, drug interactions, nonadherence to medications due to lack of financial resources or misunderstandings, a decline in functional ability including incontinence and subsequent falls, decreased nutritional intake, and cognitive impairment. As patient advocates, nurses have the responsibility of assessing the older adult's medication during transitions in care and institutionalizations. A medication review needs to focus on all medications including those prescribed, over the counter, and illicit. The list of medications should be reviewed for necessity, interactions, contraindications, and overmedication or overdosing. The American Geriatrics Society Beers Criteria for Potentially Inappropriate Medication Use in Older Adults (2015) was updated to include a more comprehensive list of medications that should be avoided in the older adult population, and those medication doses that should be reduced to prevent further complications with certain diseases that should be monitored closely. This updated list also includes medications that should be dose adjusted depending on kidney function, and drug-drug interactions. This list should be considered during all medication reviews. To reduce the risk of polypharmacy, the nurse should educate the older adult to keep a complete list of all medications and include dose, route, frequency, and reason for taking the medication. The older adult's medication list should also have their pharmacy information located on it. The older adult should also keep a list of all health care providers and their contact information. A copy of these lists should be kept in a wallet or purse for accessibility.

As older adults, especially women due to decreased estrogen, are more susceptible to osteoporosis and fractures, prevention should also focus on bone health. Close to 50% of older adult women who are at high risk for osteoporosis and fractures do not use calcium supplements, vitamin D supplements, or specific osteoporosis treatment (Castro-Lionard et al., 2013). A wide range of evidence also indicates that proper nutrition and exercise can help prevent fractures related to osteoporosis. The U.S. Preventive Services Task Force (USPSTF, 2018) recommends that all women age 65 and over be screened for osteoporosis with bone measurement testing at least once, but there is no benefit to additional screening up to 8 years after the initial screening.

Secondary Preventive Measures

Secondary prevention focuses on screening or detection of early disease. The idea here is that finding a problem early allows more effective treatment. In addition, secondary prevention includes techniques of primary prevention used on older adults who already have the disease in an effort to delay progression, for example, encouraging people who have had a heart attack to stop smoking and start exercising.

Annual screening recommendations for older adults should be made on an individual basis with the use of the guidelines and evidence-based recommendations from USPSTF. Screening for prostate cancer, for example, is not recommended for men 70 years or older, and cervical cancer screening is not recommended for women after the age of 65 if they have had negative testing previously. Evidence for the need to routinely screen for ovarian or skin cancers, or cognitive impairment, is insufficient. The personal beliefs of the individual older adult and knowledge about how results will be used must be taken into account as well. Screening is not recommended for the older adult if they are unwilling to seek treatment for whatever disease they may have. In this case screening may do more physical, emotional, and financial harm than good (Table 8.4).

Screening for osteoporosis, hyperlipidemia, depression, and obesity is recommended, but evidence is lacking as to how often screening should occur. It is important to note that, at the time of this publication, many topics on the USPSTF website are currently being updated. Thus some recommendations may be outdated.

Tertiary Preventive Measures

Tertiary prevention aims to prevent or reduce long-term effects of a disease by helping patients manage their conditions and chronic symptoms. Many older adults receive tertiary care through specialists who manage complex conditions, such as a cardiologist or pulmonologist. A good example of tertiary prevention is rehabilitation after stroke or support groups, pain management programs, and follow-up examinations to identify cancer recurrence or metastatic disease. Common conditions encountered by older adults that require tertiary care include stroke, cardiopulmonary disease, chronic pain, and cancers.

THE NURSE'S ROLE IN HEALTH PROMOTION AND DISEASE PREVENTION

As health care continually changes, nurses must be vigilant to stay up to date on current trends and continue to be lifelong learners, increasing their knowledge base to a wide variety of topics, including current recommendations for health promotion and disease prevention, as well as current practices and policies and technological advances. Nurses often have many demands placed on them during their shift. This can lead to the nurse becoming task oriented. Instead, nurses need to remember to remain care oriented and maintain caring attitudes while providing individualized care for each older adult. Nursing as a caring profession is in a unique position to facilitate human changes by assisting others in self-development and the active sharing of information with vulnerable populations such as older adults.

Requisite Knowledge

The knowledge needed for health promotion and disease-prevention activities includes an understanding of basic human needs, human behavior, human growth and development, ethnic and cultural diversity in aging, economic patterns, basics of political action, and, most important, behavior change and the challenges associated with behavior change among older adults. Moreover, the nurse must have a comprehensive understanding of health policy and the effect of advocacy in obtaining needed care for older individuals. Specifically, knowing what services are covered under Medicare for older adults and understanding and participating in advocacy for appropriate services are essential to providing optimal nursing care.

Health promotion activities on behalf of older adults are performed at local, regional, or national levels. At the local level, case management is an initial step toward individualizing the needs unique to the older adults in a single community. Case management may be initiated through the case managers or social workers in acute care facilities, Area Agencies on Aging (AAAs), community centers for older adults, church groups, or the local health department. Additionally, nurses can volunteer for guest speaker opportunities or as community health nurses to spread information regarding illness prevention and health promotion.

TABLE 8.4   Advantages and Disadvantages to Health Promotion Activities

Activity	Advantages	Disadvantages
Alcohol use	Social benefit Increases high-density lipoprotein (HDL) cholesterol Decreased mortality after heart attack Decreased risk of congestive heart failure Associated with lower C-Reactive Protein levels and decreased frailty Associated with better memory	Health complications: gastrointestinal, cardiac, dermatologic, cognitive, and neurologic; impairment of nutritional state Risk of depression Risk of falls Drug interactions
Cervical smear test	Increased risk of cervical cancer occurs with age and may result in unpleasant symptoms if untreated Older women may not have had regular cervical smear tests done and may want this early screening Only pursue, as per United States Preventive Services Task Force (USPSTF) guidelines, if woman is willing to undergo treatment if disease is identified	Life expectancy after diagnosis is small in women over the age of 70. Less risk if the patient is not sexually active Testing is difficult and uncomfortable in older women, particularly those who are no longer (or never were) sexually active
Mammography	Increased risk of breast cancer occurs with age If detected, these tumors are generally estrogen-receptor positive and treatable Only pursue if woman is willing to undergo treatment if disease is identified	False-positive results can place the older adult at risk for additional harmful tests and procedures. Tumors in older women tend to be slow growing Discomfort and pain associated with mammography Stress and anxiety over investigations Multiple complications of treatment (e.g., lumpectomy, radiation, or hormone treatment)
Prostate cancer screening	Increased risk for prostate cancer occurs with age Only pursue if man is at increased risk and is willing to undergo treatment if disease is identified	With diagnosis, only a small to no reduction in mortality was found.
Fecal occult blood test (FOBT)	Early detection of a growth that could cause the older adult discomfort and affect quality of life if left untreated Easily performed at home with no discomfort and no preparation FOBT has better predictive value in older adults than in the young adult population	False-positive results may cause additional testing and anxiety for patient
Colonoscopy	Screening is infrequent Diagnostics and treatments can be performed immediately Lower colorectal cancer mortality rate Past the age of 75 should only be screened if the older adult is at increased risk and willing to undergo treatment if disease is identified	Bowel preparation can cause complications (such as dehydration and electrolyte imbalances), discomfort, and pain Risk of perforation and bleeding Risk of complications from sedation
Diet monitoring	Decreasing cholesterol with dieting reduces morbidity and mortality from cardiovascular disease Focus should be on eating a healthy diet low in fat and high in fruits, vegetables, and grains, which can facilitate maintenance of ideal weight while decreasing the risk of cancer and other diseases	Restriction in diet may affect quality of life Restricted diets can result in unneeded weight loss and failure to thrive
Reducing/Quitting smoking	Smoking is associated with increased risk of sudden cardiac death and myocardial infarction Financial incentive May decrease peripheral vascular problems and may prevent further lung disease and chronic obstructive pulmonary disease	Nicotine replacement therapy can cause major cardiovascular adverse events Electronic cigarettes (vaping) have not been extensively studied
Exercise	Positive physical health benefits Positive mental health benefits Decreased fatigue Decreased pain Maintain weight Maintain physical function	None

Regionally, the nurse may begin to get involved by contacting the state department on aging regarding rules and regulations for care for older adults. Another way to get involved is to attend and interact at state legislature meetings and hearings. Some states have set aside an annual nurse lobby day in the state capitol. Meetings with legislators may provide an opportunity for the nurse to express opinions related to health care issues.

At the national level, action may begin with personal education involving public policy. This education may include (1) becoming aware of current and changing social policy; (2) studying the facts and the opinions of leaders on all sides of an issue; (3) speaking to civic groups, political party groups, and senior citizen groups; (4) testifying before the legislature as an advocate for healthy aging; (5) being informed on the issues and knowing social and political hot buttons; (6) putting the best foot forward with lobbying; (7) studying issues and techniques of negotiation and compromise; and (8) actively supporting the role of the advanced practice nurse working with physicians as a primary provider of health care.

Assessment

When assessing the older adult, the nurse must look at potential health hazards to identify risk factors for illness or injury. Contributing risk factors include habits, lifestyle patterns, personal and family medical histories, and environmental conditions. An example of an environmental risk factor is the lack of access to opportunities to engage in enjoyable social and physical activities; other examples include the physical presence of clutter, poor lighting, and poor footwear, which put the older adult at risk of falling.

Assessment for health promotion and disease prevention begins with collecting data about the older adult. The assessment must be developed in a comprehensive manner. Subjective data are obtained through the health history. Objective data are obtained through a complete physical examination and observation. To obtain a complete, nursing-focused assessment, the nurse must have an understanding of functional health patterns of aging. Eleven of the basic functional health patterns of older adults that are important to assess are as follows:

1. Self-perception or self-concept pattern
2. Roles or relationships pattern
3. Health perception or health management pattern
4. Nutritional or metabolic pattern
5. Coping or stress-tolerance pattern
6. Cognitive or perceptual pattern
7. Value or belief pattern
8. Activity or exercise pattern
9. Rest or sleep pattern
10. Sexuality or reproductive pattern
11. Elimination pattern

The following discussion expands on these identified functional health patterns, which are based on Gordon's typology of 11 functional health patterns (Gordon, 2009). Each pattern presented includes a description and subjective and objective assessments. Within each of these patterns, the nurse needs to identify the older adult's knowledge of health promotion, ability to manage health-promoting activities, and value given to activities of health promotion.

Self-Perception or Self-Concept Pattern

Description: This pattern encompasses a sense of personal identity; body image, attitudes toward self, and view of self in cognitive, physical, and affective realms; and expressions of sense of worth and self-esteem. Perceptions of self should be explored with direct questions, asked with sensitivity. Emotional patterns may be identified during this exploration of perceptual patterns.

Subjective: Determine the older adult's feelings about his or her competencies and limitations, particularly with regard to preventive health behaviors and behavior change, withdrawal from previous activities, self-destructive actions, excessive grieving, and increased dependency on others. Assess changes in eating, sleeping, and physical activity patterns. Explore the person's perception of his or her identity, self-worth, self-perception, body image, abilities, successes, and failures.

Objective: Identify verbal and nonverbal cues related to these subjective data. Verbal cues elicit feelings about self (strengths and limitations), and nonverbal cues include a change in personal appearance. Using tools for assessing anxiety and depression is helpful.

Roles or Relationships Pattern

Description: This pattern encompasses the achievement of expected developmental tasks. Basic needs for communication and interactions with other people, as well as meaningful communications and satisfaction in relationships with others, are examined.

Subjective: Determine family structure, history of relationships, and social interactions with friends and acquaintances. Focus on health behavior beliefs and activities among his or her social network. Assess the perceived reasons for unsatisfactory relationships, and identify attempts to change patterns and outcomes.

Objective: Examine the family or friend dynamics of interdependent, dependent, and independent practices among members.

Health Perception or Health Management Pattern

Description: This pattern encompasses the perceived level of health and current management of any health problems. Determine health maintenance behaviors and the importance the older adult places on these behaviors.

Subjective: Determine the level of understanding of any treatments or therapy required for management of health deficits or activities, including the possible sources of reimbursement and concerns about costs; include assessment of performance of activities of daily living (ADLs), instrumental activities of daily living (IADLs), or both.

Objective: Observe for cues that indicate effective management of deficits, including the physical environment in which the patient resides. Assessment should include information about prior health promotion activities (e.g., mammography, vaccinations) and management during sickness and wellness. A home safety checklist should be utilized. Focus specifically on barriers to engaging in these behaviors and what has prevented them from participating in the past.

Nutritional or Metabolic Pattern

Description: This pattern encompasses evaluation of dietary and other nutrition-related indicators.

Subjective: Determine the older adult's description, patterns, and perception of food and fluid intake, and adequacy for maintaining a healthy body mass index. It may not be realistic to obtain an accurate 24-hour food and fluid recall;

however, the nurse could possibly obtain information on how meals are prepared, who prepares them, and approximately how much is eaten during a typical day. Identify any recent weight loss or gain, and identify food intolerances, fluid intake, and gastrointestinal symptoms. Consider also access to grocery stores and restaurants and opportunities for obtaining appropriate heart healthy food sources.

Objective: Observe general appearance and various body system indicators of nutritional status. Note height, weight, and fit of clothes. If possible, observe the older adult eating a meal. A nutritional examination tool may also be used.

Coping or Stress-Tolerance Pattern

Description: This pattern encompasses the patient's reserve and capacity to resist challenges to self-integrity and his or her ability to manage difficult situations. The ability to successfully tolerate stress through personal coping behaviors is important to incorporate into any health promotion plan. Of equal importance is the identification of the older adult's support systems.

Subjective: Assess ways to handle big and little problems that occur in everyday life. Determine the past and current amount of stress present in the older adult's life. Discuss any recent losses and the methods used to deal with those specific situations. Identify any stress-reducing activities that are practiced and the usual results obtained.

Objective: Observe for the use of coping skills and stress-reducing techniques, and note their effectiveness. Consider evidence of health-promoting options for stress reduction (e.g., exercise).

Cognitive or Perceptual Pattern

Description: This pattern encompasses self-management of pain, the presence of communication difficulties, and deficits in sensory function. Modes include vision, hearing, taste, smell, touch, and compensatory assistive devices used when a deficit exists. Pain should be assessed as well as how the older adult treats this pain.

Subjective: Inquire about difficulties with sensory function and communication, and assess for any cognitive changes or pain.

Objective: Assess usual patterns of communication, and note the patient's ability to comprehend. Also note the ability to read, hear the spoken word, smell, and distinguish tactile sensations and tastes. Simple screening may be done using cognitive assessments.

Value or Belief Pattern

Description: This pattern encompasses elements of values, beliefs, and spiritual well-being that the older adult perceives as important for a satisfactory daily living experience and the philosophic system that helps him or her function within society.

Subjective: Identify the older adult's values and beliefs about health and health promotion activities. Explore also for spirituality, and note any special emphasis on how this influences

health promotion behaviors (e.g., "God will take care of health promotion and disease prevention.").

Objective: Determine what is important to the older adult's life with regard to overall goals (e.g., long life versus quality of life) and to support coping strategies. Note any references made to spirituality or religious affiliation and practices, as well as choices and decisions that are determined by values, beliefs, and spiritual practices.

EVIDENCE-BASED PRACTICE

Spiritual and Religious Coping Is Correlated With Improved Quality of Life

Background
Institutionalization can be stressful, resulting in decreased quality of life, and compromising physical and mental health. Spiritual and religious coping (SRCOPE) has not been investigated regarding quality of life in nursing home patients.

Sample/Setting
Fifty-three older adults were studied from a nursing home in the State of Minas Gerais, Brazil. Ninety-five older adults were studied from a nursing home in Santa Rita do Sapucai, Brazil. This study was undertaken in June and July 2010.

Methods
In this cross-sectional study, nursing home residents were interviewed regarding quality of life, using the WHOQOL-BREF instrument, and spiritual and religious coping, using the SRCOPE scale.

Findings
Institutionalized older adults use religious and spiritual coping strategies. SRCOPE frequently correlated with quality of life.

Implications
Encouraging religion and spirituality can help the older adult cope and adapt to health problems, while decreasing symptoms of depression.

From Vitorino, L., Lucchetti, G., Santos, A., et al. (2016). Spiritual religious coping is associated with quality of life in institutionalized older adults. *Journal of Religious Health, 55,* 549-559.

Activity or Exercise Pattern

Description: This pattern encompasses information related to health promotion that encourages the older adult to achieve the recommended 30 minutes daily of physical activity on most days of the week.

Subjective: Screen for safety related to exercise and physical activity, using screening measures such as the Exercise Assessment and Screening for You (EASY) (Chodzko-Zajko, Resnick, Barbara, & Ory, 2012). The EASY determines whether it is safe for an individual to immediately start an exercise program and, depending on comorbid conditions, matches the individual with a recommended exercise program that can be printed out from online resources, thus providing him or her with a hard copy to use. In addition, assess daily routines and activities, including patterns of exercise, leisure habits, recreation, and hobbies; and inquire about any limitations or changes in these patterns. Identify IADLs that are practiced with or without difficulty. Inquire about the older adult's typical day. Assess for pain, fatigue, and fear of falling and fall potential, and conduct a fall history.

Objective: Obtain vital signs and conduct cardiopulmonary and musculoskeletal system assessments. Assess self-care ability by observing and asking the patient about self-care activities such as bathing, dressing, toileting, and feeding, if possible. Note the use of adaptive tools or equipment. Complete the EASY with the older individual, and provide appropriate exercise resources.

Rest or Sleep Pattern

Description: This pattern encompasses the sleep and rest patterns over a 24-hour period and their effect on function. Assess rest and sleep patterns of the older adult for usual pacing of activities with consistent energy reserves that do not require immediate rest.

Subjective: Assess usual sleep patterns, including bedtime and arousal time, quality of sleep, sleep environment, and distribution of sleep hours within a 24-hour period. Inquire about episodes of insomnia and deterrents to sleep such as pain; anxiety; depression; use of pharmacologic agents such as caffeine, over-the-counter agents that may cause arousal, alcohol, and prescribed medications such as some treatments for depression; lack of exercise; and inappropriate sleep hygiene. Identify the time and circumstance for regular rest periods. Record any activities associated with a rest period.

Objective: Have the patient keep a sleep diary that includes naps and rest periods. If possible, observe daily activities and note the effects of sleep disturbance on functional ability.

Sexuality or Reproductive Pattern

Description: This pattern encompasses the older adult's behavioral expressions of sexual identity.

Subjective: Assess the patient's satisfaction or dissatisfaction with current circumstances related to sexual function and intimacy, including perceived satisfaction or dissatisfaction with sexuality or sexual experiences.

Objective: Discuss any current sexual relationship. When none is present, elicit the meaning this has for the patient's overall emotional and physical well-being.

Elimination Pattern

Description: This pattern encompasses bowel and bladder excretory functions.

Subjective: Assess lifelong elimination habits and excretory self-care routines. Inquire about the patient's perception of normal bowel and bladder functions, and explore specifically for recent changes in usual bowel and bladder functions. Assess for the effect of elimination patterns and the ability to control elimination on quality of life and on participation in health promotion activities such as exercise.

Objective: Perform abdominal and rectal examinations; external genitalia and pelvic examinations may be indicated. Note daily intake of food, particularly amount of dietary fiber, and assess total fluid intake over a 24-hour period.

A nurse's approach to completing thorough functional health assessments of older adults must be positive and reassuring. Many of the necessary assessment tools needed to complete a thorough examination of the older adult can be found at ConsultGeri.org. Permitting older adults to be active participants in this process is important to the success of gaining insight into their needs.

Planning

The role of the nurse in promoting health among older adults relies on organized planning. The planning may begin by exploring older adults' personal ideas and beliefs concerning health needs. Reading current literature provided by the U.S. Department of Health and Human Services, the National Institutes of Health, the National Institute on Aging, or the CDC will help the nurse keep abreast of the latest specific health promotion recommendations. Internet addresses for these and other information centers are provided at the end of this chapter.

Being well versed on current health policy information will safeguard patient rights. The nurse is then able to inform older adults of significant policy changes as soon as they are made at the highest (federal) level. Often, the dissemination of health policy is slow, and news reaches the recipient long after the fact. When policies are retroactive or are to be enforced on a certain date, passing the information on to older adults may be crucial to their health and well-being. Moreover, it will help establish and maintain a trusting relationship. Encouraging an older adult to engage in screening activities not covered by Medicare, for example, may cause a financial hardship for the older individual and may decrease his or her level of trust in the nurse.

Planning involves an understanding of behavior change and behavior change theories such as the theory of self-efficacy. The theory of self-efficacy states that the stronger the individual's belief that he or she can perform a behavior and the stronger his or her belief in a positive benefit to performing the behavior, the more likely he or she is to engage in the given activity. Recommendations to facilitate behavior change are shown in Table 8.5.

Implementation

Implementation may begin by adopting a proactive stance toward an action plan for health promotion of the older adult. Seeking activities, locations, and means for disseminating health promotion information to a group of older adults is an example of implementing a proactive stance. Proactive activities may have benefits as well as liabilities. The benefits include an early approach to a problem that has not been acted on previously. Annual health promotion screenings may be incorporated into programs that provide vaccinations for older adults and may include screenings for cancer, diabetes, osteoporosis, and macular degeneration, as appropriate. Likewise, monthly health talks provided in senior centers, senior housing sites, or continuing care retirement communities may be a useful way to repeatedly advocate and educate about health promotion activities such as exercise, prevention of falls, or safe medication use. Check locally for programs in a specific location within the United States.

TABLE 8.5   Interventions to Motivate Individuals to Change Behavior Using a Social–Ecologic Model

Component	Description	Example of Interventions
Intrapersonal	Demographics (age and gender)	Encouraging self-efficacy and empowerment through education of disease management and injury prevention
	Physical health and function	
	Psychosocial factors (e.g., mood, resilience), cognitive status, pain, fatigue, fear	
Interpersonal	Social support	Social support through groups of like-minded people or family and friends
	Verbal encouragement	Use of verbal encouragement to strengthen self-efficacy and outcome expectations
	Goal setting & motivation	Goal identification (e.g., losing weight, being able to walk the dog) and recognizing motivators for completing goals
	Rewards	Identifying personal rewards for completing goals
	Role models	Exposure to others engaging in similar behaviors
Environment	Physical environment	Wide range of social physical activities and safe walking areas. Accessible healthy food choices or restaurants
Policy	Disease prevention guidelines	Use of guidelines in educational interventions to encourage adherence
	Institutional policies and procedures	
	Laws	

Evaluation

Evaluation involves determining the effectiveness of your care plan. Was the older adult able to achieve the mutually established goals? The nurse should consider why these goals were or were not achieved and coordinate with the older adult to establish appropriate and realistic revised goals and realistic steps to achieve them.

SUPPORTING EMPOWERMENT OF OLDER ADULTS

Nurses can provide a bridge between the theory of health promotion and the implementation of health promotion, health protection, and preventive services. The active participation of nurses in encouraging older adults to set health promotion goals aimed at maintaining the best possible health, function, and quality of life throughout the rest of their life span is essential. Nurses can participate in collaborative interactions with other health care professionals and organizations such as the American Geriatrics Society to establish guidelines, write papers, and influence policy.

Learning about community resources and local, state, and federal programs that can provide information or services to older adults and then disseminating the information to older adults in a variety of settings are legitimate nursing roles. Health promotion programs and activities may be provided to individuals, small groups, and larger groups where older adults congregate. Many retirement centers, assisted living facilities, church groups and organizations, Salvation Army centers, and senior citizen centers look for speakers on a variety of health subjects. In most cases, the managers of these facilities welcome nursing students or registered nurse volunteers to present health promotion or disease prevention programs on a regular basis. Empowering older adults requires initiative, organization, and knowledge of the major areas of health promotion relevant to this population and governmental policies.

Nurses should ideally use an individualized approach to health promotion when working with older individuals. This approach focuses on providing appropriate education both formally in health promotion classes and informally during health care visits. The education should provide current recommendations for health promotion activities, such as receiving vaccinations and screenings, and help older patients decide what health behaviors they want to engage in. This type of individualized approach has the advantage of being cost effective in that screening is not performed if the individual does not have any intention of acting on the results; in addition, individualized health promotion increases adherence to positive health behaviors such as smoking cessation and exercise.

SUMMARY

As the older adult population in the United States continues to increase due to technology and medical advancements, emphasis must be placed on the practices of health promotion, health protection, and disease prevention in order to increase functional mobility, increase quality of life, reduce health care spending, and decrease premature mortality. Three models of health promotion activities were presented. The Transtheoretical Model provides insight to behavioral changes in stages. The Health Belief Model helps to determine behaviors that prevent participation in preventive measures. Nola Pender's Health Promotion Model presumes a collaborative effort by the participant and the health care professionals involved.

Barriers to participation in health promotion activities are complex issues involving both provider and participant. Barriers to health promotion and disease prevention programs were addressed in terms of health beliefs and factors not related to health beliefs, including a lack of transportation and financial burdens. The goals identified in the *Healthy People* initiative in regard to health protection were presented.

Primary, secondary, tertiary, and quaternary measures of disease prevention were provided. Primary prevention includes immunizations and counseling programs. Prevention counseling is aimed at healthful living, such as smoking cessation. Other areas of concern include home and medication safety. Secondary prevention focuses on detection and early treatment of disease. Tertiary prevention involves eliminating or slowing the progression of symptoms, whereas quaternary prevention deals with limiting disabilities caused by chronic conditions and overmedicalization.

The nurse's role in health promotion and protection or prevention of disease may be based on a framework of functional health patterns. Data about these health patterns are best obtained when the nurse completes a comprehensive nursing assessment of each of the areas of function using positive and reassuring communication.

The best results are achieved when the nursing process is used to assess, plan action through goal setting, and implement a plan for health promotion, behavior change related to health care activities, or disease prevention followed by evaluation. Suggested health promotion activities that offer several levels of commitment are available to nurses who wish to become involved in social policy or political action. Involvement in a proactive movement to increase health promotion is possible at local, regional, and national levels. The use of an individualized approach and the empowerment of older adults to make their own health care decisions will help them achieve their optimal level of health, function, and quality of life.

KEY POINTS

- Health promotion, health protection, and disease prevention will continue to be a national goal with the *Healthy People 2030* initiative.
- Models of health promotion are available to guide the change process in establishing a local, regional, or national effort.
- Psychosocial factors, health beliefs, environmental factors, transportation, finance, ethnic and cultural influences, and a sense of futility may be barriers to health promotion.
- Health protection targets five areas: (1) unintentional injuries, (2) occupational health and safety, (3) environmental issues, (4) food and drug safety, and (5) oral health.
- Primary prevention focuses on immunizations and health screening activities.
- Secondary prevention focuses on detection of occult disease.

- Tertiary prevention focuses on preventing the progression of symptoms while facilitating rehabilitation.
- Quaternary prevention deals with overmedicalization.
- The nurse's role in health promotion begins with a complete health assessment using the functional health patterns framework; this should incorporate an individualized approach for each patient.
- Using the nursing process in health promotion activities provides a sound foundation for success.
- Involvement in health promotion activities may be at the local, regional, and national levels.
- Using an individualized approach and empowering older adults to determine the level of health promotion and primary, secondary, tertiary, and quaternary prevention activities will help them achieve their optimal quality of life.

CRITICAL-THINKING EXERCISES

1. Several nurses have volunteered to give influenza vaccines to older adults at a senior center. When the line to receive the injections slows down, one nurse notices a table of four older women playing cards. None of the women have approached the vaccine registration table. What actions, if any, are appropriate for the volunteer nurses in this situation? Does the fact that the nurses are volunteers change any potential course of action?

2. You are caring for a stable 93-year-old woman in the acute care setting. Her 70-year-old daughter has been staying with her throughout her admission. You notice the daughter appears to be disheveled and tearful. The daughter states she has not been sleeping due to the stress of managing her mother's care at home and now her present illness. What actions would you suggest the nurse take with regard to the daughter? If an action is taken, when is it the appropriate time to do so?

REFERENCES

American Heart Association. (2015). *Alcohol and heart health.* Retrieved January 2018 from: http://www.heart.org/HEARTORG/HealthyLiving/HealthyEating/Nutrition/Alcohol-and-Heart-Health_UCM_305173_Article.jsp#.WnBzlK3MygQ.

American Heart Association. (2017). *Nearly half of U.S. adults could now be classified with high blood pressure, under new definitions.* Retrieved January 2018 from https://news.heart.org/nearly-half-u-s-adults-now-classified-high-blood-pressure-new-definitions/.

Averill. (2012). Priorities for action in a rural older adults study. *Family Community Health, 35*(4), 358–372.

Beers Criteria Update Expert Panel. (2015). American Geriatrics Society 2015 updated Beers Criteria for Potentially Inappropriate Medication Use in Older Adults. *Journal of American Geriatrics Society, 63,* 2227–2246.

Bussenius, H., Reznik, D., & Moore, C. (2017). Building a culture of oral health care. *The Journal for Nurse Practitioners, 13*(9), 623–627.

Castro-Lionard, K., Dargent-Molina, P., Fermanian, C., et al. (2013). Use of calcium supplements, vitamin D supplements and specific osteoporosis drugs among French women aged 75-85 years: patterns of use and associated factors. *Drugs Aging, 30, 1029–1038.*

CDC. (2016). *2017 recommended immunizations for adults: By age.* Retrieved January 2018 from: https://www.cdc.gov/vaccines/schedules/downloads/adult/adult-schedule-easy-read.pdf.

CDC. (2017a). *Mortality in the United States, 2016.* Retrieved January 2018 from: https://www.cdc.gov/nchs/products/databriefs/db293.htm.

CDC. (2017b). *Tables of summary health statistics.* Retrieved January 2018 from: https://www.cdc.gov/nchs/nhis/shs/tables.htm.

Chodzko-Zajko, W., Resnick, B., & Ory, M. (2012). Beyond screening: tailoring physical activity options with the EASY tool. *Translational Behavioral Medicine, 2*(2), 244–248.

Dehdari, T., Rahimi, T., Aryaeian, N., & Gohari, M. (2014). Effect of nutrition education intervention based on Pender's Health Promotion Model in improving the frequency and nutrient intake of breakfast consumption among female Iranian students. *Public Health Nutrition, 17*(3), 657–666. Retrieved July 19, 2018, from http://journals.cambridge.org/action/displayAbstract?fromPage=online&aid=8826685.

Downer, B., Jiang, Y., Zanjani, F., & Fardo, D. (2015). Effects of alcohol consumption on cognition and regional brain volumes among older adults. *American Journal of Alzheimer's Disease & Other Dementias, 30*(4), 364–374.

Fernandez, D., Larson, J., & Zikmund-Fisher, B. (2016). Associations between health literacy and preventive health behaviors among older adults: findings from the health and retirement study. *BMC Public Health, 16,* 596.

Galloway, R. (2003). Health promotion: causes, beliefs and measurements. *Clinical Medicine & Research, 1*(3), 249–258.

Golinowska, S., Groot, W., & Paviova, M. (2016). Health promotion targeting older people. *BMC Health Services Research, 16*(5), 345.

Goncalves, A., Jhund, P., Claggett, B., et al. (2015). Relationship between alcohol consumption and cardiac structure and function in the elderly: the atherosclerosis risk in communities study. *Circulation Cardiovascular Imaging, 8*(6).

Gordon, M. (2009). *Functional health topology.* Retrieved May 2009, from http://www.zwo.nhl.nl/hbov/telemark/gordon.html.

Husebo, A., & Storm, M. (2014). Virtual visits in home health care for older adults. *The Scientific World Journal, 2014.*

Kelly, J., Reidlinger, D., Hoffmann, T., & Campbell, K. (2016). Telehealth methods to deliver dietary interventions in adults with chronic disease: a systematic review and meta-analysis. *The American Journal of Clinical Nutrition, 104*(6), 1693–1702.

Prochaska, J., & Velicer, W. (1997). The transtheoretical model of health behavior change. *American Journal of Health Promotion, 12* (1), 38–48.

Steventon, A., Billings, J., Doll, H., et al. (2012). Effect of telehealth on use of secondary care and mortality: findings from the whole system demonstrator cluster randomized trial. *BMJ, 344.*

Troutman-Jordan, M., & Heath, L. (2017). The impart of health education and health promotion on management of chronic health conditions in older adults: opportunities for innovation. *Activities, Adaptation, & Aging, 41*(1), 1–13.

U.S. Department of Health Science and Human Services. (2014). *Healthy people 2020.* Retrieved January 2018 from: https://www.healthypeople.gov/2020/topics-objectives/topic/older-adults.

U.S. Preventive Services Task Force. (2017). Recommendations for primary care practice. Retrieved January 2018 from: https://www.uspreventiveservicestaskforce.org/Page/Name/recommendations.

Vitorino, L., Lucchetti, G., Santos, A., et al. (2016). Spiritual religious coping is associated with quality of life in institutionalized older adults. *Journal of Religious Health, 55,* 549–559.

World Health Organization. (2018). *Fact sheet about health benefits of smoking cessation.* Retrieved January 2018 from: http://www.who.int/tobacco/quitting/benefits/en/.

WEBSITES

AARP. http://www.aarp.org.

International Counsel on Active Aging. http://www.icaa.cc.

Administration on Aging. http://www.aci.gov/about-acl/administration-aging.

Alliance for Aging Research. http://www.agingresearch.org.

American Geriatrics Society. http://www.americangeriatrics.org.

American Society on Aging. http://www.asaging.org.

BenefitsCheckUp. http://www.benefitscheckup.org.

Centers for Disease Control and Prevention. http://www.cdc.gov.

Healthy People 2020 & 2030 documents online. http://www.healthypeople.gov.

Information on Wellness Activities. http://www.dshs.texas.gov/Wellness/Activities/.

Medicare. http://www.medicare.gov.

National Council on Aging. http://www.ncoa.org.

National Health Information Center. http://www.health.gov/nhic/.

National Institute on Aging. http://www.nia.nih.gov.

National Institutes of Health. http://www.nih.gov.

U.S. Department of Health and Human Services. http://www.hhs.gov.

U.S. Preventive Services Task Force. http://www.uspreventiveservicestaskforce.org.

PART III

Influences on Quality of Life

9

Nutrition

Neva L. Crogan, PhD, ARNP, GNP-BC, ACHPN, FAAN

http://evolve.elsevier.com/Meiner/gerontologic

LEARNING OBJECTIVES

On completion of this chapter, the reader will be able to:

1. Differentiate between the various factors that influence nutritional risk in older adults.
2. Differentiate between a nutritional screen and a nutritional assessment.
3. Identify the steps and core data collection elements of a nutritional assessment.
4. Describe the changes in nutritional requirements for older adults.
5. Describe the role of nutritional support in nutritional therapies.
6. Identify major dietary guidelines and recommendations for older adults.

WHAT WOULD YOU DO?

What would you do if you were faced with the following situations?

- You are caring for an 85-year-old older adult in a long-term care unit. The elder begins coughing while eating his lunch meal. He has a recent history of stoke. What actions do you take?
- You are making the first home health care visit to evaluate a 92-year-old older woman who lives alone. You notice that she is very thin (weighs 88 pounds), so you check the refrigerator for food options. The refrigerator has very little food in it and most of what is in there is outdated. How can you provide nutritional support to your patient?

INTRODUCTION

Food means family, togetherness, and fond memories of times past. For the older adult, food means life, comfort, and security. These factors influence an older adult's perceived quality of life (Evans, Crogan & Armstrong, 2005). Consuming a well-balanced diet in a family atmosphere leads to optimum nutritional status and enhanced quality of life. Inversely, nutritional risk, lack of food, and enjoyment of food are negatively correlated with quality of life (Edfors & Westergren, 2012). For the older adult in a nursing home or institutionalized setting, the lack of a homelike setting could negatively influence their desire to eat and ultimately lead to functional decline, weight loss, and malnutrition (Evans et al., 2005). Older adults living in the community may suffer from loneliness and depression, leading to weight gain or loss, and ultimately malnutrition. Food is an important aspect of life; eating too much or too little can negatively affect an older adult's quality of life and affect their overall health. This chapter will review those nutrition topics important to older adults and their overall health.

FACTORS INFLUENCING NUTRITIONAL RISK IN OLDER ADULTS

Many factors influence nutritional risk in older adults. These factors can be classified into three major groups: social, psychological, and biological. Social factors include isolation, loneliness, poverty, and dependency (Loreck, Chimakurthi, & Steinle, 2012), but of those, poverty is the most significant cause of weight loss and malnutrition in older adults. Even with the changes in Medicare that assist older adults to pay for expensive medication, there are still many medications that are cost prohibitive for older adults with limited incomes. Other social factors include lack of caregivers, lack of transportation, culturally determined food habits, and widowhood and bereavement (Brownie, 2013). In a 2015 population-based study of 1402 older adults, those with significantly higher nutritional risk were those who were older, female, unmarried/widowed/divorced, residing in special housing (nursing home/assisted living), and functionally impaired (Naseer & Fagerstrom, 2015). Additionally, an older adult's inability to shop, cook, or feed themselves can lead to weight loss and malnutrition (Keller, Beck, & Namasivayam, 2015).

Psychological factors that influence nutritional risk in older adults include depression, anxiety, and dementia. Of those, depression is one of the most common treatable causes of weight loss. Older adults with depression also may suffer from weakness (61%), stomach pains (37%), nausea (27%), anorexia (22%), and diarrhea (20%). Treating depression can reverse weight loss in nursing home residents (Morley, 2011).

The prevalence of dementia is increasing in older adults and is often associated with weight loss. Older adults with dementia often forget or refuse to eat. Encouraging an older adult with advanced dementia to eat can become a time-consuming process. Often, elders with advanced dementia wander excessively rather than consume food. They may express paranoid ideation, thereby refusing food because of a fear of being poisoned. Many older adults with dementia are prescribed psychotropic medications that can cause anorexia. Finally, some older adults with dementia may develop apraxia of swallowing and must be reminded to swallow after each mouthful of food (Gillen, 2016).

There are many biological factors that influence nutritional risk in older adults. Many medical conditions can cause weight loss and malnutrition by one or more of the following mechanisms: hypermetabolism, anorexia, swallowing difficulty, or malabsorption (Hajjar, Kamel, & Denson, 2004). Specific diseases that can affect an older adult's ability to eat or prepare food include stroke, tremors, or arthritis. Swallowing disorders (dysphagia) are associated with increased risk for aspiration and may result in poor food intake (Gillen, 2016). Infections are another cause of weight loss in older adults. Infections can lead to confusion, anorexia, and negative nitrogen balance (Hajjar et al., 2004).

Another disease that contributes to poor food intake is chronic obstructive pulmonary disease (COPD). Older adults with COPD experience a decrease in arterial oxygen levels when eating due to the act of eating and the brief interruption of respiration with swallowing. Frequently, older adults with COPD report they cannot eat their meals because of increased dyspnea. Additionally, their condition is further aggravated by hyperventilation and use of accessory muscles, leading to increased metabolism. Finally, hyperthyroidism and Parkinson's disease also can cause hypermetabolism, which may lead to weight loss (Hajjar et al., 2004).

DRUG–NUTRIENT INTERACTIONS

Medication use is common in older adults. There are several medications associated with poor appetite and weight loss. These include digoxin, theophylline, netformin, various antibiotics, nonsteroidal antiinflammatory drugs (NSAIDS), and psychotropic drugs such as fluoxetine, lithium, and phenothiazines (Hickson, 2006).

The interactions between nutrients and medicines may affect metabolism, absorption, digestion, or excretion of drugs. Table 9.1 lists the interactions between nutrients and drugs commonly taken by older adults. Many older patients take a variety of vitamin and herbal supplements. It is very important for the nurse to obtain an accurate assessment of all the over-the-counter therapies and drugs the patient may be taking. As the patient's drug profile changes, the nurse must continue to screen for drug–drug or drug–nutrient interactions and consult with a pharmacist or a dietitian, as needed.

DEHYDRATION

Older adults are at risk of dehydration caused by a decreased intake of fluids, loss of sodium, and increased fluid losses. Dehydration can occur quickly in an older adult, and the result

can be serious. Physiologically, the decreased intake may be related to altered thirst; older adults may not feel thirsty even when hypovolemic and often do not compensate for fluid losses during illness. Confusion, depression, and dementia also contribute significantly to reduced food and fluid intake. Dehydration takes three main forms: *Isotonic dehydration* results from the loss of sodium and water, as during a gastrointestinal illness. *Hypertonic dehydration* results when water losses exceed sodium losses. This type of dehydration is the most common and may occur from fever or limited fluid intake. *Hypotonic dehydration* may occur with diuretic use when sodium loss is higher than water loss (Weinberg & Minaker, 1995).

Dehydration can lead to electrolyte imbalances in the older adult. Hypernatremia and hyponatremia are the most common electrolyte imbalances in older adults. Risk factors include advanced age (greater than 80 years of age), female gender, residing in a nursing home, infection, and a diagnosis of dementia (Schlanger, Bailey, & Sands, 2010).

Nurses can help prevent dehydration in older adults by (Mentes, 2006):

- Providing fluids that older adults like and enjoy drinking.
- Educating older adults to drink fluids even when they are not thirsty.
- Identifying at-risk older adults.
- Identifying and treating treatable causes of dehydration, such as diarrhea and vomiting.
- Measuring fluid intake and urinary output.
- Providing appropriately sized cups and glasses for older adults to handle and straws if necessary.
- Educating caregivers to offer small amounts of fluid each time they enter the room.
- Educating caregivers to encourage the older adult to drink 8 ounces of fluids between and at each meal.
- Providing positive feedback to caregivers who provide fluid.

MICRONUTRIENT DEFICIENCY

Micronutrients, such as vitamin D, calcium, and vitamin B_{12}, are commonly found to be deficient in older adults. Even though the best way to ingest micronutrients is to eat a well-balanced diet, this may not always be possible. For those older adults found to be deficient in any micronutrient, a vitamin or mineral supplement may be necessary (Crogan, 2017).

In older adults, vitamins D and B_{12} may be difficult to gain in adequate supply. Approximately one-third of vitamin D requirements are obtained through the diet. The rest is synthesized in the skin via sunlight. This could be problematic for homebound older adults with limited sunlight exposure secondary to decreased mobility or those who reside in a nursing home or assisted living facility. Vitamin D deficiency has been linked to cancer progression, bone health (vitamin D is needed to absorb calcium), osteoporosis, and fractures. Vitamin B_{12} deficiency has been linked to pernicious anemia, bone health, and cognitive decline in older adults. Deficiencies of either vitamin can be treated with diet and supplementation (Davies, 2011).

TABLE 9.1 Sample of Drug–Nutrient Interactions*

Class	Drug	Effect
Analgesic	Acetaminophen	Decreased drug absorption with food; overdose associated with liver failure
	Aspirin	Absorbed directly through stomach; decreased drug absorption with food; decreased folic acid, vitamins C and K, and iron absorption
Antacid	Aluminum hydroxide	Decreased phosphate absorption
	Sodium bicarbonate	Decreased folic acid absorption
Antiarrhythmic	Amiodarone	Taste alteration
	Digitalis	Anorexia, decreased renal clearance in older persons
Antibiotic	Penicillins	Decreased drug absorption with food, taste alteration
	Cephalosporin	Decreased vitamin K
	Rifampin	Decreased vitamin B_6, niacin, vitamin D
	Tetracycline	Decreased drug absorption with milk and antacids, decreased nutrient absorption of calcium, riboflavin, vitamin C caused by binding
	Trimethoprim/sulfamethoxazole	Decreased folic acid
Anticoagulant	Coumarin	Acts as antagonist to vitamin K
Anticonvulsant	Carbamazepine	Increased drug absorption with food
	Phenytoin	Decreased calcium absorption; decreased vitamins D, K, and folic acid; taste alteration; decreased drug absorption with food
Antidepressant	Amitriptyline	Appetite stimulant
	Clomipramine	Taste alteration, appetite stimulant
	Fluoxetine (selective serotonin reuptake inhibitor [SSRI])	Taste alteration, anorexia
Antihypertensive	Captopril	Taste alteration, anorexia
	Hydralazine	Enhanced drug absorption with food, decreased vitamin B_6
	Labetalol	Taste alteration (weight gain for all beta-blockers)
	Methyldopa	Decreased vitamin B_{12}, folic acid, iron
Antiinflammatory	All steroids	Increased appetite and weight, increased folic acid, decreased calcium (osteoporosis with long-term use), promotes gluconeogenesis of protein
Antiparkinsonian	Levodopa	Taste alteration, decreased vitamin B_6 and drug absorption with food
Antipsychotic	Chlorpromazine	Increased appetite
	Thiothixene	Decreased riboflavin
Bronchodilator	Albuterol sulfate	Appetite stimulant
	Theophylline	Anorexia
Cholesterol lowering	Cholestyramine	Decreased fat-soluble vitamins (A, D, E, K); vitamin B_{12}; iron
Diuretic	Furosemide	Decreased drug absorption with food
	Spironolactone	Increased drug absorption with food
	Thiazides	Decreased magnesium, zinc, and potassium
Laxative	Mineral oil	Decreased absorption of fat-soluble vitamins (A, D, E, K), carotene
Platelet aggregate inhibitor	Dipyridamole	Decreased drug absorption with food
Potassium replacement	Potassium chloride	Decreased vitamin B_{12}
Tranquilizer	Benzodiazepines	Increased appetite

*Not intended to be an exhaustive or all-inclusive list. Always check pharmacology references before administering medications.
From Pronsky Z. M., & Crowe, J. P. (2012). Clinical: Food-drug interactions. In L. K. Mahan, J. L. Raymond, & S. Escott-Stump, *Krause's food and the nutrition care process* (13th ed.). St. Louis: Elsevier.

MALNUTRITION

Older age leads to a physiologic change referred to as anorexia of aging (Morley, 2013). As discussed previously, this physiologic anorexia results from alterations in taste and smell, earlier satiation, and other changes related to normal aging (Morley, 2011). Malnutrition is defined as "the state of being poorly nourished" (Hickson, 2006, p.4) and can be caused by a lack of nutrients (undernutrition) or an excess of nutrients (overnutrition). For the older adult, the cause typically is a lack of nutrients or undernutrition (Crogan, 2017). The prevalence of malnutrition is often dependent on living situation. For example, the prevalence for older adults living in the community is 15%; if homebound, it is variable at 5% to 44%. For older adults residing in a nursing home, the prevalence is 30% to 85%. If the older adult is hospitalized, the prevalence is 20% to 60% (Hajjar et al., 2004).

Two major markers of malnutrition are sarcopenia and cachexia. Sarcopenia is defined as "the decline in skeletal muscle mass that can result from physical inactivity, disuse of muscles, reduced levels of growth hormone and testosterone, neuromuscular changes, insufficient dietary protein, and impaired protein metabolism" (Brownie, 2013, p.141). Older adults can become sarcopenic after a lengthy hospitalization or illness. On the other hand, cachexia is characterized by a loss of fat and muscle mass accompanied with anorexia. It is a complex metabolic process often associated with an underlying terminal illness such as end-stage renal disease or cancer (Morley, 2011). Older adults with cachexia also will have sarcopenia, but those with sarcopenia may not have cachexia (Crogan, 2017). Older adults with sarcopenia are at increased risk for falls with injuries (see Evidence-Based Practice box).

EVIDENCE-BASED PRACTICE

Sarcopenia Influences Fall-Related Injuries in Community-Dwelling Older Adults

Background
Falls are a common occurrence for older adults. The prevalence of older adults who fall is approximately 28% to 35% worldwide. This is of concern because falls have been shown to contribute to hospitalization, nursing home placement, and functional decline. Of those who experience a fall, 80% are injured. Of those, 63% receive treatment at a hospital. Identifying the risk factors for falls could lead to earlier interventions to prevent falls in community-dwelling older adults.

Sample/Setting
Data examined were from 2848 Korean older adults aged 65 years or older who participated in the Korea National Health and Nutrition Examination Surveys (KNHANES) during 2010 to 2011.

Methods
Participants for the KNHANES were randomly sampled based on stratified regions, gender, age, and average size and price of housing. Of the 17,476 subjects who completed the KNHANES in 2010 and 2011, 3076 were 65 years or older and selected for this study. A total of 2848 subjects were included in the final analysis.

Findings
The incidence of fall-related injuries was 4.3% among the participants. After controlling for sociodemographic variables and morbidity due to chronic diseases, the incidence of fall-related injuries remained significantly elevated among older adults with sarcopenia.

Implications
Sarcopenia was found to be a significant risk factor for falls with injuries in community-dwelling older adults. To prevent falls among these persons, it is vital to implement interventions and programs that increase muscle mass.

From Woo, N., & Kim, S. (2014). Sarcopenia influences fall-related injuries in community-dwelling older adults. *Geriatric Nursing, 35,* 279-282.

ORAL HEALTH

Oral health is fast becoming a strong predictor or measure of quality of life for older adults. Poor oral health in older adults is linked to tooth loss, pain, and discomfort, and can lead to poor food intake secondary to an inability to chew (Eke, Wei, & Borgnakke, 2016). Thus oral health preventative

efforts are paramount to enhancing quality of life in our aging population.

Xerostomia, or dry mouth, is one of the most common causes of poor food intake in older adults. Individuals with xerostomia have difficulty forming a bolus, chewing, then swallowing. They will have a reduced ability to taste food and may have cracked lips or a fissured tongue, resulting in poor food intake. Additionally, xerostomia can lead to mucositis and dental caries (Stein & Aalboe, 2015). Xerostomia in the older adult is most likely drug-induced, and the risk increases with greater numbers of drugs taken (Glore, Spiteri-Staines, & Paleri, 2009).

Older adults are at increased risk for dental caries secondary to xerostomia and gingivitis. Almost 50% of older adults have dental caries affecting at least one tooth. Prevention includes the adoption of good oral hygiene and a well-balanced diet. Good oral hygiene includes the use of rotating toothbrushes, topical fluoride, daily mouth rinses, high fluoride toothpaste, and regular dental checkups that includes a fluoride varnish application (Gregory & Hyde, 2015).

Older adults with cognitive impairment are at increased risk for dental caries, oral infections, and periodontal disease (Yellowitz, 2016). Older adults with dentures should be encouraged to remove the dentures daily, inspect for damage, clean them before bed, and then return them to the mouth in the morning (Yellowitz, 2016). Cognitive-impaired older adults may need help or support completing this task. Educating caregivers is an important aspect of preventing dental caries in cognitive-impaired older adults.

As the older adult's functional abilities decline with advancing age or disease processes (arthritis), providing modified equipment such as toothbrushes with built-up handles or Velcro grips may help enhance the elder functional ability and sense of well-being (Yellowitz, 2016). Other options include the use of electric toothbrushes, specialized floss holders, or nosey cups for rinsing the mouth. Finally, frequent dental cleanings and examinations can help promote optimal oral health in at-risk older adults.

NUTRITIONAL SCREENING AND ASSESSMENT

Nutritional Screening

Nutritional screening is an abbreviated assessment of nutritional risk factors that identifies patients in need of a more comprehensive assessment and nutritional interventions. A variety of tools have been developed to conduct nutritional screening. Perhaps the most widely used of these tools is the "Determine Your Nutritional Health" screening tool developed as part of the Nutrition Screening Initiative (NSI) (Fig. 9.1).

The NSI (Dwyer, 1991), a 5-year, multifaceted national effort to promote routine nutrition screening, began in 1990 under the direction of the American Academy of Family Physicians, the American Dietetic Association (now the Academy of Nutrition and Dietetics [AND]), and the National Council on Aging. As part of the initiative, a nutritional health checklist to be used by older adults or caregivers was developed to determine risk factors associated with nutrition and health. A score of 3 or more indicates moderate to high nutritional risk and triggers the need for a more comprehensive nutritional assessment. The Level II

Screen is a tool that health care professionals use to conduct a more in-depth assessment of nutritional status (Fig. 9.2).

Other nutrition screening tools include the following:

- Mini Nutritional Assessment: A simple and reliable 18-item questionnaire that examines food intake, weight loss, body mass index, psychological stress, neuropsychological problems and mobility (Loreck, et al., 2012).

- Instant Nutritional Assessment: A simple and practical screening tool that combines three elements: lymphocyte count, albumin, and weight change (Hajjar, et al., 2004).

- Malnutrition Risk Scale (SCALES): An outpatient screening tool for malnutrition that asks about sadness, cholesterol, loss of weight, eating problems, and shopping (Morley, 1989).

The Warning Signs of poor nutritional health are often overlooked. Use this Checklist to find out if you or someone you know is at nutritional risk.

Read the statements below. Circle the number in the "yes" column for those that apply to you or someone you know. For each "yes" answer, score the number in the box. Total your nutritional score.

DETERMINE YOUR NUTRITIONAL HEALTH

	YES
I have an illness or condition that made me change the kind and/or amount of food I eat.	2
I eat fewer than 2 meals per day.	3
I eat few fruits or vegetables or milk products.	2
I have 3 or more drinks of beer, liquor or wine almost every day.	2
I have tooth or mouth problems that make it hard for me to eat.	2
I don't always have enough money to buy the food I need.	4
I eat alone most of the time.	1
I take 3 or more different prescribed or over-the-counter drugs a day.	1
Without wanting to, I have lost or gained 10 pounds in the last 6 months.	2
I am not always physically able to shop, cook and/or feed myself.	2
TOTAL	

Total Your Nutritional Score. If it's –

0-2   Good! Recheck your nutritional score in 6 months.

3-5   You are at moderate nutritional risk. See what can be done to improve your eating habits and lifestyle. Your office on aging, senior nutrition program, senior citizens center or health department can help. Recheck your nutritional score in 3 months.

6 or more   You are at high nutritional risk. Bring this Checklist the next time you see your doctor, dietitian or other qualified health or social service professional. Talk with them about any problems you may have. Ask for help to improve your nutritional health.

Remember that Warning Signs suggest risk, but do not represent a diagnosis of any condition. Turn the page to learn more about the Warnings Signs of poor nutritional health.

These materials are developed and distributed by the Nutrition Screening Initiative, a project of:

AMERICAN ACADEMY OF FAMILY PHYSICIANS

THE AMERICAN DIETETIC ASSOCIATION

THE NATIONAL COUNCIL ON THE AGING, INC.

The Nutrition Screening Initiative • 1010 Wisconsin Avenue, NW • Suite 800 • Washington, DC 20007
The Nutrition Screening Initiative is funded in part by a grant from Ross Products Division of Abbott Laboratories, Inc.

Fig. 9.1 Determine Your Nutritional Health. (Reprinted with permission from the Nutrition Screening Initiative, a project of the American Academy of Family Physicians, the American Dietetic Association, and the National Council on the Aging, and funded in part by a grant from Ross Products Division, Abbott Laboratories Inc.)

Continued

The Nutrition Checklist is based on the Warning Signs described below.
Use the word **DETERMINE** to remind you of the Warning Signs.

DISEASE

Any disease, illness or chronic condition which causes you to change the way you eat, or makes it hard for you to eat, puts your nutritional health at risk. Four out of five adults have chronic diseases that are affected by diet. Confusion or memory loss that keeps getting worse is estimated to affect one out of five or more of older adults. This can make it hard to remember what, when or if you've eaten. Feeling sad or depressed, which happens to about one in eight older adults, can cause big changes in appetite, digestion, energy level, weight and well-being.

EATING POORLY

Eating too little and eating too much both lead to poor health. Eating the same foods day after day or not eating fruit, vegetables, and milk products daily will also cause poor nutritional health. One in five adults skip meals daily. Only 13% of adults eat the minimum amount of fruit and vegetables needed. One in four older adults drink too much alcohol. Many health problems become worse if you drink more than one or two alcoholic beverages per day.

TOOTH LOSS/MOUTH PAIN

A healthy mouth, teeth and gums are needed to eat. Missing, loose or rotten teeth or dentures which don't fit well, or cause mouth sores, make it hard to eat.

ECONOMIC HARDSHIP

As many as 40% of older Americans have incomes of less than $6,000 per year. Having less -- or choosing to spend less -- than $25-30 per week for food makes it very hard to get the foods you need to stay healthy.

REDUCED SOCIAL CONTACT

One-third of all older people live alone. Being with people daily has a positive effect on morale, well-being and eating.

MULTIPLE MEDICINES

Many older Americans must take medicines for health problems. Almost half of older Americans take multiple medicines daily. Growing old may change the way we respond to drugs. The more medicines you take, the greater the chance for side effects such as increased or decreased appetite, change in taste, constipation, weakness, drowsiness, diarrhea, nausea, and others. Vitamins or minerals, when taken in large doses, act like drugs and can cause harm. Alert your doctor to everything you take.

INVOLUNTARY WEIGHT LOSS/GAIN

Losing or gaining a lot of weight when you are not trying to do so is an important warning sign that must not be ignored. Being overweight or underweight also increases your chance of poor health.

NEEDS ASSISTANCE IN SELF CARE

Although most older people are able to eat, one of every five have trouble walking, shopping, buying and cooking food, especially as they get older.

ELDER YEARS ABOVE AGE 80

Most older people lead full and productive lives. But as age increases, risk of frailty and health problems increase. Checking your nutritional health regularly makes good sense.

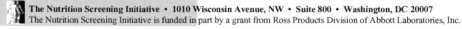

The Nutrition Screening Initiative • 1010 Wisconsin Avenue, NW • Suite 800 • Washington, DC 20007
The Nutrition Screening Initiative is funded in part by a grant from Ross Products Division of Abbott Laboratories, Inc.

Fig. 9.1, cont'd

- Malnutrition Screening Tool: A quick and reliable 2-item tool that asks about unplanned weight loss and poor apetite (Ferguson, Capra, Bauer et al., 1999).
- Food Expectations, Long Term Care: A 28-item, four-domain instrument that measures nursing home resident food satisfaction (Crogan, Evans, & Valasquez, 2004; Crogan & Evans, 2006).

Nutritional Assessment

A nutritional assessment is a comprehensive evaluation of a patient's nutritional status and typically includes data collection in each of the following areas: demographic and psychosocial data, medical history, dietary history, anthropometrics, medications and laboratory values, and a physical assessment. Nutritional assessment may be performed as a result of an identified risk on a nutritional screening or when the risk status is obvious without a preliminary screening. The American Society for Parenteral and Enteral Nutrition (ASPEN) published standards that identify nutritionally at-risk patients (Box 9.1) (ASPEN, 1998). ASPEN also identified the goals of a nutritional assessment as follows:

- Establishing baseline subjective and objective nutrition parameters
- Identifying specific nutritional deficits

- Determining nutritional risk factors
- Establishing nutritional needs
- Identifying medical and psychosocial factors that may influence the prescription and administration of nutritional support
- Setting goals for nutritional deficits; if applicable, set goals in areas of medical and psychological factors to be worked on with an interdisciplinary team

Diet History

In addition to a complete history and physical assessment, patients found to be at nutritional risk require a more specific evaluation of their dietary intake patterns. Information that is typically part of a diet history includes number of meals and snacks per day; chewing or swallowing difficulties; gastrointestinal problems or symptoms that affect eating; oral health and denture use; history of diseases or surgery; activity level; use of medications; appetite; need for assistance with meals and meal preparation; and food preferences, allergies, and aversions.

A diet history may also include a *food recall.* For accuracy and relevancy, the food recall must include specific information about the type of food ingested, the preparation method, and an accurate estimate of the amount. The patient should be asked to select days for recording typical of his or her intake patterns. It is generally best to select two weekdays and one weekend day to record the best information on intake patterns. Patients should be instructed about how to estimate portion sizes and should be given samples from which to estimate their intake (e.g., 3 ounces [oz] of meat is the size of a pack of cards; a serving of vegetables is usually half a cup). The use of food models or large specific and detailed pictures of food category serving sizes may be very

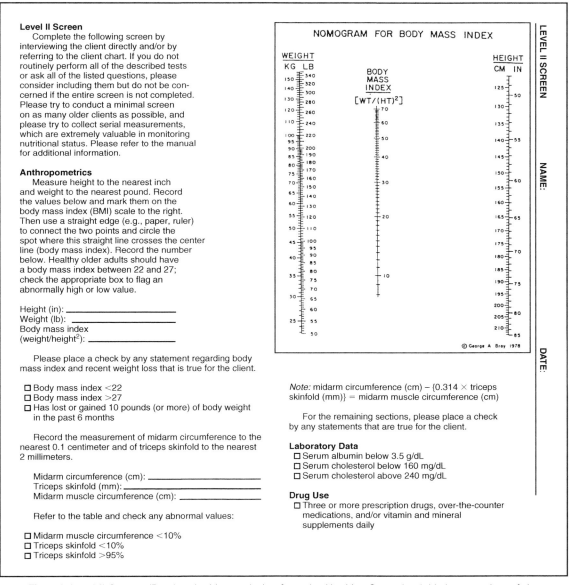

Fig. 9.2 Level II Screen. (Reprinted with permission from the Nutrition Screening Initiative, a project of the American Academy of Family Physicians, the American Dietetic Association, and the National Council on the Aging, and funded in part by a grant from Ross Products Division, Abbott Laboratories, Inc.)

Continued

Clinical Features
Presence of (check each that applies):
☐ Problems with mouth, teeth, or gums
☐ Difficulty chewing
☐ Difficulty swallowing
☐ Angular stomatitis
☐ Glossitis
☐ History of bone pain
☐ History of bone fractures
☐ Skin changes (e.g., dry, loose, nonspecific lesions, edema)

Eating Habits
☐ Does not have enough food to eat each day
☐ Usually eats alone
☐ Does not eat anything on one or more days each month
☐ Has poor appetite
☐ Is on a special diet
☐ Eats vegetables two or fewer times daily
☐ Drinks milk or eats milk products once or not at all daily
☐ Eats fruit or drinks fruit juice once or not at all daily
☐ Eats breads, cereals, pasta, rice, or other grains five or fewer times daily
☐ Has more than one alcoholic drink per day (if a woman); more than two drinks per day (if a man)

Living Environment
☐ Lives on an income of less than $6000 per year (per individual in the household)
☐ Lives alone
☐ Is housebound
☐ Is concerned about home security
☐ Lives in a home with inadequate heating or cooling
☐ Does not have a stove and/or refrigerator
☐ Is unable or prefers not to spend money on food (<$25 to $30 per person spent on food each week)

Percentile	Men 55–65 yr	Men 65–75 yr	Women 55–65 yr	Women 65–75 yr
Arm circumference (cm)				
10th	27.3	26.3	25.7	25.2
50th	31.7	30.7	30.3	29.9
95th	36.9	35.5	38.5	37.3
Arm muscle circumference (cm)				
10th	24.5	23.5	19.6	19.5
50th	27.8	26.8	22.5	22.5
95th	32.0	30.6	28.0	27.9
Triceps skinfold (mm)				
10th	6	6	16	14
50th	11	11	25	24
95th	22	22	38	36

From: Frisancho AR. New norms of upper limb fat and muscle areas for assessment of nutritional status. *Am J Clin Nutr* 1981; 34:2540–2545. Copyright 1981, American Society for Clinical Nutrition.

Functional Status
Usually or always needs assistance with (check each that applies):
☐ Bathing
☐ Dressing
☐ Grooming
☐ Toileting
☐ Eating
☐ Walking or moving about
☐ Traveling (outside the home)
☐ Preparing food
☐ Shopping for food or other necessities

Mental/Cognitive Status
☐ Clinical evidence of impairment (e.g., Folstein <26)
☐ Clinical evidence of depressive illness (e.g., Beck Depression Inventory >15, Geriatric Depression Scale >5)

Clients in whom you have identified one or more major indicators of poor nutritional status require immediate medical attention; if minor indicators are found, ensure that they are known to a health professional or to the client's own physician. Clients who display risk factors of poor nutritional status should be referred to the appropriate health care or social service professional (e.g., dietitian, nurse, dentist, case manager).

Major Indicators

Significant weight loss over time
Significantly low or high weight-for-height
Significant reduction in serum albumin
Significant changes in functional status
Significant and inappropriate food intake
Significant reduction in midarm circumference
Significant increase or decrease in skinfold
Osteoporosis or osteomalacia
Folate or vitamin B_{12} deficiency

Minor Indicators

Concurrent syndromes
  Alcoholism
  Cognitive impairment
  Chronic renal insufficiency
  Multiple concurrent medications
  Malabsorption syndromes

Symptoms
  Anorexia, nausea, or dysphagia
  Early satiety
  Change in bowel habits
  Fatigue or apathy
  Memory loss

Physical signs
  Poor oral or dental status
  Dehydration
  Poorly healing wounds
  Loss of subcutaneous fat or muscle mass
  Fluid retention

Laboratory tests
  Reduced levels of serum albumin, transferrin, prealbumin, or ascorbic acid
  Folate, iron, or zinc deficiency
  Dehydration-related laboratory phenomena

Risk Factors

Inappropriate food intake
Poverty
Social isolation
Dependency or disability
Acute or chronic diseases or conditions
Chronic medication use
Advanced age

Fig. 9.2, cont'd

BOX 9.1   Nutritionally At-Risk Patients

- Involuntary loss or gain of 10% or greater of usual body weight within 6 months, *or*
- Loss or gain of 5% of usual body weight in 1 month
- 20% over or under ideal body weight
- Presence of chronic disease or increased metabolic requirements
- Altered diets or diet schedules
- Inadequate nutrient intake for more than 7 days

Data from the American Society for Parenteral and Enteral Nutrition, Board of Directors. (2010). Standards for nutrition support: Hospitalized patients. *Nutrition in Clinical Practice, 25*(4), 403-414.

---

helpful as the typical consumer is unfamiliar with standard serving portions. The purpose of the food recall is to estimate the average number of calories and amount of protein ingested daily and to detect any deleterious food intake patterns such as overuse of fried foods or lack of vegetables or fruit. Some patients may need assistance from another person, if available, to complete the food recall.

For a more detailed picture of a patient's diet and food patterns, a 3- to 7-day food intake history is obtained. Patients are asked to keep a detailed record of everything they eat, the time at which they eat, and the amount of each type of food item consumed. In addition to recording eating habits, patients are also asked to record activities and feelings, which allow the health care professional to determine whether there are emotional issues or activities that may either interfere with or enhance eating pleasure. Seven-day diet histories may be very helpful in detecting many behavioral issues in patients; however, many individuals have difficulty recording their food intake for a continuous period.

Another way to assess dietary patterns is to look at food frequency. Food frequency questionnaires allow a health care professional to assess a particular nutrient category such as calcium or the adequacy of an individual's entire diet. A food frequency questionnaire is completed either by a medical assistant or by the patient during his or her wait in a health professional's office. Food frequency questionnaires are recommended for new patients because they allow the practitioner to collect reasonable dietary data without compromising the patient's sense of privacy about food intake and diet.

Anthropometrics

Height and weight are the mainstays of anthropometric measurements. Ideally, the patient is weighed in the morning while wearing light clothing. Height is measured, if possible. For patients who are unable to stand without assistance, height may be estimated by measuring the distance from the heel to the top of the knee (knee height) with the use of a broad-bladed caliper. Additional information and instructions on how to use a broad-bladed caliper and then estimate height using the following formula can be found at http://www.rxkinetics.com/pix/knee_height.jpg.

Females
$$\text{Height in cm} = 84.88 - (0.24 \times \text{age}) + (1.83 \times \text{knee height})$$
Males
$$\text{Height in cm} = 64.19 - (0.04 \times \text{age}) + (2.02 \times \text{knee height})$$

Measuring body surface area may help to detect those who are overweight or underweight for their heights. Body mass index (BMI) can be used to determine body fat levels, with a BMI <18.5 kg/m^2 indicating underweight and an increased risk of mortality (Loreck et al., 2012). However, in older adults, BMI may not be accurate in that height measurement may not be accurate secondary to physical changes related to aging.

Other types of anthropometric measurements include triceps skinfold (TSF) and midupper arm muscle circumference (MUAC). These measurements are of limited value when measured only one time. The MUAC is measured using a tape measure placed snugly against the skin at the midpoint of the distance between the tip of the acromial process of the scapula and the olecranon process of the ulna. MUAC was found to be a predictor of mortality in nursing home residents.

TSF is measured at the midpoint between the acromion process and the olecranon process of the upper arm using a skinfold caliper. An average of at least three measurements is used to ensure accuracy. Nutritional depletion is defined as a skinfold measure of <11.3 mm in women and <4.3 mm in men (Burr & Phillips, 1984).

Another fast, noninvasive, and highly accurate method for assessing lean tissue and bone mass is dual-energy x-ray absorptiometry (DXA). These scanning devices allow the practitioner to evaluate not only bone density at several sites but also evaluate body fat in a minimum amount of time (generally less than 20 minutes) with minimum radiation exposure (rem; less than 5 millirem [mrem]) (DXA, Hologic, Inc., Bedford, MA). The advantage of a DXA scan is that a patient is able to obtain a more reliable picture of his or her body composition (body fat versus lean body mass) compared with anthropometric measurement. The disadvantage of DXA scanning is that the patient must be mobile; however, newer models that allow for portability into homes and senior centers are now on the market.

Laboratory Values

No single laboratory test is diagnostic of malnutrition. Several tests that reflect protein synthesis may also reflect nutritional status. Serum albumin is the serum protein most frequently cited in reference to malnutrition; it reflects the liver's ability to synthesize plasma protein. Albumin has a half-life of about 21 days, so it is not always reflective of current nutritional status. Albumin values may also be affected by immune status and hydration. Given these limitations, albumin levels below 3.5 grams per deciliter (g/dL) may indicate some degree of malnutrition.

Transferrin is a carrier protein for iron and has a shorter half-life of 8 to 10 days. It is a more rapid predictor of protein depletion. Levels below 200 milligrams per deciliter (mg/dL) may indicate mild-to-moderate depletion, respectively. Levels below 100 mg/dL may indicate severe depletion.

Prealbumin is a carrier protein for retinol-binding protein and has a half-life of 2 to 3 days. It is sensitive to sudden demands on protein synthesis and is often used in the acute care setting. Prealbumin levels that range from 15 to 5 mg/dL reflect mild to moderate protein depletion. Levels below 5 mg/dL are considered reflective of severe protein depletion. Total lymphocyte count (TLC) is sometimes used as a nutritional marker. In severe or prolonged malnutrition, immune proteins are depleted and the TLC is decreased.

NURSING DIAGNOSES ASSOCIATED WITH NUTRITIONAL PROBLEMS

Nursing diagnoses are derived from an assessment of the patient during a comprehensive health history and physical examination, during a patient interview, or while carrying out nursing interventions. The nursing diagnoses subsequently become the basis for the nursing care plan and goals for nursing care. Box 9.2 lists nursing diagnoses associated with a primary nutritional problem and diagnoses that commonly have a nutritional component.

EVIDENCE-BASED STRATEGIES TO IMPROVE NUTRITION

Alterations in nutrition require a care plan that specifically addresses the nutritional problem. Nursing interventions related to nutrition include instruction and counseling regarding a diet

BOX 9.2 Nursing Diagnoses Associated With Nutritional Problems

Primary Nutritional Problem
Inadequate nutrition
Excessive nutrition
Potential for excessive nutrition

Nutritional Component
Potential for aspiration
Diarrhea
Abnormal family processes
Inadequate fluid volume
Feeding self-care inadequacy
Diminished swallowing
Potential for diminished gastrointestinal motility

adequate in a specific nutrient or nutrients, calories, and fluids. Therapeutic diets have been modified to include more or less than the recommended amounts for a specific nutrient or nutrients, and are usually prescribed to manage or treat a chronic disease or illness. Examples of therapeutic diets include those that are restricted in sodium, protein, cholesterol, total calories, fat, or gluten. Therapeutic diets also may include modifications in the texture of foods such as a low-fiber or high-fiber diet, mechanical soft diet, pureed diet, or clear liquid diet. Finally, therapeutic diets

may include specialized nutrition such as parenteral nutrition, enteral tube feeding, or oral supplements.

Oral supplements are often prescribed for patients unable to ingest adequate protein or calories because of early satiety or fatigue during eating. By adding a concentrated liquid oral supplement to the meal plan, the patient may improve protein or overall caloric intake. However, the consumption of food is always preferable to meal replacement or supplementation. If this is not possible, between-meal snacks of liquid caloric supplements can increase energy intake (Morley, 2011). Commercial oral supplements such as Ensure, Nutren, Osmolite, and Complete Modified are available at most pharmacies and grocery stores without a prescription. In addition, supplements are available as soups, nutrient bars, and smoothies. Commercial products are convenient but are often more costly than using regular food or dry powder products such as Carnation Instant Breakfast mixed with whole milk, cream soups, puddings, regular candy bars, ice cream, and powdered fortified milk.

COMPONENTS OF A HEALTHY DIET

An illustrative tool that can be used to demonstrate what constitutes a healthy diet and appropriate portion size is the United States Department of Agriculture's MyPlate method (USDA, https://www.choosemyplate.gov/). The USDA MyPlate (Fig. 9.3)

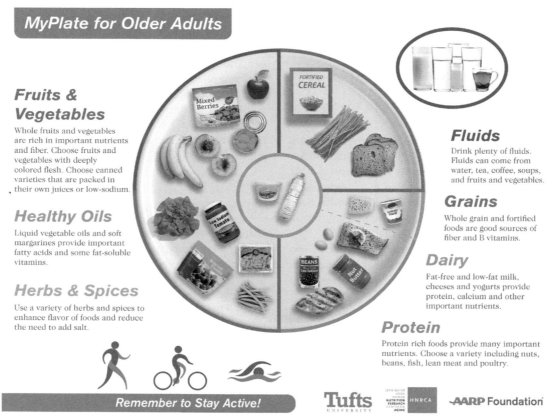

Fig. 9.3 MyPlate for Older Adults. (Copyright 2016 Tufts University. All rights reserved. "MyPlate for Older Adults" graphic and accompanying website were developed with support from the AARP Foundation. Available at http://hnrca.tufts.edu/myplate/files/MPFOA2015.pdf)

divides a plate into quarters, with one-fourth for grains, one-fourth for protein, and the remaining half for vegetables and fruits. Older adults who are not eating close to these estimations should be advised that their nutrient intake might be inadequate and action needs to be taken (Crogan, 2018).

The Department of Health and Human Services (HHS), in collaboration with the USDA, compile and publish nutritional guidelines every 5 years. The most recent guidelines were published in 2016 (Dietary Guidelines, 2016). The guidelines fit within five broad categories:

- Eat a variety of nutrient-dense foods and manage portion sizes
- Shift current food and drink choices to healthier alternatives
- Maintain a healthy diet throughout your life
- Limit caloric intake from added sugars and saturated fats, and reduce intake of sodium
- Support others in healthy eating

The guidelines pertain to all Americans. A healthy person should eat a variety of vegetables, fruits (preferably whole fruits), grains (half of which should be whole grains), fat-free or low-fat dairy, protein from a variety of sources, and a limited amount of oils. Caffeinated drinks are limited to three to five 8-ounce cups of coffee per day.

Even though the nutritional requirements of older adults are generally similar to the rest of the population, nutritional needs can become more difficult to meet because of the physiologic, psychological, and social changes associated with older age. The nurse can be instrumental in encouraging older adults to eat a well-balanced diet, thereby affecting their overall health, independence, and quality of life.

DYSPHAGIA

Dysphagia is a problem that often affects nutritional status and may occur because of a cerebrovascular accident, oral or neck cancer treatment, or a neuromuscular or neurologic disorder. Dysphagia is usually identified as either oropharyngeal or esophageal, designating the phase in which the dysfunction occurs. In the oropharyngeal phase, food is chewed and mixed with saliva and then is moved posteriorly, triggering the pharyngeal swallow reflex. This triggering moves the bolus down the pharynx. During the pharyngeal swallow, the larynx closes and the epiglottis redirects the bolus around the airway, protecting the respiratory tract. The esophageal phase begins when the bolus enters the esophagus at the cricopharyngeal juncture or upper esophageal sphincter. Peristaltic waves propel the bolus through the esophagus to the stomach (NIDCD, 2010). Because swallowing is a complex voluntary/involuntary event, the specific etiologies of dysphagia are multiple and diverse.

The nurse can play a pivotal role in the early detection of swallowing problems and then intervene to prevent complications from dysphagia. Screening for dysphagia involves determining whether the patient has signs or symptoms of dysphagia for the purpose of referral for diagnostic evaluation and treatment (Udayakumar & Eubanks, 2015; Mayo Clinic, 2014). The first clue that dysphagia may be a problem could be the development of aspiration pneumonia. Aspiration occurs when material passes into the larynx below the vocal cords. Silent aspiration refers to situations in which aspiration does not produce the typical cough or change in voice quality (Smith & Connolly, 2003). Pulse oximetry is an effective and efficient tool to detect aspiration while eating. Smith and Connolly (2003) found that a 2% drop in oxygen saturation levels from baseline detected 86% of patients with aspiration. When followed by a 10 mL water swallow test at the bedside, the ability to detect aspiration increased to 95%. If screening suggests dysphagia or aspiration, further assessment is needed, which may include a referral for diagnostic evaluation.

Dependent on the type of dysphagia, specific recommendations for care will be developed by the speech therapist (SLT) or occupational therapist (OT). Correct positioning while eating is paramount for safe eating and swallowing. An upright position with the arms and feet supported, the head midline in a neutral position, and the chin slightly tucked is recommended to prevent aspiration. The upright position should be maintained for at least 30 minutes after eating (Gillen, 2016).

The modification of food and fluids consumed is a common response to dysphagia. The Dysphagia Diet Task Force standardized food and fluid textures for the dysphagia diet. For example, the Dysphagia Pureed (NDD 1) diet consists of pudding-like consistencies. This includes pureed foods without chunks or small pieces. Patients are advised to avoid scrambled eggs or cereals with lumps. The Dysphagia Mechanically Altered (NDD 2) diet consists of moist, soft foods that are easily formed into a bolus in the mouth. Patients are advised to eat ground meats, soft vegetables, soft fruit, and slightly moistened dry cereal with little texture. No bread or foods such as peas or corn are recommended on the NDD 2 diet. The Mechanical Soft diet is the same as the NDD 2, but it allows bread, cakes, and rice. Finally, the Dysphagia Advanced (NDD 3) diet allows regular textured foods except those that are very hard, sticky, or crunchy. Patients are told to avoid hard fruit and vegetables, corn, skins, nuts, and seeds. Liquid consistencies are referred to as spoon-thick, honey-like, nectar-like, or thin (McCallum, 2003).

SPECIALIZED NUTRITIONAL SUPPORT

Specialized nutrition is used when a patient is unable to ingest, digest, or absorb nutrients. The decision to initiate an enteral tube feeding is a complicated decision made by the patient, health care provider, and family or surrogate. Common indications for enteral tube feeding include conditions in which a patient is unable to swallow foods, for example, following a cerebrovascular accident or with myasthenia gravis, amyotrophic lateral sclerosis, and multiple sclerosis (see Box 9.3).

Enteral nutrition also is used when the upper gastrointestinal tract is obstructed, as in cancer or severe esophageal stenosis. A feeding tube is placed below the area of obstruction; feeding tubes may be placed into the stomach or the intestine. The tubes are placed through the nose (nasogastric or nasointestinal), directly into the stomach (gastrostomy, percutaneous endoscopic gastrostomy [PEG], or radiology-assisted gastrostomy), or directly into the jejunum (jejunostomy or percutaneous endoscopic jejunostomy).

BOX 9.3   The Utility of Tube-Feedings in End-Stage Disease

Nasogastric Tube (NG)
- For short-term use or short-term life expectancy
- Dysphagia secondary to:
  - Cerebrovascular accident (CVA)
  - Tumors obstructing swallowing
  - Inflammatory masses
  - Medication irritation
  - Gastric esophageal reflux disease (GERD)
- Significant change of condition secondary to infection, delirium

Percutaneous Endoscopic Gastrostomy (PEG)
- For long-term use or life expectancy >6 months
- Chronic neurologic causes: multiple sclerosis, amyotrophic lateral sclerosis (ALS), Parkinson's disease, traumatic brain injury (TBI)
- Weight loss of aging, anorexia
- Severe dysphagia, unable to swallow safely
- Cognitively impaired, dementia

Enteral formulas include standard (whole protein and complex carbohydrate), modified protein (peptide), and elemental (amino acid) formulas. Some enteral formulas have added soluble or insoluble fiber. Disease-specific formulas are also available for the dietary treatment of diseases, for example, reduced protein for patients receiving renal dialysis, increased lipid percentage of total calories for patients with diabetes and pulmonary disease, and increased percentage of branched-chain amino acids for patients with hepatic disease. Specialized enteral formulas are considerably more expensive than standard formulas and should be used only when clearly indicated. Short-term enteral feeding is often used after surgery, traumatic injury, and burns.

Parenteral nutrition consists of an intravenous solution that includes dextrose, amino acids, vitamins, minerals, electrolytes, trace elements, and water. A lipid emulsion is commonly added to produce a total nutrient admixture, but it may be given by separate infusion. The dextrose and lipids provide calories to support metabolic needs, whereas amino acids are administered to meet daily protein requirements.

Parenteral nutrition is indicated when the gastrointestinal tract cannot be used for enteral feeding or cannot absorb adequate nutrients to maintain health. Diseases and conditions typically associated with the need for parenteral nutrition include severe inflammatory bowel disease, fistula, acute pancreatitis, and massive bowel resection. Parenteral nutrition is administered through a vascular access device such as a central venous catheter, tunneled catheter, peripherally inserted central catheter, or implanted port. Most parenteral nutrition solutions are hypertonic and must be administered into a large central vein.

Patients receive enteral and parenteral nutrition in various health care settings or at home. Nurses educate home care patients about the use and care of their access devices, administration of the enteral formula or parenteral solution, use of an enteral or intravenous pump, management of common problems associated with specialized feeding, and signs and symptoms of complications. Although specialized nutrition is prescribed to patients of all ages, a large percentage of the patients who receive enteral tube feeding and parenteral nutrition are older adults.

SUMMARY

Food has strong social connotations that must be recognized and assessed by the nurse when working with a patient. Nurses must understand the role of vitamins and mineral supplements in the overall diet of their patients to get a clear picture of their health and pharmaceutical history.

The older adult population is increasingly becoming the larger percentage of the total population, and the percentage of older adults will peak around 2030 with the aging of the Baby Boomer generation. Malnutrition is detected through nutritional screening and nutritional assessment. Anthropometrics, diet history, and laboratory studies are components of a nutritional assessment. Specialized nutrition therapies such as parenteral nutrition and enteral tube feeding may provide nourishment to patients unable to ingest, digest, or absorb nutrients. The nurse, along with the interdisciplinary team, plays an important role in identifying alterations in nutrition and in developing nursing interventions that restore nutritional adequacy. The nurse collaborates with the physician, the nurse practitioner, the dietitian, the pharmacist, and other members of the health care team to promote the nutritional health of patients.

KEY POINTS

- Malnutrition in older adults is a multifaceted and complex issue.
- No single tool or clinical marker accurately predicts nutritional status.
- A balanced dietary intake, based on the MyPlate and the 2015 to 2020 Dietary Guidelines for Americans, may promote nutritional health.
- Weight loss is considered clinically significant when there is a >2% decrease in baseline body weight in 1 month, a >5% weight loss in 3 months, or a >10% weight loss in 6 months.
- Nurses have the opportunity and responsibility to assess nutritional status and should collaborate with other members of the health care team to formulate a comprehensive and coordinated nutritional care plan.

CRITICAL-THINKING EXERCISES

1. A 68-year-old man with chronic obstructive pulmonary disease (COPD) has been referred to home health nursing services for medication instruction and respiratory assessment. During the nurse's first visit, the following information is obtained during history taking: overweight for height by about 30 pounds, weight loss of 10 pounds over the past 2 months, complaints of shortness of breath while eating, and unable to get to the grocery store (relies on a neighbor for assistance). How would this information relate to the development of a nursing care plan?

2. An 80-year-old woman who is 5 foot, 4 inches tall, weighs 152 pounds, and is in generally good health records the following 24-hour intake:

Breakfast: 1 glass orange juice, 2 slices whole wheat toast, 1 tablespoon butter

Lunch: ½ cup cottage cheese, 1 bag cheese curls, ½ peanut butter and jelly sandwich, 1 cup tea

Dinner: 1 cup wheat flakes cereal, ½ cup skim milk

Snack: 1 candy bar, 1 cup ice cream

Analyze this patient's diet. What conclusions, if any, can be made about her dietary status based on this 24-hour recall?

3. A 72-year-old man is a practicing vegetarian. He does not eat fish, but he does eat eggs. His physician has recommended that he ingest more protein. What recommendations can the nurse offer?

REFERENCES

Ackley, B. J., & Ladwig, G. B. (2014). *Nursing diagnosis handbook: An evidence-based guide to planning care* (10th ed.). St. Louis, MO: Elsevier.

American Society for Parenteral, Enteral Nutrition (ASPEN), Board of Directors. (1998). *Clinical pathways and algorithms for delivery of parenteral and enteral nutrition support in adults.* Silver Spring, MD: The Society.

Brownie, S. (2013). Nutritional wellbeing for older people. *JATMS, 19*(3), 140–145.

Burr, M. L., & Phillips, K. M. (1984). Anthropometric norms in the elderly. *British Journal of Nutrition, 51*(2), 165–169.

Crogan, N. (2017). Nutritional problems affecting older adults. *Nursing Clinics of North America, 52*, 433–445.

Crogan, N. (2018). Dysphagia and malnutrition. In K. Mauk (Ed.), *Gerontological nursing competencies for care* (4th ed.). Burlington, MA: Jones & Bartlett.

Crogan, N., & Evans, B. (2006). The shortened food expectations — Long-Term Care questionnaire: Assessing nursing home residents' satisfaction with food and food service. *Journal of Gerontological Nursing, 32*(11), 50–59.

Crogan, N., Evans, B., & Velasquez, D. (2004). Measuring nursing home resident satisfaction with food and food service: Initial testing of the FoodEx-LTC. *Journals of Gerontology: Medical Sciences, 59A*(4), 370–377.

Davies, N. (2011). Promoting health ageing: The importance of lifestyle. *Nursing Standard, 25*(19), 43–50.

Dietary Guidelines. Office of Disease Prevention and Health Promotion website. http://health.gov/dietaryguidelines/. Updated January 11, 2016. Accessed January 12, 2016.

Dwyer, J. T. (1991). *Screening older American's nutritional health: Current practices and future reponsibilities.* Washington, DC: Nutrition Screening Initiative.

Edfors, E., & Westergren, A. (2012). Home-living elderly people's views on food and meals. *Journal of Aging Research, 2012.* 9 pages. Access https://doi.org/10.1155/2012/761291.

Eke, P. I., Wei, L., Borgnakke, W. S., et al. (2016). Periodontitis prevalence in adults >65 years of age in the USA. *Periodontol 2000, 72*(1), 363–368.

Evans, B., Crogan, N., & Armstrong, J. (2005). The meaning of mealtimes: Connection to the social world of the nursing home. *Journal of Gerontological Nursing, 31*(2), 11–17.

Ferguson, M., Capra, S., Bauer, J., & Banks, M. (1999). Development of a valid and reliable malnutrition screening tool for adult acute hospital patients. *Nutrition, 15*(6), 458–464.

Gillen, G. (2016). *Stroke rehabilitation: A function-based approach* (4th ed.). St. Louis, MO: Elsevier.

Glore, R. J., Spiteri-Staines, K., & Paleri, V. (2009). A patient with dry mouth. *Clinical Otolaryngology, 34*, 358–363.

Gregory, D., & Hyde, S. (2015). Root caries in older adults. *Journal of the California Dental Association, 43*(8), 439–445.

Hajjar, R. R., Kamel, H. K., & Denson, K. (2004). Malnutrition in aging. *Internet Journal of Geriatric Gerontology, 1*(1), 1–16.

Hickson, M. (2006). Malnutrition and ageing. *Postgraduate Medical Journal, 82*, 2–8.

Keller, H., Beck, A., & Namasivayam, A. (2015). Improving food and fluid intake for older adults living in long-term care: A research agenda. *JAMDA, 16*, 93–100.

Loreck, E., Chimakurthi, R., & Steinle, N. I. (2012). Nutritional assessment of the geriatric patient: A comprehensive approach toward evaluating and managing nutrition. *Clinical Geriatrics, 20*(4), 20–26.

Mayo Clinic. (2014). Dysphagia. Accessed August 11, 2016 from http://www.mayoclinic.org/diseases-conditions/dysphagia/basics/causes/con-20033444.

McCallum, S. L. (2003). The National Dysphagia Diet (NDD). *Journal of the American Dietetic Association, 103*(3), 748–765.

Mentes, J. (2006). Oral hydration in older adults. *American Journal of Nursing, 106*(6), 40–49.

Morley, J. E. (1989). Death by starvation: A modern American problem? *Journal of the American Geriatrics Society, 37*, 184.

Morley, J. E. (2011). Undernutrition: A major problem in nursing homes. *JAMDA, 12*, 243–246.

Morley, J. E. (2013). Pathophysiology of the anorexia of aging. *Current Opinion in Clinical Nutrition and Metabolic Care, 1*, 27–32.

Naseer, M., & Fagerstrom, C. (2015). Prevalence and association of undernutrition with quality of life among Swedish people aged 60 years and above: Results of the SNAC-B study. *Journal of Nutrition and Health in Aging, 19*(10), 970–979.

National Institute on Deafness and other Communication Disorders (NIDCD). (2010). Dysphagia. *NIH Pub. No., 13–4307.*

Schlanger, L. E., Bailey, J. L., & Sands, J. M. (2010). Electrolytes in the aging. *Advances in Chronic Kidney Disease, 17*(4), 308–319.

Smith, H. A., & Connolly, M. J. (2003). Evaluation and treatment of dysphagia following stroke. *Topics in Geriatric Rehabilitation. 19*(1), 43–59.

Stein, P., & Aalboe, J. (2015). Dental care in the frail older adult: Special considerations and recommendations. *Journal of the California Dental Association, 43*(7), 363–368.

Udayakumar, N., & Eubanks, S. (2015). Approach to patients with esophageal dysphagia. In D. Oleynikov (Ed.), *Surgical approaches to esophageal diseases* (pp. 483–489). Philadelphia, PA: Elsevier.

Weinberg, A. D., & Minaker, K. L. (1995). Dehydration. Evaluation and management in older adults. Council on Scientific Affairs, American Medical Association. *JAMA, 274*(1), 1552–1556.

Yellowitz, J. A. (2016). Geriatric health and functional issues. In L.L. Patton & M. Glick (Eds.), *The ADA practical guide to patients with medical conditions* (2nd ed., pp. 405–422). Hoboken, NJ: John Wiley & Sons.

10

Sleep and Activity

Jennifer J. Yeager, PhD, RN, APRN

http://evolve.elsevier.com/Meiner/gerontologic

LEARNING OBJECTIVES

On completion of this chapter, the reader will be able to:
1. Identify three age-related changes in sleep.
2. Describe the features of insomnia.
3. Discuss four factors influencing sleep in older adults.
4. Discuss two sleep disorders.
5. List four components of a sleep history.
6. Describe the effects of lifestyle changes on sleep and activity in older adults.
7. Discuss the benefits of physical activity for older adults.
8. Identify three characteristics of meaningful activities for older adults with dementia.

WHAT WOULD YOU DO?

What would you do if you were faced with the following situations?
• A new patient is admitted to your hospital floor. At bedtime, she asks for "that little pill I buy at Target that helps me sleep." How would you respond?
• Following the death of his partner, your 68-year-old patient asks what he can do to remain active. How would you respond?

Sleep and activity are two universal, dichotomous functions of all human beings. Sleep is a natural, periodically recurring, physiologic state of rest for the body and mind; sleep is a state of inactivity or repose required to remain active. Activity includes the things we do while awake, for example, personal care, daily tasks, exercise, and recreation. The type, amount, and intensity of the activities pursued vary widely among individuals according to personal choice, lifestyle, and health status.

SLEEP AND OLDER ADULTS

Biologic Brain Functions Responsible for Sleep

Regulation of sleep and wakefulness occurs primarily in the hypothalamus, which contains both a sleep center and a wakefulness center. The thalamus, limbic system, and reticular activating system (RAS) are controlled by the hypothalamus and influence sleep and wakefulness. The hypothalamus consists of several masses of nuclei, interconnected with other parts of the nervous system, and is located below the thalamus, where it forms the floor and part of the lateral walls of the third ventricle. Sleep is a state of consciousness characterized by the physiologic changes of reduced blood pressure, pulse rate, and respiratory rate along with a decreased response to external stimuli.

Stages of Sleep

Normal sleep is divided into five stages: rapid eye movement (REM) sleep and four stages of non-REM sleep (NREM) (Table 10.1). NREM sleep accounts for about 75% to 80% of sleep. The remaining 20% to 25% of sleep is REM sleep. A night's sleep begins with the four stages of NREM sleep, continues with a period of REM sleep, and then cycles through NREM and REM stages of sleep for the rest of the night. Sleep cycles range from 70 to 120 minutes in length, with four to six cycles occurring in a night (Gordon, 2013).

Stage 1 of NREM sleep is the lightest level of sleep. During stage 1, an individual can be easily awakened. Sleep progressively deepens during stages 2 and 3 until stage 4, the deepest level, is reached. Muscle tone, pulse, blood pressure, and respiratory rate are reduced in stage 4. In REM sleep, pulse, blood pressure, and respiratory rate increase. The REM of this stage of sleep is associated with dreaming. When the amount of REM sleep is reduced, an individual may have trouble concentrating or may be irritable or anxious the next day (Gordon, 2013).

Variations in the REM and NREM sleep stages occur with advancing age. REM sleep is interrupted by more frequent nocturnal awakenings, and the total amount of REM sleep is reduced. The amount of stage 1 sleep is increased, and stage 3 sleep and stage 4 sleep are less deep. In the very old, especially men, the amount of slow wave sleep, as determined by electroencephalography (EEG), is greatly reduced (Kryger, Monjan, Bliwise, & Ancoli-Israel, 2004).

Sleep and Circadian Rhythm

The sleep–wake cycle follows a circadian rhythm, which is roughly a 24-hour period. The hypothalamus controls many

TABLE 10.1 Normal Stages of Sleep

Stages	Type of Sleep	Selected Characteristics
NREM Sleep (Four Stages)		
Stage 1	Light sleep	Easily awakened
Stage 2	Medium deep sleep	More relaxed than in stage 1 Slow eye movements Fragmentary dreams Easily awakened
Stage 3	Medium deep sleep	Relaxed muscles Slowed pulse Decreased body temperature Awakened with moderate stimuli
Stage 4	Deep sleep	Restorative sleep Body movement rare Awakened with vigorous stimuli
REM Sleep		
	Active sleep	Rapid eye movement Increased or fluctuating pulse, blood pressure, and respirations Dreaming occurs

REM, Rapid eye movement; *NREM*, non–rapid eye movement. Modified from Touhy, T. & Jett, K. (2012). *Ebersole & Hess' Toward healthy aging* (8th ed.). St. Louis, MO: Mosby; and Beers, M. H. & Berkow, R. (2000). *The Merck manual of geriatrics* (3rd ed.). Whitehouse Station, NJ: Merck Research Laboratories.

BOX 10.1 Age-Related Changes in Sleep

- Increased sleep latency
- Reduced sleep efficiency
- Increased nocturnal awakenings
- Increased early morning awakenings
- Increased daytime sleepiness

circadian rhythms, which include the release of certain hormones during sleep (e.g., growth hormone [GH], follicle-stimulating hormone [FSH], and luteinizing hormone [LH]). Numerous factors may gradually strengthen or weaken the sleep and wake aspects of circadian rhythm, including the perception of time, travel across time zones, light exposure, seasonal changes, living habits, stress, illness, and drug use (Hoffman, 2003). The decrease in nighttime sleep and the increase in daytime napping that accompanies normal aging may result from changes in the circadian aspect of sleep regulation (Cohen-Zion & Ancoli-Israel, 2003; Lewy, 2009).

Insomnia

Insomnia, or the inability to sleep, is a complex phenomenon. Reports of insomnia include difficulty falling asleep, difficulty staying asleep, frequent nocturnal awakenings, early morning awakening, and daytime somnolence. Insomnia may be transient, short term, or chronic (WebMD, 2017). Transient insomnia lasts only a few nights and is related to situational stresses. Short-term insomnia usually lasts less than a month and is related to acute medical conditions (e.g., postoperative pain) or psychological conditions (e.g., grief). Chronic insomnia lasts more than a month and is related to age-related changes in sleep, medical or psychological conditions, or environmental factors. Insomnia may affect the older adult's quality of life with excessive daytime sleepiness, attention and memory problems, depressed mood, nighttime falls, and

possible overuse of hypnotic or over-the-counter (OTC) drugs (Kryger et al., 2004).

Age-Related Changes in Sleep

Many older adults experience changes in sleep, which are considered "normal" age-related changes (Box 10.1). However, although some older adults either do not experience these common changes or do not consider them sources of distress, other adults find these changes problematic (Beers & Berkow, 2000). The sleep changes experienced by many older adults include increased sleep latency, reduced sleep efficiency, more awakenings in the night, increased early morning awakenings, and increased daytime sleepiness (Hoffman, 2003).

Sleep latency, a delay in the onset of sleep, increases with age. More than 30% of women report taking more than 30 minutes to fall asleep; for men, this number is under 15%. Older adults report that it takes longer to fall asleep at the start of the night and after being awakened during the night. Because the time spent awake in bed trying to fall asleep increases, sleep efficiency decreases. Sleep efficiency is the relative percentage of time in bed spent asleep. For young adults, sleep efficiency is approximately 90%. However, this percentage drops to 75% for older adults (Hoffman, 2003).

Nocturnal awakenings contribute to an overall decrease in the average number of hours of sleep. The frequency of nocturnal awakenings increases with age; older adults may wake up four or more times per night. The interruptions of sleep contribute to the perception that the amount of sleep is inadequate or of poor quality. If the person has little difficulty falling back to sleep, the decrease in the number of hours of sleep may be slight. However, some older adults report increased periods of wakefulness after nocturnal awakening. The reasons for nocturnal awakening include trips to the bathroom, dyspnea, chest pain, arthritis pain, coughing, snoring, leg cramps, restless legs syndrome (RLS), and noise (Beers & Berkow, 2000). Early morning awakening and the inability to fall back to sleep may be related to changes in circadian rhythm or to any of the reasons for nocturnal awakening.

Daytime sleepiness is often reported by older adults and may be caused by frequent nocturnal awakening or other sleep disturbances. However, in some older adults, daytime sleepiness suggests underlying disease. It is associated with functional impairment and depression, and contributes to the increased risk of motor vehicle accidents. When cognitive dysfunction is present, daytime sleepiness is a predictor of mortality and cardiovascular disease (Chasens, Sereika, & Burke, 2009). Daytime sleepiness may also be caused by drug side effects (e.g., antiarrhythmics, clonidine, selective serotonin reuptake inhibitors [SSRIs], and antihistamines).

Daytime napping is common in older adults and does not necessarily indicate problems with nighttime sleep. Naps, that is, voluntary and involuntary episodes of daytime sleep, occur throughout the day. Floyd (1995) found that no difference existed in the length of nighttime sleep between individuals who took naps and individuals who did not take naps, and the amount of nighttime sleep and the duration of naps were not correlated. Floyd concluded that the time spent napping supplemented the total daily amount of sleep.

Although some of the sleep changes experienced by older adults are related to aging, other sleep changes are associated with chronic disease and other health problems. When patterns of sleep are examined, an increase in light sleep is seen as deep sleep declines. The loss of deep sleep is associated with stages 3 and 4 of sleep (see Table 10.1). This sleep disturbance may be a normal part of aging caused by changes in the reticular formation (RF) in the brain (Friedman, 2010). When older adults describe the changes in their sleep patterns as they have aged, they offer nurses valuable clues. Their descriptions indicate health problems (actual or potential), safety concerns, and possible interventions to improve sleep quality.

Factors Affecting Sleep

Proper sleep is essential for a person's sense of well-being and health. Sleep is often defined subjectively and linked to an individual's feelings on awakening. A good night's sleep is described as one that refreshes, restores, and leaves a person ready for the coming day's activities. Feeling tired and less alert after a poor night's sleep may lead to a less active and productive day. Factors that influence sleep quality in older adults include the following, alone or in combination: environment, pain, lifestyle, dietary influences, drug use, medical conditions, depression, and dementia. Nursing interventions can modify these factors and promote a good night's sleep.

Environment

The environment can positively or negatively influence a person's quality and amount of sleep. For older adults, environments conducive to sleep include low levels of stimuli, dimmed lights, silence, and comfortable furniture (Rosto, 2001).

Home Environments. The home environment supports a good night's sleep by its very familiarity. The bed and bedding, the people, and the noises are all familiar. The routines leading up to bedtime are natural and individualized.

Hospitals and Long-Term Care Facilities. The environment of a health care institution may detract from the quality of sleep. Not only are these environments unfamiliar, they also typically have bright lights, noisy people and machines, limited privacy and space, and uncomfortable mattresses. Physical discomfort or pain may be caused by invasive procedures such as Foley catheterization, intravenous line placement, venipuncture, mechanical ventilation, and discomfort or pain from equipment such as oxygen masks, casts or traction devices, and monitors. The hospital patient or long-term care facility resident is often

awakened to receive drugs and treatments or to be assessed for changes in vital signs and condition. Nocturnal awakenings for incontinence care or for other care procedures such as repositioning and skin care interrupt the normal sequence of sleep stages (Nagel, Markie, Richards, & Taylor, 2003). Fear of the unexpected or unknown may also keep older adults awake in health care institutions. The quality of sleep in institutional settings improves as nursing interventions address (1) the scheduling of procedures and care activities to avoid unnecessary awakenings, (2) modification of environmental factors to promote a quiet, warm, relaxed sleep setting, and (3) orientation of older adults to the institutional setting.

Noise. Environmental noise potentially interferes with sleep in all health care settings. The consequences of environmental noise may include (1) sleep deprivation, (2) alteration in comfort, (3) pain, and (4) stress or difficulty concentrating, which may interfere with the enjoyment of activities. Sources of noise include personnel, roommates, visitors, equipment, and routine activities in the nursing unit. Interventions to reduce environmental noise include closing the doors of patient and resident rooms when possible, adjusting the volume control on telephones, rescheduling nighttime cleaning routines, and reminding staff and visitors to speak quietly. Some older adults may appreciate headphones to provide relaxing music and block background noise. Headphones will also reduce noise from late evening television watching. Noise reduction may include asking the facility's maintenance staff to clean and lubricate the wheels on all the unit's utility carts. Reducing environmental noise in institutions involves cooperation among employees from other departments, visitors, and nurses.

Lighting. Most individuals are accustomed to sleeping in darkened rooms. The lights in hallways and nurses' stations in some health care institutions interfere with the sleep of patients and residents. The nurse should assess environmental lighting in the institutional setting for glare, brightness, and uneven levels of illumination. Selectively dimming the institution's lights at night may promote better sleep. However, safety concerns must be considered. Nightlights in rooms, bathrooms, and hallways may be a safe compromise—promoting sleep by reducing the glare of bright lights while allowing enough light to see.

Temperature. Falling asleep and staying asleep is difficult when a person is cold. Older adults may wake during the night because of a nighttime reduction in core body temperature related to reduced metabolic rate and muscle activity. Being too warm will also disrupt sleep, but some older adults sleep better if simple measures are used to keep them warm. The ambient temperature of the bedroom should be no lower than 65° F (Worfolk, 1997). Several lightweight thermal blankets and flannel sheets (both fitted and flat) make for a warmer bed. Flannel pajamas or nightgowns, bed socks, and nightcaps help sleepers stay warm. If bed socks are worn, slippers should be used when out of bed to prevent slipping on uncarpeted floors. Heating devices such as heating pads or hot water bottles should be avoided so that the fragile skin on the feet and lower legs are not exposed to thermal injuries.

Pain and Discomfort

Body pain, acute or chronic, interferes with falling asleep and staying asleep. Nursing interventions to relieve pain begin with assessment of the location, intensity, onset and duration, quality, and any aggravating or alleviating factors. The effect of pain on older adults' lifestyle, including sleep quality, should also be assessed. Both nonpharmacologic and pharmacologic measures may be used to relieve pain. When body pain interferes with sleep, analgesics are more effective for sleep promotion than sedative or hypnotic drugs. However, alterations in pharmacokinetics common to older adults taking drugs make careful selection of analgesics important. Drugs with long half-lives linger longer in many older adults. Small initial doses that may be titrated upward to achieve analgesia may be better tolerated than generous initial doses. Attention must be paid to common side effects such as constipation.

Even without any report of body pain, some older adults find just being in bed uncomfortable. For the older individual whose discomfort prevents sleeping in a standard bed, comfortable chairs may be a solution. Reclining chairs with soft cushions may be more comfortable for individuals with heart failure or severe chronic obstructive pulmonary disease (COPD). The rhythmic motion of a rocking chair may comfort some individuals and thus promote sleep. If being out of bed is not feasible, modifying the bed with extra pillows to support painful limbs and promote comfortable body positioning or using special mattresses (e.g., air or water mattresses) may be effective. Nighttime garments should be made of a soft material such as cotton and should not be restrictive so that freedom of movement is allowed. The use of lightweight blankets avoids adding weight to sensitive body areas.

Lifestyle Changes

Loss of Spouse. Widowhood is a common life event in the older adult population. Loss of a spouse is much more common among older women than among older men. Twenty-four percent of older adults are widowed (United States Census Bureau, 2017). Loss of a bed partner may make sleep psychologically less comforting. Widowed older adults describe the strangeness of going to bed alone after many years of marriage (Felson, 2017). This change in bedtime routine may interfere with the onset of sleep. If the widowed older adult experiences depression, the depression should be treated.

Retirement. Retirement brings about changes in schedule and activities. For decades, the older adult's times for going to bed and awakening were influenced by the work schedule; retirement removes that variable. The structure of a day in retirement is not imposed by the demands of a job. The work activities that caused fatigue may have ceased. It is no longer necessary to get a good night's sleep to be restored from the day's work and prepared for the next day's efforts. The activities that remain are personal care activities, activities around the house, recreational activities, and any new activities adopted with the coming of retirement. These changes create the potential for alterations in sleep (Felson, 2017). Some retired older adults may follow the same schedule they observed while working. It is familiar; it feels comfortable. However, other retired older adults find their days and nights without structure. In the absence of old routines, sleep is disturbed. Unless other activities replace work activities, retired older adults may not feel fatigued at the end of the day or sleepy at bedtime. Sleep may also be disturbed by the uncertainties that come with retirement. Questions about family relationships, finances, and future activities may lead to sleep-disturbing stress.

Relocation. Some older adults experience relocation, or a change of residence, from their house or apartment to the home of their children or siblings, a retirement community, assisted living facility, or nursing facility. Sleep is adversely affected by the transition to these unfamiliar surroundings. Deciding to move from the familiar place of residence to another residence, even if that other residence is desirable and the relocation voluntary, engenders stress during the time of decision making, during the actual move, and during the time of adjustment to the new residence. The unfamiliar environment of the new residence also contributes to disturbed sleep. As older adults become accustomed to a new residence, sleep should improve.

Having a Roommate. Having a roommate (or a bed partner) may interfere with sleep. Some sleep-related problems occur in long-term care facilities when roommates do not get along with one another because of different interests or lifestyles. For example, one older adult may watch television to fall asleep, and the other may find this disruptive to sleep. The nursing staff must make every effort to review significant psychosocial interests with residents and to match roommates accordingly. Ideally, residents should be allowed to select roommates with whom they share common interests. The roommate or bed partner who snores loudly, sleepwalks, talks in his or her sleep, or has RLS is also a cause of sleeplessness. Treatment must be directed toward the cause of the roommate's problem; if treatment is impossible or ineffective, separate bedrooms may be needed.

Dietary Influences

Sleep is influenced by what we eat and drink. Popular caffeine-containing beverages (e.g., coffee, tea, and soda) make falling asleep more difficult for some older adults. The effects of caffeine include restlessness, nervousness, insomnia, tremors, reduced peripheral vascular resistance, increased heart rate, and relaxation of bronchial smooth muscle.

The standard advice is to avoid caffeine-containing beverages for several hours before going to bed. This diminishes the likelihood that the stimulant effect of caffeine will interfere with falling asleep and staying asleep. Other sources of caffeine include hot chocolate, chocolate candy, some OTC pain analgesics and cold remedies, and some brands of decaffeinated tea and coffee (Cochran, 2003). Some herbal products also contain caffeine. Alternative choices for late evening beverages are fruit juices, milk, and water.

Alcohol occupies an equivocal position among beverages that influence sleep. Many adults include alcohol as part of their normal lifestyle and continue to do so in their advancing years. They enjoy a glass of wine or other cocktail with an evening meal. Small amounts of alcoholic beverages may cause a slight drowsiness or a relaxation that promotes falling asleep. However, larger amounts of alcohol reduce the amount of both REM sleep and deep sleep, and impair the overall quality of a night's sleep (Burke & Laramie, 2004). The diuresis caused by alcohol-induced inhibition of antidiuretic hormone (ADH) secretion leads to nocturnal awakenings for urination. When discussing the use of alcohol with older adults, the nurse must determine how they define a "small" or "large" amount of alcohol and the circumstances of alcohol use. These details of alcohol use vary from group to group and from culture to culture.

Fluid intake in the evening and immediately before going to bed is associated with nocturia. Although nocturia may have other causes such as urinary retention related to benign prostatic hypertrophy or diuretic therapy for heart failure, many older adults reduce the kind and volume of fluid intake in the evening. However, it is important that older adults, who as a group are at risk for inadequate fluid intake and dehydration, not reduce the total amount of liquids consumed in 24 hours.

Hunger and thirst may be causes of sleeplessness. Bedtime snacks and small amounts of liquids may provide the touch of comfort that promotes sleep. Warm snacks containing protein are better at bedtime than cold snacks (Cochran, 2003). Milk, eggnog, creamed soup, or flavored gelatin may all be served hot to provide warmth and calories. Pudding, custard, or tapioca may be more palatable than crackers or graham crackers. For older adults with diabetes, bedtime snacks should be included in their special diets. Falling back to sleep after awakening during the night with a dry mouth is facilitated when a cup of water is available close to the bed.

Depression

Depression among older adults is a treatable condition that is frequently accompanied by insomnia. Patients awaken in the early morning and are unable to return to sleep. Patients may also report excessive daytime somnolence. Evaluation and treatment are essential if depression is suspected.

Dementia and Disturbed Sleep

Older adults with Alzheimer's disease or other dementias may experience disturbed sleep. Increased confusion at night, nocturnal wandering, disruptive vocalizations, and agitation have been reported. The causes of the sleep disruption may be no different from causes that disturb sleep in any older adult. However, cognitive impairment complicates assessment, intervention, and evaluation. The nurse may not receive a clear response when asking about sleep or any conditions that contribute to insomnia. Instead, nurses must anticipate the needs of older adults with dementia. Interventions include reducing confusion with an explanation of what is expected of the older adult ("Now it's time to sleep"), identification of the place for sleeping ("This is your bed"), and reassurance that going to bed is the right thing to do ("Your bed is ready for you"). Assisting older adults with dementia to perform bedtime routines redirects their behavior. Nocturnal wandering behaviors may signal a need that cannot be expressed verbally, for example, hunger, thirst, or the need to go to the bathroom. Wandering may also be an expression of pain or of a need for exercise. Once the meaning of the wandering is discerned, appropriate interventions follow naturally (Rowe, 2003). Drugs such as sedatives or antipsychotics should be avoided because of their side effects, which may worsen confusion, interfere with safe ambulation, and alter the sleep–wake cycle.

Sleep Disorders and Conditions

The two most common sleep disorders experienced by older adults are sleep apnea and periodic limb movements in sleep (PLMS). Both disorders are seen with excessive daytime sleepiness and reports of insomnia. However, PLMS is essentially a benign condition, whereas the hypoxia related to sleep apnea might lead to serious consequences.

Sleep Apnea

During sleep, individuals with sleep apnea experience recurrent episodes of cessation of respiration. These apneic episodes may last from 10 seconds to 2 minutes. The number of apneic episodes may range from 10 to more than 100 per hour of sleep (Cohen-Zion & Ancoli-Israel, 2003). The incidence of sleep apnea increases with age, and it is more common in men than in women. Complications related to sleep apnea include cardiac disease, hypertension, stroke, obesity, headaches, irritability, depression and anxiety, sexual dysfunction, daytime sleepiness, and difficulty with memory, thinking, and concentration. Persons with sleep apnea are also at increased risk for automobile or work-related accidents (Nabili, 2012).

The three major types of sleep apnea are central sleep apnea (CSA), obstructive sleep apnea (OSA), and complex sleep apnea. In CSA, a cessation of respiratory efforts, both diaphragmatic and intercostal, occurs. CSA is usually accompanied by daytime fatigue, nocturia and nighttime awakening, morning headaches, poor memory and concentration, and moodiness. Risk factors associated with CSA include heart failure, hypothyroidism, chronic kidney disease, neurologic diseases, and damage to the brainstem. Treatment consists of managing underlying associated risk factors, weight loss, avoidance of alcohol and sleeping pills, sleeping on the side, and using sprays to maintain open nasal passages. Continuous positive airway pressure (CPAP) treatment may be beneficial for those with CSA, especially those with associated heart failure (Ratini, 2012).

OSA is more common in older adults than CSA (Beers & Berkow, 2000). In OSA, air flow ceases because of complete or partial airway obstruction; respiratory efforts increase in an attempt to open the airway. Factors associated with OSA include obesity, short or thick neck, jaw deformities, large tonsils, large tongue or uvula, narrow airway, and deviated septum (Olson, Moore, Morgenthaler et al., 2003). Additionally, smoking, hypertension, and cardiac risk factors increase the likelihood of developing OSA. Older adults with OSA report daytime fatigue; waking with a headache, sore throat or dry mouth, and confusion; trouble concentrating and irritability; and sexual dysfunction. The families of older adults with OSA describe loud snoring and choking or gasping sounds during the person's sleep. Treatment consists of weight loss, avoidance of alcohol and sleeping pills, propping oneself on the side using pillows, and using sprays to maintain open nasal passages. CPAP prevents collapse of the airway during sleep (see the Nursing

⊙ NURSING CARE PLAN

Sleep Pattern Disturbance

Clinical Situation

Mr. V is a 79-year-old single white man who is admitted to the nursing facility for convalescence after a tracheotomy for obstructive sleep apnea (OSA). Before hospitalization, he was living alone on the third floor of an apartment complex for older adults. He describes himself as limited in activities such as driving, traveling, and cooking because of respiratory distress. He reports daytime fatigue associated with grooming, dressing, feeding, and toileting. He admits to sleeping poorly, with several nighttime awakenings and general fatigue all day long, which prompts him to take a daytime nap.

Medical history includes hypertension, obesity, chronic obstructive pulmonary disease (COPD), severe peripheral vascular disease with a stage II venous stasis ulcer of the lower leg, and recent tracheotomy for OSA.

While at the nursing facility, Mr. V tells you that he plans on discharging himself home in 1 to 2 weeks. He is observed to need assistance in mobility and uses a wheelchair to wheel himself around his room. He refuses to go to the dining room and requests to have a refrigerator in his room. He eats all his meals in his room and rarely socializes with any resident or staff member. His pastimes include playing solitaire in his room and watching television. He is a retired sales representative, having worked in the business for more than 40 years.

Nursing Diagnosis

Altered sleep pattern resulting from obesity and reduced activity level

Outcomes

Patient will identify personal lifestyle habits contributing to sleep pattern disturbance.

Patient will achieve weight loss of 1 pound (lb) per week.

Patient will eat a well-balanced diet, as evidenced by food diary.

Patient will participate in one group activity a day.

Patient will walk 100 feet twice daily, increasing distance to tolerance.

Patient will report increased length of uninterrupted periods of sleep.

Interventions

Teach relationship between weight and sleep pattern, and importance of losing weight to improve sleep pattern.

Explore with patient motivators to lose weight; reinforce as needed.

Teach about the USDA's food guidance system, MyPlate (http://www.choosemyplate.gov/) and assist him in identifying nutritious foods.

Teach use of food diary for self-monitoring.

Offer nutritious foods as snacks.

Encourage patient to increase level of activity on the unit by increasing mobility and engaging in nonsedentary activities; review a list of available activities with patient. Offer to accompany patient on a walk on the unit to his tolerance at least twice a day to help with wound healing and weight reduction.

Introduce patient to fellow residents on the unit who share common interests.

Encourage patient to join other residents in activities to tolerance.

Explore with patient his likes or dislikes, previous hobbies, and level of activity during middle adulthood.

Schedule an activity with the patient that will be part of his daily routine.

Discourage daytime napping; instead, replace it with a stimulating activity.

Teach patient to monitor pulse, to watch for symptoms of respiratory distress when engaging in activities on the unit, and to stop if respiratory distress occurs or an increase in heart rate causes adverse symptoms.

Offer praise and positive reinforcement when he performs a nonsedentary activity and when weight loss is achieved.

Observe patient during sleep for signs of obstructive apnea such as loud snoring or periods of apnea. Observe for daytime fatigue and somnolence.

Encourage patient to assume a side-lying position for sleep.

Discuss with patient plans for discharge, and explore alternative living arrangements, including residence on a first-floor apartment, especially if mobility is impaired.

Care Plan box). Other options include mandibular advancement devices that prevent the tongue from blocking the throat and surgery (somnoplasty, uvulopalatopharyngoplasty, mandibular or maxillary advancement surgery, or nasal surgery) (Goldberg, 2012).

Complex sleep apnea syndrome (CompSAS) occurs when persons treating OSA with CPAP are found to also have CSA during initial therapy. Persons present with excessive fatigue, sleepiness, and depression; these symptoms are secondary to unresponsiveness to CPAP. Risk factors include cardiovascular and cerebrovascular diseases, as well as use of opioid drugs. Prevalence may be as high as 20% and increases with age; it is predominant in men. Maintaining adherence to CPAP may improve CompSAS after 8 to 12 weeks. However, adherence is problematic because of poor initial response to therapy. Other methods that have been investigated include adding oxygen to CPAP, the addition of carbon dioxide to CPAP, and the use of adaptive servo-ventilation (ASV), which automatically adjusts to a person's respiration on a breath-by-breath basis (Wang, Wang, Feng et al., 2013).

Periodic Limb Movement in Sleep

Approximately 30% of older adults experience PLMS (Cleveland Clinic, 2012). In PLMS, repetitive kicking leg movements occur throughout the night, most often during non-REM sleep, and may occur every 5 to 90 seconds; each kick causes a brief disruption of sleep. Some older adults are unaware of their leg movements; others wake up and have difficulty falling back to sleep. Older adults with PLMS report insomnia and excessive daytime sleepiness (EDS). Their bed partners report being kicked during the night. Drugs such as dopamine agonists (DAs), anticonvulsants, benzodiazepines, and narcotics are accepted pharmacologic therapies for PLMS. First-line pharmacologic therapy is DAs. Additionally, patients are encouraged to eliminate caffeine-containing products (e.g., tea, chocolate, and coffee) from their diet; they should also discuss the use of antidepressants with their health care provider, as these drugs may worsen symptoms (Cleveland Clinic, 2012). If the movements are frequent, the nurse may suggest that older adults sleep alone to allow their bed partners less disturbed nights' sleep (Ancoli-Israel, 2004).

EVIDENCE-BASED PRACTICE

Natural Light on Sleep Quality of Older Adults in Nursing Homes

Background

Fifty percent of older adults report sleep problems. Typically, sleep problems are treated with pharmacologic and nonpharmacologic interventions. Nonpharmacologic interventions have included stimulus control, sleep hygiene education, sleep restriction, relaxation techniques, cognitive behavior therapy, and light therapy.

Sample/Setting

The sample encompassed 61 older adults (30 in experimental group; 31 in control group) residing in the Social Security Institution Narlidere Municipal Nursing Home in Turkey. Subject ages ranged from 75 to 84; 63.3% were female, 53.3% were widowed, and 56.7% were high school graduates.

All subjects were given the Pittsburgh Sleep Quality Index (PSQI) at baseline. The PSQI has 18 scorable questions, which are grouped into seven components. Each question can receive a score of 0 to 3. The sum of the component scores is the total PSQI score, ranging from 0 to 21; the higher the score, the poorer the sleep quality.

Methods

Experimental group subjects were taken to the garden of the nursing home for exposure to natural sunlight between 8 AM to 10 AM each morning for 5 days. They remained in the garden for at least 30 minutes but no longer than 120 minutes. Experimental subjects were provided brochures on health sleep habits. After 5 days, the experimental subjects repeated the PSQI.

The control subjects remained in their rooms, the canteen, or the nursing home living rooms while the experimental subjects were in direct sunlight. They, too, retook the PSQI after 5 days and received a copy of the healthy sleep habits brochure after retaking the PSQI.

Findings

Significant differences were found between the experimental group and control group across most of the components of the PSQI (subjective sleep quality, sleep latency, sleep duration, sleep activity, sleep disturbance, and daytime function) between baseline and day five ($p < 0.001$). A strong positive relationship was found between sunlight exposure time and sleep duration, regular sleep activity and daytime dysfunction ($p < 0.001$). There was no significant difference in global sleep quality score for those in the sunlight at least 30 minutes versus those in the sunlight at least 100 minutes.

Implications

Natural sunlight therapy can significantly improve sleep quality. This nonpharmacologic intervention is effective and has the potential to help prevent polypharmacy in nursing home residents with insomnia.

From Duzgun, G., & Akyol, A. D. (2017). Effect of natural sunlight on sleep problems and sleep quality of the elderly staying in the nursing home. *Holistic Nursing Practice, 31*(5), 295-302. doi: 10.1097/HNP.0000000000000206.

Components of the Sleep History

A complete sleep history begins with the patient's report of his or her sleep pattern and sleep-related problems (Box 10.2). The quality of sleep is usually described along a continuum of poor, fair, good, or excellent. The quantity of sleep refers to the amount of sleep in a 24-hour period, including daytime naps. Quantity may be difficult to calculate, especially for the patient with frequent nocturnal awakenings who cannot recall whether sleep occurred after awakening. The nurse should determine

---

BOX 10.2 Sleep History Components

- Sleep quality
  - The self-report of the older adult, described as poor, fair, good, or excellent
- Sleep quantity
  - The number of hours asleep per 24 hours, including daytime naps
- Bedtime routines
- Place of sleep
- Characteristics of the bed, bedding, and bedroom environment
- Food and fluid intake in the evening and at bedtime
- Use of alcohol and caffeine-containing beverages
- Drugs (prescription and nonprescription)
- Characteristics of the sleep disturbance
  - Difficulty falling asleep
  - Difficulty staying asleep
  - Frequent nocturnal awakenings
  - Early morning awakening
  - Daytime sleepiness
- The older adult's account of the reasons for the disturbed sleep

---

when the patient retires for bed, falls asleep, and usually awakens. The number of nocturnal awakenings and length of time awake at night are important to review with the patient. If a patient retires at 9 PM, does not fall asleep until 11 PM, arises at 4 AM, and takes a daytime nap from 4 to 5 PM daily, this individual has slept a total of 6 hours. Information about a person's typical bedtime rituals or practices should also be obtained.

The older adult is likely to seek additional help in achieving satisfaction with sleeping habits. If the older adult is too tired or fatigued to perform normal activities, the sleep problem may be viewed as disruptive to the daily routine and may require further evaluation. The nurse should ascertain whether the older adult experiences daytime sleepiness or has a strong desire to nap.

A patient's activities before bedtime and his or her exercise and activity pattern provide additional information about sleep habits. In general, strenuous activity should be avoided at least 2 hours before bedtime. The nurse should identify what the patient does to relax before bedtime, for example, reading or drinking a warm beverage. The nurse should question the patient having difficulty with sleep about the consumption of alcohol, caffeinated beverages, sedative-hypnotics, OTC drugs, and other practices before bedtime.

Questions about the type of bed in which the person sleeps are also important. Does the patient sleep in the same bed every night? Is it comfortable? Is the mattress soft, or does it provide adequate support? Some individuals who are unable to sleep in a recumbent position because of medical problems may be able to sleep in a semirecumbent position in a lounge chair or recliner. Patients who are unable to fall asleep in the supine position and who need several pillows or cushions in bed require further medical evaluation for heart failure, pulmonary disease, or musculoskeletal problems (Spieker & Motzer, 2003). Common problems that cause pain and discomfort in bed include COPD; rheumatologic problems such as osteoporosis; degenerative joint disease of the spine, hips, or neck; and rheumatoid arthritis. Nocturia occurring several times in the course of one night must be further evaluated. Older men with prostate enlargement need to urinate several times during the night. Older adults with congestive heart failure or urinary tract infections may also have nocturia.

Further Assessment of Sleep

A sleep diary kept by the older adult is helpful in recalling the amount of sleep, bedtime routines, and possible symptoms of disturbed sleep over a 24-hour period. The type and quantity of activities are also noted in the diary for the same 24-hour period. To complete the sleep diary, the older adult may need the assistance of a family member or the nurse. The nurse may suggest measures to help patients enter information in the diary, for example, tape-recorded entries for patients with visual impairment or difficulty writing.

Sleep laboratories specialize in treating patients with primary sleep disorders. Patients are asked to spend the night so that a sleep study can be administered. This often includes polysomnography, which provides data about the stages of sleep and ventilation, and an EEG for graphic tracing of the variations in the brain's electric force. Physicians specially trained in sleep disorders evaluate the history and objective findings, including a review of basic sleep hygienic measures, to arrive at a diagnosis and treatment plan.

Additional information about sleep may be collected with the use of questionnaires. The Epworth Sleepiness Scale (ESS) (Fig. 10.1) measures feelings of sleepiness or tiredness at specific times. The ESS also measures sleepiness, but it measures it in terms of sleep propensity, the likelihood of falling asleep at a particular time. The person completing the ESS considers certain situations and indicates the likelihood (low to high) that he or she would fall asleep in those situations (Cochran, 2003). Another instrument is the Pittsburgh Sleep Quality Index, which subjectively measures sleep quality and includes five additional questions for the bed partner. In addition to instruments that only address sleep, other instruments that have questions about sleep may be used (Cohen, 1997).

Getting a Good Night's Sleep

Whether sleep is disturbed by the environment, diet, drugs, lifestyle changes, or sleep disorders, the first step in developing interventions to improve the amount and quality of sleep is taking a thorough sleep history. Supplementing the sleep history are measurement tools to assess sleep quality and quantity, direct observation of the older adult during sleep, a sleep diary, and diagnostic studies such as EEG monitoring, and sleep study

---

The Epworth Sleepiness Scale (ESS)

How likely are you to doze off or fall asleep in the following situations, in contrast to feeling just tired? This refers to your usual way of life in recent times. Even if you have not done some of these things recently try to work out how they would have affected you. Use the following scale to choose the **most appropriate number** for each situation:

0 = would **never** doze

1 = **slight chance** of dozing

2 = **moderate chance** of dozing

3 = **high chance** of dozing

SITUATION	CHANCE OF DOZING (0–3)
Sitting and reading	
Watching television	
Sitting inactive in a public place (e.g. a theater or meeting)	
As a passenger in a car for an hour without a break	
Lying down to rest in the afternoon when circumstances permit	
Sitting and talking to someone	
Sitting quietly after a lunch without alcohol	
In a car, while stopped for a few minutes in the traffic	
TOTAL SCORE	

SCORE RESULTS:

1–6	Congratulations, you are getting enough sleep!
7–8	Your score is average
9 and up	Very sleepy and should seek medical advice

Fig. 10.1 Epworth Sleepiness Scale. (From Johns, M. W. [1991]. A new method for measuring daytime sleepiness: The Epworth Sleepiness Scale. *Sleep, 14,* 540-545.)

evaluation. After assessment, interventions to improve sleep usually begin with basic sleep hygiene measures.

Sleep Hygiene

Basic sleep hygiene includes those activities that foster normal sleep and that can be practiced by individuals on a routine basis. The goal of sleep hygiene measures is to achieve normal sleep. The various measures reinforce habits, routines, and attitudes that promote sleep and advocate changes in habits and routines that do not contribute to a good night's sleep (Kirkwood, 2001). Sleep hygiene measures emphasize stable schedules and bedtime routines, a sleep-friendly environment, avoidance of any substances that would interfere with sleep, regular exercise (but not immediately before trying to sleep), and stress reduction.

Retiring at the same time every night and awakening at the same time every morning help establish a routine. A patient may condition himself or herself to such a routine over time. Likewise, limiting the amount of time spent in bed to only the time spent sleeping establishes a routine for sleep. Retiring to the same location such as the bedroom, and not a couch or chair on some nights, also helps solidify the routine. If unable to fall asleep, the person should get up and move to another area to perform other activities until sleepy. Eliminating noise and creating a darkened environment promotes sleep. Limiting daytime napping and having warm beverages and light nutritious snacks at bedtime are additional measures that promote sleep.

Avoiding caffeinated beverages, sleeping pills, and alcohol may reduce the chances of sleep-related breathing disorders (SBDs). The basic measures to help reduce episodes of sleep apnea include losing weight, sleeping on one's side or stomach, avoiding central nervous system (CNS) depressants such as sedative–hypnotics and alcohol, and treating any obvious nasal or upper airway diseases.

Fostering Normal Sleep in Homebound Older Adults

It is important for the nurse to assess risk factors (e.g., environment, pain, or equipment such as a Foley catheter) that predispose homebound older adults to sleep disturbances. Review all drugs to identify those that may interfere with sleep patterns. Instruct caregivers and homebound older adults on activities that foster normal sleep, for example, avoidance of caffeinated beverages and alcohol. Assist with environmental changes that foster normal sleep, such as using a rocking chair or taking a warm bath. It must be kept in mind that worry and anxiety concerning safety and welfare may be obstacles to sleep in older adults. A system of notification and monitoring to link older adults living alone with the outside world is important to promote their sense of security.

Nonpharmacological Therapies to Promote Sleep

In addition to sleep hygiene measures, the American Academy of Sleep Medicine recommends other nonpharmacologic interventions to promote sleep. Among these measures are relaxation therapies, stimulus control therapy, and sleep restriction therapy and cognitive behavioral therapy. Relaxation therapies reduce either somatic arousal or cognitive arousal. Progressive muscle relaxation is one example of a therapy to reduce somatic arousal. Cognitive arousal is reduced by attention-focusing

therapies such as guided imagery or meditation. Stimulus control therapy attempts to reestablish the bedroom environment as the stimulus for sleep by banning activities from the bedroom that are not related to a good night's sleep. Examples of such activities include eating and watching television. Stimulus control therapy is helpful for individuals with sleep-onset insomnia. Sleep restriction therapy limits the amount of time spent in bed. Individuals stay in bed only for the number of hours they estimate as their average time asleep, plus 15 minutes. Cognitive behavioral therapy helps the person with insomnia to address factors, such as stress, that interfere with sleep (Siebern, Suh, & Nowakowski, 2012).

Drugs Used to Promote Sleep

Although nonpharmacological measures are the treatment of choice of insomnia, drug therapy may be necessary for a short time. Most drugs traditionally used to promote sleep (tranquilizers and sedative hypnotics) are listed as drugs to avoid on the updated 2015 Beers Criteria for Potentially Inappropriate Medication Use in Older Adults. These drugs carry the risk of physical dependence, increased risk of cognitive impairment, delirium, and falls. Additionally, the nonbenzodiazepine receptor agonist hypnotics are also drugs to avoid in older adults due to the high risk for delirium falls and increased emergency department visits and hospitalizations. One antihistamine, diphenhydramine, which is a component of many OTC sleep aids, also makes the 2015 Beers Criteria for Potentially Inappropriate Medication Use in Older Adults. This drug should be avoided in older adults as tolerance develops when used as a hypnotic, and users face an increased risk of confusion and reduced clearance, which can lead to toxicity (American Geriatrics Society, 2015).

Doxepin should not be used in doses higher than 6 mg per day as it is highly anticholinergic, and patients have increased risk for orthostatic hypotension. Mirtazapine and trazodone should be used with caution, as patients may experience significant hyponatremia (American Geriatrics Society, 2015). Two drugs, ramelteon (a melatonin agonist) and suvorexant (an orexin receptor antagonist), currently have no restrictions for use in older adults; however, these drugs carry the same side effect profile as other sleep aids. Ramelteon is indicated for use in patients who have difficulty falling asleep; suvorexant helps patients both fall asleep and stay asleep (Mayo Clinic Staff, 2018) (see Patient/Family Teaching Box). Pharmacologic treatment of insomnia should be short term—no more than one or 2 weeks.

🏃 PATIENT/FAMILY TEACHING

Treating Insomnia with Drugs

- Take the sleeping pill when all evening activities are completed and you are ready to go to bed.
- Only take a sleeping pill when you can get a full night's sleep (7–8 hours).
- Be aware of side effects; if you feel sleepy or dizzy during the day, call your health care provider.
- Never mix alcohol and sleeping pills.

Used with permission from Mayo Foundation for Medical Education and Research. All rights reserved. (2018). Prescription sleeping pills: What's right for you? Retrieved February 20, 2018, from https://www.mayoclinic.org/diseases-conditions/insomnia/in-depth/sleeping-pills/art-20043959.

BOX 10.3 Tips for Older Adults Using Herbal and Homeopathic Remedies

1. Before treating any symptom with a nonprescription product, make sure no conditions requiring medical attention exist.
2. Discuss the use of any nonprescription product with your physician and other health care providers.
3. Be cautious about viewing herbal or homeopathic products as a substitute for prescribed drugs.
4. Use single-ingredient products rather than combinations.
5. Observe for beneficial and harmful effects.
6. Report any possible side effects to your physician for evaluation.
7. Seek information from objective sources rather than relying on promotional materials and package information.
8. Check any warnings on the label or package, and check for information from additional sources.
9. Consider the fact that herbal and homeopathic products are not required to meet standards for safety and efficacy.
10. Be skeptical about exaggerated claims—if it sounds too good to be true, it probably is!

From Miller, C. A. (1996). Alternative healing products. *Geriatric Nursing, 17*(3), 145-146.

Complementary and Alternative Medicines

Various complementary and alternative medicines (CAM) have been recommended as aids for securing a good night's sleep. Unlike prescription drugs, the composition of these compounds is not readily available, and their side effects and interactions with prescription or OTC drugs have not been fully explored (Box 10.3). Some herbal remedies contain active ingredients that resemble prescription and OTC drugs, increasing the risk for drug–drug interaction (Cochran, 2003).

One CAM, melatonin, has undergone scientific study, demonstrating some effectiveness in healthy adults, decreasing sleep latency and increasing sleep duration when used for 3 months or less. However, as with other CAMs, it is unregulated, and caution is advised with its use (Ratini, 2017).

ACTIVITY AND OLDER ADULTS

Activity, as discussed in this chapter, includes routine daily activities, diversional activities, and physical exercise. Changes occur in the activities pursued by older adults as they age or experience acute or chronic illness. Other changes in activities occur in response to major lifestyle changes such as retirement, relocation, or loss of a spouse. Specialized activities to meet the needs of older adults with Alzheimer's disease or a related dementia are also available. Whether cared for at home or in a long-term care facility, the older adult with dementia benefits from an activity program that includes both diversional activities and activities to promote independence in activities of daily living (ADLs). Physical exercise deserves special attention because of its health-promoting benefits for all older adults. Although the activities pursued by a particular older adult are influenced by his or her preferences, situation, and health, some general considerations for activity in older adults do exist. In some settings, nurses participate in planning activities, adapting activities to the older adult's current situation, and evaluating the effects of activities on health.

Activities of Daily Living

ADLs include the things that most adults do every day, often without special attention or effort. Until something happens to interfere with normal daily routines, little thought may be given to bathing, dressing, eating, or attending to elimination needs. However, with advancing age and changes in health and circumstances, activities that once were accomplished with ease may require modified approaches or the assistance of others. In addition to providing direct assistance with ADLs, nurses assist older adults in the modification of routines and the use of assistive devices that help maintain independence. Nurses also support and advise family members and friends who assist the older adult with ADLs.

Basic ADLs include the everyday personal care tasks related to hygiene, nutrition, and elimination. Remaining independent in these activities is highly prized by older adults. Dependency in basic ADLs increases the risk of relocation to a long-term care facility or to the home of a family member. To remain independent in basic ADLs, older adults use assistive devices and modify their care routines. Handheld shower sprays, raised toilet seats, sturdy grab bars in bathrooms, plate guards, and built-up handles on toothbrushes and eating utensils are examples of assistive devices. Clothing with Velcro instead of buttons, ties that can be clipped on rather than tied, and shoes that can be slipped on rather than laced are examples of modifications to help with dressing. However, for some older adults, the amount of assistance needed with personal care exceeds their ability to modify routines and the capacity of family members and friends to help. Home care nurses may supplement the care provided by family members and friends, or relocation to a long-term care facility may be necessary.

Instrumental activities of daily living (IADLs) include activities such as driving, shopping, cooking, housekeeping, and using a telephone. Older adults modify their approaches to IADLs because of commonly experienced changes in aging such as reduced strength, impaired vision, or impaired hearing. Assistive devices make the tasks of cooking or housekeeping easier and safer. Driving may be restricted to familiar areas and daylight hours. Family members, friends, or paid caregivers may help with shopping and other tasks. During episodes of acute illness or recovery from hospitalization, additional help may be needed. If sufficient assistance with IADLs is available in the home, relocation to a long-term care facility is not necessary.

Physical Exercise

Physical activity is important for older adults to maintain health, preserve the ability to perform ADLs, and improve general quality of life. The benefits of physical activity include prevention of heart disease and diabetes, reduction in elevated blood pressure, reduced risk of osteoporosis, promotion of appropriate weight, reduction in depressed mood, reduced cancer risk, and promotion of more restful sleep (Schoenborn, Vickerie, & Powell-Griner, 2006). Exercise preserves mobility and reduces the risk of falls by promoting muscle strength and joint flexibility.

Older adults exercise for a variety of reasons (Schoenborn et al., 2006). They exercise to have fun, to socialize with friends and neighbors, and to simply feel better. Exercise is used to reduce stress, to promote relaxation, and, together with a good nutritional program, to control weight. The Centers for Disease Control and Prevention (CDC, 2015) recommends moderate-intensity aerobic exercise for 150 minutes a week. The activity may be divided into smaller segments of at least 10 minutes' duration. To measure the appropriate intensity while walking, the "talk test" may be used. The person exercising should be able to carry on a conversation while walking. Breathing may be slightly labored, but a conversation should still be possible. The walker should not be out of breath. Muscle strengthening should be done at least 2 days per week. Older adults with restricted abilities because of medical conditions should perform physical activity within their limitations.

If the older adult has not been exercising every day, starting with only 5 minutes of exercise each day and gradually working up to 20 or 30 minutes a day is appropriate (Schoenborn et al., 2006). A gradual progression in an exercise program for older adults who have been sedentary is recommended. A sedentary lifestyle is not unusual for older adults. In one study, physical activity and sedentary behavior were measured in adults over the age of 60. Results indicate older adults average 10 minutes to 106 minutes per day in moderate physical activity. Activity declines with age; those over 80 averaged 5 to 60 minutes of moderate physical activity per day. Women were more active than men. Older adults spent an average of 8.5 hours per day in sedentary behavior, with those over 80 spending the most time in sedentary behavior (Evenson, Buchner, & Morland, 2012).

In addition to recommending gradual increases in the amount of exercise time for older adults who have not been exercising regularly, the nurse may pass along other safety tips. Drinking water before and after exercise is important because of fluid loss during exercise. Clothing worn for exercise should allow for easy movement and perspiration. Athletic shoes should provide both support and protection. Outdoor exercise should be avoided in extremely hot or extremely cold weather. Enclosed shopping malls are sheltered places for walking during the extremes of weather or when there are concerns about neighborhood safety. Exercising with a partner provides both encouragement to continue exercising and safety. Nurses should advise older adults to stop exercising and seek help if they experience chest pain or tightness, shortness of breath, dizziness or lightheadedness, or palpitations during exercise (Gunnarsson & Judge, 1997).

Activity as Affected by Lifestyle Changes

Retirement, relocation, and the loss of a spouse influence older adults' activity levels and the types of activities they pursue. Many older adults directly experience these lifestyle changes; others experience them indirectly when a spouse retires or is admitted to a long-term care facility.

Retirement

Retirement represents a major lifestyle change for older adults. During most of their lives, older adults have gone to work or watched a spouse go to work each day. With retirement, the daily schedule changes. The hours spent on the job and in transit to and from the job are no longer committed. For couples where only the husband has worked, the wife's daily routine is affected by her husband being home. If the wife is still working outside the home when the husband retires, the husband finds himself at home alone. For the unmarried retired person, retirement may be a transition from a companionable work setting to a lonely, empty house. Key issues for the retired older adult are the replacement of work with meaningful activities and the replacement of work-related friends with new acquaintances.

Activities in retirement may be chosen to be meaningful and to meet socialization needs. Past interests influence choices about activities. If past interests have focused only on work-related topics, retirement choices may be restricted unless the retired older adult develops new areas of interest. Finances may also impose practical restrictions on the types of activities chosen. Health status issues such as limited mobility, limited endurance, or sensory deficits may also restrict activity choices. However, for many older adults, retirement is a time to become involved in activities that could not be pursued while working because of time and energy constraints. Many older adults volunteer in community organizations, return to school for the joy of learning, or even start second careers. Nurses are empathetic listeners to accounts of the changes retirement brings and sources of information about different activities available.

Relocation

Relocation is movement from one place of residence to another. Relocation may be from the long-time home in a cold climate to a house or apartment in a warmer part of the country. Older adults may also move from their home to the home of their children or grandchildren. Still other older adults may move to a retirement community or an assisted living or long-term care facility. Regardless of the destination, relocation is always an uprooting and a disordering of usual routines. Even when the move is from an unpleasant or unsafe situation, a risk still exists that relocation may adversely affect well-being.

Relocation disrupts usual patterns of activity. Adaptations that maintained independence in ADLs may no longer function. The walk through a familiar neighborhood for exercise may no longer be possible. The new community or long-term care facility will have different options for activities. New social networks can be established. The nurse's role during relocation is to support efforts to become accustomed to new situations and opportunities and to monitor the effect of relocation stress on health.

Activity programming in long-term care facilities is the responsibility of activity directors. A sufficient variety of activities is provided to allow residents to have choices. Although residents are encouraged to participate in a variety of activities, they always have the right to determine the degree of their participation. The activity preferences of each resident are assessed on admission. The individualized care plan includes activities that are appropriate for the resident. Individual (one-on-one activities), small group, and large group activities are typically provided (Fig. 10.2). Some facilities provide mechanisms for

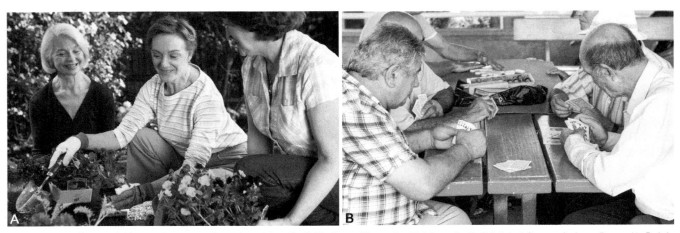

Fig. 10.2 Recreational activities are important for older adults. (**A,** © Liz Gregg/Photodisc/Thinkstock. **B,** © Michal Osmenda from Brussels, Belgium/CC-BY-2.0, via Wikimedia Commons.)

residents to participate in planning future activities and for families and friends of the residents to be part of the activity program (Box 10.4).

Loss of Spouse

The loss of a spouse disrupts both joint activities and those activities where one spouse supported the other. If death is preceded by an illness, activities are altered in advance of death. During the period of grief, activities may be reduced. For example, the older adult may not feel up to participating in an exercise class. However, part of the process of grief and recovery from grief is the adoption of a new pattern of life. That new pattern includes new activities but also includes the resumption of former activities, although these may be altered by the absence of the spouse.

Nurses assist the older adult who has experienced the loss of a spouse by listening attentively and supporting the development of new activities. Some of these new activities may require learning new skills such as handling finances, cooking, doing the laundry, or maintaining the car. Other activities may involve making new friends. Information from nurses about available programs and services may help with the acquisition of new skills and the reestablishment of social connections. During the period of adjustment after the loss of a spouse, nurses also monitor the patient's physical and mental health, remembering that stress may lead to alterations in health.

Activity Affected by Alzheimer's Disease and Other Dementias

Alzheimer's disease and other dementias affect an estimated five million people in the United States (Alzheimer's Association, 2013). As Alzheimer's disease progresses, cognitive impairment increases, which adversely affects the ability to initiate and participate in routine daily activities. The older adult with advancing dementia also loses the ability to initiate diversional activities and to participate in activities that were once enjoyed.

BOX 10.4   Examples of Activities in Long-Term Care Facilities

Exercise
Walking programs (indoor, outdoor)
Dancing (balloon, square, line)
T'ai chi (or similar disciplines)

Spectator Activities
Television (selected programming, including telecourses)
Video movies
Live performances at the facility

Participative Activities
Cards, bingo, and board games
Adapted versions of bowling and volleyball
Adaptations of TV game shows (*Jeopardy, Wheel of Fortune*)
Yard games such as croquet, miniature golf, bocce ball, and horseshoes
Field trips to museums, sports events, restaurants, shopping malls, and parks
Picnics and barbecues
Fishing

Creative Activities
Art projects (painting)
Crafts (woodworking, stitchery)
Gardening (indoor or outdoor)
Cooking or planning menus for special meals at the facility
Music (vocal or instrumental performances by residents)
Writing a newsletter for the facility

Intergenerational Activities
Visits from children's groups
Adopting (and being adopted by) a schoolroom or scout troop

Pets and Other Animals
Domestic animals kept at the facility (dogs, cats, rabbits, songbirds, parrots, fish, sheep, goats, llamas, chickens, ducks, and geese)
Other animals brought to the facility by zoos or conservation groups (owls, hawks, chimpanzees, and nonvenomous snakes)

Caregivers gradually assume more responsibility for monitoring behavior, performing basic personal care tasks, and providing opportunities for physical exercise, cognitive stimulation, and entertainment.

At the heart of planning activities for an older adult with dementia is the desire to preserve the remaining physical and cognitive abilities and to promote independence. Activities should draw on assets rather than deficits and should maximize the remaining abilities (Alzheimer's Association, 2012a). When planning activities, nurses or other caregivers must consider the extent of cognitive impairment, any concomitant physical constraints caused by aging or other diseases, and safety concerns.

Activities for older adults with dementia should be meaningful (Alzheimer's Association, 2012a). A meaningful activity has a purpose. The purpose may be to exercise arthritic joints or simply to have fun, but the activity should not be aimless. Meaningful activities are also voluntary. No one is compelled to participate. Instead, individuals are invited to participate and given encouragement and explanations of the activity. Meaningful activities foster a sense of well-being for the participants. If an older adult with dementia is stressed by the activity or indicates discomfort, that person should be allowed, or assisted, to stop or leave the activity. Activities should also be consistent with the older adult's social status and support his or her dignity. Older adults may choose to participate in an activity that appears childish, but they must also have the option to refuse to participate. Activities should promote good feelings, not feelings of embarrassment, distress, or failure. To successfully plan and implement activities for older adults with dementia, nurses and other caregivers must be flexible, patient, and sensitive to the environment (Alzheimer's Association, 2012b). Communication is enhanced when the nurse or other caregiver speaks to the older adult as one adult to another and assumes the older adult will understand. If the older adult does not understand, repetition or rephrasing may be necessary, but it is best to begin with the positive expectation that the older adult will understand. Scolding, addressing the older adult as a child, or issuing negative instructions ("Don't …") should be avoided (Alzheimer's Association, 2012b).

As cognitive impairment increases, the older adult with dementia requires more supervision and assistance with personal care activities such as bathing, dressing, grooming, toileting, oral hygiene, and eating. Personal care activities are best accomplished in regular routines that involve simple, single-step instructions and visual cues. The environment should be quiet, soothing, uncluttered, and unhurried. To promote independence and preserve functional ability, nurses should encourage older adults with dementia to do the personal care tasks, or parts of tasks, that are within their abilities.

Physical exercise for the older adult with dementia is important for general physical well-being, but exercise may also reduce agitation or wandering. The rhythmic movement of a rocking chair may reduce agitation. Going for a walk may redirect the impulse to wander. Whether the benefit is from the change of setting, the removal of the older adult from a provocative stimulus, or the physical effects of walking, the end result is often an older adult who appears more comfortable. Exercise is also important for preserving muscle strength, flexibility, and ambulation. Other activities providing physical exercise include dancing, marching in place or swinging the arms to music, and gardening.

Older adults with dementia gradually lose the ability to select diversional activities, yet when diversional activities are provided, they appear to enjoy themselves and participate to the extent of their abilities. Activities for older adults with dementia range from playing simple games to dancing to watching birds at a bird feeder. Activities may include simple housekeeping tasks such as dusting or folding towels. Activities may be one-on-one activities such as taking a walk with a caregiver or group activities such as attending a church service.

Activities that tap into the older adult's past life experiences and interests may stimulate memory. Older adults with dementia may enjoy reminiscing, in groups or individually, because long-term memory may be preserved in the early stages of dementia. Activities that involve making or growing things evoke pride in the self and in accomplishments. Even in later stages of dementia, an object or a song may evoke a memory. Song lyrics or the familiar motions of cooking, painting, or playing the piano may be remembered when many other things have been forgotten.

The benefits of activity for older adults include the promotion of health and the preservation of independence. Nurses help older adults adapt their activities to the situations that arise in the later years. Nurses also work with older adults to identify new activities. Whether the activities involve daily activities, physical exercise, or diversion, older adults and nurses should work together to design and select activities that improve the quality of life.

🏠 HOME CARE

1. Assess risk factors (e.g., environment, pain, or depression) that would predispose homebound older adults to sleep disturbances.
2. Review all drugs to identify those that may interfere with homebound older adults' sleep patterns.
3. Instruct caregivers and homebound older adults on activities that foster normal sleep, for example, avoidance of caffeinated beverages and alcohol.
4. Assist caregivers and homebound older adults with environmental changes that foster normal sleep, for example, using a rocking chair or taking a warm bath.
5. Remember that anxiety concerning safety and welfare may be an obstacle to sleep. A system of notification and monitoring to link older adults living alone with the outside world is important to promote a sense of security.

SUMMARY

Sleep and activity are two halves that make a whole day. Without sleep, we are not restored from the previous day's efforts and today's activities are slowed by fatigue. Without activities, we face going to bed without feeling the necessity of rest. Without the appropriate balance of rest and activity, we are at risk of alterations in health. Nurses, by recognizing the changes that come with age and with alterations in health status, are able to assist older adults with their sleep and activity needs.

KEY POINTS

- The sleep changes experienced by many older adults include increased sleep latency, decreased sleep efficiency, increased awakening in the night, increased early morning awakening, and increased daytime sleepiness.
- Some of the sleep changes experienced by older adults are associated with chronic disease and other health problems.
- Factors influencing sleep quality include environmental factors, pain, lifestyle changes, diet, drug use, medical conditions, depression, and dementia.
- Sleep apnea and PLMS are two common sleep disorders that may result in excessive daytime sleepiness and reports of insomnia.
- The first step in developing interventions to improve the amount and quality of sleep is a thorough sleep history.
- The sleep history includes questions about sleep amount and quality, bedtime routines, the sleep environment, activities, diet, and drugs.
- Direct observation of the older adult during sleep, reports from a roommate or bed partner, a sleep diary, measurement instruments to assess sleep quality and quantity, and diagnostic studies in a sleep laboratory may be used to supplement the sleep history.

- Sleep hygiene measures include activities that promote sleep, emphasis on stable schedules, bedtime routines, a sleep-friendly environment, avoidance of substances that interfere with sleep, exercise, and stress reduction.
- Activities pursued by a particular older adult are influenced by that individual's preferences, lifestyle, and health.
- With advancing years and changes in health and lifestyle circumstances, performance of ADLs may require modified approaches or the assistance of others.
- Physical exercise is important for older adults to maintain health, preserve the ability to perform ADLs, and improve the general quality of life.
- Safe exercise requires gradual increases in the amount of exercise for older adults who have not been exercising regularly, adequate hydration before and after exercise, and suitable clothing and footwear.
- Retirement, relocation, and the loss of a spouse influence the ways older adults are active and the types of activities that they pursue.
- The goals of activities for older adults with Alzheimer's disease and other dementias include preservation of physical and cognitive abilities and promotion of independence.

CRITICAL-THINKING EXERCISES

1. A nursing facility resident tells you she has not been sleeping well and asks you to have the doctor order a sleeping pill. What questions do you ask to assess her sleep quality and quantity? Because you are aware of the drawbacks of the use of sedatives and hypnotics, what other interventions do you suggest to improve her sleep?
2. In the clinic, you meet with an older gentleman who is accompanied by his wife. She reports that he is snoring loudly every night and is always falling asleep during the day. He denies snoring but admits that he is often very sleepy during the day. What sleep disorder do you suspect? What

reports and symptoms would strengthen your suspicion? What recommendations do you make to the patient?
3. You are checking blood pressures at a senior citizen health fair. After you check the blood pressure of an older woman, she asks you about starting an exercise program. She has not been exercising, but some of her friends have told her that she should start to exercise regularly. What recommendations do you give her? What precautions do you include in your recommendations?

REFERENCES

Alzheimer's Association. (2012a). *Activities at home: Planning the day for a person with dementia.* Retrieved from https://www.alz.org/national/documents/brochure_activities.pdf.

Alzheimer's Association. (2012b). *Behaviors: How to respond when dementia causes unpredictable behaviors.* Retrieved from http://www.alz.org/national/documents/brochure_behaviors.pdf.

Alzheimer's Association. (2013). *2013 Alzheimer's disease facts and figures [Annual report].* Retrieved from http://www.alz.org/downloads/facts_figures_2013.pdf.

American Geriatrics Society. (2015). *American Geriatrics Society 2015 updated Beers Criteria for potentially inappropriate medication use in older adults.* Retrieved from https://guideline.gov/summaries/summary/49933/American-Geriatrics-Society-2015-updated-

Beers-Criteria-for-potentially-inappropriate-medication-use-in-older-adults.

Ancoli-Israel, S. (2004). Sleep disorders in older adults: a primary care guide to assessing 4 common sleep problems in geriatric patients. *Geriatrics, 59*(1), 37.

Beers, M. H., & Berkow, R. (2000–2006). *The Merck manual of geriatrics* (3rd ed.). Whitehouse Station, NJ: Merck Research Laboratories.

Burke, M. M., & Laramie, J. A. (2004). *Primary care of the older adult* (2nd ed.). St. Louis: Mosby.

Centers for Disease Control and Prevention. (2015). *How much physical activity do older adults need?* Retrieved February 20, 2018 from https://www.cdc.gov/physicalactivity/basics/older_adults/index.htm.

Chasens, E. R., Sereika, S. M., & Burke, L. E. (2009). Daytime sleepiness and functional outcomes in older adults with diabetes. *The Diabetes Educator, 35*(3), 455–464.

Cleveland Clinic. (2012). *Periodic limb movement disorder.* Retrieved January 19, 2014, from http://my.clevelandclinic.org/disorders/periodic_limb_movement_disorder/hic_periodic_limb_movement_disorder.aspx.

Cochran, H. (2003). Diagnosis and treatment of primary insomnia. *Nursing Practice, 28*(9), 13.

Cohen, F. L. (1997). Measuring sleep. In M. Frank-Stromborg & S. J. Olsen (Eds.), *Instruments for clinical health-care research* (2nd ed.). Sudbury, Mass: Jones & Bartlett.

Cohen-Zion, M., & Ancoli-Israel, S. (2003). Sleep disorders. In W. R. Hazzard, J. P. Blass, J. B. Halter, et al. (Eds.), *Principles of geriatric medicine and gerontology* (5th ed.). New York: McGraw-Hill.

Evenson, K. R., Buchner, D. M., & Morland, K. B. (2012). Objective measurement of physical activity and sedentary behavior among US adults aged 60 years or older. *Preventing Chronic Disease, 9.* https://doi.org/10.5888/pcd9.110109.

Felson, S. (2017). *How to sleep better as you get older.* Retrieve February 20, 2018 from https://www.webmd.com/sleep-disorders/guide/aging-affects-sleep#2.

Floyd, J. A. (1995). Another look at napping in older adults. *Geriatric Nursing, 16,* 136.

Friedman, S. (2010). Pain, temperature regulation, sleep, and sensory function. In K. L. McCance, S. E. Huether, V. Brashers, & N. Rote (Eds.), *Pathophysiology: the biological basis for disease in adults and children* (6th ed.). St Louis: Mosby.

Goldberg, J. (2012). *Understanding obstructive sleep apnea.* Retrieved January 19, 2014, from http://www.webmd.com/sleep-disorders/guide/understanding-obstructive-sleep-apnea-syndrome.

Gordon, A. M. (2013). *Your sleep cycle revealed.* Retrieved February 20, 2018 from https://www.psychologytoday.com/blog/between-you-and-me/201307/your-sleep-cycle-revealed.

Gunnarsson, O. T., & Judge, J. O. (1997). Exercise at midlife: how and why to prescribe it for sedentary patients. *Geriatrics, 52*(5), 71.

Hoffman, S. (2003). Sleep in the older adult: implications for nurses. *Geriatric Nursing, 24*(4), 210–216.

Kirkwood, C. (2001). *Treatment of insomnia.* New York: Power-Pak, CE Publishers. http://www.powerpak.com.

Kryger, M., Monjan, A., Bliwise, D., & Ancoli-Israel, S. (2004). Sleep, health, and aging: bridging the gap between science and clinical practice. *Geriatrics, 59*(1), 24.

Lewy, A. J. (2009). Circadian misalignment in mood disturbances. *Current Psychiatry Reports, 11*(6), 459–465.

Mayo Clinic Staff. (2018). *Prescription sleeping pills: What's right for you?* Retrieved February 20, 2018 from https://www.mayoclinic.org/diseases-conditions/insomnia/in-depth/sleeping-pills/art-20043959.

Nabili, S. T. (2012). *Sleep apnea.* Retrieved January 19, 2014, from http://www.medicinenet.com/sleep_apnea/article.htm.

Nagel, C., Markie, M. B., Richards, K. C., & Taylor, J. L. (2003). Sleep promotion in hospitalized elders. *Medsurg Nursing, 12*(5), 279.

Olson, E. J., Moore, W. R., Morgenthaler, T. I., et al. (2003). Obstructive sleep apnea-hypopnea syndrome. *Mayo Clin Pro, 78*(1545).

Ratini, M. (2012). *Central sleep apnea.* Retrieved January 19, 2014, from http://www.webmd.com/sleep-disorders/guide/central-sleep-apnea.

Ratini, M. (2017). *Natural sleep aids and remedies.* Retrieved February 20, 2018 from https://www.webmd.com/women/natural-sleep-remedies#1.

Rosto, L. (2001). Sleep and the elderly. *Advance On-line Editions for Providers of Post-Acute Care, 4*(6), 27.

Rowe, M. A. (2003). People with dementia who become lost. *The American Journal of Nursing, 103*(7), 32–39.

Schoenborn, C. A., Vickerie, J. L., & Powell-Griner, E. (2006). Health characteristics of adults 55 years of age and over: United States, 2000–2003. In *Advance data from vital and health statistics, no 370.* Hyattsville, Md: National Center for Health Statistics.

Siebern, A. T., Suh, S., & Nowakowski, S. (2012). Non-pharmacological treatment of insomnia. *Neurotherapeutics, 9*(4), 717–727. https://doi.org/10.1007/s13311-012-0142-9.

Spieker, E. D., & Motzer, S. A. (2003). Sleep-disorder in patients with heart failure: pathophysiology, assessment and management. *Journal of the American Academy of Nurse Practitioners, 15*(11), 487.

United States Census Bureau. (2017). *Facts for Features: Older Americans Month: May 2017.* Retrieved February 20, 2018 from https://www.census.gov/newsroom/facts-for-features/2017/cb17-ff08.html.

Wang, J., Wang, Y., Feng, J., Chen, B., & Cao, J. (2013). Complex sleep apnea syndrome. *Patient Preference and Adherence, 13*(7), 633–641. Retrieved from http://www.dovepress.com/complex-sleep-apnea-syndrome-peer-reviewed-article-PPA.

WebMD. (2017). *Sleep disorders health center.* Retrieved May 1, 2014 from http://www.webmd.com/sleep-disorders/guide/insomnia-symptoms-and-causes.

Worfolk, J. B. (1997). Keep frail elders warm! *Geriatric Nursing, 18,* 7.

11

Safety

Debra L. Sanders, PhD, RN, GCNS-BC, FNGNA

http://evolve.elsevier.com/Meiner/gerontologic

LEARNING OBJECTIVES

On completion of this chapter, the reader will be able to:

1. Identify the nurse's role in the promotion of safety for older adults.
2. Name various community, state, and federal safety-related resources for older individuals.
3. Identify safety hazards in the health care setting that may lead to litigation.
4. Differentiate between intrinsic and extrinsic causes of falling in older adults.
5. Identify common treatable causes of falling in older adults.
6. Implement the nursing standard of practice for patients experiencing falls.
7. Use home safety tips to prevent burns, accidental poisoning, smoke inhalation, and foodborne illnesses among community-dwelling older adults.
8. Differentiate between hypothermia and hyperthermia and the nursing needs of each.
9. Identify disaster planning resources.
10. Differentiate among the various types of elder abuse.
11. List clinical syndromes and conditions that could impair older individuals and lead to safety hazards on the roadway.
12. Describe the pros and cons of having firearms in the homes of older adults.

WHAT WOULD YOU DO?

What would you do if you were faced with the following situations?

* Your 75-year-old nursing home resident was found on the floor in a sitting position, near the foot of the bed. After determining the resident had not sustained any head trauma or change in mental status nor sustained any apparent breaks, what would be your next steps?
* Your 80-year-old patient arrives at the clinic, using a rolling walker. He is not accompanied by his caregiver, as usual. Upon questioning, you determine he drove himself to his appointment. How would you determine whether he was safe to drive? What would you do if the determination was made he should not be driving?

Feeling safe and secure in one's living environment is important for all people. With aging comes a need to maintain peace of mind while engaging in daily activities. The confidence to carry out daily tasks is affected by perceived security and safety. Safety is a broad concept that refers to security and the prevention of accidents or injuries. When working with older adults, the gerontologic nurse must provide a standard of care that promotes safety and prevents foreseeable accidents or injuries while also respecting individuals' autonomy to make decisions. This standard of care should pervade all aspects of the nurse's health care relationships with older adults.

Previous authors: Ramesh C. Upadhyaya, RN, CRRN, MSN, MBA, PhD-C, and Deb Bagnasco Stanford, MSN, RN, CCRN.

Healthy People 2020 identifies unintentional injury as one of the top 15 killers across all age groups. Violent crimes including homicide are another concern for all Americans, including older adults (U.S. Department of Health and Human Services, 2014).

Part of the nurse's role in ensuring safety is educating older adults so that they can make informed choices. Education allows one to weigh benefits versus risks and to choose the best option in the situation. In situations in which patients are unable to make informed choices, family members or significant others are sought as advocates for the patients. If patients are unable to make informed choices and no family members are available, the nurse must use nursing judgment and follow an acceptable standard of care to promote safety and security.

This chapter presents common problems that jeopardize patient safety and lead to accidents, injuries, and even death. These include falls, restraint use, accidental injuries, crime and victimization, elder abuse, vulnerability to temperature changes, disasters, and dangers in the home environment. Attention will be given to safety tips and interventions for injury prevention.

FALLS

Overview and Magnitude of the Problem

Falls are a common clinical problem affecting nearly half of older persons in the United States. In fact, every 11 seconds, an older adult is treated in the emergency room for a fall, and older adults are more likely to experience a fall-related death.

One in four older adults over age 65 fall each year, with this incidence increasing for those over age 80 (National Council on Aging, 2017; Kiel, 2016).

Falls are the leading cause of fatal and noninjuries in older adults. Fatal falls occur among people of all ages, but falling results in higher rates of morbidity and mortality among those older than 75 because of the higher incidence of frailty and a limited physiologic reserve among the aging population. After age 75, white men have the highest fall-related fatality rates, followed by white women, black men, and black women; non-Hispanics have a higher fatal fall rate compared with Hispanics (CDC, 2017). In terms of serious injury, falls are the leading cause of hip fractures, accounting for more than 271,000 occurrences annually (CDC, 2017). Thirty to fifty percent of falls in the older population result in injuries such as bruises, abrasions, and lacerations, although roughly 10% can lead to more serious injuries such as traumatic brain injuries (TBIs) (Abrahem & Chimino-Flallos). In fact, a meta-analysis of 11 studies found that severe TBIs resulted in an almost 80% fatality rate (McIntyre, Mehta, Janzen, Aubut, & Teasell, 2013). Women are three times more likely to sustain a hip fracture from a fall compared with men (National Hospital Discharge Survey [NHDS], 2013).

Falling has numerous antecedents and consequences that can be identified and managed. Most clinical research demonstrates a reduction in fall frequency as a result of intervention strategies to modify risk factors. Clinical programs targeting high-risk older adults have incorporated intervention strategies aimed at medication modification, environmental improvements, and behavioral modification. Clinical research findings demonstrate variability in the effectiveness of these interventions. Not all falls are preventable; therefore goals for individuals who fall frequently are fall reduction, prevention of serious injury, and modification of significant risk factors.

It is also important to note that because falls are multifactorial, not all individuals fall as a result of the same antecedents. For instance, an older woman may lose her balance and fall when hurrying to answer the telephone and then experience a second fall the next morning when getting up from bed too quickly. In this example, two distinct causes of falling are present, and both can be modified through education and behavioral modification. Thus, because falls tend to be multifactorial in this age group, care must be taken to perform a comprehensive assessment of individuals who have fallen; this includes a detailed history and physical examination.

Patient education is the cornerstone of fall prevention and management. The gerontologic nurse must explore patient beliefs and misconceptions about falling. Older individuals may consider falling to be a normal part of the aging process. For some, it is an expectation of growing old. Individuals who hold these stereotypes must be educated about the normal aging process, which is distinct from diseases and the adverse effects of medications. It is important to tell older adults that the etiology of falling can most often be determined by a health care professional who has expertise in fall assessment and that falls can be reduced and even prevented through some simple interventions (Box 11.1). The treatable causes of falling must also be emphasized in continuing education and staff

---

BOX 11.1 General Fall Prevention Guidelines

General Care
- Wear low-heeled shoes with small wedge platforms.
- Wear leather- or rubber-soled shoes.
- Leave nightlights on at night.
- Keep items within reach to avoid overreaching.
- Check the tips of canes and walkers for evenness.
- Have the last step painted a different color, indoors and outdoors.
- Dangle the legs between positional changes and rise slowly.
- Avoid the use of alcohol.
- Avoid rushing.
- Avoid risky behavior such as standing on ladders unaided.

Steps and Floor Surfaces
- Be careful to avoid slippery floors and frayed carpets.
- Watch for the last step when descending the stairs.
- Count the number of steps as a cue while ascending and descending the stairs.
- Install and use sturdy banisters on both sides of staircases.
- Tack down throw rugs or remove them entirely.
- Remove obstacles in the path of traffic.
- Use carpeting that has color contrast on landing surfaces.

Bathroom
- Have grab bars installed in the tub and shower and near the toilet.
- Avoid throw rugs; have carpeting installed.
- Avoid bar soaps; use liquid soap from a dispenser mounted in the shower.

---

development programs in all health care settings. Once the patients' and staff's knowledge of falling improves, the reporting of falls in an effort to seek treatment may improve.

Definition of Falling

It is crucial for the gerontologic nurse to recognize that older individuals define falling in numerous ways and are influenced by perceptions of aging and disease, and the context of the situation. For instance, older individuals may not perceive a slip that results in a fall to the floor to be an actual "fall"; rather it may be termed a *slip, trip,* or *accident,* but not a *fall.* Box 11.2 illustrates some common reasons given by older adults to explain a fall. The falling event needs to be reviewed in detail to determine whether the person fell to the lowest level (i.e., the ground). Moreover, how individuals define falling is likely to influence the reporting of falls. A fall may be anything that causes a person to move unintentionally from one level plane to another. An example of this is a sudden and unexpected drop from standing upright into a seat or onto the floor. Injuries such as bruising, sprains, strains, or fractures may result from minimal height drops.

BOX 11.2 Common Explanations for Falling Given by Older Adults

- "I think I slipped."
- "I don't remember what happened."
- "I was in a hurry."
- "I tripped."
- "I lost my balance."

Key initial assessment points include level of consciousness (determination if loss of consciousness occurred), circulation, airway, and breathing. The rapid response team should be notified if necessary. If the patient is stable, a head-to-toe assessment including all body systems should take place, including orthostatic vital signs (Lovence, n.d.). History taking should be detailed enough for the examiner to envision the details leading to the fall and incorporate a detailed drug review.

Meaning of Falling to Older Adults

Falling, in a broad sense, is a concept that holds negative connotations because it is associated with a decline, drop, or descent to a lower level. As it relates specifically to a patient falling, the same negative connotation appears to hold true, as evidenced by the plethora of research that presents the significant negative consequences of falling. However, to patients, falling may mean something entirely different. It may not be associated with an actual dropping to a lower level, such as the ground; falling might mean a perceived loss in status. In a research investigation of community-dwelling older adults' statements about falls, the extent to which the fall was attributed to a person's own limitations instead of the environment depended on self-rated health, among other variables. Thus the meaning of falling involves several related variables and most likely is determined according to an individual perception of how serious the fall is in terms of daily living.

The health care professional may equate a fall with a decline in patient health or function, or a worsening of a patient's condition. Falling may be viewed as a marker of future decline. In fact, the concept of *prodromal falling* refers to a series of falls that occurs before the onset of illness or disease, as a prelude (or *prodrome*) (Meiner, 2015). Events such as infections are classic examples of medical conditions associated with falling.

Normal Age-Related Changes Contributing to Falling

Numerous age-related changes predispose older adults to falling, especially when these changes affect functional ability and give rise to sensory impairment or gait and balance instability. This section highlights the salient age-related changes associated with falling, along with nursing interventions directed at modifying the effect of these changes to prevent falling. Normal age-related changes in organ function may contribute to an intrinsic risk for falling (Boltz, Capezuti, Fulmer, & Zwicker, 2016).

Vision

Structural changes in eye shape and crystalline lens flexibility accompany the aging of the eye. It is the latter change—inflexibility of the lens—that causes presbyopia, a reduction in the eye's accommodation for changes in depth, as when ascending or descending the stairs. If older individuals are experiencing presbyopia, instruction must be given for them to carefully watch door edges, curbs, and landing steps, which signal a change in height. Additionally, because of the tendency for the crystalline lens to become cloudy and form a cataract with advancing years, eye glare may occur and cause temporary visual disturbances. This effect is particularly evident outdoors on sunny days or indoors as bright light reflects off shiny floors. Instruction must be given to older individuals with this problem to wear wide-brimmed hats or sunglasses to shield the eyes from the glare effect and to shade indoor windows with drapes or blinds to minimize the effects of sun glare.

Hearing

An age-related change affecting the inner ear is atrophy of the ossicle in the inner ear, which causes changes in sound conduction, including a loss of high-tone frequencies, called *presbycusis*. Other age-related changes include an amplification of background noise and a decrease in directional hearing. The vestibular system is an integral part of maintaining balance and, to a large degree, is dependent on intact hearing. Therefore older individuals with hearing impairments are more susceptible to falling when feedback to the brain is altered.

Assessment of hearing difficulties begins during the initial interview. In some individuals with significant hearing loss, it becomes necessary to use alternative forms of visual cues to signal where their feet and bodies are in space so that they can maintain stability. For instance, when hearing loss cannot be corrected, one aim of the management of hearing problems is to introduce vibratory or visual cues to compensate for hearing loss. The use of bells on shoelaces causes a vibratory sense that can be felt by older adults when a foot is placed on the ground. Nursing interventions include instructing older patients to observe foot placement on the floor by literally "watching their step" and to be especially cognizant of environmental conditions such as floor surfaces.

Cardiovascular Factors

One of the most common problems facing older adults is the loss of tissue elasticity, which affects the arteries. This lack of elasticity leads to a decrease in tissue recoil, resulting in changes in blood pressure with position changes. Older adults who lie supine and then get up quickly are likely to experience the effects of lack of tissue elasticity when blood pressure drops and a feeling of lightheadedness develops. It is important to educate older individuals to change position slowly and to dangle the legs a few minutes when arising from a supine position. Older adults should be encouraged to wait between position changes and to hold onto the side of the bed or other furniture should an episode of lightheadedness occur. The use of a single bed rail specially manufactured for transferring aids older adults in getting in and out of bed.

Musculoskeletal Factors

The bones of aging individuals, particularly the weight-bearing joints, undergo "wear and tear," which causes loss of supportive cartilage. As a result, joints may become unstable and "give way," leading to a fall. In many instances, osteoarthritis occurs in the weight-bearing joints, causing pain with weight bearing and further eroding joint stability. Interventions are directed at identifying such problems and correcting them through the use of antiinflammatory agents, prescribed activity and exercise, braces, joint replacement, or all of these measures. If joint pain develops and remains untreated, it may cause older adults to become sedentary or immobile. This phenomenon of disuse and muscle atrophy contributes to muscle weakness. This cycle of pain, reduced mobility, disuse, and atrophy may become a vicious one unless interrupted by regular mobility and pain control through the use of topical or systemic medication. Nursing interventions are directed at encouraging, supervising, or assisting with regular ambulation; appropriate use of ambulation aids; joint range of motion; and modalities such as ice, hot packs, and physical therapy.

Another normal age-related musculoskeletal change is the reduction in steppage height, which may place older adults at risk for tripping, especially when door edges are not visible or carpeting is frayed. The gerontologic nurse's role is to identify these changes and offer suggestions for improvement, depending on the cause. In some cases, an assistive device may have to be employed to aid mobility and avoid further joint damage.

Neurologic Factors

One of the most universal age-related changes affecting the neurologic system is a slowing in reaction time. It takes older individuals a longer time to respond both verbally and physically to changes in position. Older adults who lose their balance are able to right themselves to an upright position, provided the musculoskeletal strength of hips, ankles, and shoulders is adequate. However, those with functional impairments and diseases, muscle weakness, or adverse effects from medications might lose their postural stability and fall. For these individuals, uneven surfaces in the environment such as steps, sidewalks, and curbs may lead to loss of footing and subsequent falls. Nursing interventions for those with impaired righting reflexes include monitoring mobility for signs of unsteadiness and offering supervision and assistance when needed. In an effort to promote autonomy, it is important to allow older patients to continue to perform their usual activities independently and safely.

When independent activity is no longer possible, older adults require a *physiatric,* or physical therapy, evaluation for the use of a walking aid such as a straight cane, stationary walker, or posterior walker. Nursing interventions also include the use of chair or bed alarms or call buttons worn around the neck to signal that assistance is needed. Shoes should be inspected for sturdy heels that are low and preferably wedgetype. Observation of an older adult patient's ability to walk is crucial. For instance, is the walking path straight, or does the patient deviate from it? Does the patient trip when walking because of inappropriate shoes? For some older adults with gait disorders, rubber soles, for example, those on sneakers, worn on high-pile carpeting may actually be a hindrance and result in shuffling or stumbling while walking. Leather soles are preferable, as are those that are low-heeled and have laces, providing extra ankle and foot support.

Fall Risk

Overall, most published research on falls and falling pertains to determining fall risk. Antecedents (e.g., diseases such as stroke, delirium, dementia, or urinary incontinence) that lead to falls have been clearly defined (Box 11.3), but many individuals with these disease-related risk factors do not fall. Thus fall risk is not determined solely on the basis of the number and kind of

---

BOX 11.3 Treatable Causes of Falling in Older Adults

- Orthostatic hypotension
- Dehydration
- Profound anemia
- Cardiac arrhythmia (e.g., bradyarrhythmia, tachyarrhythmia, sick sinus syndrome)
- Overdosing with medication or alcohol
- Urinary tract infection
- Vitamin B_{12} deficiency
- Osteoporosis
- Hypoglycemia
- Seizures
- Carotid hypersensitivity
- Carotid stenosis
- Delirium[†]

[†]Mental status is an important determinant of fall risk because changes in mental status such as those incurred with delirium may cause older individuals to have difficulty negotiating within the environment. Delirium causes individuals to misperceive sensory input as well as stimuli and objects in the environment.

---

diseases but also on how these risk factors influence an older adult's functional ability, specifically in the areas of mobility, transferring, and negotiating within the environment.

Fall risk is best determined by observation of mobility. Fall risk may be categorized according to intrinsic (illness or disease-related) or extrinsic (environmental) risk (CDC, 2017). A risk for falling according to these categories is different from the intrinsic or extrinsic causes of falling. *Risk* is determined by the clinician and is a term that reflects a judgment based on a thorough evaluation of a patient, known hazards for falling, and foreseeable events. Older patients at "risk" for falling may not experience a fall at all. Numerous extrinsic risks for falling exist, for example, lack of color contrast on curbs, poor lighting, frayed carpeting, and unsteady furniture. Intrinsic risks for falling include conditions such as orthostatic hypotension, blindness, or advanced dementia. The presence of these risk factors, however, does not mean that an older patient will actually fall—just that he or she is *likely* to fall given certain circumstances. In fact, some individuals who are at risk for falling, as evidenced by the presence of these risk factors, do not fall. Some of the circumstances that may lead to falling in older adults include unsteady gait or balance instability, delirium or side effects of medications causing unsteadiness, and an inability to right themselves when footing is lost or balance is unstable.

As mentioned, risk for falling is different from actual intrinsic or extrinsic causes of falling. In the latter case, a fall has actually occurred and is the result of either intrinsic disease, extrinsic causes in the environment, or a combination of the two. These falls are likely to occur among those deemed at "risk for falling." The workup seeks to identify the underlying cause so that it can be treated, thus ultimately preventing or reducing recurrent falling. One aim of fall management is the reduction of risk factors to promote safety while still respecting patient autonomy. Because falling is individually determined and not always preventable or predictable, it is important to avoid classifying patients according to the clinician's perception of their risk for falling (i.e., high risk versus low risk). As previously discussed, falling does not necessarily occur among individuals deemed at greatest risk. The effect of functional ability has significance as it relates to older individuals who fall. Research has shown that the individual with frailty and physical functional limitations is at greatest risk for falling.

Intrinsic Risk

Intrinsic risk for falling refers to the combined effect of normal age-related changes and concurrent disease. The most salient observations for intrinsic risk relate to gait, balance, stability, and cognition. This requires the gerontologic nurse to observe and analyze older individuals' gait and balance, and determine whether impairment exists. Measurement tools have been developed to rate both gait and balance. These tools identify key components of gait such as step length and height, step symmetry, and path. Important areas of balance assessment include sitting and standing balance, turning, and the ability to sit without loss of balance. The Tinetti Gait and Tinetti Balance instruments are measurement tools that quantitatively score gait and balance. These tools have been tested through clinical research and hold acceptable validity and reliability ratings (Fig. 11.1) (Tinetti, 1986). In addition, other assessment tools employ a combination of measures, such as gait, balance, vestibular evaluation, and functional performance (CDC, 2017; Middleton & Fritz, 2013; Nnodim & Yong, 2015; Verghese et al., 2002). Before managing gait or balance impairments with assistive aids or physical therapy, older individuals require medical workups for treatable causes of gait and balance abnormalities (Table 11.1).

Extrinsic Risk

Numerous environmental hazards, both indoors and outdoors, may predispose individuals to falling (CDC, 2017). Research has found that older persons continue to perform the same types of risk-taking behaviors in their later years of life as in their younger years. Modification of risky behaviors in the face of functional impairment may prevent accidental falls in and around the home. Because 6 out of every 10 falls occur in the home, instruction in home safety tips should be incorporated into health encounters with older individuals who suffer falls (National Institute on Aging, 2017).

The modification of environmental risk factors is also critical for fall prevention. Environmental hazards are those that contribute to accidental falls. Research has found that about 30% of falls can be prevented through environmental modification (Wentz, Wentz, & Wallace, 2011). The key areas that require evaluation for safety are steps, floor surfaces, edges and curbs, lighting, and grab rails; nursing interventions are directed at environmental assessment of the indoor living space in these key areas. Whenever possible, steps that are uneven should be repaired or at least have a sturdy handrail to hold onto for support. Floor surfaces should have low-pile carpeting in good repair. Tears should be sewn to prevent shoe heels from becoming caught. Throw rugs should be eliminated because they are a tripping hazard. Curbs and cement landing surfaces should be painted with a contrasting color to outline edges. Lighting

---

Instructions: Client is seated in a hard, armless, chair. The following maneuvers are tested:

1. Sitting balance
   0 = Leans or slides in chair
   1 = Steady and safe

2. Arise
   0 = Unable without help
   1 = Able, but uses arm to help
   2 = Able without use of arms

3. Attempts to arise
   0 = Unable without help
   1 = Able, but requires more than one attempt
   2 = Able to arise in one attempt

4. Immediate standing balance (first 5 seconds)
   0 = Unsteady (e.g., staggers, moves feet, marked trunk sway)
   1 = Steady, but uses walker or cane or grabs another object for support
   2 = Steady without walker, cane, or other support

5. Standing balance
   0 = Unsteady
   1 = Steady, but has a wide stance (i.e., medial heels >4 inches apart) or uses a cane, walker, or other support
   2 = Narrow stance without support

6. Nudge (with subject at maximum position with feet as close together as possible. Examiner pushes lightly on client's sternum three times with palm of the hand).
   0 = Begins to fall
   1 = Staggers, grabs, but catches self
   2 = Steady

7. Eyes closed (with subject at maximum position as in #6)
   0 = Unsteady
   1 = Steady

8. Turn 360°
   0 = Discontinuous steps
   1 = Continuous steps
   0 = Unsteady (e.g., grabs, staggers)
   1 = Steady

9. Sit down
   0 = Unsafe (e.g., misjudges distance, falls into chair)
   1 = Uses arms or does not use a smooth motion
   2 = Safe, smooth motion

_____ / 16 **Balance score**

Fig. 11.1 Tinetti Balance and Gait Evaluation. (From Fortinsky, R., Iannuzzi-Sucich, M., Baker, D., Gottschalk, M., King, M., Brown, C., & Tinetti, M. [2004]. Fall-risk assessment and management in clinical practice: Views from healthcare providers. *Journal of the American Geriatrics Society, 52*[9], 1522-1526. doi:10.1111/j.1532-5415.2004.52416.x.)

---

should be adequate in high-traffic and dimly lit areas. On a more global scale, a community effort to notify the local Housing Commission of areas needing improvement is an important step in the design of future homes that are safe for older adults.

Steps. The most commonly cited place where falls occur in the home is the last step of a staircase. The last step is a problem area, primarily because of visual changes or functional impairment. Handrails should be present on both sides of a staircase or series

TABLE 11.1 Treatable Causes of Gait and Balance Abnormalities

Physical Examination Finding	Possible Associated Gait or Balance Impairment
Peripheral neuropathy	Inability to feel feet on the floor
Charcot joint	Foot instability, foot pain, or both
Loss of proprioception	Foot placement on floor altered
Hemiparesis	Leaning to one side; gait instability
Hammer toe	Foot pain during weight bearing
Decreased steppage height	Shuffling gait; tripping

of steps. The handrail typically ends at the second to last step; if a person descending the stairs is using the handrail as a guide for the landing surface, it will place the individual at the second-to-last step. Interventions to correct this include educating patients about this situation, teaching individuals to count the steps (i.e., keeping a mental tally of the number of steps ascending or descending), and reinstalling handrails that meet individuals' needs. Another problem with regard to the staircase is unevenness of steps (Fig. 11.2). Observation and correction of this phenomenon may be the first step toward fall prevention in the home.

Floor Surfaces. Floors that have been waxed or polished are common slippery surfaces that are a safety risk for older adults, especially persons with visual impairments. Heels may be caught in carpeting that is frayed or torn. Throw rugs may cause tripping or sliding (if on a hardwood or tile surface). In general, it is advisable to tack down throw rugs or remove them altogether. Floor surfaces should also be clutter free, as clutter can lead to tripping and accidental falls.

Edges and Curbs. Edging that lacks a contrasting color may lead to falls because surfaces tend to blend together. In the interior of the home, carpeting on the staircase and landing surface that are the same color may lead to falling. In the exterior of the home, concrete steps that are homogeneous in color may lead to misperceptions and subsequent falling. Uneven pavement outdoors may cause falling. Curbs that are not clearly marked

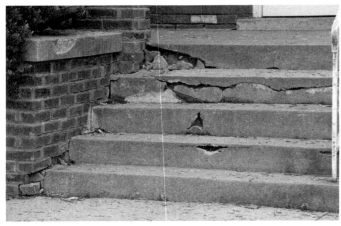

Fig. 11.2 Uneven stairs with missing handrail. (©SBSArtDept/iStock.)

with a bold contrast in color may also cause falling. Simple modifications include painting the outdoor steps a contrasting color at the landing surface and using carpet borders in a contrasting color (or adhesive tape) to distinguish changing indoor surfaces.

Lighting. Dimly lit rooms cause difficulty for aging eyes and also for those with low levels of vision or impaired vision. Bright lights may lead to glare and temporary visual impairment. Lighting should ideally be evenly distributed and have consistent brightness. Diffuse overhead lighting is often preferable to one bright light source.

Grab Bars or Rails. Grab bars and rails aid those with functional impairments and serve those who accidentally slip in the tub or shower. Grab bars to steady balance should be placed around the toilet, in the shower, or on the tub. Grab bars should be strategically placed to be most beneficial for the person with the impairment. Misplaced grab bars, which cause older persons to reach, may actually lead to falls. Tubs and showers should have adhesive mats and be well lit, and use of bar soaps should be avoided, as they may lead to slipping and accidental falls during showering.

Risk for Serious Injury

A small percentage of older individuals who fall are at the greatest risk for serious physical injury (Box 11.4). It is vital for the gerontologic nurse to identify these individuals because they possess intrinsic risk factors that can be identified and often modified to prevent serious injury. Additionally, recognition and treatment of these individuals are part of the gerontologic nurse's role in preventing foreseeable accidents. Serious injuries such as hip fractures, head trauma, and internal bleeding affect only a relatively small percentage of older individuals who fall. Although falls are the leading cause of hip fractures, only about 5% to 6% of older individuals who fall sustain them. A high mortality rate is associated with hip fractures, and the cost of their treatment places great economic strain on society for rehabilitation and other ancillary services (CDC, 2017; NCOA, 2017).

In addition, the use of physical restraints may increase the risk for serious injury. Individuals who are physically restrained may injure themselves attempting to remove the restraints. Incidents of strangulation and asphyxiation have been reported secondary to restraint use. The elevation of both side rails may cause demented or delirious older adults to fall in their attempts to climb over the side rails. These individuals are at risk for serious injury because of the height of the fall, thus the effect is greater than if the side rails had not been elevated. Physical restraint use does not prevent falls and therefore should never be employed as a "safety precaution" (American Academy of Nursing, 2018; Bradas, Sandhu, & Mion, 2012).

BOX 11.4 Conditions Associated With Greatest Risk for Serious Injury

- Mental status changes (e.g., those related to delirium and dementia)
- Osteoporosis
- Gait or balance instability
- Concurrent fractures (e.g., of the hip, pelvis, humerus, or ulna)
- Restraint use

Reducing the Risk of Serious Injury

Behavioral modification is a broad term applied to interventions that alter behavior to achieve positive outcomes. The gerontologic nurse is in a pivotal position to educate older individuals, especially those at risk for serious injury from falling, about fall prevention measures. Older individuals' knowledge base and receptivity to changing behavior are important aspects for the gerontologic nurse to assess before initiating a teaching program. Specific teaching points will vary individually, but general guidelines for fall prevention and home safety may be illustrated through a pictorial display of high-risk environmental hazards or by issuing a handout with teaching points. As they relate to those conditions most likely to result in serious injury, specific interventions can be reinforced (Table 11.2).

Behavioral modification and instruction—for example, teaching an older patient who has orthostatic hypotension to rise slowly or an individual with dizziness who moves too quickly to slow down—may not be as easy as it seems. Behavior modification first requires older patients to recognize behaviors that are contributing to problems. Often, the causes and effects of these behaviors need to be pointed out to patients in a clear and concise manner. However, this is not a foolproof method because falls might not occur while the patients are still trying to modify their behaviors. The patient's earlier behavior may thus be negatively reinforced, and he or she may feel justified in continuing to perform those same behaviors. Behavioral modification requires older patients to make conscious attempts, whenever a behavior is performed, to change or alter it. Much of what the nurse teaches must be remembered for later action; the use of notes and tape recorders as daily reminders may help.

TABLE 11.2	**Behavioral Interventions to Prevent Serious Injury**
Condition	**Patient Interventions**
Osteoporosis	Take medications prescribed for increasing bone mineral density.
	Take vitamin D and calcium supplements.
	Eat well-balanced, nutritious meals high in calcium.
	Perform moderate weight-bearing exercises on a routine basis.
	Avoid smoking.
	Avoid excessive alcohol ingestion.
	Avoid strain on the spine (e.g., heavy lifting, bending).
Gait instability	Wear footwear with nonskid soles.
	Use mobility aids and assistive devices, as prescribed.
	Make deliberate attempts to scan the environment while walking to look for possible hazards.
	Participate in an exercise program that includes muscle strengthening and gait training.
	Make environmental modifications, as needed.
Balance instability	Change positions slowly and carefully.
	Stabilize position before moving.
	Use mobility aids and assistive devices, as prescribed.
	Assume a seated position during high-risk activities such as bathing and dressing.

Disease or condition modification to reduce the risk of serious injury from falls includes appropriate treatment of the actual disease. In the case of osteoporosis, agents to prevent bone demineralization and build bone mass are prescribed and used with calcium and vitamin D supplements. The nurse plays a key role in teaching patients with osteoporosis about the importance of calcium-rich foods and ways to incorporate these foods into the diet on a daily basis. Teaching about the risk factors associated with the development of osteoporosis is also important.

In cases of delirium, condition modification includes a determination of the underlying etiology; unless the cause is identified and treated, the condition will not resolve, and patients will remain at increased risk of serious injury from a fall. It is imperative for the nurse to recognize that the etiology is often multifactorial, thus requiring a variety of interventions based on the identified causes. While the delirium resolves, injury can be prevented through additional nursing interventions, including padding of side rails, increased surveillance, assistance with activities of daily living (ADLs), and measures to promote a calm and reassuring environment.

Fall Antecedents and Fall Classification

Falling occurs when persons are upright and walking, termed *bipedal* or *ambulatory,* or when they are sitting or lying down, termed *nonbipedal.* Falls may also be considered serious or nonserious, depending on the consequences for patients. Individuals who fall but not to the lowest level (the ground) and those who catch themselves are considered to be experiencing "near falls"; those who actually fall to the ground are experiencing true falls. Falling may be classified according to the cause of the fall (intrinsic, extrinsic, or multifactorial), frequency of falling, and the timing of falling in relation to other diseases. Most falls in the older adult are *multifactorial* in etiology, that is, a combination of both intrinsic and extrinsic factors. Because so many different circumstances lead to falls in older adults, it is important to determine the type of fall according to a classification system (Box 11.5).

Isolated falling refers to a one-time event that was most likely purely accidental. The term *accidental fall* has been avoided in the literature during the last decade because most falls are not accidental but rather indicate specific disease processes or conditions.

Cluster falls may be observed among individuals with specific diseases who decompensate. The classic example is an older individual with congestive heart failure who falls with the onset of oxygen desaturation or cerebral hypoperfusion associated with overexertion. Usually, several falls occur over a short period and are markers of a decline in health.

BOX 11.5	**Fall Classification**

- Multifactorial
- Extrinsic (environmental)
- Intrinsic (illness or disease related)
- Intentional
- Isolated
- Cluster
- Premonitory
- Prodromal

Premonitory falls are those produced by specific medical illnesses. These types of falls have key symptoms that may be elicited on history taking; physical examination findings and diagnostic tests may also confirm this type of falling. Classic examples of premonitory falls are those in individuals with the new onset of stroke, seizure activity, hypoglycemia, or positional vertigo.

Prodromal falling refers to the onset of frequent falling heralding an acute medical problem; thus falling is a prodrome to later disease onset. An infectious disease typically causes this type of fall. Falls have also been associated with a clinical syndrome called *drop attack*. A drop attack has been defined as sudden leg weakness without loss of consciousness. Drop attacks are diagnosed when all other medical illness and environmental conditions have been excluded and patients continue to fall.

Intentional falls refer to falls by individuals who fall on purpose, possibly with a desire to do harm. Older patients with significant depression or suicidal ideation may throw themselves down to cause bodily harm. Other types of intentional falls include when one resident pushes another resident to the ground. This is frequently observed among residents with dementia in long-term care institutions.

Thus classifications of falls will often aid in determining the underlying causes of the falls. Box 11.6 illustrates the risk factors associated with the various types of falls. It is important to note that individuals may experience any one of these types of falls

---

BOX 11.6 The Multifactorial and Interacting Causes of Falls

Intrinsic Risk Factors
- Gait and balance impairment
- Peripheral neuropathy
- Vestibular dysfunction
- Muscle weakness
- Vision impairment
- Medical illness
- Advanced age
- Impaired activities of daily living (ADLs)
- Orthostasis
- Dementia
- Drugs

Extrinsic Risk Factors
- Environmental hazards (dim or inadequate lighting, no stair rails, slippery or uneven surfaces, no grab bars, cluttered environment or obstacles to ambulation)
- Poor footwear
- Restraints

Precipitating Causes
- Trips and slips
- Drop attack
- Syncope
- Dizziness

Modified from Rubenstein, L. Z. & Josephson, K. R. (2006). Falls and their prevention in elderly people: What does the evidence show? *Medical Clinics of North America, 90,* 807-824; and Centers for Disease Control (CDC) (2017). Risk factors for falls. Retrieved from http://www.cdc.gov.

---

singularly or in combination. If older residents experience a premonitory fall on one occasion, the next fall may be from a different cause altogether. Because falls are often unpredictable and therefore not always preventable, the clinician needs to start the evaluation with the goal of identifying and managing those falls that are treatable (Saccomano & Ferrara, 2015).

Fall Consequences
Physical Injury

The incidence of fall-related injuries spans from trivial trauma such as skin tears and sprains to serious injury such as hip fractures, internal bleeding, or subdural hematomas. Each year thousands of older Americans fall in their homes. Many of them are seriously injured, and some become disabled. It is estimated that every 19 minutes an older adult dies from a fall (CDC, 2017; NCOA, 2018). One study showed that 30.8% of home-care older adult patients had one or more falls, and 6.5% experienced falls with injury (Hnizdo, Archuleta, Taylor, & Kim, 2013). Research investigations have found that cognitive impairment, gait and balance impairment, low body mass index, and at least two chronic conditions were factors independently associated with serious injury during a fall (Tinetti, Baker, King et al., 2008). Among older adults, most injuries caused by falling are considered minor. Perhaps because of the low incidence of serious injury, older individuals often do not perceive falling to be a problem that warrants a report or a medical evaluation.

Serious injury from falling is more likely to occur among those with osteoporosis. Bones weakened by osteoporosis, particularly weight-bearing bones such as the femur, are more susceptible to breakage. Injury prevention measures to reduce the impact of falling, for example, lowering the distance an older patient might fall to the ground and even using padding over the bony prominences of the hips, are required. Undergarments such as girdles with extra padding over the high-risk bony prominences have been designed for women. Individuals with osteoporosis should also be prescribed medications to increase bone mineral density and strength over time. Exercise can aid in increasing bone mass.

Psychological Trauma

Older individuals who fall may or may not experience psychological trauma after the fall. Many factors influence the development of postfall trauma, including personality, depression, anxiety, and stress-related syndromes. Overall, little research has been done to elucidate the incidence, prevalence, and occurrence of postfall psychological trauma. One significant consequence of falling may be fear of falling again or fear of not being able to get up independently after a fall. Both these conditions have been researched more extensively than other psychological trauma associated with the postfall period. This well recognized "postfall syndrome" sets the stage for subsequent falls and resultant injury (Kiel, 2016).

Fear of falling appears to occur variably in the older adult population. Some research has shown that if older persons express a fear of falling, they may avoid activities and become physically dependent.

The gerontologic nurse's role is to determine whether fear of falling or other psychological trauma has occurred after the fall. The best time to elicit this information is during history taking with older individuals who fall. The nurse focuses attention on how confident the older adults are in performing activities that might predispose them to falling. One exception to consider, however, is an older individual who falls when nonambulatory, as in the case of a fall from bed. In this case confidence may be unaffected during mobility. Issues related to a fear of falling are presented in Box 11.7.

Defining and Measuring Fear of Falling. An older adult's fear of falling may be assessed in several ways. A simple method is to simply ask the older individual an open-ended question such as, "How do you define fear of falling, and what does it mean to you?" Responses will provide insight into the patient's perception about falling and give direction for intervention (Saccomano & Ferrara, 2015).

While interviewing an individual who falls, the nurse may also assess his or her fear of falling by simply asking the respondent to quantify fear using a visual analog scale that measures (on a 100-millimeter [mm] line) perception of how fearful the patient is during ambulation.

Some researchers have operationally defined fear of falling as low perceived self-efficacy at avoiding falls during nonhazardous ADLs. The Tinetti Falls Efficacy Tool lists a series of questions, on a Likert scale, related to how confident the person is during activities such as walking, reaching into cabinets, or hurrying to answer the telephone. This tool is based on Bandura's self-efficacy theory and is reported as a measure of fear of falling self-efficacy or confidence (Tinetti, 1986).

Jung (2006) studied the psychological effect of the fear of falling and found that an exercise regimen decreased a person's fear of falling and a previous fall increased an individual's fear of falling.

Evaluation of Patients Who Fall

History

Most often the underlying cause of falling will be identified during the health history. Because a tendency to underreport symptoms exists, the gerontologic nurse must be sure to ask about key symptoms that could be related to a treatable cause or causes of falling. At the onset of the interview, an older individual should be informed that falling is not a result of normal aging and therefore information about the fall onset, location, activity associated with the fall, and other details is essential to the evaluation. It is important to elicit the patient's own words about the circumstances surrounding the fall. Inquiries should be made about fall frequency and what usually happens immediately before a fall. The acronym SPLATT helps in further evaluation (Tideiksaar, 2009):

- **S**ymptoms at the time of the fall
- **P**revious fall
- **L**ocation of the fall
- **A**ctivity at the time of the fall
- **T**ime of the fall
- **T**rauma, postfall

A fall history depends on fall recall and intact memory. If the patient who falls suffers from dementia or delirium, it is advisable to seek additional information from witnesses or significant others. Often, a fall diary may be useful in retrieving detailed information about the fall that the individual may have forgotten. Key symptoms to inquire about are related to diseases known to cause falls. Every older adult needs to be asked about a series of key symptoms that will help to further identify the underlying cause of the fall. If these symptoms occurred at the time of the fall or precipitated the fall, it is likely that a treatable cause does exist (Table 11.3).

A postfall assessment tool can be helpful to evaluate circumstances surrounding the fall and attempt to plan for future fall prevention (Fig. 11.3).

Physical Examination

The physical examination of an individual who falls includes a focused examination based on the patient's presenting complaints in addition to the sensory, cardiovascular, musculoskeletal, and neurologic systems. Many treatable causes of falling may be identified on physical examination. Sensory input originates from visual, auditory, tactile, cardiovascular, and motor response systems. Sensory inputs from vision and hearing, proprioception of the distal lower extremities, and the peripheral sensory system all provide stimuli for the brain to process with regard to the maintenance of balance. The cardiovascular

TABLE 11.3 Key Symptoms to Elicit During History Taking From Patients Who Have Fallen

Symptom	Associated Medical Condition
Sudden onset of visual or hearing loss	Stroke
Sudden leg weakness (unilateral)	Stroke
Lower extremity weakness (bilateral)	Arthritis
Dizziness	Vertigo, labyrinthitis
Light-headedness with standing	Orthostatic hypotension
Tremors or confusion	Hypoglycemia, hypoxia
Loss of consciousness	Syncope
Involuntary loss of urinary or bowel function immediately after the fall	Seizure
Difficulty breathing or shortness of breath	Arrhythmia
Palpitations	Arrhythmia

FALLS MANAGEMENT – POST FALL ASSESSMENT TOOL

Resident		Age		Room #
Admit Date	Admit Dx		Current Dx	
Date of Fall	Day of Week		Time	AM PM
Assigned caregiver(s) (Name and title)				

1. Was this fall observed?   ❐ Yes ❐ No   *If yes*, by whom: _____
   (name and title)

2. Was the resident identified as "high risk" prior to the fall?   ❐ Yes ❐ No

3. Resident vital signs

Usual vital signs *before* the fall:	BP Lying:	Pulse:
	BP Sitting:	Pulse:
	BP Standing:	Pulse:
Vital signs *just after* the fall:	BP Lying:	Pulse:
	BP Sitting:	Pulse:
	BP Standing:	Pulse:

4. Does the resident have a history of falling?   ❐ Yes ❐ No *If yes*, list dates of all previous falls for the past 12 months:

DATE/TIME OF FALL	DATE/TIME OF FALL

5. List any life safety measures in place prior to this current fall:

6. Ask the following question of the resident "immediately" after the fall: WHY DO YOU THINK YOU FELL?

7. Ask the following questions of the resident immediately after the fall:

	Yes	No		Yes	No
Were you hungry?			Did you need to use the bathroom?		
Were you in pain?			Other:		
Were you bored?					

8. What footwear did the resident have on?

❐ Barefoot   ❐ Shoes   ❐ Slippers   ❐ Other:

9. What was the resident doing at the time of the current fall?

	Yes	No	Other:
Getting out of bed?			
Going to the bathroom?			
Looking for something?			
Getting up from a chair?			
Going to the dining room?			

Fig. 11.3 Postfall assessment tool. (From the Best Practice Committee of the Health Care Association of New Jersey. [2012]. Falls management—post fall assessment tool. In *Falls Management Guideline*. Retrieved from https://www.hcanj.org/files/2013/09/hcanjbp_fallmgmt13_050113_2.pdf.)

10. Location of this current fall (check all that apply):

Activity room	Day room	Shower	Other:
Bathroom	Dining room	Toilet	
Bed room	Hall	Transferring	
Commode	Outside	Wheelchair	

11. Was a restraint used during this fall?

None	Waist restraint	Other:
Geri Chair	Vest restraint	
Side rails	Mittens	
Wrist restraint	Lap board	

12. If a restraint was present during the fall, was it properly applied prior to the fall?   ☐ Yes ☐ No
If no, please describe:

13. Mechanical/Assistive Devices:

What *mechanical devices* were in use?	✓		Yes	No
Chair alarm		Was chair alarm working at time of fall?		
Bed alarm		Was bed alarm working at time of fall?		
Mobility monitor		Was monitor working at time of fall?		
What *assistive devices* were in use?	✓		Yes	No
Cane ☐ straight ☐ hemi ☐ quad		Was cane in good repair?		
Crutches		Were crutches in good repair?		
Walker		Was walker in good repair?		
Wheelchair		Was wheelchair in good repair?		
Geri-chair		Was Geri-chair in good repair?		
Lap board		Was lap board in good repair?		

14. Mental status of resident (check all that apply):

Mental status *prior to* the fall:	YES	NO	Mental status *after* the fall:	YES	NO
Alert			Alert		
Oriented			Oriented		
Disoriented/confused			Disoriented/confused		
Unable to follow directions			Unable to follow directions		
Other:			Other:		

15. Physical status of resident prior to the fall (check all that apply):

Physical status *prior to* fall	Yes	No	NA	Physical status *prior to* fall	Yes	No	NA
Unsteady gait				Impaired mobility/transfer			
Visual impairment				Glasses on			
Hearing impairment				Hearing aid in/working			
Weakness/fatigue				Recent acute illness			
Hearing impairment				Recent change in lab values (Hgb/Hct, blood sugar, O_2, etc.)			
Dizziness				Other:			
Pain							

Fig. 11.3—cont'd

16. Environmental status at the time of the fall (check all that apply):

Environmental status *at time* of fall	Yes	No	NA	Environmental status *at time* of fall	Yes	No	NA
Call bell within reach				Call bell on at time of fall			
Bed locked				Room light on			
Wheelchair locked				Floor wet			
Night light on				Patterned carpet/throw rugs			
Uneven floor surfaces				Power/phone/TV cords out			
Glare on floor				Other:			

17. Medication Status

	Yes	No	NA		Yes	No	NA
Diuretic				Cardiac			
Antihypertensive				Antibiotic			
Psychotropic				Other:			
Laxative							

18. List all new medications prescribed/administered to resident in the past 7 days:

19. Describe the general health of the resident in the hours, days, and weeks before the fall:

20. Is there a need to re-educate the resident, family, staff: ❐ Yes ❐ No

21. Has the resident's care/service plan been updated?   ❐ Yes ❐ No

Additional notes:

Signature/title of person completing form

Date

Fig. 11.3—cont'd

system is also critical because blood pressure regulation aids in homeostasis. Changes in apical heart rate such as bradycardia, tachyarrhythmias, or irregular rhythms may alter cerebral perfusion and thus affect balance. In particular, a drop in blood pressure when a patient goes from supine to standing may lead to falling because of cerebral hypoperfusion as blood pools in the lower extremities.

Assessment of the motor response system includes muscle strength testing, and particular attention should be paid to hip and knee extension, and ankle dorsiflexion. Several research investigations have found that poor ankle dorsiflexion affects the ability to right oneself during the phases of a fall (Tideiksaar, 2009). Manual muscle strength testing identifies weakness in particular muscle groups, which can then be targeted for exercise. Gait analysis includes evaluation of footwear, base of support, limb stability, and clearance. The neurologic examination focuses on position sense and vibratory sense, and includes the Romberg test and cranial nerve assessment. Refer to an assessment textbook for details regarding the examination of older adults.

Physical examination should identify any findings that might explain a patient's symptoms. For instance, if a patient complains of dizziness while getting up in the morning, the nurse should check orthostatic blood pressures. Other causes of dizziness for older adults include carotid artery hypersensitivity, cervical arthritis, carotid stenosis, and positional vertigo, all of which may cause dizziness with head movement and may often be reproduced during a physical examination.

Special Testing

A few tests will aid the nurse in further evaluating gait and balance. One helpful test for static balance is the sternal nudge. This is a test of the righting reflex and is done with two persons and the patient. One examiner stands in front of the patient and one behind; the examiner in front pushes on the patient's sternum to displace the patient. If the patient begins to fall, the test is considered positive. A test result is deemed "negative" when the patient is able to maintain standing balance despite the nudge. Tests of dynamic balance include observance of the patient walking and changing position. Additional tests of balance include administration of the Tinetti assessment tool for balance (see Fig. 11.1). The "timed up and go (TUG) test" is a measure of the patient's ability to arise from a seated position, walk, and sit down. The test is timed, and results are correlated with the prognosis of risk for falling. Results of less than 20 seconds have a good prognosis compared with more than 30 seconds (Kristensen, Foss, & Kehlet, 2009).

NURSING MANAGEMENT OF FALLS

The management of falls is challenging to the nurse, especially when older individuals experience multiple or recurrent falls. In these cases, it is helpful to identify a pattern, if any, to the falling. Similarities in antecedents that lead to falling or specific symptoms might help identify the underlying cause. The goals of management are to identify the underlying cause, to reduce the incidence of recurrent falling, and to prevent serious injury (Boltz, Capezuti, Fulmer, & Zwicker, 2016).

BOX 11.8   Designing a Fall Diary

1. Gather several sheets of 8½-×11-inch paper.
2. Across the longest margin, write or type the headings "Date," "Time of Fall," "Activity at the Time of Fall," "Symptoms," and "Injury."
3. Instruct patients to write, in the space underneath each heading, the information pertaining to each fall soon after the fall occurs.
4. At the bottom of the fall diary, include an "Emergency Contact Number" for patients to call in case a fall results in serious injury.
5. Instruct patients who have experienced a fall to keep a record of the fall events and to bring it to the health care provider's office at the next scheduled appointment.

Several aids for monitoring and preventing falls are available. The fall diary helps to monitor fall occurrences, injuries, and patterns. Community-dwelling older patients may use a fall diary to jot down all the important information that led to the fall, occurred during the fall, or followed the fall. This information is extremely useful in determining antecedents and consequences of falling. Fall diaries are inexpensive or may be created by the nurse simply by using a pen, paper, and ruler (Box 11.8).

For institutionalized older individuals at risk for serious injury from bed or chair falls, the use of bed or chair alarms help alert the nurse when movement is initiated. A sensor is attached to a patient and to the chair or bed via a long thin wire. When the patient attempts to get up, the wire falls off the sensor and signals an alarm. These alarms are noninvasive and do not restrict voluntary movement in any way. The alarm is fairly loud and may startle an older adult, so it is important to alert the patient and family about the noise to be expected when the alarm is triggered. In the corridors of hospitals and nursing facilities, video surveillance cameras help staff view ambulatory patients around the corner or in distant areas. These cameras are prohibited, however, in private areas such as patient rooms because of privacy laws. Other safety aids include safety belts in wheelchairs and the "lap buddy," which is a soft foam cushion that fits on the patient's lap and wraps underneath the armrests of a wheelchair. However, if a patient is unable to remove these devices voluntarily, they are considered restraining devices. If the use of these aids fits the criteria for "restraint" for a particular patient, then the clinical guidelines for restraint use must be instituted. Health care providers must ensure that the use of these aids is the least restrictive alternative available for the patient and that the aids do not replace observation or inhibit purposeful activity.

Injury epidemiology is the study of the interaction of effects of injury on the host, the environment, and the agent. The process of aging, along with the effects of disease, results in changes that affect the host. One aim of injury prevention is to alter factors that impinge on the host by maximizing patient health and functional status, reducing unnecessary medications, and altering risk-taking behaviors. These combined efforts will reduce the risk of unintentional injuries. Alterations in environment through the elimination of environmental hazards will reduce accidental injuries that occur in older patients' homes. Improved technology through research seeks to alter the transfer of energy and thus modify those agent-related factors contributing to injuries in older adults. One such example is the alteration in the transfer of energy by use of supersoft mats and floor surfaces designed to absorb the effect of a falling body and redistribute its mass. Thus when an older patient falls on a special floor surface, the rate of injury is likely to be lower than on a conventional surface.

For all older patients at risk for falls and those at risk for serious injury from a fall, it is advisable to discuss with them the possibility that falling will result in serious injury and how to reduce the potential for such injury. Patients should be given the choice of reducing mobility to prevent serious injury or continuing ambulation, knowing that the risk of serious injury is present. Patient autonomy should be promoted and respected; it is the patient's choice. In instances in which patients are demented or unable to make informed choices, discussion with the families or guardians is required. In any event, the goal of the gerontologic nurse is to promote safety.

Fall and injury prevention modalities have received much attention in recent years. Evidence suggests that certain activities and programs may improve flexibility and balance, thus preventing injury. Evidence-based fall program such as *Matter of Balance* (mainehealth.org), *Healthy Steps* (aging.pa.gov), or *Fit and Strong* (fitandstrong.org) are examples of program strategies that may improve fall prevention outcomes. Moreover, it is advisable to follow the recommendations presented in Box 11.9 and the Nursing Care Plan in an effort to reduce falling. The Emergency Treatment box gives recommendations for treating a patient who has fallen.

SAFETY AND THE HOME ENVIRONMENT

Environmental hazards in the homes of older adults are common. These hazards are found in all living areas and entrances to homes of community-living older adults. Hazards have been observed less frequently in housing that is age-restricted to older adults (Gill, Williams, Robison, & Tinetti, 1999) or has been remodeled or designed with older adults in mind. Especially injurious hazards are those associated with temperature-regulating equipment and household chemicals. The equipment

---

BOX 11.9 Fall and Injury Prevention Strategies

Physical Modifications
- Cushion the landing surface.
- Use specialized tile that absorbs the impact of falls.
- Pad the floor.
- Cushion bony prominences.
- Use padding around high-risk bony prominences.
- Gain weight (if appropriate).
- Lower the distance to the floor surface.
- Use low-rise beds.
- Use futon beds or a mattress on the floor.
- Sit during dressing and shaving, whenever possible.
- Sit in a shower chair instead of standing in a tub.
- Avoid high heels; use wedge heels or flat shoes.

Behavioral Modifications
- Slow the pace of activities.
- Avoid risk-taking behaviors such as climbing on ladders, if feeling unsteady.
- Rise slowly and dangle the legs before changing position.
- Pay attention to the environment, terrain, and uneven or slippery surfaces.

Environmental Safety
- Have the curbs and edges painted in different colors.
- Have intravenous tubing removed in the hospital setting.
- Have urinary catheter and drainage bag removed.
- Have grab bars or rails installed.
- Use the "Lifeline" for fall detection.
- Set a predetermined schedule for "checking in" with neighbors or friends.

◎ NURSING CARE PLAN

Risk for Injury: Fall

Clinical Situation

Ms. B is an 82-year-old woman admitted to the hospital from home with acute congestive heart failure secondary to aortic stenosis and new-onset pneumonia. Her medical history includes osteoporosis and a hip fracture 3 years ago. She experiences shortness of breath with minimum exertion despite a recent diuresis and the loss of 10 pounds. Ms. B is receiving intravenous diuretics and antibiotics. Vital signs include a temperature of 98° F, a pulse of 100 beats per minute at rest, respirations of 26 breaths per minute at rest, and a blood pressure of 90/60 mm Hg; her pulse oximetry while receiving 2 liters (L) of oxygen is 90%. She insists on walking by herself to the bathroom to "stay independent." As a result of the diuretic, Ms. B has to rush to the bathroom to prevent urinary incontinence. On examination, she complains of dizziness when first getting up.

Nursing Diagnosis

Potential for injury: risk for falls resulting from altered mobility, urinary urgency, and treatment modalities secondary to osteoporosis and respiratory compromise.

Outcome

Patient will maintain autonomy and independence while avoiding falls during the hospital stay.

Interventions

Observe patient during basic ADLs, instructing her regarding ways to conserve energy while still encouraging independence.

Check blood pressure and pulse, supine and standing, to determine whether orthostatic hypotension exists.

Keep immediate environment free of obstacles.

Instruct patient to dangle legs before standing up from a supine position.

Place call light within reach to encourage patient to call for assistance.

Provide temporary use of bedside commode to limit exertional activities while still encouraging independence; instruct in the use of safe transfer procedures.

Monitor electrolyte, blood urea nitrogen, and serum creatinine levels for evidence of drug-induced dehydration.

Weigh patient daily to monitor fluid status.

Monitor intake and output.

Provide nonskid slippers.

Eliminate intravenous tubing and use saline well so that tripping over clear tubing is avoided.

Don't forget to include checking for outdoor hazards: decks, sand, and uneven surfaces.

includes sources of fire, heat, and ventilation, and the chemicals include household cleaners, herbicides, and pesticides (Wentz et al., 2011).

✚ EMERGENCY TREATMENT

Mr. J is an 84-year-old man who was found lying on the floor in his bedroom in a residential care facility. He says, "I just fell down, but I feel okay." Closer examination reveals a large hematoma over the right temporal area and swelling of the right ankle and lower extremity. Mr. J's distal dorsalis pedis pulse on the right is obscured by the edema. A right lower extremity fracture is suspected. To stabilize the patient, the nurse carries out the following interventions:

1. Immobilization of the suspected fractured extremity with a splint or board and flexible bandage
2. Application of ice to the right lower extremity and right temporal area
3. Checking of the apical pulse immediately to ascertain whether an arrhythmia occurred, resulting in the fall; monitor vital signs, especially blood pressure and apical pulse
4. A neurologic assessment and inquiry about a postfall headache
5. Checking of the environment for any spills or hazards that could have led to the fall
6. Taking of health history for symptoms of medical conditions that could have led to the fall, for example, syncope, seizures, or vertigo
7. Contacting emergency transportation to move the patient to the local emergency department for radiography and evaluation

---

Burn Injuries in the Home

Burns

Residential fires are directly related to the increase in deaths of older adults as the result of burns to the body. Although hot food or beverages often cause scald burns, they do not account for the large percentage of deaths from burns. Home maintenance is associated with older adults living in older homes with limited resources for needed repairs and thus risk for fire (Tanner, 2003). The major cause of scald burns is the temperature of the hot water coming from the faucets (Harper & Dickson, 1995). Wentz and associates (2011) stated that scalds resulting from bathing or showering were caused by hot water tank temperatures in excess of 140° F (60° C). Scalds can be prevented by turning down the thermostat on the household water heater to 120° F. At temperatures of 140° F, only 3 seconds of exposure is needed to produce third-degree burns on sensitive skin (Wentz et al., 2011).

The nurse should instruct older adults to use a meat thermometer and a container with a padded or safety handle to check the hot water temperature in the kitchen and bathroom. Water should be allowed to run until steam is noted, and the container is then filled. After the thermometer registers a stable temperature, the hot water tank controls are adjusted accordingly. The temperature should not be above 120° F.

Cigarette Smoking

Home fires occur more frequently at night, and deaths are attributed to smoke injury more often than burns. Smoking materials are often the source of home fires (Touhy & Jett, 2012). Smoking in the home has been associated with the dangers of secondhand smoke for many years (Jones & McEwen, 2012). Smoking in bed

or in a chair has also resulted in the deaths of numerous older adults from unintentional home fires. The environmental hazards of cigarette smoking include the careless disposal of cigarette butts and cigarettes dropped onto cloth surfaces (e.g., stuffed furniture, curtains, carpets, and clothing). Multiple injuries and deaths have been attributed to older persons falling asleep while smoking (Markowitz, 2013; Wentz et al., 2011).

The nurse should obtain information from the National Safety Council about smoking in the home, prepare an instructional plan to offer to older adults who smoke, and review the materials with them on a quarterly basis to refresh the safety steps associated with smoking at home. These include the following instructions: (1) Never smoke in bed; (2) do not smoke in a chair when a possibility of falling asleep exists; (3) do not smoke after taking any mind-altering medications (e.g., sleeping pills, tranquilizers, or narcotic pain medicine); and (4) place all smoking debris in a container away from all combustible items (e.g., curtains, furniture, clothing, and trash). Have fire extinguishers available for use. Several types of fire extinguishers are available, but the best type for home use is a multipurpose "ABC" type extinguisher. ABC extinguishers generally use ammonium phosphate as the active chemical and are capable of putting out most common fires (National Agricultural Safety Database [NASD], 2013).

Fireplace Hazards

The risk of starting a residential fire exists when a wood or gas fireplace is used. Wood fireplaces need to be cleaned of ash and soot buildup regularly when used during winter and in geographic areas where cold weather persists for many months. When ash and other wood debris accumulate over time, the flue may become blocked, causing the smoke or flames to enter the living area instead of exiting through the chimney or vent. All chimneys, vents, and flues need to be checked annually for patency. The ash and wood debris must be removed to prevent blocking the exit of fire and smoke. If proper cleaning is not done regularly, the resulting inhalation of smoke may lead to substantial airway damage and pulmonary complications (Wentz et al., 2011).

In the past 20 years, natural gas fireplaces have replaced many wood-burning fireplaces. Although the danger of ash and wood debris is eliminated, the draft element of the fireplace must be checked regularly to ensure a patent opening for the gas fumes to escape. In many municipalities, a regulation on the use of gas fireplaces includes installation of safety valves and permanent vents to prevent the introduction of natural gas into the home (Lee-Chiong, 1999; Tearle, 1998).

The nurse should discuss fireplace safety and maintenance with older adults who acknowledge using fireplaces and suggest having the flues checked for blockages on a routine basis. Setting at least an annual date in early autumn will establish a routine.

Kitchen Hazards

Kitchen fires are frequently the result of a "dry fire" from an unattended stove with water boiling in a pan or kettle. Older adults in homes or congregate residences frequently put water on a stove to heat for instant soup, coffee, or tea. Forgetfulness concerning the boiling water is the major reason for dry fires in the homes of older adults (CDC, 2012; Wentz et al., 2011).

The nurse should instruct older adults living alone about the possibility of dry fires. Patients with mild dementia need to be evaluated for their ability to cook safely because of their forgetfulness. Instruct older adults to remember three basic rules:

1. Be on the lookout for potential hazards.
2. Doing things the right way can prevent accidents (no shortcuts).
3. Use protective equipment when needed (e.g., pot holders, oven mitts, etc.).

Space Heaters

A space heater may be overturned by accident, causing a fire that may not be noticed until it fully engulfs the home. All space heaters should have a safety mechanism that turns the unit off as soon as it changes position (e.g., falls forward or backward). This safety device can shut off the heater and prevent the ignition of a fire in carpeting, curtains, or upholstery (CDC, 2012; Wentz et al., 2011).

The nurse should recommend that older adults have home inspections; programs are often available through local fire departments. When space heaters are used, an emergency shutoff must be operable. The equipment housing and the electrical cords must be intact. The cords must be appropriate for the electrical outlets being used (i.e., a three-prong plug cannot be placed in a two-prong adapter, which negates a grounded outlet).

Fire Safety Tips

Local fire districts across the country are encouraging families to keep fire extinguishers, smoke detectors, and carbon monoxide detectors in their homes. Home fire drills are recommended for all families but especially for households with older adults. Box 11.10 lists safety tips to protect the home from the hazards of fire. Identification of exits and a plan for meeting outside the building are necessities for independent older persons or couples living alone in a private residence (Wentz et al., 2011). The nurse should instruct older adults and families with older adult members regarding prevention measures (USFA, 2008).

Common fire hazards in the home are flammable liquids (e.g., gasoline, acetone, and paint thinner), combustible liquids (e.g., lighter fluid, turpentine, and kerosene), overloaded or worn electrical circuits, rubbish and trash stored near a heat source, Christmas trees and lighting that are frayed or have poor insulation, and natural gas leaks (Touhy & Jett, 2012).

Other Injuries in the Home

Knife Injuries

The use of knives, particularly in the kitchen, provides the potential for injury. The nurse should instruct older adults in six basic rules (NASD, 2002):

1. When using knives, always cut *away* from the body and on a proper cutting surface.
2. Keep the blades sharp and clean.
3. Keep the knife grips clean.
4. Never leave knives lying in water because this may injure an unsuspecting person washing dishes.

BOX 11.10 Safety Tips to Protect the Home From Fire

- Maintain smoke alarms.
- Develop and practice a fire escape plan.
- Have home fire sprinklers installed.
- Never smoke in bed.
- Put your cigarette or cigar out at the first sign of feeling drowsy while watching television or reading.
- Use deep ashtrays, and put out your cigarettes completely.
- Do not walk away from lit cigarettes and other smoking materials.
- Never leave cooking unattended.
- Always wear short or tight-fitting sleeves when you cook. Keep towels, potholders, and curtains away from flames.
- Never use the range or oven to heat your home.
- Double-check the kitchen before you go to bed or leave the house.
- Keep fire in the fireplace by making sure you have a screen large enough to catch flying sparks and rolling logs.
- Space heaters need space. Keep flammable materials at least 3 feet away from heaters.
- When buying a space heater, look for a control feature that automatically shuts off the power if the heater falls over.

Adapted from United States Fire Administration. (2018). *Fire safety outreach materials for older adults.* Retrieved February 14, 2018, from https://www.usfa.fema.gov/prevention/outreach/older_adults.html.

---

5. When wiping blades, always point the cutting edge *away* from the hand.
6. If a knife should fall, do not try to catch it; pick it up after it has fallen.

Carbon Monoxide Poisoning

Carbon monoxide toxicity from use of heating oil or natural gas may occur during the winter months. Furnaces that do not have flues checked for patency may be one of the causes of this silent killer (Iqbal, Clower, Hernandez et al., 2012). The condition of furnace venting should be checked annually just before the furnace is turned on for the home heating season (Wentz et al., 2011).

Power interruptions during cold weather increase the risk of unintentional carbon monoxide poisoning. Often, power outages occur during severe winter storms. This may create a need for alternative heating methods. Methods associated with carbon monoxide exposure are gasoline generators, propane or kerosene heaters, and charcoal grills (Houck & Hampson, 1997; Wrenn & Conners, 1997; Yoon, Macdonald, & Parrish, 1998). Warnings regarding the use of alternative heating methods during power outages should become part of all home safety instructions.

The nurse should include a recommendation for installation of a carbon monoxide detector in all home safety programs. Box 11.11 lists ways to prevent carbon monoxide in the home.

Chemical Injuries

Inadvertent skin exposure or ingestion of household chemicals, herbicides, or pesticides has been linked to deaths or injuries requiring long-term medical care (Lee, Chen, & Wu, 1999). Reading labels and properly storing chemicals used in and around the home are essential for the protection of health

---

BOX 11.11   Carbon Monoxide Poisoning: Prevention Guidelines

- **Do** have your heating system, water heater and any other gas, oil, or coal burning appliances serviced by a qualified technician every year.
- **Do** install a battery-operated carbon monoxide (CO) detector in your home, and check or replace the battery when you change the time on your clocks each spring and fall. If the detector sounds, leave your home immediately and call 9-1-1.
- **Do** seek prompt medical attention if you suspect CO poisoning and are feeling dizzy, light-headed, or nauseous.
- **Do not** use a generator, charcoal grill, camp stove, or other gasoline or charcoal-burning device inside your home, basement, or garage or near a window when outside.
- **Do not** run a car or truck inside a garage attached to your house, even if you leave the door open.
- **Do not** burn anything in a stove or fireplace that is not vented.
- **Do not** heat your house with a gas oven.

From Centers for Disease Control and Prevention. (2017). *Prevention guidelines: You can prevent carbon monoxide exposure.* Retrieved February 14, 2018, from https://www.cdc.gov/co/guidelines.htm.

and safety. Many chemicals available for household and yard or garden use require mixing before administration. Proper ventilation during mixing and storage is mandatory for most chemicals approved for home use.

Misinterpretation of the label or visual difficulties in older persons may lead to improper mixing and storage. All home safety programs should include information related to the correct reading of labels and storage of herbicides and pesticides (Wentz et al., 2011). When labels are written in small print, older adults with visual deficits should be instructed to ask for a large print version of the label. These can usually be obtained from the manufacturer (Lanson, 1997).

To prevent accidental poisoning, all hazardous household cleaning substances should be kept in a locked cabinet. This cabinet should be made difficult to be accessed by an older adult with cognitive impairment. Some household cleaning agents (e.g., disinfectants and oven or drain cleaners) are caustic or corrosive to human skin or mucous membranes and may cause critical injuries or death if swallowed. These agents are labeled with cautions and require gloves and eye protection during use. Immediate action is required if an agent is ingested or comes into contact with the eyes or mucous membranes. Where poison centers are available, one should be contacted immediately and given the name and contents of the product that caused the injury. The emergency system (activated by dialing 9-1-1 in most areas) should be contacted for any accidental poisoning when antidotes are not immediately available in the home (Wentz et al., 2011).

Cooling Fans

Ceiling, floor, and table fan injuries occur over the summer months when air conditioning is unavailable, unused, or ineffective. Floor and table fans need to have screening surrounding the entire mechanism of the fan blade. The electric cords should be placed in no-traffic or low-traffic areas and checked monthly during use for any defect or fraying of the wires. During seasonal use of fans, cleaning should be done with floor and table fans unplugged and ceiling fans completely turned off (Potts, 1999). To avoid falls while climbing ladders to clean ceiling fans, older adults should use extension poles with dusting attachments made for fan blades (Wentz et al., 2011). If the older homeowner is unsteady on a ladder, he or she should seek assistance with ladder use or ask someone else to help with the project.

EVIDENCE-BASED PRACTICE

Social Effect of Home-Delivered Meal Programs

Background

Older adults are at increased risk of malnutrition. Roughly 8% of older adults have limited access to adequate nutrition. Home-delivered meal programs are essential for the overall well-being of homebound older adults.

Sample/Setting

This study examined 61 English-speaking older adults (≥55 years old) who were new recipients of a Meals on Wheels program in Central Florida, who completed pre- and postphone interviews. Participants received at least three meals per week from the service. Of those participating, 66% were female and 58% were Caucasian.

Methods

During a 30-minute phone interview, participants were asked questions related to nutritional status, dietary intake, mental well-being, loneliness, and food security before the start of services and again 2 months after services began. Nutritional status was determined using the Mini Nutritional Assessment Short Form (MNA-SF). This form assesses nutritional risk based on six questions including body mass index, food intake, appetite, weight loss, mobility, and psychological well-being. Dietary intake was assessed using 24-hour food recall. The Six-Item Food Security Scale was used to measure food security. Emotional well-being was measured using the World Health Organization-5 questionnaire. This questionnaire rates quality of life on a 5-point Likert-type scale. Subjective feelings of loneliness and social isolation were measured using the Three-Item Loneliness Scale, a 3-point Likert-type scale.

Findings

The study found that 58.1% of participants were "at nutritional risk" and 33.9% were "malnourished" at the start of the program based on MNA-SF results. After 2 months of meal delivery, 51% of participants had improved nutritional status. Calorie and protein intake, as determined by 24-hour recall, improved by 66% over the course of the study. General emotional health, loneliness, and well-being all improved significantly over the 2-month study. Finally, 41.2% of participants reported improved food security.

Implications

This study confirms previous findings that homebound older adults have increased risk of nutritional risk and malnutrition. Providing home delivered meals improves overall nutritional status. Additionally, the social contact afforded by home delivered meals improved overall well-being and loneliness. The results of this study provide "strong public policy implications regarding the value of nutrition programs for the health of seniors" (p. 226).

From Wright, L., Vance, L., Sudduth, C., & Epps, J. B. (2015). The impact of a home-delivered meal program on nutritional risk, dietary intake, food security, loneliness, and social well-being. *Journal of Nutrition in Gerontology and Geriatrics, 34* (2), 218-227. doi: 10.1080/21551197.2015.1022681.

Foodborne Illnesses

Food handling, preparation, and consumption behaviors associated with foodborne diseases are common in the homes of older adults. Fruits and vegetables are available all year in most parts of the United States because of the long-distance trucking industry. These foods are shipped from unknown locations, where pesticides and other sprays may have been used. Therefore washing fruits, vegetables, and hands before beginning food preparation is a must to prevent foodborne illnesses. Ground meat and ground poultry are more perishable than most foods. In the danger zone between 40° F and 140° F, bacteria multiply rapidly. Because bacteria cannot be seen, smelled, or tasted, ground meats should be kept cold to keep them safe. Safe handling and safe storage are a must when preparing ground meat and poultry (NASD, 2002).

Cleaning all surfaces before and after food preparation is essential for preventing the spread of bacteria and fungus common on raw foods. Common household bleach diluted with tap water may be sprayed and wiped off preparation surfaces after cleaning with soap and water. Cleaning procedures should be done after each different type of food is prepared (CDC, 2010).

SEASONAL SAFETY ISSUES

Older adults are at particular risk for environmental temperature-induced illnesses. Predisposing medical conditions and side effects from a variety of medications may render older persons vulnerable to heat- or cold-related symptoms ranging from weakness, dizziness, and fatigue to exhaustion, coma, and death.

The nurse should prepare seasonal information materials that deal with the dangers of hyperthermia or hypothermia for all older adults living independently. Additionally, the nurse should identify those patients at risk for illnesses associated with temperature extremes and promote ways of initiating a neighborhood watch program for dangerous climatic changes.

Health care facilities, including acute, subacute, and long-term care, need to have oversight of environmental conditions for safe patient care and living. In some areas of the United States, climatic changes may develop rapidly and unexpectedly, especially as seasons change from cold to hot or the reverse. Nurses acting as patient advocates should work with physicians and management of the health care facility to maintain environmental temperature and humidity levels conducive to patient well-being.

Hypothermia and Hyperthermia in Older Adults

With aging, thermoregulatory mechanisms undergo physiologic changes, placing the older individual at risk for inability to manage extreme temperatures. The hypothalamus is responsible for regulating the body temperature. Although no significant age-related changes occur in this organ, the hypothalamus depends on the sensory functions to transmit sensory information. These sensory functions undergo changes with aging, and older persons may be unable to effectively manage changes in temperature.

Hypothermia

Hypothermia is defined as a core body temperature of less than 95° F (35° C). The two categories of hypothermia are primary and secondary hypothermia. Primary, or exposure, hypothermia follows exposure to low temperature or immersion accidents with intact thermoregulation. Secondary hypothermia is most commonly seen in patients with chronic illnesses, alcohol or substance abuse, and extreme age (Edelstein, 2007).

Hypothermia in the United States has approximately a 21% mortality rate. This rate increases with severe hypothermia to about 40%. It is estimated that about 700 people die of hypothermia each year in the United States (Edelstein, 2007).

At rest, an individual produces 40 to 60 kilocalories (kcal) of heat per square meter of body surface area. Heat production increases with movement. Shivering increases the rate of heat production by two to five times.

The body loses heat through a variety of mechanisms. Under dry conditions, heat is lost via radiation (55% to 65%). However, evaporation is the dominant mechanism of heat loss with medical alterations in the body, especially when the person receives drugs that hinder perspiration. Conduction and convection account for about 15% of heat loss, and respiration accounts for the remainder (Edelstein, 2007). Changes in the environment drastically affect the way heat is lost. The hypothalamus controls the mechanism of thermoregulation, and alterations in the central nervous system (CNS) may impair this mechanism.

Risk Factors. Primary hypothermia is caused by environmental exposure; no underlying medical conditions contribute to this process. Secondary hypothermia is associated with an underlying medical condition that prevents the body from conducting normal thermoregulation. The causes and risk factors include the following:

- Accidental immersion in cold water
- Exposure to cold temperature
- Drastic changes in the environmental temperature
- Alcohol and substance abuse
- Excessive heat loss or impaired production
- Burns, psoriasis, or other desquamating skin conditions that contribute to heat loss
- Surgery and trauma, especially cardiac surgery
- Nutritional deficiency
- Sepsis
- Spinal cord injury with poikilothermy
- Stroke
- Anoxia
- Uremia
- Hypoglycemia
- Adrenal insufficiency and hypothyroidism
- Drugs (benzodiazepines, opiates, alcohol, barbiturates, clonidine, and lithium)

Clinical Manifestations. In its early stages, hypothermia, like other conditions in older adults, presents in a nonspecific manner. Findings include fatigue, apathy, confusion, lethargy, shivering, numbness, slurred speech, impaired coordination, and possible coma. As the core temperature drops below 95° F (35° C), the individual's clinical picture starts to appear more like a disorder. For this reason, nurses need to become familiar with clinical manifestations of hypothermia in older adults. Early signs of hypothermia include confusion, impaired gait, fatigue, lethargy, and combativeness. As the core temperature drops, the signs and symptoms worsen. When an older adult's temperature drops below 93° F (34° C), cardiac arrhythmias occur, particularly bradyarrhythmias, as well as flattening of the T or P waves and atrial fibrillation. Death is usually the result of lethal arrhythmias or respiratory arrest (Kare & Shneiderman, 2001). Peripheral vasoconstriction occurring with hypothermia may also lead to increases in kidney perfusion and a subsequent increase in urine output referred to as *cold diuresis.*

Diagnostic Findings. The most objective finding for the diagnosis of hypothermia is a measured core temperature of less than 95°F (35°C). In addition to physical findings, individuals may manifest changes in their acid–base balance. Initially the individual hyperventilates, which leads to respiratory alkalosis. As the hypothermia progresses, the metabolic rate drops, and metabolic and respiratory acidosis ensues. As a result of these stresses on the body, glucose and white blood cell levels become elevated. Coagulopathy may be seen as a result of prolonged hypothermia. Thyroid-stimulating hormone and corticotropin should also be assessed. Toxicology screening is performed to rule out the presence of opiates or illicit substances as the causative factor. Chest radiography is necessary to rule out patchy infiltrates or signs of pneumonia. Computed tomography (CT) of the head is done to rule out concomitant conditions.

Management. The therapeutic management of hypothermia depends on the core temperature. If hypothermia is mild, passive external rewarming with insulated coverings and moving the older adult to a warm environment are indicated. Active external rewarming is useful in mild to moderate hypothermia without cardiac symptoms. This rewarming includes warming blankets, covering of the head, heating lamps, and warm water immersion. Moderate to severe hypothermia requires active core rewarming techniques such as warm intravenous fluids, warm humidified oxygen, and warm gastric and bladder irrigation. Peritoneal dialysis and pleural lavage are reserved for cases with cardiac instability (Kare & Shneiderman, 2001). In older patients with comorbid conditions, the mortality rate after moderate to severe hypothermia may be greater than in the general population (by 50% or more), depending on the severity at presentation and the underlying disease (Edelstein, 2007).

Hyperthermia

Hyperthermia is defined as a disorder affecting the thermoregulatory mechanism in which patients have a core body temperature greater than 105° F (40.6° C). Hyperthermia causes severe CNS dysfunction and hot, dry skin. The most severe and life-threatening heat illness in older persons is heat stroke. This condition is most often seen in debilitated individuals and usually presents differently from the exertional heat stroke seen in the young.

To balance the core temperature, the body should have the ability to produce and dissipate heat. Core heat develops as a result of cellular metabolism. When the environmental temperature exceeds the core temperature, the body's thermoregulatory mechanism activates heat loss via dissipation. Dissipation occurs via the skin, which is one of the most important elements in body heat regulation (CDC, 2013).

In response to elevated core temperature, the hypothalamus activates efferent fibers of the autonomic nervous system to stimulate vasodilation of the skin vessels, which leads to perspiration. This form of heat dissipation is achieved via the convection and evaporation mechanisms. Heat in the body can only be generated by activity occurring in the muscular system. For body temperature to increase, the rate of heat production has to exceed the rate of heat loss. Consequently, hyperthermia occurs when excessive metabolic production of heat, excessive ambient heat, or the inability to dissipate heat overwhelms the thermoregulatory mechanism.

Risk Factors. Risk factors leading to hyperthermia are either physiologic or environmental but usually work in combination. Older individuals are unable to increase their cardiac output for heat dissipation. This condition, together with poorly ventilated homes lacking air conditioning during heat waves, increases the probability for heat stroke. Combining environmental conditions with a sedentary lifestyle, disabilities, poor hydration, and prescription medications that impair the ability to tolerate heat (e.g., diuretics, antihypertensives, neuroleptics, and anticholinergics) may also hasten the development of heat stroke (Kare & Shneiderman, 2001). Additional factors that cause or predispose older adults to hyperthermia are as follows:

- Disorders leading to excessive heat production
- Malignant hyperthermia associated with anesthesia
- Thyrotoxicosis (hormonal hyperthermia)
- Salicylic acid intoxication
- Delirium tremens
- Extensive use of occlusive clothing
- Dehydration
- Cerebrovascular accident (CVA)
- Alcohol abuse (ethanol [EtOH])
- Heat syncope and heat exhaustion

Clinical Manifestations. Anhidrosis (lack of perspiration) is the most common manifestation in hyperthermia other than a core temperature greater than 105° F (40.6° C). Most of the clinical manifestations occur as a result of altered CNS function and range from confusion to coma. Additional neurologic signs of hyperthermia include hallucinations, combativeness, bizarre behaviors, and syncope. Extensive evaluation is required to rule out possible psychiatric alterations contributing to this phenomenon.

Management. It is important to monitor core temperature and perform complete neurologic and physical assessments in older persons with hyperthermia. The main objective is to bring the temperature down immediately. Interventions used to decrease body temperature include the following:

- Spraying or sponge bathing the individual with cool water (approximately 90° F [32° C])
- Placing a fan near the patient to circulate cool air
- Decreasing the room temperature
- Placing ice packs on the groin and axillae together with cooling blankets

The nurse should use protective cream on the older adult to prevent skin burns from the cooling blanket and provide a lightweight gown and bed coverings for the individual. Bed rest should be maintained to decrease muscle activity and subsequent heat production. Antipyretic medications may be administered, as ordered, to facilitate patient comfort. It is also essential to administer oral and intravenous fluids to maintain adequate hydration.

More invasive medical techniques used in the treatment of hyperthermia include peritoneal and gastric lavage with ice water. Precautions need to be taken before conducting these interventions. The airway needs to be protected, and no surgery should be scheduled. Benzodiazepines may be used to manage shivering (Kare & Shneiderman, 2001).

By understanding the risk factors for the development of thermoregulatory disorders, the nurse is better equipped to develop strategies to prevent these alterations in older persons.

DISASTERS

Natural and human-generated disasters have become more publicized over the past decade. Floods, tornadoes, earthquakes, hurricanes, and other severe weather phenomena have frequently been brought to the attention of the public. Hurricane Katrina in 2005 was the largest natural disaster to hit the Gulf Coast of the United States. Human-made disasters such as the September 11, 2001, terrorist attacks on the United States and the 1995 bombing at the Murrah Federal Building in Oklahoma City have caused concern and initiated the development of better preparedness plans to protect the safety and health of citizens, especially older or more frail adults.

The American Association of Retired Persons (AARP, 2013) determined that more than 60% of those who suffered medical problems or died during Hurricane Katrina were frail older adults. To provide guidelines for responding to disasters involving older adults, AARP's Public Policy Institute reports, *We Can Do Better; Lessons Learned for Protecting Older People in Disasters* and *Recommendations for Best Practices in the Management of Elderly Disaster Victims,* were produced. Nurses should be knowledgeable about these materials to help prevent similar outcomes in the future.

STORAGE OF MEDICATIONS AND HEALTH CARE SUPPLIES IN THE HOME

Most older adults takes medications on a regular basis. The storage of medications at home may become a safety and drug-effectiveness issue. Some storage areas in the home are not safe for keeping medications. The windowsill in the bathroom or kitchen is frequently used to shelve medication bottles. Most drugs degrade when left in direct sunlight, with or without excessive heat. Heat changes the chemical makeup of specific compounds in the medication, and moisture is considered an undesirable element for solid-based drugs such as medications in tablet form.

The nurse should review the home conditions and instruct patients to identify those places that are undesirable areas for medication storage (e.g., kitchens, bathrooms, laundry rooms, basements, and windowsills) (Skidmore-Roth, 2013). Patients should be instructed to appropriately dispose of all outdated prescriptions when new ones are written. The most common method of disposal for outdated or unused medications is to flush them down the toilet. Instructions to older adults for throwing away old medications must explicitly direct them to dispose of them in the toilet and not in trash or garbage containers.

If health care has been delivered in the home setting, dressings and other medical supplies may remain after the treatment ends. Patients should be instructed on how to dispose of used wound dressings and needles or syringes according to local health department regulations. Dressings and bandages touched by infectious disease drainage require special disposal instructions by home care nurses. The nurse should provide and collect biohazard containers for contaminated dressings and sharp objects (e.g., needles and syringes) when home care is provided. The nurse should also prepare instructional material related to safety and the use of sharp objects that may be left with patients after home care is discontinued. These sharp objects must not be disposed of among regular paper trash in home trash collection. Arrangements for disposal should be made through the local health department or hospital.

LIVING ALONE

Fear of crime reduces the subjective well-being of older adults while also curtailing neighborhood mobility (Bazargan, 1994). The fear of crime in the home differs somewhat from fear of crime outside the home. In one study, a gender variable was identified; women were significantly more fearful of crime outside the home and much less fearful of crime inside the home. Among factors that affected the perception of personal fear was previous victimization, media exposure, trust of neighbors, and length of residence in the neighborhood (Bazargan, 1994).

Community action groups have developed neighborhood strategies to protect older adults living alone. Among those strategies are the following (Chu, 1998):
- Daily telephone calls to specific persons on a call list
- Raising and lowering window shades or curtains at specific times of the day and evening, which will be monitored by a specific person
- Mail carrier alerts when mail is not picked up daily from mailboxes of enrolled older persons

Tanner (2003) developed an evidence-based home safety assessment tool. This tool includes fall risks, injury risks, fire risks, and a crime risk assessment.

AUTOMOBILE SAFETY

Maintaining independence after retirement includes the ability to travel to shopping centers and health care providers' offices, to visit family and friends, and to participate in recreational activities. A decline in an older adult's ability to drive safely may result in the loss of driving privileges. This decline may be a result of presbyopia, decreased dark adaptation, decreased depth perception, susceptibility to glare, and the general slowing of reflexes and cognitive processing (Touhy & Jett, 2012).

Because driving is a complex skill that involves rapid cognitive and psychomotor coordination and because many older adults have age-related changes, have illnesses, or are taking medications that slow their responses to road conditions, automobile safety eventually becomes an issue. In drivers who had suffered a stroke, vision and attention essential for safe driving are often impaired. The severity of these deficits could influence driving behaviors (Fisk, Owsley, & Mennemeier, 2002).

Operating a motor vehicle often requires quick reflexes and reaction time, especially in hazardous road conditions. As response time diminishes with advancing age, health care professionals and their patients must address driving safety issues. Driving evaluations are essential for older adults with suspected dementia. Valcour, Masaki, and Blanchette (2002) identified that driving rates dropped as performances on cognitive tests declined, yet a significant percentage of older adults continued to drive with poor results on these tests.

Carr, LaBarge, Dunnigan, and Storandt (1998) established a traffic sign identification test that differentiates drivers with mild or moderate senile dementia of the Alzheimer's type from cognitively normal older adults. This test was devised to protect the driving rights of older adults while identifying those persons at risk for automobile accidents because of dementia.

Alzheimer's disease causes impaired visual–spatial ability and misperception of the environment. Because of damage to neurons and a lack of neurotransmitter substances, thinking and reflexes are slowed, impulse control and judgment are impaired, short-term memory loss occurs, and attention span is reduced. When dementia affects language function, road signs and signals may be misinterpreted or ignored. Persons suspected of having early (mild) dementia should have a driving evaluation that can determine their continued ability for safe driving (Carr et al., 1998).

Guerrier, Manivannan, and Nair (1999) found that older drivers have difficulty at intersections, especially when making left turns. Their work indicates that a deficit in information-processing abilities of older persons was responsible for accidents at intersections. The three deficits identified were in visual field dependence, visual search skills, and working memory of decision making to complete a left turn maneuver. Box 11.12 lists common reasons for pedestrian accidents.

When Finelli and Lee (1996) studied the effects of stroke and automobile accidents among older adults, visual field defect, impaired consciousness, and loss of motor control were major contributing factors to accidents. Data analysis revealed that few strokes were caused by accidents, and accidents caused by stroke were not common. When stroke survivors were questioned about driving practices, 50% reported they did not receive advice about driving, and 87% reported they did not receive any type of driving evaluation. These individuals were driving 6 or 7 days a week or 100 to 200 miles a week (Fisk, Owsley, & Pulley, 1997).

Older adults with mild to moderate Parkinson's disease have been found to have diminished driving performance (Heikkila, Turkka, Korpelainen et al., 1998). When medical treatment is effective, driving performance may improve during remission of symptoms.

BOX 11.12   Most Commonly Cited Reasons for Pedestrian Accidents

- Vehicles turning left are more dangerous than vehicles turning right. Pedestrians step off the curb before being sighted by vehicles turning left.
- Pedestrians are most vulnerable when first stepping off the curb because less time is available for the driver or pedestrian to react or respond.
- Vehicles leaving an intersection are more dangerous because they are picking up speed.
- Pedestrians or vehicles may initially be hidden from each other's view by visual screens.
- Immediate action by pedestrians often occurs as the signal turns green or changes to "Walk," often while a vehicle is still in the intersection.
- "Walk" or a green signal does not give sufficient time to allow older persons to cross safely.

From National Highway Traffic Safety Administration. (2010). *Pedestrian safety workshop: A focus on older adults.* Retrieved February 14, 2018, from https://www.nhtsa.gov/sites/nhtsa.dot.gov/files/pedsafetyworkshop-02.pdf.

Other disorders that can adversely affect driving ability are as follows (Heikkila et al., 1998):

- Vertigo
- Seizure disorders
- Stroke sequelae
- Macular degeneration or retinal hemorrhage
- Unstable cardiac arrhythmias

Nursing assessment and instruction of older patients must include inquiry about driving as a separate and independent component of a functional assessment (Gallo, Rebok, & Lesikar, 1999). When a functional assessment strongly indicates that a driving safety issue exists, discussion regarding cessation of driving may become necessary. Because an older adult's lack of driving may place a burden on other members of the family, this discussion is best done in the presence of significant others viewed as trustworthy by the patient. States laws and policies differ as to mandatory reporting of high-risk individuals and to licensing provisions. The nurse must be aware of the significance that driving has for older adults. If driving is an important quality-of-life issue for an older person and he or she wants to continue to drive, the nurse should provide the following guidelines for safe travel (Touhy & Jett, 2012):

- Preplan the route of travel.
- Bring someone else to assist in navigation.
- Maintain space between oneself and the vehicle in front.
- Avoid night driving.
- Continue to wear appropriate hearing aids and glasses while driving.
- Avoid driving in poor weather conditions (e.g., ice, snow, rain, or fog).
- Keep the automobile's maintenance records up to date.
- Avoid driving if medications warn against using mechanical devices while under the influence of the drug.

The issues of quality of life, personal autonomy, and safety dictate that older adults need to be supported in their desire to continue to drive automobiles. As the number of drivers older than the age of 70 continues to grow, new ways of evaluating driving safety while supporting personal autonomy are needed (Touhy & Jett, 2012).

ABUSE AND NEGLECT

With the estimated number of older adults suffering mistreatment by neglect or actual physical abuse reaching 2 million by the year 2020, the nurse needs to assess patients for risk factors to identify those who are most vulnerable (Bird, Harrington, Barillo et al., 1998). When signs of injury are evident, the nurse should screen for risk factors of substance abuse, familial violence, dependency needs, or stresses in the spouses, roommates, or guardians of older persons. A suggested scale for determining levels of abuse and neglect was studied by Bird and associates (1998). The four-level scale placed patients in one of the following categories:

- Low risk for abuse
- Self-neglect
- Neglect
- Abuse

A scale to rate the potential for abuse or neglect helps nursing personnel become aware of the incidence and prevalence of this tragedy. Once aware, they can initiate action to remove a patient from an abusive environment.

Older persons with physical or mental frailties are more vulnerable to abuse and neglect than independent older adults. When older adults need assistance to perform basic ADLs such as bathing, dressing, toileting, walking around the immediate living area, and eating meals, stress may overtake the caregivers (Cromwell, 1999). For older spouses or adult children with heavy financial and family responsibilities, the stress and strain of caregiving tasks is often the cause for the initial abuse or neglect (Butler, 1999; Jones, Holstege, & Holstege, 1997). Some abusive family members report the reasons that led to abuse as lack of any relief from irritable feelings or constant illnesses and fatigue. Often, they lacked knowledge about caregiving skills and community resources available to provide caregiver relief before they became abusive or neglectful (Cromwell, 1999).

Elder abuse or neglect reached such magnitude that the U.S. Congress passed the Family Violence Prevention and Services Act of 1992. The act mandated a national study, which reported that 551,000 older persons living in the community were abused or neglected in 1996 (National Center on Elder Abuse, 1998). The identified cases were broken down into six areas of abuse or neglect:

- **Neglect:** failure or refusal of a caregiver or other responsible person to provide for an older adult's basic physical, emotional, or social needs (e.g., nutrition, hygiene, clothing, shelter, and access to health care) or failure to protect them from harm (e.g., failure to prevent exposure to unsafe activities and environments)
- **Psychological or emotional abuse:** occurs when an older adult experiences trauma after exposure to threatening acts or coercive tactics (e.g., humiliation or embarrassment, controlling behavior, social isolation, disregarding needs, or destroying property)
- **Financial abuse or exploitation:** unauthorized or improper use of the resources of an older adult for monetary or personal benefit, profit, or gain (e.g., forgery, misuse or theft of money or possessions, use of coercion or deception to surrender finances or property, improper use of guardianship or power of attorney)
- **Physical abuse:** occurs when an older adult is injured, assaulted, or threatened with a weapon or inappropriately restrained (e.g., scratched, bitten, slapped, pushed, hit, burned, or threatened with a knife, gun, or other object to harm)
- **Sexual abuse:** sexual contact against an older adult's will (e.g., intentional touching directly or through clothing of the genitalia, anus, groin, breast, mouth, inner thigh, or buttocks)
- **Abandonment:** the willful desertion of an older person by a caregiver or other responsible person (National Research Council, 2003; National Vital Statistics Report, 2010; Teaster, Dougar, & Mendiondo, 2006)

In nearly 90% of abuse and neglect cases, a family member was identified as the perpetrator. The spouse or adult child of the abused or neglected older person was identified as responsible for more than 65% of the poor care. To a lesser degree, abuse or neglect is experienced at the hands of caregivers who may or may not be family members (National Vital Statistics Report, 2010).

Each state has an adult protective service (APS) agency. When geriatric assessment teams work with APS agencies, the chances of identifying the perpetrator and taking corrective action are greatly increased (Dyer, Gleason, Murphy et al., 1999; Dyer, Pickens, Burnett, 2007). The CDC's information on elder abuse (maltreatment) is available on http://www.cdc.gov/ncipc.

A newly developing nursing specialty is forensic nursing. Nurses in this specialty care for the injuries and emotional distress of the victims while collecting and preserving evidence of the crimes for the legal system. Forensic nursing represents the response of nurses to the rapidly changing health care environment and to the global challenges of caring for victims and perpetrators of intentional and unintentional injuries (American Nurses Association [ANA], 2009). Through continued support, these nurses aid the healing process and provide information to prevent further victimization.

FIREARMS

A firearm in the home may offer both benefits and risks. "Having a gun in the home might affect the risk of homicide, suicide, or unintentional firearm injury," according to Cummings and Koepsell (1998). Community training programs for the care and safe use of legal firearms have addressed gun safety issues for several decades. However, firearms are associated with high rates of suicide among older men and women (Adamek & Kaplan, 1996; American Association of Suicidology, 2010). When mortality records of three age groups of white and black men age 65 or older were examined, firearms accounted for 80% of all suicides (Adamek & Kaplan, 1996).

Contrary to myths about methods of suicide among women, firearms have become the most common suicide method among women age 65 or older. A study found that the risk of suicide by firearms varied significantly across culturally diverse groups of older women (Adamek & Kaplan, 1996). Suicide rates among older adults continue to be the highest of any age group. The age group with the highest rate of successful suicide attempt with firearms is persons age 80 or older. In one retrospective study, a large percentage of suicide victims had seen a health care provider within 6 months of their death (Purcell, Thrush, & Blanchette, 1999). Suicide is often associated with alcohol or drug dependence. In fact, in addition to advancing age in

men, alcohol and drug dependence are among the greatest risk factors.

Other dangers of firearms in the homes of older adults include the potential for accidental injury during weapon cleaning and handling. Another concern is the risk of a criminal entering a home and taking the weapon away from an older person, which often has fatal consequences.

🏠 HOME CARE

1. Assess the home environment for the presence of hazards and risk factors that predispose homebound older adults to falls.
2. Carefully assess the physical status of homebound older adults for risk factors that predispose them to falls (i.e., examine feet, gait, vision, posture, muscle control, and memory).
3. Instruct caregivers and homebound older adults on tools and techniques to maximize independent functioning.
4. Assist caregivers and homebound older adults in planning a safe environment for the older adults based on the identified risks and hazards.
5. Emphasize the value of physical therapy in assessing the home setting; determine what environmental adaptations should be made to make it safer and easier for homebound older adults.
6. Teach older adults the effects of prescribed medications, focusing on the potential risks associated with falling. Instructions to decrease the effects of orthostatic hypotension, for example, rising slowly and waiting 1 to 2 minutes before standing, are important in preventing falls.
7. For frail older adults, ascertain that emergency phone numbers are located in accessible locations throughout the home; identify emergency call buttons or boxes and alarms.
8. Assess community-dwelling older adults' homes for hazards associated with fire and heat, chemicals, food handling, storage of medications and health care supplies, and firearms, and instruct or make recommendations to promote a safe, hazard-free environment.
9. Assess the temperature of the home environment during seasons of extremely high or low temperatures. Refer homebound older adults to area energy-assistance programs, if indicated, or to other community agencies that provide heating and cooling assistance.
10. Be alert to signs of abuse and neglect of homebound older adults by caregivers. If abuse or neglect is suspected, follow the reporting laws of the given state.

SUMMARY

The concept of safety encompasses many aspects of an older person's internal and external environments. The challenge for the nurse caring for older patients is to conduct individualized safety assessments, to identify age-related risk factors that affect safety, and to develop interventions aimed at the prevention of harm and injury.

Fall-related injuries are common among older adults. It is essential to identify some of the more common risk factors before planning nursing interventions or preventive measures. Risk factors include environmental issues and existing health conditions.

Nurses must also consider non–fall-related injuries such as burns, poisoning with carbon monoxide or pesticides, seasonal

safety issues with hyperthermia and hypothermia, disasters, motor vehicle accidents, crimes and abuse, and suicide. Gerontologic nurses are on the cutting edge for developing nursing interventions and seeking research opportunities that highlight safety issues among independent older adults. Patient assessment and education concerning safety matters must be incorporated into every discharge plan and, in the case of primary care, into each clinic or office visit. The most challenging step to promoting safety in the homes of older adults is the prevention of injuries and illnesses from environmental hazards.

KEY POINTS

- Safety and freedom from harm are essential to an older adult's sense of well-being.
- A direct correlation exists between an older person's sense of autonomy and his or her sense of personal safety.
- Risk factors contributing to falls in older adults include sensory impairment, cognitive impairment, unsafe living environments (e.g., poor lighting, staircases and walkways in poor repair or without hand rails, lack of grab bars in bathrooms, unsecured or worn rugs, and unstable furniture), and a history of falls.
- Thorough and accurate assessment of the risk factors related to falls is essential.

- Methods for preventing falls in older adults may include exercise programs, alarms, and safer environmental conditions.
- As a leading cause of injury in older adults, burns may occur from scalds associated with bathing, cooking, fireplace hazards, use of space heaters, and careless smoking in the home. Chemical burns or injuries may occur when household chemicals, including pesticides and herbicides, are mixed or stored.
- Carbon monoxide poisoning is preventable through maintenance and repair of heating sources in the home and detection with properly placed carbon monoxide detectors.

- Fan injuries may occur when proper guards are not in place over the fan blade housing on floor and table fan models or during the cleaning of overhead fans. Maintenance is essential to the safe use of fans and all other electrical equipment in the home.
- Foodborne illnesses may be prevented through careful cleaning of all foods before cooking and cleaning of the food preparation area before, during, and after meal preparation.
- With aging, thermoregulatory mechanisms undergo physiologic changes, placing the older individual at risk for inability to manage extreme temperatures.
- Hypothermia is defined as a core body temperature of less than 95° F (35° C).
- Primary hypothermia is caused by environmental exposure; no underlying medical conditions contribute to this process.
- Secondary hypothermia is associated with an underlying medical condition that prevents the body from conducting normal thermoregulation.
- Hyperthermia is defined as a disorder affecting the thermoregulatory mechanism in which the core body temperature is greater than 105° F (40.6° C).
- Anhidrosis (lack of perspiration) is the most common manifestation in hyperthermia other than a core temperature greater than 105° F (40.6° C).

- Neighborhood safety programs for older adults, especially homebound persons or those living alone, should become a component of all neighborhood watch organizations.
- Operating a motor vehicle is often a basic factor in an older adult's independence. However, with this independence comes increased risk for accidents, mainly as a result of decreased visual acuity and peripheral vision.
- Many older adults are victims of abuse, usually from a relative. Risk factors include poor health, physical or mental dependency, and advanced age.
- The maintenance of firearms in the homes of older adults may present special problems. The safety of the equipment, need for its use, ability to manage firearms, and safety of others in the home must be considered.
- Suicide is a leading cause of death in older adults. It is often associated with poor physical or psychological health, alcohol or drug abuse, a history of suicide attempts, and social isolation.
- Nurses must be aware of the risk factors associated with safety hazards and injury in older adults, and they must implement the necessary methods to prevent injuries.

CRITICAL-THINKING EXERCISES

1. A 77-year-old woman is hospitalized for management of her diabetes. She has a history of functional urinary incontinence and poor vision from the diabetes. The nursing staff observes her climbing over the side rails on numerous occasions at night en route to the bathroom. She is quite agitated during this time. The nursing assistant requests that you obtain an order for a body restraint at night to prevent her from falling out of bed. Should this patient be restrained to prevent injury? Would you request the order for a body restraint? Why, or why not? What other information is relevant to this case? What nursing interventions could be tried before considering a restraint?
2. A 75-year-old woman, hospitalized on a medical–surgical unit, shares a room with another older adult. You see her sitting on the edge of her bed with her feet dangling about 2 feet from the floor. She has two intravenous lines and a Foley catheter. The Foley catheter is hanging on the floor beneath her feet as she sits on the edge of her bed. Her bed is next to a window, which is usually left open. In the middle of the night, she climbs over the side rails to get out of bed and walks barefoot to the bathroom, which is about 30 feet away. She tells you she hangs onto her intravenous pole to steady her balance and drags her Foley catheter bag alongside. What environmental hazards can you identify, and what environmental modifications could you make to improve her safety?
3. You are a home care nurse visiting a 71-year-old man in his small second-story apartment, following his discharge from the hospital after having had two toes amputated because of frostbite injuries. During your initial visit, you note that he lives in a two-room, dimly lit, musty-smelling apartment. Stacks of newspapers and old mail are scattered in both rooms. The temperature is noted to be 68° F on the wall thermostat. Cold drafts can be felt around the large window in the bedroom. List the safety hazards in this apartment, and identify nursing interventions that will improve the patient's living conditions.

REFERENCES

Adamek, M. E., & Kaplan, M. S. (1996). Firearm suicide among older men. *Psychiatric Services, 47*(3), 304.

American Academy of Nursing (2018). Physical restraints with older hospitalized patients. Retrieved from www.AANnet.org.

American Association of Retired Persons (AARP). (2013). Hurricane Katrina: 5 years later. Retrieved August 23, 2013, from http://www.aarp.org/politics-society/advocacy/katrina_what_we_have_learned/.

American Association of Suicidology. (2010). *Elderly suicide fact sheet* Retrieved April 19, 2014, from www.americanassociationsuicidology.org/resources/media-professionals.

American Nurses Association (ANA). (2009). *Forensic nursing: scope & standards of practice.* Silver Springs, Md: Nursesbooks.org.

Bazargan, M. (1994). The effects of health, environmental, and socio-psychological variables on fear of crime and its consequences among urban black elderly individuals. *International Journal of Aging and Human Development, 38*(2), 99.

Bird, P. E., Harrington, D. T., Barillo, D. J., McSweeney, A., Shirani, K. Z., & Goodwin, C. W. (1998). Elder abuse: a call to action. *Journal of Burn Care and Rehabilitation, 19*(6), 522.

Boltz, M., Capezuti, E., Fulmer, T., & Zwicker, D. (2016). *Evidence-Based Geriatric Nursing Protocols for Best Practice* (5th ed.). Springer.

Bradas, C. M., Sandhu, S. K., & Mion, L. (2012). Physical restraints. Nursing Standards of Practice Protocol: Physical restraints and siderails in acute and critical care settings. *Consult GeriRN.* Retrieved from www.consultgerirn.org.

Butler, R. N. (1999). Warning signs of elder abuse. *Geriatrics, 54*(3), 3.

Carr, D., LaBarge, E., Dunnigan, K., & Storandt, M. (1998). Differentiating drivers with dementia of the Alzheimer type from healthy older persons with a traffic sign naming test. *The Journals of Gerontology. Series A, Biological Sciences and Medical Sciences, 53*(2), 135.

Centers for Disease Control and Prevention (CDC). (2010). Preliminary FoodNet data on the incidence of infection with pathogens transmitted commonly through food – 10 states, 2009. In *MMWR, 59*(14), *418–422.* The Agency.

Centers for Disease Control and Prevention (CDC). (2012). *National Center for Injury Prevention and Control. In Web-based injury statistics query and reporting system (WISQARS), [online].* Retrieved 2013, from http://www.cdc.gov/ncipc/wisqars.

Centers for Disease Control and Prevention (CDC). (2013). *Heat stress in the elderly.* Retrieved August 29, 2013, from http://emergency.cdc.gov/disasters/extremeheat/elderlyheat.asp.

Centers for Disease Control and Prevention (CDC). (2017). Risk factors for falls. Retrieved from https://www.cdc.gov/steadi/pdf/Risk_Factors_for_Falls-print.pdf.

Centers for Disease Control and Prevention (CDC). (2017). Falls in older adults. Retrieved from https://www.cdc.gov/homeandrecreationalsafety/falls/index.html.

Chu, N. L. (1998). Environment/home. In A. S. Luggen, S. S. Travis, & S. Meiner (Eds.), *NGNA core curriculum for gerontological advanced practice nurses.* Thousand Oaks, Calif: Sage.

Cromwell, S. (1999). Social issues: abuse and violence. In D. L. Robinson (Ed.), *Core concepts for advance practice nursing.* St Louis: Mosby.

Cummings, P., & Koepsell, T. D. (1998). Does owning a firearm increase or decrease the risk of death? *JAMA, 280*(5), 471.

Dyer, C. B., Gleason, M. S., Murphy, K. P., Pavlik, V. N., Portal, B., et al. (1999). Treating elder neglect: collaboration between a geriatrics assessment team and adult protective services. *Southern Medical Journal, 92*(2), 242.

Dyer, C. B., Pickens, S., & Burnett, J. (2007). Vulnerable elders: when it is no longer safe to live alone. JAMA, *298*(12), *1448–1450* (Sep 26).

Edelstein, J. A. (2007). *Hypothermia.* Retrieved May 18, 2009, from http://emedicine.medscape.com/article/770542-overview.

Finelli, P., & Lee, N. (1996). Stroke and automobile accidents. *Connecticut Medicine, 60*(3), 145.

Fisk, G. D., Owsley, C., & Mennemeier, M. (2002). Vision, attention, and self-reported driving behaviors in community-dwelling stroke survivors. *Archives of Physical Medicine and Rehabilitation, 83*(4), 469–477.

Fisk, G. D., Owsley, C., & Pulley, L. V. (1997). Driving after stroke: driving exposure, advice, and evaluations. *Archives of Physical Medicine and Rehabilitation, 78*(12), 1338.

Fit and Strong. Retrieved at www.fitandstrong.org.

Fortinsky, R., Iannuzzi-Sucich, M., Baker, D., Gottschalk, M., King, M., Brown, C., et al. (2004). Fall-risk assessment and management in clinical practice: views from healthcare providers. *Journal of the American Geriatrics Society, 52*(9), 1522–1526. (2004). https://doi.org/10.1111/j.1532-5415.2004.52416.x.

Gallo, J. J., Rebok, B. W., & Lesikar, S. E. (1999). The driving habits of adults aged 60 years and older. *Journal of the American Geriatrics Society, 47*(3), 335.

Gill, T. M., Williams, C. S., Robison, J. T., & Tinetti, M. E. (1999). A population-based study of environmental hazards in the homes of older persons. *American Journal of Public Health, 89*(4), 553.

Guerrier, J. H., Manivannan, P., & Nair, S. N. (1999). The role of working memory, field dependence, visual search, and reaction time in the left turn performance of older female drivers. *Applied Ergonomics, 30*(2), 109.

Harper, R. D., & Dickson, W. A. (1995). Reducing the burn risk to elderly persons living in residential care. *Burns, 21*(3), 205.

Healthy Steps. Retrieved at www.aging.pa.gov.

Heikkila, V. M., Turkka, J., Korpelainen, J., Kallanranta, T., & Summala, H. (1998). Decreased driving ability in people with Parkinson's disease. *Journal of Neurology, Neurosurgery and Psychiatry, 64*(3), 325.

Hnizdo, S., Archuleta, R. A., Taylor, B., & Kim, S. C. (2013). Validity and reliability of the modified John Hopkins Fall Risk Assessment Tool for elderly patients in home health care. *Geriatric Nursing, 5*(11), 1–5. https://doi.org/10.1016/j.gerinurse.2013.05.011.

Houck, P. M., & Hampson, N. B. (1997). Epidemic carbon monoxide poisoning following a winter storm. *The Journal of Emergency Medicine, 15*(4), 469.

Iqbal, S., Clower, J. H., Hernandez, S. A., Damon, S. A., & Yip, F. Y. (2012). A review of disaster-related carbon monoxide poisoning: surveillance, epidemiology, and opportunity for prevention. *American Journal of Public Health, 102*(10), 1957–1963.

Jones, J. S., Holstege, C., & Holstege, H. (1997). Elder abuse and neglect: understanding the causes and potential risk factors. *The American Journal of Emergency Medicine, 15*(6), 579.

Jones, L., & McEwen, A. (2012). Reducing secondhand smoke exposure at home. *British Journal of School Nursing, 7*(8), 389–393.

Jung, D. (2006). *A prediction model of fear of falling in older adults living in a continuing-care retirement community.* Baltimore: University of Maryland, CINAHL Plus with Full Text, EBSCOhost (accessed August 22, 2013).

Kare, J. A., & Shneiderman, A. (2001). Hyperthermia and hypothermia in the older population. *Topics in Emergency Medicine, 23*(3), 39.

Kiel, D. P. (2016). Falls in Older Adults: Risk factors and evaluation. In *Up To Date.* Retrieved from www.uptodate.com.

Kristensen, M., Foss, N., & Kehlet, H. (2009). Factors with independent influence on the 'timed up and go' test in patients with hip fracture. *Physiotherapy Research International, 14*(1), 30–41. (2009). https://doi.org/10.1002/pri.414.

Lanson, S. (1997). Pesticide poisoning: an environmental emergency. *Journal of Emergency Nursing, 23*(6), 516.

Lee, H. L., Chen, K. W., & Wu, M. H. (1999). Acute poisoning with a herbicide containing imazapyr (arsenal): a report of six cases. *Journal of Toxicology - Clinical Toxicology, 37*(1), 83–89.

Lee-Chiong, T. L. (1999). Smoke inhalation injury. *Postgraduate Medicine, 105*(2), 55.

Lovence, K. (n.d.). Post-fall care nursing algorithm. *RNJournal.* Retrieved February 14, 2018 from http://rn-journal.com/journal-of-nursing/post-fall-care-nursing-algorithm.

Markowitz, S. (2013 Aug 23). Where there's smoking, there's fire: the effects of smoking policies on the incidence of fires in the USA. *Health Economics.*

Matter of Balance, CAPABLE. *Maine Health.* Retrieved at www.mainehealth.org.

McIntyre, A., Mehta, S., Janzen, S., Aubut, J., & Teasell, R. W. (2013). A meta-analysis of functional outcome among older adults with traumatic brain injury. *Neurorehabilitation*, 32(2), 409–414. (2013). https://doi.org/10.3233/NRE-130862.

Meiner, S. (2015). *Gerontological Nursing* (5th ed.). Maryland Heights, MO: Elsevier.

Middleton, A., & Fritz, S. L. (2013). Assessment of gait, balance, and mobility in older adults: Considerations for clinicians. *Current Translational Geriatrics and Experimental Gerontology Reports*, 2(4), 205–214.

National Agricultural Safety Database (NASD). (2002). *Kitchen safety.*

National Agricultural Safety Database (NASD). (2013). Basic principles of healthy housing. Retrieved from http://www.cdc.gov/nceh/publications/books/housing/cha02.htm.

National Center on Elder Abuse. (1998). *National elder abuse incidence study: final report.* Washington, DC: American Public Human Services Association.

National Council on Aging (NCOA). (2017). *Fall standards in older adults.* Retrieved from www.ncoa.org.

National Hospital Discharge Survey (NHDS). (2013). *National Center for Health Statistics.* Retrieved August 9, 2013, from www.cdc.gov/nchs/hdi.htm.

National Institute on Aging. (2017). Fall-proofing your home. Retrieved May 27, 2018 from https://www.nia.nih.gov/health/fall-proofing-your-home.

National Research Council. (2003). Elder mistreatment: abuse, neglect, and exploitation in an aging America. In R. J. Bonne & R. B. Wallace (Eds.), *Panel to review risk and prevalence of elder abuse and neglect.* Washington DC: National Academies Press.

National Vital Statistics Report. (2010). National Center for Health Statistics, vol 56(16), Hyattsville, Md. Retrieved August 2013, from http://www.cdc.gov/nchs/data/nvsr.

Nnodim, J. O., & Yong, R. L. (2015). Balance and gait assessment in older adults. Journal of Geriatrics Medical Gerontology, 1(1).

Potts, J. R. (1999). Ceiling fan injuries: the Townsville experience. *Medical Journal of Australia*, 170(3), 119.

Purcell, D., Thrush, C. R., & Blanchette, P. L. (1999). Suicide among the elderly in Honolulu County: a multiethnic comparative study (1987–1992). *International Psychogeriatrics*, 11(1), 57.

Rubenstein, L. Z., & Josephson, K. R. (2006). Falls and their prevention in elderly people: what does the evidence show? *The Medical Clinics of North America*, 90, 807–824.

Saccomano, S., & Ferrara, L. (2015). Fall prevetion in older adults. *Nurse Practitioner*, 40(6), 40–47. https://doi.org/10.1097/01.NPR.0000465117.19783.ee.

Skidmore-Roth, L. (2013). Mosby's drug guide for nurses with 2014 updates (10th ed.). St Louis: Mosby.

Tanner, E. K. (2003). Assessing home safety in homebound older adults. *Geriatric Nursing*, 24(4). 250–254 256.

Tearle, P. (1998). Fire awareness in the office and laboratory. *Communicable Disease and Public Health*, 1(4), 290.

Teaster, P., Dugar, T., Mendiondo, M., et al. (2006). The survey of state adult protective services: Abuse of adults 60 years of age and older. *Newark. In Del: National Center on Elder Abuse.* http://www.ncea.aoa.gov.

Tideiksaar, R. (2009). Chapter 8: falls. In B. Bonder, V. Dal Bello-Haas, & M. Wagner (Eds.), *Functional Performance in Older Adults* (pp. 193–214)(3rd ed.). Philadelphia, PA: F.A. Davis Company.

Tinetti, M., Baker, D., King, M., Gottschalk, M., Murphy, T., Acampora, D., et al. (2008). Effect of dissemination of evidence in reducing injuries from falls. *The New England Journal of Medicine*, 359(3), 252–261.

Tinetti, M. E. (1986). Performance oriented assessment of mobility problems in elderly patients. *Journal of the American Geriatrics Society*, 34, 199.

Touhy, T. A., & Jett, K. (2012). *Ebersole & Hess' Toward healthy aging: Human needs & nursing response* (8th ed.). St. Louis: Mosby/Elsevier.

U.S. Department of Health Science and Human Services. (2014). *Healthy People 2020.* Retrieved May 17, 2018, from https://www.healthypeople.gov/2020/topics-objectives/topic/older-adults.

US Fire Administration(USFA). (2008). Fire safety facts for people 50-plus. Emmitsburg, Md: National Center for Prevention & Injury Control.

Valcour, V. G., Masaki, K. H., & Blanchette, P. L. (2002). Self-reported driving, cognitive status, and physician awareness of cognitive impairment. *Journal of the American Geriatrics Society*, 50(7), 1265–1267.

Verghese, J., Buschke, H., Viola, L., Katz, M., Hall, C., Kuslansky, G., et al. (2002). Validity of divided attention tasks in predicting falls in older individuals: a preliminary study. *Journal of the American Geriatrics Society*, 50(9), 1572–1576.

Wentz, M., Wentz, D., & Wallace, D. K. (2011). *The Healthy Home: Simple Truths to Protect Your Family from Hidden Household Dangers.* New York: Vanguard Publishing.

Wrenn, K., & Conners, G. P. (1997). Carbon monoxide poisoning during ice storms: a tale of two cities. *The Journal of Emergency Medicine*, 15(4), 465.

Yoon, S. S., Macdonald, S. C., & Parrish, R. G. (1998). Deaths from unintentional carbon monoxide poisoning and potential for prevention with carbon monoxide detectors. *JAMA*, 279(9), 685.

12

Sexuality and Aging

Jennifer J. Yeager, PhD, RN, APRN

http://evolve.elsevier.com/Meiner/gerontologic

LEARNING OBJECTIVES

On completion of this chapter, the reader will be able to:
1. Identify myths surrounding sexuality and aging.
2. Explore the possible reasons for a nurse's hesitancy in talking with older adults about their need for sexuality and intimacy.
3. Describe the normal changes of aging in male and female urogenital systems.
4. Describe pathologic problems of the aging male and female urogenital systems.
5. Identify issues surrounding persons with dementia and expression of sexuality.
6. Discuss barriers to older adults' sexual expression and the ways to overcome these barriers.
7. Conduct an assessment related to an older adult's sexuality and intimacy.
8. State two nursing diagnoses applicable to older adults' sexual expression.
9. Plan nursing interventions to assist older adults in fulfilling their need for sexuality and intimacy.

WHAT WOULD YOU DO?

What would you do if you were faced with the following situations?
- Your 76-year-old mother confides in you she has started a new relationship with a gentleman in another state that she met through an online dating service. She wants to fly to his home to meet him. What do you do?
- A nearby nursing home has recently developed a protocol concerning sexuality among residents. You have been asked to develop an in-service on sexuality and aging for their employees. What would you do?
- Your 82-year-old patient—a recent widower—shyly tells you about his new relationship with a 67-year-old widow in his retirement complex. He states dating at his age is freer, as they do not need to worry about pregnancy. How do you respond?

OLDER ADULT NEEDS FOR SEXUALITY AND INTIMACY

Sexuality is an important aspect of health, general well-being, and quality of life. Human sexuality includes intimate activity as well as sexual knowledge, beliefs, attitudes, and values. Not only does sexual activity provide pleasure for older adults, it may also help maintain a healthy self-esteem, an aspect of life often diminished after retirement. Sexual activity can help each partner express love, affection, and loyalty. It can also enhance personal growth, creativity, and communication. Older persons, especially older women, who feel desirable and attractive often feel younger as well (Locklainn & Kenny, 2013; Syme & Cohn, 2016).

Sexuality is an important component of successful aging (Flynn & Gow, 2015); older adults face barriers to sexual expression, including problems arising from low desire, disease, drug therapy, societal beliefs, and changes in social circumstances (Syme & Cohn, 2016). Nurses play a key role in the assessment of age-related changes, along with changes caused by disabling medical conditions and drugs, and can intervene at an early point to enhance sexuality in older adults.

THE IMPORTANCE OF INTIMACY AMONG OLDER ADULTS

Despite evidence supporting not only the need for, but the importance of, sexual expression in older adults (Flynn & Gow, 2015), health care professionals carry out few interventions to facilitate older adults' expression of sexuality. One reason for this is that society continually equates sexuality with sexual intercourse. However, according to the World Health Organization (2015),

Sexuality is a central aspect of being human throughout life and encompasses sex, gender identities and roles, sexual orientation, eroticism, pleasure, intimacy, and reproduction. Sexuality is experienced and expressed in thoughts, fantasies, desires, beliefs, attitudes, values, behaviors, practices, roles, and relationships. Although sexuality may include all of these dimensions, not all of them are always experienced or expressed. Sexuality is influenced by the interaction of biologic, psychological, social, economic, political, cultural, ethical, legal, historical, religious, and spiritual factors. (p. 5)

If sexuality among older adults is viewed as a need for intimacy, society and health care professionals may be more comfortable in helping older adults meet those needs.

Women outlive men. The Administration on Aging (2016) reports women reaching age 65 have an additional 20.6 years life expectancy and men an additional 18 years. The ratio of older women is 126.5 women for every 100 men. This often leaves older women without sexual partners. The loss of a partner does not necessarily mean that older women do not have continuing sexual needs. The National Survey of Sexual Attitudes and Lifestyles conducted in 2013 demonstrated 42% of women and 60% of men between the ages 65 and 74 were sexually active (Flynn & Gow, 2015). Among older adults, the benefits of sexual expression include increased happiness, energy, and relaxation; decreased pain; improved cardiovascular health; decreased depressive symptoms; increased self-esteem; and improved satisfaction with relationships (Flynn & Gow, 2015; Syme, 2014). Considering this information, it is imperative health care professionals value the sexual needs of older adults.

Almost half of the older adult population experiences some sexual dysfunction ranging from erectile dysfunction (ED) and premature climax among men, and lack of desire, decreased vaginal lubrication, pain, and inability to reach orgasm among women. Older adults may be afraid to discuss the topic due to embarrassment, lack of understanding, and societal stigma related to sexuality and aging (Syme, 2014; Syme & Cohn, 2016). However, research has shown older adults are willing to discuss sexual matters when their health care provider initiates the conversation. Health care providers can initiate the conversation by asking questions about intimacy during the review of systems (Locklainn & Kenny, 2013).

Dating is an important social activity for older adults: 14% of single, older adults are in dating-type relationships (27% men; 7% women). Social connections, economic status, educational attainment, and health status all influence the older adults' ability to date (Brown & Shinohara, 2013). Although men may seek out new relationships due to the "domestic help that comes with being married" (Wion & Loeb, 2015, p. 26), older women tend to avoid marriage for this very reason (Wion & Loeb, 2015).

Technology has become a familiar tool for adults over 65, many of whom are Baby Boomers; 70% report daily Internet usage. Technology, particularly smartphones, is considered *freeing* by 82% of older adults (Anderson, 2015). Familiarity with technology has afforded many older adults the option of online dating to find a partner. In a study conducted by AARP (David, 2013), respondents identified the following as the top reasons for trying online dating:
- Able to meet a broader range of people
- No pressure; do not have to reply or talk to people they don't want to
- Recommended by a friend

The same study identified that the majority (48%) of older adults using online dating were looking for a serious relationship. Older adults recognized the risks associated with online dating, and those who indicated they did not use the services stated it was because online dating was too risky or did not fit their lifestyle (David, 2013).

Older adults participate in a variety of sexual practices depending on functional ability, including foreplay, kissing, embracing, holding hands or cuddling, masturbation, and vaginal intercourse (Syme, 2014). Masturbation is a method through which both men and women may feel sexually fulfilled in the absence of partners. The literature has established that in addition to older adults' ongoing need to express their sexuality through traditional sexual methods, the human need to touch and to be touched must also be fulfilled. A person's need for intimacy and closeness to another does not end at any age. It is known that touch is an overt expression of closeness and intimacy (Syme, 2014).

Touch is an important component of nursing care and should be incorporated into nursing interventions to achieve quality outcomes. Touch is part of nonverbal communication. It can express empathy, comfort, and reassurance, and can promote trust. Touch is important to a person's well-being and sense of self. However, the perception of touch and the need for touch varies between individuals and cultures. Touch may also have different meanings based on a person's past experiences. Touch can be interpreted as disrespectful, sexual, patronizing, or threatening. When touching, whether to provide nursing care or comfort and reassurance, ask permission. If the older adult is unable to express their wishes concerning touch, ask family his or her preferences. Always avoid touching in a manner that can be misinterpreted (Catlin, n.d.).

For older adults who reached young adulthood before 1959, sexuality was hidden behind closed doors for much of their lives. Therefore assessment of an older adult's sexuality may be the first opportunity they have to openly discuss sexuality. Embarrassment, shyness, and apprehension in this area are common. In addition, the patient may view the normal changes of aging as embarrassing or indicative of illness and may be reluctant to discuss these matters with a nurse. Some older adults are misinformed about sexuality and may refuse to discuss issues about which they harbor feelings of guilt and shame (Butler & Lewis, 2000; National Council on Aging, 1998). Understanding attitudes and myths about aging will help the nurse assess and intervene to sensitively promote the older adult's need for sexuality and intimacy.

NURSING'S RELUCTANCE TO MANAGE THE SEXUALITY OF OLDER ADULTS

One of society's pervasive myths regarding sexuality in older adults is that it is undignified. Nurses often share society's ageist beliefs about the asexuality of older adults, which may lead to nurses discouraging sexual activity (Messinger-Rapport et al., 2003).

In long-term care settings, including assisted living facilities, a resident's attempt at sexual expression is often viewed as a "problem" behavior (Rheaume & Mitty, 2008). However, residents of long-term care facilities still have their sexual identity, so their need to express themselves sexually and intimately should be encouraged, not extinguished. Educational programs for facility staff may help dispel myths related to aging and sexuality, thus encouraging environmental change designed to enhance resident expression of sexuality and intimacy (Benbow & Beeston, 2012; Katz, 2013).

Older adults may face difficulties with sexual expression. More than 70% of older adults experience difficulties with sexuality and intimacy (Santos-Iglesias, Byers, & Moglia, 2016). In their study, Santos-Iglesias et al. reported 42% of respondents felt "turned off," while others expressed a lack of interest in sex (41%) or difficulties with arousal (40%). Others experienced difficulty maintaining arousal (37%), or experienced inhibited orgasm (37%), anorgasmia (29%), or premature orgasm (25%).

Nurses are in a key position to address newly developed or potential sexual dysfunction during patient interactions. However, because of discomfort, myths, ageism, and lack of training in sexual health, these problems are often ignored. The result is that the needs of older adults with newly developed or chronic sexual dysfunction are ignored.

NORMAL CHANGES OF THE AGING SEXUAL RESPONSE

Nurses must understand the normal urogenital changes associated with aging. Knowledge about these normal changes helps nurses to work more confidently with older adults, enabling them to compensate for these changes, assisting them to understand these changes, and recognizing when possible pathologic changes occur.

To assess sexual function in older adults, health care providers need to understand the sexual response cycle, which is a psychophysiologic cascade of events leading to orgasm (Wise & Crone, 2006). The cycle includes the excitement phase, plateau phase, orgasmic phase, and resolution phase. Sexual dysfunctions include sexual desire disorders, sexual arousal disorders, ED, premature ejaculation, orgasm disorders, and sexual pain disorders.

Physiologic Changes

The orgasm response changes with aging. Dysfunctions include anorgasmia, premature ejaculation, and retarded ejaculation. In addition, a longer period of stimulation is typically required for both men and women to reach orgasm. The refractory period after orgasm is also longer for both men and women.

In older adults, the reduced availability of sex hormones in both genders results in less rapid and less extreme vascular responses to sexual arousal (Wise & Crone, 2006). Although some older adults view this gradual slowing as a decline in function, others do not consider it an impairment because it merely results in them taking more time to achieve orgasm (Butler & Lewis, 2000).

Common physiologic changes associated with aging men are an erection that is less firm and of shorter duration, less preejaculatory fluid, and semen that is less forceful at ejaculation (Butler & Lewis, 2000; Messinger-Rapport et al., 2003). The refractory period between ejaculations is long. Andropause (male menopause) has several physical, sexual, and emotional symptoms. Disagreement exists about which term should be used to accurately describe the phenomenon. Most endocrinologists now use the term *ADAM*, an acronym for *androgen*

decline in the aging male (Blackwell, 2006). A decline in the concentration of testosterone is believed to be the cause of ADAM (Blackwell, 2006). Serum sex hormone-binding globulin (SHBG) concentrations gradually increase as a function of age, making less free testosterone. Testosterone levels diminish with age from a reduction in both testosterone production and metabolic clearance. These hormonal changes lead to a loss of libido, decreased muscle mass and strength, alterations in memory, diminished energy and well-being, an increase in sleep disturbance, and possibly osteoporosis secondary to a decrease in bone mass. Testosterone appears to influence the frequency of nocturnal erections; however, low testosterone levels do not affect erections produced by erotic stimuli (Kaiser, 2000; Messinger-Rapport et al., 2003). Despite these physiologic changes, aging men may still experience orgasmic pleasure (Messinger-Rapport et al., 2003).

An instrument such as the ADAM Questionnaire, created by Morley (2000), is a helpful screening tool that should prompt further workup, including determination of the testosterone level. Other laboratory studies should include luteinizing hormone (LH), follicle-stimulating hormone (FSH), prolactin, thyroid stimulating hormone (TSH), and free T4.

ED is the inability to develop and maintain an erection long enough for sexual intercourse. Causes of ED include increasing age, structural abnormalities of the penis, the adverse effects of drugs, psychological disorders, substance use disorders, surgery, trauma and radiation of the pelvis, and vascular, neurologic, and endocrine disorders. It is most common to have more than one cause of ED. ED is treatable (Ellsworth, 2017).

The use of medications such as phosphodiesterase 5 (PDE 5) inhibitors (e.g., sildenafil citrate, tadalafil, and vardenafil hydrochloride) has increased public awareness of the prevalence of ED among men in the United States. These medications may be effective in treating ED in older men when appropriately prescribed and therefore may enhance the quality of life in older adults.

Up to 85% of postmenopausal women experience sexual dysfunction. Sexual dysfunction in older women encompasses loss of sexual desire, problems with arousal, inability to achieve orgasm, and painful intercourse. Issues leading to sexual dysfunction include physiologic changes with aging, functional decline, the adverse effects of drugs, and vascular, neurologic, and endocrine disorders (Ambler, Bieber, & Diamond, 2012).

Genitourinary Syndrome of Menopause

Genitourinary syndrome of menopause encompasses the changes in the genitourinary tract related to menopause. Genital symptoms include dryness, burning, and irritation; sexual symptoms include decreased lubrication, thinning of the vaginal wall, decreased elasticity, and decreased vaginal rugae, leading to pain, and bleeding during intercourse. Urinary symptoms include urgency, dysuria, and recurrent urinary tract infections (Ambler et al., 2012; Gass, 2016; Kim, Kang, Chung, Kim, & Kim, 2015).

Women experience a decline in both ovarian hormones and adrenal androgens after menopause, which may contribute to a diminished sense of well-being, loss of energy, loss of bone mass, and decrease or loss of libido (Gass, 2016). As women age, circulating levels of testosterone decrease; this combined with a decrease in estrogen and progesterone, and an increase in gonadotropins, may play a role in the decrease or loss of libido (Ambler et al., 2012).

Many older women experience *dyspareunia,* painful intercourse or pain with attempted intercourse, which may result in a decreased desire to participate in sexual activity. Forty percent of sexually active women between the ages of 55 to 75 experience painful sexual intercourse. The main cause of dyspareunia is dry, fragile vulvovaginal tissues. Vaginismus, involuntary painful contraction (spasm) of the lower vaginal muscles, may be experienced by older women, again decreasing their desire to participate in sexual activity. It may be triggered by the anticipation of pain during intercourse (Gandhi et al., 2016).

PATHOLOGIC CONDITIONS AFFECTING OLDER ADULTS' SEXUAL RESPONSES

Illness, Surgery, and Medication

Sexual function is a process that depends on the neurologic, endocrine, and vascular systems. It is also influenced by psychosocial factors, including family and religious beliefs, the sexual partner, and the individual's self-esteem (Merghati-Khoei, Pirak, Mansoureh, & Rezasolani, 2016). Many chronic illnesses common to older adults can affect sexual function (Box 12.1).

Surgeries may also affect an older adult's sexual responses. Some of these surgeries include coronary artery bypass surgery, hysterectomy, mastectomy, prostatectomy, orchiectomy, and removal of the anus and the rectum. In addition, many drugs adversely affect sexuality (Table 12.1).

Human Immunodeficiency Virus

Adults over the age of 50 account for 45% of those living with human immunodeficiency virus (HIV). In 2015 17% of persons newly diagnosed with HIV were over the age of 55. When older adults are found to be HIV-positive, they tend to be diagnosed later in the course of illness (Centers for Disease Control and Prevention [CDC], 2017b). Additionally, older adults living with HIV have a higher incidence of comorbid cardiovascular disease, kidney and hepatic disease, osteopenia, and endocrine and metabolic disorders than non-HIV-positive older adults (Pilowslay & Wu, 2015).

The availability of drugs to treat ED has extended the sexual lives of many men. Increasingly larger numbers of older adults have substance use disorders (e.g., alcohol, illicit drugs, and recreational use of prescription drugs). These factors combined with an underestimation of personal risk mean many older adults engage in behavior that puts them at risk for HIV infection. As many as 20% of older men and 24% of older women fail to use condoms when participating in sexual activity (Pilowslay & Wu, 2015).

Age-related changes also increase the risk of HIV infection. For example, age-related thinning of the vaginal mucosa and the subsequent vaginal tissue disruption, as well as age-related reductions in immune function, place older adults at increased

---

BOX 12.1 Conditions That Affect Sexual Function

Cardiac Conditions
Congestive heart failure
Myocardial infarction
Angina
Arrhythmias
Hypertension

Endocrine Conditions
Diabetes mellitus
Hypothyroidism

Genitourinary Conditions
Prostatitis
Cystitis and urethritis
Chronic renal failure
Incontinence

Immune Conditions
Human immunodeficiency virus (HIV) infection and acquired immunodeficiency syndrome (AIDS)
Cancer

Musculoskeletal Conditions
Arthritis
Chronic pain

Neurologic Conditions
Parkinson's disease
Dementia
Stroke
Depression

Respiratory Conditions
Chronic emphysema
Bronchitis
Sleep apnea

Surgery
Hysterectomy
Mastectomy
Prostatectomy

From Merghati-Khoei, E., Pirak, A., Mansoureh, Y., & Rezasoltani, P. (2016). Sexuality and elderly with chronic diseases: A review of the existing literature. *Journal of Research in Medical Sciences, (21),* 136.

---

risk for HIV infection. Older adults who do contract HIV are more likely to be diagnosed late in disease and experience progression more quickly; death from AIDS comes sooner after diagnosis than in their younger counterparts (Mpondo, 2016).

Malignancies

Breast cancer, one of the leading cancers affecting older women, has clear implications for self-esteem and sexual functioning. Dysphoria from the disease, fears of death, and disfigurement may diminish sexual desire before treatment begins. The presence of medical illnesses as well as myths about sexuality and the benefit of treatment to older adults often prevent clinicians from aggressively treating older women with breast cancer (Wang et al., 2013).

TABLE 12.1	**Drugs Affecting Sexuality**	
Drug Class	**Example**	**Effect on Sexuality**
Diuretics	Thiazide diuretics Potassium sparing diuretics	Decreased libido Erectile dysfunction Decreased vaginal lubrication
Antihistamines	Diphenhydramine Chlorpheniramine	Erectile dysfunction
Histamine blockers	Cimetidine Ranitidine	Decreased libido Erectile dysfunction
Antipsychotics	Phenothiazines First-generation antipsychotics Atypical antipsychotics	Decreased libido Erectile dysfunction
Antidepressants	Tricyclic antidepressants Selective serotonin reuptake inhibitors Monoamine oxidase inhibitors	Decreased libido Decreased ejaculate Delayed ejaculation
Antihypertensives	Alpha-blockers Beta-blockers Centrally acting agents	Decreased libido Erectile dysfunction Lack of orgasm Decreased ejaculate
Alcohol		Erectile dysfunction Decreased sexual response in women
Antianxiety medications	Benzodiazepines	Decreased libido Erectile dysfunction
Anticonvulsants		Decreased libido Erectile dysfunction
Hormones	GnRH analogs Estrogen	Decreased libido
Tobacco		Erectile dysfunction Decreased vaginal lubrication
Medical marijuana		Erectile dysfunction
Drugs for BPH	Finasteride	Decreased libido Erectile dysfunction Abnormal ejaculation
Opioids		Decreased libido

BPH, Benign prostatic hyperplasia; *GnRH,* gonadotropin-releasing hormone.
Data from Cleveland Clinic. (2017). *Medications that affect sexual function.* Retrieved January 18, 2018, from https://my.clevelandclinic.org/health/articles/9124-medications-that-affect-sexual-function; Health.com. (2015). *Low libido? 11 drugs that affect your sex drive.* Retrieved January 18, 2018, from http://www.health.com/health/gallery/0,20788030,00.html#libido-killing-drugs; and Conaglen, H. M., & Conaglen, J. V. (2013). Drug-induced sexual dysfunction in men and women. *Australian Prescriber, 36*(2), 42–45.

Prostate cancer is the most common cancer in men and the second leading cause of death from cancer in men in the United States (CDC, 2017a). The risk of developing prostate cancer increases with age. When cancer has not spread outside of the prostate, a radical prostatectomy may be performed; it involves removal of the prostate gland and some surrounding tissue, leading to a disruption of surrounding nerves, veins, and arteries. In 25% to 90% of men, radical prostatectomy results in impotence in up to 90% of men (Bratu et al., 2017); additionally, roughly 50% experience incontinence. The introduction of robot-assisted laparoscopic techniques has reduced sexual dysfunction; however, men may need to wait 2 to 3 years for maximum function to return. Phosphodiesterase inhibitors, prosthetic devices, and other treatment options are available to treat ED after treatment for prostate cancer (Tutolo et al., 2012).

Colorectal cancer is the third most common cancer in the United States, and the second leading cause of cancer death. Although prevalence of sexual dysfunction after surgery varies, colorectal cancer survivors experience significant sexual dysfunction due to autonomic nerve damage causing ED and ejaculation difficulties in men; women experience difficulties with vaginal dryness, dyspareunia, and decreased libido (Donovan, Thompson, & Hoffe, 2010).

Dementia

The need for companionship and intimacy does not fade just because a person is diagnosed with dementia. As dementia progresses and changes in cognition and judgment occur, some individuals experience a decrease in sexuality, whereas others may experience sexual disinhibition. Many older adults with dementia long for physical closeness and seek out physical touch; however, their intentions may be misinterpreted as sexual in nature. Masturbation continues to be a source of pleasure for both men and women with dementia, but a lack of privacy in institutional settings may lead to a public display, and the behavior is labeled as inappropriate. Inappropriate sexual behavior can be distressing for caregivers (both family and members of the health care team). Some actions labeled as inappropriate may be caused by confusion or misidentification, such as undressing in public, or kissing and touching a caregiver (Bronner, 2015).

Other persons with dementia may express sexually disinhibited behaviors, which include sexually explicit or suggestive language, exhibitionism, repeated attempts to have sex, or aggressive sexual demands. Nonpharmacologic interventions should be used to diffuse the situation (Bronner, 2015):

- Reduce overstimulation in the environment
- Separate the person from the individual who "triggers" the behavior
- Firmly state "That is not acceptable."
- Redirect the person (i.e., take them for a walk or involve them in a game)
- Leave the area or room
- Provide an alternative (i.e., give them privacy for masturbation)

Psychotherapy and cognitive behavioral therapy might be beneficial in assisting caregivers and family to cope with sexually disinhibited behaviors and reorient the person with dementia to acceptable social expression of sexuality. Pharmacologic interventions may become necessary when the behaviors become harmful or detrimental to safe care. Selective serotonin reuptake inhibitors, gabapentin, carbamazepine, beta-blockers, and cholinesterase inhibitors have been used for their known side effects of decreased libido and ED, with varying degrees of success. Hormonal agents (e.g., antiandrogens and estrogens) have been successful in treating some persons with dementia with sexually disinhibited behavior, but controversy surrounds their use as it is considered *chemical castration* (De Giorgi & Series, 2016).

ENVIRONMENTAL AND PSYCHOSOCIAL BARRIERS TO SEXUAL PRACTICE

Sexual dysfunction may signal other psychosocial disorders such as depression, delirium, and dementia. Sexuality may also be affected by anxiety concerning partner availability and lifestyle issues. Substance use disorders, including smoking, alcohol, and illicit or recreational drug use, is often associated with sexual dysfunction. Many older individuals may be self-medicating with alcohol and drugs as a way of managing depression or anxiety symptoms, coping with loneliness or loss, or dealing with pain, which can affect sexual function (*John Hopkins Special Report on Depression and Anxiety in Older Adults,* 2009; Lesser et al., 2005).

Patients with dementia should be given special attention to ensure their safety when they decide to engage in sexual relationships. Health care professionals working with cognitively impaired older adults need to determine whether the individual is consenting to a sexual activity. If the person is unable to consent to participation in a sexual activity and has a surrogate decision maker, that person should be involved with judgments regarding the benefits or potential harm associated with that person's sexual expression (Cornelison & Doll, 2012).

LESBIAN, GAY, BISEXUAL, AND TRANSGENDER OLDER ADULTS

Lesbian, gay, bisexual, and transgender (LGBT) older adults have spent much of their lives hiding their sexual preference and gender identity, not just from family and the rest of society, but from their health care providers as well. Older adults who are LGBT face many health disparities, including victimization, psychological distress, disability, discrimination, and lack of access to appropriate health services. They are also more likely to experience chronic illness and disability (e.g., cancer, obesity, hypertension, hypercholesterolemia, arthritis, cardiovascular disease, and diabetes), and delay treatment for health issues compared with older adults who are heterosexual. Older adults who are LGBT are more likely to live alone and less likely to have adult children for support and assistance (Foglia & Fredriksen-Goldsen, 2014; Hillman & Henrichsen, 2014).

Despite stereotypes, it is important for nurses to recognize that LGBT as acceptable expressions of sexuality for both men and women. Nurses should examine their own personal beliefs about LGBT practices and ensure they do not prevent older adults from fulfilling their sexual needs. Self-examination will allow nurses to enter into a therapeutic relationship with older adults who are LGBT without the interference of personal feelings. The patients' partners should be encouraged to participate in the sexual assessment and planning when appropriate. Nurses should also remember that no information about the sexual orientation of patients should be shared with a patient's family unless permission has been given. See Box 12.2 for questions that can be added to an assessment.

BOX 12.2   Questions on Sexuality

- Are you currently sexually active? If so, with one or more than one partner?
- Male or female partner?
- Are your sexual desires being met?
- Do you have any questions or concerns about your sexual function? About your partner's sexual function?
- What kind of information would you like?

NURSING MANAGEMENT

Assessment

Sexual health may have a direct effect on the well-being of individuals with chronic illnesses (Douglas & Fenton, 2013). Therefore it is essential to obtain a sexual history (Table 12.2); however, one of the greatest obstacles in assessing the sexuality of older

---

TABLE 12.2   Evaluating Sexual Risk in Older Adults

Normalizing the discussion	• I discuss sexual activity with all my patients because it is an important part of their medical care.
Broaching the topic	• Tell me about your sex life. • When you say you have had sex, what exactly do you mean? • Do you have sex with men, women, or both?
Asking about partners	• Tell me about the number of sex partners within the past 3 months. • Where do you meet your partners? • Have you ever gone online to meet partners for sex? • How well do you know your sexual partners? • What do you know about the human immunodeficiency virus (HIV) status of your partners? • How does your partner's HIV status affect your sexual behavior? • Have you noticed symptoms in your partner that are causing you concern?
Asking about sexual activity	• What sexual activities do your sexual partners engage in? • Do you have oral sex? Vaginal sex? Anal sex? • Do you select partners on the basis of HIV status? • Do you ever get drunk or high before you have sex?
Asking about prevention methods	• What do you do to protect yourself during sex? • Do you use condoms when having sex? How often? With what types of sex? • What has been your experience with using condoms? • What factors or situations get in the way of using condoms?

Adapted from Centers for Disease Control and Prevention (CDC); Health Resources and Services Administration; National Institutes of Health; HIV Medicine Association of the Infectious Diseases Society of America. (2003). Incorporating HIV prevention into the medical care of persons living with HIV. Recommendations of CDC, the Health Resources and Services Administration, the National Institutes of Health, and the HIV Medicine Association of the Infectious Diseases Society of America. *MMWR Recommendations Report, 52*(RR-12), 1-24. Retrieved February 21, 2018, from http://www.cdc.gov/mmwr/preview/mmwrhtml/rr5212a1.htm.

adults occurs at the beginning of the assessment. Getting started with the sexual history becomes easier with experience. One challenge nurses face is to help older adults develop and sustain the intimate relationship they desire. This involves active assessment, including actively reviewing health concerns and conditions that affect sexual functioning. Although discomfort in this area is understandable, increased proficiency comes with experience. Healthy sexuality depends on good communication between the health professional and the patient. Nurses are in a pivotal position to begin this communication. The PLISSIT model has been used to assess and manage the sexuality of adults since 1976. PLISSIT is an acronym for **P**ermission, **L**imited **I**nformation, **S**pecific **S**uggestions, and **I**ntensive **T**herapy. The model offers suggestions for initiating and maintaining a discussion of sexuality with older adults. It was first used with young adults but has also been successful in use with older adults (Omole, Fresh, Sow, Lin, Talwo, & Nichols, 2014). A simple sexual history performed by nurses may include questions such as those found in Box 12.2.

Some nurses are more comfortable than others in completing a sexual assessment; however, being able to do the following will help develop the necessary skills (Association of Reproductive Health Professionals [ARHP], 2010):

- Be a sympathetic listener.
- Reassure the patient who has sexual concerns that strategies for addressing those concerns do exist.
- Make an appropriate referral, if needed.

The health care provider should complete a detailed sexual history. The goal of the assessment, regardless of the model used, is to gather information that allows patients to express sexuality safely and feel uninhibited by normal or pathologic problems.

It is common for nurses and nursing students to feel uncomfortable and embarrassed when assessing the sexual desires and functions of older patients. Nonetheless, a sexual assessment should be performed as a routine part of the nursing assessment. Knowledge, skill, and a sense of comfort are necessary for the nurse to assess the sexuality of older adults. Nurses may take

several steps to create a nonthreatening environment conducive to communication:

- Provide a quiet, private meeting place and avoid interruptions during the discussion.
- Sit at eye level with the patient and ask questions in a manner that is not threatening.
- Avoid using terms that may suggest they are making assumptions about sexual behavior or orientation.
- Avoid medical terminology and the use of slang words.

Other components of the sexual history taking include reviewing medications and medical conditions that may contribute to a sexual dysfunction. In addition, the nurse should review the older adult's early experiences, if they are willing to share. A physical assessment, including examination of the breasts and genital tissue, is an essential part of the sexual assessment. Laboratory tests may be useful in determining reductions in hormone levels that may contribute to decreased libido or ED. Box 12.3 lists laboratory tests relevant to a sexual assessment of older adults.

BOX 12.3 Laboratory Tests to Guide Sexual Assessment

- Total serum testosterone
- Serum luteinizing hormone
- Serum prolactin
- Prostate-specific antigen (after risk and benefits have been reviewed)
- Chemistry panel
- Thyroid-stimulating hormone
- Hemoglobin A1c
- Lipid profile
- Urinalysis
- Complete blood count
- Estradiol
- Follicle-stimulating hormone
- Vitamin B_{12} and folate

EVIDENCE-BASED PRACTICE

Exploration of Knowledge, Attitudes, and Experiences With Sexual Expression in Nursing Homes

Background

The Baby Boomers were part of the 1960s sexual revolution and consider sexuality and sexual expression of vital importance. By 2030, 58 million of the Baby Boomers will be between the ages of 66 to 84, and increasing numbers of them in need of nursing home services. This systematic review of the literature was conducted to "explore the knowledge, attitudes, and experiences of administrators, care staff, relatives, community-dwellers, and residents toward older people's sexuality and sexual expression in nursing homes" (p. 471).

Sample/Setting

The cumulative Index to Nursing and Allied Health Literature (CINAHL) and PubMed databases were searched for quantitative studies, using the keywords sexuality *or* intimacy, and older people *or* older age *or* residents, and long-term care *or* nursing home, and attitudes *or* knowledge *or* experience. Articles were limited to those published between January 2000 and November 2106, and excluded if not written in English. Twelve research articles met selection criteria.

Methods

The Preferred Reporting Items for Systematic Reviews and Meta-Analysis (PRISMA) was used to help summarize the selection process and compare data.

Findings

Sexual expression in older adults is a need that should be supported in nursing homes. Positive attitudes toward sexuality in the nursing home environment was correlated with increased knowledge of sexuality and aging. Positive predictors among care providers included age, level of education, and years of experience. Barriers to addressing the sexual needs of residents included lack of privacy and staff discomfort.

Implications

Failure to thoroughly assess the sexual needs of older adults, and include it in the treatment plan, can lead to lack of intimacy and loneliness. Health care personnel must meet the needs of nursing home residents and accommodate their values and expectations.

From Aguilar, R. (2017). Sexual expression of nursing home residents: Systematic review of the literature. *Journal of Nursing Scholarship, 49,* 5, 470-477.

The nurse should also obtain information on sexual preferences. This should be followed by an assessment of the patient's living environment. The nurse should determine where the patient plans to engage in sexual activity. In acute and long-term care settings, the environment should be assessed for privacy and safety. This enables older adults to proceed with sexual activity safely and comfortably. In the community setting, the environment should be assessed for safety and the availability of adaptive equipment such as side rails, medical trapeze, and specialized beds, which may be needed to enable older adults to participate in sexual activity safely within the home.

The nursing staff should be cognizant of indications of sexual interest in older adults. Overt gestures of sexuality in public areas or hints of sexual interest during conversations with patients should not be ignored or punished; they should be viewed as an indication of sexual interest between two older adults.

Among older adults, an added risk factor is cognitive impairment, which may hinder a patient's decision-making abilities. Before a sexual relationship commences, it may be appropriate for the nurse to meet with both patients individually, and together discuss their intentions and expectations regarding the sexual relationship. In so doing, the patients' fears and apprehensions may be expressed, and their questions answered. In addition, such a discussion may reveal whether one patient is being coerced into the relationship or is not mentally competent to decide to enter such a relationship.

A cognitive assessment, such as Montreal Cognitive Assessment, should be performed as part of the assessment of older adults. The information gained from this assessment is useful if the nurse suspects that patients are cognitively impaired and unable to make decisions to participate in sexual relationships. If the cognitive assessment does not provide sufficiently clear information regarding patients' decision-making abilities, a more thorough assessment by a psychologist may be necessary to prevent anyone from taking advantage of these patients.

Diagnosis

Several nursing diagnoses are appropriate for older adults experiencing actual or potential sexual problems. Sexual dysfunction is an appropriate diagnosis for older adults who express concern about meeting their need for sexuality and intimacy. Factors related to this diagnosis include fear, lack of opportunity, misconceptions, pain, and embarrassment (see Nursing Care Plan on Sexual Dysfunction: Medication).

Sexual dysfunction would also be an applicable diagnosis for an aging woman experiencing dyspareunia or decreased or absent sexual desire (see Nursing Care Plan on Sexual Dysfunction: Privacy).

Other potential appropriate nursing diagnoses include:
- Anxiety
- Reduced sexual expression
- Need for health teaching
- Discomfort
- Reduced self-concept

Planning and Expected Outcomes

The nurse should develop an individualized care plan that includes the information elicited during history taking, physical assessment, and discussion about specific sexual relationships. This plan should (1) compensate for the physical disabilities of older adults, (2) prevent the spread of infection, (3) provide for the emotional well-being of older adults, (4) satisfy the needs of family members when possible, and (5) ensure patient safety. Expected outcomes of the care plan should result from specific, time-limited goals aimed at restoring or promoting the patient's sexual satisfaction.

Expected outcomes include but are not limited to the following:
1. The patient attains a satisfactory level of sexual activity as evidenced by resumption of sexual activity at a level acceptable to the patient.

NURSING CARE PLAN

Sexual Dysfunction: Medication

Clinical Situation
Mr. B, a 76-year-old retired brick layer, comes to the clinic complaining of headaches that have been increasing in severity over the past several months. His initial assessment shows severe hypertension. During the nursing assessment, it is revealed that Mr. B is a widower and lives alone. However, he has a female friend who visits him often, and they have sexual intercourse every 1 to 2 weeks. To date, he has not experienced any problems with his sexual performance. He was prescribed a beta-blocker to control his hypertension.

Nursing Diagnosis
Reduced sexual expression resulting from potential side effects from antihypertensive medication.

Outcome
The patient will not experience a disruption in meeting his need for sexuality and intimacy.

Interventions
Instruct the patient on the normal aging changes in sexual functioning.
Instruct the patient that ED is not a normal aging change and may be a side effect of his antihypertensive medication.
Instruct the patient to notify his health care provider if ED or any other sexual problem is noticed.
Instruct the patient concerning the proper and consistent use of condoms to prevent sexually transmitted infections.

◎ NURSING CARE PLAN

Sexual Dysfunction: Privacy

Clinical Situation

Mr. J is a 74-year-old retired boxer who has resided at a nursing facility for 3 years. He has Parkinson's disease and uses a walker. He is generally happy and pleasant. Mrs. H is an alert 75-year-old widow, who was admitted to the facility 1 month ago after a stroke left her wheelchair-bound and unable to perform her activities of daily living (ADLs) independently. She was upset when she arrived at the nursing facility and had some difficulty adjusting to her new home.

Over the past 2 weeks, a close relationship has developed between these two residents. Mrs. H has been happier than she was on admission, and both residents appear to have a new sense of energy and enthusiasm for life. Recently the nursing staff has noticed sexual expression and signs of intimacy between the two in public areas.

Nursing Diagnosis

Reduced sexual expression resulting from lack of privacy.

Outcome

Patients will be free to pursue their sexual relationship in private.

Interventions

Perform a sexual assessment of both patients.

Provide a climate in which both can openly discuss the situation and respond with trust and confidence.

Pay close attention to verbal and nonverbal cues while listening. Provide reassurance, as needed.

Meet with both patients individually to assess each one's desire regarding sexual activity and each one's degree of competence.

Assess the level of comfort in discussing the topic and issues, alone or with each other present; provide opportunity for both.

Provide teaching on normal changes of the aging sexual system (see Box 12.1 and the Patient/Family Teaching boxes).

Compensate for any physical disabilities assessed.

Implement precautions against the spread of sexually transmitted infections.

Find a safe, private location for the couple to pursue their sexual interests.

---

2. The patient verbalizes their sexual concerns and discusses them with their significant other.
3. The patient explores various sexual activities and practices to attain sexual satisfaction.
4. The patient verbalizes their feelings about sexual performance.

Intervention

Older adults should be provided information, education, and direction to assist them in creating and sustaining intimate relationships. Education starts with discussing changes associated with aging. Teaching and reassurance by the nurse that some changes are a normal part of aging helps patients understand their bodies and feel comfortable learning how to compensate for these changes (see Patient/Family Teaching boxes). Teaching regarding coital positioning for couples with physically disabling conditions is often a necessary intervention (Fig. 12.1).

ᨁ PATIENT/FAMILY TEACHING

Normal Changes of the Aging Female Sexual System

Instruct female patients that, with aging, the following occur:
* Vaginal secretions diminish; the use of an artificial water-based lubricant helps decrease discomfort.
* The vagina becomes shorter and does not expand to accommodate the penis. Some discomfort may be experienced, so the use of alternative positions for intercourse (see Fig. 12.1) may help decrease discomfort.
* Orgasmic contractions are fewer and may be accompanied by painful uterine contractions. However, these generally do not indicate pathologic problems.
* Vaginal irritation and clitoral pain are common and do not signify illness.
* The breasts lose tone, and the areolar area does not enlarge as much.
* Infrequent rectal sphincter contractions, which do not interfere with orgasm, and postcoital need to void may be experienced.

ᨁ PATIENT/FAMILY TEACHING

Normal Changes of the Aging Male Sexual System

Instruct male patients that, with aging, the following occur:
* The penis may take longer to become firm and may not be as firm as at a younger age; therefore a longer period of foreplay should be planned.
* Ejaculation may take longer to achieve, may be less expulsive, and may be shorter in duration. The patient should conserve strength and not work hard at the beginning of intercourse, which could result in tiring before climax.
* The erection diminishes more quickly after climax, so if condoms are being used, the patient should plan to withdraw immediately after climax.
* It takes longer to achieve a second orgasm, so the patient should plan to resume foreplay or use this time to touch or talk.
* Rectal sphincter contractions may be experienced, but these do not interfere with orgasm.

When sexual intercourse is not the preferred method of intimacy or is not possible for an older couple, the couple may be taught alternative methods of intimacy in the form of touch. Touch is a means of expressing intimacy and closeness that may fulfill older patients' sexual needs and desires. Touch is best fulfilled by finding a comfortable environment in which an older adult couple can expose parts of their bodies to each other as they feel comfortable. A shower or bath may be enjoyable. The couple should be taught to move their fingertips slowly or lightly over each other's skin while enjoying the closeness of the other person. Massage therapy, books, and videos may provide older adults with a way of touching that results in the fulfillment of sexual desires. Soft music may make the environment more conducive for older couples.

Proper precautions need to be implemented to prevent sexually transmitted infections. Low-risk behaviors such as practicing monogamous relationships, reduction in number of partners, and consistent use of condoms (male and female types) should be encouraged (see Box 12.4).

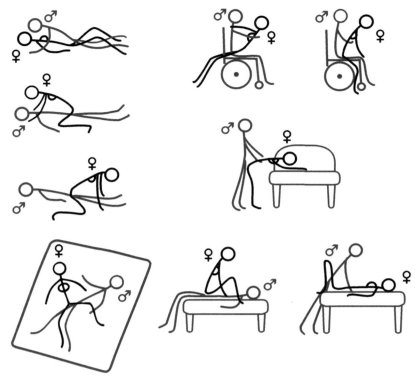

Fig. 12.1 Coital positioning for older couples.

BOX 12.4   **Actions to Prevent Spread of Human Immunodeficiency Virus Among Older Adults**

- Implement specific education programs for older adults on the transmission and prevention of human immunodeficiency virus (HIV) infection.
- Hold workshops and training sessions devoted to basic information on HIV and acquired immunodeficiency syndrome (AIDS), including safe sexual practices, all in relationship to aging.
- Fund and support more research pertaining to older adults' sexual behaviors.
- Educate health care professionals on high-risk behaviors for HIV infection, symptoms of HIV infection, misdiagnoses, testing technologies, treatments, support groups, case management, and the importance of being actively involved in the health and well-being of their older patients.
- Increase media and social marketing campaigns, which may help raise awareness of HIV and AIDS among older people and reinforce the need for educational programs while promoting respect and validation for older adults as a group.

From National Association on HIV over Fifty. (2009). *Educational tip sheet: HIV/AIDS and older adults.* Retrieved May 25, 2009, from http://www.hivoverfifty.org/tip.html; and AIDS Action. (2001). *Older Americans and HIV/AIDS.* Retrieved April 28, 2004, from http://www.aidsaction.org.

If an older adult is concerned about their family's feelings regarding a sexual relationship, further counseling should be provided and should include the family, when possible. At this time, family members may bring forth their concerns regarding the relationship, and the older adult may answer them with a nurse present. It is important for the older adult's family to understand and accept their decisions about any relationships. However, if no amenable agreement to both the older adult and family can be reached, the older adult's needs must be the nurse's primary consideration.

As discussed previously, older adults with cognitive impairment may display inappropriate sexual behavior, such as exposure or advances toward other patients and staff. It is important for the nurse to manage these behaviors while maintaining the dignity of these older adults. Ignoring the behavior or punishing the older adult does not curtail the behavior. A thorough assessment of mental status and sexuality is necessary to isolate the cause of the behavior. Inappropriate behavior is best managed by determining the root cause of the behavior (e.g., pain, discomfort, or hyperthermia) and redirecting the older adults' sexual interest toward socially acceptable behaviors, which may be accomplished by provision of a quiet place for masturbation and viewing sexually explicit materials (magazines or videos).

Acute and long-term care facilities should make proper arrangements for privacy during older adults' sexual experiences. The physical facilities within each setting vary. The ideal situation is to set up a room with a pleasant environment, which can be used for a variety of activities but may also be reserved by older adults for private visits with a spouse or partner. In most settings, this may not be possible; thus patient rooms may be used if the nursing staff gains permission from the patient's roommate and plans alternate activities for them.

In any setting, patient safety should be maintained. The call lights should be easily accessible. Side rails on the bed should be used, if necessary, and the room should be situated such that the nursing staff is aware when it is in use. Although the patients' privacy is important, they should not be left alone in any situation in which they may injure themselves.

In the community setting, adaptive equipment such as hospital beds, side rails, or a medical trapeze may be needed to allow patients to function safely. Based on the information gathered from assessment, the nurse may assist patients in acquiring the equipment. The nurse may also need to demonstrate safe transfer processes to ensure that patients are able to transfer, as well as to function, independently or with the help of the partner. See Box 12.5 for strategies that may enhance sexual function in older patients.

BOX 12.5   Strategies to Enhance Sexual Function in Older Adults

Dietary Strategies
Avoid alcohol or tobacco.
Consult with a registered dietitian about well-balanced meals.

Medication Strategies
Take pain medications before sexual activity, if needed.
Discuss with a primary care provider (medical doctor or nurse practitioner) discontinuing medications that may impair sexual function.

Environmental Adaptations
Plan for sexual activity when most rested.
Consider conjugal visits or home visits.
Acquire a pet; pets provide sensory stimulation.
Older adults with dementia should be offered objects to touch, fondle, and hold, for example, dolls or stuffed animals.

Psychological Strategies
Communicate desires to partner.
Discuss fears and concerns with a primary care provider.
Consider routine visits to hairdresser to promote self-esteem and well-being.
Join a support group.
Use relaxation techniques.

Physical Strategies
Improve exercise tolerance by participating in a supervised exercise program.
Use touching, kissing, and hugging.
Use pillows under painful joints.
Take a warm shower before activity.
Get regular checkups.

Modified from Nusbaum, M., Hamilton, C., & Lenahan. P. (2003). Chronic illness and sexual functioning. *American Family Physician, 67,* 347; Mosley, R. & Jett, K. (2007). Advance practice nursing and sexual functioning in late life. *Geriatric Nursing, 28*(1), 41-42; Arena, J. & Wallace, M. (2008). *Sexuality issues in aging. Nursing standard of practice protocol: Sexuality in older adults.* Retrieved May 4, 2009, from http://www.consultgerirn.org/topics/sexualiity_issues_in_aging/want_to_know_more; and Rheaume, C. & Mitty, E. (2008). Sexuality and intimacy in older adults. *Geriatric Nursing, 29*(5), 342-349.

Staff education about the sexuality and intimacy of older adults should include recognition of cues, desires, and interest in sexual activity and intimacy. Staff should recognize that older adults may use and have access to pornographic material, especially through the Internet. Education of nursing staff also needs to address eliminating stereotypes. Open discussion of attitudes and sexual issues among staff may help increase comfort in dealing with older patients' sexual issues. Case studies and other learning tools such as trivia games may be effective means of education. Education should also be available to the family. The training should begin by discussing and dispelling the myths surrounding older adults' sexual desires and activity. The training should include normal changes associated with older men and women and how to compensate for specific physical disabilities. A more positive attitude toward the sexual expression of older adults may develop with increased knowledge and may allow such expression to become a natural part of the aging process (Cornelison & Doll, 2012).

Training should conclude with discussion groups to allow staff and family to discuss their own feelings about sexuality and its role in the life of older adults. Role-playing may be an effective technique to gain understanding of the effect of the staff and family's personal values on older adults.

Evaluation

Evaluation of concerns related to sexuality and intimacy are based on patient achievement of established expected outcomes. Older adults may attain a satisfying level of sexual activity that is compatible with functional capacity with the help of sound, sensitive nursing interventions. When sexual functioning cannot be restored, alternatives should be explored. The use of touch and massage may be an alternative to sexual intercourse and may help older adults achieve sexual satisfaction. Although many stereotypes hinder the ability of professionals to promote sexuality among older adults, older adults can and should be allowed to achieve satisfactory sexual outcomes with the full support of health care professionals. Proper documentation is important to communicate the interventions and progress toward meeting the expected outcomes.

🏠 HOME CARE

1. Assess sexual patterns in homebound older adults who have chronic conditions.
2. Provide information regarding sexual positions or sexual function to accommodate environmental barriers (e.g., a Foley catheter) to both homebound older adults and their partners.
3. Foster a supportive environment for homebound older adults and their partners to discuss sex-related fears, concerns, and feelings.
4. Explain pathologic conditions that may adversely affect sexuality (e.g., diabetes).
5. Teach safe sexual practices to homebound older adults and their partners.
6. Teach alternative methods of intimacy to both homebound older adults and their partners based on identified sexual dysfunctions or alterations.

SUMMARY

The need for sexuality and intimacy continues throughout a person's life span. It is the nurse's role to dispel societal myths surrounding sexuality and aging, to enable older adults to reach their sexual potential. After thorough assessment and management of the normal and pathologic changes in the aging urogenital system, older adults are able to pursue sexuality as desired, resulting in the highest quality of life attainable.

KEY POINTS

- Sexual desire and interest persist throughout the life span of people into older adulthood.
- Nurses are often influenced by myths surrounding the sexual practices of older adults, and many lack the knowledge and training to work with older adults who experience sexual dysfunction.
- Normal, age-related changes in the urogenital system may interfere with an older adult's expression of sexuality.
- Pathologic problems with the aging sexual response are often related to illnesses and medication.
- Older adults with dementia may display inappropriate sexual behavior and may not be competent to participate in sexual relationships.
- Environmental barriers in the home, as well as in acute and long-term care settings, may prevent older adults from meeting their needs for sexual intimacy.

- All older adults should receive a sexual assessment so that normal and pathologic changes can be identified.
- Older adults should be taught about the normal changes of aging in the urogenital systems, and the means to compensate for these changes (i.e., topical estrogen to relieve the symptoms of vaginal atrophy).
- Interventions used to assist older adults in adapting to age-related changes include manipulation of the environment and procurement of assistive equipment and devices needed to continue to function sexually.
- Touch is an alternative to sexual intercourse and provides the intimacy needed by some older adults.

CRITICAL-THINKING EXERCISES

1. A 73-year-old female patient confides that she is embarrassed because her 75-year-old male friend wants to know why he is having difficulty getting an erection. She confesses she is very uncomfortable and does not know how to help her friend. What suggestions can you offer in dealing with this sensitive but important matter?
2. A married couple resides in the long-term care facility where you are employed. The husband is ambulatory, but his wife needs a great deal of assistance with her daily care. One afternoon as you enter their room with medication, you find the couple in bed together, and it is obvious they are attempting to have sex. How should you respond? Discuss your feelings about this situation.

REFERENCES

Administration on Aging. (2016). *A profile of older Americans 2016.* Retrieved from https://www.giaging.org/documents/A_Profile_of_Older_Americans__2016.pdf.

Aguilar, R. (2017). Sexual expression of nursing home residents: Systematic review of the literature. *Journal of Nursing Scholarship, 49*(5), 470–477.

Ambler, D. R., Bieber, E. J., & Diamond, M. P. (2012). Sexual function in elderly women: A review of current literature. *Reviews in Obstetrics and Gynecology, 5*(1), 16–27. https://doi.org/10.3909/riog0156.

Anderson, M. (2015). For vast majority of seniors who own one, a smartphone equals 'freedom'. Retrieved January 21, 2018 from http://www.pewresearch.org/fact-tank/2015/04/29/seniors-smartphones/.

Association of Reproductive Health Professionals (ARHP). (March 2010). *Talking With Patients About Sexuality and Sexual Health.* Retrieved January 20, 2018, from http://www.arhp.org.

Benbow, S. M., & Beeston, D. (2012). Sexuality, aging, and dementia. *International Psychogeriatrics, 24*(7), 1026–1033.

Blackwell, J. (2006). Androgen and the aging man. *Advance for Nurse Practitioners, 14*, 39–42.

Bratu, O., Oprea, I., Macrau, D., Spinu, D., Niculae, A., Geavelete, B., ... Mischianu, D. (2017). Erectile dysfunction post-radical prostatectomy – a challenge for both patient and physician. *Journal of Medicine and Life, 10*(1), 13–18.

Bronner, G. (2015). Addressing sexuality in dementia: A challenge for healthcare providers. *Journal of Alzheimers Disease & Parkinsonism, 5*, 180. https://doi.org/10.4172/2161-0460.1000180.

Brown, S. L., & Shinohara, S. K. (2013). Dating relationships in older adulthood: A national portrait. *Journal of Marriage and Family, 75*, 1194–1202. https://doi.org/10.1111/jomf.12065.

Butler, R., & Lewis, M. (2000). Sexuality. In M. Beers & R. Berkow (Eds.), *The Merck manual of geriatrics*. Rahway, NJ: Merck.

Catlin, A. (n.d.). How skilled human touch can transform person-centered dementia care. Retrieved January 21, 2018 from https://

www.nhqualitycampaign.org/files/Compassionate_Touch_White_Paper.pdf.

Centers for Disease Control and Prevention. (2017a). *Cancer among men*. Retrieved January 20, 2018 from https://www.cdc.gov/cancer/dcpc/data/men.htm.

Centers for Disease Control, Prevention. (2017b). HIV among people aged 50 and over. Retrieved January 21, 2018, from https://www.cdc.gov/hiv/group/age/olderamericans/index.html.

Cornelison, L. J., & Doll, G. M. (2012). Management of sexual expression in long-term care: Ombudsmen's perspectives. *The Gerontologist, 53*(5), 780–789. https://doi.org/10.1093/geront/gns162.

David, P. (2013). AARP online dating survey. Retrieved January 21, 2018 from https://www.aarp.org/research/topics/life/info-2014/online-dating-sites-survey.html.

De Giorgi, R., & Series, H. (2016). Treatment of inappropriate sexual behavior in dementia. *Current Treatment Options in Neurology, 18*, 41. https://doi.org/10.1007/s11940-016-0425-2.

Donovan, K. A., Thompson, L. M., & Hoffe, S. E. (2010). Sexual function in colorectal cancer survivors. *Cancer Control, 17*(1), 44–51. Retrieved from https://moffitt.org/File%20Library/Main%20Nav/Research%20and%20Clinical%20Trials/Cancer%20Control%20Journal/v17n1/44.pdf.

Douglas, J. M., & Fenton, K. A. (2013). Understanding sexual health and its role in more effective prevention programs. *Public Health Reports, 128*(Suppl 1), 1–4. https://doi.org/10.1177/00333549131282S101.

Ellsworth, P.I. (2017). Erectile dysfuncton (ED, impotence). Retrieved January 13, 2018 from https://www.medicinenet.com/erectile_dysfunction_ed_impotence/article.htm.

Flynn, T. J., & Gow, A. J. (2015). Examining associations between sexual behaviours and quality of life in older adults. *Age and Ageing, 44*, 823–828. https://doi.org/10.1093/ageing/afv083.

Foglia, M.B., & Fredriksen-Goldsen, K.I. (2014). Health disparities among LGBT older adults and the role of nonconscious bias. *Hastings Center Report, 44*(0 4), S40–S44. https://doi.org/10.1002/hast.369.

Gandhi, J., Chen, A., Dagur, G., Suh, Y., Smith, N., Cali, B. … Hhan, S. A. (2016). Genitourinary syndrome of menopause: An overview of clinical manifestations, pathophysiology, etiology, evaluation, and management. *American Journal of Obstetrics and Gynecology, 215*(6), 704-711. https://doi.org/10.1016/j.ajog.2016.07.045.

Gass, M. (2016). Menopause. Retrieved January 13, 2018 from http://www.merckmanuals.com/professional/gynecology-and-obstetrics/menopause/menopause#v1062799.

Hillman, J., & Henrichsen, G. A. (2014). Promoting and affirming, competent practice with older lesbian and gay adults. *Professional Psychology: Research and Practice, 45*(4), 269–277. https://doi.org/10.1037/a0037172.

John Hopkins special report on depression and anxiety in older adults. Retrieved May 4, 2009, from http://www.johnshopkinshealthalerts.com/reports/depression_anxiety/2943-1.html.

Kaiser, F. (2000). Sexual dysfunction in men. In M. Beers & R. Berkow (Eds.), *The Merck manual of geriatrics.* Rahway, NJ: Merck.

Katz, A. (2013). Sexuality in nursing care facilities. *American Journal of Nursing, 113*(3), 53–55.

Kim, H. K., Kang, S. Y., Chung, Y. J., Kim, J. H., & Kim, M. R. (2015). The recent review of the Genitourinary Syndrome of Menopause. *Journal of Menopausal Medicine, 21*(2), 65–71. https://doi.org/10.6118/jmm.2015.21.2.65.

Lesser, J., Hughes, S., & Kumar, S. (2005). Sexual dysfunction in the older woman. Complex medical, psychiatric illnesses should be considered in evaluation and management. *Geriatrics, 60*(8), 18–21.

Lochlainn, M. N., & Kenny, R. A. (2013). Sexual activity and aging. *Journal of the American Medical Directors Association, 14*, 565–572.

Merghati-Khoei, E., Pirak, A., Mansoureh, Y., & Rezasoltani, P. (2016). Sexuality and elderly with chronic diseases: A review of the existing literature. *Journal of Research in Medical Sciences, 21*, 136. https://doi.org/10.4103/1735-1995.196618.

Messinger-Rapport, B., Sandhu, S., & Hujer, M. (2003). Sex and sexuality: Is it over after 60? *Clinical Geriatrics, 11*(10), 45.

Morley, J. (2000). Validation of a screening questionnaire for androgen deficiency in aging males. *Metabolism, 49*(9), 1239–1242.

Mpondo, B. C. T. (2016). HIV infection in the elderly: Arising challenges. *Journal of Aging Research, Article ID, 2404857*, 10 pages. https://doi.org/10.1155/2016/2404857.

National Council on Aging. (1998). *Sex after 60; a natural part of life.* Washington DC. Retrieved June 14, 2010, from http://www.ncoa.org/assets/files/pdf/Economic-Security-Trends-for-older-adults-55-to-65supplement.

Omole, F., Fresh, E. M., Sow, C., Lin, J., Talwo, B., & Nichols, M. (2014). How to discuss sex with elderly patients. *The Journal of Family Practice, 63*(4), E1–E4.

Pilowskey, D. J., & Wu, L. T. (2015). Sexual risk behaviors and HIV risk among Americans aged 50 years or older: A review. *Substance Abuse and Rehabilitation, 6*, 51–60. https://doi.org/10.2147/SAR.S78808.

Rheaume, C., & Mitty, E. (2008). Sexuality and intimacy in older adults. *Geriatric Nursing, 29*(5), 342–349. https://doi.org/10.1016/j.gerinurse.2008.08.004.

Santos-Iglesias, P., Byers, E. S., & Moglia, R. (2016). Sexual well-being of older men and women. *The Canadian Journal of Human Sexuality, 25*(2), 86–98. https://doi.org/10.3138/cjhs.252-A4.

Syme, M. L. (2014). The evolving concept of older adult sexual behavior and its benefits. *Generations – Journal of the American Society on Aging, 38*(1), 35–41.

Syme, M. L., & Cohn, T. J. (2016). Examining aging sexual stigma attitudes among adults by gender, age, and generational status. *Aging & Mental Health, 2*(1), 36–45. https://doi.org/10.1080/13607863.2015.1012044.

Tutolo, M., Briganti, A., Suardi, N., Gallina, A., Abdollah, F., Capitanio, U., & Montorsi, F. (2012). Optimizing postoperative sexual function after radical prostatectomy. *Therapeutic Advances in Urology, 4*(6), 347–365. https://doi.org/10.1177/1756287212450063.

Wang, F., Chen, F., Huo, X., Xu, R., Wu, L., Wang, J., & Lu, C. (2013). A neglected issue on sexual well-being following breast cancer diagnosis and treatment among Chinese women. *PLoS ONE, 8*(9). e74473. https://doi.org/10.1371/journal.pone.0074473.

Wion, R. K., & Loeb, S. J. (2015). Older adults engaging in online dating: What gerontological nurses should know. *Journal of Gerontological Nursing, 41*(10), 25–35. https://doi.org/10.3928/00989134-20150826-67.

Wise, T., & Crone, C. (2006). Sexual function in the geriatric patient. *Clinical Geriatrics, 14*(12), 17–26.

World Health Organization. (2015). *Sexual health, human rights and the law.* Retrieved from http://apps.who.int/iris/bitstream/10665/175556/1/9789241564984_eng.pdf?ua=1.

13

Pain

Joanne Alderman, MSN, APRN-CNS, RN-BC, FNGNA

http://evolve.elsevier.com/Meiner/gerontologic

LEARNING OBJECTIVES

On completion of this chapter, the reader will be able to:

1. Define the concept of pain, including types and sources.
2. Describe the consequences of unrelieved pain in older adults.
3. Discuss the goals of pain management in older adults.
4. Identify barriers that affect the assessment of pain or its management in older adult patients.
5. Describe the effect of pain on the quality of life of older adult patients.
6. Identify factors that may affect older adults' pain experiences.
7. Use a pain assessment tool to rate patients' pain intensity.
8. Describe the use of pharmacologic and nonpharmacologic therapies for older adults with pain.

WHAT WOULD YOU DO?

What would you do if you were faced with the following situations?

* You are on a memory unit with 13 residents. You were told in the report that all residents have been calm, purposefully wandering, eating, and drinking fluids well today. At dinner, one resident begins crying when brought from her room and continues to become more upset as she walks. What would you do?
* On a skilled Long-Term Care (LTC) Unit of 16 residents, a gentleman who recently had a knee replacement presents as being confused, different from his normal presentation of alertness. As the day progresses, he becomes increasingly confused and meets criteria for being delirious. He will not allow anyone to examine him and retreats to his room. What would you do?
* You check on your mother every day, and each day she begins to present differently. Today, she does not want to go with you to the park, and you notice dishes are in the sink, her bed is not made, and she cancelled a bridge game with her friends yesterday. You notice she is walking hesitantly and you ask if she is in pain. She says, "A little." What do you do?

Pain is a common experience for many older adults. Adults aged 85 and older, are the fastest-growing segment of the U.S. population. Aging has demonstrated increases in the risk of pain secondary to high rates of chronic and acute conditions; 45% of older adults on Medicare have at least four chronic conditions (Horgas, 2017). Before the mid-1990s, little "attention was paid to geriatric pain in the clinical of empirical literature" (Horgas, 2017). However, significant efforts since that time "have been undertaken to address and improve the assessment and management of pain in older adults" (Horgas, 2017). "Assessment and management of pain is a responsibility of all

health professionals and is within the scope and standards of an RN's practice" (Arnstein, Herr, & Butcher, 2017, p. 21).

Pain has long been recognized as a symptom of something else in the body. Although pain has often been referred to as the *fifth vital sign*, in 2016 The Joint Commission specifically stated they DO NOT endorse this concept, preferring to encourage nonpharmacologic individualized interventions and appropriate prescribing of pharmacologic measures, in accordance with the patient's care, treatment, and services (The Joint Commission, 2016).

When all body systems are working together well, pain should not be felt. These are facts, whereas pain, as an expectation of aging, is a myth. Persistent, chronic pain is "prevalent, costly, and frequently disabling in later life" (Makris, Abrams, Gurland, & Reid, 2014). When approaching pain management in the older adult, health care providers need to communicate a clear understanding of the patient's treatment goals and expectations, comorbidities, cognitive and functional status, available community resources, and available family support to facilitate an integrated pain management approach (Makris et al., 2014).

Pain is underrecognized, highly prevalent, and undertreated in older adults, especially in those with impaired cognition. After age 60, the incidence rate of pain more than doubles. Many health care practitioners have encountered older adults only in an emergency room or in hospitals, where they need unusually intense medical or nursing treatment; this is not a good way to understand that the conditions of these patients/residents are not representative of normal aging. However, older adults are at high risk for pain-inducing situations during their life span. Degenerative changes, musculoskeletal changes, and pathologic and comorbid conditions from disease or injury lead to pain in older adults (Herr, Bursch, Ersek, Miller, & Swafford, 2010).

Previous authors: Jacqueline Kayler DeBrew, PhD, MSN, RN; and Ramesh C. Upadhyaya, RN, CRRN, MSN, MBA, PhD-C.

UNDERSTANDING PAIN

Definition

McCaffery (2000) further stated that pain is "whatever the experiencing person says it is, existing whenever he or she says it does." Booker and Haedtke (2016) identify uncontrolled pain as a rational reason for an older adult's hospital admission. The definition by Aronoff (2002) is more specific: "a subjective, personal, unpleasant experience involving sensations and perceptions that may or may not relate to bodily or tissue damage." Pain is also defined as an unpleasant sensory and emotional experience (Merskey & Bogduk, 1994). The literature on pain agrees that pain is (1) a complex phenomenon derived from sensory stimuli or neurologic injury and modified by individual memory, expectations, and emotions (Leo & Huether, 2010; Sternbach, 1978) and (2) usually associated with injury or a pathophysiologic process that causes an uncomfortable experience. Pain has been identified as an emerging Geriatric Syndrome (Booker & Haedtke, 2016). These authors clearly noted that pain is individual and may be very different for different persons with the same disease or injury.

Pain Classification

Pain may be classified as *acute* or *chronic*. Acute pain is defined by rapid onset and relatively short duration, and a sign of a new health problem requiring diagnosis and analgesia. Treatment usually involves treating the underlying disease or injury and short-term use of analgesics. In contrast, chronic or persistent pain continues after healing or is not amenable to a cure. This pain usually has no autonomic signs and is associated with long-standing functional and psychological impairment. The older adult is most likely to suffer from chronic, or persistent pain, rather than acute pain (Jansen, 2008). The American Geriatrics Society (AGS, 2009) advocates the use of the term *persistent pain* rather than *chronic pain*, which may be associated with negative images and stereotypes.

The AGS Panel on Persistent Pain identified four categories of pain that encompass most syndromes (Box 13.1) (AGS, 2009):

1. *Nociceptive pain* may be visceral (internal organs; Wiggins, 2017) or somatic (musculoskeletal tissue and skin; Wiggins, 2017), and is usually a result of stimulation of pain receptors. It may arise from tissue inflammation, mechanical deformation, ongoing injury, or destruction of tissue. This type of pain usually responds well to common analgesic medication and nonpharmacologic strategies.
   - **Somatic pain** is usually well defined. Movement may aggravate it. It is the most common pain in older adults due to *articular disorders* (e.g., compression fractures, hip fractures, muscle strains or sprains). Patients describe this type of pain as deep and aching; it may be sharp.
   - **Visceral pain** is caused by organ stretch, inflammation, or ischemia. Frequently, it is diffuse and not well defined. It may be accompanied by nausea and vomiting. Visceral pain may be *referred*, or pain that roams. It has been defined as intense pressure, a deep squeeze, or dullness (e.g., pancreatitis, cholecystitis, appendicitis, or diverticulitis).

2. *Neuropathic pain* results from a pathophysiologic dysfunctional process involving the peripheral or central nervous system (CNS) (e.g., diabetic peripheral neuropathy, postherpetic neuralgia, and sciatica). These types of pain do not respond as predictably to analgesic therapy as nociceptive types of pain do. Neuropathic pain normally includes parasthesias (the tingling, *pins and needles* sensation), burning, and lancinating (stabbing, cutting, shooting) (Wiggins, 2017). Neuropathic pain may respond to unconventional analgesic drugs such as tricyclic antidepressants (TCAs), anticonvulsants, or antiarrhythmic drugs.
3. *Mixed* or *unspecified pain* has mixed or unknown mechanisms. Treatment is unpredictable and may require more trials of different or combined approaches.
4. Other types of pain may be caused by rare conditions such as conversion reaction or psychological disorders. Persons with these disorders may benefit from specific psychiatric treatments, but traditional medical interventions for analgesia are not indicated. Age-associated changes in pain perception have been observed in some older persons with unusual manifestations of common illnesses. An AGS panel concluded that age-related changes in pain perception are probably not clinically significant (AGS, 2009).

Scope of the Problem of Pain

Even though pain is *not* part of normal, healthy aging, pain is a common problem among older adults, and persistent physical pain is widespread in the older population (AGS, 2009). It is estimated that 25% to 50% of community-dwelling older adults experience significant pain problems (Park & Hughes, 2012; Reid et al., 2011). Adults 65 to 85 years old are at a higher risk of developing persistent pain, especially when enduring severe, acute pain. This risk supports the importance of focused assessments, focused prevention, and prompt treatment of pain in older adults (Arnstein & Herr, 2017). Pain is even greater in older adults in nursing homes, where it has been shown that 70% to 80% of residents have substantial pain that is undertreated (AGS, 2009; Robinson, 2010; Shoefield, 2010).

Stereotyping older persons as having less pain because of their age contributes to less frequent pain assessment and consequently less appropriate and effective treatment for the pain. Older adults commonly report less pain because they do not want to be complainers, fear having to undergo more tests and medical treatments, and fear losing their independence (AGS, 2009). In addition, older adults have been told that they will have pain sometime in their later years. Thus they become resigned to the experience of pain. The fear that pain will be seen as a reason for having to give up independent living is associated with a reluctance to express pain freely to nonfamily members. Older adults may be ambivalent about the benefit of any action for their pain. Some of these responses by older persons may be attributed to health care practitioners saying, "What do you expect at *your* age?" which supports the belief that nothing can be done to control or stop the pain.

Compounding this problem is the fact that older patients have been systematically excluded from clinical trials of analgesic drugs despite the fact that they are more likely to experience the side effects of analgesic medications. Research groups do not want comorbid conditions confounding the findings of a single medication or treatment.

Consequences of Unrelieved Pain

"Persistent intense pain can harm an individual's mind, body, spirit, and social interactions, resulting in disability, financial hardships, despair, and medical frailty" (Arnstein et al., 2017). Consequences of persistent pain are numerous. Depression, anxiety, decreased socialization, sleep disturbance, decreased or impaired ambulation, prolonged recovery periods, increased use of health care resources, premature death, and increased health care use and costs have all been documented with the presence of pain in older patients (AGS, 2009). Unrelieved pain has been shown to result in decreased ambulation, impaired posture, sleep disturbance, anxiety, and impaired appetite in nursing home residents (Leo & Huether, 2010). Pain may make getting to the bathroom so difficult that it leads to incontinence. Constipation may also be related to unrelieved pain when the person changes diet plans, decreases activity, and has difficulty getting to a toilet before the urge passes (Jansen, 2008). Untreated pain may result in the older person being unable to participate in self-care activities or health promotion activities (Bishop & Morrison, 2007). Pain combined with cognitive

impairment, feeling as if they are a burden to others, and pain-related disability may drive the older adult to consider or attempt suicide (Arnstein et al., 2017). Pain may go untreated if the older adult has dementia or other cognitive impairment (Herr, Bjororo, & Decker, 2006).

The assessment and management of pain in older adults pose unique challenges to health care professionals. The nurse caring for older adults in pain must understand the special needs of this diverse population. Although older adults are at risk for chronic disease (45% of Medicare beneficiaries have at least four chronic conditions [Horgas, 2017]) and the often-painful conditions that accompany those ailments, their pain is often underrecognized and untreated, leading to poor outcomes (Arnstein et al., 2017). Therefore accurate and ongoing assessment is essential for effective pain management in older adults. Goals for pain management in older adults include the following:
- Listening to the older adult and paying close attention
- Relief from pain
- Control of chronic disease conditions causing pain
- Maintenance of mobility and functional status
- Promotion of self-care and maximum independence
- Improved quality of life

These goals can be achieved through education of patients, families, and health care professionals, and through good nursing care.

PATHOPHYSIOLOGY OF PAIN IN OLDER ADULTS

Pain has multiple components that affect one's physical and psychosocial functioning. Although older adults develop more chronic diseases as they age, pain does not need to be an expectation of normal aging. An understanding of pain physiology and pain theories is essential to effective pain management in older adults.

The three major components of the nervous system that cause the sensation and perception of pain are (1) the afferent pathways (reception), (2) the CNS (perception), and (3) the efferent pathways (reaction). The afferent pathways have nociceptors and are found on the skin. Pacinian corpuscles that mediate sensation, including pain, pressure, and itching, are the nerve endings distributed in the skin. Stimulation of these nerve endings by vibrations from massage or sound waves may reduce the perception of pain in conditions such as chronic rheumatoid arthritis. The free nerve endings of nociceptors are sensitive to mechanical, thermal, electrical, or chemical stimuli, and are responsible for transmitting sensory pain information. This stimulation flows through peripheral sensory nerves (afferent pathways) to the spinal cord. A painful stimulus (e.g., a pinprick) sends an impulse to a nociceptor (a receptor for painful stimuli) along a peripheral nerve fiber, which enters the gray matter of the spinal cord. Nociceptors terminate in the spinal cord (McCaffery & Pasero, 1999). Here, the nociceptor stimulation flows to the brain through a series of relay neurons.

When the pain stimulus or signal reaches the CNS, it is evaluated and interpreted in the limbic system, reticular formation, thalamus, hypothalamus, medulla, and cerebral cortex. The brain's interpretation is based on both physical and psychological factors. Modulation of the pain stimulus may occur in the gray matter, the dorsal horn of the cord. Here, transmission occurs from the nociceptor to the spinothalamic tract neuron. Substance P, a neurotransmitter, facilitates transmission of the stimulus from the afferent (peripheral) neuron across the synapse to the spinothalamic tract neuron. Uninhibited by drugs or other modalities, the pain impulse travels to the cerebral cortex of the brain, where the brain interprets the quality of pain, processing past experiences with pain, knowledge of pain, and cultural associations related to pain perception. The interpretation is relayed back through the peripheral nervous system (efferent) pathways that are made up of fibers connecting the reticular formation, midbrain, and substantia gelatinosa. Pain modulation takes place in the efferent neural pathways and may involve chemical factors of neuropeptides, which may increase the sensitivity of the afferent pain receptors to noxious stimuli. These pathways result in the sensation and perception of pain (McCance & Huether, 2010).

Perception of Pain in Older Adults

It is accepted, although not completely understood, that pain perception differs in older adults, compared with younger people (McCleane, 2008). Atkins (n.d.) summarized alterations in pain pathways, noting a decrease in the density of peripheral nerves with aging, accompanied by degeneration of sensory neurons, a decrease in norepinephrine and serotonin, and a decrease in neurons in the cerebral cortex. However, how these changes truly affect pain perception is in question. Lautenbacher, Peters, Heesen, Scheel, and Kunz (2017) noted in their meta-analysis that pain thresholds increase with pain, but the only alteration in pain perception supported in the literature was to heat

stimulation (nociception in superficial tissues). This change predisposes older adults to bruising, injury, and burns.

BARRIERS TO EFFECTIVE PAIN MANAGEMENT IN OLDER ADULTS

Eighty percent of older adults experience chronic conditions resulting in pain (Horgas, Yoon, & Grall, 2012). Many barriers impede the assessment and management of pain in older adults. Some of these barriers are related to nursing care, some related to efforts on the part of the prescriber, and some related to the older adult and their beliefs about pain and aging. Although not considered a normal part of aging, many health care professionals, as well as older patients and their family members, continue to believe that pain is a natural occurrence of aging and chronic disease. This belief may lead to underreporting of pain and may prevent accurate pain assessment and appropriate use of pain relief measures. Effective treatment of pain (acute or chronic) is essential for this population, as unrelieved pain may lead to altered immune function, functional decline, postoperative complications, cognitive impairment, depression, and sleep disturbance (Horgas, 2017; Fig. 13.1).

Accurate assessment and pain management is also inhibited when older patients underreport their pain. Older patients may underreport pain because they believe that stoicism and refusal to "give in" to the pain are appropriate behaviors or attitudes. Pain assessment may also be hindered by older patients who do not report pain because they "don't want to bother anyone" or they believe their report of pain will not be believed.

Older adults with cancer may fear the meaning of pain and its implications of worsening disease and possible death. Patients

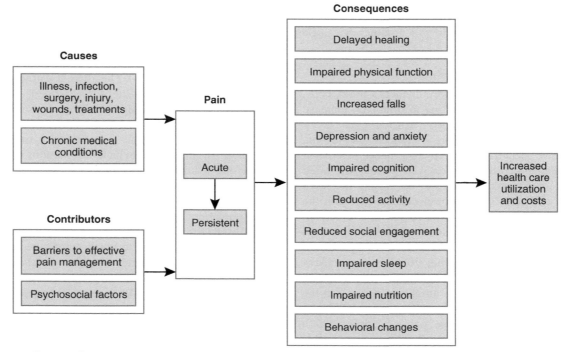

Fig. 13.1 Conceptual model of the causes and consequences of pain in older adults. (From Horgas, A. L. [2017]. Pain assessment in older adults. *Nursing Clinics of North America, 52*[3], 377).

experiencing cancer-related pain may believe that this is a natural outcome of cancer and cannot be relieved. These patients and their family members needlessly suffer from the patients' experiences of pain. Inadequate access to diagnostic services is another barrier to appropriate pain assessment for older residents of nursing facilities and frail older adults in the community. Often, it is difficult to schedule appointments and arrange transportation so that a family member or health care professional can accompany the patient to a diagnostic testing facility. Furthermore, many older adults do not have children who live near them and have lost their social networks (Robinson, 2010).

The nurse's lack of knowledge regarding adequate pain assessment is viewed as a barrier as well. Nurses should be knowledgeable of assessment techniques, how to adapt these techniques, as well as standardized tools to utilize when assessing an older adult's pain. When using any pain assessment tool, the nurse must evaluate each patient's ability to give accurate responses with that tool. The use of a second tool may help confirm the value obtained with the first tool. The Hartford Institute for Geriatric Nursing (2012) has found that commonly used pain assessment tools, such as the Faces Pain Scale–Revised (FPS-R Scale), are valid and reliable for use with older adults, even those with mild to moderate cognitive impairments. The AGS (2009) found that the most accurate and reliable indicator of pain intensity and experience is the patient's self-report.

However, the compromised ability of people with moderate to severe dementia to clearly or consistently report on their pain is challenging. Persons with dementia are consistently undermedicated. The Pain Assessment in Advanced Dementia (PAINAD) scale developed by Warden, Hurley, and Volicer (2003) is a simple, valid, and reliable tool for assessing pain in people with dementia in both community and hospital settings (Gabrick, 2016) (Table 13.1). PAINAD assesses the person with dementia in the following categories on a 0 to 10 scale:

1. Breathing
2. Negative vocalization
3. Facial expression
4. Body language
5. Consolability

Additionally, the person with dementia should be asked if they have pain, and the nurse should ask the family if their family member's behavior is customary or a change. A change in behavior could indicate pain (Horgas, 2017).

PATIENT/FAMILY TEACHING

Controlling Pain Through a Team Approach

The best way to control pain is through a team approach involving the patient, the family, and the nurse and physician. In the Long-Term Care and LTC Skilled areas, inclusion of the Social Worker and Department of Therapy would be beneficial to the resident. In addition to a patient telling the others the extent of his or her pain, he or she should be asked the following:

* Where is your pain located?
* When did the pain start?
* Describe the pain. Is it sharp? Dull? Throbbing? Burning?
* Does the pain come and go, or is it constant?
* What makes the pain worse?
* What makes the pain better?
* What medications are you taking for the pain?
* Are you using any other methods such as relaxation, a heating pad, or a cold pack to relieve your pain? Do they seem to help?

Always ask about the presence of pain when examining an older adult.

Collaborate with patient/resident, family, and staff regarding probable atypical presentations of pain inclusive of changes in function or gait, increased confusion, new behavior of withdrawal, and new or increased agitation.

PAIN ASSESSMENT

Pain assessment begins when the nurse accepts the person's report of pain and takes that report seriously. Assessment is

TABLE 13.1 Pain Assessment in Advanced Dementia (PAINAD)				
Items	**0**	**1**	**2**	**Score**
Breathing (independent of vocalization)	Normal	Occasional labored breathing Short period of hyperventilation	Noisy labored breathing Long period of hyperventilation Cheyne-stokes respirations	
Negative vocalization	None	Occasional moan or groan Low level of speech with a negative or disapproving quality	Repeated troubled calling out Loud moaning or groaning Crying	
Facial expression	Smiling or inexpressive	Sad, frightened, frown	Facial grimacing	
Body language	Relaxed	Tense Distressed pacing Fidgeting	Rigid Fists clenched Knees pulled up Pulling or pushing away Striking out	
Consolability	No need to console	Distracted or reassured by voice or touch	Unable to console, distract, or reassure	
TOTAL				

From Warden, V., Hurley, A. C., Volicer, L. (2003). Development and psychometric evaluation of the Pain Assessment in Advanced Dementia (PAINAD) scale. *Journal of the American Medical Directors Association, 4*(1). 9–15.

TABLE 13.2   Assessment of Pain in Older Adults

History	Physical Examination	Assessment of Other Variables
Medical History Acute illnesses Chronic illnesses Previous surgeries Timed events leading to present pain complaint	**Routine Examination**	**Pertinent Laboratory Data and Tests** Depression Scales Beck Depression Inventory Zung Self-Rating Scale Geriatric Depression Scale
	Musculoskeletal Examination Neuromuscular: Weakness Hyperalgesia Numbness	**Cognitive Assessment** Mini-Mental State Examination Short Portable Mental Status Questionnaire Philadelphia Geriatric Center MSQ
Pain History Intensity Character Frequency Pattern Location Precipitating factors Relieving factors Alleviating factors	**Signs of Trauma** Bruises Inflammation Tenderness Guarding Swelling	**Functional Assessment** Katz Activities of Daily Living Lawton Instrumental Activities of Daily Living Stanford Health Assessment Questionnaire Barthel Index Fulmer SPICES
History of Trauma Recent falls Other injuries	**Functional Performance** Range of motion Up-and-Go Test Tinetti Gait and Balance Test	**Psychosocial Assessment** Finances Social networks Dysfunctional relationships
Medication History Prescription Over-the-counter Herbal or natural Side effects		**Pain Assessment Scales** Visual analog scale Word descriptor scale Numeric scale Faces scale
Pain Medications Drugs that worked Drugs that did not work Prescription or over-the-counter Natural remedies Side effects		**Quality of Life Measures** Dartmouth COOP Project Profile of Mood States Pain/Quality of Life Scale
Previous Pain Experiences		

From American Geriatrics Society. (2001). The management of persistent pain in older persons. *Journal of the American Geriatrics Society, 50*(6), S205–S224.

essential in differentiating acute life-threatening pain from longstanding chronic pain (Herr, 2002). Otherwise, disease progression and acute injury may go unrecognized and be attributed to preexisting disease or illness. Table 13.2 identifies components of the clinical assessment of pain in older adults.

Pain assessment should include a thorough history and a physical examination. These assessments are especially important for older persons because effective pain management often depends on the appropriate treatment of underlying disease or illness. When the underlying disease is unknown, multidisciplinary consultation is indicated (AGS, 2009; Linton & Lach, 2007).

Some of the following are general principles on pain assessment from the AGS Panel on Persistent Pain in Older Persons (2009):

- No biologic markers for the presence of pain exist.
- The patient's report is the most accurate and reliable evidence of pain and its intensity.
- Patients with mild to moderate cognitive impairment may be assessed using simple questions and screening tools.
- Older adults may be reluctant to report pain despite substantial impairments.
- Older adults may expect pain with aging.

- Older adults may use words such as *discomfort, aching,* and *hurting,* rather than *pain.*
- Older adults may see pain as a metaphor for serious disease or death.
- Older adults may feel pain represents "God's will" or atonement for "bad" deeds.
- Assess patients for evidence of chronic pain.
- Recognize pain that significantly affects functional ability or quality of life as a significant problem.
- For patients with cognitive or language impairments, observe nonverbal pain behaviors, recent functional changes, and vocalizations (e.g., groans and cries).
- For patients with cognitive or language impairments, seek caregiver reports and input. Seek specialist consultation for patients with debilitating psychiatric problems, substance abuse problems, or intractable pain.
- Monitor patients with chronic pain by recording pain intensity, medication use, response, and associated activities in a pain log or diary.
- Reassess all patients with chronic pain regularly for improvement, deterioration, positive or negative effects of medications, and complications of treatment. Use the same pain instruments at each patient visit.

Pain Assessment and Culture

Pain is an individual experience. Patients' pain intensity and pain distress are related to factors such as culture, past pain experiences, individual attributes, and pain threshold. Nurses need to take an individual approach with each patient, incorporating his or her cultural beliefs and practices when assessing and managing pain. It is vitally important our pain assessments are culturally sensitive and that pain management is provided in a culturally competent manner. The U.S. Census Bureau predicts that diverse cultural groups will increase "from 30% of the U.S. population as reported in the 2000 census to 54% in 2050" (Narayan, 2010). Culture aspects of pain management affect the provider, the nurse, and the patient as they all are met with the challenges of assessment and management of pain while trying to understand language and communication nuances. Narayan (2010) has identified a series of questions to help nurses determine their cultural norms concerning pain (Box 13.2).

Culture affects the experience of pain. Some cultural beliefs include being stoic and not being explicit regarding location or quality of the pain. Being perceived as weak promotes a denial of pain. Some cultures believe they must scream to cope with the pain. Descriptions of pain also differ among cultures (Narayan, 2010). It is important for us to be aware of cultural differences related to management of pain. It is essential to "recognize that these beliefs and behaviors may arise from the social and cultural contexts in which the person lives rather than from a lack of willingness to confront pain" (Narayan, 2010).

An assessment tool that provides a procedure to grasp the effects of cultural standard(s) regarding a patient's pain experience is the Explanatory Model approach. A list of these interview questions is provided in Box 13.3.

BOX 13.2   Self-Assessment Questions to Help Nurses Determine Their Cultural Norms Concerning Pain

When you were a child, how did those who cared for you react when you were in pain?

- How did they expect you to behave when you had a minor injury?
- How did they encourage you to cope when you had severe pain?
- How did they encourage you to behave during an injection or procedure?

When those who cared for you as a child were in pain, how did they react?

- What words did they use to describe the pain?
- How did they cope with their pain?
- Do you tend to follow their example?

Consider a painful experience you've had as an adult (for example, childbirth, a fracture, a procedure).

- How did you express (or not express) your pain?
- Did the pain cause you fear? What were you afraid of?
- How did you cope with the pain?
- How did you want others to react while you were in pain?

Have you ever felt "uncomfortable" with the way a patient was reacting (or not reacting) to pain?

- What did the patient do that concerned you?
- Why did you feel that way?

Do you have "feelings" (make value judgments) about patients in pain who

- behave more stoically or expressively than you would in a similar situation?
- ask for pain medicine frequently or not often enough?
- choose treatments you don't believe are effective or with which you are unfamiliar?
- belong to a cultural group (ethnic, linguistic, religious, socioeconomic) different from your own?

Do you tend to feel certain reactions to pain are "right" or "wrong"? Why? What about these reactions makes them seem right or wrong?

- Are some expressions or verbalizations of pain "right" or "wrong"?
- Some descriptions of pain?
- Some treatments for pain?

From Narayan, M. C. (2010). Culture's effects on pain assessment and management: Cultural patterns influence nurses' and their patients' responses to pain. *American Journal of Nursing, 110*(4), 38–47.

BOX 13.3   Explanatory Model Interview for Pain Assessment

- What do you think is causing your pain?
- When did it start? Why do you think it started when it did?
- What do you fear most about the pain?
- What problems does it cause you?
- What have you used to help you with the pain? How does it help?
- Who else have you consulted about the pain? Family members? A traditional healer?
- What treatments do you think might help you with the pain?
- Who helps you when you have pain? How do they help?

Compiled from Lasch, K. E. (2000). Culture, pain, and culturally sensitive pain care. *Pain Management Nursing, 1*(3 Suppl 1), 16–22; and Kleinman, A., & Benson, P. (2006). Anthropology in the clinic: The problem of cultural competency and how to fix it. *PLOS Medicine, 3*(10), e294. In Narayan, M. C. (2010). Culture's effects on pain assessment and management: Cultural patterns influence nurses' and their patients' responses to pain. *American Journal of Nursing, 110*(4), 38–47.

Health care professionals should include educational materials on pain developed in collaboration with a specified cultural group. The health care professionals must understand the difference between what is culturally sensitive versus what is linguistically appropriate. Culturally sensitive materials consider the subtle nuances of culture; they go beyond simple translation (Lasch, 2000).

"Respecting cultural norms promotes a feeling of being valued" (Narayan, 2010). One model that provides a collaborative way to educate the patient is the LEARN model. Separated into its individual letters, this mnemonic represents:

Listen: Ask questions to help you understand why a certain practice is meaningful or important.

Explain: If a certain practice is harmful, explain why.

Acknowledge: Discuss differences and similarities between practices; be careful not to disparage cultural practices.

Recommend: Recommend a course of action that meets both your patient's needs and health care standards.

Negotiate: Assess learning needs and provide effective education to reach a mutually agreeable plan of care.

Pain Assessment Tools

Pain assessment tools assist health care professionals in objectively and accurately measuring a patient's report of pain and any relief or change in that pain. Pain assessment tools include numeric pain rating scales, such as a 0-to-10 scale, where 0 means no pain and 10 means the worst pain; visual analog scales; descriptive pain intensity scales, using descriptions such as "no pain," "a little pain," "a lot of pain," and "too much pain"; pain diaries; and pain logs. An example of a pain diary is illustrated in Fig. 13.2. A patient's report of pain should also be evaluated for its intensity and the amount of distress it causes. Pain intensity is a measure of the amount of pain that the patient is experiencing and is measured by a numeric pain rating scale, such as the 0-to-10 scale. The numeric pain rating scale translates the patient's report of pain into a number that provides the health care professional with an objective description of the patient's pain. This measure of pain can then be used to gauge relief, given the assumption that the number is lower after treatment of the pain. These measures should be recorded in the patient's pain log or chart.

The use of standardized tools when assessing pain in the older adult provides a consistent approach to managing pain, especially in the cognitively impaired older adult. Using pain assessment tools assists the nurse in planning the appropriate intervention for the severity and type of pain the older adult has and promotes care and comfort more promptly (Jett, 2012).

When it is used in the posttreatment period, a pain scale that relies on the level of activity rather than a subjective rating of pain alone can provide more specific data that are helpful in assessing the level of pain and the effectiveness of pain interventions (Table 13.3). Using other terms in addition to the word *pain* has been shown to more accurately reflect how many older persons view their discomfort or pain.

History

The nurse should carefully question and thoroughly assess a patient's report of pain. This is especially important in older adults because of their tendency to have multiple sources of pain from multiple chronic problems simultaneously. Acute pain is often attributed to chronic illness, but it should be evaluated with the knowledge that older adults often demonstrate an altered presentation of common acute illnesses, including "silent" myocardial infarctions and "painless" intraabdominal emergencies. In addition, chronic pain is characterized by variable intensity and character, and thus is often overlooked.

Linton and Lach (2007) suggested that questions should address the onset (acute or chronic), location (localized, referred, subcutaneous, or visceral), duration (constant or intermittent), intensity (have the older adult rate the pain on a standardized scale), characteristics (stabbing, shooting, sore, grinding, gnawing, achy, lightening, burning, etc.), aggravating and alleviating factors, and self-treatment (use of heat, cold, immobilization, elevation, or medication) or other prescribed treatments that either helped or did not help. A variety of physical assessment books recommend using the mnemonic "P, Q, R, S, T, U" to assist in remembering how to ask questions regarding pain. The root word for the mnemonic may differ from text to text, but the meaning is similar: P for the pattern of pain; Q, quality of the pain; R, what relieves the pain; S, what stimulates the pain; T, the timing, duration, and frequency; and U, what do you do that has worked and what have you not tried that was suggested or tried that did not work.

Physical Examination

Pain assessment for older adults includes a comprehensive physical examination of body systems, as many older adults experience painful traumatic and degenerative problems. Additionally, a thorough neurologic assessment includes an evaluation for autonomic, sensory, or motor deficits; these may indicate neuropathic conditions or nerve injuries. Depression and cognitive screening should be included as well.

Evaluation for Functional Impairment

Impaired functional status is a major problem for older adults. An evaluation of an older adult's level of function is important so that mobility and independence can be maximized. Evaluation of functional status includes the assessment of activities of daily living (ADLs), ambulation, psychosocial well-being, and overall quality of life. Standardized tools are available to assess functional status and have been proven effective with older adults. These include tools such as the Katz Activities of Daily Living Scale and Fulmer SPICES (Wallace & Fulmer, 1998). Functional activities may be restricted by the presence and intensity of pain. A functional evaluation includes an assessment of factors that contribute to or help alleviate pain. Functional status can be significantly improved through aggressive pain management. It is important to assess for new or different causes of pain; it should not be assumed that increased pain represents an exacerbation of a previous diagnosis. It is also imperative that the nurse assesses the older person for the cause

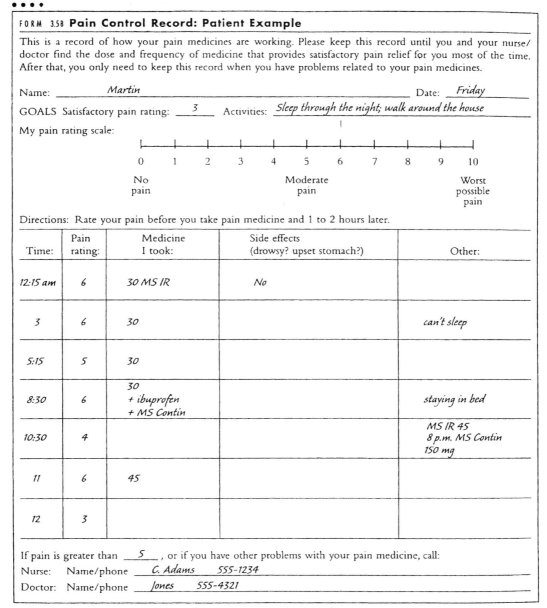

• • • •

FORM 3.5B Pain Control Record: Patient Example

This is a record of how your pain medicines are working. Please keep this record until you and your nurse/doctor find the dose and frequency of medicine that provides satisfactory pain relief for you most of the time. After that, you only need to keep this record when you have problems related to your pain medicines.

Name: _____ Martin _____   Date: _____ Friday _____

GOALS Satisfactory pain rating: ___3___   Activities: _Sleep through the night; walk around the house_

My pain rating scale:

| 0 | 1 | 2 | 3 | 4 | 5 | 6 | 7 | 8 | 9 | 10 |

No pain   Moderate pain   Worst possible pain

Directions: Rate your pain before you take pain medicine and 1 to 2 hours later.

Time:	Pain rating:	Medicine I took:	Side effects (drowsy? upset stomach?)	Other:
12:15 am	6	30 MS IR	No	
3	6	30		can't sleep
5:15	5	30		
8:30	6	30 + ibuprofen + MS Contin		staying in bed
10:30	4			MS IR 45 8 p.m. MS Contin 150 mg
11	6	45		
12	3			

If pain is greater than ___5___ , or if you have other problems with your pain medicine, call:

Nurse: Name/phone ___C. Adams   555-1234___

Doctor: Name/phone ___Jones   555-4321___

May be duplicated for use in clinical practice. From McCaffery M, Pasero C: *Pain: Clinical manual*, p. 88. Copyright © 1999, Mosby, Inc.

FORM 3.5B Patient example. This patient has been receiving the following analgesics ATC every day: ibuprofen, 400 mg qid; amitriptyline, 100 mg HS; MS Contin, 100 mg q12h (8 AM and 8 PM). His supplemental (breakthrough, rescue) dose is morphine immediate release (MS IR), 30 mg PO q2h. He usually takes two supplemental doses a day. This has relieved his pain to a 3 or less, and he has been able to sleep through the night uninterrupted by pain and walk around his home. The record reveals that his pain ratings now are greater than 3 and that he is taking supplemental doses every 3 to 4 hours. Pain keeps him awake and he stays in bed. The patient talks with the nurse at 10:30 AM. The nurse contacts the physician and the decision is to increase his morphine doses by 50% to 45 mg MS IR q2h and to MS Contin 150 mg q12h. (This dose of MS Contin requires five 30-mg tablets. However, depending on the tablet strength the patient has on hand, the MS Contin dose may be slightly more or less than 150 mg.) When an opioid dose is safe but ineffective, a 50% increase will usually produce a moderate increase in pain relief. When the patient takes more than two supplemental doses during a 12-hour period, the controlled-release should be increased.

Fig. 13.2 Daily pain diary. (From McCaffery, M., & Pasero, C. [1999]. *Pain: Clinical manual* [2nd ed.]. St. Louis, MO: Mosby.)

of a complaint of pain and not simply attribute it to age. Aging does not cause pain; disease and injury do.

Evaluation of Quality of Life

Pain is not an isolated phenomenon; it is an experience that influences all dimensions of an individual's quality of life. Pain assessment should include an evaluation of the effect of pain on a patient's quality of life. Practitioners can make a quick assessment of their patient or resident's quality of life by asking "How is life for you?" "Are you doing and enjoying what you want to do and enjoy?" and "Has there been a recent change in your life activities?" Such questions may be as effective and accurate as more scientific tools that are not practical for use in daily practice.

TABLE 13.3	Functional Pain Scale
Score	**Description of Pain by Patient Function**
0	No pain
1	Tolerable (and does not prevent any activities)
2	Tolerable (but does prevent some activities)
3	Intolerable (but can use telephone, watch TV, or read)
4	Intolerable (cannot use telephone, watch TV, or read)
5	Intolerable (and unable to verbally communicate because of pain)

From Gloth, F. M., Scheve, A. A., Stober, C. V., Chow, S., and Prosser, J. (2001). The Functional Pain Scale (FPS): Reliability, validity, and responsiveness in a senior population. *Journal of the American Medical Directors Association, 2*(3), 110–114.

Evaluation for Depression

Pain assessment of older adults also includes an evaluation for depression. A high incidence of depression is associated with chronic pain. Persistent depression affects a person's ability to cope with the pain, so it must be treated. Anxiety may also affect the management of chronic pain, especially if the outcome of the chronic problem is uncertain. The Geriatric Depression Scale is a valid and reliable tool that can be used to screen for depression in an older adult.

NURSING CARE OF OLDER ADULTS WITH PAIN

Pharmacologic Treatment

As the administrators of drugs, nurses play a major role in ensuring that older adults have their pain treated in a safe, effective, and efficient way. Nurses must be knowledgeable about the physiologic changes of aging that may alter drug absorption, metabolism, and excretion in the older adult. Changes that require ongoing assessment of a patient's response to a drug, with subsequent adjustments in dose and dosing intervals or prescribed drug, are as follows:
- Changes in physiologic factors such as decreased gastric acid production and gastrointestinal motility
- Changes in body composition such as decreased total body water, lean body mass, and serum protein and increased body fat
- Changes in organ function such as decreased hepatic blood flow and reduced glomerular filtration rate

These changes, especially those in liver and renal function, may increase the risk of accumulation of lipid-soluble drugs such as fentanyl and may slightly delay the onset of action and increase the risk for accumulating agents used to control pain (AGS, 2009). Age-related changes in absorption, distribution, metabolism, and elimination demand that prescribers be conservative, especially as recommendations for age-adjusted doses are rarely available for most analgesics (AGS, 2009).

Analgesic drugs may be classified into two categories: (1) nonopioid analgesics and (2) opioid analgesics. Additionally, many adjuvant drugs are useful in the management of pain in the older adult.

The World Health Organization has recommended a three-step approach when considering pharmacologic interventions for cancer pain (Groninger & Vijayan, 2014). This widely

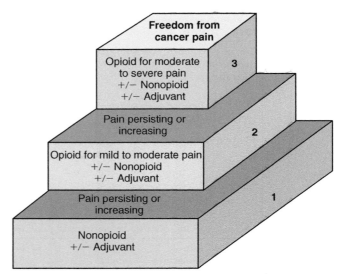

Fig. 13.3 World Health Organization's pain relief ladder. (From World Health Organization. WHO's pain relief ladder. Retrieved from http://www.who.int/cancer/palliative/painladder/en/.)

accepted practice model helps guide nurses' decisions when determining how to medicate an older adult in pain after a pain assessment has been completed. If pain occurs, drugs should be orally administered promptly in the following order: nonopioids; followed, as necessary, by mild opioids (codeine); and finally strong opioids such as morphine, until the patient is free of pain. Adjuvant drugs should be added when the person is anxious or needs more relief (Fig. 13.3). Guidelines state that pain medications should be given around the clock in anticipation of the patient's pain, rather than waiting for the patient to ask for it. The WHO has found that this three-step approach of administering the right drug in the right dose at the right time is inexpensive and 80% to 90% effective (Groninger & Vijayan, 2014; http://www.who.int/cancer/palliative/painladder/en/).

Nonopioid Analgesics

Analgesics are used as a first-line approach to pain management. Acetaminophen, ibuprofen, and naproxen are examples of nonopioid analgesics. These drugs block pain by inhibiting pain reception at the local level. As with all medications, their use by older adults must be continuously monitored. Acetaminophen seems to be well tolerated by older adults and does not affect platelet function. It is the drug of choice for relieving mild to moderate musculoskeletal pain (AGS, 2009). The maximum dosage of all consumed acetaminophen is 3000 milligrams (mg) in 24 hours unless under the care of a health care provider. Acetaminophen has few side effects and is probably the safest nonopioid for most people. Acetaminophen is as effective as aspirin in its analgesic and antipyretic properties but less effective than aspirin in its antiinflammatory properties. Although acetaminophen has not been associated with renal or gastric problems, it may result in hepatic toxicity in patients with a history of alcohol abuse or after the ingestion of persistently high doses. Older adults should be cautioned to be aware of "hidden" acetaminophen in over-the-counter products such as cold remedies or sleep aids.

Nonsteroidal antiinflammatory drugs (NSAIDs) are especially effective for treating mild to moderate arthritic pain and other inflammatory disorders. NSAIDs have been associated with a variety of adverse side effects in older adults, including stomach ulcers, renal insufficiency, and a tendency to bleed. The most common complaint associated with NSAIDs is indigestion. Indigestion may be reduced with antacid use or food consumption timed to coincide with analgesic intake. However, the health care professional must remember that gastrointestinal irritation may occur without symptoms. Severe ulceration may result in perforation and extensive bleeding. An older adult's response to the medication must be evaluated closely. NSAIDs should be avoided in high doses, for long periods, in patients with abnormal renal function, and in patients with a history of ulcer disease or bleeding (AGS, 2009).

Opioid Analgesics

Opioids are usually prescribed for patients with mild to moderate pain that is poorly tolerated or cannot be adequately managed with a nonopioid analgesic. Clinical experience suggests that older adults are particularly sensitive to the effects of opioid analgesics because they experience a higher peak and longer duration of pain relief (AGS, 2009).

Because older adults may be more sensitive to opioids, clinicians should follow the advice to "Start low, and go slow" and monitor patients until the drug is titrated for adequate pain relief. Problems with opioids usually involve those with long half-lives such as methadone or levorphanol. The half-life of an opioid is defined as the time it takes for the drug to decrease to half its initial plasma concentration. Plasma levels of drugs that have long half-lives rise slowly over several days after the initiation of a dosing schedule. Thus the risk of delayed toxicity is much greater with these drugs than with drugs having shorter half-lives. Codeine, hydromorphone, and morphine, in appropriate doses, can be used safely in older adults with pain (see Nursing Care Plan box).

Moderate-to-severe pain may be relieved with opioids such as hydrocodone, oxycodone, hydromorphone, oxymorphone, or immediate-release morphine.

◎ NURSING CARE PLAN

Prostate Cancer With Bone Metastases

Clinical Situation

Mr. K is a 77-year-old retired telephone company executive who has been admitted to the local hospital-based home care program. Mr. K had always been in good health until diagnosed with prostate cancer 2 years ago. He and his wife have enjoyed an active social life. His four adult children live in cities throughout the United States. The couple does not have any church affiliation. Mr. and Mrs. K have been married for 10 years and live in a mobile home park in the desert. They also own a condominium in the city but do not have any resources for support in that neighborhood. Three years ago, they acquired a puppy named Max. Up until the last 2½ months, Mr. K had taken morning and evening walks with Max throughout the neighborhood and local park.

In the last 2 months, Mr. K has complained about a great deal of pain in his legs and back. He has lost 35 pounds in the past month. He tires easily and is unable to walk outside his home or for distances longer than 25 feet without resting. Mr. K's first wife had died 20 years ago from breast cancer. Mr. K relates how she suffered intensely from the effects of chemotherapy and severe pain. He had refused all treatment for his cancer until 6 months ago, when he started receiving hormone therapy. He has refused to take the long-acting opioid prescribed by his physician because he does not want "to get hooked." Mr. K rates his pain as a 9 on a scale of 0 to 10, with 0 meaning no pain and 10 meaning the worst pain. Mrs. K is having difficulty caring for him and dealing with his impending death.

Nursing Diagnoses

Chronic pain resulting from inadequate knowledge of pain management

Potential for constipation resulting from analgesic use

Reduced mobility resulting from pain

Outcomes

The patient will report decreased pain (between 0 and 3) at rest and with activity, as evidenced by self-report.

The patient will continue his usual bowel elimination pattern: a soft, formed stool every day.

The patient will maintain ADLs and other physical activities, as he is able.

Interventions

Discuss general pain content information with the patient and his wife.

Elicit the patient's description of his pain, including the quality of the pain, its location, and its precipitating and relieving factors.

Identify the intensity of the patient's pain by using a pain assessment tool.

Identify the distress the patient experiences in relation to his pain.

Evaluate the patient's current use of pharmacologic and nonpharmacologic pain relief methods.

Discuss the patient's fear of addiction and the need to maintain control of his life and remain alert and functional.

Implement the use of a self-care pain management log, including the use of a pain rating scale.

Instruct the patient and his wife about around-the-clock scheduling for analgesics.

Discuss the current pain management regimen and plans for further treatment with the patient's physician.

Identify the patient's current fecal elimination pattern.

Explain the physician's prescription for a stool softener.

Discuss the use of a mild laxative if bowel movement has not occurred after 2 days.

Encourage a fluid intake of at least eight glasses of water each day.

Modify the patient's diet to increase his intake of high-fiber foods.

Discuss the effect of analgesics on fecal elimination with the patient.

Reinforce the fact that although constipation is an expected side effect of opioids, it can be prevented.

Instruct the patient to take analgesic medications on a regular basis.

Identify activities important to the patient that he would like to maintain.

Encourage him to take short walks with his dog and sit in the dining room for his meals.

Encourage use of a self-care log.

Instruct the patient about energy conservation and about the need to space activities with periods of rest.

Evaluate the environment to determine the need for equipment for ambulation or other activities.

Side Effects. Common side effects of opioids include nausea, vomiting, constipation, and urinary retention, especially in individuals with prostatic hypertrophy. Older adults are more sensitive to sedation and respiratory depression, probably because of altered distribution and excretion of medications. This is especially true in opioid-naïve patients, that is, those who have not had earlier exposure to opioids. Fentanyl patches should never be given to patients who are opioid-naïve because of the high risk for severe adverse reactions. If oral opioids are not successful and higher doses have been tried without success, a smaller dose of fentanyl may be tried with upward titrations until the correct level is found. Most nurses will never be involved in this titration determination but may be involved in the assessment of the pain response after the provider makes an increase.

Constipation as a side effect of opioid use is of particular concern in older patients because many of them have preexisting bowel conditions. It is good practice to start a patient on a bowel program when initiating opioid treatment (see Patient/Family Teaching box). Careful assessment of bowel habits, including the use of stool softeners and laxatives and the dietary intake of high-fiber foods, is essential when a patient is using opioids. The health care professional must emphasize to the patient and his or her family the importance of being proactive, that is, preventing the occurrence of constipation rather than waiting for it to occur. To deal with the side effect of constipation, the Oncology Nursing Society recommends the following (Woolery et al., 2008):

- Increase fluid intake.
- Modify diet; add high-fiber foods (see Nutritional Considerations box).
- Maintain or increase activity levels.
- Strive to maintain a daily bowel movement schedule that considers when gastrocolic reflexes are most active.
- Take medications such as stool softeners, expanders, or natural laxative mixtures, avoiding pharmaceutical laxatives when possible.

PATIENT/FAMILY TEACHING

What Can You Do for Constipation?

Opioid analgesics cause constipation in most people. The following suggestions help prevent constipation from becoming a problem and causing discomfort:

- Eat foods high in fiber, for example, uncooked fruits and vegetables, and whole grain breads and cereals.
- Add 1 or 2 tablespoons of unprocessed bran to foods.
- Drink plenty of liquids—8 to 10 glasses per day.
- Eat foods that have helped relieve constipation in the past.
- Plan your bowel movement for the same time each day, if possible.
- Try to use the toilet or bedside commode for fecal elimination.
- Have a hot drink about 30 minutes before the planned time for a bowel movement.
- Consult with a physician about using a bulk laxative such as psyllium (Metamucil) or any other laxative or stool softener.

Modified from American Cancer Society and National Cancer Institute. (2014). Pain control: Support for people with cancer. Retrieved from https://www.cancer.gov/publications/patient-education/pain-control.

NUTRITIONAL CONSIDERATIONS

High-Fiber Foods to Relieve Constipation

- Oatmeal, bran, whole wheat, rye
- Apples, pears, strawberries, peaches, plums, citrus
- Beans, dry beans
- Peas, cabbage, root vegetables, fresh tomatoes, green beans, carrots

Although nausea and vomiting caused by opioid use usually disappear after a few days of taking the medication, it is critical that clinicians take a preventive approach in treating these side effects. As with all medications, antiemetics must be evaluated for their effectiveness in controlling nausea and vomiting in older adults as well as for side effects such as sedation. The nurse should advise patients and family members that sedation may occur because of the antiemetic. If nausea persists beyond a few days of starting the opioid, a new opioid should be tried (AGS, 2009).

Sedation and impaired cognitive performance should be anticipated when starting opioids (AGS, 2009). The sedation usually decreases in 1 to 3 days. In case it does not, the patient needs to be informed orally and in writing that the health care provider should be notified. Sedation may also be related to sleep deprivation resulting from unrelieved pain. A fact that must be stressed is that sedation may occur without adequate pain relief. This type of rest does not result in the expected rejuvenation offered by sleep. Nurses should monitor for respiratory depression (<8 breaths per minute or oxygen saturation of <90% [AGS, 2009]), especially during rapid, high-dose escalations. Table 13.4 identifies analgesics that should be avoided in older adults.

Adjuvant Medications

Adjuvant medications, defined as drugs without intrinsic analgesic properties, are helpful in treating certain types of chronic pain. Adjuvant drugs include anticonvulsants, antidepressants, and some sedatives. The treatment of underlying depression or mood disorders may enhance other pain management strategies.

Anticonvulsants, drugs usually used to treat seizures, are often helpful in controlling painful conditions such as postherpetic neuralgia, diabetic neuropathy, and phantom limb pain. An anticonvulsant useful in the treatment of older adult patients that has few side effects is gabapentin. Medications in this category include zonisamide, tiagabine, pregabalin, and milnacipran. Anticonvulsants may cause blood dyscrasias; therefore laboratory data must be obtained on a regular basis. For older adults, some sedatives or tranquilizers may cause side effects such as increased confusion and constipation. Thus the use of these drugs in older adults must be continuously monitored. TCAs have been found to be useful in treating neuropathic pain but do not seem to be effective in the case of musculoskeletal pain; higher doses are needed for therapy superimposed on cancer pain. Desipramine hydrochloride seems to be better tolerated by older adults with fewer anticholinergic side effects compared with certain other drugs such as amitriptyline.

TABLE 13.4 Opioids to Avoid in Pain Management of Older Adults

Drug	Precautions	Potential Solutions
Meperidine	Metabolite (normeperidine) may accumulate and cause confusion, agitation, and seizure activity, especially among patients with renal impairment.	No advantages to either oral or parenteral meperidine exist over other opioid drugs.
Pentazocine	Mixed opioid agonist or antagonist activity often leads to central nervous system excitement, confusion, and hallucinations.	Avoid all use in frail older adults.
Levorphanol	The optimal analgesic dose varies widely among patients. Doses should be titrated to treat pain or for prevention. Use with caution in patients with hypersensitivity reactions to morphine, hydrocodone, hydromorphone, oxycodone, or oxymorphone.	For use in relief of moderate-to-severe pain.

Modified from American Geriatrics Society. (2015). American Geriatrics Society 2015 Updated Beers Criteria for Potentially Inappropriate Medication Use in Older Adults. *Journal of the American Geriatrics Society, 63,* 2227–2246. doi: 10.1111/jgs.13702.

However, TCAs may cause constipation, blurred vision, dry mouth, urinary retention, and sedation; those with glaucoma and benign prostatic hypertrophy should avoid them. TCAs have been known to cause arrhythmias, cognitive changes, orthostatic hypotension, and falls. Selective serotonin reuptake inhibitors (SSRIs) seem to have relatively low side effect profiles. Newer combination drugs of selective norepinephrine reuptake inhibitors (SNRIs) and SSRIs are helping to achieve better results in additional pain relief and antidepressant effects. These drugs appear to block pain transmission pathways (AGS, 2009).

Adjuvant drugs alter or modulate the perception of pain. They may be used alone or with other pain drugs (Touhy & Jett, 2012). It is important that the nurse notify patients and their family members when these adjuvant drugs are being used to treat the patient's pain. Clinical experience has shown that a patient may discontinue the analgesic when an adjuvant drug is added. The patient/resident may also take an adjuvant drug such as an antidepressant without realizing that it is being used in conjunction with the analgesic to treat pain. As with all analgesics, the nurse must continue to assess the patient/resident's reports of pain and the effectiveness and side effects of the adjuvant drug.

The combined use of pharmacologic and nonpharmacologic pain management therapies works well in older adults. Individually, most of the nondrug therapies work well only with mild pain. With moderate pain, drug therapy must complement the other therapies. Clinical experience suggests that many of these techniques are effective in individual cases. As with all treatment modalities, the individual response must be evaluated.

Complementary and Alternative Medicine

Complementary and alternative medicine (CAM), as well as integrative medicine, is gaining new ground in health care. These terms, however, may be confusing and are often used interchangeably, even though they have different meanings. The National Center for Complementary and Alternative Medicine (NCCAM) suggests using the term to describe products and practices used in addition to mainstream medical practices (http://nccam.nih.gov/health/whatiscam). These practices fall into two subgroups: (1) natural products and (2) mind and body practices. Natural products include herbals and botanicals, as well as vitamins and minerals. Capsicum is commonly used for pain control, particularly because it can be used as a cream and applied directly to painful areas (http://www.cancer.org/treatment/treatmentsandsideeffects/complementaryandalternativemedicine/herbsvitaminsandminerals/capsicum). Mind and body practices include such things as acupuncture, massage therapy, meditation, movement therapies, relaxation techniques, spinal manipulation, t'ai chi, healing touch, and yoga. Nurses should be aware of these alternative therapies and assess their use and effectiveness in their patients.

Heat and Cold

Heat is useful in decreasing pain and discomfort. It increases blood flow to the skin and superficial tissues, increases oxygen and nutrient delivery, and decreases joint stiffness by increasing the elasticity of muscles (DerSarkissian, 2016). Heat is delivered by hot water bottles, heating pads, compresses, tub baths, soaks, and heat lamps. Patients and caregivers need to be cautious of thermal burns when using these items. Temperature and length of use is important to determine before use.

Cold reduces inflammation, edema, and pain, especially after an acute injury such as a fall. It may reduce muscle spasms not relieved by heat therapy (DerSarkissian, 2016).

Visualization or Imagery

This is a state of pleasure and peace achieved by creating a vivid picture in one's mind. This picture might be the setting sun, a serene forest, or rolling waves of water. It might be recalled from the past or a new experience imagined. It transports the patient to another place and uses all five senses (Giacobbi, Stabler, Stewart, Jaeschke, Siebert, & Kelley, 2015).

Progressive Relaxation

This can include an alternate contraction and relaxation of the various muscle groups. It is usually done lying down in a quiet, often darkened room. It can be accomplished with soft music in the background. Relaxation tapes can be found in many bookstores (DerSarkissian, 2017).

Distraction

Distraction can be almost anything that takes one's mind off of pain. They can include radio, television, videos, music, memories, pet therapy, or projects such as games or puzzles. This is usually used with mild pain, but it can be used in conjunction with pain medication.

Exercise

Exercise and physical therapy prevent stiffness, maintain function, relieve muscle spasms, and increase the sense of well-being. Medical consultation should be obtained for patients/residents before instituting physical therapy. Many patients/residents need pretreatment analgesic medication shortly before starting the regimen.

Peripheral Nerve Stimulation

Peripheral nerve stimulation (transcutaneous electrical nerve stimulation [TENS]) is a technique for the management of chronic pain in which electrical leads are placed subcutaneously into the area of a person's pain. It may be used to treat a variety of painful conditions such as neuralgia, migraines, and orthopedic pain. Kouroukli et al. (2009) found that peripheral nerve stimulation was effective in relieving the pain of two older adults who suffered from postherpetic neuralgia for a range of 2 to 10 years.

Music Therapy

Music therapy may be incorporated into many other therapies presented here. Furthermore, it is one therapy that has been used extensively in clinical practice with older adults (Clair, 2008). The music used should be the kind appreciated by the patient and at a volume that the patient can control.

Hypnosis

Hypnosis includes some of the other cognitive modalities such as deep concentration, imagery, and breathing exercises. Self-hypnosis and imagery begin with developing a relaxed state, closing the eyes, focusing on the pain, and visualizing its color, shape, and size. Then the pain is projected out into space. It is made bigger, then smaller, and then allowed to be any size. Its color is changed and then put back as it was. Finally, the eyes are reopened.

Education

Education is a cognitive therapy that involves teaching a patient about pain and the role of cognition in pain perception. The patient learns to track the pain and record episodes of pain and distress. The nurse helps the patient/resident interpret the thoughts that accompany pain. Relaxation is incorporated to divert attention from the pain of the body. The goal is to help a patient/resident develop some mastery over his or her pain.

Planning Pain Relief

The primary consideration in selecting pain relief methods is individualized planning. Patients vary greatly in their medication requirements, choices of nonpharmacologic interventions, and prior pain experiences. Patients should be involved in choosing pain management methods and should share responsibility for implementing pain relief measures. Active involvement of patients/residents and family caregivers is essential to the successful implementation of pain management regimens. This applies to both pharmacologic and nonpharmacologic pain relief measures.

▌SUMMARY

Pain continues to be underrecognized and undertreated in older adults despite dramatic increases in the knowledge of pain and pain management. Pain in patients in nursing facilities is a large problem. Older adults suffer many painful chronic illnesses such as arthritis and cancer. When conducting assessments, the practicing nurse must look for pain in older adult patients/residents and be alert for chronic diseases that may cause pain. Many excellent pharmacologic treatments for pain and many routes of

EVIDENCE-BASED PRACTICE

Role of Nursing Assistants in Pain Management

Background
Nursing assistants provide much of the direct care to residents in nursing homes. Due to their frequent contact, they develop specialized knowledge of each resident's pain experience that enables them to play a key role in pain management. However, little research is available on this important topic.

Sample/Setting
Forty-nine nursing assistants were recruited from 12 nursing homes; 92% were female, 44.9% were between 36 and 45 years of age, and 24.49% were between 26 and 35 years of age. All had completed 7 weeks of training before becoming nursing assistants.

Method
This is a descriptive, exploratory, qualitative study, 12 nursing assistants participated in semistructured individual interviews. Another 37 nursing assistants participated in 8 semistructured focus groups. All interviews followed the same interview guide. Data was recorded and transcribed verbatim.

Findings
Through qualitative content analyses, nursing assistants were found to play four roles in the pain management process: (1) pain assessor, (2) reporter, (3) subordinate implementing prescribed medications, and (4) instigator implementing nonpharmacologic interventions.

Implications
Nursing assistants play a key role in successful pain management in the nursing home. However, their scope of practice results in them being continually undervalued by other health care professionals. In-service training and the use of standardized pain management protocols may facilitate a team approach to pain management in nursing homes.

From Liu, J. Y. W. (2013). Exploring nursing assistants' roles in the process of pain management for cognitively impaired nursing home residents: A qualitative study. *Journal of Advanced Nursing, 70*(5), 1065–1077. doi: 10.1111/jan.12259.

HOME CARE

1. The nurse caring for homebound older adults should know the effects pain has on functional status and quality of life.
2. The home care nurse should evaluate a patient's/resident's pain at each home visit.
3. The nurse should assess factors that may influence effective pain control in homebound older adults (e.g., motor, cognitive, and functional impairments).
4. When using a pain assessment tool, a home care nurse must evaluate a homebound older adult's ability to use the tool.
5. Caregivers are an important source of information to the nurse when he or she assesses homebound older adults with pain.
6. The nurse should instruct homebound older adults and their caregivers on adjunctive therapies that can be used with analgesics to enhance pain management.
7. The nurse should assess and identify barriers for homebound older adults and caregivers related to pain and its management.
8. The nurse should encourage around-the-clock pain management to provide optimal pain control.

administration are available today; thus it is possible to individualize care for each patient. Although pharmacology is the main therapy for most chronic illnesses, many alternative and complementary therapies are available that will benefit the nurse's older adult patients/residents. For further information, see the list of websites at the end of this chapter.

KEY POINTS

- Pain often remains underrecognized and undertreated in older adults, mainly because of limited gerontologic pain research. Therefore nurses must have a special understanding and conduct an accurate and ongoing assessment of the needs of this population regarding pain.
- Goals for pain management in older adults include control of chronic disease conditions that cause pain, maintenance of mobility and functional status, promotion of maximum independence, and improvement of quality of life.
- Barriers to effective pain management in older adults include the misconception that intolerance to pain is age related, underreporting of pain, lack of access to diagnostic services, cognitive and functional impairment, the inability to communicate pain effectively through pain behavior scales, fear of addiction, and inadequacies in pain education.
- Accurate and ongoing assessment, as well as a thorough understanding of pain physiology, is essential for effective pain management in older adults.
- The nurse's clinical assessment of older adults' pain includes many important components: medical history; pain history; history of trauma, medications, and previous pain experiences; physical examination; examination for signs of trauma; musculoskeletal system examination; assessment of range of motion; and assessment of functional impairments. A variety of tools and scales are available for these assessments.

- The quality-of-life assessment is a vital part of pain assessment in older adults. This assessment may include sleeping, ADL function, pain, social relationships, and other areas as deemed pertinent. Different areas will have different values based on an individual's preferences.
- Pharmacologic pain management includes the use of analgesics, opioid analgesics, and adjuvant drugs. Nonpharmacologic therapies include methods using cold or heat, relaxation or distraction, imagery, TENS, and hypnosis. For the pain management to be effective, the nurse must continually assess a patient's/resident's response to pain when employing any of these methods.
- A standard assessment scale that differentiates between pain intensity and pain distress in older adult patients/residents is a useful tool for nurses when planning successful pain interventions. Consistent use of this tool, coupled with accurate record keeping, helps promote effective pain management.
- Family members often play an integral role in the pain management of older adults. Family members may provide insight into older adult's pain experiences by offering the nurse information that the patients may not be willing or able to share accurately.

CRITICAL-THINKING EXERCISES

1. A 91-year-old woman with a small bowel obstruction is admitted to the hospital from a long-term care facility. She also has a history of dementia and is incoherent. Discuss how you would revise your assessment and evaluation techniques in managing her pain.

2. What criteria should you use to determine whether an older adult patient requires an adjustment in dose or dosing interval or a change in the drug prescribed for pain management?

REFERENCES

American Geriatrics Society. (2009). The management of persistent pain in older persons. *Journal of the American Geriatrics Society, 57,* 1331–1346. https://doi.org/10.1111/j.1532-5415.2009.02376.x.

Arnstein, P. A., Herr, K. A., & Butcher, H. K. (2017). Persistent pain management in older adults. *Journal of Gerontological Nursing, 43*(7), 20–31.

Aronoff, G. (2002). Drawing the line between pain management and addiction. *Psychopharmacol Update, 12*(9), 1.

Atkins, C. (n.d.). Older adult and pain [PowerPoint]. Retrieved February 14, 2018 from https://www.pharmac.govt.nz/assets/ss-pain-3-older-adult-and-pain-claire-atkins.pdf.

Bishop, T., & Morrison, R. (2007). Geriatric palliative care—part 1: pain and symptom management. *Clinical Geriatrics, 15*(1), 25–32.

Booker, S. Q., & Haedtke, C. (2016a). Controlling pain and discomfort, part 1: Assessment in verbal older adults. *Nursing, 46*(2), 65–68.

Booker, S. Q., & Haedtke, C. (2016b). Controlling pain and discomfort, part 2: Assessment in non-verbal older adults. *Nursing, 46*(5), 66–69.

Clair, A. A. (2008). *Therapeutic uses of music with older adults* (2nd ed.). Baltimore: Health Professional Press.

DerSarkissian, C. (2016). *Consider heat or ice.* Retrieved February 14, 2018 from https://www.webmd.com/pain-management/try-heat-or-ice.

DerSarkissian, C. (2017). *Stress relaxation and natural pain relief.* https://www.webmd.com/pain-management/guide/stress-relief-for-pain.

Gabrick, J. (2016). PAINAD scale offers alternative to assessing pain in the dementia patient. *Journal of Emergency Medical Services.* Retrieved from http://www.jems.com/articles/print/volume-41/issue-40/features/painad-scale-offers-alternative-to-assessing-pain-in-the-dementia-patient.html?c=1.

Giacobbi, P. R., Stabler, M. E., Stewart, J., Jaeschke, A. M., Siebert, J. L., & Kelley, G. A. (2015). Guided imagery for arthritis and other rheumatic diseases: A systematic review of randomized controlled trials. *Pain Management Nursing, 16*(5), 792–803. https://doi.org/10.1016/j.pmn.2015.01.003.

Groninger, H., & Vijayan, J. (2014). Pharmacologic management of pain at the end of life. *American Family Physician, 90*(1), 26–32.

Hartford Institute for Geriatric Nursing. (2012). *Pain assessment for older adults.* Retrieved April 20, 2014, from www.consultgerirn.org/uploads/File/trythis/try_this_7.pdf.

Herr, K. (2002). Chronic pain: challenges and assessment strategies. *Journal of Gerontological Nursing, 2,* 20.

Herr, K., Bjororo, K., & Decker, S. (2006). Tools for assessment of pain in nonverbal older adults with dementia: a state of the science review. *Journal of Pain and Symptom Management, 31,* 170.

Herr, K., Bursch, H., Ersek, M., Miller, L. L., & Swafford, K. (2010). Use of pain behavioral assessment tools in the nursing home: Expert consensus recommendations for practice. *Journal of Gerontological Nursing, 36*(3), 18–29. https://doi.org/10.3928/00989134-20100108-04.

Horgas, A. L. (2017). Pain assessment in older adults. *Nurs Clin N Am, 52,* 375–385.

Horgas, A. L., Yoon, S. L., & Grall, M. (2012). *Nursing standard of practice protocol: Pain management in older adults.* Retrieved February 14, 2017 from https://consultgeri.org/geriatric-topics/pain.

Jansen, M. P. (2008). Pain in older adults. In M. P. Jansen (Ed.), *Managing pain in the older adult.* New York.

Jett, K. (2012). Pain and comfort. In T. Touhy & K. Jett (Eds.), *Ebersole & Hess' toward healthy aging: Human needs & nursing response* (8th ed.). St. Louis: Mosby/Elsevier.

Kouroukli, I., Dionissios, N., Panareto, V., Zompolas, V., Papastergiou, D., Sanidas, G., et al. (2009). Peripheral subcutaneous stimulation for the treatment of intractable postherpetic neuralgia: two case reports and literature review. *Pain practice: the official journal of World Institute of Pain, 9*(3), 225–229.

Lasch, K. E. (2000). Culture, pain, and culturally sensitive pain care. *Pain Management Nursing,* (1), 16–22. 3, Suppl 1 (September).

Lautenbacher, S., Peters, J. H., Heesen, M., Scheel, J., & Kunz, M. (2017). Age changes in pain perception: A systematic-review and meta-analysis of age effects on pain and tolerance thresholds. *Neuroscience and Biobehavioral Reviews, 75,* 104–113. https://doi.org/10.1016/j.neubiorev.2017.01.039.

Leo, J., & Huether, S. E. (2010). Pain, temperature regulation, sleep, and sensory function. In K. McCance & S. Huether (Eds.), *Pathophysiology* (3rd ed.). St Louis: Mosby.

Linton, A. D., & Lach, H. W. (2007). *Matteson & McConnell's gerontological nursing: concepts and practice.* St Louis: WB Saunders.

Makris, U. E., Abrams, R. C., Gurland, B., & Reid, M. C. (2014). Management of persistent pain in the older patient. *Journal of the American Medical Association, 312*(8), 825–836.

McCaffery, M. (2000). *Pain: nursing management of the patient with pain* (3rd ed.). Philadelphia: Lippincott Williams & Wilkins.

McCaffery, M., & Pasero, C. (1999). *Pain: clinical manual* (2nd ed.). St Louis: Mosby.

McCance, K. L., & Huether, S. E. (2010). *Pathophysiology: The biologic basis for disease in adults and children* (6th ed.). St Louis: Mosby.

McCleane, G. (2008). Pain perception in the elderly patient. *Clinics in Geriatric Medicine, 24*(2), 203–211.

Merskey, H., & Bogduk, N. (Eds.). (1994). *Classification of chronic pain.* (2nd ed.). Seattle: IASP Press.

Narayan, M. C. (2010). Culture's effects on pain assessment and management. *American Journal of Nursing, 110*(4), 38–47.

Park, J., & Hughes, K. (2012). Nonpharmacological approaches to the management of chronic pain in community dwelling older adults: a review of empirical evidence. *Journal of the American Geriatrics Society, 60*(3), 555–568.

Reid, M. C., Bennett, D. A., Chen, W. G., Eldadah, B. A., Farrar, J., Ferrell, B., … Zacharoff, K. L. (2011). Improving the pharmacologic management of pain in older adults: identifying the research gaps and methods to address them. *Pain Medicine, 12*(9), 1336–1357.

Robinson, P. (2010). Pharmacological management of pain in older persons. *The Consultant Pharmacist, 25*(suppl a), 11.

Shoefield, P. (2010). "It's your age": The assessment and management of pain in older adults. *Continuing Education in Anaesthesia, Critical Care & Pain, 10,* 93.

Sternbach, R. A. (1978). Clinical aspects of pain. In R. A. Sternbach (Ed.), *The psychology of pain* (p. 223). New York: Raven Press.

The Joint Commission. (2016). *Joint Commission Statement on Pain Management.* Retrieved February 14, 2018 from https://www.jointcommission.org/joint_commission_statement_on_pain_management/.

Touhy, T. A., & Jett, K. (2012). *Ebersole & Hess' Toward healthy aging: human needs & nursing response* (8th ed.). St. Louis: Mosby/Elsevier.

Wallace, M., & Fulmer, T. (1998). Fulmer SPICES: An overall assessment tool for older adults. *Try This: Best Practices in Nursing*

Care to Older Adults. Retrieved October 29, 2017, from https://consultgeri.org/try-this/general-assessment/issue-1.

Warden, V., Hurley, A. C., & Volicer, L. (2003). Development and psychometric evaluation of the Pain Assessment in Advanced Dementia (PAINAD) scale. *Journal of the American Medical Directors Association, 4*(1), 9–15. https://doi.org/10.1097/01.JAM.0000043422.31640.F7.

Wiggins, S. A. (2017). *Pain in older adults: Overview, assessment, and management.* University of Kansas Medical Center. Retrieved October 29, 2017, from http://classes.kumc.edu/coa/education/AMED900/PainOlderAdults.htm.

Woolery, M., Bisanz, A., Lyons, H., Gaido, L., Yenulevich, M., Fulton, S., … McMillan, S. C. (2008). Putting evidence into practice: evidence-based interventions for the prevention and management of constipation in patients with cancer. *Clinical Journal of Oncology Nursing, 12*(2), 317–337.

WEBSITES

American Academy of Hospice and Palliative Medicine. http://aahpm.org.

American Academy of Pain Medicine. http://www.painmed.org.

American Geriatrics Society. https://www.americangeriatrics.org.

American Pain Society. http://americanpainsociety.org.

International Association for Hospice and Palliative Care. https://hospicecare.com/home/.

National Hospice and Palliative Care Organization. https://www.nhpco.org.

International Association for the Study of Pain. https://www.iasp-pain.org.

World Health Organization. http://www.who.int/en/.

14

Infection and Inflammation

Jennifer J. Yeager, PhD, RN, APRN

ⓔ http://evolve.elsevier.com/Meiner/gerontologic

LEARNING OBJECTIVES

On completion of this chapter, the reader will be able to:

1. Describe alterations in the immune system related to aging.
2. Describe nutritional factors that influence immune status.
3. Describe psychosocial factors that influence immune status.
4. Describe the effect of lifestyle factors on immune status.
5. Describe the effect of drugs on immune status.
6. Identify strategies to prevent nosocomial infections, community-acquired infections, or both.
7. Incorporate nutritional, psychosocial, and lifestyle factors into a nursing care plan.

WHAT WOULD YOU DO?

What would you do if you were faced with the following situations?

* Following a review of facility weights, you determine your 72-year-old resident has lost more than 5% of their weight in the past 6 months. What effect does weight loss have on the older adult's immune system? Knowing this, what would you do?
* You are discharging your patient home and ask if they have had their influenza shot yet. They respond, "No, I don't get that anymore; it doesn't help anyway." How should you respond?

The importance of investigating infections in older adults cannot be overstated. Infection is one of the 10 most common causes of death in patients older than age 65 (Kane, Ouslander, Abrass, & Resnick, 2009). Infections in older adults are often masked in their presentation, which may lead to delayed treatment. The immune system enables the body to defend itself against disease-causing microorganisms and other foreign bodies; it is vital to human survival. However, this system exhibits a diminished ability to provide such protection with aging (Newson, 2007). Considering the immune system's fundamental importance to maintaining health, a clear understanding of age-related changes is crucial.

The immune system has two primary functions: (1) to discriminate between that which is self and that which is nonself and (2) to remove from the body that which is recognized as nonself. This system comprises antibodies, cells, chemicals, and proteins, as well as lymphoid tissue, bone marrow, and the spleen (Porth, 2004). Furthermore, this system interacts with the neurologic and endocrine systems in a highly complex manner to modulate the human immune response. Immunologic function may be mediated by psychological and behavioral factors. Awareness of the effect of mood, activity level, stress,

and nutrition on the capacity of this system to provide optimal protection is increasing.

This chapter examines age-related changes in the immune system, and the influence of other factors such as psychosocial and nutritional status on the immune status of older adults. Cancer, autoimmune diseases, human immunodeficiency virus (HIV), and significant nosocomial pathogens are also discussed.

THE CHAIN OF INFECTION

For an infection to occur, a reservoir of an infectious disease, a portal of entry, and a susceptible host must be present. The source of an infectious disease is the reservoir or substance from which the infectious agent was acquired. The source may be a person's own microbial flora (endogenous) or something in the environment (exogenous) such as water, air, food, soil, or another person. Infectious diseases passed from other animal species to humans are called *zoonoses,* for example, cat-scratch fever and rabies. Infections acquired in the hospital are called *nosocomial infections,* and those acquired outside the health care facility are called *community-acquired infections.* The source of transmission may be feces, blood, and body fluids. Infections may be transmitted from person to person through shared inanimate objects (fomites) contaminated by infected body fluids. Examples of infections transmitted through this mechanism include *Clostridium difficile* infection from a commode or other contaminated surface and HIV infection from the use of shared needles by intravenous drug users.

The portal of entry is the way a pathogen enters the body and gains access to tissues, where it may multiply and cause disease. The portal of entry may be penetration of the skin, direct contact, ingestion, or inhalation. Any disruption or penetration in the integrity of the skin and mucous membranes is a potential portal of entry. The break may be accidental (e.g., an abrasion or burn), the result of a medical procedure (e.g., surgery or catheterization), or the result of direct inoculation from animal or arthropod bite (e.g., Lyme disease or malaria). In direct contact, pathogens are transmitted directly from infected tissues or secretions to exposed intact mucous membranes. Sexually transmitted diseases (STDs) such as gonorrhea and chlamydia are examples of direct contact transmission. The oral cavity and gastrointestinal tract are the most efficient portals of entry. Pathogens are ingested and successfully compete with normal bacterial flora to cause infection. Cholera, food poisoning, and hepatitis A are examples of diseases that occur through ingestion. Pathogens must be able to survive the low pH and enzymes of the gastric acid secretions to establish infection. People with reduced gastric acidity (because of disease or drugs) are more susceptible to this mode of infection.

Many pathogens invade the body through the respiratory tract and cause diseases such as influenza, the common cold, and bacterial pneumonia. The portal of entry does not limit the site of infection. Ingested pathogens may penetrate the mucosa, disseminate through the circulatory system, and cause disease in other organs (Porth, 2004). Hepatitis A and vancomycin-resistant enterococci (VRE) are examples of ingested pathogens causing infection in the liver and the bloodstream, respectively. Genetic, constitutional, and other nonspecific factors in the host determine whether a pathogen will succeed in causing infection and clinical disease.

AGE-RELATED CHANGES IN THE IMMUNE SYSTEM

Some researchers believe that much of the illness seen in older adults may be the direct consequence of changes in "both cell-mediated and antibody-mediated immune response" (Townsend, 2008). Alterations in immune status may be responsible for infections, cancer, and autoimmune processes, all of which may be life-threatening (Porth, 2004). Scientists have tried to determine whether the diminished immunocompetence noted with age is a result of decreased numbers of immune cells or merely decreased functioning of the cells. However, because immunocompetence is affected by numerous other factors, it has been difficult to isolate changes related to age alone. Atrophy of the thymus, which occurs naturally with aging, affects T-lymphocyte function. Diminished cellular (T-cell–mediated) and humoral (B-lymphocyte) immunity have both been associated with aging. Box 14.1 summarizes age-related changes in the immune system (Townsend, 2008).

Cell-mediated immunity is the ability of the host to differentiate between self and nonself. Diminished cell-mediated immunity in older adults is generally associated with diminished T-cell response (Goldman & Ausiello, 2004). With aging, B cells demonstrate reduced antibody response (Frasca & Blomberg, 2011).

As age increases, so does the production of autoantibodies. This predisposes older adults to an increase in autoimmune diseases. The mechanism underlying this issue is felt to be

---

BOX 14.1 Age-Related Changes in the Immune System

Lymphocytes
No change in total number of lymphocytes
No change in number of B cells
No change or increase in T-helper cells
Decrease in suppressor T cells
Decreased T-cell responsiveness
Decreased CD_4 and CD_8 cells

Polymorphonuclear Leukocytes
Reduced migration ability

Antibody
Decrease of T-cell–dependent antibody responsiveness
Decreased primary response to new antigens
Maintenance of secondary response to antigens
Increased globulins associated with secondary response and autoimmunity
Increased incidence of antibodies to self-antigens

Lymphoid Tissue
Involution of thymus
Atrophy of thymic cortex
Atrophy or hypertrophy of some lymph nodes

Mechanical Barriers
Changes in skin and mucous membranes, resulting in reduced effectiveness of physical barriers

---

alteration in both T-cell and B-cell function (Agrawal, Sridharan, Prakash, & Agrawal, 2012). The skin is the largest immunologically active system of the body and the body's first line of defense. Normal microbial flora on the skin (e.g., *Propionibacterium acnes* and *Staphylococcus aureus*) prevent pathogenic bacteria from flourishing ("Immune system," 2013). With aging, the skin becomes more fragile and prone to breakdown or abrasion, thus disrupting the defensive mechanisms and providing a portal of entry for bacteria.

FACTORS AFFECTING IMMUNOCOMPETENCE

Nutritional Factors

Nutritional and dietary status is of critical importance to immune function. This is especially true in the older adult population. Older adults are at high risk for nutritional deficits; at least one-third of individuals older than age 65 have nutritional deficiencies. Risks associated with the development of a nosocomial infection include poor nutrition, unintentional weight loss, low serum albumin levels, decreased fluid intake, poor oral hygiene, and altered mental status. Factors contributing to this tendency toward inadequate nutrition include altered taste, social isolation, physical inability to prepare food, altered absorption, and poverty. Older adults should consult with their health care providers and have a thorough assessment of their dietary intake done before beginning nutritional supplementation. When adequate amounts of vitamins and minerals are consumed in the diet, supplementation is unnecessary and may lead to toxicity.

Malnutrition

Significant deprivation of protein, calories, or other vitamins and minerals has been shown to result in altered immune function. Along with other age-related changes in the immune system, this deprivation results in increased susceptibility to infectious disease. Restoring nutritional balance can improve older adults' immune status (Nowson, 2007).

Iron and Trace Element Deficiency

The effects of iron deficiency on immunocompetence and susceptibility to infection have not yet been fully determined. Low levels of iron also decrease the number of circulating T cells. Iron deficiency contributes to decreased functioning of neutrophils, macrophages, and B and T cells. In addition, iron deficiency contributes to a delayed responsiveness to antigens.

Zinc is thought to be associated with immune function. A prolonged zinc deficiency leads to impaired cell-mediated immunity, wound healing, and protein synthesis. Patients with decreased zinc levels experience an increase in the number of infections and an increase in the needed healing time (Nowson, 2007).

Psychosocial Factors

Awareness is growing of the potential effect of psychosocial factors on immune status. These factors include chronic and acute stress, depression, bereavement, and social relationships. Recognition that such factors influence immune status is relatively recent, and our understanding of the nature of these relationships is constantly changing. Therefore, the clinical relevance of these changes remains a source of investigation and controversy.

Older adults experience many psychosocial changes that potentially effect immune status and must be taken into consideration. Older adults work through bereavement as they lose family and friends. Additionally, they experience a shrinking sphere of social relationships and exhibit a high incidence of depression.

Depression

Depression has also been associated with decreased immune function. This is significant because approximately 6% of community-dwelling older adults are diagnosed with depression (Akincigil et al., 2011). Furthermore, adults older than 65 years represent more than 15% of the population (U.S. Census Bureau, 2017) but make up nearly 17% of all suicides (American Association of Suicidology, 2018). Some evidence suggests that the negative effect of depression on the immune system increases with age. Thus older adults who are depressed may be at risk for greater immune deficiencies than younger individuals with depression.

Drugs

A variety of drugs may affect the immune system; these include immunosuppressants and immunoenhancers. Many drugs given for therapeutic purposes have an immunosuppressant effect. Some of these drugs include corticosteroids, cyclosporine, and chemotherapeutics for cancer. Corticosteroids such as prednisone are given for a variety of reasons, including treatment of autoimmune processes (e.g., rheumatoid arthritis [RA]). Individuals receiving corticosteroids, those taking cyclosporine following transplantation to reduce the risk of organ rejection, or individuals taking anticancer drugs have an altered immune response and are at higher risk for infection.

Complementary and Alternative Medications

Some individuals take complementary and alternative medications (CAM) to bolster their immune system (e.g., *Echinacea*, garlic, ginger, St. John's wort). However, CAM products are not thoroughly tested and have significant variability based on growing conditions and methods of harvest. Additionally, some CAM are harmful and may negatively affect the immune system (e.g., *Bupleurum,* glucosamine, red yeast rice, and cascara sagrada) or interact with prescription drugs. Patients should be advised to discuss all herbal supplementation with their health care provider.

COMMON PROBLEMS AND CONDITIONS

The immune deficits seen so often in older adults make this population more vulnerable to both infection and cancer. As people age, the likelihood of autoimmune antibodies being found in serum increases, which suggests an increased likelihood of autoimmune processes. However, whether such autoimmune processes are age related is still being debated (Kane et al., 2009).

Individuals with diminished immune function are susceptible to numerous infections. Some of the more common infections in older adults include influenza, pneumonia, tuberculosis, urinary tract infections (especially in women), and shingles (herpes zoster). Medical management of infections consists primarily of determining the source of the infection and prescribing the appropriate antibiotic or antiviral drug.

Influenza and Pneumonia

Pneumonia and influenza are ranked as the seventh-leading causes of death in older adults (Administration on Aging [AOA], 2012). More deaths from influenza occur in the 65 or older age group than in any other age group (Eliopoulos, 2005). The predominant portal of entry is inhalation of small droplets transmitted through sneezing, coughing, or talking. Closed populations such as those in long-term care facilities provide an ideal setting for the spread of influenza. The social environment in these institutions also facilitates transmission of influenza through group activities, communal dining rooms, and rehabilitation activities.

The most effective measure to control influenza is the vaccination of persons at high risk. Influenza vaccination is a Medicare-covered benefit for older adults, yet only 63.4% of the population 65 years or older was vaccinated during the 2015 to 2016 season; this number is down more than 3% from the previous year (Centers for Disease Control and Prevention [CDC], 2017). Every adult over the age of 65 should receive the influenza vaccination annually, unless they have had a serious reaction to a previous vaccination or are allergic to eggs (Wallace, 2008). Other strategies to control the nosocomial spread of influenza include the early identification and grouping of infected patients, careful hand washing, and the use of barrier precautions when handling bodily substances, especially respiratory secretions.

Community-acquired pneumonia is caused by multiple pathogens, the most common being *Streptococcus pneumoniae, Haemophilus influenzae,* atypical bacteria (i.e., *Chlamydia pneumoniae, Mycoplasma pneumoniae, Legionella sp*), and viruses (Sethi, 2017). Early recognition and treatment of bacterial pneumonia leads to recovery, although antibiotic resistance is becoming a problem. The pneumococcal vaccine is recommended for everyone over the age of 65; in 2008, 67% of older adults were vaccinated ("Pneumonia Fact Sheet," n.d.).

The major host factor associated with community-acquired pneumonia is advanced age (Wachtel & Fretwell, 2007). Smoking, excessive alcohol intake, chronic lung disease, recent history of viral upper respiratory tract infection, and neurologic disease (which may contribute to microaspiration of secretions from the oropharynx) are other contributing factors. Changes in lung function that come with aging enable inhaled microorganisms to survive and multiply. Social environments such as congregate housing, communal dining rooms, churches, crowded shopping centers, adult day care centers, or nursing facilities place older adults at risk for exposure and infection. However, social isolation is not recommended because of its negative psychological consequences. Older adults should be encouraged to select activities that reduce the risk of infection during the colder months.

Infection-control measures should be in place to reduce the risk of illness. Hand washing, monitoring fluids and nutritional intake, and proper disposal of bodily secretions help to manage the spread of infection when it does occur (Eliopoulos, 2005). Older adults and their families should be instructed to seek early medical attention for subtle changes that may signal the onset of infection. For example, pneumonia may be signaled by confusion or tachypnea, with no other findings. Many older adults present with atypical or diminished signs and symptoms. Nursing care of older patients must be attentive to ensure early detection of subtle changes (Eliopoulos, 2005).

Cancer

Neoplasms occur with greater frequency in older adults. Common types include lung cancer, breast cancer, and prostate cancer. However, the potential for numerous other forms of cancer should not be overlooked.

The presence of cancer reveals the presence of decreased immune response. Cancer cells are normally detected by the immune system and eliminated after being recognized as abnormal cells. It is only when the immune system fails to carry out this function that cancer occurs. However, the cancer and treatment for cancer may induce additional immune deficits.

For example, cancer is often accompanied by a decrease in appetite, which increases the possibility of malnutrition. Furthermore, anticancer drugs often deplete immune cells, causing further debilitation of the immune system. Because many of these drugs have their greatest effect on rapidly dividing cells, the rapidly dividing immune system cells are attacked concurrently with the cancer cells. Each patient's response to treatment is individual; decisions about treatment need to be personalized. The prognosis for cancer is highly variable depending on the time of diagnosis, the patient's general health, and the type of cancer.

Autoimmunity

Older adults may have autoimmune diseases such as RA; however, these cannot be considered solely age associated. Older adults with autoimmune diseases are more likely to take immunosuppressant drugs as treatment, and they still risk the immune deficits that accompany aging. Therefore, these older adults carry higher risks for infection compared with older adults without autoimmune disease. Criteria for identifying autoimmune disease include (1) evidence of autoimmune reaction, (2) determination that immunologic findings are not secondary to another condition, and (3) lack of other identified causes for the disorder.

Systemic Lupus Erythematosus

Systemic lupus erythematosus (SLE) may affect many parts of the body, including the joints, skin, kidneys, heart, lungs, blood vessels, and brain. The most common symptoms are extreme fatigue, painful or swollen joints, unexplained fever, skin rashes, and kidney problems. The antinuclear antibody (ANA) test is one of the more specific tests for SLE. There is no cure for SLE. The management objective is to control the severity of symptoms and prevent a flare. The warning signs of a flare are increased fatigue, pain, rash, fever, stomach discomfort, headache, and dizziness. Patients must monitor their health and learn to recognize symptoms of disease activity. Avoiding the sun, exercising, complying with drugs, limiting stress, and having regular health care visits are important.

Rheumatoid Arthritis

RA is characterized by inflammatory polyarthritis of unknown cause. Symptoms include morning stiffness lasting for hours, tenderness, pain on motion, limited range of motion, and joint deformity in the small joints of the hands and feet. Extraarticular signs are pulmonary (e.g., pleuritis and pneumonitis), cardiac (e.g., pericarditis and myocarditis), renal (e.g., amyloidosis), and ocular (e.g., scleritis); rheumatoid (subcutaneous) nodules also develop. The course of RA is highly variable; most people develop progressive functional limitation and physical disability. Patients with RA have a higher mortality rate compared with the general population. In addition to physical therapy, first-line drugs for RA are nonsteroidal antiinflammatory drugs (NSAIDs). These drugs reduce inflammation, pain, and swelling. During arthritis flare-ups or when NSAIDs are ineffective, patients may be treated with short bursts of corticosteroids. Because of their side effects, corticosteroids should not be used for long periods in high doses. Patients with RA also need drugs to slow joint destruction. These second-line drugs are known as *disease-modifying antirheumatic drugs* (DMARDs) and may take months to demonstrate an effect.

HUMAN IMMUNODEFICIENCY VIRUS INFECTION IN OLDER ADULTS

HIV infection is an underrecognized problem among the older adult population; 31% of persons living with HIV and 17% of newly diagnosed cases are in those over the age of 50 ("Older Adults and HIV/AIDS," n.d.). Many erroneously believe that the incidence of acquired immunodeficiency syndrome (AIDS) in older adults can be attributed to blood transfusions. However, the spread of HIV and AIDS is a multigenerational crisis. The low clinical suspicion of HIV infection and delayed recognition of AIDS-defining infections contributes to the poor prognosis of HIV infection in older adults. In older adults, only a short interval exists from HIV infection to the development of AIDS and death. The aging immune system is not able to eliminate the HIV residing in macrophages, lymphoid tissue, or the brain. Because the immune system's regenerative capacity is diminished and not all replacement cells are fully functional, the disease progresses more rapidly (Eliopoulos, 2005). The proportion of AIDS cases among older adults attributed to heterosexual transmission and intravenous drug use has continued to rise since 1988. Only a small proportion of older adults participating in risky sexual behavior reported the use of condoms.

These findings hold major implications for nursing practice. In assessing older adults, nurses must complete a sexual history. Nurses need to discuss HIV and risk behaviors for acquiring HIV. Older adults should be taught the proper use of condoms and how and when to get tested for HIV.

SIGNIFICANT NOSOCOMIAL PATHOGENS

Clostridium difficile

C. difficile is a nosocomial pathogen. The presence of *C. difficile* alone does not indicate infection. Disease occurs when this organism is present and the normal flora of the bowel are disturbed. *C. difficile* produces toxins, which cause hemorrhaging and cellular damage, resulting in fluid accumulation in the intestines. The hallmark diarrhea is caused by a motility-altering factor that stimulates muscle contractions.

C. difficile is transmitted person to person, primarily from the hands of health care workers. It has also been transmitted indirectly through contaminated equipment such as rectal probes and electronic thermometers. Consistent hand washing between contacts with patients and the use of gloves when handling body substances such as feces are imperative. Patients with *C. difficile* should be placed in private rooms with their own bathrooms or commodes.

Treatment begins with discontinuing current antibiotic therapy, then treatment with oral vancomycin or fidaxomicin. For patients who experience recurrent *C. difficile* infections that do not respond to antibiotics, fecal microbiota transplant should be considered (Nogrady, 2018).

Vancomycin-Resistant Enterococcus

VRE was first identified in the United States in 1989 (Wachtel & Fretwell, 2007). Multiple factors predispose a person to infection with VRE, but colonization precedes most infections (Wachtel & Fretwell, 2007). Vancomycin use has increased dramatically in the past 20 years because of many factors, including increases in the incidence of methicillin-resistant *Staphylococcus aureus* (MRSA). Risk factors for VRE acquisition include an age of more than 65 years, antimicrobial therapy, chronic kidney disease, serious illness, and prolonged hospitalization (Wachtel & Fretwell, 2007).

VRE is transmitted from person to person via the hands of health care workers. VRE is also transmitted by contaminated medical devices, including electronic thermometers, fluidized beds, and environmental surfaces (Wachtel & Fretwell, 2007). To control transmission of VRE, health care workers must perform a meticulous 15-second hand washing with an antimicrobial soap. Dedicated equipment (e.g., stethoscopes) is required for infected patients. Colonized and infected patients should be isolated in private rooms or grouped with other infected patients in the acute care setting. Barrier precautions, gloves, and gowns should be implemented for patient care. Antibiotics are not used in persons with colonization but no symptoms; symptomatic patients should be treated with antibiotics indicated through culture and sensitivity.

Methicillin-Resistant *Staphylococcus aureus*

In the early 1940s, when penicillin first became available, *S. aureus* was highly susceptible to antibiotic treatment. By the early 1950s, 80% of nosocomial *S. aureus* was resistant to penicillin. Methicillin became available in the 1960s, and by the mid-1970s, MRSA became a significant problem.

MRSA is transmitted from patient to patient via the hands of health care workers; transmission often occurs when patients are transferred from institution to institution, especially nursing homes (Wachtel & Fretwell, 2007). MRSA may also be transmitted via contaminated equipment, especially in burn units. Risk factors for acquiring MRSA are insulin-dependent diabetes mellitus, chronic hemodialysis, illicit intravenous drug use, prolonged hospitalization, prolonged antibiotic therapy, stays in intensive care or burn units, and rooming next to a patient colonized or infected with MRSA. Control of MRSA focuses on health care worker hand washing to reduce transmission. Health care workers should wear gloves for all contact with patients who are either colonized or infected. MRSA-positive patients should be placed in private rooms. Antibiotics are not used in persons with colonization but no symptoms; symptomatic patients should be treated with antibiotics indicated through culture and sensitivity.

NURSING MANAGEMENT

Assessment

With such a spectrum of possible infections, clinical assessment varies widely. However, health care workers must keep in mind some crucial aspects to assessing older adults for the presence of infection (Box 14.2). Older adults with

---

> **BOX 14.2** **Assessment of Individuals at High Risk for Infection**
>
> **Subjective**
> Take history:
> - Previous infections
> - Predisposing illnesses
> - Drugs
> - Vaccinations
> - Living environment
> - Lifestyle factors (e.g., smoking, activity level, and chemical exposures)
> - Social support system
>
> **Objective**
> Assess for signs and symptoms of infection:
> - Fever: high grade or low grade
> - Inflammation: pronounced or slight
> - Pain: slight or severe
> - Malaise, fatigue
> - Turbidity, odor, and amount of body fluids
> - Complete blood cell (CBC) count with differential

decreased immune function may not exhibit classic symptoms of infection. Diminished inflammatory response may lead to false-negative results for skin tests used in the diagnosis of disease, for example, the purified protein derivative (PPD) skin test for tuberculosis (Eliopoulos, 2005). Similarly, redness, swelling, or inflammation may be reduced with infections. These reduced responses are even more likely to occur in people who have diseases or drug treatments that further suppress the immune system, for example, patients with cancer or those taking immunosuppressants.

Another classic example of a reduced response to infection is the absence of fever. With an infection, local or systemic fever is provoked by the immune response. In younger adults, an elevated temperature is an indicator of infection. However, in older adults with decreased immune function, temperature increase may be limited or no increase may occur at all (Newson, 2007). Symptoms of pain may also be reduced or absent. Thus infection in these older adults may progress to the life-threatening stage before it is detected.

Because of this reduced immune response, mild symptoms such as a low-grade fever must be taken seriously. Close observation is needed to detect subtle symptoms. Changes in the behavior of patients (e.g., increased malaise or fatigue, especially combined with other symptoms) may indicate the onset of infection. Fever and inflammation may be reduced, whereas the white blood cell (WBC) count may still reflect an increased value (Wachtel & Fretwell, 2007). However, if immunosuppression is present from drug treatment for diseases such as cancer or AIDS, elevations in WBC counts may not be seen, even with severe infection.

In addition to observed data, subjective and historical data are valuable when evaluating older adults with infection. A history of previous episodes of infection, including the timing, nature, and severity of the infection, is important. Infections in older adults often recur. Information regarding exposure to others with infections may also be helpful. Older adults are more susceptible to infection, especially if they are living in environments conducive to the spread of pathogens. Such environments include nursing facilities, hospitals, and crowded environments, where strict hygiene standards are difficult to maintain. Immunization records also provide important information that needs to be kept on file.

It is also important to determine other disease processes for which patients may currently be receiving treatment. Persons with cancer may be experiencing assaults on their immune systems from the disease and from treatment. Older adults with autoimmune diseases may be receiving antiinflammatory and immunosuppressant drugs. Individuals with HIV infection experience an extreme assault on their immune system. All of these make older adults more prone to a variety of infections.

A thorough drug history is necessary to detect the potential for drug-related immunosuppression. This record should include both prescription and over-the-counter drugs, herbs, and other dietary supplements. Patients receiving drugs with immunosuppressant qualities are more prone to infections. In addition, information on the use of alcohol, tobacco, and other drugs, as well as exposure to toxic substances, should be obtained.

Knowledge about a patient's lifestyle may provide invaluable information in developing a care plan. Information should include a thorough nutritional history as well as activity and exercise habits. An understanding of an individual's social support system should be acquired, and indicators of life stressors should be elicited. A classic life stressor is bereavement, especially the loss of a spouse. However, the loss of friends and other family members should not be overlooked. Even the loss of a home or relocation to another place may result in a sense of bereavement.

Diagnosis

Several nursing diagnoses may be applicable to older patients who either have infections or are at high risk for developing infections. The risk factors determined during the assessment indicate potential nursing diagnoses. For example, many older adults are either inadequately or inappropriately nourished. Thus a diagnosis of "inadequate nutrition" is likely. People with cancer may be malnourished because of lack of appetite or side effects resulting from drugs. Poor nutrition may also be attributed to self-care deficit in preparing and eating food; older adults sometimes have difficulty preparing their own meals. These difficulties may be related to a variety of problems such as visual deficits, arthritis, or depression. Regardless of the cause, if these self-care deficits result in poor nutrition, the older adults are then at higher risk for infection.

The diagnosis "potential for infection" is applicable to those at risk for developing an infection and those with existing infections. The presence of an infection indicates the immune system is already challenged. This increases the likelihood of a secondary infection. For instance, it is not unusual for an individual with viral influenza to later develop a secondary bacterial infection of pneumococcal pneumonia.

A diagnosis of "need for health teaching" is also a possibility. Knowledge deficits may be in the areas of (1) immunizations,

(2) nutrition, or (3) protection against infection from oneself or others. Patients may be unaware of their nutritional needs or the relationship between nutritional and immune status. If they have this knowledge, older adults may be more likely to consume appropriate foods. Similarly, older adults may be unaware of available vaccinations or the benefit such vaccinations may hold for them. Older individuals need information on ways to reduce their risk for developing infections.

Finally, "reduced social interaction" may be a relevant diagnosis associated with the individual at risk for infection because social support has also been associated with immune status.

Planning and Expected Outcomes

In planning care for older patients, the health care team and patients must set goals together. Goals must be congruent with realistic expectations and with patients' desired outcomes. For individuals at increased risk for infection, goals include (1) avoiding primary or secondary infection and (2) maintaining or improving immune status. A careful assessment of patient knowledge in areas related to infection prevention, maintenance of immune status, and health practices determines the goals for patient teaching.

In setting nutritional goals, nurses might find a consultation with a registered dietitian appropriate. They must consider patients' dietary preferences and financial ability to buy food (if not in an institutional setting). An outcome might be that a patient consumes a well-balanced, high-calorie diet daily. Patients with cancer may have even more extreme nutritional needs. An outcome for these individuals might be that they stabilize body weight and then gradually increase it at a rate of 1 pound every 3 weeks. Another outcome may be that a patient performs self-care activities with minimum energy expenditure and risk of injury. For patients with activity deficits, an appropriate goal might be to participate in 15 minutes of moderate exercise three times a week. The exact target goal for exercise should be established in consultation with the primary care provider and possibly achieved through physical therapy.

Intervention

Nursing management of older adults with alterations in immunity focuses on the prevention of infections. Interventions addressing this goal are targeted at (1) preventing exposure to infections and (2) enhancing the immune system to enable patients to better resist infections. Totally preventing exposure to pathogens is impossible, especially because one source of pathogens is the body's own natural flora. However, exposure can be minimized for individuals with diminished immune capacity. During times of epidemics such as during the influenza season, the patient should try to avoid places with crowds of people. In an institutional or home setting, visitors should be screened for respiratory infections. If contact is unavoidable, infected visitors may be given a mask to wear to minimize potential contamination of the patients. Any catheters, intravenous fluids, or similar therapeutic devices should be carefully assessed for pathogen growth. Teaching patients to drink at least 2000 milliliters (mL) of fluids a day, unless contraindicated, will aid in preventing urinary tract infection and constipation. In addition, teaching stress

management techniques to promote immune system function may be indicated. Finally, hygiene standards should be rigorously maintained, especially for patients experiencing treatment-induced immune suppression, as is seen with some anticancer drugs. In addition to normal bathing, careful attention should be paid to oral and perineal care. Both patients and caregivers should be alert for changes in the color, consistency, and odor of body fluids to detect the onset of infections.

Nutritional Interventions

Other measures may be taken to strengthen the immune system to better enable patients to resist infection. As previously mentioned, optimal nutritional status is important. Although all nutritional needs for healthy older adults may be met through normal dietary intake, many older adults have dietary deficiencies. In patients with cancer, the nutritional deficits may be extreme. After assessment, efforts should be made to resolve detected deficiencies. In institutional settings, dietary supplements and frequent meals may be supplied. Food may be prepared specifically to suit the patients' tastes and needs. For older adults in the community, it is helpful to have services such as Meals on Wheels, assistance with food preparation, or the ability to visit a senior center nutrition site. Liquid food supplements or over-the-counter vitamins are other alternatives. However, these may be beyond the financial resources of some patients.

The inability to feed oneself is another barrier to proper nutrition. Individuals feeding patients, either in the home or institutional setting, must ensure that the patients receive a balanced, nutritional diet. Family members or nonprofessional care providers may need special instruction on how best to accomplish this with patients.

Psychosocial Interventions

A variety of modalities based on the relationships between psychosocial factors and immunity are available, and their use may enhance immunocompetence. These include (1) relaxation and visualization, (2) social support, and (3) exercise.

Exercise programs should be tailored to suit individual abilities. For patients with physical debility, exercise programs should be tailored to meet their specific needs and interests. Possible exercises include walking, dancing or dancelike movements, water exercises, or swimming. It is important to develop exercise programs that are moderately difficult rather than strenuous for older individuals.

As the relationships between immune status and psychosocial variables are explored, new treatment modalities are developed. Modalities currently being explored include biofeedback, therapeutic touch, and hypnosis.

Evaluation

Monitoring the success of interventions is based on patients' responses in meeting their goals and outcomes. One standard for evaluation is whether a patient contracts an infection, either through contact with others or by his or her own flora. Improving or at least maintaining immune status may be more difficult for some patients because the understanding of both the immune system and the concomitant changes that occur

EVIDENCE-BASED PRACTICE

Effect of Probiotics on C. difficile *Infection*

Background

Clostridium difficile is a leading cause of infectious diarrhea. The incidence has tripled in the last decade. *C. difficile*-associated diarrhea leads to increased morbidity, mortality, longer hospitalizations, and increased cost.

Sample/Setting

Following specified inclusion and exclusion criteria, five studies were selected for inclusion in the systematic review. Inclusion criteria included participants 60 years or older, patients in acute and postacute care facilities on, or intending to start, antibiotics therapy. Additionally, participants took probiotic capsules or probiotic-containing food products compared with placebo. In total, the five studies included 3,461 participants, whose mean age was over 70 years.

Method

Two independent reviewers assessed the selected experimental designed studies for methodological quality using critical appraisal instruments from the Joanna Briggs Institute (JBI). Data were extracted from the papers using the standardized data extraction tool from the JBI Meta-Analysis of Statistics Assessment and Review Instrument.

Findings

Of the five studies, only one found statistically significant results between participants receiving probiotics and those receiving placebo. The other studies demonstrated no effect on the incidence of *C. difficile* infection. However, across the studies, the type of probiotic treatment was inconsistent, as well as the strain of bacteria, method of administration and dose.

Implications

Probiotics were not found to be more effective than placebo for reducing *C. difficile* infection in hospitalized older adults. More studies need to be completed examining dose, frequency, method of administration, length of administration and number of strains of bacteria administered. Nurses should strive to be knowledgeable about the treatments with the best supporting evidence for their patients.

From Vernaya, M., McAdam, J., & Hampton, M. D. (2017). Effectiveness of probiotics in reducing the incidence of Clostridium difficile-associated diarrhea in elderly patients: A systematic review. *JBI Database of Systematic Reviews and Implementation Reports, 15*(1), 140-164. doi: 10.11124/jbisrir-2016-003234.

with aging is incomplete. Furthermore, many individuals are enduring severe assaults on their immune systems. Persons with cancer receive anticancer drugs that may literally destroy the immune response. In persons with AIDS, the immune system is directly targeted by viral attack. Interventions such as diet, exercise, and psychosocial enhancement are rarely sufficient in overcoming such odds, although unexplained recoveries have been known to occur. For most situations, it may be unreasonable to expect a return to normal status for immunocompromised individuals. However, any improvement in immune status, or even maintenance, may allow older patients to live better lives (see the Nursing Care Plan boxes).

◎ NURSING CARE PLAN

Pneumococcal Pneumonia

Clinical Situation

Mrs. C is an 80-year-old woman admitted to the hospital for treatment of pneumococcal pneumonia, which she developed while she had influenza. She lives alone in a low-rent housing development in a large city, having moved there 2 years ago after the death of her husband. Without his income, she was unable to afford the rent on her previous home. Her nearest family member, a niece, lives 75 miles away and rarely visits. Her former neighbors, who live across town, are unable to visit because of the distance and because of their own debilities. Mrs. C is 20% underweight for her height and is anemic. Her WBC count is high. Her blood values are as follows: red blood cell count, 3.7/milliliter (mL); hematocrit, 34%; hemoglobin, 10.8; WBC count, 18,200/mL; and serum albumin, 2.6 grams per deciliter (g/dL).

Nursing Diagnoses

Potential for infection resulting from compromised immune status

Inadequate nutrition resulting from low income, transportation difficulties

Reduced social interaction resulting from loss of friends and limited contact with family

Need for health teaching resulting from influenza and pneumococcal vaccination because of new experience

Outcomes

The patient will not experience additional infections as evidenced by (1) WBC count returning to normal limits, (2) afebrile state, and (3) other vital signs being within normal limits.

The patient will verbalize knowledge of infection prevention strategies.

The patient will have adequate nutrition as demonstrated by (1) weight gain of half-pound per week, (2) an increased hemoglobin level, and (3) an increased serum protein level.

The patient will consume a well-balanced, sufficient-calorie diet, as evidenced by (1) calorie counts showing an intake of at least 1,800 calories per day and (2) consumption of food from all food groups, including protein sources, breads, fruits and vegetables, and dairy products.

The patient will acquire social contacts desirable to her, as evidenced by (1) spending time each week with others and (2) voicing satisfaction with social contacts.

The patient will identify the advantages of the influenza and pneumococcal vaccines.

Interventions

Screen all visitors with infection who may come into direct contact with the patient.

Provide family and visitors with information on transmission of infection.

Teach the patient that she is at risk for additional infections because of her depressed immune status and should limit her exposure to additional pathogens. Observe for slight increases in temperature every 4 hours or more often, as needed.

Be aware that the patient may develop subtle or undetected signs and symptoms of infection and that slight changes in temperature may be highly significant.

Observe for increased respiratory difficulty.

Auscultate the patient's lungs at every shift.

◎ NURSING CARE PLAN—CONT'D

Have the patient report any sore throat.

Monitor dietary intake using calorie counts.

Teach what constitutes a well-balanced diet that is high in protein.

Ensure adequate intake of vitamins and trace minerals through diet or supplements.

Encourage the patient to eat foods that include vitamins and minerals, as well as trace minerals such as zinc and magnesium.

Provide vitamin and mineral supplements in addition to the high-protein diet, if needed.

Arrange for Meals on Wheels on discharge or facilitate attendance at a nutrition site to provide better nutrition after discharge.

Contact churches or other organizations to include the patient in their social gatherings to help her reestablish a social support system.

Assess the patient's level of stress to determine whether an easily accessible, low-exertion relaxation program is indicated. (A relaxation program may provide an easily accessible, low-exertion intervention with an immune benefit.)

Plan a program of graduated exercise designed to fit the patient's tolerance.

Contact social services or a local senior citizen center to identify center activities and transportation.

Contact area organizations or churches for information about activities.

Provide information to the patient and develop a plan of action with her.

Provide information for the patient regarding the influenza vaccine: (1) influenza could be a serious, life-threatening condition in older people; (2) yearly immunization (in early fall) is important to protect her from getting influenza; (3) the signs and symptoms of influenza are weakness, coughing, headaches, a sudden increase in temperature, aches, chills, and occasional vomiting; and (4) pneumonia is a common complication of influenza.

Refer the patient to her primary care provider for specific advice regarding recuperation time before taking the vaccine.

Provide information for the patient on the pneumococcal vaccine—primarily that she should be immunized once in her lifetime.

Inform her that the vaccine should not be administered soon after having pneumonia.

Refer the patient to her primary care provider for the specific timing of administration after her illness.

◎ NURSING CARE PLAN

Effects of Chemotherapy

Clinical Situation

Mrs. M is a 68-year-old woman who is receiving chemotherapy after a modified radical mastectomy for breast cancer. Although she was previously well nourished, chemotherapy has diminished her appetite and stomatitis has made eating painful. In addition, the chemotherapy has decreased her WBC count to 2000. Mrs. M lives with her husband in their home. She receives her chemotherapy on an outpatient basis but is visited daily by a home health nurse to maintain her Hickman catheter.

Nursing Diagnoses

Potential for infection resulting from suppressed immune system

Inadequate nutrition resulting from inability to eat secondary to side effects of chemotherapy

Outcomes

The patient will not develop an infection, as evidenced by (1) no temperature elevation, (2) no elevation in WBC count, (3) no sore throat or mouth, and (4) no redness or irritation around wounds, intravenous tubes, or catheters.

The patient will have adequate intake of proteins, vitamins, and minerals, as evidenced by (1) calorie counts of at least 2000 calories per day and (2) maintenance of body weight.

Interventions

Teach the patient to minimize exposure to pathogens and to screen visitors with contagious infections.

Explain the need to maintain careful hygiene (e.g., daily shower and proper oral, foot, and perineal care).

Use sterile technique when working with Hickman catheter.

Monitor the patient's mouth and throat for signs of infection such as white patches or redness; teach the patient to report the same to the nurse.

Auscultate the lungs at each visit.

Teach the patient to monitor body fluids for alterations in color, odor, or consistency.

Encourage fluid intake of at least 2000 milliliters per day unless otherwise indicated.

Teach the patient to eat small, frequent meals, rich in protein, vitamins, and minerals.

Teach the patient about food sources high in calories, protein, vitamins, and minerals.

Have the patient take food supplements to increase intake, if needed.

Teach the importance of eating nutrient-dense foods (e.g., those with high nutritional content in small volumes).

Acquire an oral anesthetic to treat stomatitis.

Teach the patient how to prepare bland foods of moderate temperature.

▌SUMMARY

This chapter explored age-related changes in the immune system. The influences of other factors, such as psychosocial influences and nutrition, on the immune status of older adults were also discussed. Discussions on cancer, autoimmune diseases, HIV, and significant nosocomial pathogens in older adults were also presented.

A key role of the nurse in caring for older adults in all settings is to recognize the potential for infection in this population and develop care plans to prevent infection and promote its early detection. Because of the increased risk of morbidity and mortality associated with infection in this age group, immunizations and interventions specific to various body systems should be implemented for those identified as susceptible to infection.

HOME CARE

1. Assess nutritional and dietary status to ensure proper immune functioning in homebound older adults.
2. Instruct older adults and caregivers about the need to receive a balanced nutritional diet and the role of vitamin supplements in promoting proper immune functioning.
3. An altered emotional state may lead to decreased immune functioning in homebound older adults.
4. Vaccinations are imperative for homebound older adults (e.g., annual influenza vaccine and pneumococcal vaccine [Pneumovax]).
5. Assess and report any signs of impaired immunity (e.g., fever and changes in white blood cell [WBC] count).
6. Bedridden or immunocompromised older adults are at high risk for infections. Instruct older adults and caregivers about ways to protect the older adults from infection from themselves and others.
7. Tailor an exercise program for homebound or bedridden older adults to enhance their immune system and to prevent infection.
8. Assess how homebound older adults manage personal hygiene and teach them the importance of hand washing.
9. Practice appropriate cleaning and maintenance of humidifiers, catheters, respiratory equipment, and other devices used in home care–related treatment.
10. Develop a plan for alternative care in case a caregiver develops an infection.

KEY POINTS

- With aging, the immune response diminishes.
- The diminished immune response reduces the normal responses to infection, such as fever, which makes infection in older adults more difficult to detect.
- Nutrition, especially regarding protein, energy, vitamins, and trace minerals, has a substantial effect on immune status.
- Activity has a substantial effect on immune status. Even moderate amounts of daily exercise may enhance immune status.
- Interventions dealing with infection and decreased immune response must address nutrition, exercise, mood, stress, and physical protection.

CRITICAL-THINKING EXERCISE

1. Your neighbor is a 72-year-old woman whose husband died last year. Since his death, she has become sedentary and withdrawn. Feeling concerned about her, you decide to stop by to see her. She explains that she has been ill off and on for the past few weeks and does not understand why she keeps getting sick. She says she is losing faith in her doctor. Recognizing that her depression and sedentary lifestyle may have altered her immune response, how might you intervene to help her?

REFERENCES

Administration on Aging. (2012). *A profile of older Americans: 2012.* Retrieved from http://www.aoa.gov/AoARoot/Aging_Statistics/Profile/index.aspx.

Agrawal, A., Sridharan, A., Prakash, S., & Agrawal, H. (2012). Dendritic cells and aging. Retrieved from *Expert Review of Clinical Immunology, 8*(1), 73–80. http://www.medscape.com/viewarticle/755539.

Akincigil, A., Olfson, M., Walkup, J. T., Siegel, M. J., Kalay, E., Amin, S., & Crystal, S. (2011). Diagnosis and treatment of depression in older community-dwelling adults: 1992–2005. *Journal of the American Geriatrics Society, 59*, 1042–1051. https://doi.org/10.1111/j.1532-5415.2011.03447.x.

American Association of Suicidology. (2018). *Facts & statistics.* Retrieved May 27, 2018 from http://www.suicidology.org/resources/facts-statistics.

Centers for Disease Control and Prevention. (2017). *Flu Vaccination Coverage, United States, 2015-16 Influenza Season.* Retrieved February 28, 2018 from https://www.cdc.gov/flu/fluvaxview/coverage-1516estimates.htm#age-group-adults.

Goldman, L., & Ausiello, D. (2004). *Cecil textbook of medicine* (22nd ed.). Philadelphia: W.B. Saunders.

Eliopoulos, C. (2005). Immunity. In C. Eliopoulos (Ed.), *Gerontological nursing.* Philadelphia: Lippincott.

Frasca, D., & Blomberg, B. B. (2011). Aging affects human B cell responses. *Journal of Clinical Immunology, 31*, 430–435. https://doi.org/10.1007/s10875-010-9501-7.

Immune system, skin microbiome "complement" one another, finds Penn medicine study. (2013). Retrieved from http://www.uphs.upenn.edu/news/News_Releases/2013/08/grice/.

Kane, R., Ouslander, J., Abrass, I., & Resnick, B. (2009). *Essentials of clinical geriatrics* (6th ed.). New York: McGraw-Hill.

Newson, P. (2007). Presentation of illness in the elderly patient. *Nursing Residential Care, 9*(5), 218–221.

Nogrady, B. (2018). *New C. difficile guidelines recommend fecal microbiota transplants.* Retrieved February 28, 2018 from https://www.mdedge.com/internalmedicinenews/article/158669/gastroenterology/new-c-difficile-guidelines-recommend-fecal.

Nowson, C. (2007). Nutritional challenges for the elderly. *Nutrition and Dietetics, 64*(Suppl 4), S150–S155.

Older adults and HIV/AIDS. (n.d.). Retrieved January 22, 2014, from http://www.aoa.gov/AoARoot/AoA_Programs/HPW/HIV_AIDS/.

Pneumonia fact sheet. (n.d.). Retrieved January 22, 2014, from http://www.lung.org/lung-disease/influenza/in-depth-resources/pneumonia-fact-sheet.html.

Porth, C. M. (2004). *Pathophysiology: concepts of altered health state* (7th ed.). Philadelphia: Lippincott Williams & Wilkins.

Sethi, S. (2017). *Community-acquired pneumonia*. Retrieved February 28, 2018 from http://www.merckmanuals.com/professional/pulmonary-disorders/pneumonia/community-acquired-pneumonia.

Span, P. (2013, August 7). Suicide rates are high among the elderly. *The New York Times*. Retrieved on January 24, 2014 from http://newoldage.blogs.nytimes.com/2013/08/07/high-suicide-rates-among-the-elderly/?_php=true&_type=blogs&_r=0.

Townsend, M. C. (2008). *In Essentials of psychiatric mental health nursing* (4th ed., pp. 581–609). Philadelphia: FA Davis.

United States Census Bureau. (2017). *The nation's older population is still growing, census bureau reports [Press Release CB17–100]*. Retrieved from https://www.census.gov/newsroom/press-releases/2017/cb17-100.html.

Wachtel, T., & Fretwell, M. (2007). *Practical guide to the care of the geriatric patient* (3rd ed.). Philadelphia: Mosby/Elsevier.

Wallace, M. (2008). *Essentials of gerontological nursing*. New York: Springer Publishing Company.

PART IV

Diagnostic Studies and Pharmacologic Management

15

Laboratory and Diagnostic Tests

Jennifer J. Yeager, PhD, RN, APRN

e http://evolve.elsevier.com/Meiner/gerontologic

LEARNING OBJECTIVES

On completion of this chapter, the reader will be able to:

1. Identify key laboratory values that increase or decrease with aging.
2. Describe the effect of aging on the erythrocyte sedimentation rate.
3. Name two medications that can interfere with potassium excretion and affect serum potassium levels.
4. Explain the difference between serum creatinine concentrations in younger adults and older adults.
5. Explain the relationship between bacteria in urine and urinary tract infections in older adults.
6. Relate the significance of troponin levels in diagnosing cardiac emergencies.
7. Explain the relationship of the brain natriuretic peptide to heart failure.
8. Discuss the role of laboratory tests in determining thyroid function in older adults.
9. Describe the nurse's role in interpreting laboratory values in older adults.

WHAT WOULD YOU DO?

What would you do if you were faced with the following situations?

- Your 68-year-old patient has been taking nitrofurantoin 100 mg orally twice a day for 3 days for a urinary tract infection (UTI). Your patient calls the office reporting of abdominal pain and malaise. Before a follow-up appointment, labs are drawn and show an AST of 118 units/L and an ALT of 150 units/L. What would you do?
- Your new admit to the nursing home, an 88-year-old female, comes in with routine, baseline laboratory work, which includes a urinalysis that is nitrite negative, leukocyte esterase negative and 80,000 colony-forming units per milliliter of bacteria. What would you do?

Diagnostic testing in older adults takes on a different meaning than testing in younger adults. The nurse must realize that laboratory values are classified into three general groups regarding aging: (1) those that change with aging; (2) those that do not change with aging; and (3) those for which it is unclear whether aging, disease, or both change the values (Sarkozi, 2002).

The gerontologic nurse must consider the effect of laboratory and diagnostic testing on an older adult's overall health and well-being. For example, with aging, subcutaneous tissue is decreased, and the fragility of veins is increased. Consequently, a frail older adult is more likely to have increased bruising and discomfort after a venous blood drawing. It is also important for the nurse to know what tests have been ordered to be able to provide an explanation to an anxious older adult; the patient's anxiety may range from concerns about the cost of tests, to a concern for privacy, to concerns about the test results.

The gerontologic nurse should have a basic understanding of the purpose of commonly ordered laboratory and diagnostic tests, the importance of selected hematologic and blood and urine chemistry components in the body's overall function, and the relative reference ranges for younger and older adults. These reference ranges may vary from institution to institution as well as in the literature (Table 15.1). Because of the scant research conducted on older adults, geriatricians and gerontologists may disagree as to whether changes are related to aging or disease (Beers & Berkow, 2000). When interpreting laboratory values and deciding the best course of treatment, the older adult should be viewed holistically; signs, symptoms, and test results should all be considered.

COMPONENTS OF HEMATOLOGIC TESTING

Blood is composed of cells (erythrocytes and leukocytes), specialized cell fragments (platelets), and a fluid matrix called *plasma*. The cells and cell fragments are suspended in the plasma, which is the largest component of the body's extracellular fluid (Thibodeau & Patton, 2003).

Red Blood Cells

Red blood cells (RBCs), or erythrocytes, are nonnucleated biconcave disks that carry molecules of hemoglobin. Hemoglobin allows the transport and exchange of oxygen and carbon dioxide. The average life span of an erythrocyte is 120 days. Although aging does not affect the life span of an erythrocyte,

TABLE 15.1 Hematology Test

Name	Adult Normals	Older Adult Normals	Significance of Deviations
Red blood cells (RBCs)	4.2–6.1 million/unit	Unchanged with aging	*Low:* hemorrhage, anemia, chronic illness, kidney failure, pernicious anemia *High:* high altitude, polycythemia, dehydration
Hemoglobin	12–18 grams per deciliter (g/dL)	Values may be slightly decreased	*Low:* anemia, cancer, nutritional deficiency, kidney disease *High:* polycythemia, heart failure (HF), chronic obstructive pulmonary disease (COPD), high altitudes, dehydration
Hematocrit	37%–52%	Values may be slightly decreased	*Low:* anemia, cirrhosis, hemorrhage, malnutrition, rheumatoid arthritis *High:* polycythemia, severe dehydration, severe diarrhea, COPD
White blood cells (WBCs) (total)	5.0–10.0 thousands/cubic millimeter (mm^3)	Unchanged with aging	*Low:* drug toxicity, infections, autoimmune disease, dietary deficiency *High:* infection, trauma, stress, inflammation
Neutrophils	55%–70%	Unchanged with aging	*Low:* dietary deficiency, overwhelming bacterial infection, viral infections, drug therapy *High:* physical and emotional stress, trauma, inflammatory disorders
Eosinophils	1%–4%	Unchanged with aging	*Low:* increased adrenosteroid production *High:* parasitic infections, allergic reactions, autoimmune disorders
Basophils	0.5%–1%	Unchanged with aging	*Low:* acute allergic reactions, stress reactions *High:* myeloproliferative disease
Monocytes	2%–8%	Unchanged with aging	*Low:* drug therapy (predisposition) *High:* chronic inflammatory disorders, tuberculosis, chronic ulcerative colitis
Lymphocytes	20%–40%	Unchanged with aging	*Low:* leukemia, sepsis, systemic lupus erythematosus, chemotherapy, radiation *High:* chronic bacterial infection, viral infections, radiation, infectious hepatitis
Folic acid	5–25 nanograms per milliliter (ng/mL)	Unchanged with aging	*Low:* malnutrition, folic acid anemia, hemolytic anemia, alcoholism, liver disease, chronic kidney disease *High:* pernicious anemia
Vitamin B$_{12}$	160–950 picograms per milliliter (pg/mL)	Unchanged with aging	*Low:* pernicious anemia, inflammatory bowel disease, atrophic gastritis, folic acid deficiency *High:* leukemia, polycythemia, severe liver dysfunction
Total iron-binding capacity (TIBC)	250–460 micrograms per deciliter (mcg/dL)	Unchanged with aging	*Low:* hypoproteinemia, cirrhosis, hemolytic anemia, pernicious anemia *High:* polycythemia, iron deficiency anemia
Iron (Fe)	60–180 mcg/dL	Unchanged with aging	*Low:* insufficient dietary iron, chronic blood loss, inadequate absorption of iron *High:* hemochromocytosis, hemolytic anemia, hepatitis, iron poisoning
Uric acid	4–8.5 mg/dL	May be slightly increased	*Low:* lead poisoning *High:* gout, increased ingestion of purines, chronic kidney disease, hypothyroidism
Prothrombin time (PT)	11–12.5 seconds (sec)	Unchanged with aging	*High:* liver disease, vitamin K deficiency, warfarin ingestion, bile duct obstruction, salicylate intoxication
Partial thromboplastin time (PTT)	60–70 sec	Unchanged with aging	*Low:* early stages of disseminated intravascular coagulation, metastatic cancer *High:* coagulation factor deficiency, cirrhosis, vitamin K deficiency, heparin administration
D-dimer	<0.4 mcg/mL (<0.4 mg/L SI units)	Unchanged with aging	*High:* deep vein thrombosis, disseminated intravascular coagulation, pulmonary embolism, recent surgery, sepsis
Platelets	150,000–400,000/mm^3	Unchanged with aging	*Low:* hemorrhage, thrombocytopenia, systemic lupus erythematosus, pernicious anemia, chemotherapy, infection *High:* malignancy, polycythemia, rheumatoid arthritis, iron deficiency anemia

Adapted from Pagana, K. D., & Pagana, T. J. (2018). *Mosby's manual of diagnostic and laboratory tests* (6th ed.). St. Louis, MO: Elsevier.

replenishment after bleeding may be delayed because of a decrease in hematopoietic tissue occupying marrow of the long bones (McCance & Huether, 2014).

RBCs are necessary for maintaining oxygen and carbon dioxide transport. A reduction in the number of circulating RBCs, a decrease in the quality or quantity of hemoglobin, a decrease in the volume of packed cells (hematocrit), or a combination of these factors is classified as anemia. Anemia may be attributed to (1) impaired erythrocyte production, (2) blood loss, (3) increased erythrocyte destruction, (4) dietary deficiency, (5) genetic disorders, or (6) a combination of these causes. Anemia is a clinical sign, not a disease process itself. Signs of anemia may go unnoticed if the anemia is mild, or the patient may experience overt symptoms such as fatigue, shortness of breath, and paresthesia (McCance & Huether, 2014). In addition, clinicians may miss signs of anemia, even in markedly anemic older patients (Ham, Sloane, & Warshaw, 2001). The combination of vague symptomatology and vague clinical presentation may lead the health care provider to attribute an older adult's complaints to "old age" and fail to investigate adequately.

Other conditions involving erythrocytes are related to increased cell numbers and abnormality in the cells themselves. Overproduction of RBCs is known as *polycythemia.* This may occur secondarily because of hypoxia caused by chronic pulmonary disease or heart failure (HF). In sickle cell anemia, the RBCs become abnormal in shape and surface composition because of a genetic defect in the hemoglobin.

Hemoglobin

Hemoglobin is an important iron-containing protein carried on RBCs that makes up about one-third of the weight of the RBC. Hemoglobin is necessary for the transport of oxygen; a reduction in hemoglobin may result in a decrease in oxygen content and an increase in fatigue. Rarely, genetic mutations occur producing abnormal hemoglobin, which may result in sickle cell disease and thalassemia.

Hematocrit

The hematocrit is the percentage of total blood volume that represents erythrocytes. This is determined in the laboratory by centrifuging a sample of blood, causing the heavier red cells to sink to the bottom of the tube while the less dense plasma rises to the top. The percentage of cells to liquid is calculated, giving the hematocrit reading. An increase in the hematocrit may signal volume depletion. A decrease in hematocrit may be a result of disease or dietary deficiencies. Hematocrit and hemoglobin values decline slightly after the age of 90 (Pagana & Pagana, 2018).

White Blood Cells

White blood cells (WBCs), or leukocytes, are another type of cell present in blood. Their major function is defense against foreign substances. WBCs function mainly in the interstitial fluid. Leukocytes consist of neutrophils, lymphocytes, monocytes, eosinophils, and basophils. A decrease in leukocytes in older adults may be related to drugs or severe infection. Drugs that may cause a decrease in leukocytes include antibiotics, anticonvulsants, antihistamines, antimetabolites, cytotoxic agents, analgesics, phenothiazines, and diuretics (Pagana & Pagana, 2018).

An increase in leukocytes is generally seen in the presence of infections. However, a WBC count may be only moderately elevated in older adults when an infection such as pneumonia is present. Other typical symptoms of infection such as fever, pain, and lymphadenopathy may be minimal or absent in older adults with infections (Mouton, 2001).

Consequently, the nurse must be alert for other signs and symptoms of infection such as the sudden onset of confusion or lethargy. Pharmacologic agents have also been associated with an increase in leukocytes. These drugs include allopurinol, aspirin, heparin, steroids, and triamterene (Pagana & Pagana, 2018).

Neutrophils, eosinophils, and basophils are produced in the bone marrow and possess similar structures of segmented nuclei and many membrane-bound granules. Their primary function is phagocytosis (i.e., ingestion and destruction of invading microorganisms and cellular debris). In addition, the basophil's cytoplasmic granules contain powerful chemicals such as heparin, histamine, bradykinin, leukotrienes, and prostaglandins, which contribute to activation of the inflammatory response (McCance & Huether, 2014). The monocyte, the largest of the leukocytes, is produced in bone marrow and differs in appearance from neutrophils, eosinophils, and basophils. The monocyte has a single nucleus and can destroy large bacterial organisms and virally infected cells by phagocytosis (Pagana & Pagana, 2018).

Lymphocytes, the smallest of the leukocytes, are classified into two types: B and T. Lymphocytes have large nuclei and relatively little cytoplasm. Originating in bone marrow and the thymus, lymphocytes are housed in the lymph nodes, spleen, and tonsils. Lymphocytes do not act as phagocytes but rather produce antibodies and other specific defenses against antigens (Thibodeau & Patton, 2003).

Aging does not appear to affect the function of neutrophils, although the ability of bone marrow to release and store these cells is reduced. Lymphocytes of older adults have shown impaired function in vitro and are suspected to be the cause of a reduction in antibody response in later life (Rothstein, 1999). It is suspected there is a decline in monocyte function, given the increased susceptibility to infections and increased incidence of malignancies in older adults. The remaining leukocytes, eosinophils, and basophils have shown no evidence of being affected by aging.

Leukocytes are necessary for the body's resistance and response to infections, cancers, and other foreign substances. The nursing implications regarding infections and malignancies include recognizing subtle and sometimes altered responses to infections and diseases in older adults. Educating older adults about the importance of participating in cancer screening programs and maintaining immunization status throughout life is essential.

Folic Acid

Folic acid is one of the eight B vitamins that make up the B-complex group. Folic acid is a water-soluble vitamin that functions as a *coenzyme,* which means it is inactive unless linked to an enzyme. Folic acid is necessary for the normal functioning of RBCs and WBCs. A decrease in folic acid may indicate macrocytic anemia, megaloblastic anemia, and liver and renal disease. Alcohol and various other drugs are known to interfere with the absorption of folate. Some drugs have also been shown to decrease folic acid levels. These include anticonvulsants, antimalarials, and methotrexate (Pagana & Pagana, 2018).

However, the effect of aging on folate is still debatable because of differences in defining the lower limits of "normal" and the different methods used to determine folate levels (Gilleece & Dexter, 2002).

Because of the relationship of nutrition and alcohol consumption to folic acid levels, it is important for the gerontologic nurse to assess nutritional intake, including alcohol consumption habits. Elevated levels of folic acid may be seen in people with pernicious anemia who do not have an adequate amount of vitamin B_{12} to metabolize folic acid. Therefore the folic acid levels should be tested in conjunction with assessment of vitamin B_{12} levels (Pagana & Pagana, 2018).

Vitamin B_{12}

Vitamin B_{12}, or cobalamin, is a water-soluble vitamin that is part of the B-complex group of vitamins. Vitamin B_{12} deficiency is present in nearly a quarter of older adults. Common causes of deficiency include malabsorption secondary to gastric bypass, pancreatic disease, ileal resection or inflammation, and prolonged use of certain medications such as proton pump inhibitors, colchicine, cholestyramine, histamine 2 (H_2) blockers, or metformin. Strict vegetarian or vegan diets may also lead to vitamin B_{12} deficiency (Bryan, 2010; Orton, 2012). Malabsorption of vitamin B_{12} may be caused by the effect of antibodies on gastric parietal cells and a decrease in intrinsic factor, the underlying cause of pernicious anemia. The prevalence of pernicious anemia increases significantly with aging (Chatta & Lipschitz, 1999).

Vitamin B_{12} is important for normal erythrocyte maturation (McCance & Huether, 2014) and acts as a coenzyme with folic acid. The synthesis of nucleic acids, and therefore the structure of deoxyribonucleic acid (DNA), depends on adequate vitamin B_{12} intake (Grodner, Long, & DeYoung, 2004). Vitamin B_{12} deficiency may lead to demyelination of the dorsal and lateral spinal columns, which, in turn, may lead to paresthesias of the feet and disequilibrium, and loss of vibratory sensation in the fingers (Bryan, 2010; Gaspard, 2002). Low vitamin B_{12} levels may also lead to fatigue, weakness, and memory loss (Orton, 2012).

Total Iron Binding Capacity

Total iron binding capacity (TIBC) measures the amount of iron and the amount of available transferrin in the serum (McCance & Huether, 2014). Transferrin is a protein in the plasma that collects iron and transports it to the bone marrow for incorporation into hemoglobin. Increased TIBC and transferrin levels may indicate iron deficiency anemia; decreased levels may indicate anemia caused by chronic disease.

Iron

Iron is found in the hemoglobin of the RBCs. When iron-containing foods are ingested, iron is absorbed by the small intestine and transported to the plasma (Pagana & Pagana, 2018). Iron is necessary for controlling protein synthesis in the mitochondria and for generating energy in the cells (Freedman & Sutin, 2002). Serum iron levels show progressive decreases in both genders with advancing age, although the ability to absorb iron appears to remain intact (Hall & Wiley, 1999).

Iron deficiency anemia is the most common form of anemia seen in older adults. However, despite the decreases in serum iron levels seen with aging, anemia in older adults is not a normal consequence of aging. The gerontologic nurse should assess older adults for poor dietary intake of iron-containing foods and occult or chronic blood loss (Ahluwalia, Sun, Krause, Mastro & Handte, 2004).

Uric Acid

Uric acid is a product of purine catabolism and is excreted by the kidneys. Age-related changes in uric acid levels are significantly different between the genders. Because estrogen is thought to promote the excretion of uric acid, elevated levels are rarely seen in women before the onset of menopause (McCance & Huether, 2014).

Problems with uric acid may be a result of faulty excretion (e.g., kidney disease), overproduction of uric acid, or the presence of other substances that compete for excretion sites (e.g., ketoacids) (Pagana & Pagana, 2018). Elevated uric acid levels are seen in patients with gout. Gout, a common condition in older adults, involves a disturbance in the body's control of uric acid production or excretion. Excess uric acid accumulates in the body's fluids, especially blood and synovial fluids, forming crystals in high concentrations. These crystals deposit in the connective tissue of the body, causing painful, inflamed joints. Thiazide diuretics, caffeine, low-dose aspirin, and antiparkinsonian drugs are also a common cause of increased uric acid levels in older adults (Pagana & Pagana, 2018).

Prothrombin Time

Prothrombin is a plasma protein that is converted to thrombin in the first step of the clotting cascade. Clotting is necessary to prevent the loss of vital body fluids that occurs when blood vessels rupture (Thibodeau & Patton, 2003). In addition to measuring prothrombin time (PT), health care professionals also measure the activity of fibrinogen and coagulation factors V, VII, and X. The results of the PT laboratory test reveal how effectively the vitamin K–dependent coagulation factors of the extrinsic and common pathways of the coagulation cascade are performing (McCance & Huether, 2014). An increased PT is seen in liver disease, vitamin K deficiency, bile duct obstruction, and salicylate intoxication. Some medications, including allopurinol, cephalothins, cholestyramine, clofibrate, and certain antibiotics, may also cause an increase in a patient's PT. Digitalis and diphenhydramine may cause decreased PT levels (Pagana & Pagana, 2018).

Older adults are often prescribed the drug warfarin after open-heart surgery and in cases of chronic atrial fibrillation. Warfarin interferes with the production of vitamin K–dependent coagulation factors, thereby decreasing the chance of thrombus formation. Warfarin may interact with many medications, especially those often taken by older adults (Pagana & Pagana, 2018). Gerontologic nurses should help patients understand the importance of keeping their appointments for PT checks and consulting their health providers before taking any over-the-counter (OTC) medications or supplements.

Monitoring a patient's PT level can assess the adequacy of warfarin therapy. The PT value is traditionally reported in seconds and includes a value called the *international normalized ratio* (INR). INR is a mathematic "correction" of the results of the one-stage PT and was created to standardize results caused by a variation in laboratory reagents. The INR should be between 2.0 and 3.0 for most thrombosis and embolus conditions, and between 3.0 and 4.0 for patients with a history of recurrent thromboembolism or mechanical heart valves (O'Neill, 2002) (see Nutritional Considerations box).

NUTRITIONAL CONSIDERATIONS

Vitamin K is used in emergency situations to counteract the increased coagulation times that sometimes occur when patients receive warfarin. The nurse should be aware that foods high in vitamin K may affect clotting times and counteract the prescribed therapy. Foods such as turnip greens, broccoli, cabbage, spinach, and liver, which are high in vitamin K, should be eaten in moderate amounts while receiving anticoagulant therapy.

From Grodner, M., Long, S., & DeYoung, S. (2004). *Foundations and clinical applications of nutrition: A nursing approach.* St. Louis, MO: Mosby.

Partial Thromboplastin Time

Partial thromboplastin time (PTT) refers to the measurement of the common pathway of clot formation. Heparin may inactivate prothrombin, so the PTT is a good indicator of the adequacy of anticoagulation therapy. The effect of heparin on the body is faster than that of warfarin, but the effects are shorter. Nursing considerations include monitoring for bleeding and correct administration of the heparin dosage.

D-dimer Test

D-dimer is a fragment produced during the degradation of a clot. The D-dimer test may be ordered when a person has symptoms of thrombus, embolus, or disseminated intravascular coagulation. Results are interpreted when combined with clinical information and other laboratory data. Age, vascular disease, and kidney or hepatic disease may affect test results.

Erythrocyte Sedimentation Rate

The erythrocyte sedimentation rate (ESR) test measures the time that RBCs take to settle in normal saline over 1 hour. The measured values are reported in millimeters (mm). The test does not relate to one specific condition or disorder but does indicate the presence of inflammation, so it is useful in monitoring the course of inflammatory activity in autoimmune diseases, infections, and cancers. Kane, Ouslander, and Abrass (1999) report that mild elevations may be associated with advancing age. Because of the nonspecific nature of ESR values, it is important to interpret the results in older adults in conjunction with subjective and objective findings on physical examination (Calkins, 1999).

C-Reactive Protein

C-reactive protein (CRP) is a marker present in the acute phase of an inflammatory response. CRP is useful in assessing patients with tissue injury (e.g., myocardial infarction), autoimmune diseases, or bacterial infections. CRP does not usually rise with viral infections (Pagana & Pagana, 2018). Point-of-care CRP testing has been shown to reduce antibiotic prescribing in patients with lower respiratory infections and rhinosinusitis without compromising recovery (Chaplin, 2015).

Platelets

Platelets are small, irregular bodies, also known as *thrombocytes,* which are essential for clotting. They are formed in bone marrow and stored in the spleen. When an injury occurs to a blood vessel, platelets are released and become "sticky," forming a plug at the site and triggering the clotting cascade (Thibodeau & Patton, 2003).

Decreases in platelet counts (to less than 100,000 per cubic millimeter [mm^3]) require investigation. In a condition known as *myelodysplastic syndrome* (MDS), pancytopenia is noted in more than half the patients diagnosed. Pancytopenia is present when the levels of RBCs, WBCs, and platelets are all below normal. Most often, individuals diagnosed with MDS are older than 60. Treatment consists of managing symptoms, preventing infection and bleeding, and slowing disease progression. This condition has been known to progress to acute leukemia (Gilleece & Dexter, 2002). At platelet levels below 20,000/mm^3, the nurse should observe for spontaneous bleeding. If the patient's levels are 40,000/mm^3 or below, prolonged bleeding may occur after certain procedures (Pagana & Pagana, 2018).

In assessing patients for potential or hidden blood losses, nurses have traditionally questioned patients about the color and consistency of their stools. The gerontologic nurse, however, must recognize that older adults who take iron supplements have changes in bowel habits and stool color, which may not necessarily indicate the presence of occult blood. When preparing older adults for fecal occult blood testing, it is important to instruct them to stop iron supplements 3 days before testing.

COMPONENTS OF BLOOD CHEMISTRY TESTING

Blood chemistry testing determines levels of circulating electrolytes, glucose, and various other blood components. Although many of these tests are done in groups, others may be ordered individually to diagnose or monitor a specific condition. Current terminology labels these chemical analyses with names such as "basic metabolic profile" and "complete metabolic profile," but these names may vary from institution to institution. Nurses should learn the terminology specific to their workplace and be able to identify the individual tests contained in each package.

Electrolytes

Electrolytes are inorganic substances that include acids, bases, and salts. In solutions, electrolytes break up to form positively or negatively charged particles known as *ions.* Positively charged ions are known as *cations;* negatively charged ions are called *anions.* Compounds formed from acids and bases are known as *salts.* Blood testing may include measurement of the amount of an electrolyte in the circulating blood. Although many types of electrolytes may be tested, only the most common are discussed here.

Older adults may have serious problems with electrolyte imbalance. Dehydration is the most common form of electrolyte disorder that occurs in older adults, and it is usually attributed to excess loss of water or altered fluid intake. Excess water loss may be caused by infections such as pneumonia and cystitis or environmental conditions. Altered fluid intake may result from age-related decrease in thirst sensation in older adults or a result of decreased functional ability that limits the intake of fluids (Davis & Minaker, 1999).

Sodium

The test for sodium (Na^+) measures the amount of sodium in circulating blood and is an index of body water deficit or excess. Sodium regulation is important for the maintenance of blood pressure, transmission of nerve impulses, and regulation of body fluid levels in and out of the cells. This movement of sodium affects blood volume, which is tied to the thirst mechanism and total body fluids (Grodner et al., 2004). Although sodium is also present in intracellular fluid, the majority resides in extracellular fluid, which makes it the major cation of extracellular fluid. Serum sodium levels describe the balance between ingested sodium and that excreted by the kidneys (Pagana & Pagana, 2018). Aging changes in the kidney, such as decreased glomerular filtration rate (GFR) and a decrease in the number of functioning nephrons, can mean that an older adult has difficulty in maintaining homeostasis in the presence of sodium depletion or overload (Table 15.2). Because of the intrinsic loss in function, kidneys have a decreased renin–angiotensin–aldosterone response and may not respond appropriately; thus further sodium losses may occur (Musso & Oreopoulos, 2011). A normal sodium level is necessary for maintaining the extracellular fluid balance (osmolarity).

TABLE 15.2   Blood Chemistry

Test Name	Adult Normals	Older Adult Normals	Significance of Deviation
Sodium	136–145 milliequivalents per liter (mEq/L)	Unchanged with aging	*Low:* decreased intake, diarrhea, vomiting, diuretic administration, chronic kidney disease, heart failure (HF), peripheral edema, ascites *High:* increased intake, Cushing syndrome, extensive thermal burns
Potassium	3.5–5 mEq/L	Unchanged with aging	*Low:* deficient intake, burns, diuretics, Cushing syndrome, insulin administration, ascites *High:* excessive dietary intake, kidney failure, infection, acidosis, dehydration
Chloride	98–106 mEq/L	Unchanged with aging	*Low:* overhydration, CHF, vomiting, chronic gastric suction, chronic respiratory acidosis, hypokalemia, diuretic therapy *High:* dehydration, Cushing syndrome, kidney dysfunction, metabolic acidosis, hyperventilation
Calcium	9–10.5 milligrams per deciliter (mg/dL)	Tends to stay the same or decrease	*Low:* kidney failure, vitamin D deficiency, osteomalacia, malabsorption *High:* Paget disease of the bone, prolonged immobilization, lymphoma
Phosphorus	3–4.5 mg/dL	Slightly lower	*Low:* inadequate dietary ingestion, chronic antacid ingestion, hypercalcemia, alcoholism, osteomalacia, malnutrition *High:* kidney failure, increased dietary intake, hypocalcemia, liver disease
Magnesium	1.3–2.1 mEq/L	Decreases 15% between third and eighth decade	*Low:* malnutrition, malabsorption, alcoholism, chronic kidney disease *High:* chronic kidney disease, ingestion of magnesium-containing antacids or salts, hypothyroidism
Fasting glucose	70–105 mg/dL	Increase in normal range after age 50	*Low:* hypothyroidism, liver disease, insulin overdose, starvation *High:* diabetes mellitus, acute stress response, diuretic therapy, corticosteroid therapy
Amylase	60–120 Somogyi units/dL	Slightly increased in elderly	*High:* acute pancreatitis, perforated bowel, acute cholecystitis, diabetic ketoacidosis
Glycosylated hemoglobin (HbA$_{1c}$)	2.2%–4.8%	Unchanged with aging	*Low:* hemolytic anemia, chronic kidney disease *High:* newly diagnosed diabetes, poorly controlled diabetes, nondiabetic hyperglycemia
Total protein	6.4–8.3 grams per deciliter (g/dL)	Unchanged with aging	*Low:* liver disease, malnutrition, ascites *High:* hemoconcentration
Albumin	3.5–5 g/dL	Decreases slightly with aging	*Low:* malnutrition, liver disease, overhydration *High:* dehydration

Continued

TABLE 15.2 Blood Chemistry—cont'd

Test Name	Adult Normals	Older Adult Normals	Significance of Deviation
Blood urea nitrogen (BUN)	7–22 mg/dL	May be slightly higher	*Low:* liver failure, overhydration, malnutrition *High:* hypovolemia, dehydration, alimentary tube feeding, renal disease
Creatinine	0.7–1.5 mg/dL	Decrease in muscle mass may cause decreased values	*Low:* debilitation, decreased muscle mass *High:* reduced renal blood flow, diabetic neuropathy, urinary tract obstruction
Creatinine clearance	87–107 milliliters per minute (mL/min)	Values decrease 6.5 mL/min/decade of life due to a decline in glomerular filtration rate (GFR)	*Low:* chronic kidney disease, HF, cirrhosis *High:* high cardiac output syndromes
Cholesterol (total)	>200 mg/dL	Increases until about middle age but decreases thereafter (or can increase abruptly in women)	*Low:* malabsorption, malnutrition, cholesterol-lowering medication, pernicious anemia, liver disease, myocardial infarction *High:* hypercholesteremia, hyperlipidemia, hypothyroidism, uncontrolled diabetes mellitus
High-density lipoprotein (HDL)	>45 mg/dL	Unchanged with aging	*Low:* familial low HDL, liver disease, hypoproteinemia *High:* familial HDL lipoproteinemia, excessive exercise
Low-density lipoprotein (LDL)	60–180 mg/dL	Increases with aging after menopause	*Low:* hypolipoproteinemia *High:* hypothyroidism, alcohol consumption, chronic liver disease, Cushing syndrome
Alkaline phosphatase	30–120 units/L	Slightly higher	*Low:* hypothyroidism, malnutrition, pernicious anemia *High:* cirrhosis, healing fracture, Paget disease
Aspartate transaminase (AST)	0–35 units/L	Values slightly higher	*Low:* acute kidney disease, diabetic ketoacidosis, chronic kidney dialysis *High:* myocardial infarction, hepatitis, cirrhosis, multiple trauma, acute hemolytic anemia
Creatine kinase (CK)	30–170 units/L	Unchanged with aging	*High:* diseases or injury affecting heart muscle, skeletal muscle, and brain

Adapted from Pagana, K. D., & Pagana, T. J. (2018). *Mosby's manual of diagnostic and laboratory tests* (6th ed.). St. Louis, MO: Elsevier.

The occurrence of hyponatremia (a low sodium level) increases with age. Most cases are related to the kidneys' inability to excrete free water because of decreased basal levels of renin and aldosterone. Vague symptoms such as malaise, confusion, headache, and nausea may also progress to coma and seizures. It is important, however, to determine whether an older adult has low sodium level but normal osmolarity; this is known as hypertonic hyponatremia. In these cases, the osmolarity remains normal or high because of excess amounts of other osmolites in blood, for example, glucose, triglycerides, or plasma proteins. By determining the underlying cause and providing appropriate treatment, the health care provider can take steps to ensure return of the sodium level to normal (Simon, 2018).

It is essential that gerontologic nurses understand the goal of treatment for patients with fluid and sodium disorders. In patients with fluid deficiencies, the nurse can help identify reasons for a given condition, for example, restrictions in mobility, visual disturbances, urinary incontinence, and swallowing disorders. Hypernatremia (a high sodium level) may be caused by infusion of high-sodium solute fluids, excessive water loss, prolonged diarrhea and vomiting, and decreased oral intake. Hypernatremia is often seen in hospitalized older adults; some cases are present on admission, whereas some are the consequence of hospitalization. Symptoms are similar to those of hyponatremia, and the most common neurologic signs are those of lethargy and weakness, progressing to altered consciousness and coma. The pathophysiology behind the neurologic signs is thought to be neuronal cell dehydration and brain shrinkage (Semenovskaya, 2017).

Potassium

Potassium (K^+) is present in both the intracellular and extracellular fluid. Most potassium is found within the cell and minute amounts in the extracellular fluid. This extracellular amount is measured by serum testing. Potassium imbalances in older adults are caused by the same changes in the renal system as those affecting sodium. Salt substitutes, used by many older adults with hypertension or HF, are high in potassium and should be used with caution. Many medications such as potassium-sparing diuretics, angiotensin-converting enzyme inhibitors (ACEIs), and angiotensin receptor blockers (ARBs) used in conjunction with potassium supplements may cause hyperkalemia in older adults. In addition, nonsteroidal antiinflammatory drugs (NSAIDs) interfere with potassium excretion (El-Sharkawy, Sahota, Maughan, & Lobo, 2014). Hypokalemia may be caused by gastrointestinal loss and the use of diuretics. Potassium imbalance may predispose older adults to tachyarrhythmias and potentiate digitalis toxicity (Golzari, 2008). Because OTC medication use has increased, it is important for the gerontologic nurse to carefully assess an older adult's prescription, OTC, and complementary and alternative medication history (see Emergency Treatment box).

✚ EMERGENCY TREATMENT

Abnormal Laboratory Values: Potassium

Hypokalemia
* If asymptomatic, may repeat test before treatment.
  * K^+ between 3 mEq/L to 3.5 mEq/L is seldom symptomatic.
* Monitor for neuromuscular and cardiac effects of hypokalemia:
  * Skeletal muscle weakness
  * Smooth muscle atony
  * Dysrhythmias
* Observe for signs of digitalis toxicity.
* Maximum oral replacement is 40 to 80 mEq/day if renal function is normal.
* The maximum safe rate for intravenous replacement is 20 mEq/hr.
  * Maximal concentration of 40 mEq/100 mL should be used with an infusion pump.
* Repeat K^+ level after replacement therapy and until values are normal.

From McCance, K. L. & Huether, S. E. (2014). *Pathophysiology: The biologic basis for disease in adults and children* (7th ed.). St. Louis, MO: Mosby.

Potassium, like sodium, maintains cell osmolarity, muscle function, and the transmission of nerve impulses, and it regulates acid–base balance. Cardiac muscle is particularly sensitive to serum concentrations of potassium. Hyperkalemia may cause muscle twitching, arrhythmias, and gastrointestinal symptoms (McCance & Huether, 2014). Hypokalemia may occur because of excessive loss of potassium through the gastrointestinal tract, usually by vomiting. Symptoms include muscle weakness, confusion, and absence of bowel sounds. When replacing potassium in older adults, the nurse must take care to prevent hyperkalemia.

Chloride

Chloride (Cl^-) is mostly present in the fluid outside the cell; it is the major anion in the extracellular fluid. Chloride is closely tied to sodium; losses and excesses in sodium affect chloride levels (Pagana & Pagana, 2018). Chloride levels have not been shown to change with aging (see Table 15.2).

Calcium

The serum calcium (Ca^{++}) level measures only the amount of calcium in blood, which is about 1% of the body's total calcium. Approximately 99% of the body's calcium is found in bones and teeth (Lewis, 2016a). Changes in calcium regulation occur with aging; however, due to homeostatic mechanisms within the body, there is no resultant alteration in serum calcium levels. The loss of calcium from bone maintains the normal level of calcium in blood, but the resulting bone loss secondary to calcium leaching may lead to osteoporosis (Veldurthy, Wei, Oz, Dhawan, Jeon, & Christakos, 2016). Calcium is important in blood clotting, conduction of nerve impulses, enzyme activity, and especially muscle contraction and relaxation (Lewis, 2016a). Calcium levels measure free calcium as well as calcium that is protein bound with albumin. Therefore any change in albumin level also affects calcium (Pagana & Pagana, 2018).

Calcium metabolism is one of the factors that determines phosphorus levels; an inverse relationship is present. A decrease in calcium may cause an increase in phosphorus and vice versa. Parathyroid hormone (PTH) also affects phosphorus levels by affecting the resorption of phosphorus in the kidneys (Pagana & Pagana, 2018). PTH acts on plasma membrane receptors of the nephrons of the kidneys to increase the resorption of calcium and to decrease the resorption of phosphorus (McCance & Huether, 2014).

Phosphorus

Phosphorus (phosphate) is a mineral found mostly in bone in combination with calcium. Phosphorus is generally well absorbed from the small intestine in the presence of vitamin D. Long-term use of antacids, which bind to phosphorus, may interfere with absorption. Additionally, the kidneys excrete excess phosphorus from blood; in the setting of kidney disease, hyperphosphatemia may develop. Phosphorus plays an important role in the maintenance of homeostasis (as a component in DNA and ribonucleic acid [RNA]); the metabolism of fats, carbohydrates, and proteins; and the transfer of energy stored as adenosine triphosphate (ATP) (Ehrlich, 2015). In older adults, phosphorus levels are slightly decreased in comparison with younger adults (see Table 15.2).

Magnesium

Magnesium plays a significant role in the enzymatic processes needed for energy production. The most important sites of function are muscles and nerves. Approximately one-half of the body's magnesium is contained in bones (Lewis, 2016b). With aging, gastrointestinal absorption of magnesium decreases and excretion of magnesium by the kidneys increases; these changes, coupled with lower dietary intake of magnesium, put the older adult at risk of hypomagnesemia (Office of Dietary Supplements, 2016) (see Table 15.2).

Glucose

Glucose is used for energy by the cells. Blood glucose tests are evaluated on the basis of the time blood was drawn and the duration of fasting. The American Diabetes Association updated diabetes management guidelines in 2016 (Table 15.3).

In addition to patient symptoms, four methods of diagnosing diabetes are as follows:

1. *Fasting plasma glucose.* Blood is drawn after fasting for 8 hours. A fasting plasma $\geq$126 mg/dL is indicative of diabetes.
2. *Oral glucose tolerance test.* A person fasts for at least 8 hours; then, 2 hours after the person drinks a liquid containing 75 grams of glucose dissolved in water, blood sugar is tested.

TABLE 15.3 Diagnosis and Classification of Diabetes

	HbA$_{1c}$	Fasting Plasma Glucose	Oral Glucose Tolerance Test
Diabetes	$\geq$6.5%	$\geq$126 mg/dL	$\geq$200 mg/dL
Prediabetes	5.7–6.4%	100–125 mg/dL	140–199 mg/dL
Normal	<5.7%	<100 mg/dL	<140 mg/dL

HbA$_{1c}$, Glycohemoglobin; *mg/dL*, milligrams per deciliter.
From American Diabetes Association. (2016). Standards of medical care in diabetes—2016. *Diabetes Care, 39*(suppl 1), S1-S106.

This test is typically used to diagnose gestational diabetes; a 2-hour plasma glucose ≥200 mg/dL is indicative of diabetes.

3. *Glycohemoglobin (hemoglobin A_{1c}; HbA_{1c}).* This is a blood test that checks the amount of glucose bound to hemoglobin. Test is used to diagnose diabetes and monitor therapy. It provides an average of blood glucose levels over the previous 2 to 3 months. An A_{1c} ≥6.5% is indicative of diabetes.

4. *Random blood sugar.* This test measures blood glucose without fasting. A random glucose measurement ≥200 mg/dL, combined with symptoms of hyperglycemia, is indicative of diabetes.

Glucose metabolism alters with aging; older adults develop reduced insulin effectiveness and islet cell dysfunction. This results in a higher incidence of diabetes in older adults (Kalyani & Egan, 2013). In older adults with diabetes, hypoglycemia is harder to recognize. Neurologic symptoms of hypoglycemia (e.g., dizziness and visual disturbances) are more common than autonomic symptoms (e.g., palpitations and sweating) (Abdelhafix, Rodriguez-Manas, Morley & Sinclair, 2015).

Amylase

Amylase is an important enzyme in the catabolism of carbohydrates in the intestine. The acinar units of the pancreas produce it. Amylase levels are tested to aid in the diagnosis and management of pancreatitis and other pancreatic diseases. Elevated levels may occur secondary to damage to or disease of the pancreas, or obstruction of the pancreatic duct. Elevated amylase levels also may be seen in nonpancreatic disorders such as perforated ulcer, perforated or necrotic bowel, or secondary to medications. Decreased amylase levels may be found with chronic pancreatitis, pancreatic insufficiency, or cystic fibrosis (Pagana & Pagana, 2018) (see Table 15.2).

Total Protein

Protein makes up a significant portion of vascular osmotic pressure. Protein is also a major component in muscle, enzymes, hormones, transport vehicles, and hemoglobin. Total protein testing measures the amount of albumin and globulin in the plasma. This test is performed to identify nutritional problems (Pagana & Pagana, 2018).

Albumin and Prealbumin

Serum albumin levels are used to monitor nutritional status, and liver and kidney disease. Albumin levels decrease with age. Low albumin levels (<3.5 grams per deciliter [g/dL]) have been associated with increased mortality in hospitalized patients (Akirov, Masri-Iraqi, Atamna & Shimon, 2017). Additionally, when albumin is insufficient to sustain sufficient colloidal osmotic pressure to counterbalance hydrostatic pressure, edema develops. Low albumin levels are also associated with chronic disease including diabetes, hyperthyroidism, and HF. Research is conflicting concerning the relationship between serum albumin levels and pressure injury or wound healing, with some research indicating little connection (Lizaka, Sanada, Matsui et al., 2011) and other research indicating a relationship between albumin and wound healing (Amir, Liu & Chang, 2012; Serra et al., 2012). Finally, low levels of albumin are found in patients with burns, HF, acute infection, and thyrotoxicosis. High albumin levels are associated with blood loss and dehydration.

Prealbumin is also used to assess nutritional status. It is the measurement of protein status over the short term and is a more accurate measurement of malnutrition because of its short half-life of 1.9 days. Plasma prealbumin level is useful in monitoring therapy with total parenteral nutrition (Pagana & Pagana, 2018).

Blood Urea Nitrogen

Measurement of urea in blood is known as the blood urea nitrogen (BUN) test. Urea is a major waste product of protein catabolism and a result of ammonia conversion in the liver. Urea is excreted from the body by the kidneys. BUN levels are indicative of both liver and kidney function. Values for older men are slightly higher than the adult normal levels of 7 to 22 milligrams per deciliter (mg/dL). In older women, BUN levels are also increased but less than in older men (Pagana & Pagana, 2018) (see Table 15.2).

Creatinine

Creatinine is another end-product of protein metabolism. A rise in a patient's BUN and creatinine levels is indicative of kidney disease. The physiologic decline in the GFR in older adults is not generally accompanied by a rise in the creatinine level secondary to a decrease in muscle mass with aging. Therefore the creatinine level in an older adult should not be considered an independent indicator of renal function as it would be in a younger individual. It should, instead, be used to calculate the creatinine clearance for a more realistic indication of renal function in older adults (Pagana & Pagana, 2018).

Creatinine Clearance

Creatinine clearance is the measure of the GFR, estimated from serum creatinine (SCr) and urine creatinine levels. A 24-hour urine test is required along with a serum level within the same 24-hour period. To allow for changes with aging that are not reflected in the creatinine level, many primary care providers use the Cockcroft and Gault formula to estimate creatinine clearance:

$$\text{Creatinine clearance (milliliters per minute [mL/min])}$$
$$= \frac{140 - \text{Age (in years)} \times \text{Weight (in kilograms [kg])}}{72 \times \text{Serum creatinine (\%mg/dL)}}$$

(For women, multiply the result by 0.85.)

An alternative method of calculating creatinine clearance is the Modification of Diet in Renal Disease (MDRD) formula:

$$\text{MDRD} - \text{GFR} = 186(\text{SCr})^{1.154}$$
$$\times (\text{age})^{0.203}(0.742 \text{ if female})(1.210 \text{ if black})$$

Neither method of calculating GFR is without variation; however, the MDRD is currently the method of choice. The gerontologic nurse should recognize the importance of creatinine clearance as a reflection of an older adult's overall health status. Creatinine clearance decreases an average of 6.5 mL/min each decade of life after age 20. The older adult's response to medications, especially newly prescribed drugs, should be monitored because impaired renal function may precipitate side effects that could otherwise be overlooked (Pagana & Pagana, 2018).

Triglycerides

Triglycerides are the principal lipids found in circulating blood bound to a protein; they are transported by low-density lipoproteins (LDLs) and very-low-density lipoproteins (VLDLs). Triglycerides are produced in the liver from glycerol and fatty acids found in blood. When the triglyceride level in blood reaches its peak, the excess is deposited in the fatty tissue for release later for energy between meals (Pagana & Pagana, 2018). The American Heart Association (AHA) recommends an optimal triglyceride level of 100 mg/dL or lower.

Total Cholesterol

Cholesterol is a steroid compound that helps stabilize the membranes of the body's cells. It is also the major lipid associated with cardiovascular disease. The liver metabolizes cholesterol and binds it to LDLs and HDLs for transport in the bloodstream (Pagana & Pagana, 2018). Total cholesterol levels are a combination of LDL and HDL levels in the bloodstream. The National Cholesterol Education Program recommends total cholesterol levels be kept at less than 200 mg/dL. However, it is important to evaluate cholesterol in relationship to HDL, LDL, and triglyceride levels, not in isolation.

High-Density Lipoprotein

HDL, referred to as "good cholesterol," carries greater amounts of protein and lesser amounts of lipids, hence the term *high density*. HDL's role is to take cholesterol to the liver for degradation. A high HDL level (>60 mg/dL) is considered healthy; it is protective against heart disease (Pagana & Pagana, 2018).

Low-Density Lipoprotein

LDL, referred to as "bad cholesterol," carries cholesterol from the liver to the body. The LDL level is calculated from the total cholesterol level, HDL level, and fasting triglycerides with the use of the following equation:

$$\text{LDL cholesterol} = \text{Total cholesterol} - \text{HDL cholesterol} - (\text{Triglyceride level} \div 5)$$

Patients with established heart disease and another risk factor such as smoking are recommended to have the LDL cholesterol level at less than 70 mg/dL. Those at high risk but without established disease are recommended to have the LDL level at less than 100 mg/dL. Patients considered at moderate risk for heart disease should maintain the LDL level at less than 130 mg/dL, and those at low risk for heart disease should have the LDL level at less than 160 mg/dL (Pagana & Pagana, 2018).

Brain Natriuretic Peptide

The brain natriuretic peptide (BNP) is a neurohormone secreted from the cardiac ventricles in response to ventricular stretching and pressure overloading. This test helps diagnose and treat patients with HF. Studies have shown that an elevated BNP level is highly sensitive and specific for the diagnosis of HF. Plasma levels of BNP are significantly elevated in patients with HF and left ventricular dysfunction; however, the values cannot be used to differentiate between systolic and diastolic HF (Pagana & Pagana, 2018).

Alkaline Phosphatase

Alkaline phosphatase (ALP) is an enzyme found in many tissues, although it has its highest concentrations in the liver and bone. Testing for ALP is used to identify liver and bone disorders. Testing of the ALP level in older adults is often used in the biochemical assessment of Paget disease and other bone diseases (Pagana & Pagana, 2018) (see Table 15.2).

Aspartate Aminotransferase

Aspartate transaminase (AST) measures the enzyme of the same name, which is found in muscles and in the liver and kidneys. It is primarily used to diagnose liver disease. A threefold to fivefold increase in AST may be indicative of hepatotoxicity from drugs such as isoniazid, rifampin, ethambutol, and pyrazinamide (Pagana & Pagana, 2018).

Creatine Kinase

Creatine kinase (CK) is present in cardiac and skeletal muscles, and in the brain and lungs. CK-BB is primarily found in the lungs and brain, whereas CK-MB is associated with cardiac muscle cells. CK-MM is normally found in circulating blood, and the level rises with damage to skeletal muscle. CK levels rise and peak at specific intervals during myocardial infarction, and these levels may be used to determine the amount of myocardial damage; however, this test has largely been replaced by troponin. CK may also be ordered when a person has experienced physical trauma such as crushing injuries or extensive burns, or to diagnose rhabdomyolysis (Pagana & Pagana, 2018).

Lactate Dehydrogenase

Lactate dehydrogenase (LDH) is an enzyme found in the muscles, brain, liver, kidneys, and RBCs. LDH may be isolated into five isoenzymes. These isoenzymes help clarify the site of release of the LDH and assist the nurse in assessing and monitoring specific complications related to the site of injury. Patterns of LDH elevation can be used to monitor injury to the heart, lungs, and liver (Pagana & Pagana, 2018).

Troponin

The troponin test measures the levels of certain proteins in the blood that are released when cardiac muscle has been damaged. Troponins (troponin I or troponin T) are the preferred tests for a suspected heart attack because they are more specific for detecting heart injury compared with other tests. These indices appear 2 to 8 hours after a decrease in the oxygenation of cardiac muscle caused by occlusion of the cardiac vessels. Levels may remain elevated up to 2 weeks after a myocardial infarction. This test may also be ordered when a patient has worsening angina or acute coronary syndrome without ST elevation (Pagana & Pagana, 2018).

Thyroid Function Tests

Testing of thyroid function includes the assessment of two hormones secreted by the thyroid gland: thyroxine (T_4) and triiodothyronine (T_3). Thyroid function tests are a means of screening for hypothyroidism or hyperthyroidism and for monitoring the effectiveness of thyroid suppression or hormone replacement therapy. T_4 and T_3 are generally elevated in hyperthyroidism and decreased in hypothyroidism. Thyroid-stimulating hormone (TSH), a hormone secreted by the pituitary gland, is also usually tested when thyroid function is investigated; TSH is elevated in hypothyroidism and decreased in hyperthyroidism (Table 15.4). Higher-than-normal TSH levels are most often caused by an underactive thyroid gland (hypothyroidism), which may result from autoimmune disease, treatment for hyperthyroidism, radiation therapy or thyroid surgery, or certain medications (e.g., lithium). Lower-than-normal levels may be caused by an overactive thyroid gland (hyperthyroidism), which may result from Graves' disease, toxic nodular goiter, thyroiditis, or certain medications (e.g., glucocorticoids and opioid) (Pagana & Pagana, 2018).

Prostate-Specific Antigen

The prostate-specific antigen (PSA) test measures the amount of PSA, a protein produced in the prostate and found in blood. High levels of PSA may indicate the presence of prostate cancer. However, other conditions such as an enlarged or inflamed prostate may also cause an increase in PSA levels. Before any prostate screening is initiated, the gerontologic nurse needs to ensure that the patient understands the risks and benefits associated with the results: Would diagnosis and treatment of the prostate cancer improve or worsen the person's quality of life? Would he want treatment in the event cancer was found? The risk of prostate screening may outweigh the benefit in men aged over 75 and in those with less than 10 years' life expectancy (Pagana & Pagana, 2018).

URINALYSIS

Urinalysis (UA) includes testing for the presence of protein, glucose, bacteria, blood, ketones, and leukocytes in the urine. It also involves studying the sample for properties of specific gravity and pH. Urine is a waste product formed by the kidneys and consists of 95% water. The composition of urine may inform the health care professional of the status of many body systems. When blood passes through the kidneys, water, nitrogen compounds, toxins, and electrolytes are filtered, reabsorbed, and secreted. The amounts retained or excreted affect the body's homeostasis.

Protein

Protein in urine (proteinuria) is considered an abnormal finding and indicates damage to the kidneys' glomeruli (Table 15.5). Its presence warrants further investigation to determine the presence of kidney disease, amyloidosis, or multiple myeloma.

Glucose

Normally, glucose is not present in urine. When the blood sugar levels exceed 180 mg/dL, the kidneys release some of the excess glucose from blood into urine. Glucose may also be found in urine when the kidneys are damaged or diseased.

Bacteria

Although occasional trace amounts of bacteria (bacteriuria) may normally appear in urine, significant amounts, defined as greater than 100,000 colony-forming units (CFU) per milliliter of urine, indicate infection. The gerontologic nurse should assess older adults for symptoms of urinary incontinence, flank pain, fever, voiding frequency, burning, and suprapubic or low back pain. However, common symptoms may be absent in most of the older adults, and symptoms such as confusion, new onset of incontinence, lethargy, nocturia, and anorexia may be the first indication of underlying UTI. Women are more prone to lower UTIs compared with men because of the shorter urethra and its proximity to the vagina and anus. Significant numbers of older adults are asymptomatic, even when bacteria are found in urine (Pagana & Pagana, 2018).

TABLE 15.4	**Thyroid Testing**			
Test Name	**Adult Normals**	**Older Adult Normals**	**Significance of Deviations**
Thyroxine (T_4)	4–12 micrograms per deciliter (mcg/dL)	Slightly decreased	*Low:* hypothyroidism, malnutrition, kidney failure, cirrhosis *High:* hyperthyroidism, hepatitis
Triiodothyronine (T_3)	75–220 nanograms per deciliter (ng/dL)	Slightly decreased	*Low:* hypothyroidism, pituitary insufficiency, protein malnutrition, kidney failure, liver diseases *High:* hyperthyroidism, hepatitis, hypoproteinemia
Thyroid-stimulating hormone (TSH)	2–10 microunits/mL	Unchanged with aging	*Low:* pituitary dysfunction, hyperthyroidism *High:* primary hypothyroidism

Adapted from Pagana, K. D., & Pagana, T. J. (2018). *Mosby's manual of diagnostic and laboratory tests* (6th ed.). St. Louis, MO: Elsevier.

TABLE 15.5 Urine Chemistry

Test Name	Adult Normals	Older Adult Normals	Significance of Deviations
Color	Yellow; amber	Same	Straw-colored urine indicates dilution.
Appearance	Clear	Same	Cloudy urine may indicate presence of pus, casts, blood, and bacteria.
Specific gravity	1.005–1.030	Values decrease with aging	*Low:* overhydration, kidney failure, diuresis, hypothermia *High:* dehydration, water restriction, vomiting, diarrhea
pH	4.6–8.0	Same	*Acidic urine:* diarrhea, metabolic acidosis, diabetes mellitus, respiratory acidosis, emphysema *Alkaline urine:* respiratory alkalosis, metabolic alkalosis, vomiting, gastric suctioning, diuretic therapy, urinary tract infection (UTI)
Protein	1–8 milligrams per milliliter (mg/mL)	Same	*Positive:* diabetes mellitus, heart failure (HF), systemic lupus erythematosus, malignant hypertension
Glucose	Negative	Same	*Positive:* diabetes mellitus, Cushing syndrome, severe stress, infection, drug therapy
Ketones	Negative	Same	*Positive:* uncontrolled diabetes mellitus, starvation, excessive aspirin ingestion, high-protein diet, dehydration
Blood	Negative	Same	*Positive:* kidney trauma, kidney stones, cystitis, prostatitis
Leukocyte esterase	Negative	Same	*Positive:* possible UTI
Bacteria	Negative	May be seen in older adults without symptoms; evaluate for pyuria and symptoms	*Positive:* UTI

Adapted from Pagana, K. D., & Pagana, T. J. (2018). *Mosby's manual of diagnostic and laboratory tests* (6th ed.). St. Louis, MO: Elsevier.

Leukocyte Esterase

The presence of leukocytes in urine (pyuria) is more indicative of UTI, and a positive leukocyte esterase indicates the need for microscopic examination, urine culture, and sensitivity testing (Pagana & Pagana, 2018).

Nitrites

The nitrite test is used, in conjunction with leukocyte esterase, in the diagnosis of UTI. Nitrites occur when certain bacteria (e.g., *Escherichia coli, Proteus spp.,* and *Klebsiella pneumoniae*) produce the enzyme *reductase,* which converts urinary nitrates to nitrites. If the test is positive, a urine culture should be obtained (Pagana & Pagana, 2018).

Ketones

The presence of ketones, the result of fatty acid breakdown, in urine is another abnormal finding. When overaccumulation of ketones occurs in blood, the excess is excreted in urine. Causes of ketones in urine include diabetic ketoacidosis, a low-carbohydrate diet, starvation or fasting, and severe vomiting (Pagana & Pagana, 2018).

pH

The pH of the urine sample indicates the acid or base value of urine, which reflects the body's homeostatic state. The normal range for urine pH is 4.6 to 8.0. Drugs that increase urine pH include acetazolamide, potassium citrate, and sodium bicarbonate; drugs that may decrease urine pH include ammonium chloride, thiazide diuretics, and methenamine. Urine pH can be helpful in the identification of renal calculi, which are acid or base in origin, depending on the underlying substances that form the stones: acidic urine is associated with xanthine, cystine, uric acid, and calcium oxalate stones; and alkaline urine is associated with calcium carbonate, calcium phosphate, and magnesium phosphate stones. Prevention and treatment of calculi are aimed at changing the urine to the reverse pH of the stone's composition (Pagana & Pagana, 2018).

Blood

The presence of blood in urine (hematuria) is always an abnormal finding. The cause may be renal obstruction from calculi, trauma to the kidneys, inflammation, infection, or malignancy. Blood may be grossly apparent or occult, giving urine a cloudy or pink hue on visual inspection.

COMPONENTS OF ARTERIAL BLOOD GAS TESTING

Arterial blood gas (ABG) testing involves drawing a sample of blood from an artery, usually from the radial or brachial artery. Components of ABG testing are pH, oxygen, and carbon dioxide content; oxygen saturation; and bicarbonate level (Table 15.6). It is important that the health care provider and laboratory personnel be aware of supplemental oxygenation at the time of blood draw (i.e., the type of air being breathed [room air or other], the amount of oxygen support, and the type of oxygen delivery device). Pulse oximetry is a reliable alternative to ABG testing when the percentage of oxygen saturation in blood needs to be determined. The use of pulse oximetry is less painful and less expensive, and results are immediately available (Pagana & Pagana, 2018).

TABLE 15.6   Arterial Blood Gases

Test Name	Adult Normals	Older Adult Normals	Significance of Deviations
pH	7.35–7.45	Same	*Low:* respiratory or metabolic acidosis *High:* respiratory or metabolic alkalosis
PaO_2	80–100 mm Hg	Decreases 25% between 30 and 80 years old	*Low:* cardiac or respiratory disease
$Paco_2$	35–45 mm Hg	Same	*Low:* respiratory alkalosis *High:* respiratory acidosis
O_2 saturation	95%–100%	95%	*Low:* impaired gas exchange
HCO_3^-	21–28 mEq/L	Same	*Low:* metabolic acidosis *High:* metabolic acidosis

HCO_3, Bicarbonate; *mEq/L,* milliequivalents per liter; *mm Hg,* millimeters of mercury; *Paco₂,* partial pressure of arterial carbon dioxide; *PaO₂,* partial pressure of arterial oxygen.
Adapted from Pagana, K. D., & Pagana, T. J. (2018). *Mosby's manual of diagnostic and laboratory tests* (6th ed.). St. Louis, MO: Elsevier.

EVIDENCE-BASED PRACTICE

Reducing the Treatment of Asymptomatic Bacteriuria

Background
Nearly 50% of women and 40% of men in long-term care have bacteria in their urine on testing. The presence of bacteria does not confirm diagnosis of UTI. However, it is difficult to determine whether the presence of bacteria in urine is a UTI warranting treatment with antibiotics or asymptomatic bacteria.

Sample/Setting
The sample encompassed nurses and other care providers at a 182-bed complex-care facility in Parksville, British Columbia, Canada.

Methods
The intervention included a self-learning package with information on risk factors for UTIs, signs and symptoms of UTIs, actions to help prevent UTIs, and practice points for assessing an older adult with suspected UTI. The intervention also included a clinical pathway to help care providers in the assessment and management of residents with a suspected UTI, which was made available to staff on all units in the facility.

Findings
At the 1-year point following implementation, the number of facility UTIs treated with antibiotics decreased by 36%; the number of UTIs treated based on inadequate assessment (i.e., based on the results of urine dipstick alone) decreased from 62% to 38%. Communication improved between facility nurses and care providers concerning management of suspected UTIs.

Implications
Implementation of the self-learning package and pathway improved overall care of the older adults suspected of having a UTI. Improved management led to a decrease in inappropriate antibiotic prescribing. The changes implemented at the Parksville facility set a model for other facilities to follow.

Adapted from Leduc, A. (2014). Reducing the treatment of asymptomatic bacteriuria in seniors in a long-term care facility. *Canadian Nurse, 110*(7), 25-30.

Partial Pressure of Oxygen

Age-related changes such as a decrease in chest wall recoil, decrease in alveolar surface area, and less effective oxygen-to-carbon dioxide (CO_2) exchange all contribute to potential changes in oxygenation with aging. In the absence of disease, however, respiratory function remains adequate in older adults.

Partial pressure of oxygen (PaO_2) indirectly measures arterial oxygen content. It can be used to monitor the effectiveness of oxygen therapy (Pagana & Pagana, 2018).

pH of the Blood

pH measures the hydrogen ion (H^-) concentration in the bloodstream. A pH of less than 7.0 is called *acid pH,* and a pH greater than 7.0 is called *basic pH* (alkaline). pH is influenced by vomiting, diarrhea, lung function, endocrine function, and kidney function (see Table 15.6).

Bicarbonate

Carbon dioxide (CO_2) in blood exists in the form of bicarbonate (HCO_3^-); therefore the CO_2 blood test really is a measure of blood bicarbonate level. The HCO_3^- test is used to monitor conditions that affect blood bicarbonate levels, including kidney diseases, lung diseases, and metabolic conditions. The normal adult range is 21 to 28 mEq/L.

Oxygen Saturation

Oxygen saturation (O_2 sat %) measures how much of the hemoglobin in the RBCs carry oxygen. The normal adult value for oxygen saturation is greater than 95%. Levels below 90% are low. Conditions affecting lung function (e.g., pneumonia, chronic obstructive pulmonary disease [COPD]) alter oxygen saturation.

THERAPEUTIC DRUG MONITORING

Therapeutic drug monitoring measures the blood level of certain drugs at specified intervals to monitor the therapeutic drug concentration. Individuals absorb, metabolize, and excrete drugs at different rates based upon their age, gender, diet, general state of health, genetic makeup, and other drugs they are taking. Therapeutic drug monitoring is typically used with drugs that have a narrow therapeutic index (Laboratory Tests Online, 2018); individual variations may result in toxicity in drugs with a narrow therapeutic index.

Therapeutic drug monitoring is performed in older adults receiving drugs such as digoxin, theophylline, valproic acid, and phenytoin. Drug trough monitoring is performed in older adults receiving antibiotics (e.g., aminoglycosides and glycopeptides).

SUMMARY

In providing age-specific and age-appropriate health care, providers must recognize that individuals do not respond in the same way to similar experiences. Although many laboratory values compensate for age-related changes in older adults, an older adult must be considered within the total context of a person with unique responses to diseases. Laboratory tests and their results should be considered an adjunct to the detection and treatment of illness, not in isolation from the presenting clinical picture.

🏠 HOME CARE

1. Home health nurses must know the purpose of the tests ordered and must explain the reasoning for the tests to both caregivers and homebound older adults.
2. Home health nurses should assess the homebound older adults' cultural values and beliefs regarding diagnostic testing.
3. Home health nurses must realize that laboratory values in homebound older adults may be altered because of aging or medication regimens.
4. Home health nurses must be able to differentiate normal versus abnormal laboratory results for homebound older adults, and the nurse must know when to notify the health care provider.
5. Home health nurses should instruct caregivers and homebound older adults about what is required before laboratory testing (e.g., nothing by mouth from midnight the night before until the procedure).

KEY POINTS

- The ESR rises approximately 10 to 20 mm in older adults; this is considered a normal age-related change.
- Potassium-sparing diuretics and NSAIDs may interfere with potassium excretion.
- Older adults may have hyponatremia in the presence of normal osmolarity, indicating the presence of other osmolarities in excess in blood.
- Renal and hepatic system functioning may be reflected in the BUN level.
- Hypokalemia may potentiate digitalis toxicity in older adults.
- Comparable serum creatinine levels in younger adults and older adults are not indicators of comparable kidney function.
- Urine testing for glucose in older adults is considered unreliable in view of age-related changes in renal function.
- Thyroid disease may be present in older adults without the overt symptoms typically seen in younger adults with thyroid disorders.
- Older adults may be asymptomatic in the presence of bacteriuria.
- Pyuria is more indicative of symptomatic UTI than the presence of bacteria in the urine of older adults.
- The "normal" oxygen saturation in older adults may be 95% or greater in arterial blood.

CRITICAL-THINKING EXERCISES

1. When evaluating the laboratory data for a 73-year-old man, you note that his ESR and serum creatinine level are slightly elevated, and his serum magnesium level is decreased. What conclusion, if any, can be drawn from these findings? Should the data be reported to the physician?
2. You are making home visits to an 82-year-old woman recovering from a fractured femur. During your last three visits, she consistently complained of being cold, even though it is summer, and her house is very warm. In addition, she has had frequent complaints of constipation, has not felt like eating, and has been tired. She has a bottle of hand lotion next to her chair for her dry skin. What is your assessment, and is any action warranted on your part?

REFERENCES

Abdelhafiz, A. H., Rodriguez-Mana, L., Morley, J. E., & Sinclair, A. J. (2015). Hypoglycemia in older people – a less well recognized risk factor for frailty. *Aging and Disease, 6*(2), 156–167. https://doi.org/10.14336/AD.2014.0330.

Ahluwalia, N., Sun, J., Krause, D., Matro, A., & Handte, G. (2004). Immune function is impaired in iron deficient home-bound, older women. *American Journal of Clinical Nutrition, 79*(3), 516–521.

Akirov, A., Masri-Iraqi, H., Atamna, A., & Shimon, I. (2017). Low albumin levels are associated with mortality risk in hospitalized patients. American Journal of Medicine, 130(12), 1465. e11–1465. e19. https://doi.org/10.1016/j.amjmed.2017.07.020.

Amir, O., Liu, A., & Chang, L. S. (2012). Stratification of highest-risk patients with chronic skin ulcers in a Stanford retrospective cohort includes diabetes, need for systemic antibiotics, and albumin levels. *Ulcers, 2012.* 7 pages, Article ID 767861.

Beers, M. H., & Berkow, R. (2000). *The Merck manual of geriatrics.* Rahway, NJ: Merck.

Bryan, R. H. (2010). Are we missing vitamin B12 deficiency in the primary care setting? *Journal for Nurse Practitioners*, *6*(7), 519–523.

Calkins, E. (1999). Autoimmune rheumatic diseases in the older patient. In W. R. Hazzard, et al. (Eds.), *Principles of geriatric medicine and gerontology* (4th ed.). New York: McGraw-Hill.

Chaplin, S. (2015). CRP testing could reduce antibiotic prescribing. *Prescriber*, *26*(18), 29–30. https://doi.org/10.1002/psb.1387.

Chatta, G. S., & Lipschitz, D. A. (1999). Anemia. In W. R. Hazzard, et al. (Eds.), *Principles of geriatric medicine and gerontology* (4th ed.). New York: McGraw-Hill.

Davis, K. M., & Minaker, K. L. (1999). Disorders of fluid balance: dehydration and hyponatremia. In W. R. Hazzard, et al. (Eds.), *Principles of geriatric medicine and gerontology* (4th ed.). New York: McGraw-Hill.

Ehrlich, S.D. (2015). Phosphorus. Retrieved January 23, 2018 from http://pennstatehershey.adam.com/content.aspx?productId=107&pid=33&gid=000319

El-Sharkawy, A. M., Sahota, O., Maughan, R. J., & Lobo, D. N. (2014). The pathophysiology of fluid and electrolyte balance in the older adult surgical patient. *Clinical Nutrition*, *33*, 6–13. https://doi.org/10.1016/j.clnu2013.11.010.

Freedman, M. L., & Sutin, D. G. (2002). Blood disorders and their management. In R. C. Tallis, et al. (Eds.), *Brocklehurst's textbook of geriatric medicine and gerontology* (6th ed.). Edinburgh: Churchill Livingstone.

Gaspard, K. J. (2002). The red blood cell and alterations in oxygen transport. In C. M. Porth (Ed.), *Pathophysiology: Concepts of altered health states.* (6th ed.). Philadelphia, PA: JB Lippincott.

Gilleece, M. H., & Dexter, T. M. (2002). Aging and the blood. In R. C. Tallis, et al. (Eds.), *Brocklehurst's textbook of geriatric medicine and gerontology* (6th ed.). Edinburgh: Churchill Livingstone.

Golzari, H. (2008). Use of digitalis in older adults: A recent update. *Clinical Geriatrics*, *16*(2).

Grodner, M., Long, S., & DeYoung, S. (2004). Foundations and clinical applications of nutrition: a nursing approach. St. Louis: Mosby.

Hall, K. E., & Wiley, J. W. (1999). Aging of the gastrointestinal system. In W. R. Hazzard, et al. (Eds.), *Principles of geriatric medicine and gerontology* (4th ed.). New York: McGraw-Hill.

Ham, R. J., Sloane, P. D., & Warshaw, G. A. (2001). *Primary care geriatrics* (4th ed.). St Louis: Mosby.

Kalyani, R. R., & Egan, J. M. (2013). Diabetes and altered glucose metabolism with aging. *Endocrinology and Metabolism Clinics of North America*, *42*(2), 333–347. https://doi.org/10.1016/j.ecl.2013.02.010.

Kane, R. L., Ouslander, J. G., & Abrass, I. B. (1999). *Essentials of clinical geriatrics* (4th ed.). New York: McGraw-Hill.

Lab Tests Online. (2018). Therapeutic drug monitoring. Retrieved January 28, 2018 from https://labtestsonline.org/tests/therapeutic-drug-monitoring.

Lewis, J.L. (2016a). Overview of disorders of calcium concentration. Retrieved January 22, 2018 from http://www.merckmanuals.com/professional/endocrine-and-metabolic-disorders/electrolyte-disorders/overview-of-disorders-of-calcium-concentration#v1150111.

Lewis, J. L. (2016b). Overview of disorders of magnesium concentration. Retrieved January 23, 2018 from http://www.merckmanuals.com/professional/endocrine-and-metabolic-disorders/electrolyte-disorders/overview-of-disorders-of-magnesium-concentration.

Lizaka, S., Sanada, H., Matsui, Y., Furue, M., Tachibana, T., Nakayama, T., & Miyadi, Y. (2011). Serum albumin level is a limited nutritional marker for predicting wound healing in patients with pressure ulcer: two multicenter prospective cohort studies. *Clinical Nutrition*, *30*(6), 738–745.

McCance, K. L., & Huether, S. E. (2014). *Pathophysiology: The biologic basis for disease in adults and children* (7th ed.). St Louis, MO: Mosby.

Mouton, C. P. (2001). Common infections in older adults. *American Family Physician*, *63*(2), 257–268.

Musso, C. G., & Oreopoulos, D. G. (2011). Aging and physiological changes of the kidneys including changes in glomerular filtration rate. *Nephron Physiology*, *119*(suppl 1), 1–5. https://doi.org/10.1159/000328010.

Office of Dietary Supplements. (2016). Magnesium: Fact sheet for health professionals. Retrieved January 23, 2018 from https://ods.od.nih.gov/factsheets/Magnesium-HealthProfessional/.

O'Neill, P. A. (2002). Venous thrombotic disease and varicose ulcers. In R. C. Tallis, et al. (Eds.), *Brocklehurst's textbook of geriatric medicine and gerontology* (6th ed.). Edinburgh: Churchill Livingstone.

Orton, C. C. (2012). Vitamin B12 (Cobalamin) deficiency in the older adult. *The Journal for Nurse Practitioners*, *8*(7), 547–553.

Pagana, K. D., & Pagana, T. J. (2018). *Mosby's manual of diagnostic and laboratory tests* (6th ed.). St. Louis, MO: Elsevier.

Rothstein, G. (1999). White cell disorders. In W. R. Hazzard, et al. (Eds.), *Principles of geriatric medicine and gerontology* (4th ed.). New York: McGraw-Hill.

Sarkozi, L. (2002). Biochemical tests. In R. C. Tallis, et al. (Eds.), *Brocklehurst's textbook of geriatric medicine and gerontology* (6th ed.). Edinburgh: Churchill Livingstone.

Semenovskaya, Z. (2017). Hypernatremia in emergency medicine. Retrieved January 21, 2018 from https://emedicine.medscape.com/article/766683-overview.

Serra, R., Caroleo, S., Buffone, G., Lugara, M., Molinori, V., Tropea, F., ... de Franciscis, S. (2012). Low serum albumin level as an independent risk factor for the onset of pressure ulcers in intensive care unit patients. *International Wound Journal*, *11*(5), 550–553 https://doi.org/10.1111/iwj.12004.

Simon, E.E. (2018). Hyponatremia clinical presentation. Retrieved January 21, 2018 from https://emedicine.medscape.com/article/242166-clinical.

Thibodeau, G. A., & Patton, K. T. (2003). *Structure and function of the body* (12th ed.). St Louis: Mosby.

Veldurthy, V., Wei, R., Oz, L., Dhawan, P., Jeon, Y. H., & Christako, S. (2016). Vitamin D, calcium homeostasis and aging. *Bone Research*, *4*, 16041. https://doi.org/10.1038/boneres.2016.41.

16

Drugs and Aging

Jennifer J. Yeager, PhD, RN, APRN

ⓔ http://evolve.elsevier.com/Meiner/gerontologic

LEARNING OBJECTIVES

On completion of this chapter, the reader will be able to:

1. Describe the characteristics of drug use in older adults.
2. List at least four classes of drugs best avoided in older adults.
3. Identify potential risk factors for adverse drug reactions.
4. Describe the pharmacokinetic and pharmacodynamic changes associated with aging and the implications for drug therapy and misuse.
5. Recognize significant drug–drug, drug–food, and drug–disease interactions, giving specific examples for each.
6. State the effect that drugs may have on an older adult's quality of life.
7. Describe issues related to the optimum use of antipsychotics, sedatives, hypnotics, cardiovascular agents, and antimicrobials.
8. Anticipate the effects of increased availability of nonprescription and herbal remedies on patient self-management.
9. Identify risk factors for nonadherence and suggest strategies to improve adherence.
10. List the key components of assessing older adults for substance use disorder.
11. Identify the key multidisciplinary and nursing interventions for older adults with substance use disorder.

WHAT WOULD YOU DO?

What would you do if you were faced with the following situations?

- Your resident is in the Alzheimer's unit at your facility. Your resident has been having issues with insomnia and agitation. The following drugs are prescribed:
  - Docusate 240 mg PO every HS (constipation)
  - Melatonin 3 mg PO every day (insomnia)
  - Trazodone 75 mg PO every HS (depression)
  - Mirtazapine 15 mg PO every HS (depression)
  - Sertraline 100 mg PO once daily (depression, obsessive compulsive disorder, and anxiety)
  - Singular 10 mg PO three times per day (asthma)
  - Gabapentin 600 mg PO three times per day (neuropathy)
  - Acetaminophen 650 PO every 6 hrs (PRN (headache))

  Are any of the drugs prescribed for your resident on the Beers list? What are the drug–drug interactions your resident may be experiencing, if any?
- You are precepting a 20-year-old nursing student. When reviewing the admission history they completed on a new 78-year-old patient, you notice questions about substance use disorder were omitted. When questioned, the student states, "I didn't feel comfortable asking the questions; they are elderly, so I doubt it's an issue with them anyway." How would you respond?

OVERVIEW OF DRUG USE AND PROBLEMS

Demographics of Drug Use

Drugs have an important role in the management of conditions and the maintenance of well-being in older adults. At least 94% of community-dwelling adults aged 65 to 74 take prescription or over-the-counter (OTC) drugs. Of these, 81% regularly take prescription drugs, 46% take OTC drugs, and 52% take dietary supplements. The prevalence of drug use increases in those 75 years or older (Qato, Alexander, Conti et al., 2008).

Drugs may be vital contributors to health and well-being, but all drugs carry risks. For older adults, these risks may be dangerous and even life-threatening. To ensure optimal health outcomes, it is important to understand how aging and conditions associated with aging affect drug processes and actions.

Changes in Drug Response With Aging

Aging alters the dynamic processes drugs undergo to produce therapeutic effects. These alterations involve pharmacokinetics (what the body does to the drug) and pharmacodynamics (what the drug does to the body).

Pharmacokinetic Changes: What the Body Does to the Drug

When a drug is taken, it begins a journey of four phases: (1) absorption, (2) distribution, (3) metabolism, and (4) excretion. What the body does to the drug during the four phases of this journey is known as *pharmacokinetics*. The normal physiologic changes that occur with aging alter pharmacokinetics. This section explores pharmacokinetic changes that occur with aging. A summary of important age-related physiologic alterations that affect pharmacokinetics is presented in Table 16.1.

Absorption refers to the movement of a drug from the site of administration to the systemic circulation. Primary alterations

TABLE 16.1   Age-Related Changes in Pharmacokinetics

Variable	Result	Consequence
Absorption		
Gastric pH increased	Alters absorption of drugs requiring acidic environment	Decreased absorption of calcium carbonate
Decreased small bowel surface area		
Slowed gastric emptying		Early release of enteric coated drugs
Distribution		
Decreased serum albumin	Increased volume of distribution for highly lipophilic drugs (e.g., diazepam)	Increase in drug elimination half-life
Increased alpha-1-acid glycoprotein		Increased serum levels of unbound drug
Increased body fat	Rapid decreases in serum albumin may enhance drug effects (e.g., phenytoin and warfarin)	
Decreased total body water		
Hepatic Metabolism		
Decreased hepatic metabolism via cytochrome P-450 enzyme system	Drug clearance may decrease by 30%–40%	May lead to higher circulating drug levels (e.g., nitrates, propranolol, phenobarbital, nifedipine)
Decrease in first pass metabolism (decreases 1%/year after age 40)		
Renal Excretion		
Decreased creatinine clearance (average roughly 8 mL/minute/1.73 m² / decade)	Serum creatinine typically stays the same due to decreased muscle mass and decreased physical activity	Dosage may need to be decreased or frequency of dosing decreased (e.g., levofloxacin, nitrofurantoin, hydrochlorothiazide)

From the Merck Manual, edited by Robert Porter. Copyright 2014 by Merck Sharp & Dohme Corp., a subsidiary of Merck & Co, Inc, Kenilworth, NJ. Available at http://www.msdmanuals.com/professional. Accessed February 14, 2018.

in absorption occur with drugs taken orally or via feeding tubes. Drugs administered orally first need to enter the stomach and intestines. With aging, the risk for decreased secretion of gastric acid, slowed gastric emptying, and decreased gastrointestinal motility exists. Although these effects may *slow* the absorption of oral drugs, they do not substantially affect the *amount* of drug absorption that occurs; therefore age-related changes in the absorption of most drugs are usually insignificant (Ruscin & Linnebur, 2014); however, the first dose of a new drug may take longer to take effect (Hutchison & O'Brien, 2007). Topical drugs also face barriers to absorption. Reduction in subcutaneous fat associated with integumentary changes of aging alters topical

drug absorption. These changes may result in impaired absorption of some drugs administered as lotions, creams, ointments, and patches (Flammiger & Maibach, 2006).

Distribution refers to movement of the drug from systemic circulation to the site of action. Distribution is affected by relative amounts of total body water, fat content, and protein binding. Total body water decreases with aging; decreased total body water results in higher concentrations of water-soluble drugs. Water-soluble drugs tend to stay in the circulation longer, leading to higher drug concentration levels. To decrease the risk of toxicity, smaller doses of water-soluble drugs such as digoxin, lithium, atenolol, and aminoglycosides may be needed for older adults (Aymanns, Keller, Maus, Hartmann, & Czock, 2010). Older adults have decreased lean body mass and increased percentage of fat compared with young adults. The increase in fat composition offers increased storage capability for fat-soluble drugs. As a result, fat-soluble drugs such as benzodiazepines and certain anesthetics (e.g., halothane and thiopental) may have extended half-lives (Ruscin & Linnebur, 2014). A final area of concern regarding distribution involves drugs that are highly protein bound. Drugs of this type, for example, warfarin, phenytoin, furosemide, and naproxen, tend to bind primarily to albumin, a protein in the plasma, and only become active when unbound. With age, particularly for malnourished or frail adults, albumin levels may drop as much as 15% to 25% (Kaufman, 2013), resulting in increased free drug available for action. Decreased protein available for binding may result in toxicity and difficulty maintaining stable drug levels (Ruscin & Linnebur, 2014).

Metabolism refers to the biotransformation of drugs into metabolites that are more easily excreted. Less commonly, metabolism will convert inactive drugs, known as *prodrugs,* to an active form. Metabolism is accomplished through either phase I reactions (oxidation, reduction, demethylation, or hydrolysis via the cytochrome P [CYP] 450 enzyme system) or phase II reactions (glucuronidation, acetylation, conjugation, or sulfation). Recent research has demonstrated that aging does not appear to affect phase II processes. Furthermore, although some isoenzymes (e.g., CYP2C19, which has a role in metabolizing diazepam, naproxen, omeprazole, and propranolol) are reduced with aging, others remain unchanged, are variable, or affect only those older adults who are malnourished or frail (Hutchinson & O'Brien, 2007). Additionally, with aging, a decrease in hepatic blood flow occurs (Hutchison & O'Brien, 2007). This is particularly relevant in relation to first-pass metabolism. *First-pass metabolism* is a process in which drugs absorbed from the stomach or intestines first enter the portal circulation of the liver and a portion are metabolized (inactivated) before reaching the systemic circulation. A decrease in hepatic blood flow may result in a decrease in the amount of a drug inactivated before entering the systemic circulation, resulting in a greater amount of active drug and thus increasing the risk that standard doses of drugs may result in toxic effects (Hutchison & O'Brien, 2007; Ruscin & Linnebur, 2014). The implications of these alterations are that the metabolism of some drugs may be slowed, leading to a prolonged drug half-life and an increased risk of drug accumulation and toxic effects; however, this cannot be generalized to all older adults. Individualization of drug regimens and close monitoring for signs and symptoms of toxic effects and complications is necessary while dosing is adjusted.

Excretion, the elimination of drugs from the body, occurs primarily via the kidneys. When renal function is decreased, half-life increases, and drugs may accumulate to toxic levels. This has important implications for older adults as renal function typically decreases with aging, especially for those who have conditions such as hypertension or heart disease (Shi, Mörike, & Klotz, 2008). Renal function varies from patient to patient, so it is important to evaluate renal function on an individual basis. A serum creatinine level is commonly used as a screening test for renal function; however, serum creatinine is affected by nutritional status, protein intake, and muscle mass (Ruscin & Linnebur, 2014). Therefore in older adults, the best indicator of renal function is the glomerular filtration rate (GFR). Two methods of calculating GFR are deemed acceptable for use in older adults: (1) the Modification of Diet in Renal Disease 6 (MDRD6) formula and (2) the Cockcroft and Gault formula (CG). The MDRD6 slightly overestimates GFR and includes albumin in its calculation; the CG slightly underestimates GFR and is easier to calculate (Chauvelier, Pequignot, Amzal Hanon, & Belmin, 2012). The prescriber may then use information gleaned from the GFR to adjust drug dosing based on renal function.

Nursing management associated with altered pharmacokinetics rests primarily on careful patient monitoring to assess the adequacy of the drug level to achieve the desired effect, and identify adverse drug reactions and events creating problems for the patient. Each drug manifests toxicity in different ways, so it is essential the nurse become familiar with signs and symptoms of toxicity for each drug a patient takes so toxicity can be detected in the early stages. It is also important for the nurse to understand therapeutic drug monitoring. For some drugs (e.g., digoxin), a serum drug level is measured; other drugs (e.g., warfarin) are monitored through diagnostic tests evaluating drug effects (e.g., international normalized ratio [INR]). If evidence of toxicity exists, the nurse will need to assess the patient and promptly notify the provider. The nurse should anticipate adjustment in the drug dosage.

Pharmacodynamic Changes: What the Drug Does to the Body

Physiologic changes associated with aging may also alter how the older adult's body responds to drugs. *Pharmacodynamics,* that is, what the drug does to the body, is the term used to explain the body's response to a drug. Age-related changes affect all substances involved in pharmacodynamics: enzymes, receptors on cell surfaces, carrier molecules, and protein transporters in cell membranes (Kaufman, 2013; Shi et al., 2008). As a result, drug sensitivity may be either increased (e.g., increased anticholinergic effects of tricyclic antidepressants [TCAs]) or decreased (e.g., decreased response to beta-blockers [BBs]). In both respects, the altered sensitivity is unrelated to the drug level. Furthermore, the bodily processes that maintain homeostasis (autonomic control and reflex activity) become less responsive; consequently, the older adult may be less able to tolerate certain drugs. As with nursing actions related to pharmacokinetics, it is

imperative that the nurse assess individual responses to drugs so they can be adjusted to optimize patient outcomes.

Inappropriate Drugs for Older Patients

Because of age-related changes in pharmacokinetics and pharmacodynamics, some drugs and drug classes are less likely to be tolerated by older adults. To identify problematic drugs, expert panels developed screening tools and lists detailing inappropriate drugs for older adults. The most well known of these is the *Beers Criteria for Potentially Inappropriate Medication Use in Older Adults* originally formulated in 1991 (Beers, Ouslander, Rollinger et al., 1991). The most recent update was made by the American Geriatrics Society (AGS) Beers Criteria Update Expert Panel in 2015 (AGS, 2015). The National Committee for Quality Assurance recently made changes to the *Healthcare Effectiveness Data and Information Set (HEDIS): Use of High-Risk Medications in the Elderly and Potentially Harmful Drug-Disease Interactions in the Elderly* to maintain alignment with the 2015 revised Beers Criteria (http://www.ncqa.org).

The Beers list is quite extensive. Readers are asked to review this list directly from the source (https://guideline.gov/summaries/summary/49933/American-Geriatrics-Society-2015-updated-Beers-Criteria-for-potentially-inappropriate-medication-use-in-older-adults). It is not included in this text.

The Beers list has been widely disseminated in the literature since its initial development; however, the use of potentially inappropriate drugs in older adults remains a significant problem. A systematic review conducted by Opondo et al. (2012) revealed that 20% of older adults in the community setting continue to be prescribed potentially inappropriate drugs despite recent attention to the problem. The most widely prescribed potentially inappropriate drugs were doxazosin, diphenhydramine, and amitriptyline. A separate study determined that 48% of older adults admitted to the hospital were taking potentially inappropriate drugs (e.g., benzodiazepines, aspirin, and opiates); additionally, they determined that 27% of admissions were related to potentially inappropriate drugs (Dalleur, Spinewine, Henrard, Losseau, Speybroeck, & Boland, 2012).

Although the Beers Criteria provide important information regarding potentially inappropriate drugs, it is important to recognize that drugs considered appropriate and frequently prescribed for older adults may also carry serious drug-related risks. For example, a retrospective review of more than 175,000 emergency department visits for adverse drug events (ADEs) by older adults revealed that a third of the visits were in response to problems caused by insulin, warfarin, and digoxin (Budnitz, Shehab, Kegler, & Richards, 2007). Of these, only digoxin is included in the Beers Criteria, where it is categorized as moderate risk. Thus it is important to remember that all drugs are potentially harmful and must be weighed in terms of benefit versus risk.

Drugs and Quality of Life

In addition to evaluating drugs in terms of benefit versus risk, it is also important to weigh them in terms of desired versus undesired outcomes. It is natural to assume that a drug is appropriate if it achieves the desired outcome. For example, if an antihypertensive drug such as atenolol adequately maintains blood pressure within normal parameters or if a prokinetic drug such as metoclopramide promotes adequate gastric emptying to decrease gastroesophageal reflux, they would generally be perceived as appropriate drugs. However, if atenolol caused erectile dysfunction or if metoclopramide caused tardive dyskinesia, the patient's quality of life may be decreased compared with the extent of the benefit provided by the drug.

Drugs may have various detrimental effects on cognition, emotion, ambulation, continence, and other essential functions. These negative effects on an older patient's quality of life must be carefully considered as part of pharmacologic therapy. Some patients may prefer to endure a condition rather than suffer an adverse effect for the treatment of it. Generally, alternative drugs or interventions may be used. If one uses the earlier example, an angiotensin-converting enzyme inhibitor (ACEI) will be less likely to cause erectile dysfunction compared with the BB, and the patient's gastroesophageal reflux may be managed with drugs that decrease acidity. For this reason, if a patient refuses a drug, rather than simply charting a drug as refused, the nurse should elicit the patient's perspective so that a more appropriate intervention can be implemented. When other options are not advisable, it is generally important to honor the patient's wishes. Patient-centered therapeutic management considers the patient's beliefs and goals regarding quality of life to be tantamount to those of the provider and is necessary to ensure optimal outcomes.

Pharmacologic Contributors to Risk

Many factors may increase the risk of poor outcomes for older adults who require pharmacologic therapy. Among the most important risk factors are drug interactions, polypharmacy, and substance misuse.

Drug Interactions

Drugs may interact with other drugs and with food. Some drugs may even interact with disease processes. It is important for the nurse to be aware of potential interactions so that harmful patient outcomes can be avoided.

Drug–drug interactions occur in a variety of ways. Perhaps the most common interaction is the result of altered metabolism via the CYP450 hepatic enzyme system. Some drugs can induce or inhibit the activity of various CYP isozymes, which results in increased or decreased biotransformation of drugs. If the biotransformation is accelerated, the affected drug will be inactivated prematurely; however, if the biotransformation is decelerated, the drug may accumulate to toxic levels. Drugs may also interact indirectly through opposing or antagonistic actions. For example, in the patient who has both asthma and hypertension, a BB given to control hypertension may oppose the actions of a beta-agonist given to dilate bronchi. Some drug–drug interactions occur in other ways. For example, some laxatives may cause rapid transit of an orally administered drug through the gastrointestinal system so that it is not adequately absorbed. Drugs may also interact chemically. This is more readily seen in intravenous (IV) solutions in which incompatible drugs may crystallize when mixed; however, it may also occur when certain oral drugs are taken together. Table 16.2 lists examples of significant drug–drug interactions.

TABLE 16.2 Common Drug–Drug Interactions in Older Adults

Drug–Drug Combination	Potential Effect
Warfarin and aspirin	Increased risk of bleeding
Digoxin and quinidine sulfate	Increased risk of digoxin toxicity
Cimetidine and propranolol	Decreased propranolol clearance, increased risk of bradycardia
Hydrochlorothiazide and glyburide	Increased risk of hypoglycemia
Levodopa and clonidine	Decreased antiparkinsonian effect
Hydrochlorothiazide and NSAIDs	Decreased diuretic and antihypertensive effects of thiazides
Lithium and furosemide	Increased risk of lithium toxicity
Lovastatin and gemfibrozil	Increase risk of myopathy, rhabdomyolysis, and other adverse effects
Prednisone and phenobarbital	Decreased steroid effect
Ginkgo with aspirin	Increased bleeding risk

NSAIDs, Nonsteroidal antiinflammatory drugs.

Drug–food interactions are less common than drug–drug interactions but still increase risk. Drug metabolism or effects may be altered when combined with certain foods. For example, potentially dangerous interactions may occur when certain drugs are taken with grapefruit juice because a chemical found in grapefruit juice inhibits metabolism by 3A4 isoenzymes of the CYP450 enzyme system. The 3A4 isoenzymes are responsible for first-pass metabolism of many drugs; therefore, as a result of inhibited metabolism, drugs normally metabolized by 3A4 isoenzymes, for example, calcium channel blockers (CCBs), may accumulate to high or even toxic levels. See Table 16.3 for examples (Kiani & Imam, 2007).

Drug–disease interactions may exacerbate patients' conditions or hinder healing. These drugs are generally contraindicated in patients with coexisting underlying disease. For example, 13% of African American men and 20% of African American women are carriers of a gene that may cause a deficiency in the enzyme glucose-6-phosphate dehydrogenase (G6PD). If a patient with this deficiency takes certain drugs such as sulfonamides or aspirin, erythrocyte hemolysis may occur (Lilley et al., 2007). Table 16.4 lists examples of drug–disease interactions.

Education is an essential component of any risk prevention program. Nurses should provide patients with information regarding the risk of potentially dangerous interactions among all of the drugs they are taking: prescription, OTC, and complementary and alternative drugs. It may be helpful to provide the patient with a list of acceptable OTC drugs for common problems such as mild pain or constipation. A "safe OTC drug list" may be a useful tool for health care providers to review with patients before completing the office visit (Table 16.5).

Polypharmacy

Polypharmacy is "giving drugs without a clear indication, giving two similar drugs for the same indication, giving drugs that are

TABLE 16.3 Common Drug–Food Interactions in Older Adults

Food	Drug	Potential Effect
Caffeine	Theophylline	Increased potential for theophylline toxicity
Vitamin K foods: broccoli, Brussels sprouts, kale, parsley, spinach	Warfarin	Decreased effect of drug, inhibiting anticoagulation
Food	Many antibiotics	Reduced absorption rate of drug
Dairy products	Tetracycline	Prevent the body from absorbing calcium
Tyramine foods: aged cheese, wines, pickled herring, chocolate	Monoamine oxidase inhibitors (MAOIs) (phenelzine, tranylcypromine, St. John's wort)	May precipitate hypertensive crisis
Grapefruit juice	Benzodiazepines, calcium channel blockers, cyclosporine, estrogen, statin drugs	Altered metabolism and elimination can increase concentration of drug

TABLE 16.4 Common Drug–Disease Interactions in Older Adults

Disease	Drug	Potential Effect
Chronic Kidney Disease	NSAIDs	Worsening kidney function
Heart failure	First-generation CCBs (e.g., verapamil) NSAIDs	Cardiac decompensation; fluid retention
Dementia	Anticholinergics Benzodiazepines TCAs Barbiturates	Worsening memory due to decreased acetylcholine transmission
Diabetes	Corticosteroids	Hyperglycemia
Falls	Benzodiazepines TCAs Typical antipsychotics Sedative hypnotics SSRIs	Increased risk of fall with fracture
Parkinson's disease	Metoclopramide Prochlorperazine	Worsening Parkinson's symptoms
Peptic ulcer disease	Aspirin NSAIDs	Increased risk of bleeding
Seizures	Bupropion	Decreased seizure threshold
Constipation	Anticholinergics	Worsening constipation
Benign prostatic hypertrophy	Anticholinergics	Urinary retention

CCBs, Calcium channel blockers; *NSAIDs,* nonsteroidal antiinflammatory drugs; *SSRIs,* selective serotonin reuptake inhibitors; *TCAs,* tricyclic antidepressants.

contraindicated, and/or giving drugs where the dosage is either too high or too low" (Alexander-Magalee, 2013) (see Evidence-Based Practice box). Older adults are vulnerable to polypharmacy because many have one or more chronic conditions requiring multiple drugs (Fig. 16.1). To complicate matters, patients may see more than one provider and may have prescriptions filled at more than one pharmacy (Emmons, 2008). Additional contributors to polypharmacy include the use of OTC and alternative medicines or supplements in the treatment of conditions (Qato et al., 2008). As a result, the patient may end up taking duplicate drugs, similar drugs from the same drug class, and drugs that are contraindicated when taken together.

EVIDENCE-BASED PRACTICE

Management of Potentially Inappropriate Drugs in Vulnerable Populations

Background
Nearly 40% of Medicare beneficiaries have four or more chronic illnesses, leading to duplicate testing, conflicting treatments, and poor coordination of drug therapy. African Americans face a higher incidence of chronic disease than Caucasians.

Sample/Setting
The sample encompassed 400 community-dwelling, underserved, older adults who self-identified as African Americans in Los Angeles County. The mean age was 73.5 years; 20% were over the age of 80. The majority (65%) were women. Few were married or lived with a companion (20%). Participants averaged five comorbid diseases; 19% reported at least eight comorbidities.

Methods
Polypharmacy is defined by a number of drugs prescribed for participants for a "single, or several, coexisting diseases" (p. 2). Participants were recruited from 16 predominantly African American churches. They were asked to bring all OTC and prescription drugs used over the previous 2 weeks. The 2012 Beers for Potentially Inappropriate Medications (PIM) was used to identify PIM for each participant. Pain was evaluated using the Short-Form McGill Pain Questionnaire-2, scoring pain on a 0 = none to 10 = worst imaginable scale. Comorbidity was identified by self-report. The number of health care providers and drug cost were identified by self-report. Participants were also asked to self-identify alcohol and tobacco use.

Findings
Most participants (92%) had a primary care provider and averaged seven scheduled visits over the previous 12 months. Many had more than one prescriber (38%) and used more than one pharmacy (28%). Of the participants, 23% took at least eight drugs per day; 37% took five to seven drugs per day; and 40% took zero to four drugs per day. Twenty-seven percent took drugs classified as "avoid" on the Beers list; 43% took drugs classified as "use conditionally." Women were prescribed more drugs (81% taking five or more drugs) than men (65% taking five or more drugs).

Implications
Polypharmacy and use of PIM is an issue among underserved African Americans, particularly among women. Innovative strategies to improve coordination among multiple providers and pharmacies is necessary to improve the quality of care provided to underserved populations.

From Bazargan, J., Smith, J., Movassaghi, M., Martins, D., Yazdanshenas, H. Mortazavi, S. S., ... Orum, G. (2017). Polypharmacy among underserved older African American adults. *Journal of Aging Research,* Article ID 6026358, 8 pages. doi: 10.1155/2017/6026358.

TABLE 16.5   A List of Safe Over-the-Counter Drugs

If You Have	Generally, Avoid Over-the-Counter Medicines Containing	Examples	Because	Safer Alternatives
Asthma or lung disease	Ephedrine Epinephrine Extra theophylline Pseudoephedrine Caffeine	Bronkaid Primatene Bronkaid Sudafed NoDoz, DeWitt's pills	May cause insomnia, nervousness, irregular heartbeats, especially when taking prescription asthma medicines	Ask your doctor
	Aspirin/salicylates (if you have aspirin allergy)	Ecotrin	May cause allergic reaction (e.g., wheezing, itching, hives)	Acetaminophen
	NSAIDs (if you have aspirin allergy)	Nuprin		
Blood clots (and are taking blood thinners)	Aspirin/salicylates	Ecotrin, Vanquish, Alka-Seltzer, Pepto-Bismol	May cause bleeding	Acetaminophen
	NSAIDs	Nuprin	May cause bleeding	
Heart problems (high blood pressure, heart failure, abnormal heartbeat)	Sodium, salt Phenylpropanolamine Ephedrine Epinephrine/pseudoephedrine Caffeine	Alka-Seltzer, antacids Dexatrim Bronkaid Primatene, Sudafed NoDoz	May worsen your condition	Acetaminophen, nasal sprays, nonmedicated throat lozenges
Diabetes	Liquid or syrups containing alcohol or sugar	Emetrol, many cough or cold syrups	May alter blood sugar	Sugar-free, sugarless, or alcohol-free liquids
	Phenylpropanolamine	Dexatrim, Acutrim	May increase blood sugar	Nonmedicated nose sprays, throat lozenges
	Ephedrine Epinephrine	Bronkaid Primatene		
	Aspirin/salicylates	Ecotrin, Pepto-Bismol	May decrease blood sugar if taking oral diabetes pills to lower sugar	Acetaminophen
Seizures	Aspirin/salicylates		May change levels of prescription seizure medicines	Acetaminophen
	Antihistamines (depressant medicine)	Benadryl, Unisom	May add to drowsiness caused by prescription seizure medicines	Ask your doctor
	Theophylline	Bronkaid	May change levels of prescription seizure medicine	
Stomach ulcers	Aspirin/salicylates NSAIDs	Ecotrin Nuprin	May worsen your ulcers	Acetaminophen
	Theophylline	Bronkaid	May have more side effects from theophylline if taking certain prescription ulcer medicines	Ask your doctor

Note: These are general suggestions and should be discussed with your doctor. He or she may want to change this list or may add suggestions to fit your individual needs. *Always* read the label on nonprescription (over-the-counter) medicines before purchasing, and have a pharmacist assist you if you are not sure what choice to make.
NSAIDs, Nonsteroidal antiinflammatory drugs.

Although only advanced practice nurses can prescribe drugs, other nurses play a vital role in decreasing the number of drugs taken by older adults. Whenever an older patient is seen with a new symptom, the nurse should consider whether the new problem could be caused by a drug the patient is taking (Korc, 2008). If the problem is significant, the prescriber may prefer to discontinue the drug causing the problem rather than prescribe another drug to treat the problem. The nurse may also employ nonpharmacologic interventions, whenever possible. For example, methods such as relaxation therapy and chronotherapy (an intervention combining wake therapy, bright-light therapy, and sleep scheduling) have been shown to be effective nonpharmacologic interventions for management of insomnia in older adults (Joshi, 2008). Lifestyle changes such as weight loss, dietary modifications, and an exercise plan may reduce the need for additional drugs to control hypertension (Moser, Franklin, & Handler, 2007).

Drug Errors: Human and Economic Burdens

The Centers for Disease Control and Prevention (2016) reports that 1 million emergency department visits and more than 280,000 hospitalizations occur each year in the United States

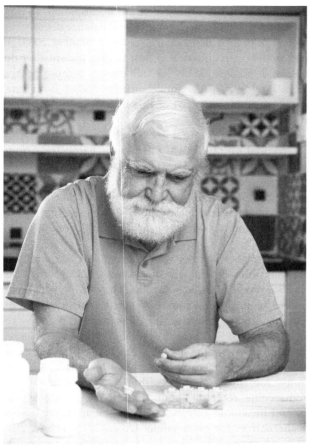

Fig. 16.1 Older adults' concurrent use of many prescription drugs may lead to polypharmacy. (©DragonImages/iStock/Thinkstock.)

secondary to drug errors, resulting in $3.5 billion in added medical costs. Older adults are disproportionately affected. They identified the following as potential causes:

- New drug development
- New uses for older drugs
- Aging American population
- Increased use of drug therapy for disease management and prevention
- Expansion of insurance coverage for prescription drugs

The U.S. Food and Drug Administration (FDA, 2017) uses the National Coordinating Council for Medication Error Reporting and Prevention (NCCMERP) definition of a medication error:

> " a medication error is any preventable event that may cause or lead to inappropriate medication use or patient harm while the medication is in the control of the health care professional, patient, or consumer. Such events may be related to professional practice, health care products, procedures, and systems, including prescribing; order communication; product labeling, packaging, and nomenclature; compounding; dispensing; distribution; administration; education; monitoring; and use."

Because this definition is both comprehensive and complex, examination of its component parts may help best understand it.

The first part of the definition—"A medication error is any preventable event that may cause or lead to inappropriate medication use or patient harm …"—speaks to the outcome of a drug error. The injuries resulting from patient harm are commonly referred to as adverse drug events.

The second part of the definition—"… while the medication is in the control of the healthcare professional, patient, or consumer"—addresses the person who manages the drug storage, dosage, schedule, and disposal. Of concern to older adults are findings of a 20-year study in which researchers identified a marked increase in fatal drug errors among those who take their drugs at home (Spiesel, 2008). This has increased, in part, because of a trend toward shorter hospital stays. As a result, patients are taking drugs at home that were previously closely monitored in a hospital setting. Additionally, development of new drugs has resulted in an increase in drugs prescribed, and this has resulted in an increase in the number of prescriptions for drugs (Spiesel, 2008) as well as an increase in OTC drugs. When patients take OTC drugs, they may not be aware of allergies, contraindications, or interactions with prescribed drugs. Further, many patients may keep drugs long after they have expired rather than disposing of them (Wendling, 2006).

The final part of the definition—"Such events may be related to professional practice, healthcare products, procedures, and systems, including prescribing; order communication; product labeling, packaging, and nomenclature; compounding; dispensing; distribution; administration; education; monitoring; and use"—details the various means by which a drug error may occur. Nurses are involved in processes related to order communication and drug administration, education, monitoring, and use. Errors in order communication commonly occur when verbal orders are poorly communicated or misunderstood (Wakefield, Ward, Groath et al., 2008). Errors in administration involve what has often been referred to as the six *rights of drug administration:* (1) the right drug, (2) in the right dose, (3) at the right time, (4) via the right route, (5) to the right patient, (6) with the right documentation (Lehne, 2013). Drug errors related to education may occur when education is insufficient or unclear. The nurse's role in drug monitoring involves assessing the patient's response for both therapeutic and adverse effects (Lehne, 2013); therefore, errors attributable to monitoring may include a failure to assess for inadequate therapeutic effect or, more likely, a failure to identify when a new problem is attributable to an adverse effect of a drug. Finally, errors related to drug use occur when drugs are not used as indicated; for example, drug misuse occurs when a prescribed opioid analgesic is given for sedation to aid sleep rather than for pain.

Interventions to decrease drug errors are receiving increased importance after the Institute of Medicine's (IOM) report on preventing drug errors (IOM, 2007). Strategies to reduce errors include use of barcoded drug labels, error tracking, and public education. Additionally, the FDA reviews drugs for look-alike or sound-alike names before marketing and has mandated standardized labeling for both prescription and OTC drugs (FDA, 2013).

COMMONLY USED DRUGS

Antipsychotics

Antipsychotic drugs are often prescribed for older adults despite evidence demonstrating their "limited efficacy and significant adverse effects" (Carnahan et al., 2017, p. 554). These drugs have been prescribed for hitting, yelling, and screaming; refusing care and wandering; and inconsolable crying, agitation, and aggression. However, research has demonstrated that these drugs do not help persons with dementia become more involved in their care, interact better with others, or stop inappropriate behavior. In fact, prescribing these drugs led to an increased risk for falls, fractures and breaks, incontinence, strokes, and death (http://www.ahcancal.org). In 2008, the FDA instituted boxed warnings for antipsychotics due to the increased risk of stroke and death in older adults with dementia (Yan, 2008). In 2012, the Centers for Medicare and Medicaid Services (CMS) collaborated with the nursing home industry to reduce inappropriate prescribing of antipsychotic drugs for residents. Since the inception of this initiative, antipsychotic prescribing has decreased from 23.9% in 2012 to 15.7% in 2017 (34.1% decrease in prescribing). CMS has called for an additional decrease of 15% by 2019 (CMS, 2017; Jaffe, 2018). The Improving Antipsychotic Appropriateness in Dementia Patients educational program (IA-ADAPT) and CMS Partnership to Improve Dementia Care programs instituted in nursing homes provided evidence-based training and treatment algorithms for the implementation and documentation of nonpharmacologic interventions to manage older adults with behavioral and psychological symptoms of dementia (BPSD). Decreasing antipsychotic use in nursing homes has not been associated with an adverse effect on BPSD (Carnahan et al., 2017).

Anxiolytics and Hypnotics

Insomnia and anxiety are problems that plague older adults. Many drugs used to treat these problems have the potential for bothersome and potentially dangerous adverse effects when used in older adults. Because insomnia and anxiety often occur secondary to drug side effects or secondary to medical conditions such as dementia, thyroid abnormalities, or depression, proper diagnosis and treatment of underlying causes of insomnia or anxiety may decrease the inappropriate use of these drugs. Nonpharmacologic interventions are often effective but tend to be underused (Adis International, 2007; Moon, 2009); therefore, a trial of nonpharmacologic treatment is preferred before initiation of pharmacologic therapy in older adults.

Barbiturates have been prescribed for both insomnia and anxiety in the past, but their use has declined. These drugs are not recommended for older adults because of their narrow margin of safety and the risks of significant drug interactions and dependence.

Benzodiazepines, which are often prescribed for insomnia and anxiety, also carry concerns for older adults. Benzodiazepines with long half-lives, for example, diazepam, should be avoided because of increased risk for toxicity; in addition, all benzodiazepines, including shorter-acting ones such as lorazepam, may cause excessive sedation, impaired memory, decreased psychomotor performance, and balance disturbances, and may lead to drug dependence (Calleo & Stanley, 2008). If a benzodiazepine is required, it is best to give the smallest dose possible and monitor closely for side effects. Because benzodiazepines should not be used for extended periods, it is important to assess for continued need of these drugs and discontinued them in a timely manner.

First-generation antihistamines, such as diphenhydramine, have been used for indications other than allergy, for example, treatment of insomnia and anxiety. Antihistamines are potentially inappropriate drugs for use in older adults because these patients are more sensitive than younger patients to the anticholinergic adverse effects such as dry mouth, urinary retention, sedation, and even delirium (Nichols, Alper, & Milkin, 2007).

Optimal treatment rests with alternative pharmaceuticals. For anxiety, non–central nervous system (CNS) depressants such as buspirone are effective agents. They take approximately 4 weeks to demonstrate a clinical response, so a benzodiazepine may be required for short-term management if the anxiety is severe (Lehne, 2013). These drugs avoid many of the adverse effects and dependence potential of the benzodiazepines. Similarly, when sleep-hygiene and other nonpharmacologic interventions for insomnia fail, short-term treatment with benzodiazepine receptor agonists (BZRAs), pyrazolopyrimidines, and melatonin receptor agonists are appropriate short-term alternatives for older adults (AGS, 2015; Lehne, 2013). BZRAs such as zolpidem have demonstrated decreased residual sedation and a decreased risk of falls compared with benzodiazepines, as have pyrazolopyrimidines such as zaleplon. The melatonin receptor agonist ramelteon, which is nonsedating, carries the least risk of falls; however, it may not be effective in some patients (Lehne, 2013; Sherman, 2007).

Antidepressants

Most antidepressants are effective for managing depression in older adults; however, some are better tolerated than others. Older TCAs have been used to treat depression as well as insomnia and neuropathic pain; however, significant side effects occur even in low doses and well before therapeutic levels are reached. As a treatment for insomnia, the TCAs are generally too sedating and may cause daytime somnolence. Additionally, TCAs possess anticholinergic side effects that may create problems for many older adults.

Selective serotonin reuptake inhibitors (SSRIs) are the antidepressants of first choice for older adults because these agents are better tolerated; however, they are not without risks. They may cause dose-related gastrointestinal disturbances, including gastrointestinal bleeding, and CNS arousal effects. Fortunately, most of the side effects of the SSRIs last only a few days.

Selection of an antidepressant is often based on side effect profiles, which differ among available agents (Table 16.6). For instance, mirtazapine has more potential for sedation compared with some of the SSRI antidepressants. It may also reduce anxiety and increase appetite; therefore if the patient suffers from depressive symptoms of anxiety, insomnia, and lack of appetite,

TABLE 16.6   Antidepressants: Comparative Profiles

Drug	Avoid in Older Adults	Anticholinergic Side Effects in Older Adults	Sedation	Orthostatic Hypotension
Tricyclics: Tertiary Amines				
Amitriptyline	√	++++	++++	++
Clomipramine	√	+++	+++	++
Doxepin	√	++	+++	++
Imipramine	√	++	++	+++
Trimipramine	√	++	+++	++
Tricyclics: Secondary Amines				
Amoxapine	√	+++	++	+
Desipramine	√	+	+	+
Nortriptyline	√	++	++	+
Protriptyline	√	+++	+	+
Phenethylamines				
Venlafaxine		0	0	0
Tetracyclics				
Maprotiline	√	++	++	+
Triazolopyridines				
Trazodone		+	++	++
Aminoketones				
Bupropion		++	++	++
Selective Serotonin Reuptake Inhibitors				
Fluoxetine		0/+	0/+	0/+
Paroxetine		0	0/+	0
Sertraline		0	0/+	0
Citalopram		0/+	0/+	0/+
Escitalopram		0/+	0/+	0/+
Fluvoxamine		0/+	0/+	0
Miscellaneous				
Nefazodone		0/+	++	+
Mirtazapine		++	+++	

Data from *Drug facts and comparisons* (59th ed.). (2005). St. Louis, MO: Facts & Comparisons.
+++, Strong; ++, moderate; +, weak; 0, none.

then mirtazapine may be an appropriate choice to help the patient sleep while also increasing appetite and reducing anxiety. A patient exhibiting depressive symptoms such as increased sleepiness, decreased affect, and decreased socialization may benefit from a more stimulating antidepressant such as sertraline or venlafaxine. Thus the side effect profile of an antidepressant may be used to identify the most appropriate drug for a patient's depressive symptom pattern.

Cardiovascular Drugs

Heart disease remains the number one cause of death among older adults; stroke is the third leading killer. Nearly a third of persons over age 65 have hypertension. In the United States, the Joint National Committee on Prevention, Detection,

Evaluation, and Treatment of High Blood Pressure (JNC) is the foremost provider of evidence-based clinical guidelines to guide the management of hypertension. The drugs recommended for the management of hypertension are also used in the management of many other cardiovascular conditions.

The Eighth Report of the Joint National Committee on Prevention, Detection, Evaluation, and Treatment of High Blood Pressure (JNC 8) has been published to offer guidance for the management of hypertension. Lifestyle modification is advised as a primary method for preventing and treating hypertension: "weight loss for overweight or obese patients with a heart healthy diet, sodium restriction, and potassium supplementation within the diet; and increased physical activity with a structured exercise program. Men should be limited to no more than

2 and women no more than 1 standard alcohol drink(s) per day" (Whelton et al., 2017, part I #6).

If a pharmacologic agent is needed to treat hypertension, the JNC 8 recommends chlorthalidone as first-line therapy for most patients based on outcome data from clinical trials (Whelton et al., 2017). The addition of a second drug is often determined by the drug's inherent benefits and risks. Those most commonly used for older adults are BBs, ACEIs, angiotensin receptor blockers (ARBs), and CCBs.

BBs have demonstrated improved mortality rates for patients with a history of cardiovascular disease. They decrease angina symptoms, cardiac workload, and oxygen demand through reduction of heart rate, cardiac output, and atrioventricular conduction. This provides a cardioprotective effect for patients with a history of ischemia or myocardial infarction.

CCBs have a beneficial effect in decreasing cardiac workload through decreasing peripheral resistance. For this reason, they are an alternative for patients with severe reactive airway disease or with a high degree of heart blockage where a BB might be contraindicated.

ACEIs and ARBs also have demonstrated value in decreasing the chance of cardiac mortality in patients with heart failure. They also confer renal protection, which is particularly beneficial for patients with diabetes.

Because older adults are likely to have more comorbidities (e.g., diabetes, reduced kidney function, and heart disease), the JNC 8 recommends selecting hypertensive treatment based on comorbid conditions or compelling indications (Whelton et al., 2017). For example, a 70-year-old patient with hypertension and diabetes would benefit from thiazide-type diuretics and an ACEI or ARB, but if the patient had hypertension with ischemic heart disease, the optimal management may be with a thiazide diuretic with a BB.

The main concerns with the use of antihypertensive drugs in older adults are an increased risk of orthostatic hypotension and dehydration, especially with volume-depleting agents and vasodilators. The older adult might have reduced kidney function and a decreased ability to maintain fluid and electrolyte balance. In addition, some older adults may have decreased appetite and sense of thirst resulting in decreased oral intake of food and fluids, and increased risk of dehydration. Subsequently, it is not surprising that dehydration is common among older people and is a frequent reason for admission to the hospital. Assessing for the adverse effects of antihypertensive therapy is essential in maintaining the health of older adults and reducing complications and hospitalizations.

In addition to drugs used in the management of hypertension and related disorders, many older adults are prescribed digoxin. Digoxin is sometimes used to treat heart failure because it increases the force of cardiac contraction, thereby increasing cardiac output; however, research has shown that it does not necessarily reduce morbidity and mortality (Ahmed, Rich, Fleg et al., 2006). For this reason, its use in management of heart failure has become controversial, and it is no longer considered first-line therapy. However, digoxin remains a beneficial agent for the management of atrial tachyarrhythmias because it slows heart rate, allowing for adequate ventricular filling.

Antimicrobials

Infections in older adults may result in devastating health events because of decreased physiologic reserves. Urinary tract infections (UTIs) and respiratory infections (especially pneumonia and exacerbations of chronic lung diseases) are common and often lead to hospital admissions. A frail older person with UTI may experience significant mental status changes, weakness, and sepsis, and may require extended hospitalization and weeks of rehabilitation to return to baseline functional status.

Pharmacologic treatment of infections has the potential to achieve cures, but problems related to their use persist. Because many older adults have reduced renal function, dosage adjustments may be needed for certain antibiotics such as fluoroquinolones. Antibiotic resistance, an increasing problem, may hinder finding the right treatment mix for complicated infections. Common antibiotic side effects such as diarrhea may create significant and even dangerous shifts in fluids and electrolytes in the older adult. Nausea may result in decreased intake, further contributing to this problem.

Nonprescription Agents

Older adults are the largest consumers of nonprescription drugs (Francis, Barnett, & Denham, 2005). They often use these drugs believing if they are available over the counter, they are safe; however, many of the prescription drugs that have been reclassified to nonprescription status (e.g., nonsteroidal antiinflammatory drugs [NSAIDs] and sedating antihistamines) have a potential for significant harm in older populations.

Older adults might not volunteer information about the use of OTC drugs (Francis et al., 2005). As a result, opportunities for drug-related education and checks for interactions with prescribed drugs or effects that may worsen the patient's current health status are missed. This need for education is complicated by the realization that many older adults have decreased visual acuity, cataracts, macular degeneration, and other visual problems that limit the ability to read finely printed labels and instructions (Pawaskar & Sansgiry, 2006). Further, one nationwide study found that 46% of patients taking prescription drugs also take nonprescription drugs, thus increasing the potential for drug–drug interactions (Qato et al., 2008).

The first challenge for nurses regarding nonprescription drugs is to remain informed about *all* drugs patients are currently taking. It is necessary to verify that no contraindications or significant interactions with prescribed drugs exist. It is also important to caution patients against certain products that may interact negatively with other drugs or with their medical condition(s).

Dietary Supplements

Dietary supplements are an overarching category of drugs that include vitamins, minerals, herbal remedies, and alternative medicines. The use of dietary supplements is an established practice among many older adults. According to a recent study, almost half (49%) of older adults living in the United States take some sort of dietary supplement on a regular basis (Qato et al., 2008). The same study identified that more than half (52%) of older adults who take prescription drugs also take supplements, and this increases the potential for drug–drug interactions. The most common dietary supplements identified in this study were vitamins or minerals and system-specific remedies such as omega-3 fatty acids, garlic, and coenzyme Q-10 for cardiovascular problems; glucosamine–chondroitin for joint problems; and saw palmetto for prostate problems. Additional frequently used supplements identified in a separate 6-year retrospective review of supplement use in older adults include ginkgo biloba, black cohosh, borage, evening primrose, flaxseed oil, dehydroepiandrosterone (DHEA), grapeseed extract, hawthorn, and St. John's wort (Wold, Lopez, Yau et al., 2005). A particularly troubling finding was the identification of supplement–drug interactions with 10 of the supplements and the potential of 142 interactions over the 6-year period.

Many additional concerns exist with regard to the use of dietary supplements. They are not regulated for safety and efficacy by the FDA in the same manner as prescription drugs, which undergo a rigorous drug approval process. As a result, predictability of product quality and potency is lacking. Many herbs are available in their natural unprocessed state, further complicating predictability. Beyond these concerns, the use and safety of these products in older adults, especially in older adults with comorbidities, have not been adequately studied.

As with any drug, dietary supplements have inherent adverse effects, particularly when taken in large doses. Although many may be beneficial, or at least not harmful, they may also interact with certain diseases and normal physiologic processes, which may lead to delayed improvement.

Unfortunately, information regarding dietary supplements is often nebulous and misleading. To address the need for scientific research and authoritative information, the National Center for Complementary and Alternative Medicine (NCCAM) was established under the umbrella of the National Institutes of Health (NIH). NCCAM provides information to health care professionals as well as to the lay public on its website at http://nccam.nih.gov.

DRUG ADHERENCE

Drug regimens are carefully planned so that optimal dosing and scheduling will prevent drug interactions and other complications while promoting optimal well-being. Many patients, however, may omit drugs at times or may alter drug dosages or schedules. This failure to stick to the agreed-on drug regimen is called *nonadherence*. Although nonadherence occurs in all age groups, it is likely to create more problems in older adults, who tend to have chronic and often multiple illnesses requiring drug therapy.

The most common reasons for nonadherence in older adults include the cost of drugs (Briesacher, Gurwitz, & Soumerai, 2007), side effects or fear of side effects (Ferdinand, 2009), complex scheduling (Bibbens-Domingo & DiMatteo, 2006), age-related changes such as visual or cognitive impairment (Kairuz, Bye, Birdsall et al., 2008; Stoehr, Lu, Lavery et al., 2008; Windham, Griswold, Fried et al., 2005), and a belief that the drugs are either ineffective or unnecessary (Chia, Schlenk, & Dunbar-Jacob, 2006; Proulx, Leduc, Vandelac et al., 2007). Other contributors to nonadherence include cultural factors (Chia et al., 2006; Wen-Wen,

Wallhagen, & Froelicher, 2007) and health literacy issues (Davis, Wolk, Bas et al., 2006; Maniaci, Heckman, & Dawson, 2008). By understanding the reasons for nonadherence, nurses are better equipped to identify adherence risks and take specific risk-targeted action to decrease this common problem.

In approximately one-third of older adults, prescription-related costs contribute to nonadherence (Briesacher et al., 2007). Drugs may be expensive, and many older adults are on fixed incomes requiring tight budgets. Even those with insurance to deflect the cost may not be able to afford the required deductible. Although resources exist to provide pharmacy assistance to low-income patients, many are unaware of these programs or do not know how to access assistance (Federman & Safran, 2008). To cope with high drug costs, some patients decrease or skip doses to make a prescription quantity last longer. Others resort to decreasing money spent on food or other needs so that they can afford drugs. For many, however, the costs are so high that prescriptions for necessary medicines are left unfilled (Madden, Graves, Zhang et al., 2008).

Side effects and the fear that side effects may occur are other common reasons for nonadherence. If the side effects are perceived as significant or if they interfere with daily activities, patients may be tempted to avoid these effects by omitting the drug that causes them. Side effects are especially relevant if drug benefits are not obvious. Indeed, the patient's perception of drug effectiveness and necessity of the drug plays an important role in adherence. Many of the drugs prescribed for chronic illnesses serve to keep the conditions from progressing but do not cure the illness. Patients who do not feel better may perceive that the drug is ineffective. If a drug is given to cure an illness such as an infection, the patient may stop the drug prematurely once the symptoms resolve because of the erroneous belief that it is no longer needed.

Age-related changes that contribute to nonadherence may be functional or cognitive. Vision changes that occur with aging may affect the ability of the patient to read labels on drug containers or to distinguish one drug from another. Stiffness of joints coupled with decreased hand strength or tremors may make it difficult to open drug bottles. Swallowing difficulties are exacerbated by large tablets. For some older adults, mental status changes that affect the ability to think clearly and make reasoned judgments contribute to unintentional nonadherence. Similarly, memory impairment and forgetfulness increase the likelihood that drugs will not be taken as prescribed.

For older adults with complex or multiple chronic illnesses requiring several drugs, drug schedules may be complex. For example, some drugs should be taken on an empty stomach, whereas others should be taken with food. Some drugs should not be taken together because drug–drug interactions may occur. Still others require scheduling to coordinate with certain times of the day (e.g., at bedtime). Keeping up with complicated schedules, particularly when they conflict with everyday activities, may increase the probability of nonadherence.

Assessing for Risk Factors

Because the effects of nonadherence can be devastating, it is important for the nurse to be proactive in preventing nonadherence. Prevention begins with an assessment of risk factors. A simple checklist may be used to help identify areas of primary concern.

- Are the prescribed drugs costly, or does the cost of drugs present a substantial burden to the patient?
- Do the prescribed drugs have the potential for significant side effects, or does the patient experience troublesome side effects?
- Are drug schedules cumbersome, or do they interfere with the patient's daily activities or sleep?
- Does the patient have any conditions that would make opening bottles, manipulating individual tablets, or swallowing drugs difficult?
- Does the patient have difficulty reading and comprehending instructions?
- Does the patient believe that any of the prescribed drugs are ineffective or unnecessary?
- Does the patient have any cultural beliefs that would cause them to avoid reliance on drugs or regard certain drugs as inappropriate?

Each item checked indicates a potential contributor to nonadherence. For those items, the nurse needs to work further with the patient to correct any misunderstandings, to establish necessary support services or networks, and to advocate for patient-centered adjustments in the drug regimens.

Strategies for Improving Adherence

Many patients do not share information regarding nonadherence, so it is a mistake to assume that the patient takes drugs as prescribed or recommended. In clinic settings, the nurse should have the patient bring in all prescription and OTC drugs and any dietary supplements at the initial visit and at least every 6 months thereafter (Korc, 2008; Pham & Dickman, 2007). Nurses working in hospitals should adopt this policy for every admission or emergency department visit ("Get a better med history," 2009). When reviewing drugs, the nurse should ask the patient how each drug is taken and compare this information with the prescription label or to the drugs listed in the patient's record to see whether nonadherence is a concern.

Patient teaching is an essential intervention for addressing the problem of drug nonadherence; however, studies show that teaching alone is rarely sufficient to evoke change (Ruppar, Conn, & Russell, 2008). To adequately address issues of drug nonadherence, nurses need to understand the factors that contribute to a patient's failure to take drugs as directed and to develop risk-specific assessments and interventions individualized to the patient. Interventions should also consider resources available in the region where services are provided. For example, if the patient has difficulty paying for drugs, the nurse may provide the patient with a resource list of pharmacies offering low-cost generic discounts. If generic drugs are not available for a proprietary drug that is ordered, the nurse may need to check for patient assistance programs for the drug in question.

The nurse should encourage all patients to have prescriptions filled at the same pharmacy each time because this provides an extra way to discover problems. The nurse should also tailor the drug regimen to the patient's home schedule to cause the least disruption in daily life and give the patient a sense of control over the drugs. The regimen should be simplified as much as possible; multiple daily doses should be avoided where appropriate and feasible.

Reviewing the Drug List for Problems

Nurses confronted with a complex drug regimen for an older patient should determine the answers to the following questions:

- Is a documented and appropriate indication for each drug present?
- Is a drug dosage appropriate for the patient's age, weight, and renal or liver function?
- Does the patient have a documented drug allergy to a drug?
- Are doses of a drug being scheduled appropriately?
- Is the duration of treatment appropriate?
- Is a chosen drug the best one for the patient?
- Are two or more similar drugs prescribed (i.e., therapeutic duplication)?
- Is the patient experiencing an adverse drug reaction?
- Is a potential drug–drug interaction present?
- Does a medical indication exist for the use of a drug when none is currently prescribed?
- Is the patient using OTC drugs appropriately?
- What herbal or alternative therapies are being used by the patient? Is the patient's health care provider aware of these?
- Is the patient adherent?

🏠 HOME CARE

1. During each home visit, assess both prescription and nonprescription drugs being taken by the homebound older adult.
2. Document and notify the primary health care provider of the homebound older adult's drug regimen and of multiple physician sources for drugs if present.
3. Teach the side effects and interactions of all OTC drugs to homebound older adults and their caregivers.
4. Collaborate with social workers to identify community resources for financial assistance with pharmaceutical needs.
5. Monitor drug levels and other appropriate laboratory values as appropriate (e.g., potassium or sodium).
6. Teach the homebound older adult to set up a daily or weekly schedule for drugs using a method or tool that fosters safe, independent administration.
7. Reduce the chance of drug errors by labeling or color-coding drug bottles.
8. Keep an accurate record of the homebound older adult's weight.
9. Teach drug safety in the home environment by instructing patients to do the following:
   - Keep drugs in original, labeled containers.
   - Follow appropriate guidelines for drug disposal; never dispose of drugs in the trash within reach of children.
   - Never "share" drugs with friends or family members.
   - Always finish a prescribed drug; do not save it for a future illness.
   - Read labels carefully and follow all instructions.
10. Instruct older adults who have difficulty opening childproof containers to ask their health care providers for non–child proof containers when writing prescriptions.

SUBSTANCE USE DISORDERS

Many older adults enjoy leisure activities as a result of decreased work schedules and retirement. However, some are unable to enjoy leisure activities because of the emotional, physical, social, and economic effects of growing older. Use of illicit drugs such as cocaine, opiates, and marijuana, previously thought to be a problem among young adults, has become more prevalent in older adults as Baby Boomers, with a history of being more tolerant of such practices, reach retirement age. Among older persons, misused substances include alcohol, prescription and nonprescription drugs, and tobacco. Marijuana and cocaine are included in the category of nonprescription drugs.

More than a million older adults had a substance use disorder (SUD) in 2014 (978,000 with alcohol use disorder [AUD] and 161,000 with illicit drug use disorder). SUD has become a public health concern among older adults. The number of older adults with SUD is expected to reach 5.7 million by 2020. The emergence of SUD as a public health concern among older adults reflects, in part, the relatively higher drug use rates of the Baby Boomers compared with previous generations. Older adults with SUD experience increased "physical and mental health issues, social and family problems, involvement with the criminal justice system, and death from drug overdose" (Mattson, Lipari, Hays, & Van Horn, 2017, para. 1) and adverse drug interactions with prescription and OTC drugs.

Frequently, the symptoms of SUD are subtle or atypical, or they mimic symptoms of other age-related illnesses and remain undiagnosed. A patient's presenting symptoms may be erratic changes in affect, mood, or behavior; malnutrition; bladder and bowel incontinence; gait disturbances; and recurring falls, burns, and head trauma (Morris, 2001; Videbeck, 2004). Many older adults began to misuse alcohol late in life because of bereavement, retirement, loneliness, or physical and emotional illnesses. Denial is more intense in older adults because of cognitive and memory problems and shame. The most frequently misused prescription drugs are opioids, benzodiazepines, sedatives, tranquilizers, and stimulants, which may result in ataxia, falls and accidents, and cognitive impairments such as attention and memory problems (Kuerbis, Sacco, Blazer, & Moore, 2014).

Definitions and Common Usage

Nurses must understand definitions associated with SUD to correctly assess it and plan appropriate interventions for older adults. The *Diagnostic and Statistical Manual of Mental Disorders, Fifth Edition* (DSM-5) published by the American Psychiatric Association (APA, 2013) is used by physicians as an aid in diagnosing patients. The DSM-5 defines SUD as "occur(ing) when the recurrent use of alcohol and/or drugs causes clinically and functionally significant impairment, such as health problems, disability, and failure to meet major responsibilities at work, school, or home. ... [A] diagnosis of substance use disorder is based on evidence of impaired control, social impairment, risky use, and pharmacologic criteria" (Substance Abuse and Mental Health Services Administration [SAMHSA], 2015).

Difficulty in Identification of Substance Use Disorder

The physiologic, psychological, and sociologic changes associated with aging make the identification and treatment SUD in older adult patients difficult. Age-related psychological and sociologic changes and symptoms may be subtle or atypical and may mimic symptoms of SUD (Mohundro & Ramsey, 2003; Videbeck, 2004). Often, clinicians and family members are hesitant to ask whether the older adult is having problems with use or misuse of prescription drugs. Traditionally accepted ways of detecting problems with substances (e.g., time lost from work, legal problems, or decreased participation in important social activities) are not helpful in older adults because they generally have fewer activities and obligations (Trevisan, 2008).

Physiologic Changes

Patients with early-onset AUD appear to have a more severe course of illness. They make up about two-thirds of older adults with AUD, are predominantly male, and have more alcohol-related medical problems and psychiatric comorbidities. Patients with later onset AUD tend to have a milder clinical picture and fewer medical problems because of the shorter exposure to alcohol. They are more affluent, include more women, and are likely to begin their alcohol use after a stressful event such as loss of a spouse, job, or home (Trevisan, 2008).

Nurses should be aware of age-related physiologic changes of absorption, distribution, plasma protein binding, hepatic metabolism, and elimination or clearance of a drug. The assessment of these changes in relation to substance use is essential in planning interventions to prevent or halt substance use and misuse in the older adult population.

Psychological Changes

Psychological changes in older adults result primarily from the numerous losses this age group experiences in a relatively short period. Roughly 6% of persons over the age of 65 drink heavily. Heavy drinking is often in response to bereavement, retirement, loneliness, relationship stress, and physical illness (Fig. 16.2).

Nurses should be aware of the misconception that select prescribed or OTC substances may help the patient deal with unmet psychological needs. For example, an older adult may become anxious if sleep has decreased to less than 8 hours and may seek sedatives. In addition, some older adults tend

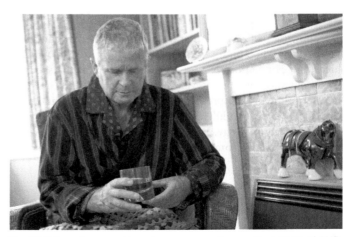

Fig. 16.2 Loneliness and hopelessness may be manifestations of AUD. (©BananaStock/Thinkstock.)

to use certain substances to mask negative feelings about themselves; they may eventually attribute some of their positive personality characteristics to substances. Examples of such substances include alcohol and benzodiazepines (e.g., diazepam). Patients who are prescribed benzodiazepines by a physician for a limited period may become dependent on the drug. An older adult who has become dependent may find another physician to prescribe the drug when the original physician discontinues it.

The nurse must also assess older adults for suicidal ideation. Patients should be asked whether they have had thoughts of harming themselves and whether they have a plan to carry out these thoughts. Advancing age and substance misuse are among the greatest risk factors for suicide. Suicide rates tend to increase with age in white men, and it should be noted that suicide is the 13th leading cause of death in older adults.

Sociologic Changes

Sociologic changes such as decreases in finances, transportation, and social support tend to place older adults at risk for SUD. Because of decreased finances and transportation, many older adults fill prescriptions through mail-order pharmacies. Mail-order pharmacies tend to increase the potential for drug misuse because of prescription errors, late arrivals, and large quantities of drugs. Social conditions such as low income, difficulty shopping, and lack of socialization tend to affect the nutrition of older adults. The nurse should educate older adults about the dual effects of poor nutritional status and drug metabolism.

Sociologic changes are based on the cultural values and attitudes about substance misuse behaviors passed from one generation to another. A lower incidence of SUD is seen in cultures whose religious and moral values prohibit or limit their use. Older adults are targeted by advertisements for prescription and nonprescription drugs because they experience minor aches, pains, and major health problems. SUD are symptomatic of the larger social problems among minority groups (e.g., poverty, substandard housing, inadequate health care, and lack of power). The lack of culturally competent care is an additional barrier to care for the older adult with SUD.

ASSESSMENT

The following section is a general overview of the key concepts in assessing and planning nursing interventions for SUD in the older adult population. Nurses should be aware of the specific assessment and nursing intervention strategies for AUD, misuse of prescription and nonprescription drugs, illicit drugs, and nicotine. SUDs in older adults are challenging in that they require expertise in gerontology, geriatrics, psychiatric mental health, and the specific presentation and management of disorders in this population.

Substance Use History

The DSM-5 criteria for SUD are developed for the general population, not specifically for the older adult population. Therefore it is essential for the nurse to assess patients' medical and psychological histories. After history taking is completed, the nurse should identify the key medical and psychological manifestations of SUD.

Screening Tools

Many screening tools are available to assess alcohol use. The two most commonly used tools are the CAGE (**C**utdown, **A**nnoyed by criticism, **G**uilt about drinking, and **E**ye-opener drinks) (Mayfield, McLeod, & Hall, 1974) and the Michigan Alcoholism Screening Test (MAST) (Selzer, 1971). The Brief Michigan Alcoholism Screening Test (BMAST) is a modified form of the MAST (Pokorny, Miller, & Kaplan, 1972). Frederick Blow developed the MAST–Geriatric Version (MAST-G) (Morton, Jones, & Manganaro, 1996). Results indicate that the MAST-G is an instrument that is more reliable and valid in the older adult population compared with the MAST (Knight & Mjelde-Mossey, 1995). Even though further research is required to validate the use of these tools for the assessment of SUD besides AUD, positive clinical results have been demonstrated with the use of these tools, substituting the words *substance* or *prescription medication* for *drink*.

Patients undergoing detoxification from AUD should be assessed with the use of the Clinical Institute Withdrawal Assessment tool on an ongoing basis. The tool measures the severity of alcohol withdrawal based on 10 common signs and symptoms: (1) nausea and vomiting; (2) tremor; (3) paroxysmal sweats; (4) anxiety; (5) agitation; (6–8) tactile, auditory, and visual disturbances; (9) headache; and (10) orientation. The maximum score is 67, and patients who score higher than 20 should be admitted to a hospital (Fontaine, 2003).

Nursing Caveats

In assessing older adults for SUD, the nurse must be aware of his or her own perceptions and attitudes regarding SUD in the older adult population. Many health care providers overlook the possibility that the presenting symptoms in an older adult may be related to SUD. It is important to have a healthy collaborative relationship with patients, showing respect for their values and choices.

Inherent changes in tissue and organ function are highly variable and individual. Hence the response to drug therapy is just as variable and as unpredictable in this population. The guiding principles are to "start low and go slow" when prescribing drugs; change or add only one drug at a time; review each drug to see whether the patient is still taking it; and determine the dose, frequency, and time.

NURSING DIAGNOSES

The following list identifies nursing diagnoses that may be used for older adults with SUD:
- Inadequate family therapeutic management
- Anxiety
- Inadequate thermoregulation
- Confusion
- Inadequate coping
- Disrupted family routines

- Inadequate nutrition
- Reduced self-care ability (bathing, dressing, feeding, or toileting)
- Reduced body image
- Reduced sleep pattern
- Reduced social interaction
- Potential for self-directed violence
- Potential for outward-directed violence

NURSING MANAGEMENT

Interventions

Multidisciplinary interventions are appropriate for all individuals overcoming SUD because no single intervention is appropriate. Effective interventions attend to the multiple needs of individuals, not just their drug or substance use. Interventions must address medical, nursing, psychological, social, vocational, and legal problems.

Interventions and treatment options include brief therapy, intensive outpatient or inpatient treatment, and residential treatment. Brief therapy is usually provided by a trained professional in a community drug treatment center. Goal-setting, self-monitoring, and identifying high-risk situations are specific learned behaviors that help stop or reduce patients' substance misuse. Intensive outpatient programs allow patients to remain at home and continue working while they participate in treatment in an unrestricted setting for 4 to 5 hours every day. Intensive inpatient treatment is provided in the emergency department or acute care inpatient units to patients at risk of severe withdrawal symptoms, those who are psychiatrically disabled, and those who have not responded to less intensive treatment efforts. Residential treatment programs are downsizing and closing because third-party reimbursement is rapidly decreasing. Traditionally, treatment lasted 7 to 21 days and offered a safe and structured environment to those who lacked social and vocational skills and drug-free social supports to be abstinent in a less restricted setting (Fontaine, 2003).

Older adults resist referrals to SUD programs and are more comfortable in senior-oriented programs. Some are unable or unwilling to leave their homes, thus programs should be specific for older adults and use special approaches such as slow-paced and emotionally supportive therapy instead of the confrontational style used with younger adults.

Acupuncture has been used to treat SUD. It eases the symptoms of withdrawal, decreases the intensity of cravings, and decreases the number of relapses. Acupuncture is a safe and relatively low-cost form of treatment. However, more research is necessary before acupuncture or other complementary and alternative therapies can be recommended as treatment modalities for SUD (Behere, Muralidharam, & Benegal, 2009).

Evaluation

The evaluation of the treatment of older adults with SUD consists of the assessment of safe detoxification, adherence to the sobriety treatment plan, and outpatient support. Detoxification is safe if a patient has been weaned from the misused substance without seizures, delirium tremens (DTs), changes in vital signs, or other complications of withdrawal. Adherence is measured by noting if the patient is abstaining from substance use and attending meetings (e.g., Alcoholics Anonymous [AA] or Narcotics Anonymous [NA]) and individual or family group sessions. Finally, outpatient support is assessed to determine whether the patient is maintaining the relationship with a sponsor. A *sponsor* is someone who can be a mentor and support the patient during abstinence.

COMMONLY MISUSED SUBSTANCES IN OLDER ADULTS

Alcohol

Prevalence

AUD is difficult to assess because of the drug's legal status and socialization as a recreational activity in the United States. The difficulty in identifying AUD notwithstanding, the incidence of AUD identified in the older adult population in health care settings is 22%. The prevalence rate of alcohol misuse is projected to increase as more Baby Boomers reach retirement age (Kuerbis et al., 2014).

Some heavy drinkers with early-onset AUD survive into old age; others are late-onset drinkers, who may have started drinking in late middle age and began to exhibit health problems related to AUD as they moved into older adulthood. Older adults who have used alcohol in the past without misuse may experience problems with alcohol consumption as changes occur in their bodies as a result of normal aging (e.g., decreased liver function or changes in body composition) (Morris, 2001).

Assessment

Older adults with AUD may display symptoms of anxiety, nervousness, memory impairment, depression, blackouts, confusion, weight loss, and falls. In addition, physical examination of an older adult may indicate the effects of alcohol on the various body systems. Table 16.7 shows age-related and alcohol-related changes in select body systems of older adults. The nurse should assess carefully for the following signs and symptoms: impaired sensations in the extremities, poor coordination, confusion, facial edema, alcohol on the breath, liver enlargement, jaundice, ascites, trembling or fidgeting, lack of attention to personal hygiene, and poor eating habits. Secondary problems may include malnutrition, cirrhosis, compromised hepatic function, osteomalacia because of compromised metabolism of vitamin D, cardiomyopathy, atrophic gastritis, and a decline in cognitive status, especially with regard to memory and information processing. Laboratory evaluation should include assessment of liver function and levels of electrolytes, glucose, and magnesium, as well as electrocardiography (ECG) (Videbeck, 2004).

AUD may not be accurately assessed in older adults also because many AUD symptoms such as falls, bruises, cardiovascular problems, hypertension, and memory problems may resemble other disease processes. Therefore if an older adult displays these symptoms, it is imperative the nurse assess for

TABLE 16.7   Age- and Alcohol-Related Changes in Body Systems of Older Adults

Age-Related Changes	Corresponding Alcohol-Related Changes
Decline in liver function	Hepatotoxicity
Delayed neurologic conduction	Increase of Parkinson's disease symptoms, altered balance
Idiopathic tremors	Tremors related to withdrawal
Predisposition to falls	Predisposition to falls
Loss of short-term memory	Impairment of short-term memory
Decreased glucose tolerance	Inhibition of glycogenesis
Decreased secretion of hydrochloric acid	Impaired absorption of nutrients
Slowed peristalsis	Impaired absorption of nutrients
Decreased saliva production	Impaired absorption of nutrients
Increase in cholesterol levels and cardiovascular disease	Increased plasma triglyceride levels
Less efficient cardiovascular function	Risk of congestive heart failure
Increased incidence of arthritis and gout	Increased uric acid levels
Decline in immunologic competence	Increased susceptibility to infection

Developed from Coffey, C. E. & Cummings, J. L. (1994). *Textbook of geriatric neuropsychiatry*. Washington, D.C.: American Psychiatric Press; Solomon, K., Manepalli, J., Ireland, G. A., & Mahon, G. M. (1993). Alcoholism and prescription drug abuse in the elderly: St. Louis University Grand Rounds. *Journal of the American Geriatric Society, 41*, 57-69.

the possibility of alcohol misuse in addition to medical illness and disease.

After obtaining a health history and conducting a physical examination, the nurse should begin to assess specifically for AUD. The CAGE, MAST, MAST-G, or BMAST screening tools may help the nurse determine the amount and frequency of alcohol consumption. Input from family and friends should also be obtained. Family and friends may deny the problem; therefore it is imperative that the nurse obtain the history of alcohol use in a detail-oriented, nonjudgmental manner (Pokorny et al., 1972; Knight & Mjelde-Mossey, 1995).

The nurse should be able to distinguish alcohol intoxication from alcohol withdrawal to apply the appropriate nursing interventions. Signs associated with alcohol intoxication include the scent of alcohol on the breath, slurred speech, lack of coordination, unsteady gait, nystagmus, impairment in attention or memory, and stupor or coma (APA, 2013). Assessment of the signs and symptoms of alcohol withdrawal is essential in providing the appropriate treatment and preventing DTs and seizures. Indications of alcohol withdrawal are elevated blood pressure, elevated pulse, and autonomic hyperactivity. In addition, fever; increased hand tremors; insomnia; nausea and vomiting; transient visual, tactile, or auditory hallucinations or illusions; psychomotor agitation; anxiety; and grand mal seizures may occur (APA, 2013). Withdrawal symptoms begin 4 to 12 hours after alcohol use has been stopped or reduced. Symptoms tend to peak 48 to 72 hours after a patient's last drink (APA, 2013).

It is important to assess older patients for the possibility of alcohol withdrawal if agitation, hallucinations, anxiety, or seizures develop 2 or 3 days after hospitalization (see Emergency Treatment box).

✚ EMERGENCY TREATMENT

Delirium Tremens

The following nursing interventions should be implemented for patients who experience delirium tremens (DTs):
1. Assessment of vital signs
2. Provision of a safe environment (padded side rails, decreased stimulation)
3. Close observation
4. Administration of prescribed drugs such as benzodiazepines, BBs, clonidine, and anticonvulsant drugs

Interventions

Nursing interventions for older adults with AUD vary, depending on whether the patient is in detoxification or rehabilitation. Nurses should observe and document signs of withdrawal, provide an environment of low stimulation (e.g., dim lights and a quiet atmosphere), and initiate seizure precautions (e.g., padded side rails and the bed in lowest position) during the detoxification process. In addition, the nurse should administer drugs, such as benzodiazepines, BBs, and anticonvulsants, which are used to reduce symptoms of withdrawal and prevent complications. During the rehabilitation stage, recommended nursing interventions include patient education; continued administration of drugs; group, individual, and family therapy; and introducing the patient to the 12-Step Program. The nurse supports the patient with (1) education on the harmful effects of alcohol on the body and the effects of alcohol taken with prescription and nonprescription drugs, (2) various methods to overcome potential triggers for future substance misuse, and (3) plans to maintain sobriety in the community setting. The nurse should also educate family members on the potential changes in family dynamics resulting from the patient's sobriety. In addition, the nurse should encourage the recognition that SUD is a "family disease" and abstinence is affected by the family process. All family members need education to help identify triggers to avoid relapse and strategies for dealing with triggers (Fontaine, 2003; Mahgoub, 2009).

Many pharmacologic interventions have been used to inhibit drinking behaviors, with varying results. Drugs for recovery may include disulfiram, naltrexone, acomprosate, or topiramate. Disulfiram, when taken with alcohol, causes vomiting; naltrexone interferes with the pleasure derived from drinking; acomprosate reduces the craving for alcohol; and topiramate may alter the stimulating effects of alcohol. Thiamine may have to be added to improve nutritional status.

Evaluation

The evaluation of the treatment of an older adult patient with AUD includes safe detoxification, adherence to a treatment plan for sobriety, and outpatient support. Safe detoxification consists of weaning from alcohol without seizures, DTs, or other withdrawal complications. The nurse also assesses whether the patient is adhering to the sobriety protocol of abstinence and attendance at AA meetings and individual or family therapy. In addition, a continued relationship with the patient's sponsor and the patient's progress as reported by home health nurses provide the opportunity for evaluation of the patient's transition back into the community (Fontaine, 2003).

Prescription Drugs

Prevalence

The prevalence of misuse of prescription drugs among older adults is high. The number of drugs prescribed is directly correlated to the risk of their inadvertent misuse. As a result, the possibility of polypharmacy is high. Prescription drugs commonly used by independent older people are cardiovascular drugs, benzodiazepines, diuretics, cathartics, antacids, thyroidal drugs, and anticoagulants. Opioid and benzodiazepine dependence is a common occurrence, and the drugs may have been prescribed for long periods (Kuerbis et al., 2014). The nurse may be the person who recognizes the possible existence of prescription drug misuse. The rapport between the nurse and the patient allows the patient to feel comfortable discussing drug use. Therefore it is imperative that the nurse assess for prescription drug misuse in older adults.

Assessment

Nursing assessment for prescription drug misuse in older adult patients is like the assessment used for AUD. The nurse should begin the assessment by taking a careful history using the CAGE, MAST, BMAST, or MAST-G screening tools (Morton et al., 1996). The nurse should remember to substitute the term *prescription drugs* for *alcohol*. In addition, the nurse should assess for a tendency to repeatedly lose prescriptions or pills (e.g., "I threw it away by accident," "I didn't think I would use them so I flushed them down the toilet"), prescriptions from multiple physicians, frequent emergency department visits, strong preferences for particular drugs (e.g., "Only X drug works for pain for me," "I'm allergic to Y, so I can only take X"), and above-average knowledge about drugs, as well as the severity of the complaint matching the clinical presentation. Finally, the nurse should assess the patient for signs associated with withdrawal, for example, anxiety, irritability, insomnia, fatigue, headache, tremors, sweating, dizziness, decreased concentration, nausea, depression, and visual or tactile hallucinations (Fontaine, 2003; Neushotz & Fitzpatrick, 2008).

Interventions

The interventions for prescription drug misuse are like the interventions associated with alcohol misuse. First, if prescription drug misuse is suspected, the nurse should ask the patient or a family member to bring in all drugs the patient is currently using and inform the physician so that a plan for safe detoxification can be established. The patient should be informed that, by bringing in all drugs currently being used, they are ensuring that the health care team can develop a comprehensive care plan to address the patient's needs. This also enables the health care provider to prevent any untoward drug interactions resulting from prescribing a new drug contraindicated because of an existing prescription. The

nurse should document any signs of withdrawal, provide an environment of low stimulation, and implement seizure precautions. In addition, the nurse should administer, on a planned reduction schedule, any drugs prescribed to minimize withdrawal symptoms. Nutritional support interventions should also be implemented for patients with compromised nutritional status. Agents used to treat opioid dependence are methadone, buprenorphine, naloxone, and clonidine. Although these harm-reduction pharmacologic treatments are widely used for persons with Opioid Use Disorder (OUD), no studies of the use of these drugs in the older adult population have been performed (Trevisan, 2008). Finally, after discussion within the multidisciplinary team, concerns about prescription drug misuse and treatment options such as AA, NA, or individual or group therapy should be presented to the patient and family members in a patient-care conference (Fontaine, 2003).

Evaluation

The evaluation of nursing interventions for prescription drug misuse includes assessment of safe detoxification, participation in a rehabilitation treatment plan, and decreased drug-seeking behaviors. The nurse should also observe and document the patient's response to any teaching regarding appropriate drug use and the effects of drug misuse on the body.

Nicotine

Prevalence

Tobacco use disorder (TUD) is the single greatest cause of preventable disease and disability in the United States. TUD is a risk factor in 6 of the 13 leading causes of death in older adults. In the United States alone, approximately $50 billion is spent annually on medical costs attributed directly to tobacco use. Many tobacco users 50 years or older express the desire to quit; however, only those older adults with chronic illnesses tend to have the motivation to do so. Older adults who stop tobacco usage may improve quality of life and possibly increase life expectancy.

Assessment

The nurse should thoroughly assess a patient's tobacco use pattern and assess for signs of nicotine withdrawal. The CAGE questionnaire can be modified, substituting the word *smoking* for *alcohol* (Rustin, 2000). The patient's responses allow the nurse to plan appropriate interventions. Older adult patients should be monitored for signs of nicotine withdrawal such as depressed mood, insomnia, irritability, frustration, anger, anxiety, difficulty concentrating, restlessness, decreased heart rate, and increased appetite (APA, 2013).

Interventions and Evaluation

Nursing interventions for older adults with TUD include monitoring for signs of withdrawal, administration of nicotine replacement, behavior modification, and education. The type of nicotine replacement used is determined by the health care provider; options include gum, inhaler, lozenge, nasal spray, or patch. The replacement period lasts from 6 weeks to several months and reduces the craving for cigarettes by weaning the patient from nicotine and preventing withdrawal symptoms.

Patients who do not tolerate nicotine replacement may respond to bupropion or varenicline.

PATIENT/FAMILY TEACHING

Safe Use of Drugs

Know the name, amount, type, frequency, purpose, and side effects of both the prescription and nonprescription drugs that you are taking.

If you see more than one care provider, always bring all your drugs to every provider visit you make.

Never borrow drugs from anyone else or share your drugs with anyone else.

Make sure your family members can safely self-administer drugs; adequate vision, memory, judgment, and coordination are all essential.

Supervise drug administration for those people who cannot safely self-administer. Talk to the health care provider about simplifying the drug regimen by using a daily dosing schedule set for once or twice a day.

Never mix alcohol with *any* drug.

Use a single pharmacy for filling all prescriptions to reduce the potential for interactions as well as misuse.

Sustained-release bupropion is an effective aid in smoking cessation. The nurse should obtain a detailed patient history regarding the existence of any seizure disorder because bupropion is contraindicated in such cases and another drug or technique should be recommended. Furthermore, the nurse must carefully assess the bupropion candidate for any history of alcohol misuse; these patients are at increased risk for seizures. Varenicline, along with education and counseling, is also effective in helping people stop smoking. Varenicline is in a class of drugs called *smoking cessation aids*. It works by blocking the pleasant effects of nicotine on the brain. Some people have experienced changes in behavior, hostility, agitation, depression, suicidal ideation, and worsening of preexisting psychiatric illness while taking varenicline (American Cancer Society, 2017).

Evaluation of nursing interventions includes assessing for decreased use of tobacco, adherence to a plan to reduce tobacco use, and understanding of the effects that tobacco and nicotine have on the body.

FUTURE TRENDS

Current figures indicate as many as 7.2% of older adults use illicit drugs; prevalence is expected to increase as more Baby Boomers reach retirement age (Kuerbis et al., 2014). Older adults should be screened for drug misuse. A simple, one-question screen, "How many times in the past year have you used an illegal drug or used a prescription drug for nonmedical reasons?" has been shown to accurately identify individuals using drugs in the outpatient setting; however, a trial has not been conducted in older adults (Smith, Schmidt, Allensworth-Davies, & Saitz, 2010).

🏠 **HOME CARE**

1. Obtain a prescription drug inventory, including the physician sources of all prescriptions.
2. Mail-order prescription suppliers send large quantities of drugs to homebound older adults, which predisposes them to drug wasting, overdosing, and other misuse.
3. Assess the number of caregivers involved with drug administration to prevent overdosing and other administration errors.
4. Drug use patterns of homebound older adults, including the administration of prescription drugs, OTC drugs, and home remedies, are influenced by cultural and ethnic health practices.
5. During assessment of homebound older adults, include an inventory of the use of caffeine, nicotine, and alcohol.
6. Assess high-risk factors (e.g., social isolation and depression) that may predispose homebound older adults to SUD.
7. Assess for signs of SUD in homebound older adults.
8. Encourage caregivers to attend support groups such as Alcoholics Anonymous (AA) to ease the burden of caring for a homebound older adult with SUD.

▌SUMMARY

Achieving positive therapeutic outcomes and reducing ADEs requires knowledge of age-related alterations that determine how older adults react to drugs, an understanding of the unique problems attributable to aging, and an awareness of resources to address problems and concerns related to drug use. Nurses must accept this responsibility if improved patient outcomes are to be realized.

The prognosis for untreated SUD in older adults is poor because of physiologic and psychological consequences. It is essential that nurses identify SUD in older adults and examine their own attitudes about SUD in this population. Early identification and intervention are essential for preventing misdiagnosis and ineffective, costly treatments. Nurses should recognize that older adults who misuse substances can be treated effectively. The first step in effective treatment is identification. After a problem is identified, a cost-effective treatment may be initiated to help an older adult return to a healthy lifestyle.

▌KEY POINTS

- Older adults consume a large proportion of pharmaceutical products. The use of inappropriate drugs results in significant morbidity and mortality, and adds an economic burden to patients and health care systems.
- Older adults may be at risk for adverse drug reactions because of age-related changes, multiple chronic illnesses, polypharmacy, nonadherence, and lack of knowledge.
- A reduction in drug dosage is often required for older adults whose ability to excrete drugs is decreased or in whom renal or hepatic function is reduced.

- Knowledge of clinically important drug interactions is essential in planning alternative drug regimens and preventing potentially serious ADEs.
- Drug problems should always be suspected in patients experiencing overt or subtle changes in cognitive or physical function.
- Antipsychotic drugs should not be used in older adults with dementia.
- The nurse can play a key role not only in assessing patients for risk factors that may reduce adherence but also in developing strategies to reduce or to eliminate these risks.
- For most drugs prescribed for older adults, it is necessary to start low, go slow, and periodically review drug regimens.
- The age-related physiologic changes of altered absorption, distribution, metabolism, and excretion affect drug usage and place older adults at an increased risk for SUD.
- Psychological changes, primarily a result of the numerous losses older adults may experience in a relatively short time, place them at an increased risk for SUD.
- Sociologic changes such as decreased finances, transportation, and social support, as well as sociocultural factors such as gender and race, may place older adult patients at risk for SUD.
- The substances most often misused by the older adult population are alcohol, prescription drugs, nonprescription drugs, nicotine, and caffeine.
- The nurse should assess older adult patients for key medical and psychological manifestations of SUD through their health history. Some of these key manifestations are falls, hypertension, memory loss, depressed mood, and social withdrawal.
- Screening tools such as the CAGE, MAST, MAST-G, and BMAST should be used to screen for SUD in older adult patients.
- Key nursing interventions for SUD in older adult patients include assessing for signs of withdrawal, administering appropriate drugs to provide safe detoxification, providing a safe environment, educating patients regarding harmful effects, and encouraging patients to participate in AA, NA, or individual, family, or group therapy.

CRITICAL-THINKING EXERCISES

1. An 83-year-old man with a history of congestive heart failure is taking many prescription drugs, including psyllium, digoxin, phenytoin, and cimetidine. He is 5 feet, 9 inches tall, and weighs 139 pounds. Based on potential drug interactions, identify the relevant assessment priorities. What factors place this patient at risk for drug toxicity?

2. A home care nurse is seeing an 82-year-old man who is taking a complex drug regimen. He cannot remember when he last took several of his drugs, and his wife states she is confused by the recent switch of several drugs to other generic brands. What questions should the nurse ask to establish the patient's risk for nonadherence?

3. A patient's daughter wonders if she should have her dad use ginkgo and other herbals to help with his Alzheimer's disease. How would you advise her?

4. Compare nursing assessments and interventions for prescription drug, nonprescription drug, and alcohol misuse. How are they similar, and how are they different? How might assessment techniques be revised for the older adult population?

5. Analyze your own perceptions and attitudes regarding SUD in general. How do these perceptions and attitudes differ from those presented here regarding SUD in the older adult population? What factors and assumptions contribute to these perceptions?

6. How might the DSM-5 criteria for SUD be revised to specifically address the older adult population?

REFERENCES

Adis International. (2007). International: Sleep-promoting medications should be used with caution in elderly nursing home residents. *Drugs & Therapy Perspectives, 23*(4), 10–13.

Ahmed, A., Rich, M. W., Fleg, J. L., et al. (2006). Effects of digoxin on morbidity and mortality in diastolic heart failure: the ancillary digitalis investigation group trial. *Circulation, 114*(5), 397–403.

Alexander-Magalee, M. A. (2013). Addressing pharmacology challenges in older adults. *Nursing, 43*(10), 58–60, 2013.

American Cancer Society. (2017). Prescription drugs to help you quit tobacco. Retrieved February 15, 2018 from https://www.cancer.org/healthy/stay-away-from-tobacco/guide-quitting-smoking/prescription-drugs-to-help-you-quit-smoking.html.

American Geriatrics Society. (2015). American Geriatrics Society 2015 Updated Beers Criteria for potentially inappropriate medication use in older adults. *Journal of the American Geriatrics Society, 63*, 2227–2246. https://doi.org/10.1111/jgs.13702.

American Psychiatric Association (APA). (2013). *Diagnostic and statistical manual of mental disorders* (5th ed.). Washington, DC: The Association.

Anonymous. (2009). Get a better med history—a life may be at stake. *ED Nursing, 12*(5), 53–54.

Aymanns, C., Keller, F., Maus, S., Hartmann, B., & Czock, D. (2010). Review on pharmacokinetics and pharmacodynamics and the aging kidney. *Clinical Journal of the American Society of Nephrology, 5*(2), 314–327. https://doi.org/10.2215/CJN.03960609.

Beers, M. H., Ouslander, J. G., Rollingher, I., et al. (1991). Explicit criteria for determining inappropriate medication use in nursing home residents. *Archives of Internal Medicine, 151,* 1825–1832.

Behere, R. V., Muralidharam, K., & Benegal, V. (2009). Complementary and alternative medicine in the treatment of substance use disorders—a review of the evidence. *Drug and Alcohol Review, 28,* 292–300.

Bibbens-Domingo, K., & DiMatteo, M. R. (2006). Assessing and promoting medical adherence. In T. E. King, M. B. Wheeler, & A. Fernandez (Eds.), *Medical management of vulnerable and underserved patients.* New York: McGraw-Hill.

Briesacher, B. A., Gurwitz, J. H., & Soumerai, S. B. (2007). Patients at-risk for cost-related medication nonadherence: a review of the literature. *Journal of General Internal Medicine, 22,* 864–871.

Budnitz, D. S., Shehab, N., Kegler, S. R., & Richards, C. L. (2007). Medication use leading to emergency department visits for adverse drug events in older adults. *Annals of Internal Medicine, 147,* 755–765.

Carnahan, R. M., Brown, G. D., Letuchy, E. M., Rubenstein, L. M., Gryzlak, B. M., Smith, M., … Chrischilles, E. A. (2017). Impact of programs to reduce antipsychotic and anticholinergic use in nursing homes. *Alzheimer's & Dementia: Translational Research & Clinical Interventions, 3,* 553–561. https://doi.org/10.1016/j.trci.2017.02.003.

Calleo, J., & Stanley, M. (2008). Anxiety disorders in later life: differentiated diagnosis and treatment strategies. *Psychiatric Times, 25*(8), 24–27.

Centers for Disease Control and Prevention (2016). Medication safety basics. Retrieved February 15, 2018 from https://www.cdc.gov/medicationsafety/basics.html.

Centers for Medicare & Medicaid Services (2017). Data show National Partnership to Improve Dementia Care achieves goals to reduce unnecessary antipsychotic medications in nursing homes [Press Release]. Retrieved from https://www.cms.gov/Newsroom/MediaReleaseDatabase/Fact-sheets/2017-Fact-Sheet-items/2017-10-02.html.

Chauvelier, S., Pequignot, R., Amzal, A., Hanon, O., & Belmin, J. (2012). Comparison between the three most popular formulae to estimate renal function, in subjects 75 years of age or older. *Drugs and Aging, 29,* 885–890.

Chia, L. R., Schlenk, E. A., & Dunbar-Jacob, J. (2006). Effect of personal and cultural beliefs on medication adherence in the elderly. *Drugs and Aging, 23*(3), 191–202.

Dalleur, O., Spinewine, A., Henrard, S., Losseau, C., Speybroeck, N., & Boland, B. (2012). Inappropriate prescribing and related hospital admissions in frail older persons according to the STOPP and START criteria. *Drugs and Aging, 29,* 829–837.

Davis, T. C., Wolk, M. S., Bass, P. F., et al. (2006). Literacy and misunderstanding prescription drug labels. *Annals of Internal Medicine, 145,* 887–894.

Emmons, B. F. (2008). Factors contributing to polypharmacy. *American Journal of Health-System Pharmacy, 65,* 1992.

Federman, A. D., & Safran, D. G. (2008). Low levels of awareness of pharmaceutical cost-assistance programs among inner-city seniors. *JAMA, 300,* 1412–1414.

Ferdinand, K. C. (2009). Antihypertensive pharmacotherapy: adverse effects of medications promote nonadherence. *Journal of the Cardiometabolic Syndrome, 4*(1), E1–E3.

Flammiger, A., & Maibach, H. (2006). Dermatological drug dosage in the elderly. *Skin Therapy Letter, 11*(8), 1–7.

Fontaine, K. L. (2003). *Mental health nursing.* Upper Saddle River, NJ: Prentice Hall.

Food and Drug Administration. (2013). *Strategies to reduce medication errors: Working to improve medication safety.* Retrieved October 28, 2013 from http://www.fda.gov/Drugs/ResourcesForYou/Consumers/ucm143553.htm.

Francis, S. A., Barnett, N., & Denham, M. (2005). Switching of prescription drugs to over-the-counter status: is it a good thing for the elderly? *Drugs and Aging, 22*(5), 361–370.

Hutchison, L. C., & O'Brien, C. E. (2007). Changes in pharmacokinetics and pharmacodynamics in the elderly patient. *Journal of Pharmacy Practice, 20*(1), 4–12.

Institute of Medicine. (2007). *Preventing medication errors: quality chasm series.* Washington, DC: The National Academies Press.

Jaffe, I. (2018). Risky antipsychotic drugs still overprescribed in nursing homes. Retrieved from https://www.npr.org/sections/health-shots/2018/02/05/583435517/risky-antipsychotic-drugs-still-overprescribed-in-nursing-homes.

Joshi, S. (2008). Nonpharmacologic therapy for insomnia in the elderly. *Clinics in Geriatric Medicine, 24*(1), 107–119.

Kairuz, T., Bye, L., Birdsall, R., et al. (2008). Identifying compliance issues with prescription medicines among older people: a pilot study. *Drugs and Aging, 25*(2), 153–162.

Kaufman, G. (2013). Prescribing and medicines management in older people. *Nursing Older People, 25*(7), 33–41.

Kiani, J., & Imam, S. Z. (2007). Medicinal importance of grapefruit juice and its interaction with various drugs. *Nutrition Journal, 6*(33), 33.

Knight, B. G., & Mjelde-Mossey, L. A. (1995). A comparison of the Michigan Alcoholism Screening Test and the Michigan Alcoholism Screening Test–Geriatric Version in screening for higher alcohol use among dementia caregivers. *Journal of Mental Health and Aging, 1*(2), 147.

Korc, B. (2008). Polypharmacy raises risks of side effects, skipped pills. *American Medical News, 51,* 20.

Kuerbis, A., Sacco, P., Blazer, D. G., & Moore, A. A. (2014). Substance abuse among older adults. *Clinical Geriatric Medicine, 30*(3), 629–654. https://doi.org/10.1016/j.cger.2014.04.008.

Lehne, R. A. (2013). *Pharmacology for nursing care* (8th ed.). St. Louis MO: Elsevier Saunders. 2006.

Lilley, L. L., Harrington, S., & Snyder, J. S. (2007). *Pharmacology and the nursing process* (5th ed.). St. Louis: Mosby-Elsevier.

Madden, J. M., Graves, A. J., Zhang, F., et al. (2008). Cost-related medication nonadherence and spending on basic needs following implementation of Medicare Part D. *JAMA, 299,* 1922–1928.

Mahgoub, N. (2009). An 80-year old woman with alcohol problems. *Psychiatric Annals, 39*(1), 17.

Maniaci, M. J., Heckman, M. G., & Dawson, N. L. (2008). Functional health literacy and understanding of medications at discharge. *Mayo Clinic Proceedings, 83,* 554–558.

Mattson, M., Lipari, R.N., Hays, C., & Van Horn, S.L. (2017). A day in the life of older adults: Substance use facts. Retrieved February 15, 2018 from https://www.samhsa.gov/data/sites/default/files/report_2792/ShortReport-2792.html.

Mayfield, D., McLeod, G., & Hall, P. (1974). The CAGE questionnaire: validation of a new alcoholism screening instrument. *The American Journal of Psychiatry, 131,* 1121.

Mohundro, M., & Ramsey, L. (2003). Pharmacologic considerations in geriatric patients. *Advance for Nurse Practitioners, 11*(9), 21.

Moon, M. A. (2009). Elderly with anxiety respond well to CBT. *Family Practice News, 39*(9), 18.

Morris, D. L. (2001). Geriatric mental health: an overview. *American Family Physician, 7*(6), 82.

Morton, J. L., Jones, T. V., & Manganaro, M. A. (1996). Performance of alcoholism screening questionnaires in elderly veterans. *The American Journal of Medicine, 101*(2), 153–159.

Moser, M., Franklin, S. S., & Handler, J. (2007). The nonpharmacologic treatment of hypertension: how effective is it? An update. *Journal of Clinical Hypertension, 9,* 209–216.

Neushotz, L. A., & Fitzpatrick, J. J. (2008). Improving substance abuse screening and intervention in a primary care clinic. *Archives of Psychiatric Nursing, 22*(2), 78.

Nichols, J., Alper, C., & Milkin, T. (2007). Strategies for the management of insomnia: an update on pharmacologic therapies. *Formulary, 42*(2), 86–98.

Opondo, D., Eslami, S., Visscher, S., de Rooij, S. E., Verheij, R., Korevaar, J. C., et al. (2012). Inappropriateness of medication prescriptions to elderly patients in the primary care setting: a systematic review. *PloS One, 7*(8), 1–9.

Pawaskar, M. D., & Sansgiry, S. S. (2006). Over-the-counter medication labels: problems and needs of the elderly. *Journal of the American Geriatrics Society, 54,* 1955–1956.

Pham, C. B., & Dickman, R. L. (2007). Minimizing adverse drug events in older patients. *American Family Physician, 76,* 1837–1844.

Pokorny, A. D., Miller, B. A., & Kaplan, H. B. (1972). The brief MAST: a shortened version of the Michigan Alcoholism Screening Test. *The American Journal of Psychiatry, 129,* 342.

Proulx, M., Leduc, N., Vandelac, L., et al. (2007). Social context, the struggle with uncertainty, and subjective risk as meaning-rich constructs for explaining HBP noncompliance. *Patient Education and Counseling, 68*(1), 98–106.

Qato, D. M., Alexander, G. C., Conti, R. M., et al. (2008). Use of prescription and over-the-counter medications and dietary supplements among older adults in the United States. *JAMA, 300,* 2867–2878.

Ruppar, T. M., Conn, V. S., & Russell, C. L. (2008). Medication adherence interventions for older adults: literature review. *Research and Theory for Nursing Practice, 22,* 114–147.

Ruscin, J.M., & Linnebur, S. (2014). Pharmacokinetics in the elderly. Retrieved February 15, 2018 from http://www.merckmanuals.com/professional/geriatrics/drug-therapy-in-the-elderly/pharmacokinetics-in-the-elderly.

Rustin, T. A. (2000). Assessing nicotine dependence. *American Family Physician, 62*(3), 579–584.

Selzer, M. L. (1971). The Michigan Alcoholism Screening Test: the quest for a new diagnostic instrument. *The American Journal of Psychiatry, 127,* 1653.

Sherman, C. (2007). Insomnia in elderly: medicate with care. *Clin Psychiatry News, 35*(10), 27.

Shi, S., Mörike, K., & Klotz, U. (2008). The clinical implications of ageing for rational drug therapy. *European Journal of Clinical Pharmacology, 64*(2), 183–199.

Smith, P. C., Schmidt, S. M., Allensworth-Davies, D., & Saitz, R. (2010). A single-question screening test for drug use in primary care. *Archives of Internal Medicine, 170,* 1155–1160.

Spiesel, S. (August 27, 2008). Medication error death rate up 500 percent [Radio broadcast episode]. In A. Chadwick (Editor and Host), *Health & Science.* Washington, DC: National Public Radio.

Stoehr, G. P., Lu, S. Y., Lavery, L., et al. (2008). Factors associated with adherence to medication regimens in older primary care patients. *The American Journal of Geriatric Pharmacotherapy, 6*(5), 255–263.

Substance Abuse and Mental Health Services Administration. (2015). Substance use disorders. Retrieved February 15, 2018 from https://www.samhsa.gov/disorders/substance-use.

Trevisan, L. A. (2008). Baby boomers and substance abuse: an emerging issue. *Psychiatric Times, 25*(8), 28.

US Food and Drug Administration. (2017). Medication errors related to drugs. Retrieved February 15, 2018 from https://www.fda.gov/Drugs/DrugSafety/MedicationErrors/default.htm.

Videbeck, S. (2004). *Psychiatric mental health nursing.* Philadelphia: Lippincott, Williams & Wilkins.

Wakefield, D. S., Ward, M. M., Groath, D., et al. (2008). Complexity of medication-related verbal orders. *American Journal of Medical Quality, 23*(1), 7–17.

Wendling, P. (2006). Doctors need to educate patients on proper disposal of old drugs. *Internal Medicine News, 34*(4), 50.

Wen-Wen, L., Wallhagen, M. I., & Froelicher, E. S. (2007). Hypertension control, predictors for medication adherence and gender differences in older Chinese immigrants. *Journal of Advanced Nursing, 61*(3), 326–335.

Whelton, P.K., Carey, R.M., Aronow, W.S., Casey, D.E., Collins, K.J., Himmelfarb, C.D., … Wright, T.T. (2017). 2017 Guideline for high blood pressure in adults. Retrieved from http://www.acc.org/latest-in-cardiology/ten-points-to-remember/2017/11/09/11/41/2017-guideline-for-high-blood-pressure-in-adults.

Windham, B. G., Griswold, M. E., Fried, L. P., et al. (2005). Impaired vision and the ability to take medications. *Journal of the American Geriatrics Society, 53,* 1179–1190.

Wold, R. S., Lopez, S. T., Yau, C. L., et al. (2005). Increasing trends in elderly persons' use of nonvitamin, nonmineral dietary supplements and concurrent use of medications. *Journal of the American Dietetic Association, 105*(1), 54–64.

Yan, J. (2008). FDA extends black-box warning to all antipsychotics. Retrieved from https://psychnews.psychiatryonline.org/doi/10.1176/pn.43.14.0001.

PART V

Nursing Care of Physiologic and Psychologic Disorders

17

Integumentary Function

Jennifer J. Yeager, PhD, RN, APRN

http://evolve.elsevier.com/Meiner/gerontologic

LEARNING OBJECTIVES

On completion of this chapter, the reader will be able to:

1. Discuss the primary functions of the integumentary system.
2. Identify normal age-related skin changes.
3. Discuss common skin problems and conditions experienced by older adults and their associated nursing implications.
4. Describe common skin cancers that affect older adults.
5. Describe the risk factors for pressure injury development.
6. Identify five pressure injury preventive strategies endorsed by the National Pressure Ulcer Advisory Panel (NPUAP) and the Agency for Healthcare Research and Quality (AHRQ) clinical guidelines.
7. State three principles necessary for successful wound healing.
8. Conduct an assessment for a patient with impaired skin integrity.
9. Determine when to appropriately use antiseptics.
10. Describe the indications, contraindications, advantages, and drawbacks of various wound dressings.
11. Distinguish between arterial and venous lower extremity ulcers.

WHAT WOULD YOU DO?

What would you do if you were faced with the following situations?

- You are caring for an older adult patient in the critical care unit. The admitting diagnosis is heart failure; the patient also has a history of diabetes type 2 and hypertension. The patient is ambulatory with standby assistance. How would you determine your patient's risk for pressure injury? What is your patient's risk?
- Your obese 68-year-old female patient with a history of chronic obstructive pulmonary disease is admitted with pneumonia and is prescribed levofloxacin and prednisone. Your patient is at risk for developing what acute skin conditions? How would the acute skin conditions be treated?

The integumentary system is the largest organ of the body. The primary function of the skin is to serve as a barrier against harmful bacteria and other threatening agents, which makes the skin the first line of defense for the immune system. Other major functions of the integumentary system include (1) preventing fluid loss or dehydration, (2) protecting the body from ultraviolet (UV) rays and other external environmental hazards, and (3) protecting underlying organs from injury. In addition, the skin provides thermal regulation of body temperature. Radiation, conduction, convection, and evaporation are facilitated by sensory perceptions that occur in the skin's nerve endings. The skin also assists in the regulation of blood pressure through "local regulation of cutaneous blood flow and salt and water metabolism" (Johnson, Titze, & Weller, 2016, p. 1). The integumentary system reveals emotions such as anger, fear, or embarrassment through vasodilatation, which reddens the skin tissue. In the presence of the sun's UV rays, the skin synthesizes vitamin D, which is then used by other parts of the body. Subcutaneous fat, the deepest layer of the integumentary system, provides insulation and acts as a caloric reservoir. Hair serves as body insulation and provides unique physical characteristics through its varying textures, shades, patterns, and colors.

A careful and thorough assessment of the integumentary system is essential when a physical assessment is performed on a patient. Skin assessment helps determine hydration status, potential for or actual infection, and other information about the individual (e.g., sun exposure, attention to personal appearance, and scars). Palpation of the skin identifies tender areas, nodules, and masses.

The value of the integumentary system is demonstrated by the high morbidity and mortality rates associated with extensive burns when all functions of the skin are greatly compromised. The overall state of health is affected by physical or emotional insults to this system, for example, loss of thermal regulation or fluid, impaired barrier protection, and other catastrophic changes in physical appearance and functioning.

AGE-RELATED CHANGES IN SKIN STRUCTURE AND FUNCTION

The integumentary system reflects changes associated with aging, which include graying hair, increased number and depth

Previous author: Sabrina Friedman, EdD, DNP, FNP-C, PMHCNS-BC.

- Loss of thickness, elasticity, vascularity, and strength that may delay the healing process and increase the risk of skin tears and bruising
- Increased lentigines (brown-pigmented spots, or age spots)
- Loss of subcutaneous tissue causing wrinkling and sagging of the skin, which may affect self-esteem, temperature control, and drug efficacy
- Loss of hair follicles along with thinning and graying
- Increased hair density in the nose and the ears, particularly in men, which may clog external ear canals and impair hearing
- Thicker nails with longitudinal lines
- Decreased sebaceous and sweat gland activity, which affects thermoregulation and decreases sweating
- Higher incidence of benign and malignant skin growths

of wrinkles, loss of elasticity, and discoloration and thickening of the nails. Box 17.1 describes basic age-related skin changes.

Epidermis

The epidermis is the outermost layer of the skin. The replacement rate of the stratum corneum, the first layer of epidermis, declines by 50% as a person ages. This decline results in slower healing, reduced barrier protection, and delayed absorption of medications and chemicals placed on the skin. The area of contact between the epidermis and dermis decreases with age, which results in easy separation of these layers. Therefore skin tears occur from harmless activities such as removing a bandage or pulling an older patient up in the bed. Bruising occurs more easily because of these age-related skin changes. A thinner epidermis allows more moisture to escape and may compound previously existing skin problems. The number of melanocytes, which provide pigment and hair color, decreases with age, giving older adults less protection from UV rays, paler skin, and graying hair. Melanocytes also produce uneven pigmentation, causing the development of solar lentigos (or lentigines), also known as *age spots* or *liver spots*.

Dermis

The dermis decreases in thickness by approximately 20% with aging. It consists of strong connective tissue that contains the sweat glands, blood vessels, and nerve endings. With aging, sweat glands, blood vessels, and nerve endings decrease in number. These changes lead to diminished thermoregulatory function and inflammatory responses, decreased tactile sensation, reduced pain perception, and development of wrinkles and sagging skin because of loss of underlying tissue. Collagen, a fibrous protein that provides tensile strength within the dermis, stiffens and becomes less soluble.

Subcutaneous Fat

Aging results in a decreased amount of subcutaneous tissue and a redistribution of fat to the abdomen and thighs. Breast tissue also changes and becomes more granular and atrophic. Because of a loss of padding supplied by subcutaneous tissues, the risk for hypothermia, skin shear (see Pressure Injuries, later in this chapter, for the definition and adverse effects of shear), and blunt trauma injury is greater. The loss of this protective padding increases vulnerability of pressure points. Topical

medication and dermal medication patch absorption may increase because of the changes in the subcutaneous tissue.

Dermal Appendages

With aging, fewer eccrine glands (sweat glands of the palms, feet, and forehead) and apocrine sweat glands (sweat glands of the axilla, scalp, face, and genital areas) exist, resulting in decreased body odor and reduced evaporative heat loss because of decreased sweating. The need for antiperspirants and deodorants is reduced. However, older adults are at greater risk of heat stroke because of a compromised cooling mechanism. Older adults should avoid heat exposure over long periods and in areas of high humidity. Hats with wide brims and cool, light, breezy clothing should be worn when outdoors. It is important that older adults drink adequate fluid to maintain adequate hydration; however, exact hydration guidelines are not available at this time (Scherer, Maroto-Sanchez, Palacios, & Gonzalez-Gross, 2016).

Sebum oils the skin and provides an antimicrobial property. The sebaceous glands and pores become larger with aging. Nevertheless, many older adults experience dry skin, which places them at a greater risk of infection because of an impaired immune response.

Hair thins, and its growth declines. A progressive loss of melanin occurs, resulting in graying of the hair. Heredity influences the onset of the graying process. Older women may have increased lip and chin hair while experiencing thinning of hair on the head, axilla, and perineal area. Men lose scalp and beard hair and experience increased growth over the eyebrows and in the ears and nostrils. The increased hair in ears predisposes men to cerumen impaction, which leads to impaired hearing. Changes in the patterns of hair growth and distribution as a person ages are thought to be hormone related. Nails grow more slowly with age and become thicker, brittle, and dull, developing longitudinal striation with ridges (Blume-Peytavi et al., 2016). These changes may affect a person's body image and self-concept (see Cultural Awareness box).

Dermatoporosis

Nearly 35% of older adults experience chronic skin fragility. This fragile skin is called *dermatoporosis*. The identifying

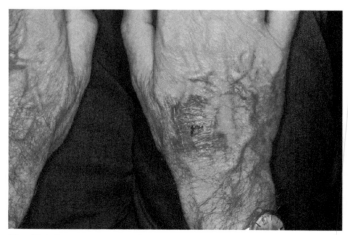

Fig. 17.1 Dermatoporosis. (From Wallach, D. [2013]. Dermatologie pour les gériatres. *NPG Neurologie – Psychiatrie – Gériatrie, 13*[78], 303-315.)

features of dermatoporosis include atopic changes, actinic purpura, and white pseudoscars (Fig. 17.1). The skin appears nearly translucent. It occurs on sun-exposed areas of the extremities. Individuals with dermatoporosis frequently experience skin lacerations associated with increased bleeding and delayed healing (Dyer & Miller, 2018).

🌐 CULTURAL AWARENESS

Skin Assessment in Darkly Pigmented Skin

Prioritize assessment of:
* skin temperature
* edema
* change in tissue consistency in relation to surrounding tissue

Assess localized pain as part of every skin assessment:
* Use natural light or halogen versus fluorescent, which gives illusion of bluish tint.
* May not distinguish blanching; look for areas darker than surrounding skin, or taut, shiny, indurated areas.
* Light from a camera flash may enhance visualization.
* Check for localized changes in skin texture and temperature.
* Erythema may cause hyperpigmentation with no redness visible.
* May appear dark bluish-purple.
* Should be able to detect heat over an area of localized inflammation.
* Injured skin may have nonpitting edema with or without color changes.

From Goldberg, M. (2015). Preventive skin care. National Pressure Ulcer Advisory Panel. Retrieved from https://www.npuap.org/wp-content/uploads/2015/02/2.-Preventive-Skin-Care-M-Goldberg.pdf.

COMMON PROBLEMS AND CONDITIONS

Benign Skin Growths

Cherry Angiomas

Cherry angiomas are common, bright red, 1- to 5-millimeter (mm) superficial vascular lesions that begin around age 30 and increase in number with age. The cause of these lesions is unknown. They are red or deep purple dome-shaped papules (Fig. 17.2). Although they are most commonly found on the trunk, they may be located anywhere on the body and vary in number. Because cherry angiomas are new growths, patients are often concerned that they are malignant or indicate a serious

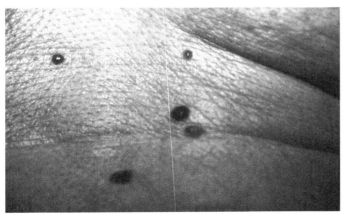

Fig. 17.2 Cherry angiomas. (From Ignatavicius, D. D., Workman, M. L., & Rebar, C. R. [2018]. *Medical-surgical nursing: Concepts for interprofessional collaborative care* [9th ed.]. St. Louis, MO: Elsevier.)

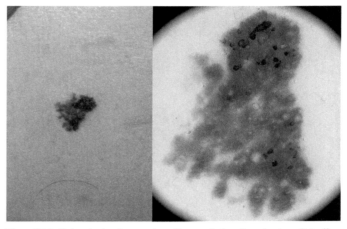

Fig. 17.3 Seborrheic keratosis. (From Bolognia, J. L., Schaffer, J. V., Duncan, K. O., & Ko, C. J. [2014]. *Dermatology essentials.* Philadelphia, PA: Elsevier Saunders.)

health problem. Patients need to be reassured that cherry angiomas are benign growths resulting from increased vascularity in the dermis and occur in most people.

Seborrheic Keratoses

Seborrheic keratoses are benign lesions more commonly seen in the older adult. These are scaly growths that have a "stuck-on," crumbly appearance that varies in color from tan to brown to black (Fig. 17.3). The lesions may be elevated and range in diameter from 2 to 3 mm. Characterized by slow growth, these lesions begin to appear later in life. The borders may be round and smooth or irregular and notched. To the untrained eye, these lesions may resemble a malignant melanoma, particularly when dark brown or black. They have a greasy feeling and often occur in sun-exposed areas (face, neck, or trunk) but may appear anywhere on the body. The growths may be removed for cosmetic reasons (often related to self-esteem) or if irritated. If the lesion is "picked off," it will recur. Therefore it is best to have a physician remove the growth if it is bothersome to a patient. Cryotherapy is effective, and the lesion usually sloughs off in a few weeks. Patients should be reassured that the growths are benign and are a commonly occurring skin manifestation.

Skin Tags (Acrochordons)

Skin tags are common stalk-like, benign tumors often found on the neck, axilla, eyelids, and groin, although they may occur anywhere on the body (Fig. 17.4). Beginning as early as age 20, these are tiny, flesh-colored or brown excrescences that develop into a long, narrow stalk (up to 1 centimeter [cm]). As they mature, they can be easily removed with scissors, electrocautery, or liquid nitrogen. Skin tags are usually excised only on the request of the patient, usually for cosmetic reasons.

Inflammatory Dermatoses

Seborrheic Dermatitis

Seborrheic dermatitis is a common, chronic inflammation of the skin. The scalp, ear canals, eyebrows, eyelashes, nasolabial folds, axilla, breasts, chest, and groin are common sites (Fig. 17.5). The

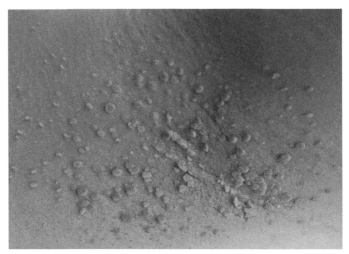

Fig. 17.4 Skin tags. (From Bolognia, J. L., Schaffer, J. V., Duncan, K. O., & Ko, C. J. [2014]. *Dermatology essentials.* Philadelphia, PA: Elsevier Saunders.)

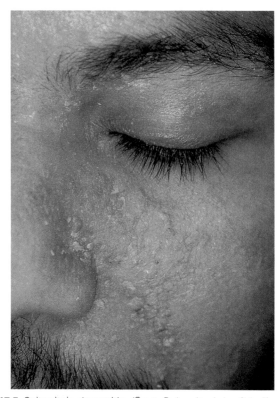

Fig. 17.5 Seborrheic dermatitis. (From Bolognia, J. L., Schaffer, J. V., Duncan, K. O., & Ko, C. J. [2014]. *Dermatology essentials.* Philadelphia, PA: Elsevier Saunders.)

usual pattern of distribution begins with the scalp and moves down toward the eyebrows, progressing to the chest with a bilateral, symmetric presentation. It is more common in patients who have Parkinson's disease or who have suffered a stroke.

In differentiating between dandruff and seborrheic dermatitis, it should be noted that *dandruff* is scaling without inflammation, and *seborrheic dermatitis* is an inflammatory response sometimes associated with scaling. With inadequate management, dandruff may evolve into seborrheic dermatitis. Seborrheic dermatitis appears as a white or yellow scale with a plaque-like appearance. An erythematous red base, indicating an inflammatory process, is *always* present. Mild itching is not uncommon. Medicated shampoos containing ketoconazole, ciclopirox, selenium sulfide, zinc pyrithione, coal tar, and salicylic acid are effective for seborrheic dermatitis of the scalp. Low-potency topical corticosteroids, such as hydrocortisone, desonide, and mometasone furoate, are effective for facial seborrheic dermatitis (Gomez, 2017).

Intertrigo

Intertrigo is a "superficial inflammatory dermatitis occurring on two closely opposed skin surfaces because of moisture, friction, and lack of ventilation. Bodily secretions, including perspiration, urine, and feces, often exacerbate skin inflammation" (Kalra, Higgins, & Kinney, 2014, p. 1). It is usually found in the armpits, inner aspects of the thighs, skin folds of the breasts, and abdominal folds. The area is erythematous and may itch. Intertrigo occurs more often in aging patients who are obese or have diabetes. Medical management includes appropriate use of an antimicrobial agent (antifungal or antibacterial), a low potency topical steroid, and keeping the skin clean and dry.

Psoriasis

Psoriasis is an autoimmune condition that affects 2% to 3% of the world's population and approximately 2.2% of the U.S. population (World Health Organization, 2016). The condition may affect persons of any age, although it often begins during early adulthood. Psoriasis is often associated with other diseases such as cardiovascular disease, metabolic syndrome, hypertension, dyslipidemia, and Crohn's disease. Obesity and tobacco use are independent risk factors for developing psoriasis. Approximately one-third of patients with psoriasis have a first-degree relative affected by the disease; those developing the disease before age 40 have a stronger genetic component (World Health Organization, 2016). Once psoriasis begins, there are periods of remission and relapse with varying degrees of intensity. Currently, no known cure exists.

Clinically, psoriatic lesions are typically seen as well-circumscribed, pink plaques covered with silver-white, loosely adherent scales. These scaly plaques result from the accelerated replication of the dermis and epidermis over certain parts of the body. Psoriasis frequently affects the skin of the elbows, knees, scalp, lumbosacral areas, intergluteal cleft, and genitals. Changes in the nails occur in approximately 30% of patients and consist of yellow-brown discoloration with pitting, dimpling, separation of the nail plate from the underlying bed (oncolysis), thickening, and crumbling. Psoriasis is a reactive disorder. Triggers such as infection, smoking, climate, and hormonal factors may exacerbate an attack; other factors such as sunlight may decrease the severity of an attack. There are multiple forms of psoriasis including plaque, nail, guttate, pustular, inverse, erythrodermic, and psoriatic arthritis.

NURSING MANAGEMENT

Assessment

Nursing assessment consists of recognizing the inflammatory dermatitis and noting its location, degree of erythema, itching, and scaling. The dermatitis should be examined for an erythematous base with yellow, white, or silvery scales or plaques. The nurse should inquire about itching, usual hygienic habits, and steps the patient has taken to control the scaly, erythematous dermatitis. Bedbound individuals are more prone to develop seborrheic dermatitis; therefore targeting these patients for assessment, in addition to thorough cleansing of scalp, hair, and skin, is a preventive strategy.

Diagnosis

Nursing diagnoses for a patient with inflammatory dermatitis include the following:

- Reduced skin integrity resulting from immunologic deficit (psoriasis)
- Reduced skin integrity resulting from bedbound state (seborrheic dermatitis)
- Reduced skin integrity resulting from the physiologic disease process (intertrigo)
- Distorted body image resulting from the psoriatic lesions

Planning and Expected Outcomes

The goal of nursing management is control of the inflammatory process with maintenance therapy using topical agents and shampoo, as prescribed. Patient comfort is evidenced when medical treatment is done according to advice. Expected outcomes include the following:

1. Skin lesions will remain free from infection.
2. The patient will experience resolution of the inflammatory process.
3. The patient will demonstrate increased knowledge of the condition, as evidenced by:
   - Verbalizing the rationale for regular and consistent skin care.
   - Verbalizing knowledge of maintenance therapy.
   - Verbalizing triggers to inflammatory dermatitis.
   - Demonstrating accurate application of topical medications.

Intervention

One crucial aspect of nursing management is to ensure proper use of an antiseborrheic shampoo containing zinc pyrithione, selenium sulfide, or ketoconazole. One successful strategy is to wet the hair, chest, axilla, and affected areas; apply the shampoo; and then proceed with the rest of the bath or shower. After cleansing the affected areas, the patient should apply prescribed steroid cream, which decreases the inflammation and irritated red appearance of the skin. After inflammation and scaling have resolved, the patient should continue using selenium shampoo on the scalp twice weekly as preventive maintenance therapy.

Nursing interventions for a patient with psoriasis consist of reinforcing the directions of the health care provider to optimize treatment and identify patient-specific triggers that may

be avoided to decrease the severity of flare episodes. Because psoriasis varies in type and severity, treatment plans may use both prescription and over-the-counter (OTC) topical ointments. As with seborrheic dermatitis, a common therapy used to treat psoriasis is a topical steroid. Topical steroids, which may be OTC or prescription-strength creams, are not recommended for use on the face. Coal tar has been used topically for many years to relieve the itching and scaling in minor cases of psoriasis. These compounds are messy and may make the skin more sensitive to UV rays and sunlight. A topical vitamin D_3 ointment, calcipotriene skin ointment, is used to treat moderate cases of psoriasis. It is available by prescription only and has few known side effects. Calcipotriene ointment should not be used on the face, as photosensitivity is likely. Tazarotene is a *retinoid,* a group of drugs related to vitamin A. It should be applied only to the affected areas, and contact with the eyes, eyelids, and mouth should be avoided. Because the medication may result in photosensitivity, exposure to sunlight should be avoided.

Light therapy using ultraviolet B (UVB) rays has been shown to be beneficial when used in prescription light boxes. It is currently thought that ultraviolet A (UVA) light therapy used in combination with psoralen (an oral or topical medication) is the preferred method (called *PUVA*). The UV dosage is carefully monitored for exposure because the total exposure time has a set limit. With UVA light therapy, it is important to be aware of the potential risk of developing skin cancer. Many reports suggest that foods may trigger psoriasis attacks; therefore approaches to diet modification and other homeopathic remedies abound in patient resource literature. Patients should be encouraged to discuss with their health care team all remedies used. The nurse should teach the older adult patient, family members, and staff the causes of inflammatory dermatitis to alleviate anxiety and misconceptions. An explanation of treatment measures and the importance of follow-through will increase adherence and involvement in care. Symptom management is an area where nurses can have a positive effect on an older adult's quality of life.

Evaluation

Nursing accountability and evaluation are supported through accurate, comprehensive charting that describes physical assessment and maintenance interventions. A weekly assessment of the lesions with a description of the response to treatment, including maintenance therapy, is recorded. In addition, the nurse should address the response to teaching (e.g., verbalized understanding) as measured by patient, family, or staff adherence with treatment.

Pruritus

Pruritus is another term for itching so intense that it causes the patient to scratch the offending area. The most common cause of itching is dry skin, or xerosis. Atopic eczema, contact or other forms of dermatitis, urticaria, psoriasis, or bullous pemphigoid are other suspects of pruritus. Infections and drug reactions can also be causative agents.

The mechanism of itching is not fully understood, but histamine is a known mediator of pruritus. Heat, sudden temperature changes, sweating, clothing, cleaning products such as soap, fatigue, and emotional stress may precipitate itching, and it may be more severe in the winter (Touhy & Jett, 2012). Pruritus may be related either to a skin disorder or systemic disease; therefore the complaint should not be dismissed and warrants a complete assessment. Pruritus may occur with other dermatologic conditions and with systemic disorders such as liver, kidney, hematologic, diabetes, and thyroid conditions (Cassano, 2010).

NURSING MANAGEMENT

Assessment

A full skin assessment is warranted when a patient complains of pruritus. The patient is interviewed to determine the location, intensity, and onset of itching. The nurse should inquire about any patterns of behavior that precipitate itching (e.g., anxiety, environmental exposures, or friction [rubbing the skin with a towel]) and obtain information about bathing practices and kinds of soaps, detergents, and skin products used (Feramisco, Berger, & Steinhoff, 2010). The nurse should also look for rashes, vesicles, scaling, and erythema; any of these suggests a skin disorder.

Diagnosis

Nursing diagnoses for a patient with pruritus include the following:
- Potential for reduced skin integrity resulting from scratching
- Pain resulting from persistent burning and itching
- Anxiety resulting from role strain, family crisis, or other sources of patient's anxiety
- Potential for infection resulting from impaired skin integrity

Planning and Expected Outcomes

The goal of nursing management is resolution of pruritus without injury from scratching. Time should be planned to teach the patient and family about etiologic factors and the importance of not scratching. Expected outcomes include the following:
1. The skin will remain intact.
2. The patient will experience adequate periods of rest without symptoms of scratching.
3. The patient will obtain adequate pain relief, as evidenced by verbalization of comfort and pain relief.

Intervention

Nursing interventions are influenced by the cause of the pruritus. If dry, scaly skin (xerosis) is present with no lesions or erythema, the nurse should suggest that the patient apply emollients (e.g., Lubriderm, Moisturel, or Eucerin lotion or cream), which have more lanolin or oily substances than many commercial lotions. Emollients should be applied at least twice daily and immediately after bathing to trap moisture. The patient should gently pat the skin dry and avoid brisk drying with a towel. If the patient is unable to apply lotion, the nurse should instruct the caregiver in its use. The patient should decrease the frequency of baths or showers to a maximum of every other day (see Patient/Family Teaching box). Antihistamines may be needed to relieve

itching and to prevent tissue breakdown from scratching but are to be used with caution because of adverse effects in older adults.

> ### ⚙ PATIENT/FAMILY TEACHING
> #### Prevention and Treatment of Dry Skin (Xerosis)
> - Take short (no more than 5 to 10 minutes) baths or showers daily with warm (not hot) water.
> - Use gentle fragrance-free cleansers.
> - Gently pat (rather than rub) the skin dry.
> - Apply skin moisturizer immediately after drying; use ointment or cream rather than a lotion.
> - Skin care products should be unscented and alcohol free.
> - If needed, use a humidifier to add moisture in the air of the home.
> - Apply sunscreen daily, especially when going outdoors.
> - Wear fabrics such as cotton that allow the skin to breathe, and use hypoallergenic laundry detergent.
> - Stay hydrated by drinking at least 8 glasses of water daily, if not contraindicated by a medical condition (e.g., heart failure or renal disease).

Modified from Terrie, Y. C. (2013). Itchy, scratchy skin: Preventing and managing xerosis. Retrieved February 12, 2018, from http://www.pharmacytimes.com/publications/issue/2013/june2013/itchy-scratchy-skin-preventing-and-managing-xerosis.

A diagnostic workup may be conducted to identify any systemic cause for persistent pruritus (e.g., cancer or diabetes). Anxiety or stress may be the source of itching. If so, the nurse should assess the patient's self-esteem and coping strategies, and identify any family or role strain or other factors that may lead to anxiety. The nurse should also discuss stress management strategies and assist the patient in determining effective ones. A referral to a community agency or counseling may be needed for continued support and guidance.

The older patient, family members, and staff need to be taught the management of pruritus and the need to prevent skin trauma from scratching. Treatment measures should also be explained to increase adherence and involvement in care. The causes of pruritus may be difficult to determine, and the expected effects of topical agents may be diminished because of the delayed absorption of medications placed on aging skin.

Evaluation

Evaluation of interventions focuses on symptom relief, prevention of secondary complications, and, when possible, identification of the source of the pruritus. Nursing accountability is demonstrated through documentation of physical presentation such as erythema and intact skin with no lesions, hives, or rash; response to treatment measures; patient comprehension of teaching; and other nursing interventions.

Candidiasis

Candidiasis is an inflammatory process of the epidermis caused by the yeastlike fungus *Candida albicans. C. albicans* is a normally occurring flora in the mouth, vagina, and gut (moist habitats). Pregnancy, oral contraception, antibiotics, diabetes, topical and inhalant steroids, skin maceration, and immunocompromised conditions create an environment that fosters the development of yeast infections such as candidiasis. Candidiasis is most commonly seen in diaper-clad infants, patients with incontinence, and bedbound individuals, and in the moisture-prone areas of the body (e.g., skin folds and axillae).

Candidiasis is characterized by erythematous, denuded, or raw skin usually surrounded by satellite papules or pustules. Satellite lesions are a helpful diagnostic clue. Red, erythematous areas on the buttocks, perineum, or intertriginous areas of incontinent patients also have diagnostic significance. Scaling may also be present, usually at the borders (Playford, Lipman, & Sorrell, 2010).

NURSING MANAGEMENT

Assessment

Nursing assessment includes inspection of the skin, particularly under any fat folds, where moisture will accumulate. A hallmark of candidiasis is a bright red erythema with satellite papules or pustules. Any breaks in the skin, which place the patient at greater risk for infection or further breakdown, should be noted. The patient may be the one to alert the nurse to the infection. The nurse should conduct a medication assessment to identify any medications that may have precipitated this fungal infection, for example, antibiotics or steroids. If the patient has diabetes, hyperglycemia may be present; therefore the nurse should conduct a diet assessment to evaluate adherence and should check the blood sugar level. In some individuals with diabetes mellitus type 2, candidiasis infection may be the first clinical manifestation of hyperglycemia. Therefore a thorough health history is warranted when a candidiasis infection is present.

Diagnosis

Nursing diagnoses for a patient with candidiasis include the following:
- Reduced skin integrity resulting from poor control of moisture
- Inadequate toileting self-care
- Inadequate urinary elimination

Planning and Expected Outcomes

The goals of nursing management are prevention and resolution of candidiasis and, consequently, increased patient comfort. Expected outcomes include the following:
1. Skin lesions will be without evidence of infection and will be healing.
2. The patient will perform self-care practices (within limitations) for keeping the skin dry and clean.
3. The skin will regain its usual appearance without evidence of candidiasis.

Intervention

The main nursing intervention is keeping the skin dry, especially the intertriginous areas. A patient's discomfort, costs, and nursing time are minimized through use of preventive strategies such as drying the skin well (particularly the skin folds) after bathing or sweating episodes, and changing the sheets as soon as possible after an episode of incontinence. After changing linens, the nurse should cleanse and dry the skin well and apply a zinc-based cream (such as Desitin or Calmaseptine) to the buttocks and perineal area. Cornstarch or powder,

whether medicated or scented, is not recommended because of clumping. Creams are much more effective and efficient.

The nurse should teach the older adult patient, family members, and support staff to pat the skin dry; the nurse should also educate the staff and provide the scientific rationale for changing linen, cleansing the affected area, and using a moisture barrier such as zinc oxide or Desitin. The importance of prompt delivery of care after an incontinent episode must be stressed. It is important to keep topical antifungal agents on the infected area until healing is complete, which may take 2 to 3 weeks. If the yeast infection does not improve, the health care provider should be informed so that an alternative agent can be considered.

Management protocols may be developed and approved by the employee's institution and medical and nursing staff with the intent of empowering the professional nurse to act immediately when candidiasis is present. This promotes high-quality care, patient comfort, a sense of professional pride, and a team approach. Nursing management is key in resolving a candidiasis infection.

Evaluation

Evaluation of nursing management focuses on treatment efficacy and the rate of recurrence. The nurse must document how the infection responds to medical treatment and the maintenance therapy of keeping the skin dry and applying a moisture barrier. The effectiveness of patient care is supported with positive outcomes, adherence with preventive actions, and verbalized comprehension. If little improvement is seen in 2 weeks, the nurse should ensure that moisture control and application of antifungal cream are being maintained. Consultation with the health care provider is needed when response to therapy is poor; another agent may need to be prescribed.

Herpes Zoster (Shingles)

Herpes zoster, also known as *shingles,* is caused by the reactivation of latent varicella zoster (chickenpox) virus. The virus remains in the dorsal nerve endings after an episode of chickenpox, which is usually experienced in childhood. The main reason for recurrence is decreased immunity. Conditions that may impair the immune system are advanced age, stress or emotional upset, fatigue, or radiotherapy. An immunocompromised state caused by disease (e.g., human immunodeficiency virus [HIV], lymphoma, leukemia, and other malignancies) or drugs (e.g., chemotherapy and steroids) may also activate the latent virus. Chickenpox is highly contagious because it is an airborne virus. Herpes zoster is not as infectious; however, it may spread through direct contact with open sores. Therefore it is not necessary to isolate a patient with herpes zoster. Cases of contracting chickenpox after personal exposure have been reported, but these have been in individuals who have not had chickenpox. Consequently, only health care personnel who have had chickenpox or have positive serum varicella titers should care for patients with herpes zoster (Centers for Disease Control and Prevention [CDC], 2018). As always, universal precautions should be followed.

Approximately 50% of herpes zoster cases involve the thoracic region, 15% involve the cranial dermatomes, and 10% affect the cervical and lumbar regions. Ophthalmic herpes zoster is referred to an ophthalmologist for evaluation and treatment because blindness could result from corneal scarring.

Herpes zoster often has prodromal symptoms of tingling, hyperesthesia, tenderness, and burning or itching pain along the affected dermatome. Vesicles follow the prodromal symptoms with an erythematous base occurring within 3 to 5 days. A unilateral, bandlike, erythematous, maculopapular rash first occurs along the involved dermatome and rarely crosses the midline of the body. The rash develops into clustered vesicles (usually on an erythematous base) that become purulent, rupture, and crust. Debilitated older adults may have a prolonged and difficult course. For them, the eruption is typically more extensive and inflammatory, occasionally resulting in hemorrhagic blisters, skin necrosis, secondary bacterial infection, or extensive scarring, which is sometimes hypertrophic or keloidal (CDC, 2018). These vesicles are prone to secondary bacterial infections. This occurs more often in older adults. It may take up to 1 month for the crusting lesions to heal; mild cases resolve in 7 to 10 days. The average duration for herpes zoster is 3 weeks. Scarring and permanent or temporary pigment discoloration may occur, especially in severe cases. Lymphadenopathy and occasional temperature elevation are not uncommon. Postinfection paresthesia and meningoencephalitis may occur for 2 to 4 weeks when motor neurons and the central nervous system (CNS) are involved (Brizzi & Lyons, 2014).

The incidence of herpes zoster increases with age, most likely because of diminishing immune function. The older adult is also at a greater risk of developing postherpetic segmental pain. Dissemination is often seen in older adults or immunosuppressed patients. Disseminated herpes zoster, which is rare and occurs in only 2% to 5% of patients, is more serious because of its systemic nature. In disseminated herpes zoster, satellite lesions appear outside the affected dermatome within 4 to 6 days after the initial eruption. Dissemination may be associated with fever, lymphadenopathy, headache, neck rigidity, and increased risk of serious complications such as encephalitis, hepatitis, and pneumonitis (Habif, 2004).

One of the major complications from this acute viral infection is postherpetic neuralgia, which is pain that persists along the affected dermatome after resolution of vesicular lesions. Postherpetic neuralgia may last less than 1 year, but it may last a lifetime with little pain relief. It affects approximately 33% of patients age 40 or older, and by age 70 the risk increases to 74%. Postherpetic neuralgia is more common in persons with trigeminal nerve involvement (CDC, 2018).

NURSING MANAGEMENT

Assessment

Nursing assessment begins with interviewing the patient to identify prodromal symptoms such as burning, itching, or tingling along a dermatome before rash development. The nurse should obtain a pertinent health history that addresses chickenpox history, medications, diabetes, malignancy with recent chemotherapy or radiotherapy, and HIV and other immuno-compromised states. The nurse should also identify persons with whom the patient has had close physical contact who have not had chickenpox or the chickenpox vaccine because they may be at risk of infection. The nurse should inspect the area of discomfort for the characteristic unilateral, bandlike,

erythematous, maculopapular rash that may have clustered vesicles. Initially, the area may be a raised, erythematous rash before the vesicles appear. Intense pain is often associated with the rash, particularly in older adults. Based on the lesions and prescribed treatments, the nurse must determine the effect on the patient's mobility and capacity for activities of daily living (ADLs). Recommended treatment measures may require the assistance of another person.

Diagnosis

Nursing diagnoses for a patient with herpes zoster include the following:
- Reduced skin integrity resulting from immunologic deficit
- Potential for infection resulting from impaired skin integrity
- Disrupted sleep pattern resulting from impaired skin integrity or pain
- Pain resulting from inadequate pain relief from analgesia
- Need for health teaching resulting from lack of previous exposure to disease process and treatment

Planning and Expected Outcomes

The goals of nursing management are pain relief and the prevention of secondary infection and scarring. Local skin care treatments may need to be taught to the patient or caregiver. The nurse must be alert to the possibility of long-term pain (postherpetic neuralgia) and the resulting depression. Expected outcomes include the following:
1. Skin lesions will remain free from necrotic tissue and infection.
2. The patient will experience adequate periods of restful sleep, as evidenced by:
   - No requests for pain medication during the night
   - Reports of uninterrupted sleep during the night and feeling well rested on arising
3. The patient will obtain adequate pain relief, as evidenced by:
   - Verbalizing comfort and pain relief after taking an analgesic
   - Augmenting analgesic pain relief with the use of relaxation exercises, music diversion tapes, or guided imagery
4. The patient will demonstrate increased knowledge of his or her condition, as evidenced by:
   - Verbalizing significant and reportable signs and symptoms of infection
   - Verbalizing the rationale for regular, consistent use of analgesics
   - Correctly performing a return demonstration of lesion care and dressing change procedure

Intervention

Nursing interventions consist of notifying the health care provider as soon as the characteristic rash and vesicles are identified, especially if they follow a dermatomal pattern. After a diagnosis is made, follow-through with medical and nursing management is paramount to patient comfort. Lesions should be monitored closely for the development of secondary bacterial infections, as evidenced by erythema, tenderness, or a purulent discharge. If satellite lesions develop outside the dermatome, especially if the patient is also experiencing headaches, neck rigidity, or pulmonary congestion, the health care provider must be notified immediately because this is indicative of disseminated herpes zoster (Dasgupta, 2009).

The nurse should teach the older adult patient, family members, and staff the cause of shingles so that anxiety and misconceptions may be alleviated, and the nurse should explain the treatment measures to increase adherence and involvement in care. Herpes zoster may be very painful, so prompt administration of pain medications is crucial for patient comfort. For optimal pain control, patients should be instructed to inform the nurse when they experience the initial onset of pain, before the pain becomes well entrenched. Effective pain management is one area in which nurses may have a positive effect on a patient's quality of life. If postherpetic neuralgia occurs, antidepressants are used as adjuncts to analgesics for control of pain.

Evaluation

Evaluation of interventions focuses on pain control, with documented results of analgesics and adjunct therapies, and on prevention of secondary infection by frequent monitoring of the site. Many barriers to effective pain management in older adults exist, leading to frequent underrecognition and undertreatment of pain. If pain is not relieved, the health care provider should be consulted to obtain an alternative analgesic agent or adjunct drug therapy. The inflammatory response in an older adult may be diminished, even in the presence of severe infection, so the nurse should be alert to even slight symptoms of a secondary bacterial infection. If evidence of cellulitis is noted, the health care provider should be informed to implement topical or oral antibiotic therapy. Documentation of assessment, the response to treatment measures, patient comprehension of teaching, and other nursing interventions demonstrates nursing accountability (see Nursing Care Plan: Herpes Zoster).

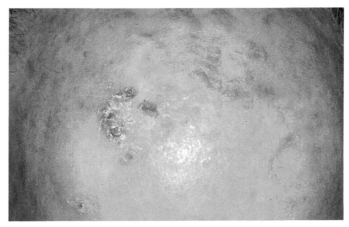

Fig. 17.6 Actinic keratosis. (From Bolognia, J. L., Schaffer, J. V., Duncan, K. O., & Ko, C. J. [2014]. *Dermatology essentials.* Philadelphia, PA: Elsevier Saunders.)

PREMALIGNANT SKIN GROWTHS: ACTINIC KERATOSIS

Actinic keratosis is a premalignant lesion of the epidermis caused by long-term exposure to UV rays. This precancerous lesion is more common in individuals with light complexions and occurs most commonly on the dorsum of the hands, scalp, outer ears, face, and lower arms. Treatment should be aggressive, and patients should be monitored closely to prevent progression to squamous cell carcinoma (SCC) (Spencer, 2017).

Actinic keratosis begins in vascular areas as a reddish macule or papule that has a rough, yellowish-brown scale that may itch or cause discomfort (Fig. 17.6). During assessment, the nurse should be attuned to the rough surface of the lesion and its location, and be particularly alert if a suspicious lesion occurs

---

⊚ NURSING CARE PLAN

Herpes Zoster

Clinical Situation

Mr. F. is a 72-year-old man who lives with his daughter and her husband. He has severe rheumatoid arthritis and hypertension. He takes ibuprofen, amlodipine, and atorvastatin. He has had both knees replaced in the past 5 years.

Mr. F. began to experience a burning with pain 2 days ago and this morning awoke with clustered vesicles on the left side of his torso extending from the mid-back around to the midline of the anterior aspect of his chest. He went in to see his primary care physician. The provider ordered acyclovir, analgesics as needed for pain, and a topical antibiotic to prevent secondary infection.

Nursing Diagnosis

Potential for infection resulting from herpes zoster and open lesions

Outcome

The patient will experience no secondary infection, as evidenced by no fever and other vital signs within normal limits and will practice habits that decrease the risk of infection.

Interventions

Instruct the patient not to scratch or rub the affected area so as not to break vesicles, which would increase the risk of secondary infection.

Assess vital signs, mental status, and skin lesions every shift to identify signs of infection (e.g., fever, tachycardia, erythema, tenderness, purulent discharge, and confusion).

If the patient is febrile, ensure adequate hydration because a fever increases hydration needs.

Tachycardia could precipitate heart failure (HF) from decreased cardiac output; monitor for shortness of breath, rales, edema, and other signs of cardiovascular compromise.

If vesicle lesions rupture, implement topical treatment, noting the response.

Ensure adequate nutrition to foster healing.

Monitor food and fluid intake and ensure food preferences are being met.

Be alert for vesicles outside of the involved dermatome, which could indicate disseminated herpes zoster; if vesicles appear, contact the physician or nurse practitioner immediately.

Teach the patient, staff, and visitors the value of hand washing and proper disposal of dressing and treatment material as an infection control standard.

Identify staff and visitors who have no known history of chickenpox or vaccine and inform them that they are not able to provide care for the patient because they may not have immunity to the varicella virus; isolation is not required. The infection control strategy is to take universal precautions.

on a sun-exposed area. Patients should be cautioned to avoid sun exposure from 10 AM to 3 PM, wear protective clothing, and use sunscreen. Medical treatment of actinic keratosis is topical fluorouracil 5% cream and imiquimod 5% cream, topical 3% diclofenac gel, ingenol mebutate 0.015% or 0.05% topical gel, and aminolevulinic acid 10% topical gel (Spencer, 2017).

NURSING MANAGEMENT

Assessment

Nursing assessment begins with the patient interview to determine risk factors such as the frequency of activities with sun exposure and the use of preventive practices (e.g., wearing a hat and long sleeves while outside). The skin should be inspected, and any rough lesions palpated and noted for location and texture. If hand lotion is used frequently, roughness will not be present; therefore the nurse should look for an erythematous macule or papule. The nurse should refer patients to their primary care provider whenever a suspicious lesion is found. The nurse should also explain the value of treating skin cancer early, which may minimize scarring and disfigurement.

Diagnosis

Nursing diagnoses for a patient with actinic keratosis include the following:

- Reduced skin integrity resulting from removal of a lesion
- Potential for infection resulting from a break in skin integrity
- Distorted body image resulting from disfigurement and scarring resulting from removal of lesion

Planning and Expected Outcomes

The goals of nursing management after the removal of premalignant lesions are the prevention of secondary infection and assistance in coping with any body image disturbance. Expected outcomes include the following:

1. The site of lesion removal will heal without evidence of secondary infection.
2. The patient will demonstrate no changes in body image perception.
3. The patient will demonstrate behavior change through adoption of preventive skin care practices.

Intervention

Nursing intervention consists of reinforcing the treatment regimen with the patient and family, monitoring the treated site to prevent secondary infection, providing support, and teaching preventive strategies. To lower a patient's anxiety and assist with body image changes, the nurse should explain the treatment, stressing that erythema and crusting are temporary. The resulting body image trauma from treatment of many facial lesions may isolate an individual. The nurse should identify the patient's fears and discuss them in an open, reassuring manner.

Wounds should be assessed for development of a bacterial infection, as evidenced by increased tenderness, increasing erythema around the treated site, purulent discharge, and possibly fever. Topical management with an antibiotic ointment may be implemented prophylactically.

The nurse should teach older adult patients and family members the strategies necessary to prevent recurrence and stress the need to wear hats with wide brims and long-sleeved shirts to protect the skin from sun exposure. If an individual is going to be exposed to the sun, a sunscreen with a sun protection factor (SPF) of at least 15 should be applied (Habif, 2004).

Evaluation

Evaluation of nursing management is supported with documentation addressing treatment progress, which includes a physical description, patient comprehension of educational information, and identification of and coping with any body image disturbances.

MALIGNANT SKIN GROWTHS

Basal Cell Carcinoma

Basal cell carcinoma (BCC) is the most common skin cancer and is more prevalent in fair-skinned, blond, or red-headed individuals with extensive previous sun exposure. It occurs more often in men than in women; however, this gender difference has decreased in recent years. BCC is most commonly found on the face and scalp, less often on the trunk, and rarely on the hands. It may also arise from scars or burns, particularly in older adults who have experienced chronic sun damage. BCC usually does not metastasize, but if left untreated it may metastasize to the bone, lungs, and lymph nodes (Bader, 2017).

Typically, BCC appears as a pearly papule with a depression in the center, giving the lesion a doughnut-shaped appearance with telangiectasia on or around the lesion (Fig. 17.7). BCC may also appear as a blue-black pearly nodule (pigmented basal cell) or a red, scaly, or eczematous-appearing macule usually on the thoracic area (superficial spreading BCC).

Squamous Cell Carcinoma

SCC is skin cancer arising from the epidermis found most often on the scalp, outer ears, lower lip, and dorsum of the hands. SCC may also develop in chronic leg ulcers or open fractures and has a 20% incidence of metastasis, generally to regional lymph nodes. SCC accounts for 90% of lip lesions and occurs along the vermillion border of the lower lip. The etiologic factors of SCC may be UV rays, chemical carcinogens, and x-rays. SCC

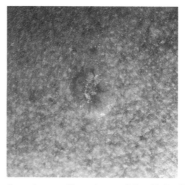

Fig. 17.7 Basal cell carcinoma. (From Ignatavicius, D. D., & Workman, M. L. [2018]. *Medical-surgical nursing: Concepts for interprofessional collaborative care* [9th ed.]. St. Louis, MO: Elsevier.)

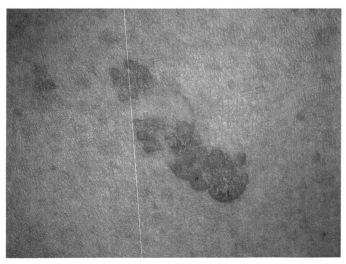

Fig. 17.8 Squamous cell carcinoma. (From Bolognia, J. L., Jorizzo, J. L., & Schaffer, J. V. [2018]. *Dermatology* [4th ed.]. St. Louis, MO: Saunders. © Yale Residents' Slide Collection.)

is more common in men and older adults, and the incidence increases with geographic proximity to the equator. Although SCC is less common in black persons, "it carries a higher mortality rate, perhaps due to delayed diagnosis, because tumors are more likely to occur in sun-protected areas in these individuals" (Najjar, 2017).

SCC usually presents as a firm, elevated lump; it may have a thick, adherent scale with a center that is often ulcerated or crusted (Fig. 17.8). At first glance, SCC may even look like a wart. The base may be inflamed and red, and it usually bleeds easily. SCC may arise from actinic keratosis, which supports early detection and removal of such lesions. If tumors are ignored or left unattended, they may enlarge, creating significant disfigurement after surgical excision.

Melanoma

Melanoma is a malignant neoplasm of pigment-forming cells capable of metastasizing to any organ of the body, even before the lesion is noted; therefore early detection is crucial. Invasive

melanoma is the fifth most common cancer in men and the sixth most common cancer in women. If detected and treated before spreading to the lymph nodes, there is a 99% 5-year survival rate (American Academy of Dermatology [AAD], n.d.).

The incidence of melanoma has doubled in recent years. Ninety-five percent of melanomas can be attributed to UV exposure. A genetic predisposition to melanoma also exists: 10% of patients have a parent or sibling with a history of melanoma. Individuals with a family history of melanoma should perform monthly skin self-examinations and have a professional skin evaluation at regular intervals (AAD, n.d.).

Individuals at high risk are fair-skinned, and their skin tends to burn rather than tan; have red or blond hair; have multiple nevi; and tend to freckle. African Americans, Asians, and dark-skinned whites are at less risk of developing melanoma; however, most melanomas found in these populations occur in skin areas not exposed to the sun, especially the periungual, palmar, and plantar surfaces. An individual with one melanoma is at risk for having another (AAD, n.d.).

Melanoma's clinical hallmark is an irregularly shaped nevus (mole), papule, or plaque that has undergone a change, particularly in color. The characteristic signs of most malignant melanomas are referred to as the *ABCDs*: Asymmetry, Border irregularity, Color variation (red, white, blue), and Diameter greater than 6 mm (Tan, 2018). *E* has been added by some providers, to indicate Elevation or Evolution (Fig. 17.9). The lesion may itch or bleed; however, this is usually a later sign. A dermatologist or family physician should examine any mole or lesion that has irregularly shaped borders and has had a color change, usually to a darker color (AAD, n.d.).

Of the four types of melanoma, the most common is the *superficial spreading melanoma*, which is slower growing. Superficial spreading melanoma accounts for 70% of all melanomas, occurring most commonly on the trunk in males, the extremities in females, and upper back in both. The mean age of diagnosis is the mid-40s. Superficial melanoma is a slow-growing, flat, slightly elevated, pigmented papule or patch that has irregular borders and varied colors within the lesion (Psaty, 2010).

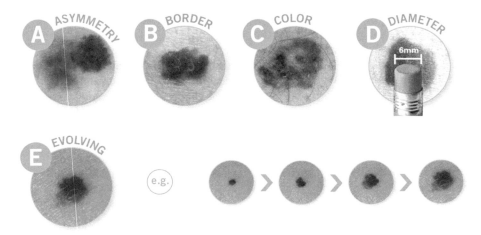

Fig. 17.9 ABCDE of melanoma. (Reprinted with permission from the American Academy of Dermatology, 2018. All rights reserved.)

Nodular melanoma occurs in 10% to 15% of patients with melanoma and has the worst prognosis because it usually invasive by the time it is diagnosed. Nodular melanoma is most often found on the trunk, legs, and arms; it may also occur on the scalp in men. The mean age at diagnosis is the fifth or sixth decade of life. Nodular melanoma is a hard, usually dark nodule arising from a preexisting mole (Habif, 2004).

Lentigo maligna occurs most often in the elderly. Lentigo maligna melanoma is a brown-tan macular lesion with varied pigmentation and highly irregular borders. It is found most often on chronically sun-exposed skin of the face, ears, arms and upper trunk, and remains superficial for some time, before becoming invasive (Habif, 2004).

Acral-lentiginous melanoma usually occurs on the palms of hands and soles of feet, as well as under finger/toe nails. It is more common in older adults, and the mean age is 60 at the time of diagnosis. It is the most common melanoma found in blacks and Asians; therefore careful inspection of the foot soles, palms, and hands is warranted when caring for black and Asian American patients. Acral-lentiginous melanoma resembles lentigo melanoma with its flat, irregular, discolored borders. It spreads superficially before becoming invasive (Habif, 2004; Rigel, Russak, & Friedman, 2010).

NURSING MANAGEMENT

Assessment

Nursing assessment begins with interviewing the patient to determine how long the lesion(s) have been present and to identify risk factors such as chronic sun exposure and family history. The nurse should inspect and palpate the suspicious lesion, surrounding tissue, and lymph nodes (to identify possible metastasis). A magnifying glass may be useful for closely examining any lesion. When a suspicious lesion is identified, the nurse should promptly refer the patient to the primary care provider. The nurse should also explain that early treatment lessens the extent of scarring and possibly intervenes before metastasis. Additionally, the nurse should discuss the patient's feelings and fears about cancer.

Diagnosis

Nursing diagnoses for a patient with skin cancer include the following:
- Reduced skin integrity resulting from removal of a cancerous lesion
- Fear of cancer, pain, or death resulting from having a cancerous skin lesion
- Potential for infection resulting from a break in skin integrity and a surgical wound
- Distorted body image resulting from disfigurement and scarring resulting from removal of a cancerous lesion

Planning and Expected Outcomes

The goals of nursing management are to facilitate the referral of patients for treatment and removal of suspicious lesions, prevent secondary infections and metastasis, and address

fears and feelings related to cancer; referrals to community resources should be made as indicated. The nurse must discuss the patient's and family's feelings about having a cancerous lesion so that any need for a community referral or educational material can be identified. Expected outcomes include the following:
1. The site of excision will heal without evidence of infection.
2. The patient will verbalize fears related to the diagnosis and actively seek information and clarification.
3. The patient will identify community resources for support and additional information.
4. The patient will verbalize understanding of the treatment plan.
5. The patient will demonstrate increased knowledge of the condition, as evidenced by adoption of preventive strategies.

Intervention

Nursing management includes reinforcement of the treatment regimen by monitoring the wound for secondary infection (e.g., erythema, tenderness, and purulent discharge) and reinforcement of the caring component of nursing by discussing the patient's and family's feelings related to cancer. The nurse should identify and discuss the patient's and family's feelings about having a cancerous lesion and refer the patient to appropriate community resources if they are having difficulty coping or have a high level of anxiety. The nurse should also explain that a risk of metastasis exists and refer the patient to the American Cancer Society (https://www.cancer.org/), appropriate Internet resources, or the local library for additional information.

The nurse should teach the patient or family dressing care and signs of infection. Removal may result in scarring, especially if the lesion was large. Consequently, reassurance must be provided, and feelings related to body image changes should be addressed; the focus is on comfort, education, and emotional support. Preventive strategies such as wearing hats with wide brims, wearing long sleeves, and using sunscreen should also be taught to both the patient and family. In addition, the patient and family members should have annual skin assessments because a hereditary tendency for occurrence exists.

Evaluation

Evaluation of nursing interventions focuses on monitoring for infection, the effectiveness of pain control measures, comprehension of patient education, and discussions related to body image changes and fears about cancer. If there is poor pain control or development of an infection, the health care provider should be contacted for an alternative strategy. Documentation of assessment, the response to treatment measures, patient comprehension of teaching, and other nursing interventions demonstrates nursing accountability.

LOWER EXTREMITY ULCERS

Chronic leg ulcers are a common problem in older adults, occurring primarily from three causes: arterial insufficiency, venous hypertension, and diabetic neuropathy (Table 17.1). A

TABLE 17.1   Leg Ulcer Differentiation

Type	Primary Cause	Characteristics
Arterial ulcers	Arterial insufficiency; peripheral vascular disease	Located on toes, feet, or lower third of leg; irregularly shaped wound; thin, shiny, cool skin with cyanotic hue, loss of hair, thickened toenails; pain with activity, rest, or at night
Venous ulcers	Venous hypertension	Located on medial aspect of lower third of leg; irregularly shaped wound; either flat or shallow crater; discoloration, varicosities, edema, and exudate; pain relieved with activity
Diabetic foot lesion	Neuropathy	Located on plantar surface of foot; circular, often deep wounds; decreased or absent vibratory sensation; painful; paresthesia

brief overview of each etiologic factor and treatment follows. Greater emphasis is placed on venous ulcers because these are more prevalent in older adults and more challenging because of their chronicity.

Arterial Ulcers

Arterial or ischemic ulcers result from arterial insufficiency. Arterial insufficiency is also referred to as peripheral vascular disease (PVD). Arteriosclerosis—thickening and hardening of the arterial wall—is the primary cause for the decreased blood flow that results in ischemia and eventually tissue death. Several risk factors, including obesity, diabetes, hyperlipoproteinemia, and hypertension, may lead to arterial ulcers.

Pain with exercise, at night, or while resting is the most common sign of arterial insufficiency. Pain at rest indicates severely restricted arterial blood flow. The area proximal to (above) the painful area is usually the site of restricted blood flow. Pulses distal to the restriction may be present because of collateral circulation. The patient may also complain of cramping, burning, or aching. As the disease advances, the extremity develops a cyanotic hue and becomes cool. The skin becomes thin, shiny, and dry, and has an associated loss of hair and thickened nails, all of which results from the diminished blood supply. Tissue anoxia leads to necrosis and poor healing. Arterial ulcers are usually located on the outer ankle, feet, and toes. The ulcerated area appears "punched out," with well-defined wound margins. The causes must be corrected so that oxygen and other nutrients are available to promote healing of necrotic wounds. Treatment is usually surgical intervention with revascularization; if the disease is too advanced, amputation may be necessary.

Venous Ulcers

Venous ulcers, also known as stasis ulcers, are thought to arise secondary to chronic venous insufficiency. Venous ulcers affect roughly 1% of the general population, and a higher incidence is seen in older adults. Chronic venous leg ulcers usually have an onset in early adulthood; however, peak prevalence is seen in people ages 70 or older. Venous ulcers occur more often in women than in men. Epidemiologic studies have revealed that 57% to 80% of all lower leg ulcers are related to venous insufficiency, and 10% to 25% have a combination of venous and arterial insufficiency.

Venous hypertension is the primary cause of venous ulcers. Valvular incompetence of the deep or perforating veins of the lower leg is present in most venous ulcer cases. Venous hypertension leads to a tortuous capillary system, which causes an accumulation of fibrinogen, leukocytes, and erythrocytes. The accumulation of erythrocytes in the tissue produces a brownish skin discoloration caused by the release of hemoglobin. Often, the discoloration and thickening of the skin (lipodermatosclerosis) is the first indication of venous hypertension. Capillary occlusion caused by trapping of white blood cells (WBCs) results in the release of proteolytic enzymes, which foster fibrinogen leakage. The fibrin cuff creates a barrier that prevents or delays exchange of oxygen and other nutrients, resulting in cell death. Anoxia and trapping of growth factors are the primary causes of ulceration and poor healing. The fibrin cuff is irreversible, which sets the stage for frequent recurrence and makes venous ulcers a chronic disorder (Vasudevan, 2014).

The diagnosis of venous ulcer is commonly based on clinical presentation. Venous ulcers are usually on the medial aspect of the lower leg, with flat or shallow craters and irregular borders, accompanied by varicosities, lipodermatosclerosis, hemosiderin deposit (reddish brown pigmentation), and itching. Venous ulcers generate a large amount of exudate and are usually surrounded by erythema and edema. Although it may be difficult, it is important to differentiate between venous ulcers and cellulitis.

It is well recognized that venous ulcers heal with prolonged elevation of the affected extremity; however, adherence is difficult. Research has demonstrated that compression therapy of at least 30 to 40 mm Hg at the ankle and distal lower leg decreases edema by compressing fluid through the fibrin cuff (Slone-Rivera & Wu, 2012). The most common cause of recurrence is nonadherence with compression therapy. It is important to remember that compression therapy is intended for ambulatory patients. The older adult with dependent edema, not primary venous disease, does not tolerate compression well. Compression therapy is not a management option for arterial insufficiency; pain and cyanosis will occur from further impaired circulation.

Diabetic Foot Lesions

Risk factors for developing diabetic foot lesions are peripheral neuropathy, foot deformity, peripheral arterial disease, and history of previous foot lesions. Adequately offloading footwear are a protective factor (Waaijman et al., 2014). Older adults who live alone or who have mental confusion are at an increased risk for foot lesions because they may not have the means to recognize a diabetic foot lesion or to follow up with appropriate treatment. A risk factor for lower extremity amputation is neuropathy, which is implicated in approximately 90% of diabetic foot lesions. This sensory loss is associated with a 15.5% relative risk of amputation. Therefore individuals with diabetes and neuropathy are at risk of developing lower leg lesions, which may lead to an amputation.

Pain and temperature are usually the first sensations affected by neuropathy. The loss of the peripheral sensory feedback system impairs the patients' ability to feel tissue damage, inflammation, or injury. Lesions resulting from diabetic peripheral neuropathy tend to be bilateral, symmetric, and located on the plantar surface of the foot. Patients usually complain of pain and paresthesias; however, they also have diminished or absent vibratory and temperature sensation of the affected extremities. Pain relieved by walking is one diagnostic sign of neuropathy. Neuropathic lesions are usually well perfused, yet a patient with diabetes may have arterial insufficiency, which compromises healing abilities.

Treatment varies, depending on the etiologic factors and wound condition. Patient education regarding how to minimize the risk of chemical, thermal, and mechanical trauma is the first line of defense against diabetic foot lesions. Physical examination of the foot should include testing for neuropathy and the identification of high foot pressures. An easy and inexpensive device for establishing neuropathy is the Semmes-Weinstein monofilament. Inability to feel the 5.07 monofilament indicates the patient is at risk for lesion development and needs orthotics (specially fitted shoes designed to prevent ulcers and decrease callous formation by redistributing weight) to offload pressure (Baraz, Zarea, Shahbazian, & Latifi, 2014). The nurse should stress to patients with diabetes, particularly if they have PVD, that any trauma to the lower leg, ankles, or feet may lead to a lesion and possible amputation. They must protect their feet and lower legs with proper shoes and foot care. Orthotics may be helpful in preventing mechanical trauma. When an ulcer is present, a total contact cast may be applied to redistribute weight and minimize trauma but is contraindicated with cellulitis or excessive drainage. Some physicians use hyperbaric oxygenation in hopes of increasing oxygenation to the affected area; however, this treatment is controversial because of its questionable effectiveness in wounds with compromised circulation, for example, diabetic foot lesions. The success of this strategy depends on the amount of circulation present in the affected area.

NURSING MANAGEMENT

Assessment

Nursing assessment begins with the determination of the location and characteristics of lower leg ulcers and lesions. The nurse should determine wound dimensions, depth, and amount of exudate; palpate popliteal pulses at least every day if the patient is in acute care and at every visit if they are in an ambulatory or home setting; and note any discoloration and edema. The nurse should also ascertain if the patient experiences any pain or itching and how it has been managed. A nutritional assessment should be conducted, which includes the patient's weight, 24-hour diet recall, chewing abilities, and food preparation abilities. The nurse should determine whether shopping assistance is needed.

Diagnosis

Nursing diagnoses for a patient with lower extremity ulcers and lesions include the following:

- Reduced skin integrity resulting from altered circulation
- Potential for infection resulting from open, chronic wounds

Planning and Expected Outcomes

The goal of nursing management is to facilitate healing without infection by promotion of treatment adherence and by provision of patient education regarding the disease process and treatment; the nurse should inform patients with venous ulcers that these ulcers are a chronic process. Time for patient education will be needed. Expected outcomes include the following:

1. Skin lesions will remain free from necrotic tissue and infection.
2. Edema in lower extremities will be controlled.
3. Skin lesions will heal with minimum scarring.
4. The patient will be able to maintain a healed state for at least 6 months.

Intervention

Nursing interventions consist of keeping the legs elevated; implementing compression therapy; administering wound care; and educating the patient about the causes of lower extremity ulcers and lesions, the strategy of compression therapy, and specific wound care. The nurse must stress the need to maintain compression therapy to facilitate healing of venous ulcers and avoid further breakdown. Infection is difficult to determine because lower extremity ulcers and lesions often have erythematous bases with induration; however, if the patient develops a fever and tenderness surrounding the wound, the health care provider should be contacted. The nurse should determine whether any community services such as home-delivered meals, grocery shopping assistance, and other support services are needed. They should also identify and discuss the patient's feelings regarding chronic illness and body image changes; teach the patient with venous ulcers that they generate a large amount of exudate and instruct on dressing changes.

Evaluation

Evaluation of nursing interventions focuses on prevention of further wound deterioration and infection, as well as the effectiveness of patient education. A return demonstration of compression therapy application and wound care is a concrete evaluation and ensures patient comprehension. Nursing accountability is demonstrated by documentation of assessment, the response to treatment measures, patient comprehension of teaching, and other nursing interventions.

PRESSURE INJURIES

Pressure injuries (previously referred to as *pressure ulcers*) have plagued humans for centuries. Hippocrates devised a debridement treatment with healing by secondary closure. Ambroise Paré, a sixteenth-century surgeon, published strategies for healing skin wounds that challenged the existing practice of pouring hot oil on the wound. These included increased nutrition and mobility, debridement, and application of dressings (Levine, 1992).

It was not until the twentieth century that scientific research began to determine the cause and appropriate management of pressure injuries. In 1930, Landis determined that the average capillary pressure before which ischemia occurs is below 32 mm Hg. In the 1950s, Kosiak (1958) found that pressure applied to rabbits' ears over 2 hours would result in ulceration. Thus the universal recommendation of turning every 2 hours was established. The first pressure injury risk assessment tool was designed and tested by Doreen Norton (1989) in the late 1950s but not disseminated until 1962 when she presented study findings at a conference.

In 1962, researchers first demonstrated that moisture, applied with occlusive dressings, increases epithelialization (the healing process) (Krasner, 1991). In 1972, a plastic occlusive dressing was shown to cut epithelialization time in half, which led to film dressings, followed by hydrocolloidal dressings.

This information explosion has resulted in varied terminology and beliefs. As a result, leading experts in pressure injury management and research formed the National Pressure Ulcer Advisory Panel (NPUAP) in 1987, with the intent of improving prevention and management through education, legislation, standardization of staging criteria, and identification of research needs. The NPUAP held consensus conferences beginning in May 1988, the outcome of which included standardized staging criteria endorsed by the International Association for Enterostomal Therapists and the Agency for Healthcare Research and Quality (AHRQ). Also, to standardize terms and to more accurately reflect the cause of pressure injury, NPUAP decreed that *pressure injury* is a more appropriate term than *pressure ulcer* or *decubitus*. Therefore the term *pressure injury* is used throughout this discussion.

Pressure injury prevention and management is one of four costly adverse events addressed in AHRQ's *Safety Program for Nursing Homes: On-Time Prevention*. The AHRQ has developed tools for nursing homes with electronic health records, designed to improve clinical decision making and prevent adverse events. For further information, see https:// www.ahrq.gov/professionals/systems/long-term-care/resources/ index.html.

Epidemiology of Pressure Injuries

The epidemiology of pressure injuries has been difficult to quantify and varies depending on sample size, definition of terms, and type of facility. Despite methodologic limitations, incidence (new cases) and prevalence (over a specific period) rates of pressure injuries are sufficiently high to generate concern.

Pressure injuries affect 2.5 million hospital patients a year, amounting to a cost between $9 and $11 billion per year; each pressure injury adds more than $43,000 per hospitalization (AHRQ, 2014). Several groups have been identified as high risk for the development of pressure injury while hospitalized: quadriplegic patients, older patients with hip fractures, orthopedic patients who are immobile, and critical care patients.

The prevalence rate of pressure injuries in long-term care facilities is roughly 7.5%, resulting in an annual cost of $3.3 billion. Incidence rates vary among nursing care facilities because of the heterogeneous case-mix and staffing patterns. Better data are needed to determine the degree of the problem in long-term care.

Etiology of Pressure Injuries

Pressure on soft tissue over bony prominences or other hard surfaces is the primary causative factor in pressure injury formation. However, other contributing factors exist and explain why the tissue of some individuals breaks down within 30 minutes of lying in the same position, whereas that of others does not break down for hours.

Pressure injuries begin at the point of contact between soft tissue and a hard surface (e.g., bone). Consequently, an inverted-cone-shaped wound develops, with the largest area of breakdown being near the bone. Common bony prominences susceptible to pressure injury development are the sacrum, ischial tuberosity (especially in an upright sitting position in a chair or bed), lateral malleolus, trochanter, and heels (Fig. 17.10).

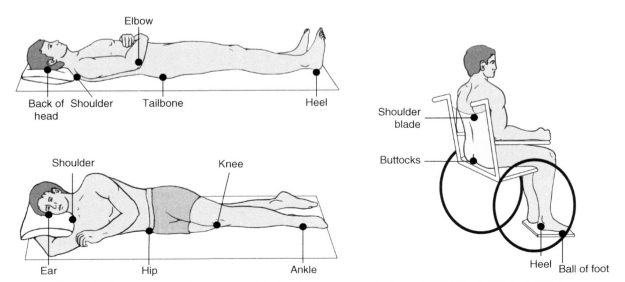

Fig. 17.10 Pressure points where pressure injuries often occur. (Adapted from deWit, S. C., & O'Neill, P. [2014]. *Fundamental concepts and skills for nursing* [4th ed.]. St. Louis, MO: Saunders.)

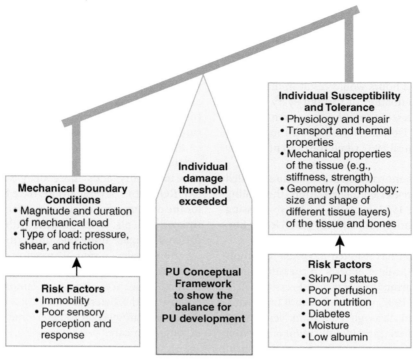

Fig. 17.11 Pressure ulcer conceptual framework. *PU*, Pressure ulcer. (From Coleman, S., Nixon, J., Keen, J., et al. [2014]. A new pressure ulcer conceptual framework. *Journal of Advanced Nursing, 70*[10], 2222-2234.)

The intensity of pressure that leads to capillary closure, compounded by the duration of pressure and tissue tolerance, results in tissue anoxia, ischemia, edema, and eventually tissue necrosis. Immobility, decreased activity, and decreased sensory perception place individuals at risk for unrelieved pressure that generates tissue ischemia and death. Tissue tolerance is influenced by extrinsic factors—moisture, friction, and shearing—and intrinsic factors—poor nutrition, advanced age, hypotension, emotional stress, smoking, and skin temperature (Agrawal & Chauhan, 2012). The development of pressure injuries is a complex, synergistic phenomenon that makes prevention a challenge (Fig. 17.11).

Capillary pressure ensures the movement of blood through the capillary membrane, maintaining oxygenation and tissue nutrition. Capillary collapse may result from prolonged pressure, which leads to tissue anoxia, ischemia, reactive hyperemia (erythema), leakage of plasma into interstitial tissue, and microvascular hemorrhaging observable by nonblanchable erythema. If the pressure persists, tissue death will result. External pressure of 33 mm Hg, depending on the location and individual, may be enough to impair circulation (Agrawal & Chauhan, 2012).

People with sensory impairment (paralysis or sedation) do not have a normal protective reflex, which is shifting weight in response to discomfort from capillary closure and tissue anoxia. This inability may explain the higher incidence of pressure injuries among individuals with paralysis or those undergoing long surgical procedures. Patients with altered mental

status because of disease (e.g., dementia) or medication may have decreased pain or tissue anoxia perception. These individuals are at risk for pressure injury development.

Tissue tolerance, another major contributing factor in the development of a pressure injury, is defined as the ability of the skin and supporting structures to endure the effects of pressure. It is apparent, then, that poor tissue tolerance makes one more vulnerable to pressure intensity and duration, thus increasing the response to pressure. Shearing, friction, age-related changes in the integumentary system, low blood pressure, and nutritional status all influence tissue tolerance.

Shearing, which is the sliding of parallel surfaces, causes stretching and occlusion of the arterial supply, usually of the fascia and muscle. Shearing forces may decrease the blood supply, leading to tissue ischemia and necrosis (Fig. 17.12). The most common position for shearing is when the head of the bed is elevated, causing the body to slide downward. Resistance keeps the skin in place while gravity pulls the body toward the foot of the bed (Agrawal & Chauhan, 2012).

Friction, the rubbing of skin against another surface, primarily affects the epidermal and dermal layers, causing a superficial abrasion (e.g., sheet burn) (Agrawal & Chauhan, 2012). Restless patients or those with persistent movements are at risk for friction injuries. However, when friction occurs concurrently with gravitational forces, shearing is the outcome.

Moisture from incontinence or profuse sweating may decrease tensile strength, alter skin resiliency to external forces,

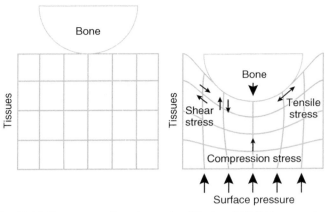

Fig. 17.12 Shear stress. (From International Review. [2010]. Pressure ulcer prevention: Pressure, shear, friction, and microclimate in context. A consensus document. London, UK: Wounds International. Retrieved from http://www.woundsinternational.com/media/issues/300/files/content_8925.pdf.)

and exacerbate friction and shearing forces (Agrawal & Chauhan, 2012). Efforts should be made to keep the skin dry.

As many studies have revealed, nutritional status greatly influences the development of pressure injuries. Protein deficiency weakens tissue tolerance (i.e., the spring between the skin surface and bony prominences), making soft tissue more susceptible to breakdown when pressure intensity is prolonged. Hypoproteinemia changes osmotic equilibrium, which leads to edema. Consequently, sluggish oxygenation and transportation create an environment for tissue breakdown and poor healing. Serum albumin levels below 3.5 grams per deciliter (g/dL) have a correlation with pressure injury development and poor wound healing (Bluestein & Javaheri, 2008). Proteins are also needed for collagen formation, granulation tissue formation, and immunologic response.

The incidence of pressure injuries is increased in older adults, particularly in those older than age 70. With aging, the epidermis thins, elasticity decreases, and vessels degenerate, resulting in reduced blood flow. These age-related changes impair the early warning sign of erythema, delay crucial early immunologic responses, and impede the healing process, thereby making older adults at risk for pressure injury development.

Low blood pressure and dehydration may reduce circulation, especially in the microvasculature, which eventually leads to tissue ischemia. Systolic blood pressure below 90 mm Hg has been found to be a risk factor for pressure injury formation, presumably because of decreased peripheral circulation and subsequent ischemia (Cox, 2017). Another factor associated with pressure injury formation is elevated temperature, especially in older adults, possibly caused by increased oxygen demands in anoxic tissue (Coleman et al., 2013).

The formation of a pressure injury is a complex process involving many variables within the nurse's control (e.g., pressure, shearing, and moisture), as well as variables out of the nurse's control (e.g., malnutrition, low blood pressure, and paralysis). The principal mechanisms of injury are loss of microcirculation through pressure compressing the microvessels or intrinsic factors causing soft tissue to become more vulnerable to lost blood supply.

Risk Assessment Tools

The success of pressure injury prevention depends on early identification of at-risk patients. As recommended by the AHRQ clinical guidelines, a valid, research-based assessment tool should be used. For consistency and accuracy to be established, there should be written protocols specifying how to use the risk assessment tool, when to use it, and which health care team members should use it. A risk assessment should be conducted on all individuals who are bedbound, chairbound, incontinent, frail, disabled, or nutritionally compromised, or who have demonstrated altered mental status (AHRQ, 2014). An assessment should be conducted on patients admitted to an acute care facility, rehabilitation hospital, nursing facility, home care agency, or other health care facility. Identified high-risk individuals should be reassessed at regular intervals if mobility or activity is impaired. The risk assessment should be repeated and the care plan modified accordingly whenever a patient's condition changes. Examples of these changes include decreased mobility, eating less, a change in the serum albumin level or other abnormal laboratory findings, and mentation changes.

Numerous instruments have been designed to identify patients at risk for pressure injury formation. However, many tools have not been subjected to vigorous evaluation of reliability and validity testing. The Braden and Norton risk assessment tools, according to AHRQ clinical guidelines, have undergone the most extensive evaluations.

The Norton Risk Assessment Scale was the first such tool designed for use in a study investigating geriatric nursing problems in hospitals. Consequently, it has set the stage for more comprehensive assessment tools. The study began in the late 1950s, but results were not disseminated until a conference in 1962. At that time, it was believed that pressure injuries were the result of poor nursing care; however, additional research has revealed the problem to be much more complex. The Norton scale is simple to use and has only five assessment categories. Although the original research assessed nutritional status, it was not included in the scale because it was believed that the patient's general health reflected nutritional status. Norton (1989) indicates that nutritional status, including eating behaviors, would have been an important parameter to include. Patients with a score of 16 or lower on the Norton scale are at risk for pressure injury development (Fig. 17.13).

The Braden Scale for Predicting Pressure Sore Risk has been shown to be highly reliable when used by registered nurses and is the most rigorously tested risk assessment tool (AHRQ, 2014). The Braden scale assesses sensory perception rather than mental status. Assessing sensory perception is thought to be a more precise risk indicator because impaired sensation prevents an individual from sensing the need to change positions, which, in turn, would decrease pressure intensity (Braden & Bergstrom, 1987). As a rule, a patient scoring below 18 on the Braden scale is at high risk for skin breakdown (Fig. 17.14).

NORTON SCALE

	PHYSICAL CONDITION	MENTAL CONDITION	ACTIVITY	MOBILITY	INCONTINENT	
	Good 4 Fair 3 Poor 2 Very bad 1	Alert 4 Apathetic 3 Confused 2 Stupor 1	Ambulant 4 Walk/help 3 Chairbound 2 Bedrest 1	Full 4 Slightly limited 3 Very limited 2 Immobile 1	Not 4 Occasional 3 Usually/urine 2 Doubly 1	TOTAL SCORE
Name	Date					

Fig. 17.13 Norton risk assessment scale. Total score over 18: low risk; between 14 and 18: medium risk; between 10 and 14: high risk; less than 10: very high risk. (From Norton, D., McLaren, R., Exton-Smith, A. N. [1962]. *An investigation of geriatric nursing problems in the hospital.* Center for Policy on Ageing. Reproduced with permission from the Centre for Policy on Ageing [formerly NCCOP], London, UK.)

Braden Scale
FOR PREDICTING PRESSURE SORE RISK

Patient's Name _____   Evaluator's Name _____   Date of Assessment

SENSORY PERCEPTION Ability to respond meaningfully to pressure-related discomfort	**1. Completely Limited:** Unresponsive (does not moan, flinch, or grasp) to painful stimuli, due to diminished level of consciousness or sedation. OR limited ability to feel pain over most of body surface.	**2. Very Limited:** Responds only to painful stimuli. Cannot communicate discomfort except by moaning or restlessness. OR has a sensory impairment which limits the ability to feel pain or discomfort over 1/2 of body.	**3. Slightly Limited:** Responds to verbal commands, but cannot always communicate discomfort or need to be turned. OR has some sensory impairment which limits ability to feel pain or discomfort in 1 or 2 extremities.	**4. No Impairment:** Responds to verbal commands. Has no sensory deficit which would limit ability to feel or voice pain or discomfort.
MOISTURE Degree to which skin is exposed to moisture	**1. Constantly Moist:** Skin is kept moist almost constantly by perspiration, urine, etc. Dampness is detected every time patient is moved or turned.	**2. Very Moist:** Skin is often, but not always moist. Linen must be changed at least once a shift.	**3. Occasionally Moist:** Skin is occasionally moist, requiring an extra linen change approximately once a day.	**4. Rarely Moist:** Skin is usually dry, linen only requires changing at routine intervals.
ACTIVITY Degree of physical activity	**1. Bedfast:** Confined to bed	**2. Chairfast:** Ability to walk severely limited or non-existent. Cannot bear own weight and/or must be assisted into chair or wheelchair.	**3. Walks Occasionally:** Walks occasionally during day, but for very short distances, with or without assistance. Spends majority of each shift in bed or chair.	**4. Walks Frequently:** walks outside the room at least twice a day and inside room at least once every 2 hours during waking hours.
MOBILITY Ability to change and control body position	**1. Completely Immobile:** Does not make even slight changes in body or extremity position without assistance.	**2. Very Limited:** Makes occasional slight changes in body or extremity position but unable to make frequent or significant changes independently.	**3. Slightly Limited:** Makes frequent though slight changes in body or extremity position independently.	**4. No Limitations:** Makes major and frequent changes in position without assistance.
NUTRITION Usual food intake pattern	**1. Very Poor:** Never eats a complete meal. Rarely eats more than 1/3 of any food offered. Eats 2 servings or less of protein (meat or dairy products) per day. Takes fluids poorly. Does not take a liquid dietary supplement. OR is NPO and/or maintained on clear liquids or IV's for more than 5 days.	**2. Probably Inadequate:** Rarely eats a complete meal and generally eats only about 1/2 of any food offered. Protein intake includes only 3 servings of meat or dairy products per day. Occasionally will take a dietary supplement. OR receives less than optimum amount of liquid diet or tube feeding.	**3. Adequate:** Eats over half of most meals. Eats a total of 4 servings of protein (meat, dairy products) each day. Occasionally will refuse a meal, but will usually take a supplement if offered. OR is on a tube feeding or TPN regimen that probably meets most of nutritional needs.	**4. Excellent:** Eats most of every meal. Never refuses a meal. Usually eats a total of 4 or more servings of meat and dairy products. Occasionally eats between meals. Does not require supplementation.
FRICTION AND SHEAR	**1. Problem:** Requires moderate to maximum assistance in moving. Complete lifting without sliding against sheets is impossible. Frequently slides down in bed or chair, requiring frequent repositioning with maximum assistance. Spasticity, contractures or agitation leads to almost constant friction.	**2. Potential Problem:** Moves feebly or requires minimum assistance. During a move skin probably slides to some extent against sheets, chair, restraints, or other devices. Maintains relatively good position in chair or bed most of the time but occasionally slides down.	**3. No Apparent Problem:** Moves in bed and in chair independently and has sufficient muscle strength to lift up completely during move. Maintains good position in bed or chair at all times.	

Key: at risk, 15-18; Moderate risk, 13-14; High risk, 10-12; Severe risk, 9.   Total Score

Fig. 17.14 The Braden Scale for Predicting Pressure Sore Risk. *IVs,* Intravenous feedings; *NPO,* nothing by mouth; *TPN,* total parenteral nutrition. (Copyright by Barbara Braden and Nancy Bergstrom, 1998. All rights reserved. Printed with permission.)

EVIDENCE-BASED PRACTICE

Critical Care Nurse Knowledge Related to Prevention and Staging of Pressure Injuries

Background

Pressure injuries in critical care are a continued challenge, often resulting from pressure, shearing forces, and bony prominences in susceptible individuals.

Sample/Setting

The sample encompassed 32 registered nurses (RNs) employed in medical intensive care/coronary care or surgical intensive care units at Veterans Affairs hospitals in the Midwestern United States.

Methods

Following a 2-year educational initiative, nurses on two critical care units were asked to complete the 72-item Pieper-Zulkowski Pressure Ulcer Knowledge Test (PZ-PUKT). The PZ-PUKT measures knowledge concerning wound descriptions, prevention/risk assessment, and staging. The test is true/false.

Findings

The mean age of participants was 44.8 years, and they were predominantly female. Overall mean subscale score for items focusing on pressure injury staging was 81%. The overall mean score for the prevention subscale was 70%. The cumulative mean score for all scales was 72%. Participants with 5 to 10 years' experience scored higher than those with 20 years or more experience, although this was not statistically significant.

Implications

Pressure injury knowledge was assessed in a small cohort of critical care nurses practicing in the Midwestern United States. Nurses participating in the study scored higher in pressure ulcer staging compared with pressure ulcer risk assessment and prevention. This study highlights the need for continued education to reduce gaps in nursing knowledge throughout a nurse's career.

From Miller, D. M., Neelon, L., Kish-Smith, K., Whitney, L., & Burant, C. J. (2017). Pressure injury knowledge in critical care nurses. *Journal of Wound, Ostomy, and Continence Nurses, 44*(5), 455-457. doi:0 10.1097/WON.0000000000000350.

Preventive Strategies

Prevention is the first line of defense against pressure injuries, which are costly health care problems that adversely affect a patient's quality of life. The professional nurse has a responsibility to identify patients at risk for pressure injuries and to implement research-based preventive strategies. Nurses as front-line providers and managers of care are key health care team members who can influence the prevalence of pressure injuries and enhance the patient's quality of life. Nurses should mobilize the health care team when needs are identified by seeking a dietary consultation and alerting the health care provider when a patient is not eating sufficiently or when a patient develops nonblanchable erythema. Written preventive protocols endorsed (and embraced) by the health care team and institution empower the professional nurse to act independently and immediately when vulnerable patients are identified.

All at-risk individuals identified through use of a risk assessment tool should have a daily skin inspection with close attention to bony prominences as recommended by AHRQ clinical guidelines. The NPUAP guidelines also recommend assessment for localized heat, edema, or induration. These signs are recommended as warning signs of pressure injury development on darkly pigmented skin because redness is not always possible to see. This routine assessment should be documented to demonstrate professional accountability and so that preventive strategy outcomes can be evaluated. Another skin-related activity recommended by AHRQ clinical guidelines is to cleanse the skin of a patient with incontinence with a mild, nonirritating cleanser using warm—not hot—water at the time of soiling to minimize skin irritation and dryness. Moisturizers such as emollient lotions should be used to keep the skin from drying and cracking. It is best to apply the lotion immediately after bathing to increase the moisture absorbed by the skin. Skin should not be rubbed or massaged over bony prominences because it may cause further deep tissue damage, especially if erythema is present (which already indicates injury) (AHRQ, 2014; NPUAP, 2014).

Proper turning and placement reduce the effects of pressure but not the intensity. It has been standard practice to turn patients a minimum of every 2 hours, which was endorsed in the AHRQ clinical guidelines. However, capillary closing pressure varies with each individual; therefore the ideal strategy is to determine the turning schedule based on development of erythema, which may precede ischemia. Currently, there is no strong evidence to support a 30-degree oblique angle versus side-lying 90-degree angle to prevent pressure injury (Gillespie et al., 2014) (Fig. 17.15). To decrease pressure intensity on the heels, a patient should have a pillow or pillows under the calves to lift the feet and heels off the bed. Commercial devices also exist to suspend the heel, maintain or correct foot-ankle position, and protect the patient from neurosensory damage.

At-risk individuals should be placed on a pressure-reducing device in hopes of preventing the development of a pressure injury by decreasing pressure intensity. Pressure-reducing support surfaces such as mattress overlays, chair cushions or overlays, and specialized beds redistribute weight over a larger area and reduce tissue-interface pressure. Tissue-interface pressure is the amount of pressure between the skin and resting surface

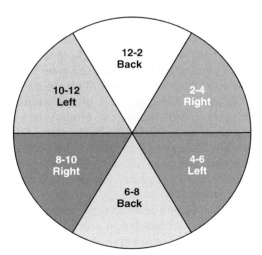

Fig. 17.15 Turning schedule for pressure injury prevention and treatment. (From Bryant, R., & Nix, D. [2016]. *Acute and chronic wounds: Current management concepts* [5th ed.]. St. Louis, MO: Elsevier.)

(e.g., mattress). It has been thought that if the tissue-interface pressure is 32 mm Hg or lower, capillary closure will not occur. However, this logic may be questioned because capillary closing pressures vary from one individual to another.

Mattress overlays reduce pressure, are usually economical with only a one-time charge, and are accessible in most environments. Overlays may be static (e.g., foam, gel, water, air, and low air loss) or dynamic (e.g., alternating air). Because the overlays are placed on top of a mattress, the height of the bed is increased, making it more difficult for patients to get in and out of the bed, which is a common patient and nurse complaint. The overlay may also decrease the protective height of bedside rails because the effective mattress height has increased. Some mattress overlays trap moisture and heat, which may be uncomfortable. Foam overlays should have a base height of at least 4 inches from the bottom to the *beginning* of the convolutions, not to the peak, and a stiffness of 25% of indentation load deflection (AHRQ, 2014). Foam overlays must also be examined regularly to assess for continued effectiveness (i.e., no obvious sagging) because their use is limited. Static air and water overlays must be checked regularly for proper inflation and must be cleaned periodically.

Specialty beds such as air-fluidized beds or low-air loss beds are generally used for individuals who have multiple stage III and IV pressure injuries or who are at high risk after posterior grafts or flap procedures. These beds may, in fact, overheat a patient and may elevate the body temperature if not adequately controlled. Multiple hybrids of the air-fluidized and low-air loss beds exist, which enables the nurse to better match beds with patient needs. Specialty beds do not eliminate the need for meticulous nursing care. Patients must still be repositioned, assessed, and kept clean and dry.

The presence of skin moisture (whether the result of incontinence of urine or feces, perspiration, or wound exudate) should be minimized. If necessary, absorbent undergarments may be used to maintain a dryer skin surface. However, it is important to check these absorbent pads or undergarments frequently to determine whether new products are needed after significant wetting or any soiling. Topical barriers such as zinc oxide may be applied after cleansing and gently drying the skin (AHRQ, 2014). Indwelling Foley catheters should be used only on a short-term basis or avoided, if possible, because of the risk of urinary tract infections. Thought must be given to the reason for a catheter and whether the benefit of placement outweighs the risk of infection. Although most orders are for turning and repositioning every 2 hours, the primary care provider may need to be contacted to implement consistent scheduled checks before the 2-hour intervals. With implementation of regular checks to keep skin clean and dry and the use of absorbent pads and topical barriers, catheter placement can be avoided, thus reducing patient risk.

Skin injury from friction or shearing forces can be avoided by using proper turning techniques and proper placement. Using proper transfer techniques and a draw sheet can prevent friction injuries. Lubricants, topical barrier creams, film or hydrocolloid dressings, or protective padding may be used to reduce damage when skin moves across a coarse or hard surface. Shearing results when the body shifts and slides downward; therefore most shearing injuries can be eliminated with proper placement. For example, not elevating the head of the bed greater than 30 degrees and elevating the knees slightly when the head is elevated prevent slipping down in bed. When the patient is sitting in a chair, placing the feet on a stool prevents sliding downward (AHRQ, 2014).

Nutritional status must be closely monitored by assessing food intake, weight, muscle mass, subcutaneous fat stores, localized or generalized fluid accumulation, and hand grip strength (Marcason, 2017). Accurate food intake should be monitored routinely to identify both the need for changes before a compromised state develops and nutritionally at-risk patients. Hydration status is another important nutritional component because dehydration may contribute to development of a pressure injury. An older adult should drink 8 glasses of water a day, unless contraindicated such as in HF or kidney failure. The use of an air-fluidized or low–air loss bed increases daily fluid needs because insensible loss is increased. When the professional nurse recognizes a pattern of decreased food or water intake, a full assessment addressing food preferences, dentition, and swallowing difficulties is warranted. The patient should also be evaluated for constipation or fecal impaction, which decreases appetite. A more comprehensive nutritional assessment may be necessary, which may include a registered dietician consultation, occupational therapy, and a dental appointment; nutritional supplements may be needed. A person's weight typically changes slowly; therefore weighing the patient monthly is sufficient and is needed more frequently only when assessing cardiovascular status. A weight loss of 5% to 10% is significant; weight loss is associated with an increased risk of mortality (Stajkovic, Aitken, & Holroyd-Leduc, 2011).

In 2009, the Academy of Nutrition and Dietetics and the American Society of Parenteral and Enteral Nutrition collaborated to identify characteristics of malnutrition in adults. Serum proteins are no longer considered indicators of malnutrition in adults, as the evidence "shows that serum levels of these proteins do not change in response to changes in nutrient intake" (Marcason, 2017, p. 1144). The consensus panel identified the following criteria for the diagnosis of malnutrition in adults; for the diagnosis to be made, the individual must show at least two of the following (Marcason, 2017):

- Insufficient energy intake
- Weight loss
- Loss of muscle mass
- Loss of subcutaneous fat
- Localized or generalized fluid accumulation that may sometimes mask weight loss
- Diminished functional status as measured by hand grip strength

Because of multiple risk factors and their synergistic effect on pressure injury development, prevention is a nursing challenge, offering an opportunity to demonstrate the effect of nursing by recognizing at-risk patients, immediately implementing preventive strategies, and preventing a costly health care problem. Most of all, preventive measures promote high-quality patient care, which is the primary goal of nursing.

Pressure Injury Management

Nurses play a key role in pressure injury management because they are the professionals responsible for wound care and often the first team members to identify wound changes. In addition, physicians perceive the nurse, especially in long-term care, as an expert in pressure injury management. It is not uncommon for physicians to say, "Do whatever treatment you think is best." Often, the health care provider, when assessing medical management, asks the nurse to describe and evaluate the treatment. Therefore it is important for the nurse to comprehend the healing process, to understand treatment strategies, and to maintain a current knowledge base. The following discussion reviews the healing trajectory and treatment options, which include nutritional management. It is hoped that the professional nurse will become empowered, promote a positive image for nursing, and, most important, be able to deliver more successful patient care by comprehending the physiology of the healing process and the logic for treatment strategies.

Physiology of Wound Healing

An understanding of the healing process is necessary for critically analyzing pressure injury care and determining the best management strategy. Pressure injury research has expanded our understanding of the etiology of pressure injuries and the healing process. The three major stages of wound healing are (1) the inflammatory stage; (2) the proliferative, or granulation, stage; and (3) the maturation, or matrix formation, stage.

The *inflammatory stage,* characterized by redness, heat, pain, and swelling, lasts approximately 4 to 5 days. The inflammatory stage initiates the healing process by stabilizing the wound through platelet activity that stops bleeding and triggers the immune system. Neutrophils, monocytes, and macrophages arrive within 24 hours of the insult to control bacteria, remove dead tissue, and secrete angiogenesis factor (AGF) and other growth factors, which stimulate the development of granulation tissue. Bradykinin and histamine, released from injured cells, cause vasodilation, which leads to swelling. This creates the red, swollen, tender, clinical presentation often seen in wounds (Mercandetti, 2017). The inflammatory stage is crucial for successful healing, and a delayed or altered response may possibly contribute to the development of chronic, stagnant wounds if appropriate growth factors and responses were not mobilized when the patient was first injured. Medications (e.g., steroids), decreased tissue oxygenation, poor nutritional status, and age-related changes (e.g., decreased response of the immune system) may impede this stage.

The *proliferative,* or *granulation, stage* begins 24 hours after injury and continues for up to 22 days. Three significant events occur: (1) epithelialization, (2) granulation, and (3) collagen synthesis. Epithelialization, via a microscopic epithelial layer, seals and protects the wound from bacteria and fluid loss. This microscopic layer, which is fostered by a moist environment, is extremely fragile and may easily be washed away with aggressive wound irrigation or harsh wiping of the involved area. *Granulation,* also known as *neovascularization,* is the formation of new capillaries that generate and feed new tissue, creating a beefy-red tissue bed that bleeds easily. Collagen synthesis creates a support matrix that provides strength to the new tissue. Oxygen, iron, vitamin C, zinc, magnesium, and amino acids are necessary for collagen synthesis. Fibroblasts, stimulated in the first phase by AGF, are necessary for collagen production. This phase rebuilds the injured area and can easily be influenced by the effectiveness of the inflammation stage and wound environment.

The *maturation stage,* also known as the *differentiation* or *remodeling phase,* is the final stage. It does not begin until 21 days after injury and may take years to Heal. During this stage, maximum tensile strength is generated through collagen deposits that make the wound thicker and more compact. These collagen deposits contract until closure is attained. Initially, the scarred area is a dark, scarlet red that fades over time to a silvery white. Tensile strength reaches only 80% of preinjury capacity, therefore the "scarred" area is more vulnerable to breakdown or injury (Mercandetti, 2017).

Definition of Terms and Staging Criteria

A *pressure injury* is localized damage to the skin and underlying soft tissue usually over a bony prominence or related to a medical or other device. The injury can present as intact skin or an open ulcer and may be painful. The injury occurs as a result of intense and/or prolonged pressure or pressure in combination with shear. The tolerance of soft tissue for pressure and shear may also be affected by microclimate, nutrition, perfusion, comorbidities, and condition of the soft tissue (Box 17.2; NPUAP, 2016). Box 17.3 provides more definitions of relevant terms.

Basic Principles of Pressure Injury Management

Three basic principles guide successful pressure injury management:
1. Eliminate or minimize precipitating factors such as pressure, friction, shearing, and poor nutrition.
2. Provide nutritional support and monitor nutritional status.
3. Create and maintain a clean, moist wound environment with adequate circulation and oxygenation.

Pressure injury preventive strategies must be implemented, or wound care efforts are futile (Box 17.4). Through institutional policy and protocol, the nurse should apply an appropriate mattress overlay. The nurse ensures that all staff members use proper technique when repositioning a patient to minimize shearing and friction forces. As leader of the care team, the nurse is responsible for observing nursing aides and other support team members who deliver hands-on care to identify specific learning needs so that pressure, shearing, and friction are minimized. Teaching the logic for such techniques may motivate staff members to exercise more diligence in performing proper preventive actions. The nurse must rely on teaching principles such as repetition of key information in a nonthreatening manner. They should reinforce appropriate activity with positive feedback.

Nutritional status should be monitored; specifically, the health care provider should monitor weight and food consumption so that needs can be identified immediately. This also

BOX 17.2 Staging Criteria

Deep Tissue Pressure Injury: Persistent Nonblanchable Deep Red, Maroon, or Purple Discoloration

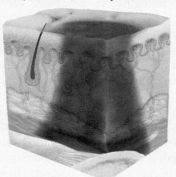

Intact or nonintact skin with localized area of persistent nonblanchable deep red, maroon, or purple discoloration, or epidermal separation revealing a dark wound bed or blood-filled blister. Pain and temperature change often precede skin color changes. Discoloration may appear differently in darkly pigmented skin. This injury results from intense and/or prolonged pressure and shear forces at the bone–muscle interface. The wound may evolve rapidly to reveal the actual extent of tissue injury or may resolve without tissue loss. If necrotic tissue, subcutaneous tissue, granulation tissue, fascia, muscle or other underlying structures are visible, this indicates a full thickness pressure injury (Unstageable, Stage 3, or Stage 4). Do not use DTPI to describe vascular, traumatic, neuropathic, or dermatologic conditions.

Stage 1: Nonblanchable Erythema of Intact Skin

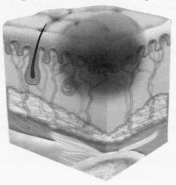

Intact skin with a localized area of nonblanchable erythema, which may appear differently in darkly pigmented skin. Presence of blanchable erythema or changes in sensation, temperature, or firmness may precede visual changes. Color changes do not include purple or maroon discoloration; these may indicate deep tissue pressure injury.

Stage 2: Partial-Thickness Skin Loss With Exposed Dermis

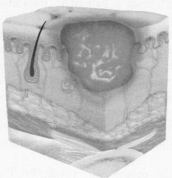

Partial-thickness loss of skin with exposed dermis. The wound bed is viable, pink or red, moist, and may also present as an intact or ruptured serum-filled blister. Adipose

(fat) is not visible, and deeper tissues are not visible. Granulation tissue, slough, and eschar are not present. These injuries commonly result from adverse microclimate and shear in the skin over the pelvis and shear in the heel. This stage should not be used to describe moisture associated skin damage (MASD) including incontinence associated dermatitis (IAD), intertriginous dermatitis (ITD), medical adhesive related skin injury (MARSI), or traumatic wounds (skin tears, burns, abrasions).

Stage 3: Full-Thickness Skin Loss

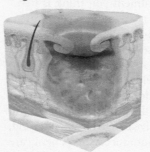

Full-thickness loss of skin, in which adipose (fat) is visible in the ulcer and granulation tissue and epibole (rolled wound edges) are often present. Slough and/or eschar may be visible. The depth of tissue damage varies by anatomic location; areas of significant adiposity can develop deep wounds. Undermining and tunneling may occur. Fascia, muscle, tendon, ligament, cartilage, and/or bone are not exposed. If slough or eschar obscures the extent of tissue loss, this is an Unstageable Pressure Injury.

Stage 4: Full-Thickness Skin and Tissue Loss

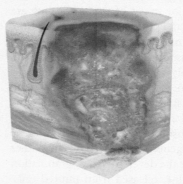

Full-thickness skin and tissue loss with exposed or directly palpable fascia, muscle, tendon, ligament, cartilage, or bone in the ulcer. Slough and/or eschar may be visible. Epibole (rolled edges), undermining, and/or tunneling often occur. Depth varies by anatomic location. If slough or eschar obscures the extent of tissue loss, this is an Unstageable Pressure Injury.

Unstageable Pressure Injury: Obscured Full-Thickness Skin and Tissue Loss

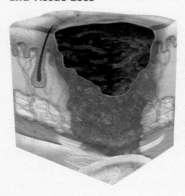

Continued

BOX 17.2 Staging Criteria—cont'd

Full-thickness skin and tissue loss in which the extent of tissue damage within the ulcer cannot be confirmed because it is obscured by slough or eschar. If slough or eschar is removed, a Stage 3 or Stage 4 pressure injury will be revealed.

Stable eschar (i.e., dry, adherent, intact without erythema or fluctuance) on the heel or ischemic limb should not be softened or removed.

From the National Pressure Ulcer Advisory Panel (2016). Reprinted with permission. Reproduction of the National Pressure Ulcer Advisory Panel (NPUAP) materials in this document does not imply endorsement by the NPUAP of any products, organizations, companies, or any statements made by any organization or company.

BOX 17.3 Definitions of Terms

Autolysis: Self-debridement of necrotic tissue by white blood cells, which is fostered by a dressing that retains moisture (e.g., transparent film); a yellowish-brown fluid is generated from the white blood cells and breakdown of tissue

Debridement: Removal of dead, damaged tissue

Epithelialization: Growth of a microscopic layer that covers an open wound, which creates a barrier that protects from fluid loss and bacterial assault and that is highly fragile and easily destroyed

Eschar: Thick, necrotic, devitalized tissue; often black but may be yellowish

Exudate: Wound discharge that may be serosanguineous, serous, or purulent

Friction: Rubbing of skin against another surface (e.g., sheets, bed, or chair)

Granulation tissue: New capillary growth that creates a beefy-red color and tissue that bleeds easily (friable)

Interface pressure: Force exerted between body and support surface (e.g., mattress)

Pressure injury: Lesion caused by unrelieved pressure that causes tissue damage and death; usually occurs over bony prominences or other pressure points (e.g., tubing, foreign material in bed)

Reactive hyperemia: Transient, blanching erythema from tissue anoxia, which generates a compensatory mechanism resulting in dilated vessels

Shearing force: Sliding of parallel surfaces when skeletal frame and deep fascia slide downward; the superficial fascia remains attached to the dermis, thus stretching or occluding the arterial supply to fascia and muscle, which may lead to tissue anoxia and damage; most common position for this occurrence is when the head of the bed is elevated and the body slides downward

Sinus tract: Vertical tunnel connecting one anatomic compartment with another

Tissue tolerance: The skin's (i.e., blood vessels, interstitial fluid, collagen, and other structures) ability to endure the effects of pressure without adverse consequences

Undermining: Separation of tissue under the dermis creating a horizontal tunnel; length can be measured by inserting a cotton-tipped applicator into the tunnel, marking length on applicator, and then placing next to a tape measure

Modified from Bryant, R. A., Shannon, M. L., Pieper, B., et al. (1992). Pressure ulcers. In R. A. Bryant (Ed.), *Acute and chronic wounds: Nursing management.* St. Louis, MO: Mosby; Agency for Health Care Policy and Research. (1992). *Pressure ulcers in adults: Prediction and prevention,* Clinical Practice Guideline No 3, Rockville, MD: U.S. Department of Health and Human Services; Sanders, S. L. (1992). Pressure ulcers, part II: Management strategies. *Journal of the American Academy of Nurse Practitioners, 4*(3), 101.

BOX 17.4 Pressure Injury Prevention Strategies

Risk Assessment

1. Consider bedfast and chairfast individuals to be at risk for development of pressure injury.
2. Use a structured risk assessment, such as the Braden Scale, to identify individuals at risk for pressure injury as soon as possible (but within 8 hours after admission).
3. Refine the assessment by including these additional risk factors:
   a. Fragile skin
   b. Existing pressure injury of any stage, including those ulcers that have healed or are closed
   c. Impairments in blood flow to the extremities from vascular disease, diabetes or tobacco use
   d. Pain in areas of the body exposed to pressure
4. Repeat the risk assessment at regular intervals and with any change in condition. Base the frequency of regular assessments on acuity levels:
   a. Acute care . . . . Every shift
   b. Long term care . . . . Weekly for 4 weeks, then quarterly
   c. Home care . . . . At every nurse visit
5. Develop a plan of care based on the areas of risk, rather than on the total risk assessment score. For example, if the risk stems from immobility, address turning, repositioning, and the support surface. If the risk is from malnutrition, address those problems.

Skin Care

1. Inspect all of the skin upon admission as soon as possible (but within 8 hours).
2. Inspect the skin at least daily for signs of pressure injury, especially non-blanchable erythema.

3. Assess pressure points, such as the sacrum, coccyx, buttocks, heels, ischium, trochanters, elbows, and beneath medical devices.
4. When inspecting darkly pigmented skin, look for changes in skin tone, skin temperature and tissue consistency compared with adjacent skin. Moistening the skin assists in identifying changes in color.
5. Cleanse the skin promptly after episodes of incontinence.
6. Use skin cleansers that are pH balanced for the skin.
7. Use skin moisturizers daily on dry skin.
8. Avoid positioning an individual on an area of erythema or pressure injury.

Nutrition

1. Consider hospitalized individuals to be at risk for under nutrition and malnutrition from their illness or being NPO for diagnostic testing.
2. Use a valid and reliable screening tool to determine risk of malnutrition, such as the Mini Nutritional Assessment.
3. Refer all individuals at risk for pressure injury from malnutrition to a registered dietitian/nutritionist.
4. Assist the individual at mealtimes to increase oral intake.
5. Encourage all individuals at risk for pressure injury to consume adequate fluids and a balanced diet.
6. Assess weight changes over time.
7. Assess the adequacy of oral, enteral, and parenteral intake.
8. Provide nutritional supplements between meals and with oral medications, unless contraindicated.

Continued

BOX 17.4   Pressure Injury Prevention Strategies—cont'd

Repositioning and Mobilization

1. Turn and reposition all individuals at risk for pressure injury, unless contra-indicated due to medical condition or medical treatments.
2. Choose a frequency for turning based on the support surface in use, the tolerance of skin for pressure and the individual's preferences.
3. Consider lengthening the turning schedule during the night to allow for uninterrupted sleep.
4. Turn the individual into a 30-degree side lying position, and use your hand to determine whether the sacrum is off the bed
5. Avoid positioning the individual on body areas with pressure injury.
6. Ensure that the heels are free from the bed.
7. Consider the level of immobility, exposure to shear, skin moisture, perfusion, body size and weight of the individual when choosing a support surface.
8. Continue to reposition an individual when placed on any support surface.

9. Use a breathable incontinence pad when using microclimate management surfaces.
10. Use a pressure-redistributing chair cushion for individuals sitting in chairs or wheelchairs.
11. Reposition weak or immobile individuals in chairs hourly.
12. If the individual cannot be moved or is positioned with the head of the bed elevated over 30 degrees, place a polyurethane foam dressing on the sacrum.
13. Use heel-offloading devices or polyurethane foam dressings on individuals at high risk for heel ulcers
14. Place thin foam or breathable dressings under medical devices.

Education

1. Teach the individual and family about risk for pressure injury.
2. Engage individual and family in risk reduction interventions.

From National Pressure Ulcer Advisory Panel. (2016). *Pressure injury prevention points.* Retrieved from http://www.npuap.org/resources/educational-and-clinical-resources/pressure-injury-prevention-points/.

---

promotes a collaborative effort among health care providers. When food intake is first noted to decrease, the nurse should identify reasons, such as not meeting food preferences, sore mouth, the patient being rushed to eat, conflict with staff, depression, or pain.

For closure of the wound, a clean, moist environment must be created and maintained. This principle is the key to successful healing and should guide the professional nurse and practitioner. Consequently, necrotic tissue must be removed and any infectious process (as evidenced by erythema, induration, and tenderness in the periwound skin; pus; or a pale wound bed) resolved to implement a dressing strategy that fosters rapid epithelialization and granulation.

It is important to know when to culture a wound because of the expense to the patient and the health care system. Also, inappropriate antibiotic use is decreased when wounds are cultured appropriately. All wounds are contaminated; therefore all cultures grow surface bacteria, and the true pathogen may not be identified. A culture is warranted only when cellulitis (e.g., erythema, induration, and tenderness) or a wound infection (evidenced by a pale wound bed, pus, increased tenderness, persistent exudate, or no new growth) exists. An accurate culture includes both anaerobic and aerobic species. To obtain the culture, the nurse should use the most accurate method, considered the gold standard for wound cultures, which is deep-tissue or punch biopsy (Spear, 2014). According to the AHRQ treatment guidelines, an ulcer is *not* to be cultured with the use of a culturette because colonized bacteria may be obtained instead of the offending pathogen. The NPUAP treatment guidelines recommend obtaining a tissue biopsy or quantitative swab technique (10-point swab culture). An infected wound is managed topically with antiseptics, or systemically, depending on the severity and risk of osteomyelitis.

NPUAP guidelines recommend the use of nontoxic topical antiseptics for a limited time to control bacterial colonization. The following antiseptics are commonly used (NPUAP, 2014):

- iodine compounds (povidone iodine and slow-release cadexomer iodine)
- silver compounds (including silver sulfadiazine)
- polyhexanide and betaine (PHMB)
- chlorhexidine
- sodium hypochlorite
- acetic acid

Antiseptic solutions are used with wet-to-dry dressings, which also provide some mechanical debridement. At times, a wound may be irrigated with the antiseptic; however, a rinse with normal saline should follow. If the nurse notices that antiseptic use has continued for longer than 1 week, a reminder or question should be posed to the health care provider.

The first step in pressure injury care is to thoroughly assess the wound to determine the most effective strategy and dressing. The nurse is usually the first person to identify a need for change; therefore this assessment should be an ongoing process. The nurse should examine the wound, noting its color; any discharge, bleeding, or odor; degree of undermining or presence of a sinus tract (may be measured using a cotton-tipped applicator); any necrotic tissue; pain or tenderness; and amount of erythema surrounding the wound edges. Limited erythema around the wound is a normal phenomenon that signifies increased circulation to provide nutrients; however, if the erythema extends, infection or candidiasis should be suspected, and the wound closely monitored. Ideally, the wound base should be a beefy-red color, which is indicative of granulation. However, some hydrogel and hydrocolloid dressings generate a pale pink wound bed, which ordinarily would mean an "ill" wound bed. If the bed is pale pink and not associated with a purulent discharge or cellulitis, the wound environment is most likely clean and should just be observed. Note that granulation tissue has a rich capillary supply and bleeds easily and profusely when disturbed (e.g., when it is irrigated or during a dressing change). Thus if a tunneling wound bleeds, it can be deduced that granulation tissue exists, although it is not visible because of the tunneling.

Patient name _____ Patient ID# _____
Ulcer location _____ Date _____

Begin paragraph as:
Directions: Observe and measure the pressure ulcer. Categorize the ulcer with respect to surface area, exudate, and type of wound tissue. Record a subscore for each of these ulcer characteristics. Add the subscores to obtain the total score. A comparison of total scores measured over time provides an indication of the improvement or deterioration in pressure ulcer healing.

Length × width	0 0 cm²	1 <0.3 cm²	2 0.3–0.6 cm²	3 0.7–1.0 cm²	4 1.1–2.0 cm²	5 2.1–3.0 cm²	Subscore
		6 3.1–4.0 cm²	7 4.1–8.0 cm²	8 8.1–12.0 cm²	9 12.1–24.0 cm²	10 >24.0 cm²	
Exudate amount	0 None	1 Light	2 Moderate	3 Heavy			Subscore
Tissue type	0 Closed	1 Epithelial tissue	2 Granulation tissue	3 Slough	4 Necrotic tissue		Subscore
							Total score

Length × Width: Measure the greatest length (head to toe) and the greatest width (side to side) using a centimeter ruler. Multiply these two measurements (length × width) to obtain an estimate of surface area in square centimeters (cm²). *Caveat:* Do not guess! Always use a centimeter ruler and always use the same method each time the ulcer is measured.

Exudate Amount: Estimate the amount of exudate (drainage) present after removal of the dressing and before applying any topical agent to the ulcer. Estimate the exudate (drainage) as none, light, moderate, or heavy.

Tissue Type: This refers to the types of tissue that are present in the wound (ulcer) bed. Score as a "4" if there is any necrotic tissue present. Score as a "3" if there is any amount of slough present and necrotic tissue is absent. Score as a "2" if the wound is clean and contains granulation tissue. A superficial wound that is reepithelializing is scored as a "1." When the wound is closed, score as a "0."

    4   **Necrotic tissue (eschar):** black, brown, or tan tissue that adheres firmly to the wound bed or ulcer edges and may be either firmer or softer than surrounding skin
    3   **Slough:** yellow or white tissue that adheres to the ulcer bed in strings or thick clumps, or is mucinous
    2   **Granulation tissue:** pink or beefy red tissue with a shiny, moist, granular appearance
    1   **Epithelial tissue:** for superficial ulcers, new pink or shiny tissue (skin) that grows in from the edges or as islands on the ulcer surface
    0   **Closed/resurfaced:** the wound is completely covered with epithelium (new skin)

Directions: Observe and measure the pressure ulcers at regular intervals using the PUSH Tool. Date and record PUSH subscale and total scores on the Pressure Ulcer Healing Record below.

Pressure Ulcer Healing Record														
Date														
Length × width														
Exudate amount														
Tissue type														
Total score														

Version 3.0: 9/15/98
© National Pressure Ulcer Advisory Panel

Fig. 17.16 The Pressure Ulcer Scale for Healing (PUSH) Tool. (From National Pressure Ulcer Advisory Panel. [1998]. Pressure Ulcer Scale for Healing [PUSH]: PUSH Tool 3.0. Retrieved from http://www.npuap.org/resources/educational-and-clinical-resources/push-tool/.)

The wound assessment should be ongoing and supported with documentation (Fig. 17.16). All new wounds should be described, including location, color, discharge, tenderness, amount of necrotic tissue or undermining, dimensions, and stage. The wound measurements should include length, width, and depth. When measuring undermining, the nurse should use a cotton-tipped applicator, marking depth on the applicator and placing it next to a tape measure to obtain dimension and to note position (e.g., 4 cm at 2 o'clock). It is not imperative that all dimensions or locations of undermining be documented. The nurse should record only the greatest length because the wound cannot be deemed healed until closed. It is recommended that facilities develop a written procedure stating how dimensions should be obtained and documented (e.g., length by width by depth and undermining) to establish continuity and minimize confusion regarding the procedure.

Debridement

Necrotic tissue provides the ideal environment for bacteria growth, which may cause inflammation and impair the body's ability to fight infection. Therefore necrotic tissue must be debrided as soon as possible, and measures (such as wet-to-dry dressings or topical antimicrobials) should be taken to resolve bacterial insults until purulent discharge has dissipated. If necrotic tissue is not debrided, the nurse's efforts are futile, and the patient's comfort and quality of life are affected.

The removal of dry, hard eschar should be considered because its presence slows the migration of epithelial cells and delays healing, except for stable heel ulcers, in which case dry eschar should be left intact (AHRQ, 2014). At times, this dry eschar may serve as an efficient and comfortable dressing, but the area must be watched for development of infection. If the patient has diabetes or has an ischemic wound with a dry, hard, intact eschar, it may be more prudent to leave the eschar in place. It serves as a barrier and does not place the patient at risk for any possible problems from frequent dressing changes (e.g., infection, skin tears, and candidiasis). However, the eschar and periwound skin must be monitored. If the eschar becomes soft and boggy, tissue liquefaction is most likely accumulating and must be removed. This is especially true if the wound is tender or has periwound erythema, indicating infection.

Various methods of debridement include mechanical, autolytic, enzymatic, conservative sharp, and surgical sharp. Mechanical debridement (continually moist gauze or pulsed lavage) is effective for removing slough that cannot be removed surgically or chemically (because of damage to viable tissue). If mechanical debridement using continually moist gauze dressings is employed, the nurse should protect wound borders from maceration with zinc oxide or stoma adhesive. Using pulsed lavage once or twice daily may mechanically debride and should be reserved for large, exuding wounds; this should be discontinued after the wound is clean or demonstrates stability. Mechanical debridement requires more nursing time, is more uncomfortable for the patient, and may destroy fragile epithelial cells. For these reasons, a more efficient method should be sought first (NPUAP, 2014).

Autolytic debridement is effective for removing eschar and slough when less than 50% of the wound bed is involved and no evidence of infection exists in the periwound skin. Autolytic debridement involves using the body's own enzymes to provide additional debriding and cleansing. Hydrocolloid or hydrogel dressings may soften and facilitate removal of eschar and slough if the wound is not infected. It should be noted that autolysis creates a larger appearing wound because debris is being removed. Autolysis generates a brownish yellow fluid that may have some pus in it because of dead cells and neutrophils. The nurse should not become alarmed unless clinical evidence of infection exists (e.g., erythema, tenderness, heat, and swelling). Autolytic debridement may be used in conjunction with mechanical methods to further shorten the time to wound cleansing.

Enzymatic debridement is costly and time consuming; however, it may be effective on small, necrotic areas or for removing yellow, tender eschar that is difficult to remove surgically. Enzymatic debridement is primarily used in the home setting or nursing facility where appropriately educated or certified professionals are not readily accessible for conservative sharp debridement at the bedside. Enzymatic debridement may save the patient from hospital admission. If used, the enzymatic agent must *not* be applied on healthy, viable tissue because the enzyme will destroy granulation tissue and epithelial cells.

If the wound has a dry, rubbery eschar, conservative sharp debridement is recommended over enzymatic debridement because enzymatic debridement takes much longer. The main principle that guides conservative sharp debridement is to stop when bleeding occurs, which indicates that viable, healthy tissue has been reached. Because the wound is dirty, aseptic technique is appropriate. To prevent "showering" of bacteria from conservative sharp debridement and to assist in cleaning up the wound, nurses should apply wet-to-dry dressings moistened with an acceptable antiseptic every shift for 1 to 3 days, depending on the wound condition.

Surgical sharp debridement is reserved for cases of suspected sepsis, for wounds with tunneling or undermining, if necrotic tissue cannot be removed by other means, or for stage III or IV wounds not healing with conservative treatment.

Wound Care Principles and Dressing Types

The wound care market is a multibillion-dollar business and has created many dressing options. Therefore the nurse must understand the healing trajectory to select the best treatment option. The major goal is to create an environment that supports healing—a clean, moist (hydrated, not wet) wound bed. If no growth is evident in weekly measurements after 2 to 4 weeks, consideration should be given to changing the dressing strategy. Table 17.2 provides a brief overview of commonly used dressing types and general treatment principles.

With each dressing change, all open wounds should be *gently* irrigated with approximately 20 to 50 mL of normal saline with the use of a catheter-tip syringe. After irrigation, the wound can be assessed.

It is prudent to always write the date and time of the dressing change on the outside of the dressing itself. This practice reflects professional accountability and assists in problem solving. For example, a wound may have more discharge or a significant change because the dressing was not changed soon enough or, inadvertently, not changed at all.

If the wound border has candidiasis, evidenced by a fire-red erythema usually with satellite lesions and denuded skin, a zinc oxide–nystatin (50/50) mixture may be applied on affected areas and then the dressing applied. Because candidiasis flourishes in a moist environment, a thorough assessment should be done to identify the reason for excess moisture. Is a moist dressing overlapping the wound edges? Is the film dressing generating so much fluid retention and maceration that candidiasis is occurring? If so, the zinc oxide–nystatin cream could be applied, and the wound monitored. It may be that the dressing type must be changed. After the candidiasis has resolved, a stoma adhesive

TABLE 17.2 Commonly Used Types of Dressings

Advantages	Drawbacks	Contraindications
Gauze		
Allows for mechanical debridement via continually moist gauze dressing method	Requires more frequent dressing changes	Do not use on healthy, granulating wound unless moistened with saline or other noncytotoxic
Protects dry, healing wounds	Requires securing with tape or film	solution; even then fragile epithelial cells may
Serves as filler dressing for dead space	Requires loose packing or it may create pressure and possibly enlarge the wound	be destroyed.
Absorbs exudate	Destroys fragile epithelial cells and slows down healing, especially if gauze dries out	Do not use on dry, necrotic tissue, unless keeping eschar in place for protection
Assists with cleaning up wound; manages exudates		(appropriate only when no signs of infection exist).
Foam Dressings		
Decreases trauma to wound base and fragile epithelial cells because does not adhere to tissue or wound base	Requires securing with tape or film	Not appropriate for mechanical debridement because it does not adhere.
Protects healing wound	Usually requires daily to every-shift dressing changes	Do not use on a healthy, granulating wound unless a topical agent (e.g., bacitracin) is used.
Has minimum to moderate absorption ability, which can prevent or decrease maceration		Do not use on dry, necrotic tissue, unless keeping eschar in place for protection
Insulates wound provides comfort		(appropriate only when no signs of infection exist).
Protects "at risk" tissue		
Transparent Film Dressing		
Retains moisture and is semipermeable and comfortable	May be difficult to apply	Do not use on infected wounds or wounds with cellulitis.
Is water resistant, thus can seal and secure other dressings	May leak	Do not use on thin, friable skin surrounding
Allows easy inspection to monitor for complications	Should not be used over enzymatic debriding agents, gels, or ointments	wound edges that cannot be protected with stoma adhesive (risk of creating other open
Fosters autolysis because of moisture retention		wounds or skin tear).
Minimizes friction injury when applied to vulnerable areas (e.g., elbows, coccyx, heels)		Do not use on exuding wounds.
Hydrocolloid Dressing		
Retains moisture, which facilitates granulation and is comfortable	Melt-out occurs, creating foul odor and possible leakage	Do not use on infected wounds or wounds with cellulitis.
Provides a water and bacteria barrier, which protects wound	Prevents visibly monitoring wound	Do not use on thin, friable skin surrounding wound edges (more damage may be created
Requires less frequent dressing changes, which promotes efficient use of nursing time and comfort to patient	May cause hypergranulation tissue (leafy, friable, beefy-red granulation tissue), which impedes healing and usually requires debridement or	when wafer removed).
Promotes removal of dry necrotic eschar when left in place for several days	removal with sharp instrument or silver nitrate	Do not use on heavy, exuding wounds.
	Is expensive but requires fewer dressing changes	
Hydrogel		
Provides moisture, which facilitates granulation	Must use another product to keep in place and secure with tape or film	Do not use on heavy, exuding wounds.
Facilitates some debridement for wounds with thin, stringy yellow eschar	May cause hypergranulation tissue (leafy, friable, beefy-red granulation tissue), which impedes	Do not use on wounds with cellulitis.
Promotes removal of dry necrotic eschar when dressing left in place for several days	healing and usually requires debridement or removal with sharp instrument or silver nitrate	Do not use on wounds with purulent discharge.
Nonadherent surface, which provides comfort to patient	Is expensive but requires fewer dressing changes	
Requires less frequent dressing changes, which promotes efficient use of nursing time and comfort to patient		

wafer may be placed around the wound to protect the skin from future problems. Stoma adhesive is recommended over a hydrocolloid dressing because tape and film dressings do not stick to the stoma adhesive barrier as they do to a hydrocolloid wafer. If no infection exists, another alternative that decreases maceration is to apply petroleum jelly or zinc oxide around the wound borders and then to apply the dressing.

Gauze dressings have been used for many years with success; however, a large amount of scientific information regarding pressure injuries and wound care has been accumulating since 1962, when moisture was first identified as a facilitator of healing. This discovery has generated many other effective, efficient, and comfortable options. Thus gauze is primarily used for debriding and cleaning up the wound bed, except when used for protecting closed surgical wounds or when the newer expensive dressings are not on the formulary. However, when a wound has tunneling or undermining, saline-moistened gauze, *loosely* packed into the wound, may maintain a moist environment.

Caution should be exercised not to pack tightly or have the moistened gauze touching the healing surface surrounding the ulcer to avoid additional damage and maceration. If gauze is being used on a clean wound, the strategy should be wet-to-moist dressing to prevent drying of epithelial cells. The nurse should slightly moisten the gauze, touching the wound bed with normal saline, and place dry gauze or an abdominal pad over the moist gauze and secure with tape; this should keep the wound moist at all times.

Some gauze is impregnated with material such as povidone-iodine, or petroleum jelly. Gauze ribbons impregnated with povidone-iodine (iodoform gauze) are effective for cleaning up a tunneling wound that has purulent or foul exudate. However, the povidone-iodine gauze should be stopped when the purulent, foul exudate has resolved so that healthy tissue is not destroyed. Petroleum jelly gauze is a good, inexpensive method for keeping a wound from drying out and protecting the wound and surrounding tissue. Petroleum jelly gauze secured with Kerlix wrapped around the extremity, changed every 2 to 4 days and as needed, is an effective strategy for healing skin tears. The petroleum jelly keeps the wound moist and protects from further insults.

Nonadherent dressings are used when the wound bed must be protected and epithelial cells left undisturbed. Nonadherent dressings are suitable for skin tears, skin grafts, or other wounds that require minimum insult. Often, an antibiotic ointment is applied to the wound bed (which keeps it moist), and then the bed is covered with a nonadherent dressing, which is changed once or twice a day.

Foam dressings, which are nonadherent, absorbent dressings, protect the wound and assist in minimizing maceration of the wound edges. Consider use of foam dressings for stage II and shallow stage III pressure injuries, exudating cavity ulcers, painful ulcers, and on body areas and pressure injuries at risk for shear injury (NPUAP, 2014). Foam dressings have also been used around tracheal tubes; they are beneficial when candidiasis exists around tracheal stomas, acting to absorb moisture. Foam dressings are secured with tape or film and may be used in combination with other topical agents or primary dressings.

Transparent films are used for stage I or II pressure injuries (superficial wounds) to secure dressings, to protect vulnerable areas (e.g., elbows) from friction, and to facilitate autolysis. Transparent films are semipermeable, thus allowing exchange of air. However, they should not be used to cover enzymatic debriding agents, gels, or ointments. Film dressings may be left on for 3 to 7 days but should be checked a minimum of once a day. Film dressings facilitate autolysis, which causes fluid buildup and may consequently lead to maceration of good tissue and dressing leakage. Petroleum jelly or zinc oxide applied around the wound edges before placement of the film may prevent maceration. A nonadherent dressing or alginate may also be used under the film to assist with exudate management.

Hydrocolloids are sticky, nonpermeable wafers containing a hydrocolloid material that eventually melts, combines with natural body fluids, and keeps the wound bed moist. The nonpermeable wafer also serves as a barrier and creates a hypoxic wound environment that stimulates granulation, if peripheral circulation provides enough oxygen. Consider the use of hydrocolloid dressings on noninfected, shallow stage III pressure injuries and to protect body areas at risk for friction injuries or at risk of injury from tape (NPUAP, 2014). Hydrocolloid dressings should not be used if candidiasis exists. Hydrocolloid wafers are usually changed every 3 to 7 days. It should be noted that the foul, sour odor generated by hydrocolloid dressings is considered normal. Infection is present when erythema, warmth, tenderness, or purulent discharge exists. Hydrocolloid dressings should *never* be applied to ulcers that are infected, have purulent discharge, or have a suspected infection. The occlusive, moist environment provides a perfect medium for bacterial growth and may worsen the infection.

Hydrogels consist primarily of water and are effective in maintaining a moist ulcer bed, which fosters healing. Hydrogel dressings may be obtained in a sheet form suitable for superficial wounds or as an amorphous gel that can be applied and spread into deep, cavity wounds. Hydrogel dressings should not be used on infected wounds because they retain humidity, thus facilitating autolytic debridement. The cover dressing should be chosen based on the health of the surrounding skin and the degree of wound exudate. Examples of cover dressings include gauze, foam, and transparent films. Dressings using a hydrogel may be left in place for 1 day or up to 5 to 7 days, depending on the setting, product, and ulcer state (see Table 17.3 and Nursing Care Plan: Pressure Injury).

TABLE 17.3   General Pressure Injury Care Guidelines

Stage	Actions	Dressing Options
1	Implement preventive strategies (e.g., mattress overlay; nutritional assessment; reinforcement of value of turning, keeping dry, and minimizing friction)	May protect with film or hydrocolloid
2 and 3	Implement preventive strategies, assess for infection, debride necrotic tissue, conduct nutritional assessment, and provide appropriate nutritional support	May use film, if clean, depending on depth; hydrocolloid; hydrogel, foam, honey-impregnated, collagen matrix, continually moist gauze dressing; if infected, manage topically with appropriate antiseptic and continually moist gauze dressing until infection is resolved
4	Same as 2 and 3; specialized bed may be considered	If clean, hydrogel, hydrocolloid paste and wafer, collagen matrix or continually moist gauze dressing; if infected, manage topically with antiseptic and continually moist gauze dressing until infection is resolved (but no longer than 5 days)

NURSING CARE PLAN

Pressure Injury

Clinical Situation

Mrs. M. is an 80-year-old female who developed stage IV pressure injury on her sacral area and right ischium while recently hospitalized for pneumonia. Her decreased appetite and poor food intake, a 10-pound weight loss, and her not being initially placed on an egg-crate mattress led to the development of the pressure injury. Mrs. M. was discharged home with home health care.

The sacral and ischial pressure injuries are clean, beginning to granulate, managed with a hydrogel, covered with a foam dressing to lessen maceration, and sealed with a transparent dressing changed every other day. It is estimated that complete healing will take 6 to 8 months as long as nutritional status and other preventive strategies are maintained.

Nursing Diagnosis

Reduced skin integrity resulting from altered nutrition, altered circulation, and immobilization

Outcome

The patient will have intact skin, as evidenced by clean, healing wounds; maintenance of circulation to skin; and laboratory values within normal limits.

Interventions

Implement pressure injury preventive strategies to create an environment that will foster healing and prevent further development of ulcers.

Place the mattress overlay on the bed and obtain an appropriate pressure-relieving chair cushion to decrease ischial pressure.

Teach the patient and family to position the patient at a 30-degree angle and support extremities with pillows when lying in bed to lessen trochanter pressure.

Teach the patient, family, and nurse's aide to avoid the use of hot baths and harsh soaps, to use moisturizers for dry skin, and not to massage over bony prominences.

Teach the patient not to sit at a 45- to 90-degree angle when in bed or on the couch to minimize shearing forces.

Assess and treat incontinence by cleansing the skin at the time of soiling; use a topical moisture barrier and (if necessary) absorbent undergarments to maintain a dry surface and decrease the risk of additional skin breakdown.

Inspect the skin during home visits, observing for any pressure points, as seen by erythema or skin breakdown. If a stage I or II injury is present but the site is not infected, apply the film or hydrocolloidal dressing to protect from further breakdown.

Assess the pressure injury when changing the dressing, noting the wound bed and border color, discharge, and general condition.

Document each assessment and measure weekly. If the wound bed is infected or has developed cellulitis as seen by erythema, tenderness, pale granulation tissue, or purulent discharge, change the dressing to wet-to-dry with an appropriate antiseptic but only until the wound is improved and no longer than 5 to 7 days to minimize damage to viable tissue.

If the wound is stagnant, as documented by serial dimensions over 3 to 6 weeks, consider changing to another dressing strategy.

Monitor nutritional status because it may influence skin integrity and the healing process.

Monitor weight gains or losses monthly.

Take a 24-hour diet recall with each visit to assess eating habits and nutritional intake.

Teach the patient and family the role nutrition plays in healing and general health status.

If weight loss is experienced, interview the patient to determine the reason (e.g., food preferences are not met, or food is cold or esthetically unappealing).

Examine the oral cavity and, if appropriate, fit for dentures.

Maintain a clean, moist wound environment to foster healing.

If necrotic tissue is present, facilitate debridement by arranging for a physician, nurse practitioner, or certified enterostomal therapist to perform bedside debridement.

If only a small amount of necrotic tissue is present, attempt chemical or mechanical debridement.

Select the most comfortable and efficient dressing, such as a hydrogel or hydrocolloidal dressing, with the intent of maintaining a moist wound environment, which fosters granulation and thus healing.

Use clean technique for dressing care; sterile technique is not necessary because the wound is dirty.

Gently irrigate the wound with normal saline to clean wound, make an appropriate assessment, and measure the wound dimensions weekly.

Teach the patient and family dressing care and changing technique to involve them in the care and to promote self-care.

Alginates are a category of exudate management dressings. The alginate dressings are manufactured from seaweed and are applied to wounds that are moderately to heavily exudative. In most cases, the alginates are safe to use on infected wounds. These dressings have excellent exudate handling properties and are useful in wounds and around drainage tubes when the wound fluid is causing periwound skin maceration.

In addition, some types of dressings are impregnated with various substances, for example, silver-impregnated dressings, which are used for infected or heavily colonized ulcers and stage II and shallow state III pressure injuries; honey-impregnated dressings, which are impregnated with medical grade honey and are used for stage II and III pressure injuries; and cadexomer iodine dressings, which are used for highly exudating wounds.

Biophysical Agents in Pressure Injury Management

Research has been conducted on the use of different energy forms in the management of pressure injuries. These include acoustic energy (ultrasound) for debridement and treatment of infected wounds and UV light therapy as adjunctive therapy to reduce bacterial colonization. Negative-pressure wound therapy may be considered as an early adjuvant for deep stage III and IV exudative pressure injuries without necrotic tissue. Last, hydrotherapy (pulsed lavage with or without suction) can be used as an adjunct for wound cleaning and to facilitate healing (NPUAP, 2014).

SUMMARY

Pressure injuries are a costly health care problem, not only in terms of dollars but also in terms of nursing time and human lives. Prevention is the first line of defense against pressure injury development. Nurses have an opportunity to demonstrate the profession's power and accountability by implementing preventive strategies, thereby having a positive effect on a patient's quality of life while preventing a costly health care problem. It is imperative that the nurse conduct pressure injury risk assessments, use mattress overlays, teach support staff prevention and management techniques, monitor the patient's nutritional status, and serve as a role model by focusing on prevention. With expanded pressure injury knowledge and the publication of the AHRQ and NPUAP clinical guidelines, preventive measures are a nurse's responsibility.

The collaborative relationship that the nurse establishes with the health care provider to utilize the most efficient and effective strategies is vital to successful healing. Collaboration develops trust and professional maturity and is necessary for growth.

Successful pressure injury management requires the application of the principles of healing, which should guide selection of treatment strategies. Frequent review of the healing trajectory, when reinforced with clinical examples, facilitates comprehension of this complex process. Pressure injury management is a science and an art that requires experience.

HOME CARE

1. Regularly assess for signs and symptoms of skin breakdown in homebound older adults who are at high risk for the development of a pressure injury.
2. Assess for and instruct caregivers and homebound older adults on factors that predispose patients to the development of a pressure injury.
3. Use the services of a wound care clinical nurse specialist in assessing, planning, and recommending appropriate wound care management techniques.
4. Prevention is the first-line strategy for pressure injury care. Teach caregivers of at-risk homebound older adults the techniques for preventing a pressure injury—focusing on preventing moisture, avoiding friction and shearing, changing position frequently, and ensuring excellent nutritional intake.

KEY POINTS

- Because of normal, age-related changes in the skin, older adults are more susceptible to skin tears and bruising caused by thinning of the skin.
- Older adults are at greater risk for hypothermia, shearing, pressure damage, and blunt trauma because of decreased subcutaneous tissue.
- Older adults may experience altered medication absorption because of an age-related decrease in fatty tissue and dermis blood supply.
- Older adults are at increased risk of heatstroke because of the compromised cooling mechanism from decreased sweating.
- The typical pattern of spreading for seborrheic dermatitis starts at the scalp margins, progresses downward to the eyebrows, the base of the eyelashes, and around the nose in a butterfly pattern, and continues to the ears and sternum.
- Psoriasis is a common disorder affecting the epidermis and the dermis. It is recognized by the presence of erythematous, scaly, and itchy patches on various parts of the body. Many triggers exacerbate the condition.
- Pruritus warrants a full skin assessment because it may be indicative of many diseases, drug reactions, and possibly cancer. The nurse should determine the location, intensity, alleviating and aggravating events, onset, and what the patient is doing to control it.
- Candidiasis, recognized by fire-red, denuded skin with satellite macules or pustules, develops in moist intertriginous areas.
- Herpes zoster is characterized by prodromal symptoms of itching or burning along a dermatome, followed by a unilateral, bandlike maculopapular rash and vesicles, which rarely cross the midline.
- The nurse should notify the health care provider if the following suspected lesions are found on assessment of actinic keratosis: BCC, SCC, or melanoma.
- Arterial ulcers are usually located on toes or feet and are associated with pain during activity, nighttime, and rest. The cause of decreased arterial blood flow must be corrected for ulcers to heal.
- Venous hypertension leads to the formation of a capillary fibrin cuff, which causes chronic edema, decreased circulation, and recurring medial lower leg ulcers.
- Diabetic foot lesions are usually located on the plantar foot and result from loss of protective sensation in the foot, which leads to abnormal gait and increased pressure on the foot. Bony deformities may develop and further change foot pressures, increasing the likelihood of trauma and subsequent ulceration.
- Pressure injuries are a costly health care problem, not only in terms of dollars but also in nursing time and human lives. Prevention is the first-line strategy for pressure injury care.
- The nurse should assess the nutritional status of patients with pressure injuries with a determination of monthly weight and laboratory variables.
- To minimize friction, the nurse should use sheets to lift and pull the patient up in bed and apply a film dressing or lotion to vulnerable areas such as elbows, coccyx, and heels.
- To minimize shearing forces, the nurse should not elevate the head of the bed greater than 30 to 45 degrees.

- Antiseptic solutions should be used only when the wound is infected; they should never be used on a clean, healthy wound because they are cytotoxic and destructive to tissue.

- Surface cultures have been shown to grow different organisms than what is in underlying tissues and blood cultures, thus routine wound cultures are not appropriate.

CRITICAL-THINKING EXERCISES

1. Outline major teaching points that would be beneficial to maintaining the integumentary health of older individuals.

2. A 78-year-old Hispanic man has a history of SCC. After having a lesion removed from his upper back 3 years ago, he has been extremely anxious about other skin lesions and skin changes. What approach would you take to help your patient reduce his anxiety and yet remain active in the prevention and early recognition of skin cancer?

3. Your 79-year-old female patient suffered a stroke 6 months ago and is cared for in her sister's home. The patient is dependent for position changes, is unable to communicate the need to be turned, must be fed, and has a stage II pressure injury on her sacral area. Develop a teaching plan for the family to ensure that the patient's needs are met.

REFERENCES

Agency for Health Care Research and Quality. (2014). *Preventing pressure ulcers in hospitals.* Retrieved February 12, 2018 from https://www.ahrq.gov/professionals/systems/hospital/pressureulcertoolkit/index.html.

Agrawal, K., & Chauhan, N. (2012). Pressure ulcers: Back to the basics. *Indian Journal of Plastic Surgery, 45*(2), 244–254. https://doi.org/10.4103/0970-0358.101287.

American Academy of Dermatology. (n.d.). Skin cancer. Retrieved February 12, 2018 from https://www.aad.org/media/stats/conditions/skin-cancer.

Bader, R. S. (2017). *Basal cell carcinoma.* Retrieved February 12, 2018 from https://emedicine.medscape.com/article/276624-overview#a6.

Baraz, S., Zarea, K., Shahbazian, H. B., & Latifi, S. M. (2014). Comparison of the accuracy of monofilament testing at various points of feet in peripheral diabetic neuropathy screening. *Journal of Diabetes and Metabolic Disorders, 13*, 19. https://doi.org/10.1186/2251-6581-13-19.

Bluestein, D., & Javaheri, A. (2008). Pressure ulcers: Prevention, evaluation, and management. *American Family Physician, 78*(10), 1186–1194.

Blume-Peytavi, U., Kottner, J., Sterry, W., Hodin, M. W., Griffiths, T. W., Watson, R. E., & Griffiths, C. E. (2016). Age-associated skin conditions and diseases: Current perspectives and future options. *The Gerontologist, 56*(S2), S230–S242. doi: 10.1093/geront/gnw003.

Braden, B. J., & Bergstrom, N. (1987). Clinical utility of the Braden scale for predicting pressure sore risk. *Decubitus, 2*(3), 44.

Brizzi, K. T., & Lyons, J. L. (2014). Peripheral nervous system manifestations of infectious diseases. *Neurohospitalist, 4*(4), 230–240. https://doi.org/10.1177/1941874414535215.

Cassano, N. (2010). Chronic pruritus in the absence of specific skin disease: an update on pathophysiology, diagnosis, and therapy. *American Journal of Clinical Dermatology, 11*(6), 399–411.

Centers for Disease Control and Prevention. (2018). Shingles (herpes zoster). Retrieved February 12, 2018 from https://www.cdc.gov/shingles/about/overview.html.

Coleman, S., Gorecki, C., Nelson, A., Closs, S. J., Defloor, T., Halfens, R., & Nixon, J. (2013). Patient risk factors for pressure ulcer development: Systematic review. *International Journal of Nursing Studies, 50*(7), 974–1003. https://doi.org/10.1016/j.ijnurstu.2012.11.019.

Cox, J. (2017). Pressure injury risk factors in adult critical care patients: A review of the literature. *Ostomy Wound Management, 63*(11), 30–43. https://doi.org/10.25270/owm.201.

Dasgupta, G. (2009). New concepts in herpes simplex virus complex vaccine development: notes from the battlefield. *Expert Review of Vaccines, 8*(8), 1023–1035.

Dyer, J. M., & Miller, R. A. (2018). Chronic skin fragility of aging: Current concepts in the pathogenesis, recognition, and management of dermatoporosis. *The Journal of Clinical and AEsthetic Dermatology, 11*(1), 13–18.

Feramisco, J. D., Berger, T. G., & Steinhoff, M. (2010). Innovative management of pruritus. *Dermatologic Clinics, 28*(3), 467–478.

Gillespie, B. M., Chaboyer, W. P., McInnes, E., Kent, B., Whitty, J. A., & Thalib, L. (2014). Repositioning to prevent pressure ulcers. *Cochrane Database of Systematic Reviews, 4.* Art. No.: CD009958 https://doi.org/10.1002/14651858.CD009958.pub2.

Gomez, J. (2017). *Seborrheic dermatitis.* Retrieved February 10, 2018 from https://www.dermnetnz.org/topics/seborrhoeic-dermatitis/.

Habif, T. P. (2004). *Clinical dermatology* (4th ed.). St Louis: Mosby.

Johnson, R. S., Titze, J., & Weller, R. (2016). Cutaneous control of blood pressure. *Current Opinion in Nephrology and Hypertension, 25*(1), 11–15. https://doi.org/10.1097/MNH.0000000000000188.

Kalra, M. G., Higgins, K. E., & Kinney, B. S. (2014). Intertrigo and secondary skin infections. *American Family Physician, 89*(7), 569–573.

Kosiak, M. (1958). Etiology and pathology of ischemic ulcers. *Archives of Physical Medicine and Rehabilitation, 40*(2), 62.

Krasner, D. (1991). Resolving the dressing dilemma: selecting wound dressings by category. *Ostomy/Wound Management, 35*(4), 62.

Levine, J. M. (1992). Historical notes on pressure ulcers: the cure of Ambrose Pare. *Decubitus, 5*(2), 23–26.

Marcason, W. (2017). Should albumin and prealbumin be used as indicators for malnutrition? Retrieved February 13, 2018 from http://jandonline.org/article/S2212-2672(17)30444-6/fulltext.

Mercandetti, M. (2017). *Wound healing and repair.* Retrieved February 13, 2018 from https://emedicine.medscape.com/article/1298129-overview.

Najjar, T. (2017). *Cutaneous squamous cell carcinoma.* Retrieved February 12, 2018 from https://emedicine.medscape.com/article/1965430-overview#a5.

National Pressure Ulcer Advisory Panel. (2014). *NEW 2014 Prevention and treatment of pressure ulcers: Clinical practice guideline.* Retrieved February 13, 2018 from http://www.npuap.org/resources/educational-and-clinical-resources/prevention-and-treatment-of-pressure-ulcers-clinical-practice-guideline/.

Norton, D. (1989). Calculation of the risk: Reflections on the Norton scale. *Decubitus, 2*(3), 24.

Playford, E. G., Lipman, J., & Sorrell, T. C. (2010). Prophylaxis, empirical and preemptive treatment of invasive candidiasis. *Current Opinion in Critical Care, 16*(5), 470–474.

Psaty, E. L. (2010). Defining the patient at risk for melanoma. *International Journal of Dermatology, 49*(4), 362–376.

Rigel, D. S., Russak, J., & Friedman, R. (2010). The evolution of melanoma cells: a 25-years beyond the ABCDs. *Cancer Journal for Clinicians, 60*(5), 301–316.

Scherer, R., Maroto-Sanchez, B., Palacios, G., & Gonzalez-Gross, M. (2016). Fluid intake and recommendations in older adults: More data are needed. *Nutrition Bulletin, 41,* 167–174. https://doi.org/10.1111/nbu.12206.

Slone-Rivera, N., & Wu, S. C. (2012). A guide to compression dressings for venous ulcers. *Podiatry Today, 25*(2). Retrieved from https://www.podiatrytoday.com/guide-compression-dressings-venous-ulcers.

Spear, M. (2014). *When and how to culture a chronic wound.* Retrieved February 13, 2018 from https://woundcareadvisor.com/when-and-how-to-culture-a-chronic-wound-vol3-no1/.

Spencer, J. M. (2017). *Actinic keratosis.* Retrieved February 12, 2018 from https://emedicine.medscape.com/article/1099775-overview.

Stajkovic, S., Aitken, E. M., & Holroyd-Leduc, J. (2011). Unintentional weight loss in older adults. *Canadian Medical Association Journal, 183*(4), 443–449. https://doi.org/10.1503/cmaj.101471.

Tan, W. W. (2018). *Malignant melanoma clinical presentation.* Retrieved February 13, 2018 from https://emedicine.medscape.com/article/280245-clinical.

Touhy, T., & Jett, K. (2012). *Ebersole and Hess' toward healthy aging: Human needs and nursing response* (8th ed.). St Louis: Mosby.

Vasudevan, B. (2014). Venous leg ulcers: Pathophysiology and classification. *Indian Dermatology Online Journal, 5*(3), 366–370. https://doi.org/10.4103/2229-5178.137819.

Waaijman, R., de Haart, M., Arts, M.L., Wever, D., Verlouw, A.J., Nollet, F., ... Bus, S.A. (2014). Risk factors for plantar foot ulcer recurrence in neuropathic diabetic patients. *Diabetes Care, 37,* 1697–1705. doi: https://doi.org/10.2337/dc13-2470.

World Health Organization. (2016). *Global report on psoriasis.* Retrieved from http://apps.who.int/iris/bitstream/10665/204417/1/9789241565189_eng.pdf.

18

Sensory Function

Beth Culross, PhD, RN, GCNS-BC, CRRN, FNGNA

ⓔ http://evolve.elsevier.com/Meiner/gerontologic

LEARNING OBJECTIVES

On completion of this chapter, the reader will be able to:

1. Describe age-related changes in the senses.
2. Distinguish between cataracts and glaucoma, including the associated nursing interventions.
3. Distinguish between retinal disorders, including the medical and nursing management of each disorder.
4. Identify nursing interventions for older adults with low vision.
5. Describe the proper method for instilling eye medications.
6. Describe common changes in the ear that affect hearing.
7. Identify nursing interventions for hearing impairment.
8. Identify nursing interventions for older patients with xerostomia.
9. Describe safety issues for older adults with diminished senses of vision, hearing, and touch.
10. Conduct a sensory system assessment and describe the normal findings.

WHAT WOULD YOU DO?

What would you do if you were faced with the following situations?

• You are caring for a 75-year-old widow who lives independently. You start noticing she is having increased difficulty in reading, she is stumbling into things, and she has told you about a recent fall. What do you do?

• The spouse of your patient states that her husband of 50 years has become withdrawn and complains that everyone mumbles when talking and can't be understood. She complains that she can't stand to be in the room when the television is on because it is so loud. What do you do?

• When assessing a 90-year-old man, you notice he is underweight. He states that family and friends are concerned over his eating habits. He does not enjoy eating because nothing seems to taste the same as he remembers, and his mouth is dry most of the time. What do you do?

The senses connect the human body to the environment. They allow individuals to be aware of and interpret various stimuli, thus enabling interaction with the environment. Sensory changes may have a dramatic effect on the quality of life of older adults. Visual and hearing impairments may interfere with communication, social interactions, and mobility, leading to social isolation. Olfactory, gustatory, and tactile deprivations may lead to nutritional problems and safety hazards. It is important to understand the sensory changes associated with aging to help older adults adapt and function as independently as possible. An emphasis on maintaining healthy senses is part of Healthy

People 2020 (U.S. Department of Health and Human Services, 2010). This is especially important with the understanding that impaired senses can be linked to increased mortality (Cacchione, 2014; Boltz et al., 2016).

The five primary sensory categories include the following: sight, hearing, taste, smell, and touch. Two additional sensory categories that are recognized are general and special. General senses include the senses of touch, pressure, pain, temperature, vibration, and proprioception (position sense). These have relatively simple receptors, which are located all over the body. These senses are further classified as somatic (those providing sensory information about the body and the environment) or visceral (those supplying information about the internal organs). Special senses are produced by highly localized organs and specialized sensory cells. These include the senses of sight, hearing, taste, smell, and balance.

Sensation is a conscious or unconscious awareness of external and internal stimuli. Perception is the interpretation of conscious sensations. The brain receives stimuli from both inside and outside the body. Conscious sensation occurs via action potentials generated by receptors that reach the cerebral cortex.

VISION

Vision plays an integral part in a person's ability to function in the environment. Visual acuity (the ability to see clearly) is an important part of performing activities of daily living (ADLs); dressing, grooming, cooking, sewing, driving, and reading are all tasks that involve the use of eyesight (Fig. 18.1).

Previous authors: Cindy R. Morgan, RN, MSN, CHC, CHPN, and Ramesh C. Upadhyaya, RN, CRRN, MSN, MBA, PhD-C.

EVIDENCE-BASED PRACTICE

Effects of Sensory Impairments in Older Adults

Sample/Setting

The sample for this study consisted of 3005 older adults living in the community. Women represented 1551 and men 1454 of the sample. The age range was 57 to 84. Respondents were from Wave 1 of the study with some additional respondents that refused Wave 1.

Methods

Interviewers from the National Opinion Research Center conducted in-home interviews to collect the following data: demographic, social, psychological, and biological measures. Sensory function was detailed and is discussed in this article.

Findings

Findings included alterations in all sensory function as follows:

Vision: Difficulties were found in driving during the day (14%), driving at night (40%), and an overall 16% stated vision as poor or fair.

Hearing: A total of 22% reported poor or fair corrected hearing; 20% stated they experienced frustration when having conversations with family and 18% stated frustrations when visiting with others. Only 12% reported limitations on personal or social life although 42% had difficulty hearing whispered words. Hearing loss was found to be a significant burden.

Touch: Results indicated a general difference in perception of touch and how appealing it is for the older adult. The indication is that changes in this perception can affect relationships between partners and activities such as exercise.

Olfaction: This was one area that had potential alterations due to 8% of respondents having a cold at the time of the interview. The decline in olfaction may reflect the inability to detect malodor and potentially provide insights into other aspects of health.

Implications

Vision and hearing impairments are highly prevalent in older adults and are related to important functional changes that include personal interactions. The effect is on relationships with family and friends and critical activities that the older adult may participate in such as driving.

Other affected areas include access to health care, personal safety, alterations in communication, and decreased social function and quality of life. This can lead to social isolation, depression, and anxiety.

From Pinto, J. M., Kern, D. W., Wroblewski, K. E., Chen, R. C., Schumm, L. P., & McClintock, M. K. (2014). Sensory function: Insights from wave 2 of the national social life, health, and aging project. *Journals of Gerontology, Series B: Psychological Sciences and Social Sciences, 69(8)*, S144-S153. DOI:10.1093/Gerontology/gbu102.

Age-Related Changes in Structure and Function

Normal age-related changes in the external and internal eye have been well documented. The eyelids lose tone and become lax, which may result in ptosis of the eyelids, redundancy of the skin of the eyelids, and malposition of the eyelids. Eyebrows may turn gray and become coarser in men, with outer thinning in both men and women. The conjunctiva thins and yellows in appearance. In addition, this membrane may become dry because of diminished quantity and quality of tear production. The sclera may develop brown spots. The cornea yellows and develops a noticeable surrounding ring made up of fat deposits, called the *arcus senilis*. The pupil decreases in size and loses some of its ability to constrict. Changes resulting from aging that decrease the size of the pupil and limit the amount of light

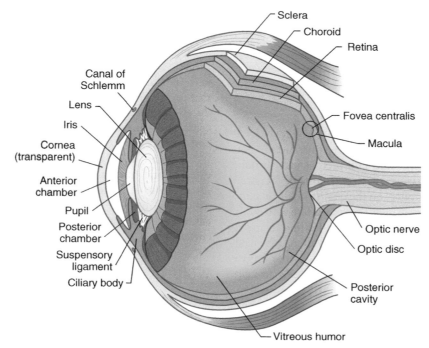

Fig. 18.1 Anatomy of the eye. (From Lewis, S. M., Bucher, L., Heitkemper, M. M., & Harding, M. M. [Eds.]. [2017]. *Medical-surgical nursing: Assessment and management of clinical problems* [10th ed.]. St. Louis, MO: Elsevier. Modified from Patton K. T. & Thibodeau G. A. [2013]. *Anatomy and physiology* [8th ed.]. St. Louis, MO: Mosby.)

entering the eye also occur in the iris. The lens increases in density and rigidity, affecting the eye's ability to transmit and focus light. Peripheral vision decreases, night vision diminishes, and sensitivity to glare increases (Boltz et al., 2016; Garrity, 2017). There may be a gradual reduction in the ability to see colors in aging along with color deficits due to multiple disease processes including diabetes, glaucoma, macular degeneration, Alzheimer's disease, and Parkinson's disease (American Optometric Association, 2017).

Ophthalmoscopic examination of the retina may reveal the following changes: blood vessels have narrowed and straightened; arteries seem opaque and gray; and *drusen,* localized areas of hyaline degeneration, may be noted as gray or yellow spots near the macula (Porter, 2017). Two common complaints of older adults, floaters and dry eyes, are discussed in the following section.

Common Complaints

Floaters and Flashers

Floaters appear as dots, wiggly lines, or clouds that a person may see moving in the field of vision. They become more pronounced when a person is looking at a plain background. Floaters occur more often after age 50, as tiny clumps of gel or cellular debris float in the vitreous humor in front of the retina. They are caused by degeneration of the vitreous gel and are more common in older adults who have undergone cataract operations or yttrium–aluminum–garnet (YAG) laser surgery.

In general, floaters are normal and harmless, but they may be a warning sign of a more serious condition, especially if they increase in number and if changes in the type of floater, light flashes, or visual hallucinations are noted. These symptoms may indicate a vitreous or retinal tear, which could lead to detachment. In addition, visual hallucinations have been associated with a brain tumor or cortical ischemia. Therefore any of these symptoms warrants a complete eye examination by an ophthalmologist.

Flashers occur when the vitreous fluid inside the eye rubs or pulls on the retina and produces the illusion of flashing lights or lightning streaks. Flashers that appear as jagged lines, last 10 to 20 minutes, and are present in both eyes are likely to be caused by a spasm of blood vessels in the brain called a *migraine.* These flashers commonly occur with advancing age, but they warrant prompt medical attention if they increase in number, if a large number of new flashers appears, or if partial loss of side vision is noted (Boyd, 2017).

The nurse should refer a patient who experiences any of these symptoms to an ophthalmologist for a comprehensive eye examination. If no cause is found for floaters and flashers, the nurse should teach the patient about the condition and how to live with it. Patients should be taught to look up and down to get the floaters out of the field of vision. In addition, the nurse should provide the patient with the printed information instruction sheet titled "Aging and Your Eyes" so that he or she may learn more about floaters and flashers (Boyd, 2017) (Box 18.1).

Dry Eyes

Dry eyes result as the quantity and quality of tear production diminish with aging. Stinging, burning, or a scratchy sensation are common complaints of the individual with dry eye. Episodes of excess tearing may occur following a period of discomfort, dryness, pain, redness, and possibly discharge in the eyes. Blurred vision and a heavy feel to eyelids may also be experienced (National Institutes of Health [NIH], 2017b).

Treatment consists of tear replacement or conservation. Tears may be replaced by instilling an over-the-counter (OTC) artificial tear preparation to lubricate the eye and replace missing moisture. This type of preparation may be used as often as necessary, especially before activities that require significant eye movement. Solid inserts that gradually release lubricants throughout the day are also available. An ophthalmologist can help conserve the naturally produced tears by temporarily or permanently closing the lacrimal drainage system. Other methods of conservation include use of a humidifier when the heat is on, wraparound glasses to reduce evaporation of eye moisture caused by wind, and avoidance of smoke (NIH, 2017b).

Common Problems and Conditions

Common problems resulting from the aging eye include presbyopia, ectropion and entropion, blepharitis, glaucoma, cataracts, retinal disorders, eye injuries, and visual impairment. Presbyopia is a normal change that occurs with aging. The other problems are eye diseases that are more prominent in older adults.

Presbyopia

The most common complaint of adults older than age 40 is a diminished ability to focus clearly on close objects (arm's length) such as a newspaper. In presbyopia, the lens loses its

---

BOX 18.1 Aging and Your Eyes: Health Promotion

1. Have an eye examination with eyes dilated annually. This will help to detect common eye diseases before the onset of signs or symptoms.
2. Be sure to use adequate lighting for the task you are completing.
3. Wear sunglasses to protect your eyes from ultraviolet (UV) radiation. Wearing a wide-brimmed hat will help as well.
4. Choose eye-healthy foods including fruits, vegetables, and whole grains. Vitamins C and E, zinc, and zeaxanthin have been shown to help eye health.
5. Quit smoking and avoid second-hand smoke to reduce the risk of eye diseases such as cataract and age-related macular degeneration. Smoking also worsens dry eye.
6. Be active and keep a healthy weight. Thirty minutes of daily exercise can help reduce the risk of eye disease that have been linked to other health issues (diabetes, hypertension, and hyperlipidemia)
7. Chronic disease maintenance. Maintaining normal blood pressure, blood glucose, and cholesterol levels will help reduce the risk of eye disease.
8. Prevent eyestrain. Blink and look away from computer screens or other electronic devices every 20 minutes. Looking approximately 20 feet away for 20 seconds will help.
9. Know the symptoms of low vision. These include finding lights are not bright enough, can't see well enough for everyday tasks, difficulty recognizing faces known to you, and trouble reading street signs.

Data from National Institutes of Health. National Institute on Aging (2017). Aging and your eyes. Retrieved from https://www.nia.nih.gov/health/aging-and-your-eyes; and Kern, D. (2014). Seven sight-saving habits for older adults to help maintain independence. *American Academy of Ophthalmology.* Retrieved from https://www.aao.org/eye-health/tips-prevention/seven-sight-saving-habits.

ability to focus on close objects. Accommodation is impaired as the lens thickens and loses its elasticity. The ciliary muscles weaken the lens's ability to contract. Treatment involves wearing reading glasses or bifocals (two-part lenses that correct near and distant vision); the prognosis for corrected vision is excellent.

Nursing care is aimed at encouraging the patient to adjust to the glasses by wearing them and following up with a visit to the ophthalmologist every 2 years. Information for patient education on vision and aging is available through the National Institute on Aging (see Box 18.1).

HEALTH PROMOTION/ILLNESS PREVENTION
The Eye

Health Promotion
- Have a yearly eye examination and screening (including a glaucoma test) for eye disease and vision problems.
- Use a bright light when sewing, reading, and cooking; avoid fluorescent light.
- Have an ultraviolet-filter coating on spectacle lenses and sunglasses for outdoor activities.

Prevention and Treatment of Disease
- See your health care provider/ophthalmologist with the occurrence of any pain, discharge, redness, swelling, or loss of vision.
- Take measures for detection and appropriate treatment of vision difficulties and eye disease (e.g., cataracts, glaucoma, diabetic retinopathy, and macular degeneration).
- Maintain prescribed corrective lenses, low-vision aids, and medications.

Blepharitis

Blepharitis is chronic inflammation of the eyelid margins commonly found in older adults. It may be caused by seborrheic dermatitis or infection. The use of antihistamines, anticholinergics, antidepressants, and diuretics may exacerbate this condition because of the drying effects of these medications. In addition, the deficiency in tear production with aging may lead to infection. The symptoms include red, swollen eyelids; matting and crusting along the base of the eyelash at the margins; small ulcerations along the lid margins; and complaints of irritation, itching, burning, tearing, and photophobia. Treatment is aimed at removing the causative bacteria and healing the affected areas. Physicians may prescribe topical antibiotics or steroids. However, the nurse can play a significant role in the treatment of this condition by teaching patients certain interventions, described later.

The patient must be taught scrupulous eye hygiene, including good hand-washing habits. Mild soap (e.g., Ivory, Neutrogena) should be used. Contact lens wearers must be taught proper cleaning and storage techniques to prevent contamination of the eye, lens, lens solution, and lens case. Because cosmetics are a common source of bacterial contamination, eye makeup products should be replaced every 3 to 6 months to avoid bacterial growth. It is also important that patients know how to apply makeup with cotton balls and cotton-tipped applicators, and understand the importance of discarding the applicators after each use. Mascara should be water resistant, free of lash-extending fibers, and not applied to the base of the lashes. Eyeliner should be a medium-hard pencil and not be applied to

the inner margin of the eyelid. Patients should avoid the use of aerosol hairsprays because these may irritate the eyes. Inflammation caused by blepharitis will be resolved and the patient's comfort level will improve after a week of these hygiene measures.

Glaucoma

Glaucoma is the second leading cause of blindness in the United States and the first cause of blindness among African Americans (especially over the age of 40). Although glaucoma may occur at any age, those most at risk are adults older than age 60, especially Mexican Americans (NIH, 2017a; Lewis et al., 2017). Glaucoma is a group of diseases that can result in vision loss and lead to blindness due to damage to the optic nerve. The most common form, open-angle, has few, if any, symptoms and may cause partial vision loss before it is detected. This major public health problem affects approximately 3 million older Americans and is associated with more than 120,000 blind older adults (Glaucoma Research Foundation, 2017).

Glaucoma results from a blockage in the drainage of the fluid (the aqueous humor) in the anterior chamber of the eye. Normally, this fluid drains through the Schlemm canal and is transported to the venous circulation system. If the fluid forms in the eye faster than it can be eliminated, intraocular pressure (IOP) increases. Pressure is then transferred to the optic nerve, where irreparable damage, possibly even total blindness, may result. Three types of glaucoma are found in older adults: chronic open-angle glaucoma, acute angle-closure glaucoma, and secondary glaucoma.

Chronic Open-Angle Glaucoma. Chronic open-angle glaucoma, the most common type (making up 90% of all primary glaucoma), develops slowly. Degenerative changes in the Schlemm canal obstruct the escape of aqueous humor, resulting in increased IOP. This type of glaucoma may damage vision so gradually and painlessly that a person is unaware of a problem until the optic nerve is badly damaged. Visual loss begins with deteriorating peripheral vision, intolerance to glare, loss of contrast perception, and difficulty adapting to the dark (Boltz et al., 2016).

Acute Angle-Closure Glaucoma. This is acute glaucoma that occurs suddenly because of complete blockage. This is a medical emergency and requires immediate medical attention to avoid severe vision loss or blindness. The following symptoms of closed-angle glaucoma occur rapidly:
- Severe eye pain
- Redness in the eye
- Clouded or blurred vision
- Nausea and vomiting
- Bradycardia
- Rainbow halos surrounding lights
- Pupil dilation
- Steamy appearance of cornea

Secondary Glaucoma. Secondary glaucoma occurs due to complications from other medical conditions or certain drug therapies. Uncontrolled diabetes or hypertension, cataracts, some types of eye tumors, uveitis or other irritation or inflammation are examples. Steroid drugs may trigger glaucoma. Serious eye injuries or surgical procedures may also lead to onset of glaucoma.

NURSING MANAGEMENT OF GLAUCOMA

Assessment

Patients with glaucoma may complain of dull eye pain, or they may experience no early symptoms. Visual field testing reveals a loss of peripheral vision (tunnel vision), and increased IOP is seen on ophthalmologic examination. Patients also may report increased difficulty seeing in low light or darker rooms and increased sensitivity to glare.

Diagnosis

Potential nursing diagnoses for the patient with glaucoma include the following:
- Need for patient teaching resulting from lack of exposure and inexperience regarding glaucoma causes and treatments
- Pain resulting from increased IOP
- Potential for infection resulting from eye drop instillation
- Decreased ability to dress self resulting from visual impairment

Planning and Expected Outcomes

Expected outcomes for the patient with glaucoma include the following:
1. The patient will have no further loss of vision.
2. The patient will follow prescribed glaucoma care guidelines daily.
3. The patient will state that eye pain is decreased.
4. The patient will be free from eye infection.
5. The patient will be able to perform ADLs safely and independently.

Intervention

Nursing management is aimed at teaching the patient that glaucoma is a chronic condition requiring lifelong medical treatment. Any current visual loss is permanent, but following the care guidelines outlined in Box 18.2 may prevent further loss. If medication fails to control rising IOP, surgical intervention may be necessary.

Trabeculoplasty is usually performed on an outpatient basis. It requires an IOP check 3 to 4 hours after surgery. A sudden rise in IOP may occur immediately after surgery. A 4- to 8-week wait is necessary to determine whether the procedure was effective. However, continual use of glaucoma medications is necessary.

Trabeculectomy requires overnight hospitalization. Postoperative nursing care for the patient who has had a trabeculectomy includes (1) routine postanesthesia care; (2) protection of the operated eye with an eye patch or a shield, proper positioning of the patient on the back or on the side of the nonoperated eye, and the use of a call light and side rails; (3) administration of pain medications and cold eye compresses to maintain comfort; (4) monitoring of the eye for increased IOP, bleeding, or infection; and (5) assistance and teaching of safe, independent performance of ADLs (NIH, 2017a).

Evaluation

Evaluation includes documentation of the achievement of the expected outcomes, no further vision loss, and the independent performance of ADLs. It is imperative that the patient and family understand the chronic nature of this disease and its treatment. The patient must be able to state the name and

BOX 18.2 The Patient With Glaucoma

1. Medical follow-up and eye medication will be required for the rest of your life.
2. Eye drops *must* be continued as long as prescribed, even in the absence of symptoms.
   a. Blurred vision decreases with prolonged use.
   b. Avoid driving for 1 to 2 hours after administration of miotics.
3. To prevent complications:
   a. Press lacrimal duct for 1 minute after eye drop insertion to prevent rapid systemic absorption.
   b. Have a reserve bottle of eye drops at home.
   c. Carry eye drops on person (not in luggage) when traveling.
   d. Carry card or wear Medic-Alert bracelet identifying glaucoma and the eye drops solution prescribed.
4. Bright lights and darkness are not harmful.
5. No apparent relationship exists between vascular hypertension and ocular hypertension.
6. Report any reappearance of symptoms immediately to the ophthalmologist.
7. If admitted to the hospital for a different medical condition, alert staff of continued need to use prescribed eye drops.
8. Avoid the use of mydriatic or cycloplegic drugs (e.g., atropine) that dilate the pupils.

Data from U. S. Department of Health and Human Services (2017). *Facts About Glaucoma*. Bethesda, MD: Author.

dosage of the prescribed eye medications and describe their daily use, even during periods of travel or hospitalization. The patient must also be able to identify significant signs and symptoms so that they can be reported to the ophthalmologist.

Cataracts

Cataracts are the most common disorder found in the aging adult. Although cataracts are considered an "age-related" condition, it can occur in individuals in their 40s and 50s but typically does not have a significant effect on vision. More than half of Americans over the age of 80 have cataracts or have had a surgical procedure for cataracts. Cataracts can occur in one or both eyes. In addition to aging, other risk factors for cataracts include smoking, prolonged exposure to ultraviolet light, and diabetes.

Changes in the lens lead to cataracts. Over time, protein meant to keep the lens clear and allow light to pass through starts to clump together behind the lens. This creates a cloud in a small area of the lens. This cloud is called a cataract. As the cataract grows, vision becomes more difficult, including reduced sharpness of images reaching the retina. The lens itself becomes discolored over time with a yellow/brown tint.

There are different types of cataracts not specifically age related. A secondary cataract may be related to other health problems such as diabetes or following surgical eye procedures. Some medications such as steroids are also linked to this. A traumatic cataract may develop after an eye injury, maybe years later. A radiation cataract may develop after radiation exposure (NIH, 2015b).

The size and location of a cataract determine the amount of interference with clear sight. A cataract located near the center of the lens produces more noticeable symptoms such as the following:
- Dimmed, blurred, or misty vision
- The need for brighter light to read

- Glare and light sensitivity
- Halo that appears around lights
- Double vision or multiple images in one eye
- Loss of color perception
- Recurrent eyeglass prescription changes

These symptoms develop slowly and at different rates in each eye.

NURSING MANAGEMENT OF CATARACTS

Assessment

Subjective complaints include having trouble reading and the necessity for constantly cleaning one's glasses (the vision difficulties are thought to be caused by dirty glasses). Lens opacity may be visible on external or internal eye examination.

Diagnosis

Nursing diagnoses for the patient with cataracts include the following:

- Anxiety resulting from uncertain surgical outcome
- Need for patient teaching about cataracts resulting from lack of exposure
- Potential for injury resulting from changes in visual acuity
- Decreased ability to dress self resulting from an inability to see the body and face clearly enough to maintain appearance of clothes and cosmetics

Planning and Expected Outcomes

Expected outcomes for a patient with cataracts include the following:

1. The patient will have cataract surgery when recommended by an ophthalmologist.
2. The patient will ask questions about preoperative and postoperative care and report satisfaction with information.
3. The patient's affected eye will be free from increased IOP, stress on the suture line, hemorrhaging, and infection.
4. The patient will verbalize appropriate home care activities to avoid and activities to do after cataract surgery.
5. The patient will demonstrate correct administration of eye drops.
6. The patient will remain injury-free by maintaining a safe environment to avoid falls or bumping into items.
7. The patient will use caution when driving before and after surgery as directed by an ophthalmologist.

Intervention

Nursing management for a patient with cataracts focuses mainly on preoperative and postoperative surgical care because surgery is the only method for treating cataracts. However, asymptomatic patients do not require referral. Most cataract surgery is performed as outpatient surgery with the administration of a local anesthetic; this makes preoperative teaching difficult because patients arrive just hours before surgery. Many ambulatory centers conduct preoperative assessment and teaching via phone calls a week before surgery. Preoperative care involves administering eye drops and a sedative, as ordered. Postoperative care requires teaching the patient and family home care procedures for the period after cataract surgery (see Patient/Family

---

BOX 18.3   Administering Eye Drops

The following steps should be followed to properly administer eye drops:

- Wash hands
- Hold the bottle upside down
- Tilt head back
- Hold the bottle in one hand and place as close as possible to the eye without touching the eye
- Use the other hand to pull down the lower eyelid to form a pocket
- Place the prescribed number of drops into the lower eyelid pocket
- Wait at least 5 minutes in between if administering more than one type of eye drop
- To keep the drops in the eye, close the eye or press the lower lid lightly with one finger for at least 1 minute; this also prevents the drops from draining into the tear duct and increasing the risk of side effects

Data from U.S. Department of Health and Human Services (2017). *Facts About Glaucoma*. Bethesda, MD: Author.

Teaching box: Home Care after Cataract Surgery). It is also important to follow the proper method for instilling eye drops (see Box 18.3). The home care instructions need to include special precautions recommended by the ophthalmologist based on the type of surgery performed. If a lens implant has not been inserted, patients need to wear contact lenses or cataract glasses. Patients wearing cataract glasses experience loss of depth perception and distorted peripheral and color vision. They need to be taught that objects are magnified by 25% and appear larger and closer than they really are; this requires home safety measures and the modification of dressing and cosmetic application after surgery (see Nursing Care Plan).

PATIENT/FAMILY TEACHING

Home Care After Cataract Surgery

What to Expect
- The affected eye may be bruised or bloodshot for up to 7 days
- May experience itching or mild discomfort for several days
- May experience some fluid discharge
- Sensitivity to light
- Eye may have a scratchy or sandlike feeling for up to 2 weeks
- May feel tired for the first 24 hours

Activity Level and Care
- No driving for 2 days or as instructed by provider
- Avoid bending at the waist or heavy lifting for 2 days
- Avoid alcohol for at least 2–4 hours
- Do not rub or press on your eye
- Sleep on back or nonoperative side for 2 nights
- Wear the bandage or eye pad as instructed
- Perform regular hand hygiene before attending to any bandage or eye pad
- Instill eye drops using a clean technique (see Box 18.3)
- Monitor pain and report if unrelieved with medication
- Recognize signs and symptoms of infection and report as soon as possible
- Follow up with provider as recommended

Modified from Lewis, S. M., Bucher, L., Heitkemper, M. M., & Harding, M. M. (2017). *Medical-surgical nursing: Assessment and management of clinical problems* (10th ed). St. Louis, MO: Elsevier; and Fairview Health Services. (2017). Discharge instructions for cataract surgery. Retrieved from https://fairview.org/sitecore/content/Fairview/Home/Patient-Education/Articles/English/d/i/s/c/h/Discharge_Instructions_for_Cataract_Surgery_83388.

NURSING CARE PLAN
Cataracts

Clinical Situation

Mrs. D, a 78-year-old retired nurse, has been admitted to the skilled nursing unit of a local hospital for rehabilitation therapy after repair of a right hip fracture. Her daughter accompanies her. Mrs. D has no significant medical history, but a fall in her home resulted in the break in her hip. She states that she has been having trouble with her eyes, and she tripped on the stairs. Since her admission to the hospital, a vision screening detected cataracts in both eyes, and surgery is recommended once she recovers. Mrs. D requires assistance with all ADLs except eating. She is unable to bear weight on her right leg, so assistance is needed to transfer to the toilet, chair, or bed. She also needs help bathing and dressing the lower half of her body because she cannot reach her legs or feet. Mrs. D states that her biggest concern is fear of falling again.

Nursing Diagnoses

Potential for injury resulting from altered visual acuity
Decreased ability to bathe self resulting from immobility
Decreased ability to dress self resulting from immobility
Decreased ability to toilet self resulting from immobility
Anxiety resulting from fear of falling

Outcomes

The patient will verbalize questions and concerns regarding cataracts and the recommended surgical treatment.
The patient will have cataract surgery, when appropriate.
The patient will not fall.
Patient will maintain a safe environment.
The patient will assist with self-care as much as possible, as evidenced by fulfilling needs for cleanliness, grooming, and toileting.

The patient will report reduced anxiety, as evidenced by a relaxed state and learning about cataract surgery.

Interventions

Provide the patient with the printed information sheet, "Aging and Your Eyes" (review Box 18.1) and the patient education sheet "Home Care after Cataract Surgery" (see Patient/Family Teaching box).
Encourage the patient and family member to speak with an ophthalmologist about the recommended surgery.
Explain preoperative and postoperative procedures resulting from the recommended surgery.
Provide a safe environment (e.g., bed in low position, side rails as needed, and call light and personal items in reach).
Assist with transfers until the patient demonstrates safe transfer while unassisted.
Assess the patient's home for factors that hinder or support vision changes.
Administer pain medication as needed before helping the patient to perform self-care.
Encourage the patient to perform as much of her own care as possible to help restore independence.
Provide assistance, supervision, and teaching with the use of assistive devices, as needed, to perform self-care. Assess factors in the patient's home that support or hinder self-care.
Encourage expression of fears of falling.
Use therapeutic communication to gain insight into the patient's fears and give realistic feedback.
Increase attention to the patient when she is feeling anxious.

Modified from Gulanick, M., & Myers, J. L. (2013). *Nursing diagnosis and intervention: Planning for patient care* (8th ed.). St. Louis, MO: Mosby; Ackley, B. J., & Ladwig, G. B. (2014). *Nursing diagnosis handbook: An evidence-based guide to planning care*. (10th ed.). St. Louis: Elsevier.

Evaluation

Evaluation includes documentation of the achievement of the expected outcomes. Patients who have had successful cataract surgery will be free from complications and will have improved vision. Additionally, they will report performance of their usual daily activities with the use of lens implants, contact lenses, or corrective glasses. The patient and family will arrange for assistance with ADLs for the first 24 to 48 hours after surgery, or they will notify the home health agency.

Retinal Disorders

Three common disorders that affect the retina of an older adult are macular degeneration, diabetic retinopathy, and retinal detachment.

Age-Related Macular Degeneration. Age-related macular degeneration (AMD) is the leading cause of blindness among people over the age of 50 in the United States. It does not cause total blindness but results in loss of central vision. AMD causes damage to the macula leading to changes in the center of the field of vision. Peripheral vision is unchanged by AMD. The cells within the macula diminish in functional ability with age, and replacement of the damaged cells is decreased, causing irreversible damage to the macula (NIH, 2015a). As a result, central visual acuity declines, which makes performance of daily tasks requiring close vision nearly impossible.

Types of AMD include the following:
- **Dry macular degeneration.** Also known as *involutional macular degeneration*, this condition is caused by breakdown

or thinning of macular tissue resulting from the aging process. Vision loss is gradual.
- **Wet macular degeneration.** Also known as *exudative macular degeneration*, this type of AMD results when abnormal blood vessels form and hemorrhage on the retina. Vision loss may be rapid and severe.

AMD is more common among Caucasians than other races. There is also an increased risk in those with a family history. Although there are no recommended genetic tests for AMD, nearly 20 genes have been identified that may affect the risk of developing this eye disorder. Smoking has been shown to double the risk of developing AMD (NIH, 2015a). Lifestyle choices can help reduce the risk of developing AMD, such as avoiding smoking, exercising regularly, eating a healthy diet rich in green leafy vegetables and fish, and maintaining a blood pressure and cholesterol within a normal range.

Symptoms of macular degeneration include the following:
- Difficulty performing tasks that require close central vision, such as reading and sewing
- Decreased color vision (i.e., colors look dim)
- Dark or empty area in the center of vision
- Straight lines appearing wavy or crooked
- Words on a page looking blurred

Diabetic Retinopathy. Loss of visual function is one of the most common complications of diabetes. Altered circulation to the eye may result in retinal edema, degeneration, or detachment. This condition is a complication of diabetes that affects the retinal capillary circulation. Ballooning of these tiny vessels leads to hemorrhaging, scarring, and blindness. These vascular changes, in and around the retina, lead to macular edema, which causes the retina to swell. No symptoms of early retinal changes exist, and no symptoms may be apparent even when the retinopathy is advanced. Early detection requires a complete ophthalmoscopic examination; therefore, patients with diabetes should have yearly examinations by an ophthalmologist.

Hypertension Retinopathy. Another form of retinopathy can be caused by uncontrolled hypertension. In this form of retinopathy, chronic hypertension will cause progressive damage to the retina with few or even no symptoms until the late advancement of symptoms. Abnormalities found include permanent arterial narrowing, arteriosclerosis, and vascular wall hyperplasia. Controlling blood pressure is the primary treatment. Laser procedures or intravitreal injections of corticosteroids may also be used in the case of vision loss (Mehta, 2017).

Retinal Detachment. Retinal detachment occurs when the sensory layer of the retina separates from the pigmented layer. Tears or holes occur in the retina because of trauma, aging (degeneration), hemorrhaging, or the presence of a tumor. When a tear occurs, fluid seeps between the layers, which causes detachment. The usual symptoms include the following:

- Light flashes
- A shower of floaters that resembles spots, bugs, or spider webs
- Loss of vision
- Veil or curtain obstructing vision

NURSING MANAGEMENT OF RETINAL DISORDERS

Assessment

There are no early symptoms of diabetic retinopathy or hypertensive retinopathy and sometimes no symptoms are observed even with advanced retinopathy. Patients with macular degeneration may complain that they are unable to thread a needle or that the words on a page look blurred, making reading difficult. Patients with retinal detachment notice flashes of light followed by floating spots before the eye with progressive loss of vision. The specific area of vision loss depends on where the detachment is located. When detachment occurs quickly and is extensive, the patient may feel that a curtain has been drawn before the eyes.

Ongoing nursing assessment involves monitoring the patient's subjective statements about changes in vision and observing for signs of anxiety. All three retinal disorders are diagnosed with ophthalmoscopy.

Diagnosis

Nursing diagnoses are determined by analysis of the patient assessment. Possible nursing diagnoses for a patient with a retinal disorder include the following:

- Need for patient teaching resulting from lack of exposure to accurate information about the effect of diabetes on eyes
- Need for patient teaching resulting from retinal detachment condition, surgery, preoperative and postoperative care, and home care after surgery
- Anxiety resulting from fear of blindness

Planning and Expected Outcomes

Expected outcomes for an older person with a retinal disorder include the following:

1. The patient will adjust successfully to vision loss by using low-vision aids.
2. The patient will state in his or her own words the effect of diabetes on the eyes.
3. The patient will see an ophthalmologist yearly.
4. The patient will ask questions about preoperative and postoperative retinal surgery care and report satisfaction with the information.
5. The patient's affected eye will be free from further retinal detachment, infection, or hemorrhaging.
6. The patient will verbalize appropriate home care activities to participate in after retinal surgery.
7. The patient will demonstrate correct administration of eye drops.
8. The patient will report reduced anxiety.

Intervention

Patients with macular degeneration and diabetic retinopathy must learn to cope with chronic, gradual vision loss. Patients with macular degeneration are often taught to self-monitor their central vision using an Amsler chart, which is a small printed grid. The appearance of an increase in waves or curves on the grid may indicate worsening disease. Patients must be taught how to obtain and use low-vision aids (Box 18.4). Teaching about the condition and encouraging yearly follow-up visits with an ophthalmologist help patients understand the disease and how it affects their eyes.

Patients with retinal detachment require the immediate care of bed rest in the proper position (i.e., retinal hole in most dependent position) and eye patches (may be prescribed for one or both eyes) until surgery is performed. Safety precautions and means of communicating are essential for the patient at this point. Postoperative care includes administration of eye medication, pain medication, antiemetics (as needed), and cough medication (as needed). Cold compresses are applied to reduce

---

BOX 18.4 Low-Vision Aids

- Magnifying devices: glasses, stand or hand magnifier, telescope, video magnifier. Some have built-in lighting.
- Audio books or electronic books
- Apps for smartphones, computers, and tablets (e.g., AMagnify, DAISY Talk, TapTapSee, Seeing AI)
- Devices with speech capability: watches, timers, blood glucose monitors, blood pressure cuffs, prescription bottles
- Large print reading material and items with large-sized numbers/letters and high-contrast colors
- Increased light: higher-watt light bulbs and number of lights indoors, adjust light to reduce glare inside and wear sunglasses or wide brimmed hat outdoors, use color to create contrast in the house, use a bold felt tip marker to makes lists or notes.
- Request a referral early to access the many low-vision aids and devices to help with daily activities. Many people will need vision rehabilitation to achieve the best possible quality of life. Examples: Light House for the Blind and Visually Impaired (http://lighthouse-sf.org/programs/skills/) or Lions Club International (http://www.lionsclubs.org/EN/how-we-serve/health/sight/index.php).

swelling and promote comfort. Patients must be instructed to avoid jerking movements of the head, as with coughing, sneezing, and vomiting. If the eyes are patched, safety precautions such as keeping call lights, side rails, and necessary items within reach must be instituted. Finally, assistance must be provided with ADLs and walking, as needed, to promote comfort and safety. Home care instructions to teach the patient and family include the following: (1) report increases in floaters or flashes of light, decreased vision, drainage, or increased pain to an ophthalmologist; (2) administer eye drops; (3) limit physical activity for 1 to 2 weeks, and resume active sports and heavy lifting as indicated by a physician; and (4) make follow-up appointments with the ophthalmologist.

Patients with any retinal disorder may experience anxiety about the loss of vision and possible blindness. The opportunity for patients to discuss their concerns needs to be provided. Nurses must also be knowledgeable about available resources.

Evaluation

Evaluation includes documentation of the achievement of the expected outcomes. Patients with macular degeneration and diabetic retinopathy will describe the condition and report use of low-vision aids. These patients will also follow up with annual visits to the ophthalmologist. Patients who have had surgery for retinal detachment will experience no complications and gradual improvement in vision. Patients will limit their physical activity for 1 to 2 weeks with the help of significant others or home health care. Patients with macular degeneration will monitor their central vision with an Amsler chart and report changes to the ophthalmologist. Patients with any retinal disorder will report reduced anxiety, as evidenced by their ability to learn about and cope with their disease.

Visual Impairment

Visual impairment is the most common sensory problem faced by older adults. The visually impaired population includes those with low vision (20/50 to 20/200) and those who are legally blind (visual acuity of 20/200 or worse in the better eye with the aid of the best possible correction with the use of spectacles or contact lens) (Lewis et al., 2017). Blindness in older adults results from diabetic retinopathy, glaucoma, cataracts, and macular degeneration, and its incidence has increased as the number of adults age 65 or older grows.

✚ EMERGENCY TREATMENT

Eye Injuries

Determine Etiology
Trauma: blunt or penetrating
Burn: chemical (acid or alkaline), thermal (direct or indirect burn)
Foreign body penetration (glass, metal, wood, plastic, ceramic)

Common Assessment Findings
* Pain
* Photophobia
* Localized or diffuse redness
* Swelling, ecchymosis, tearing
* Absent eye movement
* Fluid drainage

* Visible foreign body
* Visual loss, decreased vision, or visual field defect

Interventions
Initial:
* Determine cause of injury (etiology)
* Ensure airway, breathing, circulation
* Assess for the following: other injuries considering type of exposure, visual acuity, pain, changes around and in the eye
* Do not put pressure on the eye; instruct patient to not blow the nose
* In case of chemical exposure, irrigate the eye immediately and continue until emergency personnel arrive; if no chemical exposure, do not attempt to treat
* Stabilize foreign objects, but do not attempt to remove
* Cover eye with dry, sterile patch and protective shield
* Elevate the head of the patient to 45 degrees
* Do not provide food or drink to patient
* Administer medications/analgesia only as ordered by a provider
Ongoing Monitoring:
* Provide reassurance to the patient
* Monitor pain, changes in visual acuity, changes in or around the eye
* Prepare patient for potential surgical repair when appropriate

Modified from Lewis, S. M., Bucher, L., Heitkemper, M. M., & Harding, M. M. (2017). *Medical-surgical nursing: Assessment and management of clinical problems* (10th ed.). St. Louis, MO: Elsevier.

Sudden vision loss is considered a medical emergency and should be evaluated immediately. It may be caused by retinal detachment or an eye injury. A trained provider must evaluate this as soon as possible. The medical management of vision loss depends on the type, cause, and amount experienced. In the case of a traumatic eye injury, treatment is dependent on the type of injury (see Emergency Treatment box).

Any patient with a visual disability that cannot be improved by corrective lenses or surgery should be referred to a low-vision specialist or center. Assistive devices for low vision, including glucose monitoring instruments, large-print books, talking clocks, and computer accessories, are available and are continuing to be developed for many health issues (Turbert, 2018).

NURSING MANAGEMENT OF VISION IMPAIRMENT

Assessment

Nursing assessment of the patient with impaired vision requires an understanding of the patient's response to the vision loss. The older adult who becomes suddenly blind usually has a harder time adjusting to the disability than a person who was born blind. Loss of vision may result in a self-esteem disturbance, leading to social isolation. A self-esteem disturbance leads to decreased self-confidence, which may affect interactions with others, the ability to carry out normal daily activities, job performance, and the desire to engage in familiar hobbies. Grief and mourning occur over the loss of vision and result in reactions like those experienced with death, for example, denial, anger, guilt, hopelessness, and depression. The patient's ability to cope with the loss depends on the type, amount, and duration of the vision loss as well as the patient's support system and coping style. Over time, persons with vision loss can compensate by increasing sensitivity in other senses such as hearing, taste, touch, and balance.

Diagnosis

Potential nursing diagnoses for the patient with visual impairment include the following:

- Decreased self-esteem resulting from sudden loss of vision
- Social disengagement resulting from impaired communication
- Inadequate coping resulting from sudden loss of vision
- Decreased ability to feed/bathe/dress/toilet self resulting from visual impairment
- Decreased mobility resulting from visual impairment
- Potential for injury resulting from impaired vision

Planning and Expected Outcomes

Expected outcomes for a patient with visual impairment include the following:

1. The patient will perceive himself or herself positively, by making positive statements about self.
2. The patient will participate successfully in activities with others.
3. The patient will demonstrate increased objectivity and ability to solve problems, make decisions, and communicate needs.
4. The patient will safely provide self-care by using low-vision aids and environmental strategies.
5. The patient will demonstrate the safe and correct use of adaptive devices.

Intervention

Counseling provides an opportunity for persons who have become visually impaired to talk about their feelings, concerns, and anxieties. Once these emotions have been identified, patients may be given assistance in identifying their strengths and resources. Problem solving may lead to alternative ways to complete the tasks of everyday living and participate in recreational activities.

The nurse interacting with a visually impaired patient must rely heavily on various techniques and methods when communicating with that person. See Boxes 18.5 and 18.6 for tips and aids that facilitate communicating and caring for the visually impaired. Keep in mind that these tips can be used in any setting—home care, acute care, or long-term care.

Strategies to increase adaptation to daily living include (1) organizing the environment, (2) encouraging the use of the clock method of eating, and (3) using a sighted guide to assist in ambulation (Box 18.7). Organizing the environment means placing items of clothing in specific drawers or closets to facilitate selection and placing furniture in specific locations to facilitate mobility. Additionally, the use of color-contrast and color-coding schemes helps the patient locate items; bright, sharply contrasting colors make furniture and personal items visually distinct. For example, a bright red toothbrush shows up well against a white sink. Coding schemes that facilitate independent living include applying fluorescent tape around light switches, thermostats, and keyholes. Coding with colored paper, textured paper such as sandpaper, or rubber bands may help the patient differentiate among medication containers. The clock method assists the patient at meals because the location of food on the plate is described in terms of a clock face (e.g., beans at the top of the plate are at the 12 o'clock position; potatoes at the bottom of the plate are at the 6 o'clock position). In addition, the patient may use a piece of bread or roll to push food onto the fork. Sighted guides, who lead persons with visual impairments from place to place, can help a patient walk confidently (see Box 18.7). The use of a cane or a seeing-eye dog also help promote independence in mobility, especially when the patient is in an unfamiliar environment.

BOX 18.5   Signs and Behaviors That May Indicate Vision Problems

Patient May Report*

- Pain in eyes
- Difficulty seeing in darkened area
- Double or distorted vision
- Sudden loss of vision or blurred vision
- Flashes of light
- Halos surrounding lights

Others May Notice the Patient:

- Getting lost
- Bumping into objects
- Straining to read or not reading
- Spilling food on clothing
- Withdrawing socially
- Making less eye contact
- Displaying placid facial expressions
- Viewing the television at close range
- Suffering from a decreased sense of balance
- Mismatching clothes

*These issues should be addressed right away.
Data from U.S. Department of Health and Human Services. (2017). *Aging and your eyes.* Bethesda, MD: Author, and modified from McNeely, E., Griffin-Shirley, M., & Hubbard, A. (1992). Teaching caregivers to recognize diminished vision among nursing home residents. *Geriatric Nursing, 13*(6), 332.

BOX 18.6   Communicating With and Caring for Visually Impaired Nursing Facility Residents

- Always identify yourself clearly.
- Always make it clear when you are leaving the room.
- Make sure you have the resident's attention before you start to talk.
- Try to minimize the number of distractions.
- Whenever possible, choose bright clothes with bold contrasts.
- Check to see that the best possible lighting is available.
- Assess your position in relation to the resident. One eye or ear of the resident may be better than the other.
- Try not to move items in the resident's room. Narrate your actions.
- Try to keep the resident between you and the window or you will appear as a dark shadow.
- Use some means to identify residents who are known to be visually impaired.
- Use the analogy of clock hands to help the resident locate objects.
- Keep color and texture in mind when buying clothes.
- *Be careful about labeling residents as confused! They may be making mistakes because of poor vision.*
- Obtain and encourage the use of low-vision aids.

Modified from McNeely, E., Griffin-Shirley, M., & Hubbard, A. (1992). Teaching caregivers to recognize diminished vision among nursing home residents. *Geriatric Nursing, 13*(6), 332; and Adams-Wendling, L., & Pimple, C. (2008). Nursing management of hearing impairment in nursing facility residents. *Journal of Gerontological Nursing 34*(11), 9-17.

The home health or community health nurse can assist with referral to a social worker who has information on local, state, and federal services available. Services for persons with visual impairments include counseling, mobility training, vocational rehabilitation, self-care skills training, special education, and financial assistance. Low-vision aids such as "talking books," tapes, and tape players are available from public libraries, the National Federation of the Blind, the American Foundation for the Blind, the National Association for Visually Handicapped, the National Braille Association, and the U.S. Library of Congress. Legal blindness entitles a person to some federal assistance based on need. Blind persons can claim an additional tax deduction on their federal income tax returns. The American Council of the Blind (ACB) also has resources for the blind and visually impaired such as a directory of banks with talking ATMs, voting access guide for blind voters, and music resources (ACB, n.d.).

Evaluation

Evaluation includes documentation of the achievement of the expected outcomes, demonstrated by the patient actively participating in self-care and social activities. Patients who display signs and symptoms of depression or social isolation require further counseling to talk about their feelings, strengths, and resources. In addition, alternative visual aids and strategies will need to be identified to increase communication and promote self-care.

HEARING AND BALANCE

The organs of hearing and balance can be divided into three parts: the external ear, the middle ear, and the inner ear. The external ear and middle ear are involved only in hearing; the inner ear is involved in both hearing and balance. The external ear consists of the auricle and the external auditory canal, a passageway from the outside to the eardrum. The middle ear is an air-filled space that contains the tympanic membrane, the eardrum, and the auditory ossicles. The inner ear contains the sensory organs for hearing and balance. It is made up of interconnecting, fluid-filled tunnels and chambers in the petrous portion of the temporal bone (Fig. 18.2).

The organs of balance are located within the inner ear and are divided into two parts. The *vestibule* contains the membranous labyrinth, which consists of the utricle and saccule. This portion evaluates the position of the head relative to gravity or linear acceleration and deceleration. The second part is in the semicircular canals and is called the *kinetic labyrinth*. This labyrinth evaluates the movements of the head.

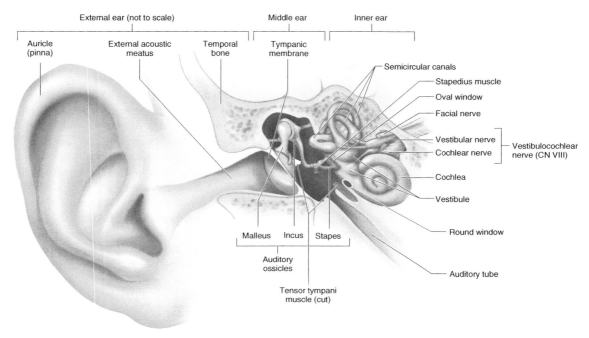

Fig. 18.2 Anatomy of the ear. (From Patton K. T., & Thibodeau G. A. [2013]. *Anatomy and physiology* [8th ed.]. St. Louis, MO: Mosby.)

Age-Related Changes in Structure and Function

Age-related changes in the external ear may be seen in the auricle, which appears larger because of continued cartilage formation and loss of skin elasticity. The lobule of the auricle becomes elongated, with a wrinkled appearance. The periphery of the auricle becomes covered with coarse, wirelike hairs. Compared with women, men have larger tragi, which are laterally situated in the external canal. These tragi become larger and coarser with age. The auditory canal narrows because of inward collapsing. The hairs lining the canal become coarser and stiffer. In addition, cerumen glands atrophy, causing the cerumen to be much drier. In the middle ear, age-related changes in the tympanic membrane cause a dull, retracted, and gray appearance. Degeneration and calcification of ossicular joints in the middle ear has also been noted. Finally, changes within the inner ear result in decreased vestibular sensitivity.

Age-related balance decline is caused by a combination of decreased sensory input, slowing of motor responses, and musculoskeletal limitations. Numerous studies comparing healthy younger and older adults have reported an increase in postural sway in older adults. Despite this increase, most healthy older adults have enough sensory function reserve to maintain postural control. However, deprivation in more than one system is likely to lower the balance threshold. In addition, under conditions in which balance is maximally stressed, for example, climbing up or down steps or curbs and getting in and out of a bathtub, maintaining balance becomes more difficult.

Common Problems and Conditions

Pruritus

Pruritus, itching within the external auditory canal, results from age-related atrophic changes in the skin. Atrophy of the epithelium and epidermal sebaceous glands results in dryness. Often, chronic pruritus of the ear canal results from an itch–scratch–itch cycle initiated by dry skin. The problem may be exacerbated by efforts to retard and remove dry earwax buildup. Several drops of glycerin or mineral oil instilled in the ear canal daily will add moisture to the external ear. Instilling steroid-containing medications in the external canal may treat more resistant conditions.

Cerumen Impaction

Cerumen impaction is a reversible, often overlooked, cause of conductive hearing loss. With increasing age, atrophic changes in the sebaceous and apocrine glands lead to drier cerumen. These changes in the cerumen coupled with a narrowed auditory canal and stiffer, coarser hairs lining the canal lead to cerumen impaction. The cerumen blockage may interfere with the passage of sound vibrations through the external auditory canal to the middle and inner ear, affecting a person's ability to hear and communicate. This impaired communication may then lead to social isolation and depression.

Common symptoms of cerumen impaction include hearing loss, a feeling of fullness in the ear, itching, and tinnitus (ringing in the ears). Identification and removal of the impaction may restore hearing acuity and relieve symptoms associated with impaction. Older adults have a decreased production of cerumen that is a drier consistency creating more risk of impaction in the ear canal (Schwartz et al., 2017).

NURSING MANAGEMENT OF CERUMEN IMPACTION

Assessment

Patients with cerumen buildup may complain of ear fullness, itching, and difficulty hearing. An otoscopic examination will show whether the external ear canal is obstructed by cerumen and whether the tympanic membrane is visible.

Diagnosis

Potential nursing diagnoses for a patient with the aforementioned assessment findings include the following:
- Social disengagement resulting from difficulty communicating with family and friends

Planning and Expected Outcomes

Expected outcomes for a patient with cerumen impaction include the following:
1. The patient will be free from cerumen impaction.
2. The patient will follow proper instillation of softening agents.
3. The patient will report a satisfactory level of involvement with family and friends.

Intervention

The nurse must assess patients for signs of hearing impairment that may indicate cerumen impaction, including (1) difficulty understanding the spoken word (patients may ask why others are mumbling or deliberately excluding them from conversation), (2) loud radio and television volume, (3) withdrawal from social activities and accompanying depression, and (4) possible confusion and paranoia. Once an otoscopic examination reveals an impaction, the nurse should follow the protocol for cerumen removal. For patients living in the community, both patients and their families should be taught how to instill the softening agent. In addition, patients should be instructed to notify their health care provider if they experience a decrease in hearing, any pain, or a ringing or a crackling in their ear.

Management of cerumen impaction (modified from Schwartz et al., 2017):
- Before attempting to remove cerumen, verify any history of ruptured tympanic membrane, tympanostomy tubes, or any recent ear surgery. These may be contraindications for cerumen removal and must be verified with a provider.
- Impaction may be resolved by instilling fluid into the ear canal. This can be an over-the-counter cerumenolytic agent (carbamide peroxide is the only treatment approved for this). Other options for this are two to three drops of baby oil or mineral oil, liquid docusate sodium, or hydrogen peroxide. Avoid hydrogen peroxide if the patient has pruritus or dry skin. The liquid should be instilled daily for 3 to 5 days to resolve the impaction. To instill, have the patient tilt the head to the side not being treated, and hold the auricle as straight as possible. Follow the directions on packaging for length of time the solution should stay in the ear. The ear may be irrigated to remove the loosened cerumen.
- Water or normal saline that has been warmed to body temperature may be used to irrigate using an ear syringe. This is used in the case where the cerumen is deeper in the ear canal

or not cleared with other methods previously listed. For irrigation, the patient should tilt the head to the side being treated with a towel or small basin to catch what is discharged from the ear. Holding the auricle as upright as possible, the irrigating solution should be administered upward in the ear to avoid pressure to the tympanic membrane.

- In cases where liquid is contraindicated or does not resolve the problem, a cerumen spoon or curette may be appropriate. For this method of removal, the patient must be able to remain still during the procedure. The cerumen should be visualized and in the lateral third of the external ear canal. A physician or advanced practice nurse performs this procedure.

Evaluation

The patient will be free from cerumen impaction and verbalize a decrease in ear fullness and an increase in the ability to hear. The cerumen removal should be documented, noting the method of irrigation, the amount and type of debris removed, and the patient's response. The patient will demonstrate the proper method to instill the softening agent. The patient will also state the ear symptoms to report to his or her health care provider.

Tinnitus

Tinnitus is a chronic combination of both conductive and sensorineural hearing loss. It is a subjective sensation of noise in the ear, defined as a ringing, buzzing, or hissing. Tinnitus occurs more frequently in whites, and the prevalence of tinnitus is almost twice as frequent in the south as in the northeast. Individuals at any age may experience tinnitus, but its prevalence increases with advancing age. About 12.3% of men and almost 14% of women age 65 and older are affected by tinnitus. For most, it is an annoying and bothersome condition, and for others, it is an indication of permanent hearing loss or a tumor (Benson, 2018).

The most common causes of tinnitus are noise or toxin damage to the hair receptors of the cochlear nerve and age-related changes in the organs of hearing and balance. Tinnitus is not a disease but a symptom associated with many diseases, conditions, and medical treatments. Tinnitus is classified as subjective or objective. Subjective tinnitus is audible only to the patient. It is characterized as ringing, buzzing, or humming. Objective tinnitus, although rare, is audible to both the patient and the examiner. It is more likely to be low pitched and is often associated with an identifiable cause such as muscle spasms or vascular and musculoskeletal cranial disorders. An additional important classification of tinnitus is whether it is bilateral or unilateral. Unilateral tinnitus is associated with more serious diseases, such as Meniere disease, tumors, or vascular problems, and requires an extensive workup (Benson, 2018).

NURSING MANAGEMENT OF TINNITUS

Assessment

The Tinnitus Screener can be used to assess the patient for the presence and level of tinnitus (Box 18.8). In addition, the patient should answer questions about the effect of the tinnitus on daily living. Tools such as the Tinnitus and Hearing Survey (Henry, Greist, Zaugg, et al., 2015) can identify the effect of tinnitus, hearing loss, and sound tolerance.

BOX 18.8   Tinnitus Screener: Interview-by-Clinician Version

During the past year:
1. Have you experienced tinnitus lasting more that 2 to 3 minutes?
   No—stop here—no tinnitus
   Yes—go to #2
2. Have you experienced tinnitus for at least 6 months?
   No—acute tinnitus
   Yes—chronic tinnitus
3. In a quiet room, can you hear tinnitus?
   Always—stop here—constant tinnitus
   Usually—stop here—constant tinnitus
   Sometimes/occasionally—go to #4
4. When you heard tinnitus this past year, was it caused by a recent event? (e.g., loud concert, head cold, allergies, drugs)
   No—go to #6
   Yes, sometimes—go to #5
   Yes, always—stop here—temporary tinnitus
5. Does your tinnitus seem to "come and go" on its own, in addition to being caused by a recent event(s)?
   No—stop here—temporary tinnitus
   Yes—go to #6
6. Do you experience tinnitus on a
   Daily or weekly basis—stop here—intermittent tinnitus
   Monthly or yearly basis—stop here—occasional tinnitus

National Center for Rehabilitative Auditory Research. (2017). Tinnitus Screener: Interview-by-clinician. Retrieved June 12, 2018 from https://www.ncrar.research.va.gov/Education/Documents/TinnitusDocuments/TinnitusQuestionnaires.asp.

Diagnosis

Potential nursing diagnoses for the patient with tinnitus include the following:

- Inadequate health maintenance resulting from a lack of knowledge about tinnitus prevention practices
- Anxiety resulting from coping with the chronic condition of ringing in the ears

Planning and Expected Outcomes

Expected outcomes for the patient with tinnitus include the following:

1. The patient will follow tinnitus prevention practices.
2. The patient will use home masking measures and a hearing aid or tinnitus masker to relieve tinnitus.
3. The patient will cope with anxiety independently by using relaxation techniques.

Intervention

Nursing interventions are outlined in Box 18.9. Patients should be taught prevention practices, including (1) treating correctable problems (e.g., cerumen impaction and ear infections) that cause tinnitus, (2) softening loud sounds through improved acoustics, (3) using protective ear plugs, and (4) avoiding foods, drinks, and drugs that contain ototoxic substances. Teach patients about the following home masking measures that produce a variety of distracting sounds:

- Portable radio tuned between stations
- Loud ticking clock
- Soft, pleasant music

BOX 18.9 Chronic Tinnitus Interventions

Mild Tinnitus (Does Not Affect ADLs)
- Reassure the older adult that tinnitus is not life-threatening.
- Instruct the patient to avoid ototoxic substances in foods, drinks, and drugs.
  - Avoid quinine, aspirin, and antiinflammatory drug compounds.
  - Avoid caffeine, sodium, chocolate, tea, and alcohol.

Moderate Tinnitus (Interferes With Sleep and ADLs)
- Teach simple home masking measures to relieve tinnitus:
  - Radio tuned between stations
  - Clocks that tick loudly
  - Soft, pleasant, distracting music
  - Semielevated head position to sleep
- Recommend evaluation for properly fitted hearing aid; may relieve tinnitus even if hearing loss is mild.
- More sophisticated, commercial tinnitus maskers and instruments may be matched to the individualized pitch of one's tinnitus.
- Use habituation therapy (exposing patients to low-level broad-band noise produced by wearable noise generators).
- Medications (e.g., amitriptyline [Elavil], zolpidem [Ambien], alprazolam [Xanax], lorazepam [Ativan], and histamines) may be used, but with caution because they may cause drowsiness and mental confusion.

Severe Tinnitus
- Refer patient for extensive counseling and education.
- Apply all moderate tinnitus interventions.
- Teach relaxation methods to cope with stress and promote sleep; combined with biofeedback, this has proved to be beneficial for long-term sufferers of tinnitus.
- Perform electrical stimulation.
- Perform acupuncture.
- Perform surgery (rare; for those patients with objective tinnitus or those who have no auditory function and perceive tinnitus as originating from the non-functioning ear).
- Contact local self-help tinnitus support groups (for information, contact the American Tinnitus Association, www.ata.org).

Data from Ross, V., Echevarria, K. H., & Robinson, B. (1991). Geriatric tinnitus: Causes, clinical treatment and prevention. *Gerontological Nursing, 17*(10), 6; Seidman, M. D., & Jacobson, G. P. (1996). Update on tinnitus. *Otolaryngological Clinics of North America, 18*(3), 455; and Ruppert, S. D., & Fay, V. (2012). Tinnitus evaluation in primary care. *The Nurse Practitioner, 37*(10), 20-26.

- Electric fan
- Sleeping with head elevated on two pillows

Recommend that patients get evaluated for aids or a specially designed masker to lessen tinnitus. Coping strategies to relieve anxiety and stress – for example, relaxation training, biofeedback, and counseling – should also be taught.

Evaluation

Patients following recommended tinnitus interventions and strategies to cope with the chronic ringing in their ears will show achievement of the expected outcomes. The Tinnitus Handicap Inventory was published in 1996 to identify the problems that individuals have with tinnitus. The 25-question inventory delves into feelings and interference with living issues (American Tinnitus Association n.d.). Some areas of interference in daily living include the ability to concentrate, frustration, stress, and problems with sleep, among others. Patients noting no improvement or increase in symptoms should be referred to a multidisciplinary team (specializing in tinnitus) composed of an otolaryngologist, audiologist, and psychiatrist for evaluation and counseling. Patients taking medications should be free from side effects. Those displaying adverse side effects should report to their health care provider for dosage modification, alternative drug therapy, or discontinuation of the medication.

Hearing Loss

Approximately 17% (36 million) of American adults report some degree of hearing loss. A strong correlation exists between age and hearing loss; however, hearing loss is not a normal part of the aging process and should be further evaluated for proper treatment. More than 30% of adults age 65 or older in the United States have some type of hearing impairment, and only one out of five people who could benefit from a hearing aid actually wears one (NIH, 2017b).

Hearing impairment is classified as conductive, sensorineural, or mixed. Conductive hearing loss results from interruption of the transmission of sound through the external auditory canal and middle ear. Conditions that may result in conductive hearing loss are cerumen impaction, otitis media, and otosclerosis (fixation of auditory ossicles).

Sensorineural hearing loss results when the inner ear, auditory nerve, brainstem, or cortical auditory pathways do not function properly so that sound waves are not interpreted correctly. Mixed hearing loss is a conductive hearing loss superimposed on a sensorineural hearing loss.

Older adults with sensorineural hearing loss are increasingly selecting cochlear implants. This implant is surgically placed in the mastoid bone (behind the ear) where it transmits electrical signals by way of the auditory nerve to the brain's hearing center (Ham, Sloane, Warshaw et al., 2013; National Institute on Deafness and Other Communication Disorders, 2016).

Presbycusis

Presbycusis, a sensorineural hearing loss, is the most common form of hearing loss in older adults. Typically, the loss is bilateral, resulting in difficulty hearing high-pitched tones and conversational speech. It affects men more than women. The cause of presbycusis remains unclear. Studies designed to identify a direct cause have proven no clear correlation. Therefore the diagnosis is one of exclusion, which involves ruling out other causes of hearing loss:
- Noise-induced hearing loss (i.e., prolonged exposure to loud noise)
- Infection
- Head injury
- Metabolic disease (of the pancreas or kidneys)
- Vascular disease
- Heart disease
- Genetic factors

Signs and symptoms displayed by the patient include the following:
- Increasing the volume on the television or the radio
- Tilting the head toward the person speaking
- Cupping the hand around one ear

- Watching the speaker's lips
- Speaking loudly
- Not responding when spoken to

NURSING MANAGEMENT OF HEARING LOSS

Assessment

Subjective data that should be obtained from an older patient with hearing loss include onset, type, and progression of hearing loss, including differences in either ear; a family history of hearing loss; the presence of other symptoms such as pressure or pain in the ears, ringing in the ear, or dizziness; a history of head injury or noise exposure; and current medications with known ototoxic effects. Objectively, the patient may display some behavioral symptoms of hearing loss (Box 18.10). A complete hearing evaluation should be conducted.

Diagnosis

Nursing diagnoses based on analysis of the patient's hearing loss include the following:
- Social disengagement resulting from difficulty with communication
- Potential for chronic low self-esteem resulting from hearing loss

Planning and Expected Outcomes

Expected outcomes for a patient with a hearing loss include the following:
1. The patient will effectively use aural rehabilitative techniques.
2. The patient will maintain satisfactory social contacts and activities with others.
3. The patient will perceive himself or herself positively, as evidenced by positive self-talk and behaviors.

Intervention

Interventions for the patient with a hearing impairment focus on aural rehabilitation and facilitation of communication. Patients often deny their hearing loss and need much encouragement and support to explore the various methods to improve hearing. The nurse should provide patients with a printed information sheet on hearing loss (Box 18.11).

Aural rehabilitation includes auditory training, speech and reading training, and hearing aids. Auditory training helps the person with a hearing impairment listen to a speaker by

---

BOX 18.10   Behavioral Clues Indicating Difficulty Hearing

- Difficulty hearing over the telephone
- Finding it hard to follow conversation when two or more persons are talking at the same time
- Turning up the volume on the television so loud that others complain
- Presence of background noise interferes with ability to hear
- Complaining about people mumbling
- Difficulty understanding women and children talking
- Asking for frequent repetition of what others are saying

Data from National Institutes of Health. National Institute on Aging (2017). Hearing loss: A common problem for older adults. Retrieved from https://www.nia.nih.gov/health/hearing-loss-common-problemolder-adults.

BOX 18.11   Hearing and Older Adults

1. Presbycusis is the normal hearing loss associated with aging. This is also called age-related hearing loss and comes on gradually. It occurs due to changes in the inner ear and auditory nerve and seems to run in families. It creates difficulty with hearing what others are saying and tolerating loud sounds. Presbycusis may most often affect both ears equally. Due to gradual onset, the individual may not recognize the hearing loss.
2. Tinnitus or ringing in the ears is another common problem for older adults. This is typically described as ringing in the ears and is a symptom, not a disease. It can be as simple as earwax causing a blockage in the ear canal or the result of numerous health conditions (such as high blood pressure or allergies), or can be a medication side effect. Tinnitus may be in one ear or bilateral and described as ringing, roaring, clicking, hissing, or buzzing. It may be constant or intermittent and can accompany other forms of hearing loss.

Data from National Institutes of Health. National Institute on Aging (2017). Hearing loss: A common problem for older adults. Retrieved from https://www.nia.nih.gov/health/hearing-loss-common-problemolder-adults.

---

differentiating among gross sounds. Speech and reading training includes lip reading and speech skills. Lip reading requires understanding of verbal communication by integrating lip movements, facial expressions, gestures, and environmental clues. This process is extremely difficult without auditory clues. Speech skills must be conserved with the reduced auditory feedback experienced by the patient with impaired hearing. Older adults who have hearing impairments must learn to work intelligently with inefficient communication and decreased speech (see Patient/Family Teaching: Strategies to Improve Communication When There Is Hearing Loss). Hearing aids amplify sound but do not improve the ability to hear. Technologic advances currently offer patients a wide variety of amplification options to suit their changing environmental needs (i.e., quiet to noisy). Patients and their families should be instructed on the basics of hearing aid use and care (see Patient/Family Teaching: Assisted-Listening Devices). All nurses and nursing assistants should have a basic understanding of how to work with a hearing aid to assist the patient unable to care for the aid. Patients and their families should be taught where to obtain and how to use assisted-listening devices (see Patient/Family Teaching Box: Hearing Aid Assessment Tool for Cleaning, Inserting, and Troubleshooting and Health Promotion/Illness Prevention: The Ear).

PATIENT/FAMILY TEACHING

Strategies to Improve Communication When There Is Hearing Loss

- Speak clearly and use a normal tone of voice. Avoid talking fast.
- Get closer to the person and make eye contact.
- Don't shout. This makes it harder for the person to understand.
- Get the attention of the person before speaking.
- Keep your hands away from your mouth.
- Choose a quieter location to talk.
- Build breaks into the conversation. It may be tiresome for the person to try to listen for long periods.

American Speech-Language-Hearing Association. (2015). Age-related hearing loss. Retrieved from http://www.asha.org/uploadedFiles/AIS-Hearing-Loss-Age-Related.pdf.

PATIENT/FAMILY TEACHING

Assisted-Listening Devices

Assistive devices or assistive technology has become more accessible and available with advancing technology. These systems allow a hearing-impaired person to communicate more effectively and function more independently.

Assisted listening devices (ALDs) help to improve sound transmission and include:
- Hearing loop systems
- Frequency-modulated systems (FM)
- Infrared systems
- Personal amplifiers

Alerting devices may connect with a sound device such as a doorbell, telephone, or smoke detectors or other alarms and add blinking lights and louder sound.

Augmentative and alternative communication devices include:
- Closed-captioned television and telephones
- Teletypewriters – less common with the new technology

Data from National Institutes of Health. National Institute on Deafness and Other Communication Disorders. (2016). Quick statistics about hearing. Retrieved from www.nidcd.nih.gov/health/statistics/quickstatistics-hearing.

PATIENT/FAMILY TEACHING

Hearing Aids Care and Troubleshooting

General care:
- Perform listening checks daily
- Perform battery checks and keep spare batteries on hand
- Clean hearing aids regularly using a soft, dry cloth
- Minimize exposure to moisture; store in a hearing aid drying container with batteries removed
- Avoid feedback; hearing aid should be securely seated in the ear and fitted to proper size

If hearing aid has weak sound or is not working:
- Be sure it is switched on
- Check battery for correct placement
- Check for any blockage in the receiver opening or vent opening with cerumen or other debris
- Check all tubing for proper connections, no bends or twists
- Check microphone for blockage

If sound is distorted or intermittent:
- Check for moisture and remove with an air blower
- Check tubing and any cords that connect the hearing aid or other assistive devices for cracks and holes; notify audiologist if these are present
- Replace battery

American Speech-Language-Hearing Association. (2015). Daily care and troubleshooting tips for hearing aids. Retrieved from https://www.asha.org/uploadedFiles/AIS-Hearing-Aids-Troubleshooting.pdf.

HEALTH PROMOTION/ILLNESS PREVENTION

The Ear

Health Promotion
- Notify physician of any pain, discharge, redness, swelling, dizziness, ringing in ears, or loss of hearing.
- See physician for early detection and appropriate treatment of hearing difficulties and ear disease (e.g., cerumen impaction, tinnitus, presbycusis, and vertigo).
- Maintain prescribed hearing aids, assistive listening devices, and medications.

Prevention of Disease
- Have a periodic ear examination and screening for ear disease and hearing problems.
- Avoid exposure to hazardous noise.
- Use protective earplugs in high-risk occupations and activities.

Evaluation

Evaluation is based on documentation of the achievement of expected patient outcomes, as evidenced by the patient using aural rehabilitation techniques and devices to enhance communication. The patient and family should demonstrate the proper use, cleaning, and troubleshooting of the hearing aid. The older patient should remain actively involved with others and the environment. Those older patients displaying signs and symptoms of depression and social isolation will require further encouragement and support to explore other methods to improve hearing.

Dizziness and Disequilibrium

Dizziness and disequilibrium are common complaints of older adults. Although a general decrease occurs in vestibular sensitivity with aging, the symptoms of dizziness or imbalance should not be considered a normal part of aging. Balance disorders contribute to deficits in ambulation that may interfere with an older person's ability to carry out normal ADLs. The five age-related conditions of disequilibrium that have been documented in older adults are as follows:

1. **Benign paroxysmal positional vertigo:** severe episodes of vertigo precipitated by a particular change in head position
2. **Ampullary disequilibrium:** vertigo or disequilibrium associated with rotational head movements
3. **Macular disequilibrium:** vertigo precipitated by a change of head position in relation to the direction of gravitational force (e.g., severe dizziness when rising from bed)
4. **Vestibular ataxia of aging:** a feeling of unbalance when ambulating
5. **Meniere's disease:** an uncommon disease seen most often in older women, characterized by severe vertigo accompanied and usually preceded by tinnitus and progressive low-frequency sensorineural hearing loss

Although the vestibular system of the inner ear is the most common source of dizziness and balance disorders, the following causes must also be considered:
- Visual disturbances
- Musculoskeletal disorders
- Neurologic dysfunctions
- Metabolic abnormalities
- Cardiovascular disease
- Medications

Signs and symptoms vary for each disorder but may include any of the following:
- Whirling dizziness when the head is moved in a certain position
- Dizziness or imbalance when the head is moved quickly to the right, left, up, or down
- Constant feeling of imbalance when walking

Meniere Disease

Meniere disease is caused by pressure within the labyrinth of the inner ear, which is a result of excessive endolymphatic fluid that causes swelling in the cochlea. What causes the excessive fluid is unclear. The three major characteristics are vertigo, tinnitus, and hearing loss. Other associated symptoms include loss of balance, nausea and vomiting, and spasmodic eye movements.

Roughly 615,000 people have been diagnosed with Meniere disease in the United States, and another 45,500 are newly diagnosed each year (NIH, 2015).

NURSING MANAGEMENT OF VERTIGO

Assessment

Subjective data include a description of vertigo episodes (including frequency and duration); a list of accompanying symptoms, such as nausea and vomiting, hearing loss, or tinnitus; a history of balance problems; and a drug history. Objective data include a complete assessment of hearing and balance.

Diagnosis

Potential nursing diagnoses for the patient with vertigo and Meniere disease include the following:
- Potential for injury resulting from acute onset of vertigo
- Need for patient teaching resulting from lack of exposure and inexperience about cause of vertigo and its treatment
- Need for patient teaching resulting from lack of exposure to preoperative and postoperative surgical care for Meniere's disease
- Anxiety resulting from uncertainty of future vertigo attacks

Planning and Expected Outcomes

Expected outcomes for the patient include the following:
1. The patient will accurately follow the prescribed medication regimen and exercise protocol.
2. The patient will safely follow measures to reduce dizziness and prevent falls.
3. The patient will state the causes and treatment of vertigo.
4. The patient will ask questions about the surgical care for Meniere disease.
5. The patient will meet his or her own self-care needs, as evidenced by reports of normal appetite, sleep, and activity.

Intervention

Pharmacologic treatment includes antivertiginous drugs such as meclizine or diphenhydramine. Meclizine may cause drowsiness; patients should be instructed to avoid alcoholic beverages while taking this drug. Patients with a history of asthma, glaucoma, or enlargement of the prostate gland must be monitored carefully while taking meclizine because of its anticholinergic action. Diphenhydramine, an antihistamine, is likely to cause dizziness, sedation, and hypotension in older patients. A diuretic such as hydrochlorothiazide (HCTZ) and a low-sodium diet help remove excess endolymphatic fluid. Older patients undergoing diuretic therapy need to be monitored for evidence of fluid or electrolyte imbalances.

Vestibular rehabilitation therapy is conducted by a physical therapist who designs an exercise program designed to help train the brain to use other senses that can substitute for the deficiencies created by a vestibular disturbance (Farrell, 2015).

Surgery may be performed for Meniere disease to prevent further damage and sensorineural hearing loss. An older patient undergoing ear surgery is given a local anesthetic. Preoperative care includes giving instructions for postoperative care and

sedating the patient. Postoperative care includes (1) positioning the operative ear up for 4 hours after surgery; (2) medicating for pain and vertigo; (3) following safety precautions (e.g., side rails up, call light in reach, and assistance with ambulation); (4) monitoring the patient for changes in hearing, vertigo, neurologic symptoms (e.g., headache), or facial paralysis; and (5) instructing the patient to keep his or her mouth open when sneezing or coughing.

No complete cure for vertigo exists. Therefore patients must be taught the following measures to reduce dizziness: (1) move slowly; (2) avoid bright, glaring lights (a quiet, darkened room is best); and (3) if vertigo occurs during ambulation, lie down immediately and hold the head still. The patient with vertigo must be taught the causes of vertigo and the pharmacologic treatment, vestibular exercises, and measures to reduce vertigo and promote safety during an acute attack.

Evaluation

Evaluation includes achievement of the expected outcomes, as evidenced by patients accurately following the prescribed medication regimen and exercise protocol. Patients displaying adverse side effects should report these to their health care provider for a modification in their medication regimen. Patients should be free from falls by following measures to reduce dizziness. Those with reported falls should be evaluated with a fall assessment tool and taught alternative safety measures.

TASTE AND SMELL

The senses of taste and smell detect the esthetics and safety of the environment. Some evidence suggests that the senses of smell and taste diminish with aging. Loss of smell and taste may affect an older person's food choices and intake, and subsequently impair nutritional and immune status, which may exacerbate disease states. A decreased sensitivity to odors puts the older person at potential risk for noxious chemicals and poisonings (e.g., a person may fail to detect the odor of smoke or leaking gas).

Age-Related Changes in Structure and Function

Age-related changes in the senses of smell and taste result from alterations in the oral mucosa and tongue, and the pathologic state of the nasal cavity. Anatomic and physiologic changes occur with aging (e.g., reductions in cell number, damage to cells, and diminished levels of neurotransmitters). In healthy older adults, olfactory losses result from normal aging, medications, viral infections, long-term exposure to toxic fumes, and head trauma. Most studies indicate a dramatic decline in sensitivity to airborne chemical stimuli with aging. Additionally, recognition of odors declines dramatically with age.

The cause of taste changes in normal aging is not fully understood. Studies of anatomic losses in the structures of the taste system in older adults report conflicting findings. Taste losses result from disease states of the nervous and endocrine systems, nutritional and upper respiratory conditions, viral infections, and medications. The most common cause of change in the sense of taste is thought to be due to xerostomia, which is discussed next (Boltz et al., 2016).

Common Problems and Conditions

Xerostomia

Xerostomia, commonly referred to as *dry mouth,* is a subjective sensation of abnormal oral dryness. Reduced salivary flow is a common complaint of older adults. Longitudinal studies have established that salivary flow from the parotid gland is unchanged with advancing age. Factors leading to a dry mouth include disease states (e.g., Alzheimer's disease, depression, Sjögren syndrome), conditions (e.g., radiotherapy of the head and neck or mouth breathing), and medications (e.g., sedatives, antihistamines, antidepressants, diuretics, chemotherapy, or anticholinergics).

Dry mouth in older adults may lead to increased risk of serious respiratory infection, impaired nutritional status, and reduced ability to communicate. Complaints of abnormal taste sensations, burning of the oral tissues and tongue, and cracking of the lips are common. The oral mucosa is dry, thin, and smooth, and the tongue may have a thick, white, foul-smelling coating. The decrease in salivary flow interferes with chewing and swallowing. Patients with dentures may complain of sore gums and tissues, and denture slippage from the loss of salivary flow, which forms a mechanical barrier.

NURSING MANAGEMENT OF XEROSTOMIA

Assessment

Subjective assessment should include a health history of factors leading to a decrease in salivary flow and the patient's oral complaints. Objective assessment of the lips of a patient with xerostomia reveals red, inflamed, cracked, and dry lips, and they may bleed. The tongue has red areas and a coated base; it appears thicker, with a prominent lingual groove and papillae. The mucous membranes of the palate and the lining of the mouth and gums appear dry, red, and edematous. The saliva is scant, ropy, and viscid. The amount of moisture in the oral cavity is assessed by running a gloved finger over the oral mucosa to evaluate stickiness, which indicates dry mucous membranes. The patient's voice may be dry and raspy, and he or she may complain of difficulty articulating words. Taste testing is performed to evaluate taste sensation, which may be diminished.

Diagnosis

Potential nursing diagnoses for the patient with xerostomia include the following:

- Inadequate oral mucous membrane resulting from changes induced by xerostomia
- Inadequate nutrition resulting from changes induced by xerostomia

Planning and Expected Outcomes

Expected outcomes for the patient with xerostomia include the following:

1. The patient will verbalize an increase in taste sensation.
2. The patient will exhibit unimpaired oral mucosa tissue integrity, as evidenced by moist, pink, smooth mucosal surfaces.
3. The patient will verbalize no oral discomfort.
4. The patient will state contributing factors, symptoms, and treatment of xerostomia.
5. The patient will demonstrate a correct oral hygiene regimen.

Intervention

Nursing interventions for the patient with xerostomia focus on attaining intact oral mucosa tissue integrity. Teaching patients about the factors leading to a decrease in salivary flow, as well as the associated symptoms, is key to the prevention and treatment of xerostomia. The treatment regimen focuses on increasing salivary flow. Patients need to be taught the basic oral hygiene of brushing teeth twice daily with a soft toothbrush and a nonabrasive fluoride toothpaste, as well as daily flossing. Fluid balance is vital for maintaining moisture in the oral cavity. Patients need to take in 2 to 3 liters (L) of fluid per day, if not contraindicated. Also, foods prepared with gravy or sauces contain moisture and should be included in the diet, if not contraindicated. Additional methods to teach patients to increase salivary flow include the use of artificial saliva, sugar-free hard candy, and gum.

Evaluation

Evaluation of the interventions is based on the appearance of the oral mucous membranes, the patient's relief of symptoms, and an increased level of comfort through effective daily treatment practices.

🏠 HOME CARE

1. Sensory changes may lead to social isolation in homebound older adults (e.g., not being able to interact effectively with family members because of visual or hearing deficits).
2. Sensory changes increase safety hazards (e.g., burning or falling) for homebound older adults.
3. Instruct caregivers and homebound older adults about signs and symptoms of age-related sensory changes. Instruct them to report to their physician or home care nurse any signs and symptoms that interfere with independent function or present safety hazards.
4. Instruct caregivers and homebound older adults about prescribed treatments or surgical procedures (e.g., preoperative and postoperative care of cataract surgery, eye drops, eardrops, and antibiotics).
5. Assist caregivers and homebound older adults in organizing the environment to accommodate any decreased sensory function (e.g., use of color contrast, bold print books, hearing aid on the telephone).

TOUCH

At birth, touch is the most developed sense. Touch involves tactile information on pressure, vibration, and temperature. Although touch, pressure, and vibration are commonly classified as separate sensations, the same types of receptors detect them. The only differences among these three are that (1) touch sensation usually results from stimulation of receptors in the skin or in tissues immediately beneath the skin; (2) pressure sensation generally results from deformation of deeper tissues; and (3) vibration sensation results from rapidly repetitive sensory signals.

Sensitivity to light touch diminishes in older adults and may result from a decreased density of cutaneous receptors for touch sensation. Tactile vibratory thresholds progressively increase with age, most likely because of changes in Pacinian corpuscle receptor sensitivity. Studies to evaluate the influence of age on thermal perception report conflicting findings. The warm–cold difference threshold increases with age.

The most common disorders affecting tactile information include cerebrovascular accident (CVA), peripheral vascular disease (PVD), and diabetic neuropathy. All three conditions involve changes in the vascular system that result in decreased blood flow to various parts of the body. Signs and symptoms of a CVA depend on the cerebral artery affected and the portion of the brain supplied by that artery. In PVD and diabetic neuropathy, the impaired blood flow manifests as a loss of sensation most commonly noted in the lower extremities.

The common thread among these disorders is the alteration of peripheral tissue perfusion. Nursing interventions are directed toward preventing accidental trauma and injury in the affected limbs. Patient education focuses on skin, leg, and foot care. The effectiveness of nursing interventions is determined by the absence of trauma, especially in the lower extremities.

SUMMARY

The senses of older adults are the key to their interaction with the environment. As these senses decline because of normal age-related changes or pathologic conditions, nurses in every setting must adapt interventions to promote the highest level of independent functioning.

KEY POINTS

- Studies have documented age-related changes in the senses of vision and hearing.
- Age-related changes in the senses of taste and smell remain questionable.
- A cataract is opacity of the lens and requires surgery for successful treatment.
- Glaucoma is caused by increased IOP and requires lifelong treatment with medications to lower the pressure.
- Retinal detachment requires immediate medical attention and can be repaired only by surgical intervention.
- Wet macular degeneration and diabetic retinopathy can be treated successfully with laser surgery.
- Creating a safe environment with the appropriate level of assistance is important for an older adult who is visually impaired to maintain independence and prevent injury.

- Hearing loss affects an older person's ability to communicate and may lead to depression, social isolation, and loss of self-esteem.
- Prevention and treatment of cerumen impaction is an important nursing function in the care of older adults.
- Vertigo and tinnitus may be chronic and annoying conditions. Each must be treated in ways to assist the older adult with management and maintaining safety.
- Xerostomia may cause pain in the oral mucosa, gums, and tongue, leading to alterations in taste. Treatment includes a daily oral care regimen and methods to increase salivary production.
- Older adults with a diminished sense of touch are at potential for injury, especially in the affected limbs.

CRITICAL-THINKING EXERCISES

1. A 69-year-old woman has tinnitus and episodes of imbalance. Her son and daughter-in-law are concerned about having to leave her alone during the day while they are at work. What strategies could you suggest to the family regarding safety measures in the home?

2. Discuss how loss of sensory function in older adults affects their self-esteem, performance of ADLs, safety, independence, and interactions with others.

REFERENCES

Ackley, B. J., & Ladwig, G. B. (2014). *Nursing diagnosis handbook: An evidenced-based guide to planning care* (10th ed.). Maryland Heights, MO: Elsevier.

American Council of the Blind. (n.d.). Resources. Retrieved June 12, 2018 from http://acb.org/resources.

American Optometric Association. (2017). Color vision deficiency. Retrieved from https://www.aoa.org/patients-and-public/eye-and-vision-problems/glossary-of-eye-and-vision-conditions/color-deficiency.

American Speech-Language-Hearing Association. (2015). Age-related hearing loss. Retrieved from http://www.asha.org/uploadedFiles/AIS-Hearing-Loss-Age-Related.pdf.

American Speech-Language-Hearing Association. (2015). Daily care and troubleshooting tips for hearing aids. Retrieved from http://

www.asha.org/uploadedFiles/AIS-Hearing-Aids-Troubleshooting.pdf.

American Tinnitus Association. (n.d.). Tinnitus handicap inventory (THI). Retrieved from https://www.ata.org/sites/default/files/Tinnitus_Handicap_Inventory.pdf.

Benson, A. G. (2018). Tinnitus. Retrieved June 12, 2018 from https://emedicine.medscape.com/article/856916-overview.

Boltz, M., Capezuti, E., Fulmer, T., & Zwicker, D. (Eds.). (2016). *Evidenced-based geriatric nursing protocols for best practice* (5th ed.). New York, NY: Springer Publishing.

Boyd, K. (2017). *What are floaters and flashers?* Retrieved from the American Academy of Ophthalmology. https://www.aao.org/eye-health/what-are-floaters-flashses.

Cacchione, P. Z. (2014). Sensory impairment: A new research imperative. *Journal of Gerontological Nursing, 40*(4), 3–5.

Farrell, L. (2015). Vestibular rehabilitation: An effective, evidence-based treatment. Retrieved June 12, 2018 from https://vestibular.org/understanding-vestibular-disorder/treatment/treatment-detail-page.

Garrity, J. (2017). Effects of aging on the eye. Retrieved from http://www.merckmanuals.com/home/eye-disorders/biology-of-the-eyes/effects-of-aging-on-the-eyes.

Glaucoma Research Foundation. (2017). Glaucoma facts and stats. Retrieved June 12, 2018 from https://www.glaucoma.org/glaucoma/glaucoma-facts-and-stats.php.

Gulanick, M., & Myers, J. L. (2013). *Nursing diagnosis and intervention: planning for patient care* (8th ed.). St Louis: Mosby.

Ham, R., Sloane, D., Warshaw, G., et al. (2013). *Ham's primary care geriatrics: A case-based approach* (6th ed.). St. Louis: Mosby.

Henry, J. A., Griest, S., Zaugg, T. L., Thielman, C. K., & Carlson, K. F. (2015). Tinnitus and hearing survey: A screening tool to differentiate bothersome tinnitus from hearing difficulties. *American Journal of Audiology, 24,* 66–77.

Kern, D. (2014). Seven sight-saving habits for older adults to help maintain independence. *American Academy of Ophthalmology.* Retrieved from https://www.aao.org/eye-health/tips-prevention/seven-sight-saving-habits.

Lewis, S. M., Bucher, L., Heitkemper, M. M., & Harding, M. M. (Eds.). (2017). *Medical-surgical nursing: Assessment and management of clinical problems* (10th ed.). St. Louis, MO: Elsevier.

McNeely, E., Griffin-Shirley, M., & Hubbard, A. (1992). Teaching caregivers to recognize diminished vision among nursing home residents. *Geriatric Nursing, 13*(6), 332.

National Center for Rehabilitative Auditory Research. (2017). Tinnitus questionnaires. Retrieved from http://www.ncrar.research.va.gov.

National Institutes of Health. National Eye Institute (NEI). (2015a). Facts about age-related macular degeneration. Retrieved from http://www.nei.nih.gov/health/maculardegen/armd_facts.

National Institutes of Health. National Eye Institute. (2015b). Facts about cataract. Retrieved June 12, 2018 from https://nei.nih.gov/health/cataract/cataract_facts.

National Institutes of Health. National Institute on Aging. (2017). Aging and your eyes. Retrieved from https://www.nia.nih.gov/health/aging-and-your-eyes.

National Institutes of Health. National Institute on Aging. (2017). Hearing loss: A common problem for older adults. Retrieved from https://www.nia.nih.gov/health/hearing-loss-common-problem-older-adults.

National Institutes of Health. National Institute on Deafness and Other Communication Disorders. (2016). Quick statistics about hearing. Retrieved from www.nidcd.nih.gov/health/statistics/quick-statistics-hearing.

National Institutes of Health. National Institute on Deafness and Other Communication Disorders. (2016). NIDCD Fact Sheet: Cochlear implants. Retrieved from https://www.nidcd.nih.gov/sites/default/files/Documents/health/hearing/FactsheetCochlearImplants.pdf.

National Institutes of Health. National Institute on Deafness and Other Communication Disorders. (2016). NIDCD Fact Sheet: Assistive devices for people with hearing, voice, speech or language disorders. Retrieved from https://www.nidcd.nih.gov/sites/default/files/Documents/health/hearing/NIDCD-Assistive-Devices-FS.pdf.

National Institutes of Health. National Institute on Deafness and Other Communication Disorders (2015). Meniere's disease. Retrieved from https://www.nidcd.nih.gov/sites/default/files/Documents/health/hearing/MenieresDisease.pdf.

Pinto, J. M., Kern, D. W., Wroblewski, K. E., Chen, R. C., Schumm, P., & McClintock, M. K. (2014). Sensory function: Insights from wave 2 of the national social life, health, and aging project. *Journals of Gerontology, Series B: Psychological Sciences and Social Sciences, 69*(8), S144–S153.

Porter, D. (2017). What are drusen? *American Academy of Ophthalmology.* Retrieved from https://www.aao.org/eye-health/diseases/what-are-drusen.

Schwartz, S. R., Magit, A. E., Rosenfeld, R. M., Ballachanda, B. B., Hackell, J. M., Krouse, H. J., ... Cunningham, E. R. (2017). Clinical practice guideline (update): Earwax (cerumen impaction). *Otolaryngology - Head adn Neck Surgery, 156*(15), S1–S29. https://doi.org/10.1177/0194599816671491.

Turbert, D. (2018). Low vision rehabilitation and low vision aids. *American Academy of Opthalmology.* Retrieved from https://www.aao.org/eye-health/diseases/low-vision-aids-rehabilitation.

19

Cardiovascular Function

Mary B. Winton, PhD, RN, ACANP-BC

e http://evolve.elsevier.com/Meiner/gerontologic

LEARNING OBJECTIVES

On completion of this chapter, the reader will be able to:

1. Explain the age-related changes in the structure and function of the cardiovascular system.
2. Identify contributing risk factors for cardiovascular disease.
3. Explain the pathophysiology and treatment regimen for common cardiovascular conditions.
4. List nursing interventions for cardiovascular conditions.
5. Implement the nursing process for cardiovascular conditions.

WHAT WOULD YOU DO?

What would you do if you were faced with the following situations?

- An older adult neighbor comes to you about his blood pressure of 154/89 mm Hg. The blood pressure was taken at a local supermarket. You know the neighbor also has type 2 diabetes mellitus and does not manage his glucose. What would you do?
- You live with an older adult male who consumes 64 ounces of beer and smokes 1.5 packs of cigarettes daily. You have also noticed that, with moderate activity, he has difficulty breathing. His feet have also been swelling in the last 15 days. What would you do?

Heart disease is the leading cause of death in the United States and is a major cause of disability. Coronary heart disease (CHD) is the principal type of heart disease. According to the Centers for Disease Control and Prevention (CDC), more than 800,000 people die of heart disease in the United States each year, which is about 30% of all U.S. deaths (Benjamin et al., 2017). Direct and indirect costs for the years 2012 to 2013 for cardiovascular related health care were $300 billion, including health care services, pharmacotherapies, and lost productivity (Benjamin et al., 2017). Risk factors for cardiovascular disease (CVD) include elevated cholesterol, hypertension (HTN), diabetes mellitus, tobacco use, physical inactivity, obesity, alcohol use, advancing age, and heredity. As individuals age, the chances of comorbid conditions increase. The reality is that atherosclerosis, the underlying cause of most clinical cardiovascular problems, is typically present for years before the onset of a clinical event such as a heart attack, or symptoms such as angina manifest (Benjamin et al., 2017).

Previous author: Ramesh C. Upadhyaya, RN, CRRN, MSN, MBA, PhD-C.

AGE-RELATED CHANGES IN STRUCTURE AND FUNCTION

Aging alters the cardiovascular system both structurally and physiologically. However, increasing evidence suggests that lifestyle and diet may modify some of these age-related changes (Aronow, 2015; Khan et al., 2013; Yancy, 2017). As people age, changes occur within the heart. For example, the heart rate decreases, the left ventricular wall thickens and results in an overall increase in oxygen demand, and there is increased collagen and decreased elastin in the heart muscle and vessel walls (Huether, McCance, Brasher, & Rote, 2017). The size of the left atrium increases, and aortic distensibility and vascular tone decrease. These changes decrease myocardial muscle contraction resulting in decreased cardiac output and cardiac reserve. Decreases occur in diastolic pressure, diastolic filling, and beta-adrenergic stimulation; increases occur in arterial pressure, systolic pressure, wave velocity, and left ventricular end diastolic pressure; and the muscle contraction, muscle relaxation, and ventricle relaxation phases are elongated (Banasik, 2013b). An S_4 heart sound commonly occurs in older adults (Huether, McCance, Brashers, & Rote, 2017), and about 50% of older adults have a grade 1 or 2 systolic murmur (Jett, 2008).

Conduction System

The sinoatrial (SA) node, atrioventricular (AV) node, and the bundle of His become fibrotic with age (Banasik, 2013b). The number of pacemaker cells located in the SA node decreases with age, which results in less responsiveness of the cells to adrenergic stimulation. Common aging changes reflected by electrocardiography (ECG) include a notched P wave, a prolonged P–R interval, decreased amplitude of the QRS complex, and a notched or slurred T wave (Banasik, 2013b).

Vessels

Calcification of vessels occurs, making them tortuous. The elastin in the vessel wall decreases, which causes thickening and rigidity, especially in the coronary arteries (Ball, Dains, Flynn et al., 2014). This increases the risk of atherosclerotic buildup, especially in those individuals with adverse lifestyle practices. Systolic blood pressure (SBP) is increased in older adults because of a loss of arterial elasticity (Emerson & Lungstrom, 2013). The diastolic blood pressure (DBP) remains the same or may be elevated slightly; thus the pulse pressure widens. Older adults are less sensitive to the baroreceptor regulation of blood pressure. This causes fluctuations in blood pressure and contributes to increased SBP. Isolated systolic hypertension (ISH) is common in the older adult population.

Response to Stress and Exercise

Decreased cardiac output and cardiac reserve diminish the older adult's response to stress. Reduced stress response plus the changes to the heart and vessels affect the body's reaction to exercise. During stress or stimulation, the heart rate increases more slowly; however, once elevated, it takes longer to return to the resting rate (Banasik, 2013b). Nonetheless, this does not exclude older adults from participating in exercise programs.

COMMON CARDIOVASCULAR PROBLEMS

CVD is the leading cause of death for both men and women in the United States, although women tend to be older when their CVD becomes apparent (American Heart Association [AHA], 2015b; Banasik, 2013a). In addition, CVD accounts for more hospital admissions than any other disease or condition. About half of the hospitalizations are attributed to CHD (also referred to as *ischemic heart disease*), and conditions such as strokes, HTN, heart failure, arrhythmias (particularly AV and bundle branch blocks), valvular conditions, and peripheral vascular disease (PVD) account for other CVDs (Banasik, 2013a).

The aging process varies among individuals, which may be attributed to factors of heredity. In addition, the effects of advancing age on cardiovascular structure and function are influenced by the presence of noncardiovascular disease and variations in lifestyle. It may not always be clear which changes in the cardiovascular system are from the normal aging process and which are caused by lifestyle choices (Banasik, 2013a). Many forms of CVD may be accelerated by unhealthy lifestyle choices such as smoking, physical inactivity, high-risk dietary behaviors, obesity, stress, and hormonal use. Chronic diseases such as HTN and diabetes mellitus also play a role in accelerating changes.

Risk Factors for Heart Disease

Risk factors are classified as nonmodifiable and modifiable (Box 19.1). Age, gender, and family history are risk factors that cannot be modified. Smoking, high blood pressure, a high-fat diet, obesity, physical inactivity, and stress are amenable to change. Research has demonstrated that the adoption of a healthier lifestyle has the potential to reduce or prevent the incidence of morbidity and death from ischemic heart disease and stroke.

BOX 19.1   Risk Factors for Cardiovascular Disease

Nonmodifiable
- Male gender
- Age (men >45 years, women >55 years)
- Heredity (including ethnicity)
- Family history of premature CVD (MI or sudden death <50 years in parent or sibling)

Modifiable
- Cigarette smoking/tobacco use
- Hypertension or on antihypertensive drug
- Physical inactivity
- Overweight/obesity
- Diabetes mellitus
- Atherogenic diet (high intake of saturated fats and cholesterol)
- Dyslipidemia

CVD, Cardiovascular disease; *kg/m^2*, kilograms per square meter; *MI*, myocardial infarction.
Modified from National Cholesterol Education Program. (2002). *Third report of the NCEP Expert Panel on Detection, Evaluation, and Treatment of High Blood Cholesterol in Adults (Adult Treatment Panel III).* Washington, D.C.: National Institutes of Health.

Diet

Elevated serum cholesterol levels are a major risk factor for CHD. A total cholesterol (TC) level of 150 milligrams per deciliter (mg/dL) is the point at which atherosclerosis begins to accelerate. Approximately 28 million adults aged 20 and over have TC of 240 mg/dL or greater (Benjamin et al., 2017). Women have a higher prevalence of hypercholesterolemia than men. Risk for CHD increases even with a modestly elevated cholesterol. The serum levels of low-density lipoprotein (LDL) and high-density lipoprotein (HDL) are also important to monitor. LDL (bad cholesterol) carries cholesterol to the walls of the arteries (a positive risk factor), and HDL (good cholesterol) removes LDL from the arterial walls and transports it back to the liver (a negative risk factor). HDL cholesterol levels should be above 60 mg/dL and LDL cholesterol levels below 100 mg/dL (Stone et al., 2013). The levels of cholesterol are taken in context with other risk factors (e.g., diabetes, smoking).

Decreasing fat content in the diet is the first step in reducing TC levels. The AHA recommends reducing the risk of CVD by limiting the intake of saturated and *trans* fat to less than 6% of total calories (AHA, 2017d) Because of the increased risk of CVD in older adults, even seemingly small improvements in risk factors (i.e., small reductions in blood pressure and LDL cholesterol level through diet and lifestyle changes) are of great benefit. However, the AHA warns that, because older individuals have decreased energy needs yet their vitamin and mineral requirements remain constant or increase, they should be counseled to select nutrient-dense choices within each food group (Lichtenstein et al., 2006).

Smoking

Smoking continues to be a major risk factor in the development of heart disease, even though a decline in tobacco use has occurred, largely as a result of health promotion campaigns, clean air environments, and peer pressure. Cigarette smoking greatly increases an individual's risk of stroke, and smokers are more likely to develop CVD than nonsmokers (Benjamin et al., 2017). Smoking increases platelet aggregation and causes coronary artery spasms. Nicotine increases blood pressure and cardiac demands. Carbon monoxide in tobacco smoke decreases the oxygen-carrying capacity of the blood.

Even smoking a few cigarettes per day greatly increases cardiac risk. Smoking cessation decreases the risk of myocardial infarction (MI). After 10 years of abstinence, an individual's risk is the same as that of a nonsmoker. Smoking cessation should be encouraged at every patient encounter. The Agency for Health Care Policy and Research has established recommendations for smoking cessation (see Chapter 20 for smoking cessation information).

Physical Activity

A sedentary lifestyle is another modifiable cardiac risk factor. The AHA (2014) recommends moderate to vigorous aerobic activity for a total of 75 to 150 minutes per week (such as brisk walking) and moderate- to high-intensity muscle-strengthening activity at least 2 days per week.

Before aerobic exercises, a 10- to 15-minute warm-up is recommended to allow for a gradual increase in heart rate and breathing. Walking is the best aerobic exercise for older adults. They may set their own pace, decide the location, and avoid injuries. Health care professionals should encourage patients to exercise and promote ways to increase activity with daily routines such as parking the car a little farther from the store or using the stairs rather than the elevator.

Obesity

Obesity is another modifiable cardiac risk factor. Obesity is usually associated with a sedentary lifestyle and a high-fat diet, which add to the individual's cardiac risk profile. A healthy body weight is currently defined as a body mass index (BMI) of 18.5 to 25 kilograms per square meter (kg/m^2). Overweight is a BMI between 25 and 29.9 kg/m^2, and obesity is BMI 30 kg/m^2 or greater. Currently, more than one-third of adults are obese (Ogden, Carroll, Fryar, & Flegal, 2015). The data from the 2011 to 2014 National Health and Nutrition Examination Survey (NHANES) revealed that 37% of adults aged 60 and over were obese (Ogden, Carroll, Fryar, & Flegal, 2015). Excess body weight increases cardiovascular risk factors (e.g., by increasing LDL, blood pressure, and blood glucose levels, and by reducing HDL levels). Benefits of any physical activity include fewer joint and muscle pains, improved sleep patterns, and reduction of developing type 2 diabetes (AHA, 2014).

Diabetes

Hyperglycemia is related to the incidence of CVDs, which include heart disease, stroke, PVD, cardiomyopathy, and heart failure (Stone et al., 2013). Individuals with diabetes mellitus are two to four times more likely to die of cardiovascular causes, and the presence of diabetes is associated with an increased prevalence of HTN and dyslipidemia (Eckel, Kahn, Robertson, & Rizza, 2006). Silent MI (asymptomatic MI) is more common in individuals with diabetes mellitus and in older adults. Thus older adults with diabetes should be monitored closely for other symptoms of CVD.

Stress

Everyone manages stress differently. Some people respond to stress by overeating, smoking, physical inactivity, or drinking. How a person reacts to stressful situations has a direct effect on health. Excessive stress can trigger asthma, and lead to HTN and irritable bowel syndrome. Excessive stress has also been linked to CHD. Our bodies respond to stressful events by triggering the *fight or flight* response (adrenaline is released, causing tachypnea, tachycardia, and HTN; AHA, 2017c).

Stress can be decreased in many ways, and much literature is available on the topic. Yoga, tai chi, meditation, relaxation tapes, visualization, positive self-talk, doing something enjoyable, and physical activity are a few of the methods used. Nurses must help older adults examine environmental issues that cause stress and work with them to find ways to manage the stress (AHA, 2017a; AHA, 2017c).

Menopause

Before menopause, estrogen is believed to have a protective effect by helping to maintain adequate levels of HDL cholesterol and relaxing the smooth muscles of arteries, which helps maintain normal blood pressure. However, it is believed that these beneficial effects are lost after menopause, and this corresponds to the time when the rate of heart disease–related death for women begins to increase (AHA, 2017b).

Hypertension

HTN continues to be the most common preventable cause of disease and death (Paul et al., 2014). Approximately one in three adults in the United States has HTN and only about 50% are under control (CDC, 2017a). Furthermore, it is estimated that nearly 80% of U.S. older adults will develop HTN by the year 2060 (Patel & Stewart, 2015). HTN contributes to CVD (such as arteriosclerosis and stroke), heart failure (HF), and end organ damage (such as kidney disease). HTN is known as the *silent killer*, and many people are unaware of having HTN because they have no warning signs, or symptoms (e.g., headache or vomiting; CDC, 2017a). Normal blood pressure is an SBP less than 120 mm Hg and/or a DBP less than 80 mm Hg. Blood pressure is categorized as normal, elevated, or stage 1 or stage 2 HTN (Whelton et al., 2017) (see Table 19.1). The BP values are on the basis of average BP taken during office visits for health care.

TABLE 19.1 Blood Pressure Categories for Adults			
BP Category	**Systolic Blood Pressure**	**and/or**	**Diastolic Blood Pressure**
Normal	<120 mm Hg	and	<80 mm Hg
Elevated	120–129 mm Hg	and	<80 mm Hg
Hypertension			
Stage 1	130–139 mm Hg	or	80-89 mm Hg
Stage 2	≥140 mm Hg	or	≥90 mm Hg

Reprinted with permission. Hypertension. 2018;71:1269-1324. ©2018 American Heart Association, Inc.

Among older adults, ISH is more common. Elevated SBP is more predictive of cardiovascular risk than the DBP (Patel & Stewart, 2015). However, it is important to note that low DBP (below 65 mm Hg) increases the risk of subtle heart damage and increases risk of death from all causes (Beddhu et al., 2017). The American College of Cardiology (ACC) and the AHA recently updated the HTN guideline. Older adults age 65 or greater should be treated for HTN with an SBP goal of less than 130 mm Hg and a DBP goal of less than 80 mm Hg. The risk of CVD in older adults has decreased with the more intensive treatment. Prevention and proper management of HTN is necessary to reduce the risk for comorbidities, such as cardiovascular, renal, and cerebrovascular diseases (Qaseem, Wilt, Rich, Humphrey, Frost, & Forciea, 2017).

EVIDENCE-BASED PRACTICE

Frailty Is Significantly Associated With Heart Failure

Sample/Setting
Two thousand eight hundred twenty-five participants aged 70 to 79 years were randomly chosen from white Medicare beneficiaries and black community residents residing in Pittsburgh and Memphis and completed the Health ABC Short Physical Performance Battery (HABC Battery) and the Gill index

Methods
Participants completed a self-reported survey for any hospitalizations and were followed up every 6 months for interim hospitalizations in addition to reviewing medical records. HABC Battery evaluates physical performance in gait speed, repeated chair stands, and tandem balance tests. HABC Battery also assessed lower extremity endurance. The Gill index categorizes participants into either nonfrail, moderately frail, or severely frail based on a combination of chair-stand and walking speed test. Inflammatory biomarkers (e.g., cytokines, interleukin-6, and tumor necrosis factor-α) were obtained after overnight fasting.

Findings
Participants classified as having moderate to severe frailty had a higher risk of developing heart failure compared with nonfrail participants. The results were comparable across age, sex, and race. During a median follow-up of 11.4 years, 466 participants developed heart failure.

Implications
Older adults should have a regular exercise regimen and maintain optimal physical function through resistance training to minimize the risk of developing heart failure. Older adults should be screened to identify individuals at increased risk for heart failure. These individuals may benefit from early interventions to improve physical functioning and quality of life.

From Khan, H., Kalogeropoulos, A.P., Georgiopoulou, V.V., Newman, A. B., Harris, T.B., Rodondi, N., … Butler, J. (2013). Frailty and risk for heart failure in older adults: The health, aging, and body composition study. *American Heart Journal, 166*(5), 887-894.

For primary prevention of CVD in the general public, the ACC and AHA recommend starting therapy drug therapy when the SBP is persistently at or above 140 mm Hg or DBP at 90 mm Hg or above (Whelton et al., 2017). Treatment for secondary prevention of recurrent CVD events should start if SBP is greater than or equal to 130 mm Hg or DBP is greater than or equal to 80 mm Hg. Other treatments include lifestyle modifications (i.e., smoking cessation, management of glucose intolerance and hypercholesterolemia), and increased physical activity.

The diagnosis of HTN is made with three different measurements on more than two office visits (Patel & Stewart, 2015). Blood pressure should be taken in both arms initially; future BP checks should be done using the arm with the highest initial BP reading (Whelton et al., 2017).

HTN has been classified into two types: primary and secondary. Primary HTN is the most common form. Although the exact cause is unknown, the contributing factors are family history, age, race, diet (e.g., foods high in saturated fats and salt or decreased potassium, magnesium, and calcium intake), smoking, stress, alcohol and drug consumption, lack of physical activity, and hormonal intake.

Secondary HTN refers to elevated blood pressure caused by underlying disease such as renal artery disease, renal parenchymal disorders, endocrine and metabolic disorders, central nervous system (CNS) disorders, coarctation of the aorta, and increased intravascular volume.

In older adults presenting with HTN, the nurse should assess all prescription and over-the-counter (OTC) drugs for possible causes of elevated blood pressure. Drug-induced HTN has occurred with the administration of amphetamines and glucocorticoids. Decongestants, phenobarbital, rifampin, and nonsteroidal antiinflammatory drugs (NSAIDs) may adversely affect the action of some drugs for HTN. NSAIDs have been found to cause elevated blood pressure (Whelton et al., 2017). Many older adults are taking NSAIDs for various musculoskeletal problems. These individuals should have their blood pressure closely monitored.

A positive correlation exists between obesity and high blood pressure. Advancing age is associated with a loss of lean body mass and an increase in adipose tissue. Excess fat in the upper body or a waist circumference of 35 inches or greater in women or 40 inches or greater in men increases the risk for HTN (excess upper body fat correlates with metabolic syndrome, which includes abdominal obesity, glucose intolerance, high triglyceride levels, and low HDL levels). A blood pressure drop of 1 mm Hg for every 1-kg weight reduction is expected with weight loss (Whelton et al., 2017).

Increased sodium intake is closely correlated to high blood pressure. A reduction in sodium to 1000 mg per day may reduce SBP by 2 to 6 mm Hg. The Dietary Approach to Stop Hypertension (DASH) diet may reduce SBP by 3 to 11 mm Hg (Whelton et al., 2017).

The pathophysiology of HTN is complex because various environmental, structural, renal, hormonal, and homeostatic mechanisms contribute to blood pressure maintenance, especially in the aging population.

HTN has been associated with arteriolar thickening, vascular smooth muscle constriction, and elevated vascular resistance. With age, peripheral vascular resistance increases significantly. The alpha-adrenergic responsiveness of the vascular smooth muscle does not change with age; however, the beta-adrenergic responsiveness declines with age with a consequent decrease in the relaxation of the vascular smooth muscle. Renal vascular resistance appears to be increased and renal blood flow appears to be decreased. Left ventricular hypertrophy occurs as an adaptation to longstanding HTN and may lead to HF. Once this occurs, there is a significant increase in cardiovascular risk, particularly for ventricular arrhythmia and sudden death.

In mild to moderate HTN, the patient may be asymptomatic. As the disease progresses, the patient may experience fatigue, dizziness, headaches, vertigo, and palpitations. In severe HTN, the patient may experience throbbing headaches, confusion, visual loss, focal deficits, epistaxis, and coma.

It is important that persons with HTN be assessed for end organ damage and symptoms. HTN may lead to damage in various organs, resulting in the following conditions:

- **Heart:** HF, ventricular hypertrophy, angina, MI, sudden death
- **CNS:** transient ischemic attack, stroke
- **Peripheral vessels:** PVD, aneurysm
- **Kidney:** serum creatinine greater than 133 mmol/L (1.5 mg/dL), proteinuria, microalbuminuria
- **Eye:** hemorrhage or exudates, with or without papilledema

Older adults are likely to have coexisting cardiac, vascular, and renal disease.

Health care providers should obtain a history regarding lifestyle factors and conduct an in-depth physical examination. The physical examination should include examination of the neck (to detect carotid bruits, jugular vein distention, or an enlarged thyroid), the heart (to detect abnormalities in rate and rhythm, heaves, lifts, murmurs, and third or fourth heart sounds), the lungs (to detect rales), the abdomen (to detect bruits, masses, and aortic pulsations), and the extremities (to detect peripheral pulses and edema).

Diagnostic tests can be beneficial in determining any effects on end organs due to HTN. The following tests should be included: hemoglobin and hematocrit to exclude anemia or polycythemia; urinalysis to investigate for proteinuria or other signs of renal failure; serum sodium, potassium, and creatinine levels; fasting plasma glucose level to determine whether antihypertensive therapy is affecting diabetes mellitus; serum TC and HDL levels to assess for hyperlipidemia; ECG; chest radiograph; and possibly echocardiography to assess left ventricular function and hypertrophy.

Pharmacologic Treatment

One of the most important considerations in drug therapy in older adults is that blood pressure should be lowered gradually, beginning with low doses of a single agent. When treating HTN in the older adult, the following should be kept in mind:

1. The goal of treatment is a blood pressure less than 130/80 mm Hg.
2. Older adults are more likely to experience an orthostatic drop in blood pressure than younger adults. Blood pressure should always be taken with the patient both sitting and standing and in both arms.
3. When pharmacologic therapy is used, dose should be lower than that recommended for younger adults.
4. Both nonpharmacologic interventions and lifestyle modifications should be employed. Older adults respond to modest sodium reduction and weight loss.
5. Select an appropriate drug with consideration for comorbidity. On the basis of clinical trials, the use of diuretics and angiotensin-converting enzyme inhibitors (ACEIs) are first-line therapy. Beta-blockers are preferred in patients with heart failure with reduced ejection fraction.
6. Increase the dose of the first drug, then add a second drug of a different class or substitute a drug from another class.
7. Concurrent use of angiotensin-converting-enzyme inhibitor (ACEI), angiotensin II receptor blockers (ARB), and/or renin inhibitors is not recommended.
8. Continue adding agents from other classes. Consider referral to an HTN specialist.

The use of antihypertensive drugs has been shown to be effective and well tolerated in older adults. The prescription is "to proceed slowly and with caution" and to monitor for adverse reactions. If this principle is adhered to, side effects will be minimal in older adults. Table 19.2 provides the classifications of antihypertensive drugs, their adverse effects, and the nursing implications.

Diuretics

The thiazide diuretics, hydrochlorothiazide and chlorthalidone, continue to be the most commonly prescribed antihypertensive agents for older adults. Initial dosing should start at 12.5 to 25 mg/day. Loop diuretics, such as furosemide, are not used unless patients have kidney disease or HF.

The primary concerns related to diuretic therapy are hypotension and hypokalemia. Patients should be carefully monitored for hypokalemia. If hypokalemia continues despite supplementing with potassium, then a potassium-sparing diuretic, such as spironolactone, may be prescribed. With potassium-sparing diuretics, hyperkalemia can occur; therefore close potassium monitoring is still warranted. Hypomagnesemia, hyponatremia, hyperglycemia, and increased uric acid may also occur. Increases in blood glucose are generally minor with low doses of a thiazide diuretic.

Beta-Blockers

Beta-blockers (BBs) are preferred in adults with heart failure with reduced ejection fraction (HFrEF) (Whelton et al., 2017). BBs are effective in lowering morbidity and mortality in older adults. Beta-adrenergic blockage decreases heart rate and contractility. This decreases cardiac workload and is cardioprotective. BBs, such as atenolol and metoprolol, are cardioselective BBs. Noncardioselective BBs include carvedilol. Cardioselective BBs may be better tolerated in older adults with lung disease or PVD. However, carvedilol is the preferred beta-blocker for patients with HFrEF (Whelton et al., 2017).

Angiotensin-Converting Enzyme Inhibitors

ACEIs inhibit the converting enzyme responsible for the formation of angiotensin II, a potent vasoconstrictor that stimulates the release of aldosterone. These drugs decrease mortality in older adults with decreased left ventricular function and preserve renal function in those with diabetes mellitus. Side effects of these drugs include rash, cough, taste disturbance, neutropenia, and proteinuria. ACEIs should not be used if acute renal failure or bilateral renal artery stenosis is suspected.

Calcium Channel Blockers

Calcium channel blockers (CCBs) inhibit the inward movement of calcium across the cell membrane of the vascular smooth muscle, which results in vasodilatation of peripheral, coronary, and renal

TABLE 19.2 Classification of Antihypertensive Drugs

Antihypertensive Drug	Adverse Effects	Precautions
Diuretics		
Thiazide Diuretics		
Chlorothiazide	Hyperglycemia	Patients with diabetes may require an increase in insulin.
Chlorthalidone	Hypokalemia	Encourage patients to restrict sodium intake and eat foods high
Hydrochlorothiazide	Hypomagnesemia	in potassium.
Indapamide	Hyponatremia	Check baseline and later levels of LDL and HDL, cholesterol,
Metolazone	Hyperuricemia	and triglycerides.
	Hypercholesterolemia	Report dry mouth, muscle weakness, cramps, drowsiness, and loss
	Sexual dysfunction	of appetite, which may be indicative of electrolyte imbalance.
	Photosensitivity	Be cautious in sunlight.
	Hypersensitivity to sulfonamides	
Loop Diuretics		
Bumetanide	Fluid electrolyte imbalance	Observe for signs of dehydration and acid–base imbalance.
Furosemide	Diuresis leading to hypovolemia, hypotension, and shock	Monitor blood pressure to detect signs and symptoms of shock.
Torsemide	May cause thromboembolism in older patients	Observe for signs and symptoms of thromboembolism.
Potassium-Sparing Diuretics		
Amiloride	Hyperkalemia	Monitor serum potassium levels.
Triamterene	May cause breast pain and amenorrhea in women	Potassium supplements should be discontinued when these drugs
	May cause renal calculi	are added to a sulfonamide diuretic regimen.
	Impotence, sexual dysfunction	Triamterene should be given cautiously to patients taking indomethacin.
Aldosterone Receptor Blockers		
Eplerenone	Hyperkalemia	Monitor electrolytes.
Spironolactone	GI bleeding or ulceration	Use K diuretics sparingly.
		Do not give NSAIDs.
Beta-Blockers		
Atenolol	Cardiac effects, including bradycardia and heart block	Report bradycardia and episodes of dizziness and syncope.
Betaxolol	Dizziness and fainting	Do not administer drugs to patients with heart failure or advanced
Bisoprolol	Fatigue, weakness, lethargy, depression, disorientation, and	degrees of heart block.
Metoprolol	hallucinations	Observe patient for any changes in physical and mental status.
Metoprolol extended release	Sexual dysfunction	Check LDL and HDL, triglyceride, and cholesterol levels.
Nadolol	Nausea, vomiting	Instruct patients to avoid abrupt discontinuation of the drug.
Propranolol	Bronchospasm in patients with asthma	
Propranolol long-acting	May mask hypoglycemia	
Timolol	May aggravate peripheral vascular insufficiency	
Beta-Blockers with Intrinsic Sympathomimetic Activity		
Acebutolol	Fatigue, dizziness, headache, urinary frequency	Avoid abrupt discontinuation of drug.
Penbutolol	May mask hypoglycemia or hyperthyroidism	Monitor weight, blood sugar, and vital signs.
Pindolol	Constipation, diarrhea	
	Insomnia	
	Safety concerns	
	Bradycardia, edema, weight gain, hypotension, syncope,	
	atrioventricular block	
	Diarrhea, nausea, hyperglycemia, abnormal vision, dyspnea	
Combined Alpha- and Beta-Blockers		
Carvedilol	Fatigue, dizziness, postural hypotension, muscle weakness,	Avoid driving during initial administration.
Labetalol	diarrhea, or constipation	Take with food.
		Report any new cough that continues.
		Report any unusual swelling of extremities.
ACEIs		
Benazepril	Tickle in throat or hacking cough	Observe patients for cough.
Captopril	Hyperkalemia	Check electrolytes for increase in potassium.
Enalapril	Rash	Observe for rash.
Fosinopril	Reversible renal failure in patients with proteinuria or renal	Check for increase in BUN or serum creatinine levels.
Lisinopril	artery stenosis	Observe for signs of dizziness, headache, and diarrhea.

Continued

TABLE 19.2 Classification of Antihypertensive Drugs—cont'd

Antihypertensive Drug	Adverse Effects	Precautions
Moexipril	Dizziness, headache, diarrhea, and fatigue	
Perindopril	Impaired sense of taste and sexual dysfunction rare	
Quinapril		
Ramipril		
Trandolapril		
Angiotensin II Antagonists		
Azilsartan	Dizziness, cough, upper respiratory infection, diarrhea,	Monitor renal function.
Candesartan	fatigue, and headache	Instruct patient to avoid alcohol, barbiturates, and narcotics.
Eprosartan	Edema, flushing, and palpitations.	Adjust insulin and antidiabetic drugs, which potentiate
Irbesartan	Serious reactions include angioedema, anaphylaxis, severe	hydrochlorothiazide, headaches, and dizziness.
Losartan	hypotension, hyperkalemia, kidney dysfunction,	Potentiated by grapefruit juice.
Olmesartan	rhabdomyolysis.	Avoid beta-blockers, digitalis, and diuretics.
Telmisartan		Do not crush.
Valsartan		Monitor liver studies in older patients.
Calcium Channel Blockers		
Nondihydropyridines		
Diltiazem extended release	Headache, dizziness, flushing, and weakness	Monitor heart rate.
Verapamil immediate release	Bradycardia	Monitor blood pressure during dose adjustment.
Verapamil extended release	Edema	Check laboratory results to assess liver and kidney function.
Verapamil-COER	Nausea	
	Constipation (especially with verapamil)	
	Gingival hyperplasia	
Dihydropyridines		
Amlodipine	Edema, fatigue, palpitations, dizziness, abdominal pain, GI	Monitor for hepatic dysfunction, CVD, and/or aortic stenosis.
Felodipine	upset, flushing	
Isradipine extended release	Drowsiness	
Nicardipine sustained release		
Nifedipine long-acting		
Nisoldipine		
Alpha₁-Blockers		
Doxazosin	Syncope with first dose, dizziness, fatigue, edema, rhinitis,	Monitor BP.
Prazosin	tinnitus, epistaxis, sexual dysfunction, polyuria, urinary	Check orthostatic blood pressure.
Terazosin	incontinence, ataxia, leukopenia, neutropenia, arrhythmia,	Limit ETOH.
	somnolence, rash, red eyes, dry mouth	
Central Alpha₂-Agonists and Other Centrally Acting Drugs		
Clonidine	Dry mouth, drowsiness, dizziness, weakness, constipation,	Monitor BP and supervise ambulation initially due to the risk of
Methyldopa	rash, myalgia, urticaria, nausea, insomnia, agitation,	orthostatic hypotension.
Reserpine	orthostatic hypotension, impotence, arrhythmias	Monitor fluid and electrolyte status.
Guanfacine		Do not stop abruptly.
Direct Vasodilators		
Hydralazine	Headache, tachycardia, angina, palpitations, nausea,	Monitor BP and HR. Monitor for signs and symptoms of lupus with
	vomiting, and diarrhea. Serious reactions include MI, severe	long-term therapy. Monitor periodic BUN, creatinine, uric acid,
	hypotension, neutropenia, blood dyscrasias, lupus-like	potassium glucose, and ECG.
	syndrome, peripheral neuritis, and hypersensitivity reaction.	
Minoxidil	Hypertrichosis, edema, tachycardia, breast tenderness,	Monitor BP and pulse. Do not stop drug abruptly as could result in MI
	weight gain, paresthesia, headache, and ECG	or CVA. Monitor fluid and electrolyte balance periodically. Monitor
	abnormalities. Serious reactions include pericarditis,	weight and report weight gain of 2 lb in 1 day. Monitor for edema
	pericardial effusion, cardiac tamponade, HF, angina,	and signs and symptoms of HF, and paradoxical pulse.
	Stevens-Johnson syndrome, and toxic epidermal necrolysis.	

ACEIs, Angiotensin-converting enzyme inhibitors; *BUN,* blood urea nitrogen; *CVD,* cardiovascular disease; *ETOH,* ethanol; *GI,* gastrointestinal; *HDL,* high-density lipoprotein; *K,* potassium; *LDL,* low-density lipoprotein; *MI,* myocardial infarction; *NSAIDs,* nonsteroidal antiinflammatory drugs.
Whelton, P. K., Carey, R. M., Aronow, W. S., Casey, D. E., Collins, K. J., Himmelfarb, C. D., … Wright, J. T. (2017). 2017 ACC/AHA/AAPA/ABC/ACPM/AGS/APhA/ASH/ASPC/NMA/PCNA guideline for the prevention, detection, evaluation, and management of high blood pressure in adults: A report of the American College of Cardiology/American Heart Association Task Force on clinical practice guidelines. *Hypertension, 70*(6), doi: https://doi.org/10.1161/HYP.0000000000000065. Retrieved November 28, 2017, from http://hyper.ahajournals.org/

arteries. They may cause orthostatic hypotension in older adults. These drugs typically have vasodilator effects such as headache, flushing, dizziness, and weakness. Constipation may also occur. CCBs are useful drugs in treating older adults and may be used when diuretics are not tolerated or are contraindicated.

Prognosis

HTN, if unrecognized and untreated, significantly increases the risk of coronary disease, heart and renal failure, and stroke. Risk increases with smoking, glucose intolerance, hyperlipidemia, left ventricular hypertrophy, male gender, black race, and increasing age. With an individualized pharmacologic and nonpharmacologic treatment program based on assessment of total cardiovascular risk, the risk of cardiovascular-related death from stroke and heart attack may be reduced. The degree of end organ damage affects overall morbidity and mortality (Whelton et al., 2017).

NURSING MANAGEMENT

Assessment

The majority of patients with HTN are asymptomatic. Subjective data are obtained through careful in-depth history. Symptoms that do occur are variable, depending on the progression of disease in target organs. Vague discomfort, fatigue, headache, epistaxis, and dizziness may be early indicators. Severe HTN may result in a throbbing headache—particularly prevalent in the morning but disappearing several hours later—as well as confusion, vision loss, focal deficits, and coma. Symptoms of heart failure such as dyspnea may be present. If the kidneys are affected, hematuria or nocturia may occur.

Objective data are obtained from a thorough assessment of blood pressure on three separate occasions. Blood pressure readings should be recorded with the patient in both the sitting and standing positions and in both arms. The patient's arms should be bared and supported at heart level. The nurse should instruct the patient not to ingest caffeine or smoke for 30 minutes before the blood pressure reading. The proper cuff size must be used. The bladder of the cuff should surround a minimum of 80% of the arm. Many older individuals will require a large cuff. If these steps are not taken, blood pressure readings may be inaccurate. If BP differs from each arm, then the higher BP should be recorded and used to diagnose HTN.

Diagnosis

Nursing diagnoses for an older adult patient with HTN include the following:

- Potential for injury
- Need for patient teaching resulting from new diagnosis of HTN, self-care management, and interventions
- Poor coping mechanisms resulting from perceived limitations of diagnosis
- Inadequate nutrition resulting from high fat, caloric, and sodium intake, and altered taste

Planning and Expected Outcomes

Expected outcomes for an older patient with HTN include the following:

1. The patient will identify personal risk factors.

2. The patient will explain the disease process and its effects on health and well-being.
3. The patient will incorporate nonpharmacologic treatment measures into daily living.
4. The patient will verbalize purpose, dose, action, and significant and reportable side effects of drugs prescribed for HTN.
5. The patient will verbalize the need to increase social interaction.
6. The patient will develop a meal plan that includes a low-fat, low-cholesterol, and reduced-sodium diet.

Intervention

Knowledge levels vary among older adults with HTN. The teaching plan should incorporate an explanation of the disease process and therapeutic (nonpharmacologic and pharmacologic) interventions. An explanation of the physical examination and appropriate tests should be given to allay anxiety. Anxiety, depression, denial, and fear are often involved in a chronic condition. Although these emotions diminish as the condition is controlled, the patient's ability to absorb this information and make the required changes is initially hampered because the patient may be in denial. For older adults, participation in community-based programs by the AHA or other agencies may be beneficial. It is crucial that any interventions take into account the physiologic changes of aging; for example, using large print and making sure that printed material is appropriate for the patient's culture and educational level.

Patient education includes providing information regarding the disease process; signs and symptoms of HTN; treatment regimen; drugs and their actions and side effects, including sexual dysfunction; and the need for frequent monitoring of blood pressure and risk factors. The nurse should explain the importance of a low-sodium, high-potassium, low-fat, reduced-calorie diet. Weight loss should be encouraged, if indicated. A dietitian may assist with meal planning, preparation, and label reading. Foods are healthier if prepared by baking, broiling, or steaming. The nurse should also discuss the importance of alcohol restriction and smoking cessation; explain the relationships between stress, anxiety, anger, and HTN; identify stressful situations at the patient's home and work; and teach meditation and relaxation techniques. Exercise is beneficial for weight and stress reduction. Exercises should include vigorous aerobic and high-intensity muscle strengthening activities. Initially, the patient should walk 10 to 15 minutes a day, gradually increasing to 1-hour walks three or four times a week. Other activities include mall-walking and water aerobics. Encourage the patient to reduce or eliminate smoking through a smoking cessation program. Prescription and over-the-counter drugs and other supports are available for smoking cessation. Other alternatives for smoking cessation include hypnotism or behavior modification. Positive reinforcement should be provided, whenever possible.

Evaluation

Evaluation consists of determining the patient's achievement of the expected outcomes. The patient's blood pressure should decrease and return to optimal levels. The patient should be able to maintain the treatment plan with minimal side effects or complications. Outcome measures related to quality of life are also important because of the chronic nature of HTN. The nurse must determine the patient's perception of any change in quality of life resulting from the prescribed therapeutic regimen. Documentation includes accurate records of blood pressure, weight, exercise, and activity patterns; 24-hour dietary intake; cholesterol levels; and any blood pressure monitoring results outside the clinical encounter.

Coronary Artery Disease

CAD, or ischemic heart disease, refers to a broad group of conditions that partially or completely obstruct blood flow to the heart muscle. Obstruction of coronary arteries may result in ischemia (an imbalance between the oxygen supply and demands of the heart) or infarction (death or necrosis) of the myocardium. Ischemia and infarction occur when the oxygen supply is unable to meet the demands of the heart. Atherosclerosis is the usual cause of CAD; angina, MI, and sudden death may be the final outcomes.

Atherosclerosis usually begins in childhood and is characterized by a local accumulation of lipid and fibrous tissue along the intimal layer of the artery. Lipids accumulate and infiltrate the area, forming a raised fibrous plaque over the site. Eventually, the plaque becomes calcified, which causes the vessel to lose its elasticity and ability to dilate. Progressive narrowing of the artery occurs, resulting in compromised blood flow to the area of the myocardium supplied by that vessel. In advanced stages of the disease, hemorrhage into the atheromatous plaque, thrombus formation, embolization of a thrombus or plaque fragment, and coronary arterial spasm may cause additional insult to the body. The incidence of atherosclerosis increases with age; the severity of this process may be accelerated with the adverse lifestyle behaviors of smoking, physical inactivity, and obesity, as well as elevated serum cholesterol levels, HTN, and diabetes mellitus. Promoting healthy lifestyles in younger and older individuals is an important aspect of care in the prevention of CAD. The adoption of healthier lifestyles by an older adult may be difficult because of long-term habits; however, healthy behavior changes may slow or halt the progression of the disease (Martin, 2016).

CAD is the major cause of morbidity, disability, and mortality in the older adult population. Alterations in cardiac function are likely to cause the older adult to feel afraid or unsure about the future. However, overwhelming fear can interfere with rehabilitation and staying well (AHA, 2015a).

Stable angina is caused by inadequate blood flow to the myocardium. The classic symptom is chest pain during activity that is relieved with rest or nitroglycerin. MI is caused by total disruption of blood flow to an area of the myocardium; it is characterized by more severe, more intense chest pain for a longer time than that associated with stable angina. Other symptoms that may accompany MI include nausea, diaphoresis, shortness of breath, dizziness, and weakness.

But, most often, older adults do not present with classic symptoms. Atypical presentation of MI in the older adult may include vague symptoms, such as fatigue, weakness, dizziness, nausea, confusion, and a decline in functional status. More often, older adults report shortness of breath rather than chest pain (Box 19.2). Possible reasons for the atypical presentation include age-related physiologic changes and loss of physiologic

BOX 19.2 Symptoms Associated With Atypical Presentation of Coronary Artery Disease in Older Adults

Shortness of breath	Dizziness or syncope
Fatigue	Confusion
Weakness	Decrease in functional status
Nausea	Abdominal or back pain

reserve, the interaction between acute and chronic conditions, and underreporting of symptoms. Women, especially older women, may not exhibit the classic signs of CAD, and the nurse needs to be aware of this to adequately assess female patients (Garcia, Mulvagh, Merz, Buring, & Manson, 2016). Because symptoms of acute coronary syndrome (ACS) or MI may be vague and atypical of textbook symptoms, older adults may not recognize their seriousness and may not seek medical attention as soon as they should. This may cause a delay in seeking medical attention. Unrecognized ACS or MI may cause permanent cardiac damage and precipitate complications of heart failure and pulmonary edema.

Diagnostic Tests and Procedures

Diagnosis is based on patient history, alterations on the ECG, and serum cardiac enzyme levels.

- 12-lead ECG should be obtained to gather information on rate, rhythm, hypertrophy, and myocardial injury (ischemia or infarction) and to assess for Q waves, ST segment elevation, ST segment depression, and T wave inversion (Zafari, 2017).
- Cardiac biomarkers/enzymes: the ACC and AHA recommend cardiac troponin should be obtained when MI is suspected. Troponin (a contractile protein released in the setting of myocardial necrosis) rises when infarction changes cell membrane permeability. Cardiac troponin T increases 3 to 5 hours after MI and remains elevated for 14 to 21 days. Cardiac troponin I rises within 3 hours, peaks at 14 to 18 hours, and remains elevated for 5 to 7 days (Zafari, 2017).
- Complete blood cell count (CBC) to determine whether angina is caused by anemia (Zafari, 2017).
- Comprehensive metabolic panel should be drawn to monitor serum electrolytes, particularly sodium, potassium, and calcium. Elevated or reduced levels of these electrolytes can lead to fluid imbalance or ventricular arrhythmias (Zafari, 2017).
- Serum lactate dehydrogenase (LDH) levels rise within 24 hours of an MI, peak in 3 to 6 days, and return to baseline in 8 to 12 days (Zafari, 2017).
- Chest radiography to determine presence of cardiomegaly, pulmonary edema, or other indications of HF (Singh, 2015).
- Color-flow Doppler transthoracic echocardiography or Doppler echocardiography is used to evaluate wall motion and ventricular performance, and detect pericardial effusion and valvular disease (Singh, 2015).
- Coronary angiography to detect the presence, location, and extent of lesions in coronary arteries (Singh, 2015).
- Exercise stress test to determine activity tolerance. Stress tests may be combined with myocardial imaging to identify changes in myocardial perfusion during exercise. In the

absence of an acute cardiac event such as MI, an exercise stress test may be troublesome for older adults with coexisting diseases such as arthritis, PVD, and chronic obstructive pulmonary disease (COPD). Pharmacologic stress tests may be a better choice in these older individuals (Garcia, Mulvagh, Merz, Buring, & Manson, 2016). For older adults not able to complete an exercise stress test, dobutamine-stress echocardiography is an option (Singh, 2015).

Pharmacologic Treatment

Treatment of CAD is directed toward restoring the balance between myocardial oxygen demand and oxygen supply. Pharmacologic therapy plays a major role. Normal changes with aging (e.g., alterations in body mass, water composition, liver size, renal system, and plasma protein concentration) alter the metabolism and excretion of many drugs, so smaller doses are generally prescribed for older adults.

Nitrates

Nitrates are used for the prevention and termination of anginal attacks and for reducing the pain associated with myocardial ischemia. These drugs decrease cardiac preloading and afterload, which reduces the myocardial demand for oxygen. These changes occur due to the vasodilating effects of nitrates on coronary arteries and peripheral vasculature. Intravenous, sublingual, and aerosol preparations have a rapid onset of action (1 to 3 minutes) and are used to prevent or terminate an anginal attack. Oral and transdermal preparations have a prolonged effect and are used to prevent anginal attacks. Tolerance to oral and transdermal nitrate preparations reduce drug effectiveness; an 8- to 12-hour nitrate-free interval can reduce tolerance (Fillit, Rockwood, & Young, 2017). Headache, flushing, dizziness, hypotension, syncope, and tachycardia are side effects attributed to the vasodilating effects. Nitrates are effective in older adults; however, aggressive therapy to reduce preload and afterload may trigger reflex tachycardia and severe orthostatic hypotension. Older adults should take rapid-acting nitrates in the sitting position or supine to prevent falls, and should sit up slowly with assistance (Julian, Aroesty, Joseph, & Kannam, 2017).

Beta-Blockers

BBs are used in patients with stable angina to decrease the frequency of angina or to reduce the size of infarction and complications of MI. Blockage of beta-adrenergic receptors in the heart decreases sympathetic nervous stimulation reducing heart rate, stroke volume, and contractility; this leads to decreased myocardial oxygen requirements. Side effects include bradycardia, hypotension, dyspnea, dizziness, syncope, gait difficulties, sexual dysfunction, heart failure, heart block, bronchoconstriction, and depression. For patients with lung disease, metoprolol and atenolol are safer drugs, as they are cardioselective. Sudden cessation of therapy may induce myocardial ischemia. Older adults are more sensitive to decreased heart rate, leading to decreased exercise performance and possible syncope (Julian et al., 2017).

Calcium Channel Blockers

CCBs are used to treat stable and variant angina and to increase coronary perfusion, reduce blood pressure, and decrease myocardial contractility in individuals with MI. CCBs slow electrical conduction through the heart (to varying degrees), decrease the force of cardiac contraction, and dilate blood vessels by blocking the entry of calcium ions into vascular smooth muscle cells, thereby decreasing myocardial oxygen demand and increasing coronary perfusion. Adverse reactions include bradycardia, constipation, hypotension, flushing, dizziness, syncope, headaches, dyspnea, palpitations, and peripheral edema. Verapamil and diltiazem are not recommended in older adults because they significantly slow electrical conduction through the heart, decreasing heart rate and increasing the incidence of heart block. Amlodipine, a dihydropyridine CCB, is recommended for older adults because it does not slow cardiac electrical conduction to the extent nondihydropyridines do (Julian et al., 2017; Whelton et al., 2017).

Fibrinolytics, Anticoagulants, and Antiplatelets

These drugs are used to prevent, reduce, and dissolve thrombi around atherosclerotic plaques by altering blood-clotting mechanisms. Fibrinolytic or thrombolytic drugs are given intravenously within 6 hours of the onset of symptoms. Patients must be observed for bleeding, arrhythmia, and allergic reactions. Older adults have an increased risk for bleeding with fibrinolytics. Heparin followed by oral anticoagulation, such as warfarin, should be administered after fibrinolytic therapy to prevent secondary clot formation.

Heparin and warfarin are anticoagulants used to prevent the enlargement of existing thrombi and new clot formation after MI. Therapeutic effects of heparin are monitored by partial thromboplastin times (PTTs); the antidote is protamine sulfate. Warfarin is monitored by the international normalized ratio (INR); the antidote is vitamin K. Patients who initially receive heparin for anticoagulation and who need oral anticoagulation for maintenance usually take both forms of drug for 3 to 5 days to develop therapeutic blood levels. As with thrombolytics, bleeding is a complication. Patients should be educated on signs and symptoms of bleeding, such as unexplained bruising, dark and tarry stools, and bleeding that is not controlled within 15 minutes.

Aspirin, an antiplatelet, decreases the mortality rate of acute MI. It inhibits platelet aggregation and facilitates fibrinolysis. Its effects on platelets occur within 20 minutes of administration. Many aspirin preparations are available. Dose for aspirin can be 81 mg or 325 mg/day.

Lipid-Lowering Drugs

Lipid-lowering drugs are used to lower serum lipid levels by preventing absorption of cholesterol and promoting its secretion. Side effects common to all lipid-lowering agents, regardless of class, include diarrhea, constipation, nausea, abdominal pain, and elevation in liver function studies. Lipid-lowering drugs are given to reduce the risk for MI and stroke. They should be prescribed if dietary and activity measures are ineffective in lowering cholesterol, triglycerides, and LDLs. Although some older adults may benefit from lipid-lowering drugs (those with established atherosclerosis), there is debate concerning their benefit for adults over 65. In adults over 75, there is concern risk of harm outweighs any benefit (Zoungas, 2017). Older adults and their families should discuss the issue with their health care providers. When taking lipid-lowering drugs, the benefits related to CAD and stroke prevention should clearly outweigh the potential risk associated with drug therapy (Banach & Serban, 2016; Zoungas, 2017).

Nonpharmacologic Treatment

At each encounter with the health care system, as appropriate, older adults should be encouraged to quit smoking (avoid second-hand smoke), eat healthily, engage in routine exercise, maintain a healthy weight, and manage stress. Improvement in each of these factors has the potential to reduce the progression of CAD.

Percutaneous Transluminal Coronary Angioplasty

Percutaneous transluminal coronary angioplasty (PTCA) is performed to open blocked coronary arteries. In this minimally invasive procedure, a balloon-tipped catheter is inserted through the femoral artery, under fluoroscopy, and advanced until it has reached the occluded coronary artery. The balloon is then inflated to compress the obstructing plaque, resulting in a larger vessel lumen and improved blood flow to the myocardium. A *stent* may be placed to keep the vessel open and maintain blood flow through the coronary artery.

Coronary Artery Bypass Graft Surgery

Coronary artery bypass graft (CABG) is a surgical procedure to improve blood flow to ischemic myocardium. During surgery, portions of saphenous vein or internal mammary artery are grafted to sites above and below the obstructed coronary artery.

Coronary Artery Disease in Women

CAD is the leading cause of death and disability in women older than 55 years. It is estimated that every minute in the United States a woman dies of heart disease (Garcia, Mulvagh, Merz, Buring, & Manson, 2016). Women have smaller coronary arteries that occlude more easily. Women have a lower hematocrit and blood volume, which decreases the oxygen-carrying capacity of the blood. Women also have a higher heart rate at rest, higher stroke volume at rest, and lower left ventricular end-diastolic pressure compared with men. Women experience atypical symptoms associated with CAD, such as epigastric pain and shortness of breath.

Differences in treatment between women and men with CAD include the following: Women experience a longer interval between emergency department admission and performance of ECG. Women are less likely to be admitted to an intensive care unit (ICU). Women are less likely to receive thrombolytic therapy. Women have a higher incidence of total occlusion after PTCA. Women have an increased incidence of CABG after PTCA. Women experience more recurrent angina, heart failure, recurrent infarction, and strokes after MI. Women are referred less often for cardiac rehabilitation. Women have poorer attendance at cardiac rehabilitation if they are referred. Women are typically 10 years older than men when diagnosed with cardiac disease and experience worse outcomes than men (Garcia, Mulvagh, Merz, Buring, & Manson, 2016). The National Coalition for Women with Heart Disease (http://www.womenheart.

org/) provides information and resource links for both health care professionals and women diagnosed with heart disease.

Prognosis

Age-related physiologic changes, longstanding unhealthy lifestyles, and chronic conditions in older adults may complicate the progress and treatment of CAD; however, advances in the medical and surgical treatments of CAD and the adoption of healthier lifestyles have the potential to positively influence disease outcomes in older adults.

NURSING MANAGEMENT

Assessment

Assessment of an older adult with CAD begins with a complete health history and physical examination. Complaints of dyspnea, fatigue, syncope, vertigo, and confusion warrant further investigation. Subjective data may have to be collected when vital signs are stable and discomfort is relieved (Box 19.3).

Specific health questions during the assessment (e.g., "Are you able to shop for groceries?") may elicit more detailed responses than open-ended questions (e.g., "What type of activities at home are difficult for you?"). When gathering objective data on older adults, nurses should keep in mind that slower heart rates, irregular heart rhythms, the presence of a third or fourth heart sound, systolic ejection murmurs, higher SBPs, and wider pulse pressures may be a result of aging, not the current ischemic episode (Ball et al., 2014).

BOX 19.3 Assessment of Patients With Chest Pain

Subjective Data
Chest pain (location, intensity, radiation, onset, and duration)
Precipitating factors (activity, emotions, rest, hot or cold exposure, and eating)
Associated symptoms (diaphoresis, dyspnea, vomiting, weakness, palpitations, and indigestion)
Relieving symptoms (rest and nitrates)
Prior hospitalization (for angina, MI, and other disorders)
Drugs
Family history (parents or siblings with CAD onset before age 50)
Modifiable cardiac risk factors (smoking, high cholesterol level, hypertension, diabetes mellitus, obesity, and physical inactivity)
Psychosocial state (denial, anxiety, fear, or anger)
Activity levels
Support systems

Objective Data
Behaviors (nervous, lethargic, rubbing chest, or grimacing)
Changes in vital signs
Changes in cardiac rhythm
Associated symptoms (diaphoresis, pallor, or cold and clammy skin)
Peripheral pulses (radial, femoral, and pedal)
Heart sounds and murmurs
Respiratory rate and breath sounds
Jugular vein distention
Diagnostic test results (cardiac enzymes, ECG, chest radiography, CBC, and electrolyte levels)

CAD, Coronary artery disease; *CBC,* complete blood cell count; *ECG,* electrocardiogram; *MI,* myocardial infarction.

Diagnosis

Nursing diagnoses common for an older patient with CAD include the following:

- Chest discomfort resulting from an imbalance between oxygen need and supply
- Ineffective cardiac output resulting from decreased pumping ability of the heart
- Decreased activity level resulting from decreased cardiac output
- Potential for nonadherence
- Anxiety resulting from fear of death

Planning and Expected Outcomes

As with all patients, older adults with CAD should be included in the planning of care. Family should also be included in the planning process; however, older adults should be consulted to determine the extent of the family involvement. Discharge planning should begin on admission to the hospital, and special attention should be given to the necessary support services in the home.

Expected outcomes for an older patient with CAD include the following:

1. The patient will verbalize pain relief.
2. The patient will maintain adequate perfusion with stable vital signs, mental alertness, urine output greater than 30 milliliters per hour (mL/hr), no ECG changes, and clear breath sounds.
3. The patient will tolerate activity without complaints of chest discomfort or dyspnea.
4. The patient will explain the disease process and therapeutic plan, including causes and risk factors for CAD; precipitating and alleviating factors for angina; and names, dosages, actions, and side effects of drugs.
5. The patient will describe actions to take in the event of chest pain.
6. The patient will express fears and have reduced anxiety.

Intervention

Interventions for an older adult with CAD focus on relieving pain, improving myocardial blood flow, decreasing myocardial workload, and educating the patient.

Cardiovascular, respiratory, kidney, and neurologic assessments should be conducted on a regular basis to detect progress and prevent complications. Diagnostic testing, especially of potassium levels because older patients are prone to hyperkalemia, should be conducted and evaluated daily, and any adverse changes in patient status should be reported to the physician.

Older adults and their family members may express concern about emergency measures such as resuscitation or life support. Nurses should be sensitive to these needs and initiate discussion with the patient, family, and health care team to establish a plan of action.

Older adults should be encouraged to participate in cardiac rehabilitation programs to restore their physical and mental health to the highest level of function. Cardiac rehabilitation promotes restoration, diminishes the effects of disease, and encourages optimal physical, psychological, and social functioning. Cardiac rehabilitation consists of three phases. Phase 1 begins in the hospital and includes early ambulation and patient and family education. Phase 2 lasts about 12 weeks and takes place in a supervised outpatient setting. Phase 3 is a maintenance phase that lasts indefinitely; it includes counseling, exercise, education, and socialization.

Exercise should be gradually increased during recovery. Older adults should be taught to monitor their pulse rate to evaluate tolerance to activity. Walking, with a progressive increase in duration and frequency, is recommended. Heavy lifting should be avoided. Activities should be paced throughout the day. Older adults may benefit from a written plan of progressive activities. Properly designed exercise programs for older adults incorporate longer times for the return to a resting heart rate after exercise. Orthostatic hypotension is more common in the older population because of decreased baroreceptor sensitivity. Thermoregulation among older adults is impaired; thus caution must be used during exercise in hot and humid environments. A heart rate of 50% to 70% of the maximum heart rate achieved at exercise testing with no discomfort during exercise is recommended (Touhy & Jett, 2012).

Activities that that build endurance, increase the level of self-care, and improve quality of life should be encouraged. Activities to suggest include walking, swimming, water aerobics, bowling, and dancing. Older adults with unstable angina should not exercise. Those who require cardiac monitoring during rehabilitation include those who have an ejection fraction of less than 39%, a resting complex ventricular arrhythmia, or decreased blood pressure during exercise. They also include those who escape sudden death, those who experience major complications due to the MI (e.g., heart failure or shock), and those who demonstrate inability to self-monitor their heart rate because of physical or cognitive impairment.

In spite of the documented benefits of cardiac rehabilitation programs, adherence to rehabilitation remains low. About 50% of patients drop out before completing the program. Reasons for this include other medical problems, lack of transportation, personal and financial factors, and conflicts with work schedules. Women have the poorest adherence to rehabilitation programs (Touhy & Jett, 2012). Interdisciplinary teams should recognize these issues and make every effort to assist patients with these problems.

Sexual activity is an important aspect of quality of life. The resumption of sexual activity should be discussed with older adults. It is generally safe to resume sexual activity within 4 to 6 weeks of MI, as long as an older adult is symptom-free during their usual daily activities. The equivalency or expenditure of energy for sexual activity correlates with the same energy expenditure required for climbing a flight of stairs or walking around the block. The pamphlet *Sex and Heart Disease* produced by the AHA may be used to supplement counseling (AHA, 2015b).

Visiting nurse programs provide education, support, and supervised activities in the home environment if older patients are unable to attend outpatient services. Home care services are usually available to assist older patients with activities of daily living (ADLs). Both programs typically require physician referral.

Local heart associations are excellent sources for learning materials and community programs on CAD. Some heart associations offer educational and support programs for patients recovering from CAD or surgery (e.g., Mended Hearts), and they usually provide direction for community programs on risk factor reduction, cardiopulmonary resuscitation (CPR), and mall-walking.

NURSING CARE PLAN
Myocardial Infarction

Clinical Situation

Mrs. S is an 84-year-old widow who was admitted to the hospital from a nursing facility with complaints of fatigue, weakness, and vertigo. Staff at the nursing facility became concerned after two episodes of syncope. Mrs. S suffered a stroke 4 years ago that left her with severe weakness in her left arm and left leg. She was unable to care for herself at home; her daughter encouraged her to enter the nursing facility. She has been following a diet low in saturated fat and cholesterol and takes enteric-coated aspirin daily, as well as levothyroxine for hypothyroidism. Mrs. S is mobile with the use of a walker.

Routine ECG showed pathologic Q waves. Cardiac enzymes were tested. Creatinine phosphokinase (CPK) levels were normal, but LDH was elevated. She was diagnosed with an inferior MI. Because she did not meet the time criteria for fibrinolytic therapy, the physician instituted prophylactic measures with oral anticoagulants (warfarin) on a daily basis. Mrs. S developed occasional premature ventricular contractions and periodic bouts of atrial fibrillation. Atenolol and nitroglycerin were added to her regimen. She became agitated in the coronary care unit about being a burden to her family and declined invasive treatment procedures. The nurse organized a meeting with the physician, daughter, and patient to discuss her anxiety, and a "no resuscitation" order was written. Lorazepam 1 milligram (mg), as needed three times a day, was added to the protocol.

Currently, Mrs. S denies having chest pain and can walk short distances with her walker. She follows a low-cholesterol, low–saturated fat diet, and she is scheduled for echocardiography later in the week. Her blood pressure is in the low to normal range, and her pulse is irregular at 102 beats per minute (beats/min).

Nursing Diagnoses

Anxiety resulting from threat of death and change in health status

Cardiac tissue injury r/t decreased cardiac tissue perfusion as evidenced by pathologic Q waves and elevated cardiac biomarkers

Dysrhythmia resulting from electrical dysfunction as evidenced by premature ventricular contractions and atrial fibrillations

Reduced stamina resulting from imbalance of myocardial oxygen supply and demand and left peripheral limb weakness

Potential for nonadherence resulting from lack of exposure to disease process and treatment plan

Outcomes

The patient will verbalize reduced anxiety, as evidenced by a slower heart rate, reduced apprehension, and participation in self-care.

The patient will obtain pain relief, as evidenced by verbal statements.

The patient will maintain adequate circulation, as evidenced by stable vital signs, mental alertness, clear lung sounds, and urine output greater than 30 milliliters per hour (mL/hr).

The patient will tolerate activity, as evidenced by stable vital signs; absence of pain, weakness, fatigue, and vertigo; and participation in activity.

The patient will demonstrate knowledge of the disease process, symptoms of ischemia with appropriate responses, and the treatment plan, as evidenced by explanation of and participation in the plan.

The patient will demonstrate an accurate pulse-taking method.

Interventions

Explain equipment, procedures, and unit routine.

Encourage verbalization of feelings.

Teach relaxation techniques and guided imagery to alleviate anxiety.

Supervise tolerance to visitation.

Offer lorazepam, as needed.

Encourage participation in care and emphasize improvements in health status.

Encourage relaying of pain sensations to the nurse.

Explain how sensations of fatigue, weakness, and vertigo may be symptoms of ischemia and that these symptoms need to be reported to the nurse.

Encourage the patient to take nitroglycerin at the onset of chest pain or at sensations of ischemia.

Obtain vital signs during episodes, and contact the physician if the drug is ineffective.

Offer oxygen, if needed.

Monitor therapeutic effects of nitrates and atenolol, observing for hypotensive effects.

Measure blood pressure, apical pulse, and rhythm every 4 hours. Auscultate heart and lungs every 8 hours.

Monitor ECG for reversion to normal sinus rhythm, INR, and digoxin and electrolyte levels.

Administer and evaluate the effects of warfarin and atenolol.

Observe for signs of hemorrhage, shock, heart failure, and emboli.

Assist with ADLs, as needed.

Remind the patient to perform leg exercises every hour and range-of-motion exercises. Apply antiembolic stockings.

Before the patient ambulates, encourage the patient to do leg exercises and sit at the bedside for 3 to 5 minutes before standing.

Gradually increase the distance and frequency of walking.

Monitor vital signs before and after activity.

Ensure that call bell and walker are within reach.

Encourage the patient to wear shoes with good support and to walk in lighted areas.

Balance activity with rest.

Teach the patient to count her own pulse.

Encourage the patient to recognize sensations of ischemia and cease activity when they occur.

Include the patient's daughter in teaching sessions.

Describe the disease and healing process of MI using pictures, models, and large printed material.

Describe the patient's sensations of ischemia, and teach the appropriate use of nitrates and rest.

Discuss and provide written information for drug dosage, purpose, side effects, and special precautions for warfarin, digoxin, and atenolol.

Encourage a progressive increase in activity.

Assess emotions and reassure the patient that depression is common.

Teach the patient to take a radial pulse and to monitor it before, during, and after activity.

Evaluation

Evaluation and documentation of the progress of an older patient with CAD focuses on the achievement of goals outlined in the planning process.

Older adults should demonstrate adequate circulation, ability to perform ADLs, and control of symptoms. Documentation should focus on the older adult's risk factor profile and progress, and measures should be aimed at reducing risks because a reduction of behaviors associated with the identified risks will reduce morbidity and mortality (see Nursing Care Plan: Myocardial Infarction).

Arrhythmia

Arrhythmia is an abnormal heart rhythm caused by a disturbance in automaticity, conductivity, contractility, or a combination of the three. Arrhythmias can originate in the atria, AV junctions, ventricles, bundle of His, or Purkinje fibers, and may result in decreased cardiac output and impaired perfusion of coronary arteries.

Older adults may develop any type of arrhythmia; however, atrial fibrillation, sick sinus syndrome, and heart block occur more often in the older population due to the loss of cardiac pacemaker cells, and deposition of fat and fibrous tissue in some pathways of the conduction system. Older adults may also have comorbid conditions that damage heart muscle (e.g., HTN or diabetes) and place them at risk for arrhythmias (National Heart, Lung, and Blood Institute, 2011). The incidence of atrial fibrillation increases with age and is the most common contributing factor for ischemic stroke in older adults. According to the AHA, the incidence of stroke due to atrial fibrillation among people age 50 to 59 is 1.5%, whereas 23.5% of people age 80 to 89 developed stroke due to atrial fibrillation (Benjamin et al., 2017). In the setting of atrial fibrillation, stroke is caused by an embolus from the heart that occludes a cerebral vessel. Atrial fibrillation is characterized by chaotic, rapid depolarization within the atria and an irregular ventricular response. It is a common complication of MI or CABG. Older adults need increased diastolic filling pressures to compensate for structural changes within the heart and to maintain cardiac output, so chaotic or quivering depolarization within the atria diminishes the atrial kick needed for adequate ventricular filling (Ball et al, 2014).

Atrial fibrillation may be triggered or made worse by emotional stress, alcohol use, caffeine, cigarettes, and stimulant drugs. Chronic atrial fibrillation tends to occur in patients with HTN, CAD, rheumatic heart disease, cardiac valve disease, HF, pericarditis, COPD and asthma, cardiomyopathy, hyperthyroidism, obesity, diabetes, sleep apnea, and viral infections (Beckerman, 2017).

Sick sinus syndrome increases the risk for developing atrial fibrillation. It is characterized by alternating episodes of bradycardia (less than 60 beats/min), normal sinus rhythm (60 to 100 beats/min), tachycardia (greater than 100 beats/min), and periods of long sinus pauses that fail to stimulate the atria or ventricles. Sick sinus syndrome tends to occur in patients with CAD, rheumatic heart disease, and HTN.

Heart block is characterized by delayed or blocked impulses between the atria and ventricles and is classified as first-, second-, or third-degree heart block; each respective classification increases in severity. First-degree block is common in older adults with or without CAD and is a common complication of MI. Digitalis preparations may also cause first-degree heart block. Second- and third-degree blocks may be caused by degeneration within the conduction system, ischemia, enhanced vagal tone, electrolyte imbalance, and effects of drugs (e.g., digoxin and beta-blockers).

Symptoms of arrhythmia are related to decreased cardiac output and include weakness, fatigue, palpitations, dizziness, shortness of breath, confusion, chest pain, and syncope, all of which predispose older patients to falls and injuries. Patients with first-degree block and sick sinus syndrome may have no symptoms, whereas patients with atrial fibrillation may have symptoms associated with rapid ventricular response.

Diagnostic Tests and Procedures

Diagnosis of arrhythmia is made by physical assessment, accompanied by ECG evaluation, Holter monitor, or patient-activated event recorder. When an arrhythmia is diagnosed, a variety of tests may be performed to determine a causative factor.

Treatment

Treatment should be limited to symptomatic patients with significant arrhythmias.

Atrial Fibrillation

The treatment of atrial fibrillation has three objectives: (1) controlling the underlying cause, (2) slowing the heart rate and/or converting the rhythm to a normal sinus rhythm, and (3) preventing stroke with maintenance anticoagulation therapy. CCBs are first-line therapy for long-term rate control. Diltiazem and verapamil are the drugs of choice. Beta-adrenergic receptor blockers are also effective for long-term rate control. Atenolol and metoprolol (both cardioselective) and propranolol (nonselective) may be used. In patients with AF and HF, digoxin is effective; when used, close monitoring of drug levels and kidney function is required. Elective cardioversion is appropriate for acute atrial fibrillation (duration of less than a few months), if pharmacologic treatment (chemical cardioversion) is not effective, and left ventricular hypertrophy is NOT present. When duration of atrial fibrillation is longer than 48 hours or duration is uncertain, anticoagulants are prescribed to reduce the risk of thromboembolic events.

Sick Sinus Syndrome

A permanent pacemaker is the treatment of choice for symptomatic patients with bradycardia. If patients have tachycardia, a BB or CCB may be effective. If BBs or CCBs are not tolerated or not effective, patients with tachycardia will require a permanent pacemaker.

Heart Block

Treatment for first-degree heart block includes correction of the causative factor (e.g., electrolyte imbalance or drug toxicity). In patients with severe bradycardia or potential to progress to a higher-degree block, a dual-chamber pacemaker may be used. With symptomatic second- and third-degree blocks, a permanent cardiac pacemaker is treatment of choice, if correction of the underlying cause does not reverse the heart block.

Prognosis

Older adults with the arrhythmias have an excellent prognosis when these arrhythmias are corrected. Patients with atrial fibrillation are at an increased risk for complications, such as ischemic stroke.

NURSING MANAGEMENT

Assessment

Older adults should be assessed for a history of CAD, heart failure, HTN, cardiac valve disease, and current drugs (e.g., cardiac drugs, diuretics, and supplemental electrolytes), which may be causing arrhythmias. Symptoms due to decreased cardiac output include weakness, confusion, palpitations, dizziness, shortness of breath, chest pain and syncope, and should be assessed for onset, duration, frequency, aggravating and alleviating factors, and home treatment remedies.

Objective data include level of consciousness, orientation, heart rate and rhythm, blood pressure, peripheral pulses, and urine output. Measuring the apical pulse for 60 seconds yields the most accurate measurement of heart rate. Apical and radial rates should be compared simultaneously to assess peripheral perfusion. Electrolyte, hemoglobin, and hematocrit values should be assessed for imbalances and anemia.

Diagnosis

Nursing diagnoses common for an older patient with arrhythmia include the following:
- Reduced cardiac perfusion resulting from altered heart rate and rhythm
- Reduced physical stamina resulting from altered heart rate and cardiac output
- Potential for injury resulting from potential thrombus and emboli formation
- Potential for nonadherence resulting from lack of information about disease process, drugs, and treatment plan

Planning and Expected Outcomes

The overall goals for a patient with arrhythmia are to maintain ADLs and adequate heart rate, sustain cardiac output, and prevent complications. Expected outcomes include the following:
1. The patient will maintain an adequate cardiac output, as evidenced by heart rate and rhythm within normal range, stable blood pressure, adequate peripheral pulses, baseline mental status, urine output of 30 mL/hr, and clear breath sounds.
2. The patient will tolerate activity, as evidenced by stable vital signs and no complaints of dizziness, fatigue, or syncope.
3. The patient will remain free from injury.
4. The patient will verbalize increased knowledge about his or her diagnosis, treatment plan, and health maintenance behaviors.

Intervention

Vital signs should be monitored every 15 to 60 minutes if the patient's condition is acute and every 4 hours if it is stable. Heart rate and rhythm should be monitored continuously by telemetry. The patient should be taught to report symptoms of weakness, dizziness, and palpitations to the nurse for correlation to telemetry readings. Cardiovascular, respiratory, and neurologic systems, as well as vital signs, oxygen saturation and intake/output measurements, should be assessed on a regular basis. Therapeutic response and side effects of prescribed drugs should be determined.

Older patients with slow or rapid ventricular responses to atrial fibrillation, long periods of sinus arrest with sick sinus syndrome, and second- or third-degree heart blocks are at risk for asystole and sudden cardiac death, so nurses should be prepared to initiate emergency measures.

Sensations of weakness, fatigue, dizziness, or dyspnea affect a patient's activity tolerance. Nurses should assist patients to

---

PATIENT/FAMILY TEACHING

Pacemaker

Maintain follow-up care with your health care provider to evaluate pacemaker function.

Watch for signs of infection at the incision site (e.g., redness, swelling, or drainage). Report any signs of infection to your health care provider.

Avoid activities that would cause direct blows to the generator site (e.g., contact sports or use of a rifle).

Avoid proximity to high-output electrical generators or to large magnets such as magnetic resonance imaging (MRI) scanners. These devices can reprogram the pacemaker.

Microwave ovens are safe to use and do not threaten pacemaker function.

Travel without restriction is allowed. The metal case of a small implanted pacemaker rarely may set off airport security alarms.

Take a radial pulse at the same time daily. Contact your health care provider if the rate is below the setting of the pacemaker.

Always carry a pacemaker identification card. Information should include the type and brand of pacemaker, Inter-Society Commission on Heart Disease code, and settings.

Sexual activity may be resumed as tolerated, and as directed by your health care provider.

Engage in normal activities of daily living.

Discuss all drugs, including herbal, prescription, and over-the-counter drugs with your health care provider.

Do not lean over gasoline engines or motors. Avoid direct contact of pacemaker generator with electrical appliances.

From Blach, D. A. (2013). Management of clients with problems of the cardiovascular system. In Ignatavicius, D. D. & Workman, M. L. (Eds.). *Medical surgical nursing: Patient centered collaborative care* (7th ed.). St. Louis, MO: Saunders; Lewis, S. L., Heitkemper, M. M., Dirksen, S. R., et al. (2014). *Medical surgical nursing: Assessment and management of clinical problems* (9th ed.). St. Louis, MO: Mosby.

---

identify factors that increase or decrease activity tolerance, and develop activity patterns that are spaced with adequate rest. Physiologic responses to activity should be monitored.

Tachycardia, bradycardia, and long periods of sinus pause reduce cardiac output and place patients at a higher risk for fainting and falls. Interventions to prevent injury include (1) having patients sit for 3 to 5 minutes before activity and (2) protecting patients from objects with sharp or protruding edges by rearranging their living area or padding objects in their environment.

Disease processes and the dosage and side effects of all drugs should be reviewed with the patient. Older patients taking anticoagulants should be taught ways to prevent injury, such as not going barefoot, using a soft toothbrush, shaving with an electric razor, having blood for coagulation studies drawn at the proper times, and taking drugs at the same time every day.

If older patients anticipate difficulty with home recovery, a home health agency may be consulted. Heart associations are excellent sources for information and community programs. The family or significant others should be encouraged to attend CPR programs. All patients should be encouraged to wear medical-alert bracelets to identify the arrhythmia, the use of a pacemaker, and any drugs they use (see Patient/Family Teaching Box: Pacemaker).

Evaluation

Older adults with arrhythmias or pacemakers should maintain a cardiac rhythm that supports adequate cardiac output. Implantable cardioverter–defibrillators (ICDs) may also be used. If the patient receives a shock from the device, they should sit or lie down immediately and contact their health care provider (Blach, 2006). The ability to resume ADLs, knowledge of the therapeutic plan, and achievement of expected outcomes define an older adult's readiness for independence in their care. Documentation should focus on the patient's response to the treatment plan, and how well symptoms are controlled. Hemodynamic stability is reflected in documented trends in the patient's vital signs.

Orthostatic Hypotension

Orthostatic hypotension is a major risk factor for syncope and falls in older adults. Orthostatic hypotension is defined as a decrease of 20 mm Hg or greater in SBP or a decrease of 10 mm Hg or greater in DBP upon standing. The decrease in blood pressure occurs due to blood shifting into the lower extremities. Symptoms associated with the fall in blood pressure include dizziness, light-headedness, confusion, and blurred vision (Higginson, 2016). Orthostatic hypotension is even more common among persons with certain risk factors such as autonomic dysfunction, low cardiac output, and hypovolemia. The use of certain drugs such as sedatives, antihypertensives, vasodilators, and antidepressants also predisposes older adults to orthostatic hypotension. A drop in SBP is sometimes more pronounced when arising in the morning because of diminished baroreceptor function after prolonged recumbence. Orthostatic hypotension in older adults may be caused by an increase in sedentary activity and blunting of autonomic reflexes.

NURSING MANAGEMENT

Assessment

Assessment of an older patient begins with taking a complete health history and physical examination. Reports of syncope, falls, and near falls should be thoroughly investigated. Assessment data should reflect drugs (prescription, OTC, herbals and supplements), environmental factors, and temporal relationship to meals. Hydration status should be evaluated along with a CBC and serum glucose level; dehydration, anemia, and hypoglycemia can cause syncope and falls.

To assess for orthostatic blood pressure changes, blood pressure and heart rate should be obtained after the patient has been supine for at least 5 minutes. Then the nurse should help the patient to a sitting position, with feet dangling or flat on the floor, and repeat the blood pressure and heart rate after 1 minute and 3 minutes. Then, if the patient can stand, the nurse should obtain a third set of blood pressure and heart rate readings, noting the differences (Higginson, 2016); document all measurements in the patient's record. If the patient complains of lightheadedness or dizziness and/or the SBP drops 20 mm Hg or more or DBP decreases 10 mm Hg or more, the findings are considered abnormal (CDC, 2017b).

All prescribed and OTC drug and herbal preparations should be reviewed carefully. Special attention should be given to drugs known to induce hypotension in older adults, such as amitriptyline, antidepressants, bromocriptine, antiarrhythmics, antihistamines, diuretics, insulin, monoamine oxidase inhibitors, narcotics, sedatives, nitrates, sympatholytics, sympathomimetics, and vasodilators.

Diagnosis

Nursing diagnoses common for an older adult with orthostatic hypotension include the following:
- Potential for reduced cardiac perfusion
- Potential for injury
- Need for health teaching resulting from positional hemodynamic changes and risk for falls

Planning and Expected Outcomes

Expected outcomes for an older adult with orthostatic hypotension include the following:
1. The patient will remain free of injury.
2. The patient will verbalize and correctly demonstrate measures to prevent symptoms of orthostatic hypotension.
3. The patient will verbalize fears and identify coping measures.

Intervention

The nurse should teach an older adult at risk for or with orthostatic hypotension to move slowly from the recumbent position to the sitting position. The patient should then remain sitting for several minutes before attempting to stand.

Exercising the lower legs and ankles facilitates venous return and raises the blood pressure. Elastic stockings help in the same way. In some instances, a higher salt diet may increase blood volume and ameliorate orthostatic changes. The nurse should work with the patient and physician to eliminate unnecessary drugs that may contribute to orthostatic hypotension; the nurse should also encourage the patient to limit alcohol intake, avoid large meals, and monitor and control diabetes mellitus, which is associated with peripheral autonomic dysfunction.

Environmental safety remains important. Grab bars, nonskid surfaces, and an uncluttered living space minimize injuries. In long-term care settings, low beds are sometimes used for cognitively impaired individuals with orthostatic hypotension and a history of falls.

Fear of falling (also referred to as postfall syndrome) produces a fear that frequently causes older adults to limit activity and potentially increases fear for further falls. In addition, caregivers may also fear injury for an older adult and feel compelled to limit the older person's freedom. This leads to a cycle of activity avoidance, increased frailty, and a concomitant increased risk of falling and decreased quality of life (Choi, Jeon, & Cho, 2017; Kapan et al., 2017). Educating patients on the proper technique of standing aids in alleviating this fear. Encouragement and support are also important means for relieving fear.

Evaluation

Evaluation is based on achievement of the expected outcomes and the safe performance of ADLs. Documentation of the patient's blood pressure trends in the three positions aids in evaluating the effectiveness of the recommended treatments.

Syncope With Cardiac Causes

Syncope is a transient loss of consciousness, usually related to decreased cerebral perfusion, with spontaneous recovery (AHA, 2017d). Causes of syncope are broadly grouped into the classes of reflex or neurally mediated (e.g., vasovagal), cardiac (e.g., arrhythmias), miscellaneous neurologic (e.g., psychogenic and cerebrovascular), and orthostatic disorders (e.g., dehydration) (Goyal & Maurer, 2016).

Vasovagal syncope occurs when fright, pain, or nausea stimulate the vagus nerve. Signs and symptoms include nausea, diaphoresis, anxiety, and a feeling of warmth. These same manifestations may also be part of the atypical presentation of MI in an older adult. Vasovagal syncope may also be caused by straining during a bowel movement and by pushing up in bed without assistance. Vasovagal attacks usually occur in the upright position, and the patient regains consciousness upon lying down (Goyal & Maurer, 2016).

Cardiac arrhythmias are often first seen as a loss of consciousness that occurs without warning. Ectopic beats, whether supraventricular or ventricular, increase in frequency with age. Specific arrhythmias include supraventricular and ventricular tachycardias and a variety of bradyarrhythmias.

Atrial fibrillation is an atrial arrhythmia recognized by the lack of a clear P wave on ECG and an irregular ventricular conduction. Because atrial fibrillation is associated with an increased risk of cerebral embolism, anticoagulation should be considered in any older adult with atrial fibrillation (Benjamin et al., 2017). Atrial fibrillation may cause syncope if the ventricular rate becomes too fast for adequate ventricular filling during diastole. In addition, the loss of atrial kick, which accounts for 30% of ventricular filling, may be enough to decrease cardiac output and thus syncope.

Ventricular tachycardia is a medical emergency. It is a tachycardia without atrial activity, a wide QRS complex, and ventricular rates of 120 beats/min and higher. The problem is inadequate ventricular filling during diastole, leading to significantly diminished cardiac output and syncope if not quickly treated. Ventricular tachycardia associated with hemodynamic instability, such as hypotension, requires immediate electrical cardioversion. Long-term control of this type of arrhythmia is accomplished through drug therapy and implantable automatic defibrillators.

Bradyarrhythmias are more common in older adults because of a dysfunction to the intrinsic conduction system. Bradyarrhythmias requiring pacemakers are AV blocks, such as Mobitz type II and third-degree heart block, and sick sinus syndrome if the bradycardia is symptomatic (Fillit, Rockwood, & Young, 2017). Structural problems of the heart such as aortic stenosis, cardiomyopathy, and acute myocardial cell death can also cause syncope.

NURSING MANAGEMENT

Assessment

The assessment of an older patient with syncope begins with a complete history and physical examination. Family members or other witnesses to the patient's syncopal episode should be asked to describe what the patient was doing just before losing consciousness. The older adult should be examined for evidence of acute infarction and arrhythmias with the use of a 12-lead ECG. The carotid arteries should be auscultated for bruits. Blood work should include CBC and complete chemistry panel, including glucose levels (Fillit et al., 2016).

Diagnosis

Nursing diagnoses for an older adult with syncope include the following:
- Reduced cardiac output resulting from inadequate left ventricular filling, arrhythmia, or orthostasis
- Potential for injury
- Anxiety resulting from near or full loss of consciousness

Planning and Expected Outcomes

Syncope with cardiac causes is often an emergency, requiring intensive care for the older adult. Communication between the medical team and family or other caregivers is very important. It is hoped that a health care proxy is available if the patient can no longer speak for himself or herself.

Expected outcomes for an older adult with syncope include the following:
1. The patient will regain a normal range of cardiac output as demonstrated by stable vital signs and alert and oriented sensorium.
2. The older adult and family will verbalize understanding of the cause of syncope and the therapeutic treatment plan.

Intervention

Emergency measures such as CPR and defibrillation should be employed, when needed, to correct life-threatening arrhythmias. Oxygen should be administered, and oxygen saturation should be evaluated.

Nurses need to help older adults identify causes of syncope such as straining during defecation. Constipation is a common complaint among older adults. Measures to avoid constipation include increasing fiber in the diet, adequate fluid intake, and exercise as tolerated. Nurses should instruct the older adult to lie down if they become dizzy or experience other prodromal symptoms.

Evaluation

Evaluation is based on achievement of the expected outcomes and a positive change in the clinical picture of the older adult. Older adults should be able to identify the cause of their syncope and methods of prevention, including methods of preventing injury if syncope occurs.

Valvular Disease

Valvular disease occurs when the cardiac valves do not completely open (stenosis) or close (regurgitation, insufficiency), which prevents efficient circulation of blood through the heart's chambers and increases the myocardial workload. Mitral and aortic valvular diseases are more common than the tricuspid and pulmonic valves.

Stenosis of the mitral valve impedes blood flow from the left atrium to the ventricle during diastole. With time, the left atrium becomes accustomed to increasing volumes and pressure, which causes dilation and hypertrophy. Stenosis of the aortic valve obstructs blood flow from the left ventricle to the aortic arch during systole. With time, hypertrophy of the left ventricle occurs because of increased pressures and volumes. Both stenotic conditions may eventually lead to hypertrophy of pulmonary vessels and decreased cardiac output.

Mitral regurgitation allows ejected blood to flow back into the left atrium from the ventricle during systole, resulting in dilation and hypertrophy of the left atrium and ventricle. Aortic regurgitation allows ejected blood to flow back into the left ventricle from the aorta during diastole, leading to volume overload that can cause dilation and hypertrophy of the left ventricle. Mitral valve prolapse (a form of valvular insufficiency) occurs when one or both cusps prolapse into the left atrium during ventricular systole. The prolapse is normally benign but may progress to severe regurgitation with ventricular dilation.

Rheumatic fever is the most common cause of valvular disease, although the incidence of rheumatic fever has declined since the introduction of antibiotics. Infective endocarditis, connective tissue disorders, and atherosclerosis are other causes of valvular disorders. Mitral regurgitation and aortic stenosis may also be attributed to degeneration or calcification of the valves.

Aortic insufficiency, mitral stenosis, and mitral valve prolapse are more common in younger adults than in older adults. Pulmonary and tricuspid valvular disorders do not often occur in older adults. In older adults, aortic stenosis and mitral regurgitation are more common because of degeneration or calcification of the valves.

Individuals with valvular disease may be asymptomatic for many years, but with the deterioration of the valves and hypertrophic changes to the atria or ventricles, symptoms become evident (Box 19.4). Exertional dyspnea is frequently the initial symptom. Other symptoms related to decreased cardiac output include dizziness, fatigue, weakness, and palpitations. Atrial

---

BOX 19.4 Examples of Clinical Manifestations of Valvular Heart Disease

Mitral Stenosis
Dyspnea on exertion, orthopnea, fatigue, loud accentuated opening snap, low-pitched rumbling, diastolic murmur heard at apex

Mitral Regurgitation
Weakness, fatigue, dyspnea, palpitations, soft S_3 often present, high-pitched pansystolic murmur with a harsh, blowing quality that radiates to the axilla

Aortic Stenosis
Angina, syncope, heart failure, soft prominent S_4, crescendo–decrescendo harsh ejection systolic murmur that radiates to carotids

Aortic Regurgitation
Exertional dyspnea; orthopnea; nocturnal angina; soft or absent S_2, S_3, or S_4; soft decrescendo high-pitched diastolic murmur; wide pulse pressure

Data from Kennedy, E. B. & Ignatavicius D. D. (2013). Interventions for clients with cardiac problems. In Ignatavicius, D. D. & Workman, M. L. (Eds.). *Medical surgical nursing: Critical thinking for collaborative care* (7th ed.). St Louis, MO: Saunders; Ott, B. B. & DeFrancesco-Loukas, M. A. (2009). Management of clients with structural cardiac disorders. In J. M. Black & J. H. Hawks (Eds.). *Medical surgical nursing: Clinical management for positive outcomes* (8th ed.). St. Louis, MO: Saunders.

---

fibrillation is often associated with mitral disorders secondary to distention of the left atria. Symptoms of angina are more common with aortic disorders because of decreased cardiac output. Symptoms of valvular disease may be difficult to recognize in older adults because symptoms may mimic those of CAD.

Diagnostic Tests and Procedures

Chest radiography and ECG are initial diagnostic tests that may suggest valvular disease or evaluate damage to the heart from valvular problems. ECG with Doppler and ultrasonography provides the most detailed information on the valve's structure, function (abnormal cusp movement), and any evidence of cardiac hypertrophy. Cardiac catheterization may be done to assess the severity of the valve disorder (i.e., valve size, pressure changes within the chamber, and pressure gradients across valves), and additional effects on the heart. Exercise stress tests may also be conducted to evaluate the patient's exercise capacity and hemodynamic response to exertion and recovery (Garcia, Mulvagh, Merz, Buring, & Manson, 2016).

Treatment

Treatment is directed toward the management of presenting symptoms and correction of the cause of the valvular disorder. Treatment for symptoms of heart failure consists of digoxin, diuretics, vasodilating agents, restricted sodium intake, and oxygen therapy. Symptoms of decreased cardiac output related to atrial fibrillation are treated with cardioversion, anticoagulants, or antiarrhythmics, such as digoxin, BBs, and CCBs. Symptoms of decreased cardiac output related to ischemia are treated with vasodilating agents. Prophylactic antibiotics before invasive procedures (e.g., surgery, invasive tests, and dental work) are recommended for all patients with valve disorders to prevent infective endocarditis. For patients with valvular disorders resulting from degenerative processes, medical treatment of symptoms tends to be unsuccessful over time, and surgical repair or replacement of diseased valves can become necessary.

Prognosis

Morbidity and mortality are higher for older adults requiring valve surgery. Older adults often have more advanced disease and multiple coexisting chronic diseases at the time of surgery. Zellner (2012) reports a 75% survival rate at 5 years and a 10-year survival rate greater than 55% for older adults undergoing mitral valve repair. Valvular surgery on older adults has steadily increased during the past decade and has increased the quality of life for older adults.

NURSING MANAGEMENT

Assessment

Assessment should include the history of prior episodes of rheumatic fever, infective endocarditis, staphylococcal and streptococcal infections, and family history of cardiac disease. Symptoms of valvular disease (e.g., fatigue, dyspnea, palpitations, dizziness, weakness, syncope, peripheral edema, distended neck veins, periods of memory loss or confusion, and chest pain) or related complications (e.g., arrhythmia, angina, and heart failure) should be noted, as well as the patient's level of fatigue, toleration of activity, and current drugs.

Objective data should be obtained primarily from cardiovascular and respiratory assessments. Cardiovascular data include blood pressure, pulse pressure, heart rate and rhythm, recent weight loss or gain, peripheral pulses, presence of peripheral edema, neck vein distention, and heart sounds. Different heart sounds are heard with each valvular disorder, and auscultation should be performed for identification of abnormalities or changes. Respiratory data include rate, depth, and breath sounds.

Aortic stenosis is the most common valvular disorder among older adults because of calcification of the valve with aging. Stenosis of this valve tends to occur without fusion of the cusps, resulting in a spray of blood through the valve rather than forceful propulsion. Physical examination may reveal softer and more musical heart murmurs that may be associated with the normal aging process rather than with a valvular disorder. Older adults may require diagnostic testing to support a diagnosis of valvular disease.

Diagnosis

Nursing diagnoses common for an older patient with valvular disease include the following:

- Reduced cardiac output, secondary to altered blood flow through the heart
- Reduced activity level, secondary to decreased cardiac output
- Anxiety, secondary to new diagnosis, treatment plan, and uncertain outcome
- Need for health teaching, secondary to lack of previous exposure to information about the disease process, drugs, and treatment plan

Planning and Expected Outcomes

Expected outcomes for an older patient with valvular disease depend on the severity and extent of the disease. Outcomes include the following:

1. The patient will maintain adequate cardiac output, as demonstrated by stable vital signs, mental alertness, urine output of 30 mL/hr or greater, and clear breath sounds.
2. The patient will tolerate a usual level of daily activity, as demonstrated by stable vital signs and no dyspnea with activity.
3. The patient will experience reduced anxiety through verbalization of decreased anxiety, the ability to express specific fears.
4. The patient will correctly explain the disease process, therapeutic plan, and preventive precautions.

Intervention

Cardiovascular and respiratory assessments should be conducted on a regular basis to detect progress and to prevent complications. Nurses should monitor patients for therapeutic and adverse reactions to prescribed drugs; monitor blood pressure, heart rate, respirations, heart sounds, breath sounds, and cardiac rhythm; ensure that the patient maintains an appropriate activity level and performs range-of-motion exercises during

bed rest to prevent complications; elevate the head of the bed to maximize thoracic excursion; and administer oxygen, as prescribed.

Nurses should also assess the older adult's activity level and balance activity with rest periods; organize care to provide rest periods and advance activity according to the patient's tolerance. Because older adults are more prone to dizziness and lightheadedness due to orthostatic hypotension, older adults should be instructed to rise slowly and stay in the sitting position for a few minutes before standing. Older adults should wear nonslip footwear, and handrails should be available for support and to prevent falls.

Older adults should understand the disease process and treatment plan, and recognize the signs and symptoms of heart failure and when to notify their health care provider. As appropriate, a low-sodium or other healthy diet should be followed. Bleeding precautions should be reviewed with patients receiving anticoagulant therapy. Patients should be taught the importance of appropriate oral hygiene and its importance in the prevention of trauma and infective endocarditis, as well as the necessity for pretreatment with antibiotics before invasive procedures, including all dental work.

For patients who do not respond to medical treatment, heart valve surgery may be necessary to improve cardiac performance. Older patients benefit more from surgery when their condition is stable, and the procedure is performed on an elective basis. Before heart valve surgery, patients should be informed of the necessity for extensive diagnostic tests and blood studies. The patient and family should also be oriented to the ICU or coronary care unit (CCU) and the equipment that will be used postoperatively. Postoperative assessment activities and treatments should be explained.

After surgery, patients will be monitored closely for complications, such as MI, heart failure, thromboembolism, hemorrhage, arrhythmia, and infection. Older patients have a greater risk for complications compared with younger adults. Older adults are also prone to the development of delirium after surgery due to multiple factors, including the stress of the procedure, drug therapy and other treatment modalities, and environmental alterations. The presence of the family and familiar belongings and the use of personal hearing aids or eyeglasses may help alleviate episodes of delirium.

Recovery from heart valve surgery is generally complete within 6 to 8 weeks; however, recovery may be delayed in older adults resulting from a higher incidence of postoperative complications. Exercise and ADLs should be gradually resumed during the first 6 weeks of recovery. Patients should be taught to monitor their pulse and respiratory rate to evaluate tolerance to activity. Patients should be encouraged to progressively increase the duration and frequency of walking. Patients should avoid lifting heavy objects. Prophylactic use of antibiotics should be explained to the patient. Anticoagulants may be prescribed for patients with prosthetic valves. Signs and symptoms of valve failure should be reviewed with the patient in case deteriorating symptoms develop that necessitate valve replacement following surgical repair of a valve; patients with valve replacements may need new valves after 10 to 15 years.

Evaluation

Evaluation of an older patient with valvular disease focuses on achievement of the expected outcomes. Older adults should demonstrate adequate cardiac output, the ability to perform ADLs within limitations, and control of symptoms. The nurse should also note the patient's and family's ability to manage the care requirements and resolve any problems appropriately. Documentation should accurately reflect the care delivered in the preoperative and postoperative periods and the older adult's response. Assessment of the progress toward self-care and the degree of functional ability must also be documented on an ongoing basis because the older adult's recovery depends in large part on returning to the prior level of functioning.

Heart Failure

Approximately 6.5 million adults in the United States suffer from heart failure (Benjamin et al., 2017). More than 900,000 new cases are diagnosed each year. Furthermore, it is estimated that the prevalence of heart failure will increase 46% by the year 2030. Even though mortality rates for heart failure have declined over the past years, mortality continues to be high with approximately 50% of people diagnosed with heart failure dying within 5 years.

Heart failure is a syndrome characterized by poor perfusion of oxygen- and nutrient-rich blood. Heart failure occurs when the heart does not function as it should, leading to decreased cardiac output (AHA, 2017e). Heart failure occurs over time and can affect either the right side, left side, or both. Left-sided heart failure can occur with reduced (systolic failure) or preserved (diastolic failure) ejection fraction (Table 19.3). Right-side heart failure prevents oxygen-poor blood from reaching the lungs to obtain oxygen, whereas left-side heart failure impedes oxygen-rich blood from leaving the heart and reaching the rest of the body. In systolic heart failure, the left ventricle is unable to effectively contract to push enough oxygen-rich blood into circulation; in diastolic heart failure, the left ventricle is unable to relax, preventing the heart from filling with oxygen-rich blood. Swelling in the body (e.g., hands, feet, abdomen, neck veins) can occur with right-side heart failure; fluid buildup in the lungs can occur with left-side heart failure. All heart failure can cause fatigue and shortness of breath.

Heart failure is classified according to symptom severity and function status. The ACCF/AHA stages of heart failure are used to determine the presence of and severity of failure (Table 19.4), whereas the New York Heart Association (NYHA) functional classification focuses on symptomatology and exercise capability (Yancy et al., 2013a&b).

The most common risk factors for heart failure include CHD, HTN, diabetes mellitus, obesity, and smoking (AHA, 2017e). Lifetime risk for heart failure is higher for males with HTN; among older adults, current and past cigarette smoking increases their risk for heart failure. The prevalence of heart failure increases as adults age. In clinical trials, approximately 50% of participants with heart failure were older adults over the age of 75 (Azad & Lemay, 2014). Hospitalization due to heart failure is higher among older adults.

TABLE 19.3　ACC/AHA Heart Failure Definitions of Heart Failure Based on Ejection Fraction

Classification	EF (%)	Comments
Heart failure with reduced ejection fraction (HFrEF) (aka: systolic heart failure)	≤40	Major reduction in systolic function. May also have diastolic dysfunction and variable degrees of LV enlargement.
Heart failure with preserved ejection fraction (HFpEF) (aka: diastolic heart failure)	≥50	Does not have a major reduction in systolic function. Patients are usually treated for underlying causes of heart failure. Risk factors include diabetes mellitus, obesity, CAD, and atrial fibrillation.
HFpEF, borderline	41–49	
HFpEF, improved	>40	

aka, Also known as; *CAD,* coronary artery disease; *EF,* ejection fraction; *LV,* left ventricle.
Adapted from Yancy, C. W., Jessup, M., Bozkurt, B., Butler, J., Casey, D. E., Drazner, M. H., … Wilkoff, B. L. (2013a&b). 2013 ACCF/AHA guideline for the management of heart failure: A report of the American College of Cardiology Foundation/American Heart Association Task Force on Practice Guidelines. *Journal of the American College of Cardiology, 62*(16): e147-239. https://doi.org/10.1016/j.jacc.2013.05.019

TABLE 19.4　ACCF/AHA Stages of Heart Failure

Stages	Description
A	Asymptomatic. At high risk for HF. No structural heart disease.
B	Asymptomatic. Has structural heart disease.
C	Symptomatic or history of symptoms. Has structural heart disease.
D	Symptomatic. Has refractory HF requiring interventions.

HF, heart failure.
Adapted from Yancy, C. W., Jessup, M., Bozkurt, B., Butler, J., Casey, D. E., Drazner, M. H., … Wilkoff, B. L. (2013a&b). 2013 ACCF/AHA guideline for the management of heart failure: A report of the American College of Cardiology Foundation/American Heart Association Task Force on Practice Guidelines. *Journal of the American College of Cardiology, 62* (16):e147-239. https://doi.org/10.1016/j.jacc.2013.05.019

Age-associated cardiovascular and renal changes that affect the clinical course of heart failure and responses to treatment include decreased renal and systemic blood flow, increased arterial stiffness and peripheral resistance, reduced ventricular compliance, and reduced maximum aerobic capacity. In a majority of people, the ideal blood pressure is less than 130/80 mm Hg. However, among older adults with heart failure or those who are at increased risk of heart failure, the optimal goal is for SBP of less than 120 mm Hg (Yancy et al., 2017). But 50% of older adults over the age of 75 with heart failure have diastolic dysfunction (Azad & Lemay, 2014). (See Evidence-Based Practice box.)

Diagnostic Tests and Procedures

The ACC and AHA guidelines recommend the following diagnostic tests for the initial and serial evaluations of patients with heart failure: complete laboratory evaluation (e.g., B-type natriuretic peptide, CBC, urinalysis, serum electrolytes, kidney function, thyroid panel, and lipid panel); 12-lead ECG, chest x-ray to assess heart size and to detect other cardiopulmonary diseases; and echocardiogram to assess cardiac function (e.g., left ventricular ejection fraction) (Yancy et al., 2013a&b). (See Evidence-Based Practice box.)

EVIDENCE-BASED PRACTICE

Heart Failure in Older Adults

Background
Frail older adults experience poor physical functioning and outcomes. Some studies have indicated an association between frailty, coronary vascular disease, and mortality in older adults.

Sample/Setting
Study participants included 2,825 community-dwelling older adults aged 70 to 79 years who lived in Pittsburgh or Memphis. U.S. participants had comorbid chronic illnesses such as CHD, diabetes mellitus, and HTN. Of the 2,825 participants, 48% were male and 59% were white. Frailty, identified by the Gill index, was present in 17.5% of study participants.

Method
Study participants were recruited from a random sample of Medicare beneficiaries and age-eligible persons living in Pittsburgh and Memphis. Frailty was determined using the Health Aging (Health ABC) and Body Composition Short Physical Performance Battery (HABC Battery), and the Gill index. The Gill index categorizes participants into nonfrail, moderately frail, or severely frail based on chair-stand and walking speed. The HABC Battery evaluates physical performance by a combination of gait speed, repeated chair stands, and tandem balance tests. Medical records for hospitalizations were reviewed at baseline and every 6 months during the longitudinal study for episodes of heart failure. Data were analyzed to determine associations between frailty, associated medical conditions, age, gender, and episodes of heart failure.

Findings
Frailty was determined to be a significant predictor for heart failure in both genders and in blacks and whites. The findings were independent of other variables.

Implications
Heart failure is one of the most common cardiovascular problems and reasons for hospital admission in older adults. Frailty has been associated with increased risk for heart failure. Screening older adults for frailty can identify those at risk for heart failure, enabling early intervention aimed at improving physical endurance, thereby improving quality of life.

From Khan, H., Kalogeropoulos, A. P., Georgiopoulou, V. V., Newman, A. B., Harris, T. B., Rodondi, … Butler, J. (2013). Frailty and risk for heart failure in older adults: The health, aging, and body composition study. *American Heart Journal, 166*(5), 887-894. https://doi.org/10.1016/j.ahj.2013.07.032

Treatment

Treatment of heart failure in older adults requires careful control of precipitating factors, a low-sodium diet, fluid restriction as appropriate, adequate rest, and exercise. Treatment of heart failure also includes drug therapy. Table 19.5 lists selected drugs for the treatment of heart failure. For adverse effects and nursing implications, see Table 19.2. The American College of Cardiology Foundation (ACCF) and the AHA (Yancy et al., 2013a&b) established the guidelines for the treatment of heart failure. Depending on the severity of heart failure, treatment consists

of nonpharmacological and pharmacologic therapy. Nonpharmacological therapies include lifestyle modifications (e.g., regular physical activity, sodium restriction, smoking cessation, and reduced alcohol intake). Pharmacologic therapy for heart failure involves several classes of drugs, depending on whether the ejection fraction is preserved or reduced.

Systolic Heart Failure (Reduced Ejection Fraction)

Diuretics are important to maintain euvolemia and are prescribed for patients exhibiting evidence of pulmonary or systemic congestion (e.g., furosemide, bumetanide, or torsemide). Kidney function and electrolytes must be closely monitored in older adults because of age-related changes in kidney function. ACEIs are first-line therapy in systolic heart failure with reduced ejection fraction, as they have been shown to reduce morbidity and mortality. The initial dose should be low; if renal function remains stable, the dose should be titrated up as tolerated. ARB is prescribed if ACEI is not tolerated due to its side effects, such as cough (The Medical Letter, 2015).

Beta-blockers (e.g., bisoprolol, carvedilol, and metoprolol succinate) given along with ACEI have been shown to reduce hospitalization and mortality. Beta-blockers are started at low doses and increased every 2 weeks to the highest dose tolerated. Patients should be told that symptoms of heart failure may worsen slightly the first 2 weeks of treatment and that full therapeutic benefits may not occur for several months (The Medical Letter, 2015).

Aldosterone antagonists (e.g., eplerenone or spironolactone) may prescribed for patients with systolic heart failure with ejection fraction of 35% or less to reduce hospitalization and mortality. However, life-threatening hyperkalemia can occur with aldosterone antagonists (The Medical Letter, 2015).

Hydralazine and isosorbide dinitrate may be beneficial for some patients, particularly African Americans who have not responded to ACEI and beta-blockers. These two drugs in a fixed dose combination have been shown to reduce mortality. Digoxin has been shown to reduce hospitalizations in patients with advanced heart failure and reduced ejection fraction. Digoxin should be prescribed at a low dose (0.125 mg; The Medical Letter, 2015).

Anticoagulation (e.g., warfarin) is indicated if atrial fibrillation is present and the older adult has risk factors for embolic events, such as HTN, diabetes mellitus, or age 75 years or greater. In hospitalized patients, sympathomimetics (e.g., dopamine and dobutamine) may be beneficial to increase the force of myocardial contraction. As with heart failure with preserved ejection fraction, exercise is encouraged. Statin drugs and CCBs are not recommended for treatment of heart failure with reduced ejection fraction.

Diastolic Heart Failure (Preserved Ejection Fraction)

The goal is to reduce ventricular filling pressure and control symptoms. The principle goal in treating heart failure with preserved ejection fraction is geared toward managing HTN with CCBs, ACEIs, or ARBs; controlling heart rate with beta-blockers or digoxin; and the use of diuretics to treat pulmonary or systemic congestion. However, overuse of diuretics leading to

TABLE 19.5 Selected Drugs for Congestive Heart Failure

Drug Classification	Adverse Reactions	Precautions
ACEIs Captopril Enalapril Lisinopril Quinapril Ramipril Trandolapril	Cough (common), skin rash, hypotension, taste disturbance, angioedema	Monitor renal function. Avoid sudden changes in position.
Aldosterone Antagonist Spironolactone	GI bleeding, sexual dysfunction, fever, urticaria, confusion, ataxia	Monitor for fluid, electrolyte imbalance, and weight. Monitor renal and hepatic levels.
Beta-Blockers Bisoprolol Carvedilol Metoprolol Metoprolol extended release	Bradycardia, shortness of breath, fatigue, dizziness, depression, diarrhea, pruritus, rash, arthralgia May mask symptoms of hyperthyroidism and hypoglycemia	Monitor heart rate. Monitor for signs of hyperglycemia.
Diuretics ***Thiazide Diuretics*** Hydrochlorothiazide Metolazone	Electrolyte depletion, hypovolemia, hyperglycemia, gastric irritation	Monitor electrolytes, especially potassium. Monitor urine output.
Loop Diuretics Furosemide Bumetanide Ethacrynic acid Torsemide	Electrolyte depletion, anorexia, diarrhea, malaise, mental confusion, ototoxicity A dramatic increase occurs in urine output	Monitor electrolytes, especially potassium. Monitor hearing.
Cardiac Glycosides Digoxin	Altered color perceptions, visual disturbances, confusion, headache, muscle weakness, nausea, anorexia, arrhythmias, bradycardia	Monitor potassium levels. Use with caution in patients with IHSS. Half-life may be longer in the elderly leading to increased risk of toxicity. Monitor vital signs.
Sympathomimetics Dopamine	Headache, tachycardia, arrhythmias, hypertension	Contraindicated in patients with IHSS or sensitivity to any sulfite.
Dobutamine	Headache, nausea, hypotension	Contraindicated in patients with IHSS or hypersensitivity to metabisulfite.
Amrinone	Headache, anorexia, hepatotoxicity, thrombocytopenia, hypotension	Use with caution in patients with CAD or recent MI. Contraindicated in patients with metabisulfite hypersensitivity.

CAD, Coronary artery disease; *GI,* gastrointestinal disease; *IHSS,* idiopathic hypertrophic subaortic stenosis; *MI,* myocardial infarction.
Data from Lehne, R. A.: (2013). *Pharmacology for nursing care* (8th ed.). Philadelphia: Saunders; Yancy, W. C., Jessup, M., Bozkurt, B., Butler, J., Casey, D. D., Drazner, ... Westlake, C. (2017). 2017 ACC/AHA/HFSA focused update of the 2013 ACCF/AHA guideline for the management of heart failure. *Journal of the American College of Cardiology, 76*(6), doi: https://doi.org/10.1016/j.jacc.2017.04.025

hypotension and electrolyte imbalance can be problematic for older adults; therefore close monitoring is warranted.

Prognosis

HF in older adults is associated with a poor prognosis; 25% of older adults with HF are readmitted to the hospital within 30 days of discharge, and 70% are readmitted within a year. Mortality is higher for older adults with systolic HF than those with diastolic HF. Mortality rates for older adults discharged to skilled nursing facilities following hospitalization are 50% at 1 year. Mortality rates increase with age; for adults 80 years and older, mortality at 5 years is roughly 50% (Benjamin et al., 2017; Dharmarajan & Rich, 2017).

NURSING MANAGEMENT

Assessment

Older adults should be assessed for a history of CAD, rheumatic heart disease, HTN, arrhythmias, cardiac valve disease, infection, diabetes, kidney disease, and current drugs. The initial physical evaluation of an older adult suspected of having HF includes measurement of blood pressure, evaluation for pitting edema of the legs and ankles, assessment of jugular venous distension, heart and lung auscultation, and percussion of the lung for effusions. Assessment for orthopnea, fatigue at rest, paroxysmal nocturnal dyspnea, and nocturnal urination are also important. Nurses should determine how symptoms have affected ADLs for older adults.

Diagnosis

Common diagnoses for an older adult patient with HF include the following:

- Reduced cardiac output resulting from decreased cardiac contractility
- Altered gas exchange resulting from pulmonary venous congestion
- Increased fluid volume resulting from increased sodium and water reabsorption
- Anxiety resulting from perceived threat to self
- Reduced stamina resulting from decreased cardiac output
- Decreased ability to cope resulting from knowledge deficit and fear of uncertain outcome
- Altered sleep pattern resulting from nocturnal dyspnea and nocturnal urination
- Need for health teaching resulting from lack of previous exposure to disease process, drugs, and treatment plan

Planning and Expected Outcomes

Expected outcomes are aimed at maximizing myocardial function and assisting with the lifestyle modifications and emotional adjustments imposed by the disease. Expected outcomes for an older adult with HF include the following:

1. Cardiac output will be maximized, as evidenced by vital signs within an acceptable range, no arrhythmia, adequate cardiac output, urine output greater than 30 mL/hr, and alert mental state.
2. Gas exchange will be improved, as evidenced by decreased or no reported dyspnea, normal respiratory rate, lungs clear on auscultation, no evidence of central or peripheral cyanosis, and a patient report of improved activity tolerance.
3. Excess fluid volume will be reduced, as evidenced by reductions in water weight, dependent edema, and abdominal girth.
4. The patient will experience less anxiety, as evidenced by communication of fears to nurse and self-report of the use of coping skills.
5. Activity will be restored to its prior level, as evidenced by fewer or no reports of fatigue with usual activities.
6. The patient will experience adequate coping, as evidenced by the naming of coping skills used in the past and a self-report of feeling positive about the future.
7. The patient will experience an acceptable sleeping pattern, as evidenced by reports of sleep uninterrupted by dyspnea and a feeling of being rested on awakening.
8. The patient will demonstrate an adequate knowledge level, as evidenced by the ability to correctly state information about the disease process; treatment plan; and drug indications, dosage, frequency, and side effects.

Intervention

It is essential for nurses to assess blood pressure, apical pulse, heart rate, heart and lung sounds, and peripheral edema to detect early signs and symptoms of altered cardiac output. The intake and output and daily weights should be monitored and recorded. The older adult should be weighed at the same time each day to accurately monitor fluid loss or retention. The older adult's activity should be increased as tolerated, and time for adequate rest provided; while in bed, the patient should maintain Fowler's position. Older adults may need more than one pillow to sleep with at night. Nurses should instruct patients to take diuretics in the morning so sleep is not disturbed by getting up to void. Nurses should encourage older adults to take slow deep breaths during dyspneic episodes and maintain a calm environment.

Nurses should instruct the older adult about restricted sodium and fluid intake. A dietitian may be consulted. Older adults should be instructed to avoid canned foods and prepared frozen meals due to their high sodium content and to use salt sparingly. A weight gain of 3 lb in 48 hours and a return of any symptoms should be reported to the health care provider immediately. Electrolyte levels, especially potassium, and signs and symptoms of electrolyte imbalance should be monitored.

Nurses should give older adults instructions on their condition, procedures, diet, and risk factors in a clear, simple manner, using proper language, appropriate reading level, and incorporating cultural considerations. When teaching, the environment should be kept relaxed and as quiet as possible; all procedures should be explained and questions answered clearly and concisely. Older adult patients and family members should be given the opportunity to verbalize their concerns.

Referral to a home health agency for assistance with ADLs and referral to Meals-on-Wheels may be necessary for some individuals. Older adults should be encouraged to enter a cardiac rehabilitation program to monitor activity tolerance in a secure environment.

Evaluation

Improved ventricular function is demonstrated by unlabored respirations, decreased or no peripheral edema, improved or no cough or orthopnea, and an increase in urine output. Patients should increase their activity levels as tolerated (i.e., without experiencing dyspnea) and should return to prior level of ADL function. Documentation of trends is critical for older adults with heart failure, especially regarding assessment findings and treatment responses (see Nursing Care Plan: Congestive Heart Failure).

Peripheral Artery Disease

Peripheral artery disease (PAD) is a narrowing of the systemic arteries that impairs tissue perfusion. PAD is associated with significant morbidity and mortality and, if left untreated, can be life-threatening (Gerhard-Herman et al., 2016). Most common causes of PAD are arteriosclerosis and atherosclerosis. Although the exact cause of atherosclerosis is unclear, several risk factors have been identified. These include advanced age, smoking, elevated serum cholesterol levels, HTN, diabetes mellitus, physical inactivity, obesity, and family history.

◎ NURSING CARE PLAN

Congestive Heart Failure

Clinical Situation

Mr. H, an 86-year-old man who is widowed and lives alone, arrives in the emergency department complaining he has had difficulty breathing, especially at night, associated with nausea, for the past week. He states that he must sleep with two pillows to breathe more easily at night and still does not get a good night's rest. He also complains of a cough that is worse at night and relieved by nothing. Mr. H is concerned he has pneumonia. Assessment of Mr. H reveals the following:

- Vital signs: temperature, 98° F; apical heart rate, 86 beats/min and irregular; respiratory rate, 36 breaths/min and labored; and blood pressure, 170/96 mm Hg
- Skin—pale, cool, and diaphoretic
- Inspiratory bibasilar crackles that do not clear with coughing
- S_3 heart sound on auscultation
- Visible jugular vein distention
- 3+ bilateral pedal edema

Twelve-lead ECG and a chest radiography (CXR) are ordered. An intravenous line (IV) is started at 30 mL/hr. Oxygen via mask is ordered. Intravenous furosemide is given, and Mr. H is admitted with a diagnosis of heart failure.

Nursing Diagnoses

Reduced cardiac perfusion resulting from ineffective myocardial contractility

Fluid overload resulting from decreased cardiac contractility

Decreased gas exchange resulting from increased fluid in pulmonary vasculature

Need for patient teaching resulting from new diagnosis of heart failure, disease process, and treatment

Outcomes

Cardiac output is maximized, as evidenced by vital signs within acceptable limits, controlled arrhythmias, clear breath sounds, fewer dyspneic episodes, decreasing edema, and alert mental status.

The patient will demonstrate normal fluid balance, as evidenced by reduced pedal and pretibial edema and a loss of water weight with a stable dry weight.

The patient will correctly verbalize prescribed sodium and fluid restrictions.

The patient will have improved gas exchange, as evidenced by increased activity tolerance, decreased episodes of shortness of breath and nocturnal dyspnea, and clearer breath sounds.

The patient will describe HF and reasons for limitations, identify his own risk factors, and explain techniques to initiate lifestyle changes.

The patient will participate in the treatment plan.

Interventions

Monitor and document heart rate, rhythm, blood pressure, respirations, and lung and heart sounds hourly and as needed.

Assess for edema and jugular vein distention every 2 to 4 hours.

Monitor intake and output hourly.

Assess skin temperature and color, and assess for the presence of diaphoresis at regular intervals.

Provide a restful environment.

Administer cardiac drugs, as ordered; document patient's response.

Monitor intake and output hourly.

Weigh daily, using the same scale at the same time of day.

Care Plan

Administer diuretics as ordered; document patient's response.

Assess levels of electrolytes, blood urea nitrogen (BUN), and creatinine, as well as symptoms of any imbalance.

Instruct the patient to elevate extremities when sitting.

Instruct the patient on sodium and fluid restrictions.

Assess respiratory status hourly and as needed (rate, rhythm, use of accessory muscles, and lung sounds).

Maintain the patient in Fowler's position to aid breathing.

Administer oxygen as ordered and monitor oxygen saturation.

Discuss the benefits of increased activity (e.g., a walking program); instruct the patient to avoid strenuous and taxing activities and to take advantage of peak energy periods.

Discuss the normal function of the heart and how HF alters heart function.

Discuss drug therapy, including indications, side effects, and specific monitoring.

Discuss specific risk factors and the patient's role in modifying them.

Review signs and symptoms that need to be immediately reported to a health care provider.

Provide an environment that allows the patient to verbalize feelings and ask questions.

Refer the patient to community resources and support groups.

Encourage the patient to obtain annual flu immunization.

Atherosclerosis involves the development of atheromatous plaques on the intimal layer of arterial vessels. These lesions progressively narrow the artery lumen and lead to the formation of thrombi, emboli, and aneurysms.

As the lumen narrows, partial or complete obstruction occurs, leading to inadequate tissue perfusion beyond the lesion and ischemia. Common sites for plaque formation are the aortoiliac vessels, femoropopliteal vessels, and popliteal–tibial arteries. Symptoms appear when the artery is unable to supply the tissues with adequate oxygenated blood flow.

Plaques may rupture or break loose and circulate through the arterial system, causing MI or stroke. The emboli also tend to block arteries at bifurcation points of the femoral and popliteal arteries. Impaired blood flow and ischemia occur at sites distal to the occlusion.

As the atheromatous plaque progresses, the medial layer of the wall calcifies and loses elasticity, which weakens the arterial wall. As the vessel wall weakens, pouches or aneurysms form. Pressure within the arteries, especially in the presence of HTN, may further dilate the aneurysm until it ruptures. Aneurysms commonly occur in large arteries such as the abdominal aorta. Multiple aneurysms may develop in the popliteal artery. Thrombi may form within the aneurysm and circulate to smaller distal vessels in the arterial system.

Signs and symptoms of arterial insufficiency depend on the site, extent of occlusion, and degree of collateral circulation. Collateral circulation often develops in the setting of gradual occlusion caused by plaque formation.

Intermittent claudication (exercise-induced reversible muscle ischemia) is one of the initial symptoms with atherosclerosis obliterans. Pain in the foot or calf is experienced with exercise and subsides with rest (AHA, 2017a). As the disease progresses, the distance walked becomes shorter before pain is felt. Burning pain in the foot at rest or during sleep indicates a severe form of the disease. Cold, numbness, and tingling may accompany the pain. The foot appears pale when elevated and dusky red in dependent positions (dependent rubor). Dry skin, thickened toenails, loss of pedal hair, and cool skin may result from poor circulation. Painful arterial ulcers may be noticed on the toes, between the toes, or on the upper aspect of the foot. Cold extremities with mottling, delayed filling of capillaries, and absent pedal pulses are indicative of acute arterial insufficiency and should be treated immediately. Care should be taken to examine both extremities for comparison. Advanced stages of ischemia lead to necrosis, ulceration, and gangrene of the toes.

The pain with arterial emboli is sudden and severe. The affected extremity appears pale and cool, and distal pulses are absent. Impaired motor and sensory function is evident. Shock may develop if large arteries are occluded.

Diagnostic Tests and Procedures

Screening all patients for asymptomatic PAD is not recommended. Patients who have increased risk for PAD should have a comprehensive history and physical assessment for clinical manifestations (Gerhard-Herman et al., 2016). SBPs should be obtained in both arms and ankles in patients with PAD and ankle-brachial index calculated. A low (≤0.90) ankle-brachial index indicates PAD:

- Mild (0.71 to 0.90)
- Moderate (0.41 to 0.70)
- Severe (≤0.40)

Other diagnostics for patients with PAD include imaging studies. Doppler ultrasound (Duplex) imaging detects and measures the velocity of blood flow through arterial segments. Angiography is performed to determine the exact location and extent of arterial occlusion. Contrast material is injected into the arterial system through a specialized catheter inserted into the brachial or femoral artery, and a series of radiographic studies trace the dye through the arterial system.

Treatment

Treatment of PAD includes lifestyle modifications, such as adopting a structured exercise regimen of swimming or biking and smoking cessation, which is crucial for patients with PAD. Pharmacotherapy should be guideline-based to reduce cardiovascular and limb-related events. Antiplatelet therapy with aspirin alone or combined with clopidogrel is highly recommended for symptomatic patients to reduce cardiovascular events, such as MI and stroke. Antiplatelet drugs inhibit the adherence and aggregation of platelets along damaged vessels. Dipyridamole and cilostazol are other antiplatelet drugs that inhibit platelet aggregation (Gerhard-Herman et al., 2016).

Statin drugs, such as simvastatin, are also indicated for patients with symptomatic PAD to improve blood flow and reduce cardiovascular events and decrease loss of limbs. Control of blood pressure with antihypertensive drugs is necessary to decrease cardiovascular events.

Surgical Procedures

Percutaneous transluminal angioplasty involves gaining access to the arterial system with a specialized balloon-tipped catheter.

The catheter is advanced under fluoroscopy to the atherosclerotic lesion and inflated over the site to compress the plaque and improve blood flow. Intravascular stents keep the vessel open. Thromboendarterectomy is the opening of the artery and removal of the plaque. Revascularization (arterial bypass and reconstruction) may be performed to increase blood flow. Advanced cases of atherosclerosis and gangrene of the extremities necessitate amputation of the limb.

Prognosis

The key to preventing or halting the progression of PAD and subsequent complications appears to be controlling the risk factors for atherosclerosis through adherence to a healthy diet, a program of exercise, weight loss if needed, and smoking cessation. If lifestyle changes are ineffective, pharmacologic therapy or surgical intervention may be necessary (see Patient/Family Teaching box: PAD).

PATIENT/FAMILY TEACHING

Peripheral Artery Disease (PAD)

Prevention is the key to the management of PAD.

Control risk factors: stop smoking; lose weight; control HTN and diabetes mellitus; eat a low-fat, low-cholesterol diet; and exercise daily by walking.

Do not cross legs while sitting; do not stand or sit for long periods.

Do not wear constricting garments.

Foot care is essential. Inspect the feet daily, and keep them clean and dry. Do not soak feet. Use mild soap and a washcloth to clean. Check water temperature with a thermometer or elbow, but do not use your toes. After bathing, dry well between toes; lubricate feet with lotion daily. Avoid walking barefoot, and wear proper-fitting footwear that is flexible yet protective.

Immediately notify the health care provider of changes in color, temperature, or sensation of the affected area or of damage to skin integrity.

From Blach, D. A. & Ignatavicius, D. D. (2013). Interventions for clients with vascular problems. In D. D. Ignativicius and M. L. Workman (Eds.). (2013). *Medical surgical nursing: Patient centered collaborative care* (7th ed.). St. Louis, MO: Saunders; Black, J. M. (2009). Management of clients with vascular disorders. In J. M. Black & J. H. Hawks (Eds.). *Medical surgical nursing: Clinical management for positive outcomes* (8th ed.). St. Louis, MO: Saunders; Morton, P. G., Fontaine, D. K., Hudak, C. M., & Gallo, B. M. (2012). *Critical care nursing: A holistic approach* (10th ed.). Philadelphia: Lippincott Williams & Wilkins; Sieggreen, M. Y. & Kline, R. A. (2011). Vascular ulcers. In S. Baranoski & E. A. Ayello (Eds.). *Wound care essentials*. Philadelphia: Lippincott Williams & Wilkins.

NURSING MANAGEMENT

Assessment

Assessment of an older adult with PAD begins with a complete history and physical examination. Assessment data should reflect the presence of acute or chronic arterial insufficiency.

Subjective and objective assessment of a patient with PAD is outlined in Box 19.5.

Diagnosis

Nursing diagnoses for older adults with PAD include the following:

- Decreased peripheral tissue perfusion resulting from decreased arterial blood flow

- Decreased activities of daily living resulting from an imbalance between tissue need and blood supply
- Potential for skin integrity issues
- Need for health teaching resulting from lack of previous exposure to disease process, drug, and treatment plan

Planning and Expected Outcomes

Older patients with PAD and their family members should be included in the planning of care. Discharge planning should begin as soon as an older adult is admitted to the hospital. Additional support services may be necessary during home recovery.

Expected outcomes for an older adult patient with PAD include the following:

1. The patient will manifest reduced signs and symptoms of arterial insufficiency, as evidenced by warm skin temperature over the affected area, the presence of pedal pulses, and decreased claudication in the affected extremities.
2. The patient will successfully participate in activities within limits imposed by the disease.
3. The patient will demonstrate protective behavior and self-care measures to prevent injury to the skin.
4. The patient will correctly describe the disease process and treatment plan, including drug actions, dosage, and side effects.
5. The patient will identify personal risk factors and methods to reduce these factors.

Intervention

Nursing interventions include the initiation of a graduated, regular exercise program. Patients should be encouraged to balance activities with rest and may need assistance to develop a schedule of paced activities. Patient education is also important for preventing injuries.

Evaluation

Evaluation of an older adult patient with PAD focuses on the achievement of expected outcomes. Short-term evaluation focuses on those interventions aimed at reducing risk factors. Long-term evaluation is based on trends in progress toward improving tissue perfusion and viability. Involvement of the older adult and their family in planning care is a crucial factor in achieving a successful outcome over time (see Nursing Care Plan: PAD).

◎ NURSING CARE PLAN

Peripheral Artery Disease

Clinical Situation

Mrs. A, a 72-year-old woman, is complaining of a decreased activity level because of pain in her right leg when walking. This has been getting worse over the past few months, and it is now difficult for her to walk to the mailbox without pain. She states that sometimes her toes tingle at night. She does not complain of chest pain or shortness of breath. She denies smoking and takes amlodipine for high blood pressure and aspirin as needed for arthritis.

  Assessment of Mrs. A reveals the following:

- Vital signs: temperature, 98.4° F; heart rate, 84 beats/min and regular; respiratory rate, 16 breaths/min and not labored; blood pressure, (left arm) 160/84 mm Hg, (right arm) 143/80 mm Hg
- Height: 5 ft, 6 in; weight: 164 lb
- Skin: warm and dry
- Right foot pale and cooler than left
- Pedal pulse: right foot 1+; left foot 2+
- Femoral pulse: 2+ bilateral
- Able to move toes equally

  Pentoxifylline is ordered, and an exercise program is prescribed. Doppler studies are scheduled.

Nursing Diagnoses

Decreased activity resulting from pain when walking
Altered tissue perfusion resulting from decreased circulation
Risk for skin breakdown
Need for health teaching resulting from lack of knowledge of the disease and the treatment plan

Outcomes

The patient will identify factors that cause pain.
The patient will participate in a plan to increase activity and decrease claudication.
The patient will demonstrate no signs of skin breakdown or impairment in skin integrity.
The patient will identify the risk factors of the disease, describe lifestyle changes, and participate in the treatment plan.

Interventions

Plan activities to include a walking program.
Encourage the patient to increase walking regimen daily, up to 30 minutes per day with intermittent rest periods if experiencing pain.
Encourage the patient and give reassurance that activity does not harm painful tissue.
Assist the patient in identifying, reducing, and eliminating risk factors (e.g., reducing weight and controlling HTN).
Assess for ischemic ulcers.
Have the patient report ulcers or darkened areas on her skin to the health care provider.
Teach foot care measures, including daily inspection, daily washing using mild soap, and drying well; the patient may use lotion but should avoid use between the toes.
Teach the patient proper nail care and to wear proper-fitting closed-toe shoes.
Explain drug therapy, including side effects and when to call the health care provider.
Identify available community resources.

Chronic Venous Insufficiency

Chronic venous insufficiency (CVI) is any disturbance that impairs tissue perfusion. The most common disorders due to CVI are (1) varicose veins, (2) venous ulcerations, and (3) venous thrombosis.

Varicose veins of the leg occur particularly in women and may be divided into primary and secondary varicose veins. Primary varicose veins are more common, and the varicosity, which occurs in the wall of the vein, may be related to weakness of the wall, incompetent valves of the saphenofemoral junction, or perforating veins. Underlying causes include obesity, estrogenic hormones, and, in older adults, a previous occupation that required long periods of standing. Varicose veins are unattractive but generally do not lead to other serious vascular disease. Complications of primary varicose veins due to CVI are venous ulcers. The superficial system is subjected to high pressure, which results in poor tissue oxygenation of the lower limbs. Venous ulcers occur on the medial side of the lower half of the leg. The ulcer is usually painful, may easily be infected, and, if left untreated, may involve the circumference of the leg. The management of venous ulceration depends on relieving the HTN occurring in the superficial system through bed rest, elevation of the limb, and single or multilayer compression dressings. A characteristic brownish discoloration of the skin develops from deposits of melanin and hemosiderin. Older adults often complain of heaviness in the legs. The signs and symptoms of varicose veins are protrusion of veins on the legs, aching, ankle swelling, night cramps, skin changes such as itching, varicose eczema, and (in extreme cases) hemorrhage. Most varicose veins may be treated with conservative therapy, including the use of compression dressings or stockings, elevation of the lower extremities when sleeping or relaxing, regular exercise, and weight reduction. In more severe cases, surgical interventions such as sclerotherapy, ligation, ablation, or phlebectomy (vein stripping) may be required.

Secondary varicose veins are the result of thrombosis in the deep system, which may subsequently occur with obstruction of the valves. Deep vein thrombosis (DVT) due to Virchow Triad (venous stasis, hypercoagulability, and intimal changes to the vessels) is a common and serious disorder. CDC estimates an annual occurrence of DVT at 300,000 to 600,000 with 34% being fatal pulmonary embolism (PE). Immobility, advancing age, obesity, hormonal usage, and cigarette smoking are contributing factors. Medical conditions predisposing individuals to DVT include blood dyscrasias, cancer, systemic infection, dehydration, heart disease, stroke, inflammatory bowel disease, and incompetent venous valves. Incidences greatly increase with age for both males and females (Benjamin et al., 2017).

Diagnostic Tests and Procedures

Indirect methods to detect obstruction include Doppler ultrasonography, plethysmography, venous duplex ultrasonography, and contrast venography. Doppler ultrasonography measures venous obstruction and reflux of blood by changes in the frequency of sound waves. Laboratory work includes a CBC, prothrombin time, PPT and activated PPT, INR, highly sensitive D-dimer, and chemistry panel.

Treatment

The therapeutic aim of treatment of more serious CVI is to preserve not only the extremity but also its function. Interventions range from palliative measures to ease symptoms to the use of pharmacologic and surgical strategies to enhance blood flow and prevent clot formation.

Palliative measures are important for maintaining comfort. Preservation of skin integrity is of prime importance in maintaining the overall health of the extremity. Pharmacologic intervention is directed at increasing blood flow and preventing clot formation. For prophylaxis, rather than treatment during the acute phase, low-molecular-weight heparins (LMWHs) such as enoxaparin sodium are used for their antithrombotic action. This class of drug has a lower risk of bleeding and does not require laboratory monitoring for therapeutic doses. Typically, LMWHs are given subcutaneously once or twice a day. Anticoagulation therapy, such as heparin and warfarin, is used to prevent further clot formation. A variety of surgical procedures may be performed to reduce the effects of CVI.

NURSING MANAGEMENT

Assessment

Assessment of an older adult with CVI begins with a complete history and physical examination. Subjective data include pain in the extremity, precipitating factors, relieving factors, modifiable risk factors, and personal and family history. Objective data include skin color, hair distribution, atrophy, edema, varicosities, petechiae, lesions, and ulcerations. Table 19.6 provides more information for the assessment of peripheral arterial and venous disease.

Diagnosis

Nursing diagnoses for an older adult with CVI include the following:

- Potential for skin integrity issues resulting from venous stasis
- Decreased peripheral tissue perfusion resulting from interruption of venous flow
- Pain resulting from inflammatory processes

Planning and Expected Outcomes

Expected outcomes for an older patient with CVI include the following:

1. Skin integrity will be maintained or improved.
2. The patient will exhibit no ulceration or signs of the inflammatory process.
3. Tissue perfusion will be improved, as evidenced by decreased edema and fewer complaints of discomfort.

Intervention

Nursing interventions for an older patient with venous disease include assessment of skin integrity (e.g., skin texture, skin temperature, pain, color, edema, and pulses). The nurse should use a Doppler sensor if pulses are absent. The affected extremity should be elevated to facilitate venous circulation, and the size of the affected limb should be measured and recorded at least daily. Elastic compression stockings may also be ordered; it is

TABLE 19.6	Differentiating Arterial and Venous Insufficiency	
Assessment	**Arterial Disease**	**Venous Disease**
Acute pain	Sudden and severe	Little or no pain; tenderness along inflamed vein
Chronic pain	Intermittent claudication; rest pain	Heaviness; fullness
Hair	Hair loss distal to occlusion	No hair loss
Nails	Thick and brittle	Normal
Sensation	Possible paresthesia	Normal
Skin texture	Thin, dry, shiny	Stasis dermatitis; veins may be visible; skin mottled
Skin color	Pallor or reactive hyperemia (pallor when limb is elevated; rubor when limb is dependent)	Brawny (reddish brown); cyanotic, if dependent
Skin temperature	Cool	Warm
Skin breakdown (ulcers)	Severely painful; usually on or between toes or on upper surface of foot over metatarsal heads or other bony prominence	Mildly painful, with pain relieved by leg elevation; usually in ankle area
Edema	None or mild, usually unilateral	Typically present (usually foot to calf); may be unilateral or bilateral
Pulses	Diminished, weak, or absent	Normal

Adapted from Lewis, S. L., et al., (2011). *Medical surgical nursing: Assessment and management of clinical problems* (8th ed.). St. Louis, MO: Mosby; Springhouse. (2007). *Cardiovascular care.* Philadelphia: Lippincott Williams & Wilkins; Centers for Disease Control and Prevention (CDC). (2012). Vital signs: Awareness and treatment of uncontrolled hypertension among adults - United States, 2003-2010. *MMWR: Morbidity & Mortality Weekly Report, 61,* 703-709.

helpful to demonstrate their application and removal and require a return demonstration to assess the patient's ability to correctly apply them. Devices are available through medical supply companies for assistance with application, if necessary. Stockings should be replaced every 3 to 6 months in the absence of any evidence of excess wear.

Bed rest versus early ambulation of patients with DVT has not been associated with increased risk of pulmonary embolism (PE; Liu, Tao, Chen, Fan, & Li, 2015). Early ambulation has also been shown to decrease pain. Instruct older adults to apply their elastic compression stockings before walking and to avoid standing or immobility for prolonged periods. Instruction on foot care is an important part of the prevention plan for venous ulcers. The skin should be inspected daily, washed gently in tepid water with a neutral soap, and patted dry with special attention paid to adequately drying between the toes. A foot cream or moisturizer, then cotton socks, should be applied after washing to aid in retaining moisture. A professional should perform nail care. Shoes should fit well and provide good support.

Evaluation

Evaluation focuses on the patient's progress in maintaining skin integrity, improving venous circulation, and reducing pain and discomfort. Documentation should include accurate recording of the skin assessment, including measurements of the affected extremity as well as the older adult's response to other nursing interventions.

Anemia

Anemia is defined as a reduction in RBC mass, decreased quantity of hemoglobin, and decreased hematocrit. The World Health Organization further defines anemia as a hemoglobin <12 g/dL in women and <13 g/dL in men. More than 20% of older adults over the age of 85 have anemia. Anemia in the older adult typically has a different etiology from anemia in younger adults; it is usually insidious in nature and an incidental finding on hematological studies. When anemia is discovered, it is important for reversible causes to be identified, as anemia in the older adult is correlated with increased hospitalizations, morbidity, and mortality (Artz, 2015; Goodnough & Schrier, 2014).

The most common causes of anemia in the older adult are iron deficiency anemia (15% to 23%), anemia of chronic disease (15% to 35%), and anemia related to CKD (8%). Vitamin B_{12} or folate deficiency accounts for as many as 14% of cases, and myelodysplastic syndromes 5%. However, up to 45% of cases of anemia go unexplained (Artz, 2015).

Symptoms vary in frequency and severity. Fatigue and weakness are frequent complaints of older adults with anemia. Pallor is another common sign. Skin color is not a good indicator of pallor because of varying pigmentation. Oral mucous membranes as well as conjunctivae and nail beds are better indicators. Headaches, dyspnea on exertion, palpitations, poor concentration, and dizziness are other common symptoms of anemia. Older adults may exhibit symptoms of anemia (e.g., fatigue and dizziness) but attribute these to the aging process or to other chronic diseases. The nurse should be aware of the nonspecific nature of symptoms so that detection and treatment can be initiated as soon as possible (Artz, 2015).

Diagnostic Tests, Procedures, and Treatment

In addition to a thorough history and physical examination, the following laboratory tests should be obtained:
- CBC with differential and peripheral smear
- Reticulocyte count
- LDH level
- Serum ferritin
- Serum iron
- Total iron-binding capacity
- Vitamin B_{12} Folate and Thyroid-Stimulating Hormone (TSH)
- Serum chemistry with estimated glomerular filtration rate (eGFR).

In iron-deficiency anemia, in addition to the serum iron level, serum ferritin is the most useful test (a ferritin level <12 ng/mL is specific for iron deficiency anemia; levels between 18 and 44 ng/mL are suggestive of iron deficiency anemia; levels over 100 mg/dL indicate adequate iron stores). Although a low mean corpuscular volume (MCV) is suggestive of iron deficiency anemia, the MCV should not be completely relied on, as microcytosis is a late finding and other factors may influence changes in red blood cell size (Artz, 2015). Stool should be tested for occult blood and, if positive, the patient should be evaluated for anemia caused by gastrointestinal blood loss. Treatment includes dietary sources of iron and supplemental intake of iron (i.e., ferrous sulfate, 325 mg, three times a day). Iron therapy should continue until ferritin levels normalize. If there is no response to oral replacement, IV iron should be tried.

Anemia of chronic disease is related to inflammatory processes; inflammation inhibits erythropoiesis. In this form of anemia, iron levels are decreased, but ferritin levels are normal or increased (Artz, 2015). Additional laboratory testing that may be useful includes C-reactive protein, fibrinogen, erythrocyte sedimentation rate, IL6, and hepcidin levels. The treatment focuses on treating the underlying disease along with administration of an erythropoiesis-stimulating agent (e.g., epoetin alfa or darbepoetin alfa) if necessary (Goodnough & Schrier, 2014).

Folate deficiency is usually the result of inadequate dietary intake or malabsorption; it also occurs in the setting of alcoholism, and the use of methotrexate, phenytoin, and trimethoprim. In addition to decreased folic acid levels in folate deficiency, serum homocysteine levels are elevated; folate deficiency is a macrocytic anemia (MCV >100 fL). In addition to the common symptoms associated with anemia, patients with folate deficiency also experience mouth sores and tongue swelling (glossitis). Treatment includes increased dietary intake (e.g., citrus fruits and dark green vegetables) of folic acid; older adults with alcoholism usually require exogenous folic acid (Waterbury, 2015).

Older adults frequently experience low vitamin B_{12} levels. A level <200 pg/mL may be indicative of malabsorption or pernicious anemia. If the B_{12} level is between 200 and 350 pg/mL, a methylmalonic acid level should be drawn; an elevated methylmalonic acid level is indicative of B_{12} deficiency (please note, methylmalonic acid levels are elevated in CKD) (Artz, 2015). Patients with B_{12} deficiency may experience paresthesia and exhibit ataxia, decreased proprioception, and decreased vibratory sensation on examination, in addition to the more common symptoms of anemia. Lifelong treatment with cyanocobalamin (vitamin B_{12}) is necessary; dosing may be oral, nasal, or by injection (SQ/IM).

Prognosis

The prognosis for anemia depends on the cause. With drugs and dietary changes, the prognosis is usually good.

NURSING MANAGEMENT

Assessment

The assessment of an older adult with anemia focuses on identifying the underlying cause and its effects on functional ability (Box 19.6).

Diagnosis

Nursing diagnoses for an older adult with anemia include the following:
- Decreased activity resulting from an imbalance between oxygen supply and demand
- Inadequate nutrition resulting from malabsorption or decreased intake of vitamins, minerals, and nutritious foods
- Need for patient teaching resulting from lack of exposure to information about condition and treatment plan

Planning and Expected Outcomes

Expected outcomes for the older adult include the following:
1. The patient will experience increases in activity without dyspnea or other previous symptoms over a period of 3 to 6 weeks.
2. The patient will consume a well-balanced diet with foods high in minerals and vitamins, as evidenced by food diary or planned weight gain.
3. The patient will verbalize an understanding of the cause of anemia and an understanding of the treatment plan.

Intervention

Nursing interventions for an older adult with anemia focus on dietary management, a balance of rest and activity to support functional ability, and education about the condition. Environmental safety issues are also important for an older patient experiencing symptoms that increase the risk of injury.

BOX 19.6 Assessment of Older Adults With Anemia

Subjective Data

History (e.g., gastric surgery, liver or kidney disease, recent blood loss, or trauma)
Current drugs (e.g., prescription, over-the-counter, vitamins and minerals, NSAIDs)
Nutritional habits (i.e., ask the older adult to give a 24-hour diet recall)
Alcohol intake
Change in bowel habits (e.g., color, consistency)
Weight loss
Complaints (e.g., fatigue, palpitations, dyspnea, paresthesia, painful tongue, dizziness, headache, or tinnitus)

Objective Data

Pallor (e.g., nail beds, conjunctivae, or oral mucous membranes)
Physical appearance
Tachycardia
Tachypnea
Crackles on pulmonary auscultation
Edema
Syncope
Systolic murmur
Confusion
Unsteady gait
Stomatitis
Vital signs (including orthostatic BP/P)
Laboratory values

NSAIDs, Nonsteroidal antiinflammatory drugs; *BP*, blood pressure; *P*, pulse.

The patient and family should be instructed about appropriate food selection and meal preparation to promote RBC formation. The nurse should provide a list of foods high in iron, folic acid, and vitamin B$_{12}$ to incorporate into the daily meal plan. The health care provider may order supplemental iron preparations and, if so, the nurse should assess the patient's tolerance of the preparation. Side effects of oral iron preparations include gastrointestinal upset, constipation or diarrhea, and green or black stools. It may be helpful to recommend taking the iron preparation after meals to minimize gastrointestinal upset.

In addition to dietary recommendations, the gerontologic nurse should ensure that the older adult patient has adequate income to purchase necessary foods, the functional ability to acquire and prepare foods, and adequate oral health, including properly fitting dentures. The nurse should also be alert to the presence of other variables that may adversely affect the older adult's ability to eat, such as loneliness, grief, depression, or alcoholism.

Older patients and their families should also be instructed to balance rest and activity. It is helpful for older adults to identify peak energy periods during waking hours and carry out desired or important activities during those times. However, patients should not carry out activities to the point of fatigue or dyspnea; rather, they should rest at intervals until activities are completed.

Evaluation

Evaluation focuses on the patient's progress toward meeting the expected outcomes. Specifically, the older patient should have fewer complaints of dyspnea, fatigue, and dizziness, and weight should be within the established norm. Normal values of the older adult's hemoglobin, hematocrit, and RBC count indicate the success of interventions. The older patient's symptoms, weight trends, and activity levels should be documented, along with any patient and family teaching.

NUTRITIONAL CONSIDERATIONS
DASH Diet

Daily Food Group	Servings	Significance of Each Food
Grains	6–8	Energy and fiber
Vegetables	4–5	Potassium, magnesium, and fiber
Fruits	4–5	Potassium, magnesium, and fiber
Low-fat or nonfat dairy foods	2–3	Calcium and protein
Lean meats, poultry, and fish	6 or less	Protein and magnesium
Nuts, seeds, and legumes	4–5 per week	Energy, magnesium, potassium, protein, and fiber
Fats and oils	2–3	The DASH study had 27% of calories as fat, including fat in or added to foods.
Sweets and added sugars	5 or less per week	Sweets should be low in fat.

DASH, Dietary Approaches to Stopping Hypertension.
Modified from National Institutes of Health, National Heart, Lung, and Blood Institute. (2006). *Your guide to lowering your blood pressure with DASH*, NIH Publication No. 06–4082. Washington, D.C.: U.S. Department of Health and Human Services.

SUMMARY

CVD remains the leading cause of death in the United States. In the older adult population, it is often difficult to clearly distinguish between CVD and normal aging. The presentation and effects of CVD may vary widely from person to person. Older adults often display atypical symptoms of CVD, enabling the disease process to advance before discovery and treatment is initiated. The challenge for the nurse is to obtain an accurate and complete assessment of the older adult patient that allows the planning and initiation of appropriate physical and psychosocial care. The nurse should focus on assisting older patients in modifying risk factors and optimizing health status.

HOME CARE

1. Homebound older adult patients, spouses, family, significant others, and caregivers should be included in all aspects of the care-planning process in the home setting.
2. Older patients value education in the home care setting, and this should continue as an important focus of care after hospitalization.
3. Older adult patients dealing with chronic disease management in the home setting often experience anxiety, frustration, and depression. This factor should be taken into consideration when providing home care services, and appropriate interagency referrals should be initiated.
4. The fear of dying is often a major factor for homebound older adults with CVD, particularly those with HF. Counseling and referral to agencies should be provided.
5. Homebound older adults have a high anxiety level about needing help and not being able to obtain it. Establishing a link with an emergency community service such as a lifeline program may alleviate some anxiety.
6. The nurse should direct teaching of homebound older adults about the anatomy and physiology of the heart, modifiable risk factors for CVD, drug regimens (especially regarding dosage and side effects), exercise tolerance, daily weight monitoring, and dietary modification (e.g., low-sodium and low-fat diets and fluid restriction).
7. Caregivers need to be educated about signs that suggest deterioration in status.
8. Assistance with ADLs may be required, especially for those homebound older adults who live alone or are responsible for household tasks. Often, these older adult patients do not request assistance, so the nurse should offer these services where appropriate.
9. Participation in a cardiac rehabilitation program or activities such as walking or swimming should be encouraged by the home care nurse.
10. Homebound older adult patients should be encouraged to wear medical alert bracelets that identify the patients' conditions and drugs.

KEY POINTS

- CVD is the leading cause of death among both men and women.
- For those older than age 65, mortality rates for CVD rise sharply, and it is anticipated that the actual number of deaths resulting from CVD will escalate as the proportion of the older adult population increases.
- Older adults who stay physically fit have twice the work capacity and a lower amount of body fat than older adults who are sedentary.
- Smoking cessation in older adults significantly reduces the risks of coronary events and cardiac death within 1 year of quitting. The risk continues to decline gradually for many years thereafter.
- Smokers have twice the chance of developing CAD and four times the chance of sudden death compared with nonsmokers.
- It is estimated that more than 45% to 50% of the population older than age 65 has high blood pressure, and the consequences are the most common causes of morbidity and mortality, including MI, CHF, and CVI.
- Older adults may have difficulty adopting healthier lifestyles because of long-term habits; however, healthy behavior changes may slow or halt the progression of disease.
- Older adults have more atypical signs of CAD.

- Older adults may not recognize the onset of ischemia. Initial symptoms may consist of sudden dyspnea, confusion, fatigue, weakness, vertigo, syncope, vomiting, and exacerbation of heart failure.
- The incidence of atrial fibrillation increases with age and is the most common contributing factor to ischemic stroke in older adults.
- Atrial fibrillation, sick sinus syndrome, and heart block appear more often in the older adult population because of fewer pacemaker cells and extensive deposits of fat and fibrous tissue throughout the conduction system.
- Orthostatic hypotension is a major risk factor for syncope and falls in older adults.
- Older adults are prone to dizziness with position changes, resulting from decreased sensitivity of baroreceptors.
- HF is the leading cause of hospitalization in the older adult population.
- Older adults may exhibit symptoms of anemia that are attributed to the aging process or to a variety of chronic diseases.
- Nursing interventions (e.g., education on the role of cardiovascular risk factors, preventive measures, and treatment regimens) may enhance the quality of life of older patients, reduce hospitalization, and positively affect the cost-effectiveness and efficiency of cardiovascular programs.

CRITICAL-THINKING EXERCISES

1. You are preparing to teach an 85-year-old woman about the actions and side effects of nitroglycerin for the treatment of angina. What aspects of teaching would you emphasize given the patient's age?
2. A 78-year-old woman has a long-standing history of atrial fibrillation. She takes digoxin 0.125 mg and warfarin 2.0 mg daily. She recently read of the advantages of taking aspirin and started taking four tablets daily. How would you intervene in this situation, and why?
3. What specific assessment findings indicate that an older adult patient being treated for HF is not responding to digoxin, furosemide, and vasodilator therapy? How would you differentiate among expected, adverse, and toxic side effects?

REFERENCES

American Heart Association. (2014). *Body Mass Index in Adults (BMI Calculator for Adults).*

American Heart Association. (2017a). *Four ways to deal with stress.* Retrieved December 18, 2017 from http://www.heart.org/HEARTORG/HealthyLiving/StressManagement/FourWaystoDealWithStress/Four-Ways-to-Deal-with-Stress_UCM_307996_Article.jsp#.WjfmHN-nGUk.

American Heart Association. (2017b). *Menopause and heart disease.* Retrieved December 18, 2017 from http://www.heart.org/HEARTORG/Conditions/More/MyHeartandStrokeNews/Menopause-and-Heart-Disease_UCM_448432_Article.jsp#.WjfnMd-nGUk.

American Heart Association. (2017c). *Stress and heart health.* Retrieved December 18, 2017 from http://www.heart.org/HEARTORG/HealthyLiving/StressManagement/HowDoesStressAffectYou/Stress-and-Heart-Health_UCM_437370_Article.jsp#.Wjfiu9-nGUk.

American Heart Association. (2017d). *The skinny on fats.* Retrieved December 18, 2017 from http://www.heart.org/HEARTORG/Conditions/Cholesterol/PreventionTreatmentofHighCholesterol/The-Skinny-on-Fats_UCM_305628_Article.jsp#.Wjfr3d-nGUk.

American Heart Association (AHA). (2017e). *Types of heart failure.* Retrieved October 2017, from http://www.heart.org/HEARTORG/Conditions/HeartFailure/AboutHeartFailure/Types-of-Heart-Failure_UCM_306323_Article.jsp#.Weet4DCQxhE.

American Heart Association. (2015a). *Coping with feelings.* Retrieved December 18, 2017 from http://www.heart.org/HEARTORG/Conditions/More/CardiacRehab/Coping-with-Feelings_UCM_307092_Article.jsp#.WjgWS9-nGUl.

American Heart Association. (2015b). *Women & cardiovascular diseases [Fact Sheet].* Retrieved December 18, 2017 from https://www.heart.org/idc/groups/heart-public/@wcm/@sop/@smd/documents/downloadable/ucm_472913.pdf.

Aronow, W. S. (2015). Blood pressure goals and targets in the elderly. *Current Treatment Options in Cardiovascular Medicine, 17*(33), 1–11. https://doi.org/10.1007/s11936-015-0394-x.

Artz, A. S. (2015). *Anemia in elderly persons.* Retrieved December 30, 2017 from https://emedicine.medscape.com/article/1339998-overview.

Azad, N., & Lemay, G. (2014). Management of chronic heart failure in the older population. *Journal of Geriatric Cardiology, 11,* 329–337. Retrieved October 2017 from https://www.ncbi.nlm.nih.gov/pmc/articles/PMC4292097/.

Ball, J. W., Dains, J. E., Flynn, J. A., Solomon, B. S., & Stewart, R. W. (2014). *Seidel's guide to physical examination* (ed 8). St Louis: Mosby.

Banach, M., & Serban, M. C. (2016). Discussion around statin discontinuation in older adults and patients with wasting diseases. *Journal of Cachexia, Sarcopenia and Muscle, 7*(4), 396–399. https://doi.org/10.1002/jcsm.12109.

Banasik, J. L. (2013a). Alterations in cardiac function. In L. C. Copestead & J. L. Banasik (Eds.), *Pathophysiology* (ed 5). St Louis: Saunders Elsevier.

Banasik, J. L. (2013b). Cardiac function. In L. C. Copestead & J. L. Banasik (Eds.), *Pathophysiology* (ed 5). St Louis: Saunders Elsevier.

Beckerman, J. (2017). *Atrial fibrillation: Causes, risks, and triggers.* Retrieved December 21, 2017 from https://www.webmd.com/heart-disease/atrial-fibrillation/causes-risks-triggers-afib.

Beddhu, S., Chertow, C. M., Cheung, A. K., Cushman, W. C., Rahman, M., Greene, T., ... Whelton, P. K. (2017). Baseline diastolic BP and effects of intensive BP control. *Circulation, 136*(24), https://doi,org/1CIR.0000000000000471/CIRCULATIONAHA.117.030848.

Benjamin, E. J., Blaha, M. J., Chiuve, S. E., Cushman, M., Das, S. R., Deo, R., & ...Muntner, P. (2017). Heart disease and stroke statistics—2017 update. *Circulation, 135*(10), e16–e603. https://doi.org/1CIR.0000000000000471/CIR.0000000000000485.

Blach, D. A., & Ignatavicius, D. D. (2013). Interventions for clients with vascular problems. In D. D. Ignatavicius & M. L. Workman (Eds.), *Medical surgical nursing: critical thinking for collaborative care* (ed 7). St Louis: Elsevier Saunders.

Blach, D. A. (2006). Management of clients with problems of the cardiovascular system. In D. D. Ignatavicius & M. L. Workman (Eds.), *Medical surgical nursing: critical thinking for collaborative care* (ed 5, pp. 676–707). St Louis: Elsevier-Saunders.

Black, J. M. (2009). Management of clients with vascular disorders. In J. M. Black & J. H. Hawks (Eds.), *Medical surgical nursing: clinical management for positive outcomes* (ed 8). St Louis: Elsevier Saunders.

Centers for Disease Control and Prevention. (2017a). *High blood pressure.* Retrieved on October 2017, from https://www.cdc.gov/bloodpressure/index.htm.

Centers for Disease Control and Prevention (CDC). (2017b). *Assessment: Measuring orthostatic blood pressure.* Retrieved on December 9, 2017, from https://www.cdc.gov/steadi/pdf/measuring_orthostatic_blood_pressure-a.pdf.

Choi, K., Jeon, G., & Cho, S. (2017). Prospective study on the impact of fear of falling on functional decline among community dwelling elderly women. *International Journal of Environmental Research and Public Health, 14*(5), 469. https://doi.org/10.3390/ijerph14050469.

Dharmarajan, K., & Rich, M. W. (2017). Epidemiology, pathophysiology, and prognosis of heart failure in older adults. *Heart Failure Clinics, 13*(3), 417–426. https://doi.org/10.1016/j.hfc.2017.02.001.

Eckel, R. H., Kahn, R., Robertson, R. M., & Rizza, R. A. (2006). Preventing cardiovascular disease and diabetes. *Circulation, 113,* 2943–2946.

Emerson, R. J., & Lungstrom, N. (2013). Alterations in blood flow. In L. C. Copestead & J. L. Banasik (Eds.), *Pathophysiology* (ed 5). St Louis: Saunders Elsevier.

Fillit, H. M., Rockwood, K., & Young, J. (2017). *Brocklehurst's textbook of geriatric medicine and gerontology* (8th ed). Philadelphia, PA: Elsevier.

Garcia, M., Mulvagh, S. L., Merz, C. N. B., Buring, J. E., & Manson, J. E. (2016). Cardiovascular disease in women: Clinical perspectives. *Circulation Research, 188,* 1273–1293. https://doi.org/10.1161/CIRCRESAHA.116.307547.

Gerhard-Herman, M. D., Gornik, H. L., Barrett, C., Barshes, N. R., Corriere, M. A., Drachman, D. E., ... Walsh, M. E. (2016). 2017 AHA/ACC guideline on the management of patients with lower extremity peripheral artery disease: A report of the American College of Cardiology/American Heart Association Task Force on clinical practice guidelines. *Circulation.* https://doi.org/10.1161/CIR.0000000000000471.

Goodnough, L. T., & Schrier, S. L. (2014). Evaluation and management of anemia in the elderly. *American Journal of Hematology, 89*(1), 88–96. https://doi.org/10.1002/ajh.23598.

Goyal, P., & Maurer, M. S. (2016). Syncope in older adults. *Journal of Geriatric Cardiology, 13*(5), 380–386. https://doi.org/10.11909/j.issn.1671-5411.2016.05.002.

Higginson, L. A. (2016). *Orthostatic hypotension.* Retrieved December 24, 2017 from http://www.merckmanuals.com/professional/cardiovascular-disorders/symptoms-of-cardiovascular-disorders/orthostatic-hypotension.

Huether, S. E., McCance, K. L., Brashers, V. L., & Rote, N. S. (2017). *Understanding Pathophysiology* (6th ed.). St. Louis, MO: Elseiver.

Jett, K. (2008). Physiological changes with aging. In P. Ebersole, T. Touhy, & P. Hess, et al. (Eds.), *Toward healthy aging: human needs and nursing response* (ed 7, pp. 65–87). St Louis: Mosby Elsevier.

Julian, M, Aroesty, M.D., Joseph, P., & Kannam, M.D. (2017). Patient education: Medications for angina (beyond the basics). Retrieved December 18, 2017 from https://www.uptodate.com/contents/medications-for-angina-beyond-the-basics.

Kapan, A., Luger, E., Haider, S., Titze, S., Schindler, K., Lackinger, C., & ...Dorner, T.E. (2017). Fear of falling reduced by a lay led home-based program in frail community-dwelling older adults: A randomised controlled trial. *Archives of Gerontology and Geriatrics, 68,* 25–32. https://doi.org/10.1016/j.archger.2016.08.009.

Kennedy, E. B., & Ignatavicius, D. D. (2013). Interventions for clients with cardiac problems. In D. D. Ignatavicius & M. L. Workman (Eds.), *Medical surgical nursing: critical thinking for collaborative care* (ed 7). St Louis: Elsevier Saunders.

Khan, H., Kalogeropoulos, A. P., Georgiopoulou, V. V., Newman, A. B., Harris, T. B., Rodondi, ... Butler, J. (2013). Frailty and risk for heart failure in older adults: The health, aging, and body composition study. *American Heart Journal, 166*(5), 887–894. https://doi.org/10.1016/j.ahj.2013.07.032.

Lehne, R. A. (2013). *Pharmacology for nursing care* (8th ed.). Philadelphia: Saunders.

Lewis, S. L., Dirksen, S. R., Heitkemper, M. M., et al. (2011). *Medical surgical nursing: assessment and management of clinical problems* (8th ed.). St Louis: Mosby Elsevier.

Lichtenstein, A. H., Appel, L. J., Brands, M., et al. (2006). Diet and lifestyle recommendations revision 2006: a scientific statement from the American Heart Association nutrition committee. *Circulation, 114,* 82–96.

Liu, Z., Xixi, T., Yuexin, Ch., Fan, Z., & Li, Y. (2015). Bed rest versus early ambulation with standard anticoagulation in the management of deep vein thrombosis: A meta-analysis. *PLOS One, 10*(4). https://doi.org/10.1371/journal.pone.0121388.

Martin, L. J. (2016). *Aging changes in the heart and blood vessels.* Retrieved December 18, 2017 from https://medlineplus.gov/ency/article/004006.htm.

Morton, P. G., Fontaine, D. K., Hudak, C. M., & Gallo, B. M. (2012). *Critical care nursing: a holistic approach* (10th ed.). Philadelphia: Lippincott Williams & Wilkins.

National Cholesterol Education Program. (2002). *Third report of the NCEP Expert Panel on Detection, Evaluation, and Treatment of High Blood Cholesterol in Adults (Adult Treatment Panel III).* Washington, DC: National Institutes of Health.

National Health and Nutrition Examination Survey III (NHANES III). (2006). Retrieved March 21, 2010, from http://www.cdc.gov/nchs/nhanes.htm.

National Heart, Lung, and Blood Institute. (2011). *Who is at risk for arrhythmia?* Retrieved December 9, 2017 from, https://www.nhlbi.nih.gov/health/health-topics/topics/arr/atrisk.

Ogden, C. L., Carroll, M. D., Fryar, C. D., & Flegal, K. M. (2015). Prevalence of Obesity Among Adults and Youth: United States, 2011–2014. *NCHS Data Brief, No. 2019, November 2015.*

Ott, B. B., & DeFrancesco-Loukas, M. A. (2009). Management of clients with structural cardiac disorders. In J. M. Black, & J. H. Hawks (Eds.), *Medical surgical nursing: clinical management for positive outcomes* (ed 8, pp. 1384–1409). St Louis: Saunders.

Patel, A., & Stewart, F. (2015). On hypertension in the elderly: An epidemiologic shift. *American College of Cardiology.* Retrieved on September 7, 2017 at http://www.acc.org/latest-in-cardiology/articles/2015/02/19/14/55/on-hypertension-in-the-elderly.

Qaseem, A., Wilt, T. J., Rich, R., Humphrey, L. L., Frost, J., & Forciea, M. A. (2017). *Pharmacologic treatment of hypertension in adults aged 60 years or older to higher versus lower blood pressure targets: A clinical practice guideline from the American College of Physicians and the American Academy of Family Physicians.*

Sieggreen, M. Y., & Kline, R. A. (2011). Vascular ulcers. In S. Baranoski & E. A. Ayello (Eds.), *Wound care essentials.* Philadelphia: Lippincott Williams & Wilkins.

Singh, V.N. (2015). Acute myocardial infarct imaging. Retrieved December 18, 2017 from https://emedicine.medscape.com/article/350175-overview#a1.

Springhouse. (2007). *Cardiovascular care.* Philadelphia: Lippincott Williams & Wilkins.

Stone, N. J., Robinson, J., Lichtenstein, A. H., Merz, C. N. B., Blum, C. B., Eckel, R. H., … Wilson, P. W. F. (2013). 2013 ACC/AHA guideline on the treatment of blood cholesterol to reduce atherosclerotic cardiovascular risk in adults. *Circulation.* https://doi.org/10.1161/01.cir.0000437738.63853.7a.

The Medical Letter. (2015). Drugs for chronic heart failure. *The Medical Letter on Drugs and Therapeutics, 57*(1460), 9–13.

Touhy, T., & Jett, K. (2012). *Ebersole & Hess' Toward healthy aging: human needs and nursing response* (ed 8). St Louis: Mosby.

Waterbury, S. (2015). Anemia in the elderly. Retrieved December 30, 2017 from http://www.netce.com/coursecontent.php?courseid=1145.

Whelton, P. K., Carey, R. M., Aronow, W. S., Casey, D. E., Collins, K. J., Himmelfarb, C. D., … Wright, J. T. (2017). 2017 ACC/AHA/AAPA/ABC/ACPM/AGS/APhA/ASH/ASPC/NMA/PCNA Guideline for the prevention, detection, evaluation, and management of high blood pressure in adults. *Hypertension, 71*(1). Retrieved from http://hyper.ahajournals.org/content/early/2017/11/10/HYP.0000000000000065.

Yancy, W. C., Jessup, M., Bozkurt, B., Butler, J., Casey, D. D., Drazner, M. H., … Wilkoff, B. L. (2013a). 2013 ACCF/AHA guideline for the management of heart failure: Executive summary. *Journal of the American College of Cardiology, 62*(16), 1495–1539. https://doi.org/10.1016/j.jacc.2013.05.020.

Yancy, C. W., Jessup, M., Bozkurt, B., Butler, J., Casey, D. E., Drazner, M. H., … Wilkoff, B. L. (2013b). 2013 ACCF/AHA guideline for the management of heart failure: A report of the American College of Cardiology Foundation/American Heart Association Task Force on Practice Guidelines. *Circulation, 128,* e240–e327. https://doi.org/10.1161/CIR.0b013e31829e8776.

Yancy, W. C., Jessup, M., Bozkurt, B., Butler, J., Casey, D. D., Drazner, … Westlake, C. (2017). 2017 ACC/AHA/HFSA focused update of the 2013 ACCF/AHA guideline for the management of heart failure. *Journal of the American College of Cardiology, 76*(6). https://doi.org/10.1016/j.jacc.2017.04.025.

Zafari, A. M. (2017). Myocardial infarction workup. Retrieved December 18, 2017 from https://emedicine.medscape.com/article/155919-workup#c14.

Zellner, W. (2012). Mitral valve repair safe for older patients. Retrieved December 26, 2017 from http://www.futurity.org/mitral-valve-repair-safe-for-older-patients/.

Zoungas, S. (2017). How old is too old for cholesterol lowering medications? Retrieved December 21, 2017 from http://theconversation.com/how-old-is-too-old-for-cholesterol-lowering-medications-78102.

20

Respiratory Function in Aging

Debra L. Sanders, PhD, RN, GCNS-BC

ⓔ www.//evolve.elsevier.com/Meiner/gerontologic

LEARNING OBJECTIVES

On completion of this chapter, the reader will be able to:

1. Describe anatomic changes in the lungs resulting from the normal aging process.
2. Describe age-related changes in ventilation.
3. Identify nursing interventions and outcomes for older adults with various respiratory alterations.
4. Discuss smoking cessation methods and interventions.
5. Identify risk factors for the development of tuberculosis in older adults.
6. List the benefits of pulmonary rehabilitation for older adults with chronic obstructive pulmonary disease.

WHAT WOULD YOU DO?

What would you do if you were faced with the following situations?

* Your 72-year-old patient comes to the clinic for their annual physical examination. During the history, your patient notes they continue to smoke 1 pack per day. Chart review indicates they have received smoking cessation counseling on their last three visits. What should you do?
* Your 68-year-old patient, newly diagnosed with sleep apnea, is struggling to wear their CPAP when sleeping. What additional measures can they take to help nocturnal oxygenation?

The respiratory system is responsible for gas exchange between the environment and blood, and involves two processes: ventilation and oxygenation. *Ventilation* is the movement of air into and out of the lungs, and consists of inhalation and exhalation. During inhalation, oxygen-rich air is moved into the lungs, and then during exhalation, carbon dioxide (CO_2)-rich air is moved out. During *oxygenation,* CO_2 is transferred from the vasculature to the pulmonary side of the lungs, and oxygen is transferred from the pulmonary side to the vasculature, where it is loaded onto hemoglobin. The process of respiration, including rate and depth, are controlled by chemoreceptors in the medulla oblongata, the arch of the aorta, and in the carotid artery, and are sensitive to oxygen levels and pH. Respiration depends on adequate structures for moving air during ventilation, an environment where oxygen and CO_2 can transfer, and chemoreceptors sensitive to the maintenance of oxygenation and pH levels.

AGE-RELATED CHANGES IN STRUCTURE AND FUNCTION

Normal aging results in changes to the ribs and vertebrae. The ribs become less mobile, and chest wall compliance decreases.

Osteoporosis and calcification of the costal cartilage lead to increased rigidity and stiffness of the thoracic cage. If kyphosis or scoliosis is present, degeneration of the intervertebral disks occurs, resulting in a shorter thorax with an increased anteroposterior diameter. Advanced cases may result in marked limitation of thoracic movement because of the rib cage resting on the pelvic bones. Such changes in the chest wall can impair respiratory compliance, leading to increased work of breathing.

Progressive loss of elastic recoil of the lung parenchyma and conducting airways and reduced elastic recoil of the lung and the opposing forces of the chest wall also are present. The lung becomes less elastic as collagenic substances surrounding the alveoli and alveolar ducts stiffen and form cross-linkages that interfere with the elastic properties of the lungs. Any and all of these structural changes make it more difficult for the older person to ventilate, leading to an increased work of breathing and heightened energy expenditure. Table 20.1 summarizes various changes in the aging respiratory system (McCance & Huether, 2014).

As muscle strength declines with age, and as respiratory muscles weaken, it becomes increasingly more difficult to exert inspiratory and expiratory forces. The combination of an increasingly stiffer skeletal structure and weaker muscles results in additional effort and energy to breathe. The diaphragm, a major respiratory muscle, flattens and becomes less efficient in patients with advancing chronic obstructive pulmonary disease (COPD). Because of this, older adults use the less efficient accessory muscles of respiration such as the abdominal, sternocleidomastoid, and trapezius muscles. As the abdominal muscles become more important to older adults, their breathing patterns may become more affected by positioning and increased abdominal pressure.

Respiratory rates generally are faster and shallower in older adults: a normal rate is 16 to 25 breaths per minute. This combination results in a relatively unchanged arterial CO_2 pressure ($PaCO_2$). However, shallow breathing patterns may result in

Previous author: Sue E. Meiner, EdD, APRN, BC, GNP.

TABLE 20.1 Age-Related Changes in the Respiratory System

Respiratory Function	Pathophysiologic Changes	Clinical Presentation
Mechanics of breathing	Increased chest wall compliance	Decreased vital capacity
	Loss of elastic recoil	Increased reserve volume
	Decreased respiratory muscle mass and strength	Decreased expiratory flow rates
Oxygenation	Increased ventilation–perfusion mismatch	Decreased PaO_2
	Decreased cardiac output	Increased A–a oxygen gradient
	Decreased mixed venous oxygen	
	Increased physiologic dead space	
	Decreased alveolar surface area available for gas exchange	
	Reduced CO_2 diffusion capacity	
Control of ventilation	Decreased responsiveness of central and peripheral chemoreceptors to hypoxemia and hypercapnia	Decreased V_T Increased respiratory rate Increased minute ventilation
Lung defense mechanisms	Decreased number of cilia	Decreased ability to clear secretions
	Decreased effectiveness of mucociliary clearance	Increased susceptibility to infection
	Decreased cough reflex	Increased risk of aspiration
	Decreased humoral and cellular immunity	
	Decreased IgA production	
Sleep and breathing	Decreased ventilatory drive	Increased frequency of apnea, hypopnea, and arterial oxygen desaturation during sleep
	Decreased upper airway muscle tone	
	Decreased arousal	Increased risk of aspiration
		Snoring
		Obstructive sleep apnea
Exercise capacity	Muscle deconditioning	Decreased maximum oxygen consumption
	Decreased muscle mass	
	Decreased efficiency of respiratory muscles	Breathlessness at low exercise levels
	Decreased reserves	
Breathing pattern	Decreased responsiveness to hypoxemia and hypercapnia	Increased respiratory rate Decreased V_T
	Change in respiratory mechanics	Increased minute ventilation

A–a, Alveolar–arterial; *IgA,* immunoglobulin A; *PaO₂,* partial pressure of arterial oxygen; *VT,* tidal volume.
Modified from Pierson, D. J. & Kacmarek, R. M. (Eds.). (1992). *Foundations of respiratory care.* New York: Churchill Livingstone.

hypoxemia and hypercapnia as the alveoli at the base of the lungs are underventilated, which, in turn, results in a decreased ventilation–perfusion ratio and less effective alveolar gas exchange. Age-related reductions in cardiac output and mixed venous oxygen content compound the effect of the ventilation–perfusion imbalance in older adults. In healthy older adults, the number of alveoli remains relatively unchanged but their structure may be altered. As a result, the number of functioning alveoli decreases. With age, alveolar supporting structures deteriorate, which leads to a progressive loss of the intraalveolar septum. As the alveolar septal walls become thinner, the alveoli enlarge because of dilation of the proximal bronchioles, but fewer capillaries are available for gas exchange. The increase in physiologic dead space is seen as the capillary structures surrounding the alveoli diminish. The result is a decrease in the surface area available for gas exchange from the normal 80 square meters (m^2) at age 20 to about 65 to 70 m^2 by age 70. As such, less surface area is available for gas exchange to take place, which contributes to the systemic reduction in the partial pressure of arterial oxygen (PaO_2) (Vaz Fragoso & Gill, 2011).

Older adults may also have a decrease in the number and effectiveness of cilia in the tracheobronchial tree, which results in increasing difficulty clearing secretions. As immunoglobulin A (IgA), which is found in the nasal respiratory mucosal surface, decreases with aging, the older adult's ability to neutralize viruses becomes hindered. This combination of decreased IgA and an increase of pooling secretions from impaired mucocilliary transport make infections more likely. With repeated respiratory tract infections or smoking, the effectiveness of the ciliary action and the number of cilia are significantly decreased, which results in an ineffective mucociliary escalator (Brashers, 2012).

One of the primary functions of the respiratory system is gas exchange. For a healthy adult, the normal PaO_2 is 80 to 100 mm Hg. However, after the age of 60, the PaO_2 drops by 1 mm Hg per year. Therefore a PaO_2 of 70 mm Hg for a 70-year-old is relatively normal, which is how the phrase "70 at 70" originated. The expected decrease in PaO_2 is most likely caused by some of the factors previously discussed—reduced tidal volume (V_T), less alveolar surface area, and increased residual volume (RV) (Sorenson, 2017).

The oxygen-carrying capacity of blood is also reduced with age. Hemoglobin is the molecule most responsible for oxygen transport to peripheral tissues, but its levels are diminished in older adults. The alveolar–arterial (A-a) oxygen gradient, a measure of the efficiency of oxygen transfer from lungs to the blood, compares the partial pressure of oxygen in alveolar air (PAO_2) with the PaO_2. With rapid diffusion in a healthy adult, the net difference is close to zero. This gradient normally increases in older adults, most likely because of the ventilation–perfusion mismatch (Brashers, 2012).

The arterial pH of the older person remains within the normal adult range of 7.35 to 7.45 unless influenced by an acute illness or comorbidity. Despite an increase in RV, $PaCO_2$ does not normally rise, primarily because of increased ventilation. However, older adults do not react as quickly to changes in either hypoxemia or hypercapnia. The normal clinical response to hypoxemia is an increase in the rate and depth of respiration as well as an increase in heart rate and blood pressure. Older patients show less increase in heart rate and a lower response to increasing CO_2. In fact, their ventilatory responses to hypoxia and hypercapnia may be diminished by as much as 50% in comparison with adults in their 20s largely as a result of a reduced sympathetic nervous system response. Therefore careful assessment is crucial. The most sensitive clinical indicator for hypoxia and hypercapnia in older adults is mental status changes and complaints of occipital headaches or forgetfulness that are not otherwise explained. Finally, dyspnea on exertion is an increasing problem because any increased oxygen demand may lead quickly to symptomatic hypoxia (Brashers, 2012; McCance & Huether, 2014).

As previously described, many of the changes in pulmonary functions in older adults are related to the changes in elastic recoil and musculoskeletal changes of the chest wall. Table 20.2 lists the lung volumes measured, the normal findings,

and alterations related to aging. The ability to determine accurate pulmonary function by testing requires patience on the part of the health care provider as an older patient may not be able to perform quickly. Ensure adequate time for this assessment of the older adult patient.

Although the total lung capacity (TLC) remains relatively unchanged, the individual volumes that comprise TLC change dramatically. V_T is decreased in older adults. Vital capacity (VC) is also decreased as a result of decreased mobility of the chest wall and altered inspiratory and expiratory capabilities. The rate of reduction of VC is greater in older men than in older women. The inspiratory capacity of older adults is affected by the decreased ability to take deep breaths. Decreased compliance of the thorax accounts for the increase in RV and expiratory reserve volume (ERV). RV is also reduced because of decreased muscle strength and a shallow breathing pattern. As a result, functional dead space ventilation is increased from one-third to as much as one-half of each breath, which results in a decrease in the volume of air that can participate in gas exchange (Brashers, 2012; McCance & Huether, 2014).

Airflow in the tracheobronchial tree is affected by the size of the airway, resistance in the airway, muscle strength, and elastic recoil. When measured in the older patient, all of these indices are decreased. Forced expiratory volume in 1 second (FEV_1) is reported to drop between 25 and 30 milliliters (mL) per year after age 30. Changes in the airflow measures are related to the stiffness of the chest wall and the loss of elastic recoil of the lungs. The decrease in thoracic muscular strength contributes to the decreased force of the air moved, and as much as a 50% reduction may occur in the maximum voluntary ventilation and FEV between ages 30 and 90.

At low V_Ts, small airways tend to close early because of the loss of elastic recoil and decreased flow rates caused by increased airway resistance, trapping air in the alveoli. Closing capacity (CC), the volume at which the smallest airways close, increases with age, and by age 65 it exceeds the functional residual capacity (FRC) when in the upright position. This contributes to early airway closure. Other factors contributing to early airway closure include increased time in a supine position and shallow breathing.

In younger adults, pulmonary vascular circulation is a relatively low pressure system with high distensibility and low resistance. As adults age, these vessels become less distensible and more fibrous, which results in increased pulmonary artery diameter and greater thickness of the vessel wall; in turn, these increases result in increased pulmonary vascular resistance and increased pulmonary artery pressure. The alveolar capillary membrane also thickens, which further reduces the surface area available for gas exchange. The number of functional capillaries declines, which results in decreased alveolar vascularity; this, in combination with a diminished cardiac output, causes a decrease in pulmonary capillary blood flow (Brashers, 2012).

FACTORS AFFECTING LUNG FUNCTION

Exercise and Immobility

Exercise has a positive effect on the respiratory and cardiovascular systems. However, the ability of older patients to perform

TABLE 20.2　Pulmonary Function Changes in Older Adults

| | | AVERAGE VALUE | |
	Description	Adult Male	Older Patient
Lung Volume			
Tidal volume (V_T)	Volume of air inhaled or exhaled per breath	5–10 (mL/kg)	Decreased
Inspiratory reserve volume (IRV)	Volume of air inhaled in addition to normal V_T	3000 mL	Decreased
Expiratory reserve volume (ERV)	Maximum volume of air that can be exhaled in addition to normal V_T	1200 mL	Decreased
Residual volume (RV)	Volume of air left in lungs after maximum exhalation	1200 mL	Increased by as much as 25%
Lung Capacity			
Functional residual capacity (FRC)	Volume of air left in lung after a normal exhalation (RV + ERV)	2400 mL	Increased
Residual volume/ total lung capacity (RV/TLC)	Ratio of RV to TLC expressed as percentage	33%	Increased
Vital capacity (VC)	Volume of air exhaled after maximal inhalation (IRV + V_T + ERV)	4800 mL	Decreased by as much as 25%
Total lung capacity (TLC)	Total volume of air in lungs after maximum inhalation (IRV + V_T + ERV + RV)	6000 mL	Unchanged

exercise is affected by the changes in cardiac output, skeletal muscle function, joint function, and overall coordination.

Increased oxygen demands during exercise periods may well exceed the abilities of older patients, and for those with COPD, activity intolerance is exacerbated. In addition, older patients are more likely to have comorbidities involving the cardiovascular and respiratory systems that may deter exercise ability. Strength and endurance may also be reduced, which leads to increased immobility and increased breathlessness when activity is attempted. Older patients with COPD and immobility may benefit from a program of regular exercise to increase strength and endurance, and decrease breathlessness as the respiratory muscles become trained (see Health Promotion/Illness Prevention box).

HEALTH PROMOTION/ILLNESS PREVENTION

The Respiratory System

- Avoid cigarette and secondhand smoke.
- Avoid environmental and air pollutants.
- Avoid allergens.
- Maintain a healthy diet.
- Exercise.
- Keep immunizations up-to-date.
- Use masks, scarves, and filters to protect against community-acquired illnesses.
- Incorporate stress management activities into daily life.
- Ensure early diagnosis and treatment of respiratory tract infections.
- Adhere to medical regimen for chronic respiratory illnesses.
- Maintain clean environment (i.e., dust regularly, change air filters in furnace and air conditioner every 3 months, change toothbrush every 3 to 4 months and after an illness).
- Maintain adequate hydration (at least 64 ounces of water daily).

Smoking

Smoking damages the lungs. Prolonged exposure to secondhand smoke has also been shown to damage the lungs of nonsmokers. Heavy smokers may demonstrate a nine-times increase in the reduction of FEV_1 over normal expected reductions. Cilia, which are paralyzed by nicotine, are unable to protect and clean the lungs, and, when coupled with the increased mucus production of goblet cells induced by tobacco, respiratory infections become more likely. Cigarette smoke also causes bronchoconstriction, increased airway resistance, and increased closing volumes, and interferes with gas exchange because carbon monoxide, a byproduct of tobacco, competes with oxygen for the hemoglobin molecule. Many medications are also affected by smoking, which decreases clearance and increases serum drug levels. Some drugs altered by the chemicals present in smoking include antidepressants, propranolol, theophylline, insulin, clopidogrel, methadone, warfarin, erythromycin, and lidocaine (Fiore et al., 2008; Sarna & Bialous, 2010; Lucas & Martin, 2013).

During an assessment of social behaviors, a smoking history needs to include pack-years, that is, the number of packs smoked per day multiplied by the number of years the patient has smoked. An example is someone who has smoked two packs per day from age 15 through age 40, but increased to three packs until quitting smoking at age 62. Subtract 15 from 40 and multiply by 2; then, subtract 40 from 62 and multiply by 3. Add the two numbers, and the total is 106 pack-years (Sarna & Bialous, 2010).

Smoking Cessation

Smoking cessation is imperative to prevent decline in lung function with aging and comorbid disease. The five components of smoking cessation, known as the "Five A's" consist of asking, advising, assessing, assisting, and arranging (Agency for Health Care Research and Quality [AHCRQ], 2012). At each encounter, the patient is asked about tobacco use. This gives the health care worker an opportunity to advise and discuss the health benefits and promote smoking cessation. When speaking to older adults, the nurse should use strong, clear, and personalized language. The nurse should assess older adults for their willingness to give up smoking and determine how soon they are ready to start the process. Then the nurse assists older adults with smoking cessation by encouraging them to set a quit date, reviewing preparations for quitting (e.g., removing associated objects such as ashtrays), recommending nicotine replacement therapy, providing advice on successful quitting (e.g., avoid constant exposure to other smokers), providing supplemental educational materials, and offering appropriate skills training and support. Finally, the nurse arranges for follow-up (Agency for Health Care Research and Quality [AHCRQ], 2012).

Many new treatments are available for older smokers to assist with quitting. These include the use of bupropion hydrochloride, varenicline, nicotine gum, nicotine patches, and nicotine inhalation systems. Bupropion hydrochloride is given for 3 days at 150 milligrams (mg) per day and then increased to 150 mg twice a day, with doses 8 hours apart and the first dose in the morning. Older patients can smoke during the first week of treatment and are encouraged to set a quit-smoking date before the end of the first 14 days of treatment. Varenicline, a nicotinic receptor partial agonist, is initiated 1 week before the quit date with dosing of 0.5mg daily, increasing to 0.5mg twice daily on the fourth day. On the actual quit date, dose is increased to 1 mg twice daily for 12 weeks. Varenicline has shown efficacy in dampening cravings for smoking, particularly when used in tandem with behavioral approaches. Nicotine inhalation systems, gums, and patches are used to replace the patient's need for nicotine. While using these nicotine substitutes, the older adult patient should not smoke. Gradually, over a 6- to 8-week period, the frequency of usage is decreased (Woo & Robinson, 2016).

Obesity

The effect of obesity on respiratory function results in a decrease in chest wall compliance and reduction in FRC, VC, and ERV because the additional weight of the relatively stiffer chest and larger abdomen creates a mechanical disadvantage to breathing and impedance to overall body movement. As a result, pulmonary functions are reduced and breathlessness increases. The combination of decreased ability to take a deep breath, early airway closure, and the increased likelihood of immobility puts the older patient at high risk of developing atelectasis and upper and lower respiratory tract infections.

Moreover, excessive weight can lead to hypoventilation with or without hypercapnia, further interfering with adequate respiratory ventilation and perfusion. Obesity is a well-recognized precursor to obstructive sleep apnea (OSA), a periodic reduction or cessation of breathing during sleep causing narrowing or occlusion of the upper airway. OSA is increasing in prevalence due to escalating obesity rates. The World Health Organization (WHO, 2018a) defines overweight as a body-mass index (BMI) equal to or greater than 25 kg/m², and obesity as a BMI equal to or greater than 30 kg/m². Even a 10% reduction in body weight can significantly improve VC and respiratory mechanics in the older adult. Nurses can play an integral role in educating older adults about obesity and the modifiable risk factors associated with weight gain and concomitant disease (Cash & Glass, 2016).

Anesthesia and Surgery

Because aging can decrease overall pulmonary reserves, older adults are more susceptible to respiratory compromise during the perioperative and postoperative periods. An older patient undergoing surgery has an increased risk of aspiration as a result of loss of laryngeal reflexes. If surgery is an emergency, this risk is increased because of the older patient's delayed gastric emptying and the potential for a full stomach. Even younger, healthier adults have the risk of postoperative atelectasis because of general anesthesia and the inability or unwillingness to cough and deep breathe because of incisions, pain, and drowsiness. In the older adult, these risks are amplified because of decreased muscle strength, a decreased cough reflex, and a greater likelihood of alterations in consciousness. Postoperative immobility decreases ventilation and increases the risk of airway clearance problems. Because a healthy adult patient can tend to be slightly "dry" after surgery in combination with a reduced thirst sensation, the older adult has an increased risk of hypovolemia and resultant thickened secretions that are difficult to clear. Promotion of deep breathing for effective pain management, adequate hydration, frequent position changes, and early mobility will decrease the risk of developing atelectasis. Furthermore, anesthetic agents used during surgical procedures can increase the risk of perioperative hypercapnia and hypoxemia as well as postoperative complications such as respiratory failure. This risk is compounded in the older adults who have cardiovascular or respiratory comorbid disease (Barnett, 2018).

RESPIRATORY SYMPTOMS COMMON IN OLDER PATIENTS

Respiratory symptoms common in older patients include alterations in breathing patterns, dyspnea, and coughing. Abnormal breathing patterns in older patients may also be indicative of other metabolic and respiratory illnesses. An early sign of respiratory problems is a change in mental status. Because the physiologic responses to hypoxemia and hypercapnia are blunted in older patients, compensatory changes in heart rate, respiratory rate, and blood pressure may be delayed and cerebral perfusion may suffer. Mental status changes may include subtle increases in forgetfulness and irritability. Older patients may also complain of an occipital headache or confusion when awakening from sleep. If these signs persist, a more in-depth evaluation of the older patient's respiratory status is indicated.

Complaints of dyspnea or breathlessness in older patients are often associated with underlying respiratory and cardiac disease. Dyspnea is a subjective perception of breathlessness that is difficult for the older patient to quantify; dyspnea may therefore be dismissed, especially when no clinical evidence can be attributed to the complaint. Older patients most often describe their breathlessness as a sensation of an inability to get enough air, difficulty taking a deep breath, breathing rapidly, or a choking or smothering feeling. Dyspnea at rest is most often associated with an acute respiratory or cardiac illness, whereas dyspnea on exertion may be related to immobility, obesity, and respiratory muscle deconditioning or an overall deconditioned state. Older patients with COPD may experience dyspnea on exertion initially and dyspnea at rest as the disease progresses. Dyspnea is a common complaint in older patients with pulmonary disease. However, older patients usually do not complain of dyspnea until it begins to interfere with their activities of daily living (ADLs) and then only if those activities are important to them. For example, it may become difficult to use the stairs; therefore an older patient may simply choose the elevator or escalator and not consider reporting the shortness of breath associated with stair climbing. It is important to determine which ADLs an older patient no longer participates in and why.

The cough mechanism in older patients is altered because of the loss of elastic recoil and decreased respiratory muscle strength. Causes of coughing in older patients include postnasal drip, chronic bronchitis, acute respiratory tract infections, aspiration, gastroesophageal reflux disease (GERD), congestive heart failure (CHF), interstitial lung disease, cancer, and angiotensin-converting enzyme inhibitor (ACEI) medications for hypertension and CHF. Because of the age-related changes that affect an older patient's coughing mechanism, it is important to recommend cough suppressants with caution. Suppression of the cough and depression of any respiratory function could lead to retention of pulmonary secretions, plugged airways, atelectasis, and aspiration.

RESPIRATORY ALTERATIONS IN OLDER PATIENTS

Chronic respiratory disease affects not only older patients but also their families (Cruz, Marques, & Figueiredo, 2017). Many patients with respiratory illness feel a loss of control over their lives because of breathlessness on exertion and at rest. They may become demanding and controlling in dealing with their families and friends. The quality of older patients' lives depends on their feelings about and control of the disease. Support groups sponsored by the American Lung Association and local hospitals are available to help patients and families deal with anger, loss of control, and hopelessness. The family, or a significant other, needs to be included in all aspects of planning and care for an older patient with respiratory illness. The patient's success in complying with the medical recommendations may depend on the assistance he or she receives in getting to the physician's office, getting to the pharmacy for medications, administering medications, and performing ADLs. Older patients with respiratory disease need a good family support system and a health care team to support both them and their families (see Evidence-Based Practice: COPD Self-Management in Ethno-Cultural Communities).

EVIDENCE-BASED PRACTICE

COPD Self-Management in Ethno-Cultural Communities

Sample/Setting
The study included 30 patients with COPD and 16 family members.

Methods
Qualitative data were collected via interviews.

Findings
Five themes emerged: current knowledge and practice of COPD self-management; trusted sources of health information; insufficient care from medical doctors; information they wish to receive; and barriers to accessing health information.

Implications
Consider diverse cultural beliefs and practices when developing educational materials; engage patients and families in development of educational materials; and ensure that education is appropriate and relevant to patient and family's ethnic and cultural beliefs and practices to facilitate adherence.

From Shum, J., Poureslami, I., Vheng, N., & Fitzgerald, J.M. (2014). Responsibility for COPD self-management in ethno-cultural communities: The role of patient, family member, care provider, and system. *Diversity and Equality in Health Care, 11*, 201–213.

Respiratory disease is divided into two categories: (1) obstructive pulmonary disease and (2) restrictive pulmonary disease. Obstructive lung diseases are characterized by changes in expiratory airflow rates and obstruction of the airway. The lumen of the airway may be decreased by mucus, edema of the airway lining, or constriction of the muscles surrounding the airway, causing bronchoconstriction. Restrictive lung disease is characterized by decreased ability to expand the chest, impaired inhalation, and decreased lung volumes. Changes in the chest wall, lung parenchyma, pleural space, and extrapulmonary factors such as body mass may result in restrictive lung disease. Examples of these diseases include bronchogenic carcinoma and tuberculosis (TB). Other respiratory diseases seen in older patients include bronchopulmonary infections, pulmonary edema, and pulmonary emboli.

OBSTRUCTIVE PULMONARY DISEASE

Asthma

Asthma is a chronic inflammatory disease that affects the airways and is characterized by reversible airway obstruction, airway inflammation, and increased airway responsiveness to a variety of stimuli. Asthma has higher morbidity and mortality rates in older adults than in other age groups. Older patients diagnosed with asthma have lower expiratory flow rates and fewer symptom-free periods. Because of other comorbidities, the provider may delay a diagnosis of asthma. Asthma occurs

in about 8.3% of older adults after age 65, and many of these older adults have asthma as a continuing chronic disorder (Global Initiative for Asthma [GINA] Guidelines, 2018).

Airway inflammation contributes to airway hyperresponsiveness; airflow limitations, including acute bronchoconstriction, airway edema, and mucous plug formation; airway wall remodeling; respiratory symptoms; and disease chronicity (GINA-Guidelines, 2018; McCance & Huether, 2014). Inflammation causes recurrent episodes of wheezing, breathlessness, chest tightness, and coughing, often at night or early in the morning. Blood vessel dilation and capillary leakage is caused by inflammation of airway mucous membranes. This leads to tissue swelling and increased secretions with mucus production (Brashers, 2012).

Recent evidence suggests that persistent abnormalities in lung function are associated with subbasement membrane fibrosis in some patients. Patients with asthma, especially older patients who may not have had this disease through most of their lives, require careful education to include self-management, how to adjust medications during exacerbations, and the correct way to prepare themselves for exposure to known triggers.

An asthma attack may be precipitated by exposure to allergens or irritants such as changes in weather, odors, or stress. In older patients, asthma is often associated with viral respiratory infections. Signs and symptoms include dyspnea, audible wheezing, cough, palpitations, tachypnea, tachycardia, use of accessory muscles of respiration, pulsus paradoxus, diaphoresis, and hypoxemia. Initially, a patient may hyperventilate and effectively blow off increasing CO_2. However, falling PaO_2 levels and pH with rising $PaCO_2$ are indicative of imminent respiratory failure. The increasing $PaCO_2$ is a result of the patient's exhaustion and inability to hyperventilate as increasing work of breathing ensues.

Prognosis

The prognosis for an older adult with asthma is relatively good. Success is based on a partnership between the patient and the health care provider to properly use prescribed medications, avoid asthma triggers, identify early signs of exacerbation, and maintain a healthy lifestyle.

Treatment

The goals of asthma therapy are to control asthma by reduction of impairment and risk, which may be achieved by (1) preventing chronic and troublesome symptoms such as coughing or breathlessness during the day, at night, or after exercise, (2) maintaining (near) normal pulmonary function, (3) maintaining normal activity levels, including exercise and attendance at work or school, (4) requiring infrequent use ($\leq$ 2 days a week) of inhaled short-acting beta$_2$-agonists (SABAs) and satisfying the patient's and family's expectations of asthma care, (5) preventing recurrent exacerbations and minimizing emergency department visits, and (6) providing optimal pharmacologic treatment with minimal or no adverse effects (GINA, 2018). A stepwise approach to pharmacologic management is recommended by the GINA (2018) clinical practice guidelines. The specific drug, dose, and frequency are dictated by the severity of the asthma attack at the time that therapy is initiated, and subsequently the drug should be stepped down to maintain long-term control with the minimum medication necessary. Medications are classified into two categories: (1) long-term control medications and (2) quick-relief medications.

Long-Term Control Medications

Long-term control medications are taken daily and include anti-inflammatory agents, long-acting bronchodilators, and leukotriene modifiers. Corticosteroids are the most potent and effective long-term control medications in the treatment of mild, moderate, or severe persistent asthma. They are well tolerated and safe when used at the recommended dosage. Most of the benefit is achieved with relatively low doses, and the potential for side effects increases with the dose. However, for asthma not controlled with maintenance doses of corticosteroids, two options are now available. The first is to combine the corticosteroids with long-acting beta$_2$-agonists (LABAs), and the second, most recent recommendation is to increase the dose of corticosteroids (GINA, 2018). The clinical response to corticosteroids is a reduction in airway inflammation, improvement in peak expiratory flow rate (PEFR), diminished airway hyperresponsiveness, prevention of exacerbations, and possible prevention of airway wall remodeling. Corticosteroids are generally inhaled twice a day.

LABAs act by relaxing the smooth muscle of the airways and stimulating beta$_2$-receptors to increase cyclic adenosine monophosphate (cAMP). They are not recommended as a monotherapy for long-term control but, rather, are often prescribed in combination with corticosteroids. The duration of action is 12 hours for a single dose. These medications are also not indicated for acute exacerbation, although they may be used to prevent exercise-induced exacerbations; however, when beta$_2$-agonists are used on a long-term basis before exercise, their effects last only 5 hours. An example of these medications is inhaled salmeterol, or formoterol.

Leukotriene modifiers are potent biochemical mediators released from mast cells, eosinophils, and basophils. They act on the lungs, causing airway smooth muscle contraction and increased mucous secretion; they also attract and activate inflammatory cells in the airways. Leukotriene antagonists improve lung function, diminish symptoms, and reduce the need for SABAs. They are an alternative, although not preferred, therapy for the treatment of mild persistent asthma. They may also be used with corticosteroids, although the LABAs are the preferred adjunct. An example of a leukotriene antagonist is montelukast or zafirlukast. These drugs block the leukotriene receptors, whereas zileuton prevents leukotriene synthesis. These drugs do not reverse symptoms during an asthma attack and should not be used as rescue medication (Woo & Robinson, 2016).

Cromolyn and nedocromil stabilize mast cells. Although they are not the preferred method of treatment, they are also an alternative therapy for mild persistent asthma and may also be used before exercise or before a known exposure to a trigger.

The immunomodulators are monoclonal antibodies that prevent the binding of IgE to the receptor cells of the basophils and mast cells. They are used for the treatment of severe persistent asthma, especially if allergies are the primary trigger. The

nurse should always be prepared and equipped to treat for anaphylaxis that may occur.

Quick-Relief Medications

Quick-relief medications are used to treat acute symptoms and exacerbations such as chest tightness, coughing, and wheezing. This group of medications includes SABAs, anticholinergics, and systemic corticosteroids. SABAs are bronchodilators that provide smooth muscle relaxation within 30 minutes and are the drug of choice for treating acute asthma symptoms and preventing exercise-induced exacerbations (GINA, 2018). Older patients who use more than one canister per month do not have adequate control and need additional antiinflammatory therapy. Daily use of SABAs is not recommended.

Anticholinergics such as ipratropium bromide may provide an additive benefit to inhaled beta$_2$-agonists in the treatment of severe exacerbations. They may also be used as an alternative to SABAs in patients who do not tolerate them well. Finally, systemic corticosteroids, although not short acting, may be used in the treatment of moderate to severe asthma exacerbations as an adjunct to the SABAs. Their onset of action is more than 4 hours, and they act by preventing progression of the exacerbation, speeding recovery, and preventing early relapse (GINA, 2018).

Asthma Medications Administered Through a Stepwise Approach

Step 1: No daily medication indicated. SABAs are used as required (prn). If they are used more than two times a week, consider long-term control therapy.

Step 2: Daily low-dose inhaled corticosteroid.

Step 3: Daily low-dose inhaled corticosteroid used in conjunction with a long-acting bronchodilator. An alternative is to increase the corticosteroid dose to a medium level without the addition of a long-acting bronchodilator. If ineffective, a leukotriene modifier may be added to a low-dose corticosteroid. SABAs are used prn. With daily or increased usage, add additional long-term control therapy.

Step 4: Daily antiinflammatory, inhaled corticosteroid (medium dose), and a long-acting bronchodilator. If ineffective, a leukotriene modifier may substitute for the long-acting bronchodilator. SABAs are used prn. Add additional long-term control therapy if SABAs are used daily or if there is an increase in use.

Step 5: Daily inhaled corticosteroid (high dose) plus a long-acting bronchodilator. Consider an immunomodulator for patients with allergies. Short-acting beta$_2$-agonists are used prn. Add additional long-term control therapy with daily or increased usage.

Step 6: Daily inhaled corticosteroid plus long-acting bronchodilator plus an oral corticosteroid. Consider an immunomodulator for patients with allergies.

(GINA, 2018; Cash & Glass, 2016).

Patient education, environmental control, and quick management of comorbidities are required at each step. An asthma specialist should be considered at Step 3 and implemented at Step 4.

In older adults, asthma management may occur alongside management of chronic bronchitis or emphysema. A trial of systemic corticosteroids is useful in determining the presence of reversible airflow obstruction (GINA, 2018). An older adult may have medical conditions such as cardiac disease and osteoporosis that are aggravated by asthma medications. Older adults with ischemic heart disease may be more sensitive to beta$_2$-agonist side effects such as tremors and tachycardia; the dosage may need to be adjusted, or different medications may need to be added as an adjunct.

Corticosteroids may cause confusion, agitation, and changes in glucose metabolism in older adults. The use of inhaled corticosteroids in older adults may predispose them to a reduction in bone mineral content, especially in the presence of preexisting osteoporosis, changes in estrogen levels affecting calcium utilization, and a sedentary lifestyle. The GINA (2018) guidelines recommend calcium and vitamin D supplements, as well as estrogen replacement therapy, when appropriate. An increased risk for adverse drug and disease interactions exists: Asthma may be exacerbated using nonsteroidal antiinflammatory drugs (NSAIDs) for arthritis, aspirin for circulation, nonselective beta-blockers for hypertension, or glaucoma eye drops that contain beta-blockers. Finally, it is imperative that older adults are carefully assessed for their ability to use prescribed medications appropriately and devices correctly as the increased risk of physical (arthritis, visual) or cognitive impairments could be challenging for them (Cash & Glass, 2016).

NURSING MANAGEMENT

Assessment

Evaluation of respiratory symptoms includes effect on ADLs, quantity of breathlessness on a scale of 1 to 10 (Stupka & deShazo, 2009), presence of asthma triggers, and frequency of the need for bronchodilator therapy. Physical assessment includes inspection of the chest for shape and symmetry, determination of respiratory rate and pattern, body position, use of accessory muscles of respiration, and amount and color of sputum production. Palpation and percussion of the chest are indicated so that increased tactile fremitus, chest wall movement, and diaphragmatic excursion can be assessed. When the chest wall is auscultated, the older adult should be given enough time to take deep breaths comfortably without becoming dizzy. Determine the presence of any wheezing, the phase of respiration in which it occurs, and whether it is present during a forced expiratory maneuver. Determination of the PEFR with a peak expiratory flow meter (PEFM) is important in determining trends of airway resistance (Fig. 20.1).

Diagnosis

Nursing diagnoses common for an older patient with asthma include the following (Malone, 2011):

- Airway obstruction resulting from bronchospasm, excessive mucus production, tenacious secretions, adventitious breath sounds, or a combination of all of these
- Decreased gas exchange resulting from alveolar–capillary membrane changes
- Need for patient teaching resulting from lack of information and education about asthma

The diagnosis of asthma is based on episodic symptoms of partially reversible airflow obstruction. Key indicators for the

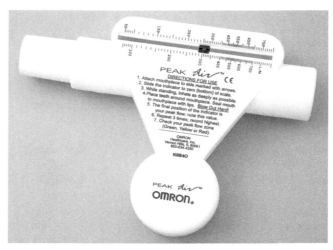

Fig. 20.1 A sample of a peak expiratory flow meter. This model displays results in colored areas: faster exhalation rates are in green, reduced exhalation rates are in yellow, and seriously reduced exhalation rates in red. (From Aehlert, B. [2011]. *Paramedic practice today: Above and beyond*. St. Louis, MO: Mosby.)

diagnosis of asthma include (1) wheezing, (2) a history of a cough that is worse at night, (3) recurrent difficulty breathing and chest tightness, (4) variation in PEFR of 20% or more, and (5) symptoms that worsen during exercise, with viral infection, in the presence of environmental irritants such as animal fur, dust mites, mold, smoke, pollen, changes in weather, airborne chemicals, or dust, during menses, or with strong emotional expression (GINA, 2018, 2016; Cash & Glass, 2016).

Pulmonary function tests (PFTs) are used to measure the presence and amount of airway obstruction. An FEV$_1$–forced vital capacity (FVC) ratio of less than 65% indicates obstruction of airflow. Measurements of FEV$_1$, FVC, and the FEV$_1$–FVC ratio before and after inhaled short-acting bronchodilators are recommended. Other diagnostic procedures include methacholine, histamine, or exercise challenge; chest radiography; allergy testing; ear, nose, and throat evaluation for nasal polyps and sinus disease; evaluation for gastroesophageal reflux; a 1- to 2-week evaluation of diurnal variation in PEFR; and evaluation for vocal cord dysfunction (GINA, 2018).

The diagnosis and management of asthma in older patients is more difficult than in younger patients. The symptoms of asthma mimic other conditions such as myocardial ischemia or pulmonary embolus. Asthma may appear as late as the eighth or ninth decade of life. Older adults with asthma may not show allergic skin sensitivity; therefore serum IgE and eosinophil levels may be more predictive. Incomplete reversibility of airflow obstruction is increasingly common. Older adult patients with asthma may achieve only a 12% improvement in their FEV$_1$, even with optimally prescribed inhaled bronchodilators. In older patients with heartburn, coughing, nocturnal symptoms occurring early in the night, and resistance to routine therapy, gastroesophageal reflux disease should be considered (GINA, 2018; Cash & Glass, 2016).

Asthma is classified into three categories according to (1) severity of symptoms, (2) frequency of nighttime symptoms, and (3) lung function (Table 20.3). Asthma also occurs as seasonal asthma, cough variant asthma, and exercise-induced asthma.

TABLE 20.3   **Classification of Asthma by Severity of Disease Before Treatment***

Characteristic	Mild	Moderate	Severe
Frequency of exacerbations	≤2 times/week; lasting less than 1 hour	>2 times/week; may last days; not frequently severe	Frequent exacerbations, often severe
Frequency of symptoms	Minimal	Often	Continuous
Exercise tolerance	Minimal	Diminished	Poor; activity limited
Frequency of nocturnal asthma	≤2 times/month	>2 times/week	Almost nightly, chest tight in morning
School or work attendance	Good	Fair	Poor
Pulmonary function: peak expiratory flow rate (PEFR)	>80%	60%–80%	<60%
PEFR variability	<20%	20%–30%	>30%
Spirometry	Minimal airway obstruction	Airway obstruction evident with reduced expiratory flow at low lung volumes	Substantial airway obstruction with increased lung volumes and marked unevenness of ventilation

*After treatment, severity is measured by the minimum medications needed to maintain good health.

From National Heart, Lung, and Blood Institute, National Institutes of Health (NIH). (2007). *Clinical practice guidelines: Guidelines for the diagnosis and management of asthma.* Retrieved April 2014 from https://www.nhlbi.nih.gov/files/docs/guidelines/asthsumm.pd.

Planning and Expected Outcomes

Older patients with asthma and their families should be included in care planning (GINA, 2018; Cash & Glass, 2016). It is important to incorporate the changes in ADLs required for ongoing monitoring and maintenance of patients with asthma. Expected outcomes include the following:
1. The patient will maintain a patent airway.
2. The patient will maintain arterial blood gas (ABG) values at baseline.
3. The patient will be able to demonstrate proper use of the PEFM.
4. The patient will be able to demonstrate relaxation techniques to control breathing.
5. The patient will be able to list the significant and reportable signs and symptoms.

Well-controlled asthma results in temporary and reversible airway changes. Poorly controlled asthma leads to chronic inflammation, which may cause damage and hyperplasia of the bronchial epithelial cells and bronchial smooth muscle (GINA, 2018).

Intervention

Interventions for patients with asthma include health maintenance, lifestyle changes, administration of medications at designated time intervals, exercise, and promotion of hydration and good nutrition. Education is started at the time of diagnosis and is integrated into every aspect of care. Emphasis is placed on asthma self-management; basic facts about asthma; roles of medications; environmental control measures; the use of inhalers, spacers, and PEFMs; and a daily written action plan for management of exacerbations (Cash & Glass, 2016). Additional topics include smoking cessation, weight gain or loss, exercise requirements, and breathing retraining.

In addition to the basic interventions already described, older patients may require special considerations. The nurse should be accommodating to any neurologic changes such as altered senses, decreased fine motor movements, and memory loss. These expected changes may be managed with a number of strategies (GINA, 2018):
- Make treatment plans simple.
- Use short explanations and easily explained graphs.
- Make sure instructional materials are in large type, and use color-coded PEFM diaries.
- Increase lighting, and speak in a low-pitched, clear voice.
- Have the patient read and then repeat the instructions.
- Allow sufficient time for instruction, demonstration, and return demonstrations.

Evaluation

Physical evaluation is based on normal breath sounds and the ability to clear secretions and maintain airways with a normal respiratory rate. The evaluation of self-management is based on the patient's success in following through with the plan. Determine the frequency of rescue inhaler use, success at avoiding triggers, and the patient's ability to monitor and address lifestyle changes. Making permanent changes rather than temporary adjustments, although initially difficult for older adults, will be more likely to be achieved after thorough education. Continue to stress the need for regular follow-up with the primary care provider. Pictures and instructions on the use of multiple inhaler devices are available for download at https://ginasthma.org/2018-gina-report-global-strategy-for-asthma-management-and-prevention/.

Chronic Bronchitis

Chronic bronchitis is a clinical syndrome characterized by excessive mucous production with a chronic or recurrent cough on most days for a minimum of 3 months of the year for at least 2 consecutive years in a patient in whom other causes have been ruled out. Hypertrophy of the bronchial mucous glands, increase in the number of goblet cells, and decrease in the effectiveness of the mucociliary escalator all occur, usually as a result of repeated infections. Cigarette smoking is the single most important factor that exacerbates chronic bronchitis. Chronic bronchitis is associated with right-sided heart failure, cor pulmonale, polycythemia, hypoxemia, and respiratory insufficiency. Clinical symptoms often include a persistent cough, dyspnea on exertion, purulent sputum, cyanosis, crackles on auscultation, tachycardia, pedal edema, unexplained weight gain, and a decreased PaO_2 with a normal or elevated $PaCO_2$ (McCance & Huether, 2014).

Emphysema

Emphysema usually occurs between ages 60 and 70 and is characterized by progressive destruction of the alveoli and their supporting structures. The alveoli distal to the terminal bronchioles become enlarged, and loss of elastic recoil leads to chronic airflow limitation. Loss of connective tissue supporting the alveoli leads to permanent obliteration of the peripheral airways. Physical signs include the classic barrel chest appearance and the use of accessory muscles of respiration. Emphysema is often associated with a history of smoking. The clinical presentation includes dyspnea on exertion or at rest, decreased weight, a chronic cough with little sputum production, digital clubbing, hyperresonance of the chest on percussion, an elevated hemoglobin level, markedly decreased breath sounds or, at times, crackles and wheezes on auscultation, and abnormal PFTs with decreased VC, increased TLC, increased FRC, increased RV, and decreased FEV_1 (McCance & Huether, 2014).

Chronic Obstructive Pulmonary Disease

COPD is characterized by progressive airflow limitation that is not fully reversible and, during the course of the disease, lung tissue that becomes abnormally inflamed. The changes manifested include peripheral airway inflammation, airway fibrosis, hypertrophy of smooth muscles, hyperplasia of goblet cells and resultant mucus hypersecretion, and, eventually, the destruction of the lung parenchyma (McCance & Huether, 2014). The two reversible components in COPD are airway diameter and expiratory flow rate. COPD is a broad term that describes two obstructive airway diseases: chronic bronchitis and emphysema. Asthma may also be included in COPD, especially if a component of airway hyperreactivity exists; however, it may be difficult to differentiate between the two, especially if a history of cigarette smoking is present.

COPD is a progressive and ultimately fatal disease. The fatality rate for COPD is more than two times higher in men than in women between the ages of 65 and 74 and three times higher between the ages of 75 and 84. The number of women with COPD has been increasing since 1991 (GOLD Guidelines, 2017), likely a result of the increase in the number of women who smoke. Risk factors for COPD include age, male gender, reduced lung function, air pollution, exposure to secondhand smoke, familial allergies, poor nutrition, and alcohol intake. COPD is often a comorbid factor in deaths from pneumonia and influenza; it accounts for increased physician visits and is preventable and treatable (GOLD Guidelines, 2017).

Signs and Symptoms

The characteristic symptoms of COPD are chronic and progressive dyspnea, coughing, and sputum production. Chronic coughing and sputum production may precede limits on airflow by many years, which provides a real opportunity for intervention before it becomes a major health problem. It is also possible that airflow limitations may develop without either a chronic cough or excess sputum production (GOLD Guidelines, 2017).

Diagnostic Tests and Procedures

A diagnosis of COPD should be considered based on a history of exposure to tobacco smoke or other occupational irritants and progressive dyspnea, a chronic cough, and chronic sputum production; the diagnosis should then be confirmed with spirometry testing. COPD is staged based on the percent of the predicted value of FEV_1 (Table 20.4).

Most patients seek medical treatment because of progressive dyspnea leading to breathlessness and anxiety. Chronic coughing is often the first sign of COPD, but the absence of coughing does not rule it out. Initially, chronic coughing is intermittent, and patients may describe "good days and bad days." As the disease progresses, the cough is present every day. Wheezing and "chest tightness" may vary from day to day and may vary throughout a single day. Once again, an absence of tightness or wheezing does not rule out COPD. Weight loss, anorexia, depression, and anxiety often accompany the pulmonary signs of COPD (GOLD Guidelines, 2017).

TABLE 20.4 Staging Chronic Obstructive Pulmonary Disease by Level of Airflow

Stage	% Predicted FEV_1	Description
I: Mild	≥80%	Mild airflow limitation. Possibly cough and sputum but possibly not. Patient may be unaware of altered lung function.
II: Moderate	≥50% and <80%	Worsening airflow. Shortness of breath especially on exertion. Cough and sputum may be present but not always. Usually the stage where people seek medical help.
III: Severe	≥30% and <50%	Further worsening of airflow. Increased shortness of breath and dyspnea on exertion. Fatigue. Repeated exacerbations that affect quality of life.
IV: Very severe	<30% or <50% plus presence of chronic respiratory failure	Severe airflow limitation. Respiratory failure is defined as PaO_2 <60 mm Hg at sea level. Cardiac complications may occur (e.g., cor pulmonale). Quality of life is appreciably affected, and exacerbations are frequent and life threatening.

FEV_1, Forced expiratory volume in 1 second; PaO_2, partial pressure of arterial oxygen.
Modified from Rabe, K. F., et al. (2007). Global strategy for the diagnosis, management, and prevention of chronic obstructive pulmonary disease: GOLD executive summary. *American Journal of Respiratory Critical Care Medicine, 176,* 532-555.

Treatment

Managing COPD focuses on increasing treatment, depending on the disease severity; the clinical status of the patient with airflow limitations provides a general guide. Treatment is focused on symptom management through education about the disease and active engagement of the older patient in care management. Aspects of management include smoking cessation, a stepwise approach to pharmacotherapy, limited occupational exposure to toxins and air pollution, and a healthy lifestyle, including regular exercise and weight control. Proper nutrition is essential for promoting efficient respiratory muscle work as COPD patients use a lot of calories and energy to breathe. Pneumococcal and annual influenza vaccinations are recommended for older patients. During peak influenza season, older patients with COPD should avoid crowds to decrease the risk of contracting influenza.

The single most important and cost-effective intervention is smoking cessation. Smoking cessation improves FEV_1 and helps relieve symptoms. Benefits to smoking cessation include reduction in the number of respiratory infections, improvement in the function of the mucociliary clearance of the lungs, decreased coughing and dyspnea, increased appetite, and decreased sputum production. Older patients with COPD should also avoid secondhand smoke, as it may also cause bronchospasm and coughing. Many pharmacotherapies are now available to help the older patient quit smoking. Nicotine replacement drugs and some antidepressants (bupropion and nortriptyline) as well as varenicline may increase smoking abstinence rates but should be used as part of an overall program of abstinence (GOLD Guidelines, 2017; Cash & Glass, 2016).

Pulmonary pharmacotherapy is recommended in a stepwise approach based on the severity of airway obstruction and patient symptoms. None of the medications modify the long-term decline of the patient and thus are only used to reduce symptoms and complications. Bronchodilators are key in managing the symptoms of COPD and are given for both long-term therapy and during acute exacerbations; they include beta-adrenergic drugs, anticholinergics, and methylxanthines. Once a patient reaches stage 3, the addition of inhaled glucocorticosteroids is appropriate. However, chronic treatment with systemic glucocorticosteroids is not recommended unless patients are thought to have a significant asthmatic component.

Bronchodilators

Bronchodilators are the central pharmacologic tool used in managing the symptoms of COPD. They may be prescribed for long-term maintenance or short-term exacerbations. Inhaled medications are preferred because the systemic complications they cause are both less severe and more rapidly reversed. However, with inhalation therapy, proper training is essential. The primary bronchodilators used are the beta$_2$-agonists, anticholinergics, and the methylxanthines. The choice of drug will depend on the patient's response.

Beta$_2$-Agonists

These sympathomimetic drugs work by stimulating the beta$_2$-receptors in the lungs, which results in bronchial dilation, increased mucociliary clearance, and possibly increased diaphragmatic function. The drugs may be administered by metered-dose inhaler (MDI) with a spacer, dry powder inhalation, or by aerosolized therapy. Beta$_2$-agonists should be used with caution in the older patient with ischemic heart disease. Examples of beta$_2$-agonists include albuterol, metaproterenol sulfate, and pirbuterol acetate.

Anticholinergics

Inhaled anticholinergics—ipratropium bromide or oxitropium bromide—are used to treat chronic bronchitis. They work by inhibiting vagal stimulation of the lungs, preventing contraction of the smooth muscle, and decreasing mucous production. A combination of an SABA and an anticholinergic results in a greater and more sustained improvement than with either drug alone (GOLD Guidelines, 2017). Tiotropium, a long-acting antimuscarinic antagonist (LAMA), which blocks the bronchoconstrictor effect of acetylcholine, has been shown to have a greater effect on exacerbations rates compared with the LABA alone.

Glucocorticosteroids

Inhaled glucocorticosteroids do not reduce the decline of the older adult with COPD, but for those patients with advanced disease (stage 3 or 4), they have been shown to reduce the frequency of exacerbations and improve overall health status. Chronic oral steroid use is no longer recommended as it may lead to steroid myopathy, which is associated with muscle weakness and respiratory failure. Steroid therapy may not be well tolerated in older patients (GOLD Guidelines, 2017).

Vaccines

Influenza vaccines reduce both morbidity and mortality rates in patients with COPD by 50% (GOLD Guidelines, 2017). Vaccines containing killed or live inactivated viruses are recommended for older adults, and the pneumococcal polysaccharide vaccine is recommended for those older than 65 years.

Oxygen Therapy

Long-term oxygen therapy increases survival rates and improves hemodynamics, exercise and lung capacity, and mental status, and can decrease long-term effects of a heart stressed by chronic hypoxemia. Supplemental oxygen therapy is indicated for patients with resting PaO_2 55 mm Hg or less or saturation of arterial oxygen (SaO_2) 88% or less with or without hypercapnia. Oxygen therapy may also be indicated if the patient's PaO_2 is between 55 and 60 mm Hg, the SaO_2 is 88% or less, or evidence of pulmonary hypertension, peripheral edema, or polycythemia (hematocrit level >55%) exists. The primary goal of oxygen therapy is to increase baseline PaO_2 to at least 80 mm Hg and SaO_2 to at least 90% (GOLD Guidelines, 2017).

Pulse oximetry recognizes hemoglobin saturation, which normally is between 95% and 100%. The pulse oximeter uses infrared light waves and a sensor placed on the finger of the patient. However, the oximeter probe may be placed on toes, earlobes, or even the nose if circumstances do not permit a finger to be used. Pulse oximetry can detect desaturation before physical appearance of dusky skin, pale mucosa, or pale nail beds are noted.

Antibiotics

No evidence suggests that the prophylactic long-term use of antibiotics has any beneficial effect. Antibiotics should be used only when concomitant bacterial infection is present.

Surgical Options

Surgical options consist of a bullectomy, which reduces dyspnea and improves lung function by allowing previously compressed lung tissue to expand. Another option is a lung volume reduction surgery, which, thus far, shows some promise for those with upper lobe emphysema and low exercise capacity. Lung transplantation is the final surgical option and does improve quality of life. All three procedures are extremely expensive and somewhat controversial because all are essentially palliative by nature (GOLD Guidelines, 2017).

NURSING MANAGEMENT

Assessment

Dyspnea is the hallmark symptom of COPD. It is the primary reason that patients seek treatment and the major cause of disability and anxiety. As such, spirometry remains the primary tool in determining the severity and staging of COPD. Evaluation of respiratory symptoms also includes assessing their effect on ADLs, quantifying breathlessness on a scale of 1 to 10, and identifying environmental and social factors that may contribute to the symptoms. The nurse also identifies the type of onset of the symptoms—whether sudden or insidious—and any precipitating factors such as exercise, temperature changes, and stress. Physical assessment includes assessment of the shape and symmetry of the chest, respiratory rate and pattern, pulse oximetry, body position, use of accessory muscles of respiration, color, temperature, appearance of extremities, and the color, amount, consistency, and odor of sputum.

To assess cyanosis in darkly pigmented older adults, the nurse should examine the patient with favorable lighting conditions (e.g., use overbed light or natural sunlight). The nurse should be attentive to factors that may mask cyanosis by causing vasoconstriction, which may include environmental conditions (e.g., air conditioning and mist tents) and patient behaviors (e.g., smoking and taking medications causing vasoconstriction). Examine the usual places in which cyanosis is found, namely the lips, nail beds, around the mouth, cheek bones, and earlobes. Be aware that the darker skin may mask the underlying cyanosis, and the region around the mouth is often darker in people of Mediterranean descent. When cyanosis is questionable, apply light pressure to create pallor. In cyanosis, tissue color returns slowly from the periphery to the center. Normally, color returns in 1 second, from below the pallid spot as well as from the periphery. Cyanosis of an extremity may become more recognizable if the elevation of an extremity is changed.

The nurse should observe for other clinical manifestations of decreased oxygenation of the brain. These include changes in the level of consciousness, increased respiratory rate, the use of accessory muscles of respiration, nasal flaring, positional changes, and other manifestations of respiratory distress.

The nurse should use palpation and percussion of the chest to assess for increased tactile fremitus, chest wall movement, and diaphragmatic excursion. When auscultating the chest wall, the nurse must give an older adult enough time to take deep breaths comfortably without becoming dizzy.

Diagnosis

The primary nursing diagnoses common for an older patient with COPD include the following (Malone, 2011):
- Airway obstruction resulting from retained secretions
- Reduced gas exchange resulting from an altered oxygen supply
- Inadequate nutrition
- Insomnia resulting from anxiety, dyspnea, depression, hypoxemia or hypercapnia or both, paroxysmal nocturnal dyspnea, and orthopnea
- Potential for infection resulting from inadequate primary and secondary defenses and chronic disease

Planning and Expected Outcomes

As with all patients, older patients with COPD should be included in the care planning. It is important to include the spouse or significant other, family, and any other caregivers in the planning process. Discharge planning should begin as soon as an older patient is admitted to the hospital. If an older patient requires special equipment for home care, such as supplemental oxygen therapy or aerosolized therapy, the patient and his or her family will benefit from learning the new skills in the acute care setting. Expected outcomes for the older patient with COPD include the following (Moorhead et al., 2008):
1. The patient will maintain a patent airway.
2. The patient will maintain a stable weight.
3. The patient will maintain ABG values at baseline.
4. The patient will maintain a balanced intake and output.
5. The patient will be able to effectively clear secretions.
6. The patient will be able to demonstrate diaphragmatic and pursed-lip breathing.
7. The patient will be able to demonstrate relaxation techniques to control breathing.
8. The patient will maintain a respiratory rate between 16 and 25 breaths per minute.
9. The patient will be able to list significant and reportable signs and symptoms.

Intervention

Interventions for patients with COPD include maximizing the effects of bronchodilator therapy, administering medications at designated intervals, and promoting hydration, good nutrition, and increased mobility (Cash & Glass, 2016). The majority of nursing care for the patient with COPD involves extensive education. Topics include normal respiratory anatomy and changes associated with the disease; medical intervention, including tests and medications; and lifestyle changes such as smoking cessation, weight gain or loss, exercise, and breathing retraining (see Nursing Care Plan: Chronic Obstructive Pulmonary Disease).

Pulmonary Rehabilitation

Patients with COPD at all stages benefit from COPD education for self-management and exercise training. Pulmonary

◎ NURSING CARE PLAN

Chronic Obstructive Pulmonary Disease

Clinical Situation

Mr. W is an 80-year-old retired truck driver admitted to the medical intensive care unit (ICU) for exacerbation of his COPD. He lives with his wife, who is 78 years old. Mr. W continues to smoke one to two packs of cigarettes per day, as he has done since the age of 15.

Over the past week, Mrs. W has noticed a decrease in Mr. W's activity level and attention span. He has a productive cough of thick tenacious sputum, averaging 1 cup per day. Over the past week, the sputum has become yellow. His appetite has decreased, and he has difficulty sleeping at night, often awakening and gasping for breath. Mr. W is having increasing difficulty in bathing and dressing.

Physical examination reveals a thin man with weight of 138 pounds (lb). He has a barrel chest and uses his accessory muscles of respiration to breathe. Auscultation of the chest reveals diminished breath sounds with scattered coarse crackles bilaterally and no wheezes. Mr. W's blood pressure is 138/68 mm Hg, his pulse is 92 beats per minute, and his respiratory rate is 35 breaths per minute. His oral temperature is 101° F (38.3° C).

Laboratory tests show arterial blood gases (ABG) measurements as follows: pH, 7.40; $PaCO_2$, 68 mm Hg; PaO_2, 58 mm Hg; SaO_2, 80%; and bicarbonate (HCO_3), 28. Mr. W has a white cell count of 12,000. Sputum cultures reveal *Haemophilus influenzae*. A diagnosis of *H. influenzae* pneumonia is made.

Because of increasing shortness of breath and decreasing oxygenation, Mr. W is intubated and begins receiving mechanical ventilation according to the couple's wishes. Intravenous antibiotic therapy is started, and bronchodilator therapy is initiated to reduce airway resistance and promote pulmonary hygiene. Mr. W receives mechanical ventilation for 6 days until he is successfully weaned off the ventilation and then transferred to the medical division.

He remains in the medical division for 10 additional days. Mr. W is sent home with home oxygen therapy and bronchodilators, and is told absolutely not to smoke.

Nursing Diagnoses

Reduced stamina resulting from decreased strength and endurance

Airway obstruction resulting from retained secretions

Reduced gas exchange resulting from alveolar hypoventilation

Reduced spontaneous ventilation resulting from infection and decreased respiratory muscle endurance

Inability to communicate resulting from endotracheal intubation

Need for patient teaching about home oxygen therapy and smoking cessation resulting from inexperience with concepts

Outcomes

The patient will be able to safely and comfortably perform ADLs.

The patient will be able to effectively clear secretions with coughing or suctioning.

The patient will be able to maintain spontaneous ventilation without mechanical assistance.

The patient will be able to effectively communicate with caregivers and family.

The patient and family will be able to demonstrate the use of the home oxygen equipment.

The patient and family will be able to verbalize oxygen safety measures.

The patient and family will be able to verbalize the need to quit smoking and techniques for achieving success.

Interventions

Provide active and passive range-of-motion exercises and early mobilization to maintain mobility.

Assess the need for supplemental oxygen to enhance activity tolerance.

Arrange for physical and occupational therapy consultation.

Pace activities to provide rest and decrease episodes of breathlessness and fatigue

Provide chest physiotherapy (CPT) to promote secretion removal and chest expansion, as tolerated.

Provide hydration to maintain fluid volume status and to decrease viscosity of secretions.

Turn every 2 hours to promote ventilation and to help drain pulmonary secretions.

Monitor ABGs, as ordered.

Monitor pulse oximetry continuously.

Provide mechanical ventilation during an acute phase if indicated for acute respiratory failure.

Suction as needed based on assessment findings; maintain patent airway.

Monitor ventilator settings every 2 hours.

Provide reassurance for the patient and family.

Provide oral care every 2 hours.

Provide rest periods.

Schedule care activities based on the patient's energy level.

Provide an alternative method of communication such as a picture board, talking board, or alphabet board.

Speak in clear, short sentences, and ask questions that require only a short response.

Provide the patient and family with information about home oxygen therapy, liter flow, and equipment for home use. Provide instruction about oxygen safety.

Instruct the patient and family in smoking cessation techniques and how this relates to oxygen safety.

Provide information about local smoking cessation programs.

Refer to outpatient pulmonary rehabilitation program for COPD education and exercise training.

---

rehabilitation programs are designed to provide the patient with exercise training, breathing retraining, education, smoking cessation, medications, ADL retraining, nutrition counseling, and group support. The exercise component should include 20 to 30 minutes of moderate intensity exercise three to five times a week, as well as strength training, and should result in increased exercise tolerance and decreased dyspnea and fatigue. It may also reduce cardiovascular disease risks, improve musculoskeletal functioning, help control weight or promote weight loss, and may help prevent bone loss in older patients (GOLD Guidelines, 2017; Garvey et al., 2016). One of the best exercises is walking or using a treadmill. It strengthens both the legs and the upper body, especially if the arms are used. Exercise on a

stationary bicycle is also useful, but it does not have the benefit of overall body conditioning that can be achieved with walking. Older patients with COPD may start a program in small increments, for example, walking or biking for 3 to 5 minutes daily. It is important to develop an exercise program achievable for an older patient. Targets are based on desired outcomes. The appropriate exercise intensity for health benefit is maintaining a heart rate of at least 55% of the maximum rate for a patient's age (i.e., a rate of 88 beats per minute [beats/min] for a 60-year-old and 80 beats/min for a 75-year-old). Adding strength training to the comprehensive exercise program can help to improve overall muscle mass, enhance muscle efficiency, and complement conditioning. Strength training can also help to reduce oxygen consumption and minimize dyspnea (Garvey et al., 2016).

Another benefit of a formal pulmonary rehabilitation program is the social aspect. Pulmonary rehabilitation classes and exercise times usually allow many patients to participate in a group setting. This group setting helps motivate older patients, provides emotional support, and offers them an opportunity for socialization and interaction. The pulmonary class sessions are often mini–support groups. Pulmonary rehabilitation may help reduce health care costs by reducing the frequency of hospitalizations, and helping older patients and their families learn to cope with the disease process (GOLD Guidelines, 2017; Garvey et al., 2016).

Smoking Cessation

Smoking cessation is the best and most cost-effective way to reduce exposure to risk factors. Older patients with COPD who continue to smoke increase their risk of repeated respiratory infections and progression of the underlying disease process. Older patients should be offered an opportunity for smoking cessation, and it should be offered at every opportunity. It is important to provide support for older patients attempting to quit smoking. Success depends in part on the support of family and friends. Many older patients find it impossible to stop smoking completely. They should be encouraged to reduce the amount and frequency of their smoking and perhaps consider nicotine replacement therapy to facilitate total cessation. Although smoking reduction is not ideal, it may help decrease some of the symptoms associated with respiratory illness. Programs are available through the American Lung Association, the American Cancer Society, and many community hospitals. The U.S. Public Health Service provides a framework for cessation (Centers for Disease Control and Prevention [CDC], 2017a; Surgeon General's report, 2014) (Table 20.5).

Nutrition

Older patients should be instructed on the benefits of eating nutritious meals. Adequate nutrition is often difficult to maintain in older patients and those with COPD have the additional problem of breathlessness. The patient should be instructed to eat frequent small meals, avoid gas-producing foods, reduce carbohydrates to only 50% of the diet (the breakdown of carbohydrates has been shown to increase the CO_2 load, thereby increasing the work of breathing, especially in those with CO_2 retention), eat high-protein foods, and reduce the intake of fat (see Nutritional Considerations box).

NUTRITIONAL CONSIDERATIONS
Respiratory System

Nutrient requirements for patients with respiratory disease are as follows:
Calories—25 to 35 kilocalories per kilogram (kcal/kg) of body weight for maintenance; 35 to 40 kcal/kg for replacement and building
Protein—1 to 1.5 grams (g)/kg of body weight for maintenance; 1.5 to 2 g/kg for replacement and building; 25% to 50% of caloric intake
Carbohydrates—50% of caloric intake; the breakdown of carbohydrates increases the CO_2 load and may increase the work of breathing, especially in older patients with CO_2 retention
Fats—20% to 25% nonprotein calories

Breathing Retraining

The goals of breathing retraining include decreasing the work of breathing, improving oxygenation, increasing the efficiency of breathing patterns, and promoting patient control of breathing. Two of the most commonly taught techniques are diaphragmatic breathing and pursed-lip breathing (Boxes 20.1 and 20.2; Figs. 20.2 and 20.3).

Diaphragmatic breathing increases the patient's awareness of breathing patterns and improves the efficiency of breathing. Pursed-lip breathing increases expiratory pressure, improves oxygenation, helps prevent early airway closure, increases

---

TABLE 20.5   How to Help the Patient Who Is Willing to Quit Smoking

ASK	Identify all tobacco users at every visit.
	For every patient, regardless of setting, tobacco usage is queried and documented.
ADVISE	Strongly urge them to quit.
	Be clear. Be caring. Be personable.
ASSESS	Determine the patient's readiness to quit.
	Ask every patient at every opportunity if he or she is willing to try to quit.
ASSIST	Help patient with a quit plan.
	Provide counsel. Provide support. Help patient obtain treatment.
	Help patient with approved pharmacotherapy.
ARRANGE	Schedule follow-up contact either in person or by phone.

Adapted from Fiore, M. C., Bailey, W. C., Cohen, S. J., et al., and The Tobacco Use and Dependence Clinical Practice Guidelines Panel, Staff, and Consortium Representatives. (2000). A clinical practice guideline for treating tobacco use and dependence: A U.S. Public Health Services report. *Journal of the American Medical Association, 283,* 3244-3254.

BOX 20.1   Diaphragmatic Breathing

1. Lie in the supine or semi-Fowler position.
2. Place one hand on the middle of the stomach below the sternum.
3. Place the other hand on the upper chest.
4. Inhale slowly through the nose. The stomach should expand. (Note the movement of the hand over the stomach.)
5. Exhale slowly through pursed lips. The stomach should contract.
6. Rest.
7. Repeat.

BOX 20.2   Pursed-Lip Breathing

1. Assume a comfortable position.
2. Inhale slowly through the nose, keeping the mouth closed.
3. Remember to use the diaphragmatic breathing technique.
4. Pucker the lips as if blowing out a candle, kissing, or whistling.
5. Exhale slowly, blowing through pursed lips (exhalation should be at least twice as long as inhalation).
6. Rest.
7. Repeat.

Inhale ⬇

Exhale ⬆

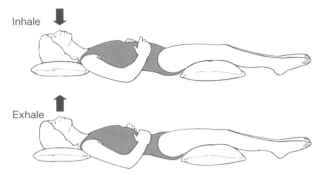

Fig. 20.2 Diaphragmatic breathing.

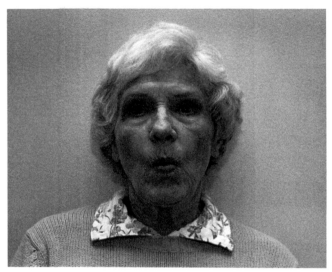

Fig. 20.3 Pursed-lip breathing. (Courtesy of Ursula Ruhl, St. Louis, MO.)

exhalation time, reduces the respiratory rate, and allows the patient to slow the breathing.

Chest Physiotherapy

Chest physiotherapy (CPT) includes chest percussion, postural drainage (PD), and vibration for patients who have difficulty clearing their own secretions. Contraindications include hemoptysis, pulmonary emboli, osteoporosis, and bleeding disorders. PD consists of positioning the patient in a head-down position after CPT to facilitate drainage of pulmonary secretions. Older patients may not tolerate the head-down position of PD or the percussion of CPT. The nurse should explain to patients that they may experience increased breathlessness as a result of the mobilization of secretions and increased coughing as they try to clear the airway. To help decrease the discomfort associated with chest percussion, the nurse should place a bath towel over the percussed area.

Pulmonary Hygiene

Pulmonary hygiene consists of hydration, deep breathing exercises, and coughing techniques (Box 20.3). Older patients are prone to dehydration and therefore are at risk for airway plugging. The nurse should encourage a volume of oral fluids of 4 to 6 quarts a day, if not contraindicated by cardiovascular disease. The nurse should also instruct older patients to sip fluids all day to decrease the chance of feeling full by drinking a large amount at one time and prevent dyspnea from bloating in the abdomen.

Medications

Patient education regarding medications includes the purpose of the medication, dosage, side effects, and schedule of administration. Medications are administered by mouth, MDI (Box 20.4), dry powder inhaler (DPI), or nebulizer. Inhaled medications are only as effective as the delivery technique. Simple human errors that affect delivery of inhaled medications include

---

BOX 20.3   Effective Coughing Techniques

Cascade Cough
1. Take a deep breath and hold it for 1 to 3 seconds.
2. Cough out forcefully several times until all air is exhaled (usually two to six coughs).
3. Inhale slowly through the nose.
4. Repeat once, if necessary.
5. Rest.
6. Repeat, as needed.

Huff Cough
1. Take a deep breath and hold it for 1 to 3 seconds.
2. Keeping glottis open, cough out several times until all air is exhaled (usually two to six coughs). Sometimes, it helps to say the word *huff* while coughing.
3. Inhale slowly through the nose.
4. Repeat, as necessary.

End-Expiratory Cough
1. Take a deep breath and hold it for 1 to 3 seconds.
2. Exhale slowly.

3. At the end of the exhalation, cough once.
4. Inhale slowly through the nose.
5. Repeat, as necessary.
6. Follow with a cascade or huff cough, in which secretions are moved from smaller to larger airways.

Augmented Cough
1. Take a deep breath and hold it for 1 to 3 seconds.
2. Perform one or more of the following maneuvers:
   a. Tighten knees and buttocks to increase intraabdominal pressure.
   b. Bend forward at the waist to increase intraabdominal pressure.
   c. Place hand flat on the upper abdomen just under the xiphoid process and press in and up abruptly during the cough or exhalation, or place hands on the lateral rib cage and quickly press in and release with each cough (this is called *rib springing*).
   d. Keep hands on the chest wall and press inward with each cough.
3. Inhale slowly through the nose.
4. Rest, if necessary.
5. Repeat, as needed.

BOX 20.4 Using a Metered-Dose Inhaler

1. Select the appropriate canister of medication.
2. Shake the inhaler 15 to 20 times.
3. Hold the inhaler directly in front of the mouth about 2 to 3 inches from the lips. When a spacer is used, place the inhaler in the spacer and place the mouthpiece directly into the mouth.
4. Take a deep breath and exhale completely.
5. Open the mouth wide. When a spacer is used, seal the lips around the mouthpiece.
6. Activate the inhaler.
7. Inhale slowly and deeply.
8. Hold breath for a count of 10.
9. Exhale slowly.
10. Wait 1 to 5 minutes between puffs. Repeat the steps for each puff ordered.

---

failure to shake the inhaler before use, failure to exhale slowly before inhaling, lack of mechanical coordination of compression of the inhaler and inhaling, rapid inhalation or lack of deep inhalation, not waiting at least 30 seconds between puffs, failure to clean the MDI periodically, holding the MDI upside down, and failure to remove the cap before spraying the medication. A spacer device can help overcome errors in delivery technique and promote better drug deposition into the lung (Woo & Robinson, 2016). The patient's inhaled medication technique should be evaluated and reviewed at every health care encounter.

Home Oxygen Therapy

Oxygen therapy decreases morbidity and mortality rates for patients with COPD when used more than 18 hours a day. A patient's acceptance of oxygen therapy and attitude about the disease determine the level of compliance with treatment. Oxygen is a medication, and patients and their families need to be taught the correct administration, which includes proper liter flow, the times that oxygen is to be used, and the proper use of the equipment.

Home oxygen therapy is available in E-cylinders, concentrators, and liquid systems. A liquid oxygen system with portability is the most easily transported and may provide older patients with more mobility. However, it is the most expensive option. The concentrator is a machine about the size of small bedside table. It is stationary and usually accompanied by an E-cylinder for limited portability. The E-cylinder, a small green tank that can be pulled on a cart like a luggage rack, is economical, although it is a little less portable because of its size.

All the persons involved in a patient's care—patient, family, physician, and nurse—should discuss the patient's level of activity and select the right oxygen system to support his or her lifestyle. Social workers may be helpful in determining the amount and type of insurance coverage the patient has available for home oxygen therapy. Many third-party payers do not cover liquid oxygen systems unless the patient is active and spends a good portion of the day out of the home. If an older patient is homebound, only leaving the home for medical appointments, the most economical system is the concentrator with an E-cylinder.

Exacerbations of Disease and Self-Monitoring

It is critical that patients with COPD are taught how to monitor their symptoms for signs of lung infection and what action to take should they suspect they are experiencing an exacerbation of disease. Knowing the signs/symptoms of infection can enable the patient to seek prompt medical attention, shorten the length of an exacerbation, and hopefully prevent worsening disease and function. Exacerbations can sometimes be managed at home; however, if symptoms are severe, hospitalization may be necessary as exacerbations can be serious enough to be fatal. Therefore early detection and treatment is essential.

Patients should discuss with their health care providers what steps or actions they should take for exacerbations; this "Action Plan" can outline specific steps and instructions at the first signs of exacerbation (Lareau, Moseson, & Slatore, 2014). Experiencing worsening shortness of breath; change in the quality, amount, or color of sputum; coughing; wheezing; and the need for increased use of inhaled medication can all be signs of lung infection. Because underlying lung infection can often cause exacerbations, antibiotics and oral corticosteroids may be necessary in an acute exacerbation (Woo & Robinson, 2016). Patients can be taught how and when to start these medications as part of their overall "Action Plan."

Although not all exacerbations can be prevented, measures like quitting smoking, getting an annual flu vaccine and updating a vaccination for pneumonia, avoiding close contact with sick individuals, and good hand washing are a few strategies that may help to minimize exacerbations.

A quick reference fact sheet on COPD exacerbations can be obtained at https://goldcopd.org/wp-content/uploads/2016/12/wms-GOLD-2017-Pocket-Guide.pdf.

Evaluation

Evaluation of an older patient with COPD focuses on airflow as measured by spirometry, the ability to accomplish ADLs, and minimization of exacerbations. Older patients may need additional caregivers in the home because the spouse or significant other is most likely of a similar age and may also have chronic health problems. Older patients may need more time to learn the educational materials; however, once taught, they should have a good understanding and be able to adapt these techniques to their lifestyle.

RESTRICTIVE PULMONARY DISEASE

Restrictive lung disease results in loss of functioning alveoli, loss of lung volume, and decreased chest wall compliance. Restrictive lung disease may be the result of extrapulmonary factors such as excessive weight and muscle mass, a chest splint, or a restrictive dressing. Mechanisms of restrictive lung disease include pleural-based diseases, impaired lung expansion, impaired neuromuscular contraction, and thoracic deformities.

Lung Carcinoma

Lung cancer is the leading cause of cancer deaths, accounting for 28% of cancer deaths. Approximately 224,210 new cases of lung cancer are reported annually in the United States. It is rare in patients younger than 44 years of age but increases in incidence between ages 60 and 70, and the average age at diagnosis is 71 years (National Cancer Institute [NCI], 2017). The increase in smoking by women has raised the rate of death from lung cancer to the point that it now exceeds the rate of death from breast cancer.

Risk factors for development of lung cancer include tobacco use; marijuana use; recurring inflammation; or exposure to asbestos, talcum powder, or minerals. Less frequently, radon exposure, heredity, vitamin A deficiency, and exposure to air pollution may be risk factors. The leading cell types of lung cancer are small-cell lung carcinoma (SCLC), which accounts for 20% of cases, and non–small-cell lung carcinoma (NSCLC), including squamous cell carcinoma and adenocarcinoma, which accounts for 79%, and other specified and nonspecified types, which account for about 1% of cases (NCI, 2017). The most lethal type of lung cancer is SCLC, which usually has a 5-year survival rate of 6.3%. SCLC is an aggressive cancer that metastasizes to the central nervous system (CNS), bones, and liver. NSCLC is a slower growing and less aggressive cancer that has a 5-year survival rate of 17.5% (NCI, 2017).

Diagnostic Tests and Procedures

Diagnosis is based on the clinical history and chest radiography. The initial workup includes a complete blood cell (CBC) count, carcinoembryonic antigen (CEA) level, chest radiography, computed tomography (CT), ABG measurements, PFTs, and an electrocardiogram (ECG). Sputum cytology is used to determine the cell type. If metastasis is suspected, additional diagnostic tests include magnetic resonance imaging (MRI) of the brain, bone scintigraphy, exercise PFTs, quantitative ventilation–perfusion scanning, treadmill exercise test, Doppler echocardiography, and carotid Doppler ultrasonography. Fiberoptic bronchoscopy is used to obtain tissue confirmation of the diagnosis. Surgical diagnosis includes cervical mediastinoscopy, mediastinotomy, and thoracotomy. PFTs are used to determine impairment in ventilation and help predict functionality if surgery is a consideration. On the basis of diagnostic testing, the stage of NSCLC involvement is determined (Table 20.6). SCLC is not staged because it is extremely aggressive and is always assumed to be systemic once diagnosed.

TABLE 20.6 Staging Of Non–Small-Cell Lung Carcinoma

Stage	Description
1a	Tumor <3 cm, localized, no lymph node involvement
1b	Tumor >3 cm, invading local areas, no lymph node involvement
2a	Tumor <3 cm, lymph node involvement on same side of chest
2b	Tumor >3 cm, lymph node involvement on same side of chest, tissue involvement of local organs
3a	Spread nearby (chest wall, pleura, pericardium) and to regional lymph nodes
3b	Extensive tumor (heart, trachea, esophagus, scalene, and supraclavicular lymph nodes
4	Distant metastasis

Adapted from National Cancer Institute. (2017). *Lung cancer*. Retrieved January 15, 2018, from http://www.cancer.gov.

Treatment

Treatment is based on histologic analysis and staging. SCLC has a median survival of 2 to 4 months from diagnosis and is very aggressive. It is much more responsive to chemotherapy and radiation therapy, but a cure is very difficult. The treatment of NSCLC depends on the staging and is basically divided into three groups of patients. The first group contains those patients with resectable cancer. Generally, this is stage 1 and 2 and some stage 3 cancers. These patients have the best prognosis. The second group of patients includes the remainder of NSCLC patients except for those with stage 4 cancer. This second group may benefit from a mixed modality of surgery, radiation therapy, and chemotherapy. The final group is those with stage 4 cancer, and they receive palliative treatment that includes chemotherapy, radiation therapy, and endobronchial laser therapy (NCI, 2017). If an older patient has significant lung disease, resection of the lung or segmental resection may not be possible. The decision to perform a surgical resection depends on the amount of functional lung tissue that would remain after the surgery.

Careful management of pain, nausea, vomiting, and chemotherapy-related side effects is important for providing as much physical comfort as possible for the patient and mental comfort for the family. Older patients may not be able to tolerate a complex medical regimen, especially with other organ involvement or underlying disease processes.

NURSING MANAGEMENT

Assessment

Assessment includes the identification of risk factors for lung cancer. The clinical presentation of lung cancer may easily be mistaken for other chronic lung diseases such as chronic bronchitis. Often, no symptoms are present, or the symptoms are ignored or attributed to smoking or a preexisting lung disease. Common early signs include coughing, chest pain, and hemoptysis. It is also important to assess the patient's and the family's understanding of the numerous diagnostic tests that will be performed shortly. An assessment of the anxiety level is also appropriate.

Diagnosis

Nursing diagnoses for lung cancer include the following (Malone, 2011):
- Reduced gas exchange resulting from altered blood flow and alveolar–capillary membrane changes
- Acute pain and chronic pain resulting from the pressure of the tumor on surrounding structures
- Inadequate nutrition
- Anxiety resulting from a lack of knowledge of the diagnosis or unknown prognosis and treatment
- Hopelessness resulting from failure or deterioration of physiologic condition and long-term stress

Planning and Expected Outcomes

Planning includes developing interventions and expected outcomes for the patient that focus on improving gas exchange, promoting airway clearance, increasing comfort, and reducing anxiety. Expected outcomes include the following (Moorhead et al., 2008):

1. The patient will be able to maintain ABG values at baseline.
2. The patient will be able to sustain spontaneous respiration.
3. The patient and family will be able to verbalize their feelings related to the diagnosis of lung cancer.
4. The patient's pain will be controlled.
5. The patient will report a decrease in the number of episodes of breathlessness.
6. The patient's lungs will be clear on auscultation.
7. The patient will maintain a stable weight.
8. The patient will report feeling a decrease in fatigue.
9. The patient will maintain a realistic level of activity.

Intervention

Nursing care of an older patient with lung cancer includes relief of pain, emotional support, counseling, and discussion of options and alternatives. The older patient may have fewer friends and family members for support. Interventions include providing factual information concerning the diagnosis, treatment, and prognosis; encouraging an attitude of realistic hope as a way of dealing with feelings of helplessness; acknowledging the patient's spiritual and cultural background; and encouraging verbalization of feelings, perceptions, and fears (NCI, 2017). The nurse needs to be sensitive to the values of older patients and how they see the diagnosis affecting their quality of life. Many older patients may be more concerned about immediate survival and quality-of-life issues than the 5-year postoperative survival rate.

Evaluation

Symptom management is evaluated by assessing how often symptoms occur, how the patient has been able to incorporate changes into his or her lifestyle, and how the symptoms alter the patient's ADLs. The nurse should determine the success of pain management and the level of patient comfort. Older adults may not have the same tolerance for pain and discomfort as younger patients. The nurse should help patients quantify their pain on a scale of 1 to 10. This will help both the nurse and the patient monitor the effectiveness of pain management. The nurse should also evaluate the older adult's use of pain medication. The main goal of pain management is to optimize function and quality of life while minimizing pain and associated side effects where possible (Boltz, Capezuti, Fulmer, & Zwicker, 2012). Many older adults are concerned about becoming addicted to their pain medication and, therefore, may not use pain medication appropriately as prescribed. Nurses should be astute to pain management protocols for older adults and employ accurate assessment and evaluation in managing the older adult's pain (Boltz, Capezuti, Fulmer, & Zwicker, 2012). The nurse should ensure that the older patient understands that the dose and frequency of medications will be carefully monitored. In addition, many older adults may become depressed after a diagnosis of cancer and should be monitored for signs of depression; a referral should be made if depression is suspected.

Tuberculosis

TB is caused by the organism *Mycobacterium tuberculosis.* TB is most often seen in populations living in crowded quarters and in those with little or no health care or preventive care. It is the number one fatal and communicable disease in the United States. TB is divided into primary and active varieties. TB is transmitted by inhalation of infected droplets aerosolized in the air from the cough or sneeze of an infected person. The body's immune system responds to the local inflammation by walling off the bacteria. When active, the patient with TB is seen with symptoms of inflammation of the airway that led to the development of a lesion and necrosis of the tissue. TB may remain inactive in the body for decades. Although TB primarily attacks the lungs, it can travel via the pulmonary lymphatics or enter the vascular system and affect the brain, kidneys, spine, bones, and joints. The bacillus infects a greater number of older adults than causes active TB. However, active TB may be present in any patient admitted with pneumonia, pleural effusion, human immunodeficiency virus (HIV) or acquired immunodeficiency syndrome (AIDS), weight loss, cancer, or alcohol or substance abuse (CDC, 2016; Cash & Glass, 2016).

In an older patient, the presence of TB may be a reactivation of a dormant organism that has been present in the individual for some time. As patients age, changes in the immune system increase the risk of reactivation of TB. Medical risk factors that substantially increase the risk of TB include silicosis, gastrectomy, jejunal bypass, weight more than 10% *below* ideal body weight, chronic renal failure, diabetes mellitus, and hematologic disorders such as leukemia, lymphomas, and other malignancies. Older residents of nursing homes and other long-term care facilities are at increased risk of developing TB; they have a two to seven times greater incidence of the disease compared with older adults in the general population (CDC, 2016).

Many older adult patients have underlying lung disease that puts them at higher risk of morbidity and mortality should they become infected. Most nursing home and long-term care facility residents are older adults. These concentrations of older adults, many of whom are infected and some of whom are immunocompromised, create high-risk situations for transmission of TB. An estimated 1.1 million (13%) of the 8.6 million people worldwide who developed TB in 2012 were HIV-positive. About 75% of these cases were in the African region (CDC, 2016; WHO, 2018b).

Diagnostic Tests and Procedures

Older patients with any of the following symptoms should alert the practitioner to a high probability of TB: night sweats, atypical pneumonia, low-grade fever, nonproductive coughing, hemoptysis, anorexia, and weight loss. However, tuberculin skin testing in older patients is an unreliable indicator of TB because they are more likely to have false-negative results because of reduced immune system activity. If skin testing is used, it is recommended that the standard 5 tuberculin unit (5 TU) Mantoux test be given and then repeated to create a booster effect. The second test may be a 5 TU or a second strength 250 TU test. If the size of the induration is 10 mm or greater (or $\geq$ 5 mm in an HIV-positive patient), the purified protein derivative (PPD) is positive. In the event of a positive PPD with symptoms, chest radiography is recommended within 72 hours (CDC, 2016; Cash & Glass, 2016).

A positive chest radiography result with the following strongly indicates TB: infiltration in the posterior and apical segments of the upper lobes or in the superior segments of the lower lobes, cavitation, nodular infiltrates, atelectasis, fibrotic scarring with retraction of the hilum, and deviation of the trachea. Older adults may show lower lobe nodular infiltrates without cavitation. Diffuse, finely nodular, uniformly distributed lesions characterize hematogenous TB. Older patients with any persistent infiltrate must be suspected as having TB. Although the previously mentioned radiographic changes are most common, TB may produce almost any form of pulmonary radiographic abnormality. Older patients should be questioned about potential exposure to TB, tested for HIV infection, and screened for other symptoms such as chronic osteomyelitis, chronic urinary tract infections, and any of the previous symptoms not present on initial examination. If a patient has a positive PPD and is asymptomatic, prophylaxis with isoniazid for 4 months is indicated (WHO, 2018b; CDC, 2016; Cash & Glass, 2016).

For older patients with a positive PPD, symptoms, and positive chest radiography, many additional laboratory tests and referrals are indicated. These include CBC count, erythrocyte sedimentation rate, chemistry panel, sputum test for AFB performed three times, and bone marrow biopsy. A referral to an infectious disease specialist is also recommended, especially if the patient has been determined to have multiple drug-resistant TB (MDR-TB) or extensively drug-resistant TB (XDR-TB).

Treatment

Treatment with the standard four-drug anti-TB therapeutic regimen will cause a rapid reduction in the number of viable mycobacteria (WHO, 2018b; CDC, 2016; Cash & Glass, 2016). A reduction in the viable organism load is seen within 2 weeks. Cultures will convert to negative within 3 months in patients compliant with therapy. Medications include a combination of bactericidal drugs. The most common drugs are isoniazid, rifampin, ethambutol, streptomycin, and pyrazinamide (CDC, 2016). Other drugs used in the treatment of TB include ethionamide, kanamycin, para-aminosalicylic acid, cycloserine, and rifabutin. Fluoroquinolones such as ciprofloxacin are also being used to treat TB.

Monitoring of liver function on a monthly basis is recommended because older adults are at greater risk of developing hepatitis. Isoniazid may lead to toxic hepatitis and peripheral neuropathy, especially in malnourished or diabetic older adults.

Because the incidence of MDR-TB has been on the rise, the CDC recommends anti-TB drug–susceptibility testing on initial *Mycobacterium tuberculosis* isolated from all patients with TB. MDR-TB is more common in patients who have spent time with someone with MDR-TB, in those who do not take their medicine regularly or do not take all their prescribed medication, in those who redevelop TB after

having been treated, and in those who come from areas high in MDR-TB incidence, come from countries with high MDR-TB burden, which include Bangladesh, China, DPR Korea, DR Congo, Ethiopia, India, Indonesia, Kazakhstan, Kenya, Mozambique, Myanmar, Nigeria, Pakistan, Philippines, Russian Federation, South Africa, Thailand, Ukraine, Uzbekistan, Viet Nam (Kanabus, 2017).

Prognosis

The prognosis for an older patient with TB is good if the patient follows the medical regimen and maintains good nutrition. The greater problems are the side effects of isoniazid and the risk of spreading TB to other vulnerable older adults.

NURSING MANAGEMENT

Assessment

Signs and symptoms include fatigue, weight loss, weakness, night sweats, low-grade fever, purulent sputum, and sputum positive for AFB. Older adults may not always manifest all the classic symptoms of TB, so the nurse should suspect TB when an older patient complains of weight loss and a chronic cough. If the disease has progressed, the patient may have hemoptysis, lung consolidation, crackles and wheezes on auscultation, upper lobe patchy infiltrates, and cavitation on chest radiography.

Diagnosis

Nursing diagnoses for an older patient with TB include the following (Malone, 2011):
- Inadequate breathing pattern resulting from decreased lung capacity
- Need for health teaching resulting from lack of knowledge about the disease process and therapeutic regimen
- Nonadherence resulting from lack of knowledge of disease process, lack of motivation, and long-term nature of treatment
- Inadequate nutrition resulting from chronic poor appetite, fatigue, and productive cough

Planning and Expected Outcomes

Planning for older patients with TB must include the patient and the family. If a patient is a resident in a nursing or extended care facility, the medical and nursing directors need to be included in planning as well. Expected outcomes include the following (Moorhead et al., 2008):
1. The patient will be able to demonstrate safe coughing techniques.
2. The patient and family will be able to verbalize the medication regimen.
3. The patient and family will be able to verbalize the side effects of the anti-TB medications.
4. The patient will be able to verbalize the need for continued medication.
5. The patient and family will be able to state how TB is transmitted.
6. The patient will be able to verbalize feelings related to social isolation.

TABLE 20.7 Tuberculosis Medications

Medication	Dosage	Adverse Reactions	Nursing Considerations
Isoniazid	Primary therapy: 5 mg/kg, PO/IM, daily up to 300 mg/day	Anemia, hepatitis, hypersensitivity, peripheral neuritis, seizures, and systemic lupus erythematosus	Therapy lasts for 6–9 months and is used in conjunction with other antituberculosis medication. Instruct patient to avoid alcohol.
Rifampin	10 mg/kg body weight (maximum 600 mg)	Decreased effectiveness of oral contraceptives, hemolysis, hepatic toxicity, increased metabolism of hepatically excreted drugs, induction of methadone withdrawal, renal failure, thrombocytopenia, orange body fluids, and rash	Monitor hepatic, renal, and hemolytic parameters. Give 1 hour before or 2 hours after meals. Monitor hepatic function (urine may become red-orange in color). Instruct patient to avoid alcohol. Usually used with one other drug.
Pyrazinamide (PZA)	15 to 30 mg/kg/day up to 2 g/day	Anorexia, arthralgia, gout (rare), hepatitis, hyperuricemia, nausea, renal failure (rare), and vomiting	Monitor platelet count and complete blood cell count (CBC). Have patient take medication with meals or snack to reduce gastric irritation. Instruct patient to report any problems with urination. Monitor liver function tests. Instruct patient regarding signs of thrombocytopenia, such as unexplained bleeding or bruising, appearance of petechiae, and nosebleeds.
Ethambutol	15 mg/kg po daily in adults with no prior anti-TB therapy Increase to 25 mg/kg po daily if previous therapy	Headache, nausea/vomiting, blurry vision, joint pain, skin rashes	May take with or without food Refrain from getting immunizations while on ethambutol Monitor renal function, hepatic function, uric acid

g/day, Gram per day; *mg/kg/day,* milligram per kilogram per day; *po,* by mouth; IM, Intramuscular.
From Centers for Disease Control and Prevention (CDC). (2016). Tuberculosis. Retrieved January 17, 2018, from http://cdc.gov; Cash, J. C., & Glass, C. A. (2016). *Adult gerontology practice guidelines.* New York: Springer.

Intervention

Nursing measures for patients with TB include education about TB and how it is transmitted. Patients and families should be educated about the measures necessary to prevent further TB transmission, the importance of continued medication administration, and good nutrition. Table 20.7 lists the most common drugs used to treat TB, their dosages, adverse reactions, and nursing considerations. The nurse should teach the patient that, if any of the adverse reactions named in Table 20.7 occur, he or she should call the doctor or nurse immediately. Patients should not drink alcohol while taking isoniazid.

Other TB drug side effects to report to the health care practitioner include skin rashes, easy bleeding, aching joints, dizziness, tingling or numbness around the mouth, easy bruising, blurred or changed vision, ringing in the ears, and hearing loss. Nurses should inform older adults that rifampin may cause urine, stool, saliva, sputum, sweat, and tears to turn red or orange, and may stain clothes or contact lenses (Vallerand & Sanoski, 2017; Woo & Robinson, 2016).

Older adults may view TB as a socially unacceptable disease. They may remember the stigma of TB in the early 1900s when a person with TB was required to be separated from family and friends and placed in a sanatorium. Finally, the nurse must address the need for psychosocial interaction and support.

Evaluation

Evaluation of an older patient with TB includes assessment of compliance because older adults may find it difficult to adhere to the lengthy medication regimen. The nurse should also evaluate compliance with public health measures such as wearing a mask in public. Evaluation also includes monitoring of hepatic and renal function and repeated sputum cultures for AFB. The patient's mood should be evaluated for depression because of social isolation.

Pneumonia

Pneumonia is an inflammation of the lung parenchyma, usually associated with the filling of the alveoli with fluid. Pneumonia may be viral, bacterial, or caused by aspiration, which occurs more frequently in older adults. In fact, for the older adult, pneumonia is an extremely serious illness that often results in death. Increased risk of mortality in the older adult is related to the normal age-related deterioration of the immune system, increased likelihood of underlying chronic illnesses, weakened cough reflex, and decreased mobility. However, the diagnosis of pneumonia in the older adult may be missed because the symptoms may be obscured by a coexisting disease or the chronic use of corticosteroids or antiinflammatory drugs. In addition to the typical pneumonia signs and symptoms, an older patient may also manifest more atypical symptoms such as altered mental status, dehydration, and a failure to thrive. The patient may require hospitalization and admission to the ICU with subsequent intubation and mechanical ventilation. The incidence of pneumonia in older adults in long-term care institutions is three times higher than it is among older adults in the community (Dobbin & Howard, 2011; Cash & Glass, 2016). The Pneumonia Severity Index Calculator (Fine, 2017) can be used to estimate risk of pneumonia mortality and help decide if the patient should be treated on an inpatient or outpatient basis.

Community-Acquired Pneumonia

Community-acquired pneumonia (CAP) is a lower respiratory tract infection that has an onset in the community or emerges within the first 2 days of hospitalization. Classic symptoms of community-acquired or bacterial pneumonia include fever, cough, sputum production, general feelings of fatigue and malaise, and shortness of breath. Older patients do not always exhibit fever and coughing but often have symptoms of dehydration, confusion, and a respiratory rate greater than 26 breaths per minute. Other signs may include tachycardia, chest discomfort, dyspnea, headache, nausea, vomiting, myalgia, arthralgia, fatigue, weakness, abdominal pain, diarrhea, and anorexia (Cash & Glass, 2016). In multiple-lobe pneumonia, chest radiography may show incomplete consolidation of the lung. Some older patients manifest dramatic symptoms, resembling septic shock or adult respiratory distress syndrome (ARDS). *Streptococcus pneumoniae* is the leading cause of CAP in older adults, accounting for approximately 25% of pneumonia cases; its associated death rate is 30% to 40% among older adults (CDC, 2017b). About 5% to 15% of cases are caused by *Haemophilus influenzae, Moraxella (Branhamella) catarrhalis,* and *Legionella pneumophila* (Table 20.8).

Health Care–Associated Pneumonia, Hospital-Acquired Pneumonia, and Ventilator-Associated Pneumonia

Health care–associated pneumonia (HCAP) is new-onset pneumonia. It is seen in a patient who (1) was hospitalized in an acute care facility after 2 days or longer within 90 days of the infection; (2) resided in a long-term care facility; (3) received recent intravenous antibiotic therapy, chemotherapy, or wound care within a month of the current infection; or (4) was seen in a hemodialysis facility. Hospital-acquired pneumonia (HAP) occurs within 48-hours or longer after hospital admission but not found to be incubating at the time of admission. Ventilator-associated pneumonia (VAP) occurs more than 48 hours after endotracheal intubation. These infections increase the incidence of death from pneumonia. The costs associated with these diagnoses and longer hospital stays are significantly higher than a direct admission for pneumonia treatment alone. A major problem with treatment for any of these diagnoses is multidrug resistance (MDR). The virulence of the organisms may significantly reduce the available and appropriate antimicrobial therapy (McCance & Huether, 2014).

Nosocomial Pneumonia

Staphylococcus aureus, Klebsiella pneumoniae, Pseudomonas aeruginosa, and *Escherichia coli* most often cause nosocomial pneumonia. Older patients have an incidence of nosocomial pneumonia three times higher than younger patients probably because of the age-related decline in the immune system and a high incidence of comorbidities. In addition, older adults are more likely to be in high-risk areas such as residential centers, hospitals, and extended care facilities for other coexisting diseases.

Viral Pneumonia

Viral pneumonia in older patients is most often associated with a history of the influenza A virus. Older adults are especially susceptible to secondary bacterial infections from *S. aureus* and *H. influenzae.*

Aspiration Pneumonia

Aspiration pneumonia is commonly associated with clinical situations such as stupor, coma, cardiopulmonary resuscitation, alcohol or drug intoxication, neurologic illness, nasogastric feeding, and general anesthesia. Aspiration of gastric contents into the airway may result in obstruction, chemical pneumonitis, or infection. Older adults are especially prone to aspiration pneumonia because of decreased coughing and gagging reflexes. In addition, positioning, feeding, and the use of a feeding tube place older patients at increased risk for aspiration pneumonia. The use of narcotic medications, alcohol, and sedatives increases the risk of aspiration.

Diagnostic Tests and Procedures

The diagnosis of pneumonia is made based on a *history* of colds and influenza and the *clinical presentation.* Signs and symptoms include fever, chills, pleuritic chest pain, crackles on auscultation, and a productive cough with purulent sputum. Atypical pneumonia is first seen with a fever, constitutional symptoms, a dry cough, and headache. Laboratory sampling includes total white blood cell (WBC) count, blood cultures, gram stain, and sputum culture. Of older patients, 20% to 25% fail to demonstrate leukocytosis, and about one-third are unable to produce a sputum sample. *Chest radiography* (posterior, anterior, and

TABLE 20.8 Criteria for Severe Community-Acquired Pneumonia (CAP)

	Minor Criteria		Major Criteria
Respiratory rate (RR) ≥30	Uremia (BUN ≥20)	Hypothermia Core temperature <96.8° F	Invasive mechanical ventilation
Multilobar infiltrate	Leukopenia (WBC <4000)	Hypotension requiring fluid resuscitation	Septic shock with a need for vasopressors
Confusion/ disorientation	Thrombocytopenia Platelets <100,000		

Note: Either one major criteria or three minor criteria qualify for intensive care unit admission. *BUN,* Blood urea nitrogen; *WBC,* white blood cell. From Mandell, L. A., Wunderink, R. G., Anzueto, A., et al. (2007). Infectious Diseases Society of America/American Thoracic Society consensus guidelines on the management of community-acquired pneumonia in adults. *Clinical Infectious Diseases, 44S,* 27-72.

lateral) is performed to identify infiltrates and assess for complications such as effusions or lung abscess. Chest radiography is the gold standard for diagnosis. If the patient is dehydrated, infiltrates may not be evident even if they are present (Bartlett, 2017; CDC, 2017b; Cash & Glass, 2016).

Treatment

Treatment consists of administration of the appropriate antibiotics, hydration, good nutrition, and rest. The length of treatment with antibiotics may range from 10 to 14 days, depending on the causative organism. The initial management of immunocompetent patients with CAP emphasizes empiric treatment instead of extensive testing because of the difficulty in determining the etiologic pathogen in the disease.

The severity of the illness, site of acquisition (e.g., community or nursing facility), age, and presence of comorbid illnesses are all considerations in determining initial antibiotic therapy. Therapy is aimed at pneumococcal and atypical pneumonia. Antibiotics used include macrolides such as azithromycin and clarithromycin for outpatients. For patients with advanced age and comorbidity, a second-generation cephalosporin such as cefuroxime or a combination agent such as trimethoprim–sulfamethoxazole is added. If an older patient is hospitalized, a second-generation or third-generation cephalosporin or a beta-lactam or beta-lactamase inhibitor is used in combination, with or without a macrolide. Patients with resistant or severe CAP may need an aminoglycoside, an antipseudomonal agent, or quinolone (CDC, 2017b; Woo & Robinson, 2016)

The American Thoracic Society Criteria for Assessing Pneumonia Severity established guidelines for ICU admission of older patients. To qualify for admission, the patient must meet either one major or at least three minor criteria (see Table 20.8), including a respiratory rate of 30 beats/min or more, PaO_2 or fractional concentration of oxygen in inspired gas (FiO_2) of 250 mm Hg or less, multilobe infiltrates on chest radiography, and hypotension requiring fluid resuscitation (Bartlett, 2017). Health care providers may use various guidelines that attempt to quantify the risk factors of individual patients when determining whether the patients should be hospitalized (Table 20.9). Some of the factors in these indexes include age greater than 65 years, presence of coexisting illness, altered mental status, chronic alcohol abuse, dehydration, malnutrition, nursing facility residency, aspiration, history of cigarette smoking, recent upper respiratory tract infection or influenza, and previous hospitalization within 1 year (Singanayagam, Chalmers, & Hill, 2009) (see Table 20.9). Clinical signs include unstable vital signs, extrapulmonary involvement, leukopenia, hypoxemia, and PaO_2 of 60 mm Hg or less.

Prognosis

Clinical improvement usually occurs between 3 and 5 days of the initiation of treatment. Patients failing to respond to therapy will require aggressive evaluation to assess for noninfectious causes, complications, or MDR causes. Pneumonia remains the most common cause of death in older adults because of the altered immune response related to aging, underlying chronic disease, and a diminished cough reflex.

NURSING MANAGEMENT

Assessment

A history of generalized fatigue, malaise, decreased appetite and fluid intake, or a recent viral infection may indicate a bronchopulmonary infection in an older adult. Fever, chills, shortness of breath, sputum production, and an abnormal chest examination suggest pneumonia. The nurse should assess the chest for decreased breath sounds, wheezing, dullness to percussion, egophony, and increased vocal and tactile fremitus. The nurse should also assess for symptoms of dehydration and confusion, and other signs and symptoms such as tachycardia, tachypnea, chest discomfort, dyspnea, headache, nausea, vomiting, myalgia, arthralgia, fatigue, weakness, abdominal pain, diarrhea, and anorexia.

The nurse must be alert to signs and symptoms suggestive of an increasing severity of illness and a potential need for intensive care. These include tachypnea (30 to 35 breaths per minute or more); severe respiratory failure (PaO_2 or FiO_2 of 250 mm Hg or less); shock (diastolic hypotension of 60 mm Hg or systolic hypotension of 90 mm Hg or less); fever (temperature over 102.6° F [39.3° C or 102.5 F]); decreased urine output (20 milliliters per hour [mL/hr]); and abnormal laboratory values for blood urea nitrogen (BUN over 20 milligrams per deciliter [mg/dL]), creatinine (over 1.2 mg/dL), WBCs (4000 or over 30,000), hemoglobin (9 grams per deciliter [g/dL]), PaO_2 (60 mm Hg), or $PaCO_2$ (over 50 mm Hg) (Bartlett, 2017; CDC, 2017b). Another sign that may indicate more intensive care is needed is a rapid change in chest

TABLE 20.9 Variables Used to Calculate Pneumonia Risk and to Determine Hospitalization

Demographics	Comorbidity	Vitals	Diagnostics	Other
Age ≥65	Neoplastic	Respiratory rate >30	pH <7.35	Altered mental status
Male	Cerebrovascular	SBP <90	BUN >10.7 mmol/L	New-onset mental confusion
Nursing home resident	CHF	Temp either <95° F or > 104° F	Sodium <130 mEq/L	
	Chronic renal	Pulse >125	Hematocrit <30%	
	Chronic liver		PaO_2 <60 mm/Hg	
			Glucose >13.9 mm Hg	
			Radiography shows effusion	

BUN, Blood urea nitrogen; *CHF,* congestive heart failure; *mEq/L,* milliequivalents per liter; *mmol/L,* millimoles per liter; *PaO₂,* partial pressure arterial oxygen; *SBP,* systolic blood pressure.
Adapted from Singanayagam, A., Chalmers, J. D., & Hill, A. T. (2009). Severity assessment in community-acquired pneumonia: A review. *Quarterly Journal of Medicine, 102,* 379-388.

radiography that consists of spreading infiltrates and extrapulmonary sites of infection. An older patient with such indications needs close monitoring, ongoing nursing care, and possibly even short-term mechanical ventilation for respiratory support.

Diagnosis

Nursing diagnoses for a patient with bronchopulmonary infection include the following (Malone, 2011):

- Airway obstruction resulting from decreased energy and tracheobronchial infection, obstruction, and secretions
- Reduced gas exchange resulting from altered oxygen supply and alveolar–capillary membrane changes
- Inadequate breathing pattern resulting from respiratory muscle fatigue
- Potential for reduced fluid volume resulting from altered intake and factors influencing fluid needs
- Acute pain resulting from inflammation as well as ineffective pain management, comfort measures, or both, as evidenced by patient report of pleuritic chest pain and presence of pleural friction rubbing and shallow respirations

Planning and Expected Outcomes

Planning for an older adult with pneumonia should include the patient and family. It is important to focus on supporting respiratory function, promoting good pulmonary hygiene, and maintaining adequate oxygenation. Expected outcomes for an older patient with a bronchopulmonary infection include the following (Moorhead et al., 2008; Cash & Glass, 2016):

1. The patient will maintain a patent airway.
2. The patient will maintain a PaO_2 of 80 mm Hg by ABG analysis or an arterial oxygen saturation (SaO_2) greater than 90% by pulse oximetry.
3. The patient will have decreased complaints of fatigue.
4. The patient will have clear lungs on auscultation.
5. The patient will be able to clear secretions effectively.
6. The patient will be able to sleep through the night without episodes of breathlessness or coughing.
7. The patient will maintain baseline vital signs and weight.

Intervention

Nursing management of an older patient with a bronchopulmonary infection includes maintenance of hydration, promotion of effective airway clearance, and proper positioning. Other interventions include monitoring fluid, monitoring vital signs and oxygenation parameters, maintaining a clean environment, and assisting the patient with airway clearance by encouraging coughing or by suctioning (CDC, 2017b; Cash & Glass, 2016). Because of the ventilation–perfusion imbalance in the lung, it is important to position the patient with the "good lung down." This technique promotes drainage of secretions from the lung with the pneumonia and increases the perfusion of the healthy lung, which results in improved oxygenation. It may be a challenge to keep the older patient positioned on the appropriate side.

The key to pneumonia prevention is early vaccination. Antibodies to most pneumococcal vaccine antigens remain elevated in healthy adults for at least 5 years. Antibody declines have been shown in older adults after 5 to 10 years (CDC, 2017b). Therefore all persons age 65 or older should receive the pneumococcal vaccine, including all persons who have not previously been vaccinated and those who have not received the vaccination within 5 years and were 65 or younger at the time of their last vaccination. Vaccination is recommended for all persons with unknown vaccination status (CDC, 2017b). Revaccination is recommended for immunocompromised patients age 65 or older, including those with HIV infection, leukemia, lymphoma, Hodgkin's disease, generalized malignancy, chronic renal failure, and organ or bone marrow transplantation, and those taking long-term systemic corticosteroids or undergoing immunosuppressive chemotherapy (CDC, 2017b).

Nurses should assess older patients for their potential for aspiration. Nursing care planned to prevent aspiration focuses on careful assessment of RVs of feedings and proper positioning of the older patient during and after eating. Minimize the use of sedatives and hypnotics if a meal will follow afterward. Provide a 30-minute rest period before eating. If assisting the older patient with meals, nurses should alternate between solid and liquid boluses. Determine the food viscosity that is best tolerated for each patient. Be aware of which patients have aspirated previously. Clinical signs of aspiration include a sudden appearance of coughing, cyanosis, or voice changes. Notify the provider if suspicion of aspiration exists.

Evaluation

Evaluation includes achievement of the expected outcomes, return of sputum to preinfection color and consistency, and return to baseline respiratory status. The nurse should monitor the patient for adequate hydration by assessing vital signs, body weight, and tissue turgor. Dehydration contributes to secretion retention and an inability to clear the airways. The effectiveness of an older adult's cough should be monitored because a weaker cough is common in older adults and ineffective coughing may contribute to fatigue and result in aspirated secretions. The nurse should also monitor the patient's lungs for adventitious lung sounds and monitor the respiratory pattern for effective breathing and use of accessory muscles of respiration.

OTHER RESPIRATORY ALTERATIONS

Severe Acute Respiratory Syndrome

The first outbreak of severe acute respiratory syndrome (SARS) initially occurred in China in 2003 and, within months, spread to Canada, North America, South America, and across Europe and Asia. The patient's history of foreign travel is imperative to determine whether he or she had exposure to or close contact within 10 days of symptoms with a person known to have or suspected of having SARS. The mortality rate has been estimated at 10% in the population at large, but some estimate that rate to be close to 50% for those older than age 64 (CDC, 2017c; McIntosh, 2017). The patient may be asymptomatic or have a mild respiratory illness. The signs and symptoms often include a temperature over 100.4° F, coughing, shortness of breath, headache, malaise, or myalgias. In fact, defining criteria include: history of recent fever or a documented fever plus one or more symptoms of lower respiratory tract infection, plus radiographic evidence of infiltrates consistent with pneumonia or ARDS (CDC, 2017c; McIntosh, 2017).

The detection of antibody to SARS coronavirus (CoV) drawn during the acute illness or 21 days after the onset of illness confirms the diagnosis. Other diagnostic tests include chest radiography, CBC, ABG analysis, clotting profile, respiratory viral panel for influenza and syncytial viruses, lactic dehydrogenase, metabolic profile, cross-reactive protein (CRP) test, and *Legionella* and pneumococcal urinary antigen testing. The patient should wear a mask, and universal precautions should be observed as the illness is thought to be spread by person-to-person contact and respiratory droplet. Care is usually supportive. No new cases of SARS have been reported since 2004.

Cardiogenic and Noncardiogenic Pulmonary Edema

Pulmonary edema (PE) is an abnormal increase in the amount of fluid in the alveoli and interstitial spaces of the lungs, and may be a complication of many cardiac and lung diseases. The most common form of PE is a result of left ventricular failure. Left ventricular failure commonly occurs in older adults, especially in persons age 85 or older, because of coronary artery disease, mitral stenosis and insufficiency, and aortic stenosis. Cardiogenic PE is the most common form of PE and is caused by the increased capillary hydrostatic pressure that results from myocardial infarction, mitral stenosis, decreased myocardial contractility, left ventricular failure, or a fluid overload. Other predisposing factors include CHF, infusion of excessive volumes or an overly rapid infusion of intravenous fluids, impaired pulmonary lymphatic drainage from Hodgkin's disease or obliterative lymphangitis after radiation, inhalation of irritating gases, left atrial myxoma, pneumonia, and pulmonary venoocclusive disease. A rise in pulmonary capillary pressure occurs because of elevated left ventricular end-diastolic filling pressure, elevated left atrial pressure, and elevated pulmonary venous pressure.

The clinical presentation of acute cardiogenic PE includes acute shortness of breath; orthopnea; frothy, blood-tinged sputum; cyanosis; diaphoresis; and tachycardia. Physical findings include crackles in the bases on auscultation, fremitus, and dullness on percussion.

Noncardiogenic PE results from a variety of noncardiac causes. Examples of noncardiogenic PE include ARDS, reexpansion PE, and neurogenic PE as well as posttraumatic head injury, salicylate toxicity, pulmonary embolus, and opioid overdose (Givertz, 2017).

Cardiogenic Pulmonary Edema
Diagnostic Tests and Procedures
Diagnosis is based on clinical presentation and diagnostic testing. ABG measurements are drawn to determine arterial PO_2, arterial PO_2 saturation, and pH. A reduced oxygen tension and saturation and a resultant acidity related to retained CO_2 would be expected with PE. The biomarker B-type natriuretic peptide (pro-BNP) may be drawn to help provide additional

data for cardiogenic versus noncardiogenic PE. Because underlying conditions that may predispose to heart failure may be etiologic factors for cardiogenic PE, other cardiac specific markers may be included in the workup (Pinto, 2017). Hemodynamic measurements often reveal decreased cardiac output, increased pulmonary artery pressure, and right-sided heart pressure in biventricular failure. Because older patients have difficulty maintaining normal hemoglobin levels, it is important to take blood samples judiciously.

Treatment
The nurse must help reduce preload and afterload, and correct the underlying process if possible. The first step is supplemental oxygen administration; mechanical ventilation should not be used unless necessary. Myocardial function is improved by reducing preload, which is the quantity of blood returned to the heart. This is accomplished through diuresis (furosemide) and pulmonary or cardiac dilation (nitroglycerin). Morphine is also a mainstay of treatment; it reduces anxiety and therefore reduces oxygen demand. Afterload (the force the heart pumps against) is reduced through peripheral vasodilation (nitroprusside, enalapril). Inotropic support may involve use of drugs like dobutamine or catecholamines (dopamine, norepinephrine) (Sovari, 2017). PE is extensive; an older patient may require transfer to the ICU, initiation of mechanical ventilation, and insertion of a pulmonary artery catheter.

Prognosis
The prognosis for a patient with cardiogenic PE is good when symptoms are easily reversed, and cardiac complications are controlled. However, older adults usually have one or more comorbidities such as underlying cardiac or lung disease, which increases their risk for complications. With extensive rehabilitation and physical therapy, older adults may be able to return to independent living and baseline ADLs.

Noncardiogenic Pulmonary Edema: Adult Respiratory Distress Syndrome
Diagnostic Tests and Procedures
The most commonly used test is the ABG, which determines the degree of hypoxia. Other tests include chest radiography, CT, CBC, and hemodynamic measurements. Older patients may need intubation and mechanical ventilation. In addition, the placement of an arterial line and pulmonary artery catheter may be indicated so that oxygenation and cardiopulmonary hemodynamics can be monitored.

Treatment
Treatment consists of supplemental oxygen therapy, ventilation support, and maintenance of hemodynamics. Neuromuscular blocking agents, sedatives, and narcotics may be used to reduce anxiety, decrease the work of breathing, decrease oxygen consumption, and increase oxygen delivery. Positive end-expiratory pressure may be added to mechanical ventilation to improve oxygenation.

A pulmonary artery catheter may be used to monitor fluid volume status. Fluids and vasopressors may be indicated for the maintenance of adequate blood pressure. If a bacterial infection is evident, antibiotic therapy may be added. Corticosteroids are reserved for ARDS caused by a chemical injury or fatty emboli.

Prognosis

Overall, the prognosis is fair to poor, and the mortality rate is approximately 30% to 60%. Comorbidity, frailty, and nosocomial infections put older adults at increased risk for complications. If an older adult does not require mechanical ventilation, the prognosis is good to fair, depending on underlying disease states and complications. Extensive rehabilitation, physical therapy, and retraining of ADLs may be necessary to return the older adult to independent living (Farley, McLafferty & Hendry, 2009).

NURSING MANAGEMENT

Assessment

The nurse should determine through the health history whether the patient has risk factors for the development of PE. Assessment begins with the evaluation of respiratory and cardiac status. The nurse should observe the older patient for signs and symptoms of PE. Nonspecific signs may include insomnia, wandering, anorexia, nausea, delirium, weakness, and weight gain.

Assessment for noncardiogenic PE involves identifying predisposing factors, which include aspiration of gastric contents, pneumonia, thoracic injury, pulmonary contusions, smoke inhalation, multiple blood transfusions, uremia, cardiopulmonary bypass surgery, fracture of long bones, and sepsis. The clinical presentation of noncardiogenic PE includes refractory hypoxemia, crackles on auscultation, hypotension, cyanosis, tachypnea, hyperventilation, and increased tracheobronchial secretions.

Diagnosis

Nursing diagnoses for an older patient with PE include the following (Malone, 2011):

- Inadequate breathing pattern resulting from decreased energy
- Reduced gas exchange resulting from alveolar–capillary membrane changes and altered blood flow
- Airway obstruction resulting from decreased energy and tracheobronchial obstruction
- Fluid overload resulting from a compromised regulatory mechanism
- Reduced spontaneous ventilation resulting from metabolic factors and respiratory muscle fatigue
- Potential for infection resulting from inadequate primary and secondary defenses
- Reduced stamina resulting from generalized weakness and imbalance of oxygen supply and demand
- Need for patient teaching resulting from a lack of previous experience with cardiogenic PE or noncardiogenic PE

Planning and Expected Outcomes

Planning includes developing interventions and expected outcomes for older patients that focus on restoration of the oxygen supply and demand balance. The patient and family must be included to help the patient achieve the expected outcomes. It is important that both the patient and the family know about expected outcomes and necessary interventions such as oxygen administration or mechanical ventilation. Expected outcomes include the following (Moorhead et al., 2008):

1. The patient will maintain ABG values within normal limits.
2. The patient will maintain oxygenation within normal values.
3. The patient will have a cardiac output within normal values.
4. The patient will be able to verbalize feelings related to the illness.
5. The patient will maintain a patent airway.
6. The patient will maintain a balanced intake and output.
7. The patient will have an alternative method of communication if receiving mechanical ventilation.
8. The patient will maintain skin integrity.
9. The patient will be able to sustain spontaneous ventilation without mechanical ventilation.
10. The patient will have stable hemodynamics.

Intervention

The effect of PE may be severe in older adults because of its associated functional disability secondary to activity intolerance, drug therapy, and frequent rehospitalizations. The nurse should be alert to these factors and plan interventions that include daily weight assessments, energy-conserving ADLs, elevation of the feet and legs, reduction in or elimination of sodium intake, and use of diuretics. The nurse should assess the patient for adventitious lung sounds, respiratory muscle fatigue and the use of accessory muscles of respiration, and airway patency. The patient should be positioned to facilitate ventilation–perfusion matching and to minimize respiratory efforts. This can be accomplished by adding pillows at the back and under the arms, and encouraging the patient to sit up straight with legs and feet elevated. The patient should be encouraged to cough effectively, which may require splinting and analgesic interventions; the patient should also be encouraged to change positions frequently and practice slow, deep breathing.

Inpatient interventions for PE include positioning the patient to improve ventilation by elevating the head of the bed 30 degrees. If the patient is producing large amounts of frothy sputum, he or she should be turned to the side to facilitate drainage; frequent suctioning then becomes appropriate. The nurse should reassure the patient and family or significant other and, if necessary, prepare them for intubation and mechanical ventilation, which may be particularly frightening for an older patient. An integral part of planning nursing care for older patients requiring intensive care is a discussion about the patient's wishes in regard to high-technology medical care. The patient and family should be asked if they have any advance medical directives (AMDs) or durable powers of attorney in case the older patient becomes unable to speak. If the patient is unaware of AMDs but expresses an interest, a family conference including the physician, nurse, social worker, and pastoral caregiver should be planned to help the older patient express his or her wishes. If the older patient has an AMD or a durable power of attorney, a copy should be filed in the medical record and reviewed with the older patient, family, physician, and any other caregivers. It is important to understand and respect the wishes of older patients and families before initiating high-technology medical care.

Interventions include supplemental oxygen, mechanical ventilation, and nursing measures to promote oxygen balance. Monitoring PaO_2 saturation helps the nurse determine which activities deplete oxygen saturation. Interventions such as suctioning, turning, and positioning have been well documented as increasing oxygen consumption and decreasing arterial and mixed venous oxygen levels. The nurse should plan care to decrease the number of interventions performed at one time so as to minimize oxygen consumption and stress. It is important to provide an alternative means of communication for older patients receiving mechanical ventilation. If a patient has a hearing aid, it may be difficult for him or her to hear over the noise of the technology in the intensive care setting.

Older patients in the ICU need astute assessment, monitoring, and interventions to help prevent ICU delirium (DiSabatino Smith & Grami, 2017). The ICU provides no cues as to day and night; therefore patients need to be continually oriented to time. Furthermore, older patients are particularly sensitive to continuous stimuli in the unit—sound, sights, smells, and textures—and may become confused and combative. The nurse should try to establish a regular nighttime routine with older patients, for example, vital sign assessment, oral care, and toileting. The lighting should then be reduced as much as possible to promote rest and sleep while allowing for safe care. This helps older patients establish a routine or pattern that they can recognize as "time to sleep." Such nursing measures can help to reduce the incidence of ICU delirium, which will only prolong hospital days and potentially lead to additional complications for the patient.

Evaluation

Evaluation is based on improvement in the clinical picture, resolution of symptoms, and prevention of further complications. The nurse should monitor the patient's vital signs, cardiac function, and oxygenation status for stability and improvement. The nurse should also monitor the older adult's reaction to frightening therapies and invasive interventions. Older adults need continual reassurance and information to reduce their anxiety. The nurse should constantly monitor the airway for effective clearance of secretions. Careful evaluation of daily weight and the patient's intake and output will help determine whether the patient is retaining additional fluids. The nurse should monitor the patient's subjective measure of dyspnea using the dyspnea scale.

Pulmonary Emboli

A pulmonary embolus is an occlusion of pulmonary arteries by a thrombus, fat, or air embolus. Often, in the older patient, the occlusion is a result of a deep vein thrombosis. The thrombosis breaks loose, becoming an embolus, and travels to the lungs through the venous system, where it is trapped in a small vessel of pulmonary circulation. Occlusion of the lung with a large embolus causes pulmonary infarction, which results in necrosis of the lung tissue. The embolus, which is composed of platelets, red blood cells (RBCs), and WBCs, releases vasoactive substances that cause bronchial constriction, ventilation–perfusion mismatch, and hypoxia. The amount of physiologic dead space—ventilation in excess of perfusion—is increased, which leads to an increase in intrapulmonary shunting and hypoxia.

Risk factors for the development of pulmonary emboli include an age older than 40 years, immobility, recent surgery, recent trauma, history of hospital or nursing home confinement, central venous catheter placement, neurologic disease with extremity paresis and a history of vascular disease, COPD, heart disease, diabetes mellitus, malignancy, and previous pulmonary emboli. Thromboembolism is more common in older patients who have a natural tendency for hypercoagulation (Farley et al., 2009).

The clinical presentation includes coughing, dyspnea at rest, hypotension, hypoxia, hemoptysis, tachycardia, anginal or pleuritic chest pain, decreased PaO_2, and S_3 or S_4 gallop (Thompson, Kabrhel, & Pena, 2017).

Diagnostic Tests and Procedures

Diagnosis is based on ventilation–perfusion lung scanning (VQ scan) or pulmonary angiography. ABG measurements may reveal hypoxemia with PaO_2 between 60 and 80 mm Hg. ECG may show a right axis deviation, right bundle branch block, tall peaked P waves, a depressed ST segment, and supraventricular tachycardia if the emboli are extensive. Massive pulmonary emboli may result in electromechanical dissociation, in which electrical conduction continues without heart muscle response or cardiac output. Chest radiography may reveal an elevated hemidiaphragm; atelectasis, consolidation, or both; and pleural effusion. Additionally, workup may include a D-dimer used in conjunction with probability assessment. The Wells score for pulmonary embolism may be helpful in classifying patients regarding predetermination of low, moderate, or high probability of a pulmonary embolus along with other diagnostic tests and symptomatology (Thompson et al., 2017).

Treatment

The patient with suspected pulmonary embolus should initially be resuscitated and stabilized, focusing on hemodynamics and oxygenation. Unless contraindicated, anticoagulation should be started. Heparin is usually the anticoagulant of choice in the inpatient setting, and unfractionated heparin levels should be monitored. Heparin can be administered subcutaneously or intravenously to achieve a prothrombin time of 1.5 to 2.5 times control. Thrombolytic therapy such as the use of streptokinase, urokinase, or tissue plasminogen activator (TPA) is used in patients with extensive pulmonary emboli who exhibit unstable hemodynamic situations. Patients with a likelihood of recurring pulmonary emboli are treated on a long-term basis with warfarin (Coumadin) and monitoring of their international normalized ratio (INR). The goal range of the INR is 2.5 to 3.0. Patients with recurrent pulmonary emboli or in whom anticoagulation is contraindicated may be good candidates for Greenfield vena cava filters.

Prognosis

The prognosis for pulmonary emboli is variable. The incidence increases with aging, and older adults treated for pulmonary emboli are more at risk for complications of the disease and anticoagulation. Furthermore, the ability to predict mortality in older adults seems to be lower than with younger populations (Polo et al., 2015).

NURSING MANAGEMENT

Assessment

Assessment begins with the identification of risk factors for the development of pulmonary emboli. In older adults, dehydration and immobility are leading causes. If an older patient has a history of recent fracture of a long bone or a pelvic fracture secondary to falling, fat emboli should be suspected. Clinical signs and symptoms may include sudden dyspnea, chest pain, restlessness, a weak and rapid pulse, tachypnea, and tachycardia.

Diagnosis

Diagnoses for an older patient with pulmonary emboli include the following (Malone, 2011):

- Reduced gas exchange resulting from altered blood flow and oxygen supply
- Potential for reduced cardiac tissue perfusion resulting from interruption of arterial flow
- Reduced spontaneous ventilation resulting from metabolic factors

Planning and Expected Outcomes

Planning includes developing interventions and expected outcomes for the older patient that are aimed primarily at improving oxygenation and reducing pain. Expected outcomes include the following (Moorhead et al., 2008):

1. The patient will maintain ABG values within normal limits.
2. The patient will maintain adequate respiratory muscle function.
3. The patient will be able to sustain spontaneous ventilation without mechanical ventilation.
4. The patient will maintain adequate oxygenation.
5. The patient will have adequate pain control.
6. The patient will maintain adequate cardiac output.
7. The patient will maintain adequate vital signs.

Intervention

The primary goals of treatment are to stop the clot from getting bigger and to prevent new clots from forming. Although treatment is focused on these goals, maintaining effective oxygenation and ventilation is paramount. The nurse should monitor tissue oxygen delivery, signs and symptoms of respiratory failure, laboratory values for changes in oxygenation or acid–base balance, and hemodynamic parameters and respiratory pattern for symptoms of respiratory difficulty. Oxygen therapy is administered to improve oxygenation and decrease breathlessness. Heparin therapy is initiated to prevent formation of future clots. Older patients need reassurance and careful monitoring of vital signs. Sedation relieves pain and anxiety, and reduces oxygen demand. If an older patient is dehydrated or has hypotension, intravenous fluids are administered. The

nurse may use vasopressors if hypotension cannot be reversed with fluids.

The patient needs to be monitored for bleeding complications from anticoagulant therapy. The nurse should observe the urine for color changes, check the stool for occult blood, and monitor for other complications including bruising, gastric bleeding, hemorrhaging, and stroke.

Because immobility is a risk factor for the development of pulmonary emboli, it is important to promote mobility as soon as medically possible. The nurse should use antiembolic compression hose and passive and active range-of-motion exercises during the acute phase. The older patient should be encouraged to move about as soon as is medically feasible.

Education topics for the older patient and his or her family include signs and symptoms of pulmonary emboli, long-term anticoagulant therapy (warfarin), and the importance of exercise and mobility. Education on anticoagulant therapy includes elimination of aspirin or NSAIDs, elimination of green leafy vegetables, cautionary use of over-the-counter medications that potentiate the anticoagulation effect, and prompt reporting of any bleeding. An electric razor is recommended for male patients. The nurse must also help the patient understand the importance of regular monitoring of the INR and the importance of taking anticoagulation medication at the same time every day.

Evaluation

Evaluation is based on successful achievement of the expected outcomes. The nurse should monitor the older patient's response to oxygen therapy, respiratory support, and effective pain management and relief by using a pain scale. The nurse should also monitor the patient for follow-up care with INR blood draws, dietary restrictions, and medication compliance. With older adults, it is especially important to evaluate the patient's ability to recall the signs of excessive anticoagulation.

Obstructive Sleep Apnea

Obstructive Sleep Apnea Syndrome (OSAS) is a disorder of breathing during sleep due to periodic reduction (hypopnea) or cessation (apnea) of breathing due to an obstruction of the upper airway (Cash & Glass, 2016; McCance & Huether, 2014). This upper airway obstruction can be associated with oxygen desaturation and hypercapnia. Pathogenic factors include intermittent hypoxemia or hypercapnia, mechanoreceptor activation during obstructed efforts, chemoreflex activation through chronic body and CNS excitability, and arousal that results from abnormal breathing (McCance & Heuther, 2014). These changes result in partial awakening of the patient with a startle response of snorts and gasps, which move the tongue and soft palate and relieve the obstruction. Chronic effects on the cardiovascular system are a result of increased sympathetic nervous system activity. During obstructive apnea, large fluctuations in intrathoracic pressure occur, causing changes in venous return, left ventricular filling, cardiac output, baroreflex, and release of volume-regulatory peptides (McCance & Huether, 2014).

Obesity is the dominant risk factor for OSAS in both men and women. OSAS is twice as common in men as in women, and the risk increases with age. Because obesity is a strong predictive factor, even a 10% reduction in weight can lead to a substantial decrease in respiratory disturbance index (RDI) (Downey, Gold, Rowley, & Wickramasinghe, 2018). Other risk factors for OSAS include family history, increased neck circumference, genetic syndrome, smoking, alcohol use, employment requiring shift rotation or sleep restrictions, tonsillar hypertrophy, craniofacial abnormalities, medications, and ethnicity (African Americans, Hispanics, and Pacific Islanders have a higher incidence of OSAS compared with whites) (Cash & Glass, 2016).

Diagnostic Tests and Procedures

The diagnosis of OSAS is made based on the history and the objective measurement in tandem with polysomnography (PSG) in the sleep laboratory. PSG is the gold standard diagnostic test for OSA and particularly important in patients with underlying cardiovascular disease, hypoventilation syndrome, stroke, and insomnia (Kapur, Auckley, Chowdhuri, Mehra, Ramari, & Harrod, 2017). Diagnostic criteria include complaints of excessive daytime sleepiness, frequent episodes of obstructed breathing during sleep, loud snoring, morning headaches, dry mouth on awakening, and falling asleep during normal awake time activities or driving. Sleep study criteria include more than five episodes of obstructive apnea longer than 10 seconds in duration per hour of sleep and one or more of the following: frequent arousal from sleep, bradycardia, tachycardia, and arterial oxygen desaturation associated with apneic episodes. Clinical practice guidelines for OSA identify other tools such as the Epworth Sleepiness Scale (ESS), a self-report scale for evaluating inclination of daytime sleepiness or dozing, and the STOP-BANG questionnaire as an OSA screening tool, which can be used to provide additional information and supplement PSG.

Treatment

Treatment starts conservatively and involves teaching the older patient to avoid alcohol or sedatives at bedtime, humidify the air, and wear a dental device to keep the jaw forward. Weight loss should also be encouraged, as overweight and obesity can be associated with increased incidence of OSAS. These interventions may be enough to may relieve sleep apnea problems in some individuals. The next line of treatment for patients with OSAS is nasal continuous positive airway pressure (CPAP) therapy. CPAP provides immediate prevention of upper airway collapse and can lead to correction of ABG derangements, improved sleep continuity, improved cognition, and reduction of sleepless symptoms. The most critical factor in the use of nasal CPAP is the patient's level of adherence to the treatment modality. It is estimated that 29% to 83% of patients are nonadherent to CPAP therapy (<4 hrs/nightly) (Weaver, 2017). Alternatives to nasal CPAP may include weight reduction, sleep position training, and avoidance of alcohol, sedative-hypnotic and narcotic medications, cigarette smoking, and sleep deprivation.

Surgical interventions include tracheotomy or uvulopalatopharyngoplasty (UVPP or UPPP). The goal of UVPP or UPPP is to remove redundant or obstructing tissue of the soft palate, uvula, and posterolateral pharynx, thereby eliminating obstruction. The procedure may eliminate snoring but may not reduce the apneic episodes (Adil, 2017).

Prognosis

The prognosis for a patient with OSAS is good. Patient commitment to medical management, such as weight loss and daily use of nasal CPAP, is essential for a good outcome. Older adults may have difficulty with weight reduction. Patients may also find the nasal CPAP machine annoying and disruptive to their sleep, and therefore not wear it consistently at night. Although surgery may be an option, comorbidity may preclude its use in some older adults.

NURSING MANAGEMENT

Assessment

The nurse should assess the patient for the presence of chronic loud snoring, gasping or choking episodes during sleep, excessive daytime sleepiness (especially when driving), automobile or work-related accidents attributed to fatigue, and personality changes or cognitive difficulties. Clinical signs include obesity, systemic hypertension, nasopharyngeal narrowing, and, in rare cases, pulmonary hypertension and cor pulmonale.

Diagnosis

Nursing diagnoses for a patient with OSAS include the following
- Fatigue resulting from increased energy required for ADLs
- Disrupted sleep pattern resulting from sensory alterations
- Inadequate breathing pattern resulting from decreased energy or fatigue

Planning and Expected Outcomes

Expected outcomes for an older patient with OSAS include the following (Moorhead et al., 2008):
1. The patient will verbalize a feeling of rest and well-being.
2. The patient will verbalize an improvement in quality of life.
3. The patient will report an absence of sleepy episodes during the day.
4. The patient will have increased ability to concentrate.
5. The patient will have increased endurance, as evidenced by ability to participate in ADLs.
6. The patient will maintain adequate vital signs.
7. The patient will maintain adequate oxygenation and ventilation during sleep, as evidenced by continuous pulse oximetry monitoring.
8. The patient will achieve or maintain appropriate body weight.

Intervention

Interventions for a patient with OSAS include monitoring the patient's sleep pattern; noting physiologic and psychological circumstances that interrupt sleep; and implementing sleep-promoting therapies and bedtime routines conducive to sleep, lifestyle modifications, and the use of CPAP (Fig. 20.4). The nurse should assist the patient with nutrition counseling, weight reduction, and exercise plans (Cash & Glass, 2016). Exercise may be especially difficult for older adults with underlying orthopedic problems and decreased activity. Exercise programs that incorporate water aerobics may be helpful for older adults with joint problems. The nurse should encourage healthy food choices such as fresh fruits and vegetables and less processed and prepackaged foods, which may be challenging for older adults who live alone and do not cook regularly.

Evaluation

Evaluation is based on achievement of the expected outcomes and improvement in the patient's perception of sleep. The nurse should evaluate the patient's daytime somnolence and ability to complete ADLs, noting the frequency of napping, and monitoring for lower extremity edema, fluid retention, and weight gain.

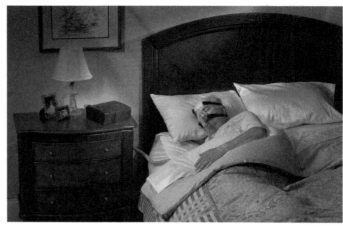

Fig. 20.4 Management of sleep apnea often involves sleeping with a nasal mask in place. The pressure supplied by air coming from the compressor opens the oropharynx and nasopharynx. (From Lewis, S. M., Dirksen, S., Heitkemper, M. M., et al. [2011]. *Medical-surgical nursing: Assessment and management of clinical problems* [8th ed.]. St. Louis, MO: Mosby.)

SUMMARY

Neurochemical control and the respiratory muscles are involved in the process of respiration. The structures of the lungs include upper and lower airways, as well as extrapulmonary and intrapulmonary structures. Age-related changes in pulmonary structure and function include elastic recoil and musculoskeletal changes of the chest wall and decreased compliance of the thorax. Asthma, chronic bronchitis, emphysema, and pneumonia are respiratory conditions common in older adults. Chronologic age and tobacco use put older patients at risk for bronchogenic carcinoma. Nursing management of older patients with respiratory alterations focuses on a complete and accurate physical assessment, minimization of risk factors for disease development, development of partnerships with the patient to successfully implement lifestyle changes and treatment regimens, and, most important, pulmonary hygiene and airway patency.

🏠 HOME CARE

1. Encourage homebound older adult patients with respiratory disease to drink 8 to 10 glasses of water a day, if not contraindicated.
2. Encourage homebound older adult patients with respiratory disease to exercise within their capacity to promote thoracic muscle conditioning.
3. Monitor homebound older adult patients for smoking and exposure to secondhand smoke. Encourage family members to refrain from smoking in the presence of the patient.
4. Encourage homebound older adult patients to use pursed-lip breathing to control breathlessness and improve oxygenation.
5. Monitor pulse oximetry to assess oxygenation.
6. Encourage frequent small meals to reduce breathlessness associated with eating.
7. If a patient is using home oxygen, assess the home environment for potential safety hazards, including the possibility of the patient tripping over oxygen tubing.
8. Assess patients for confusion, occipital headaches, and forgetfulness. These symptoms may be indicative of CO_2 retention. Teach family caregivers these signs as well.

KEY POINTS

- Changes in lung functions associated with the aging process, in the absence of primary pulmonary disease, are not associated with decreased activity or increased breathlessness.
- Older adults with chronic lung disease can lead active lives with proper medical and nursing management.
- Breathing retraining (e.g., pursed-lip breathing and diaphragmatic breathing) may result in decreased breathlessness and increased oxygenation.
- It is important to include the family in planning care for an older adult with chronic lung disease.
- An older patient with chronic lung disease may demonstrate unacceptable behavioral patterns because of the loss of control experienced with chronic illness.
- Smoking cessation may not be achievable for some older patients; interventions for these patients should focus on reducing the number of cigarettes smoked.
- Exercise plays an important part in overall lung function and has been shown to improve breathing in older patients.
- Care planning that includes the use of mechanical ventilation or other technology should include the patient and family.
- Primary nursing diagnoses for the older patient with respiratory disease focus on increasing airway clearance, decreasing breathlessness, and improving oxygenation.

CRITICAL-THINKING EXERCISES

1. How might pulmonary hygiene measures be revised for a frail older adult with a history of CHF and osteoporosis?

2. You are caring for a 71-year-old man who has a history of smoking 75 pack-years. He has COPD but continues to smoke, stating that it would be impossible to quit now and besides, "It's too late." How would you assist this patient?

3. Think about your own personal views regarding advanced life-support measures for the older adult population. What are the ethical implications of placing (or not placing) an 80-year-old person on mechanical ventilation for acute respiratory failure? How would you assist patients and/or family members faced with decisions of this nature?

REFERENCES

Adil, E. A. (2017). Uvulopalatopharyngoplasty. Retrieved June 8, 2018 from https://emedicine.medscape.com/article/1942134-overview.

Agency for Health Care Research and Quality (AHCRQ). (2015). *Quit smoking: consumer guide.* Silver Springs, MD: The Agency.

Agency for Health Care Research and Quality (AHCRQ). (2012). Five major steps to intervention(the 5 A's). Retrieved from http://www. ahrq.gov/protocols/clinicians-providers/guidelines. recommendations/tobacco/5steps.html.

Barnett, S. (2018). Anesthesia for the older adult. Retrieved January 16, 2018 from https://www.uptodate.com/contents/anesthesia-for-the-older-adult.

Bartlett, J. G. (2017). Community acquired pneumonia in adults. *UptoDate.* Retrieved January 2018 from uptodate.com.

Boltz, M., Capezuti, E., Fulmer, T., & Zwicker, D. (2012). *Pain management. Evidence-based nursing protocols for best practice* (4th ed.). New York: Springer.

Brashers, V. L. (2012). Alterations of pulmonary function. In S. E. Huether, K. L. McCance, V. L. Brashers, & N. S. Rote (Eds.), *Understanding pathophysiology* (5th ed.). St. Louis, MO: Mosby/ Elsevier.

Cash, J. C., & Glass, C. A. (2016). *Adult gerontology practice guidelines.* New York: Springer.

Centers for Disease Control and Prevention (CDC). (2017a). Cessation materials for starting tobacco control programs. Retrieved January 2018 from http://cdc.gov.

Centers for Disease Control and Prevention (CDC). (2017b). Pneumococcal disease. Retrieved January 15, 2018, from http://cdc. gov.

Centers for Disease Control and Prevention (CDC). (2017c). SARS basic facts sheet. Retrieved January 2018, from Http://cdc.gov.

Centers for Disease Control and Prevention (CDC). (2016). Tuberculosis. Retrieved January 17, 2018, from http://cdc.gov.

Cruz, J., Maarques, A., & Figueiredo, D. (2017). Impacts of COPD on family carers and supportive interventions: A narrative review. *Health and Social Care in the Community, 25*(1), 11–25. https://doi. org/10.1111/hsc.12292.

DiSabatino Smith, C., & Grami, P. (2017). Feasibility and effectiveness of a delirium prevention bundle in critically ill patients. *American Journal of Critical Care, 26*(1), 19–27.

Dobbin, K., & Howard, V. (2011). Listen closely to detect healthcare-associated pneumonia. *Nursing 2011, 41*(7), 59–62.

Downey, R., III, Gold, P. M., Rowley, J. A., & Wickramasinghe, H. (2018). Obstructive sleep apnea treatment and management. Retrieved January 11, 2018 from medscape.com.

Farley, A., McLafferty, E., & Hendry, C. (2009). Pulmonary embolism: Identification, clinical features and management. *Nursing Standard, 23*(28), 49–56.

Fine, M. J. (2017). PSI/PORT Score: Pneumonia Severity Index for CAP. Retrieved January 17, 2018, from https://www.mdcalc.com/ psi-port-score-pneumonia-severity-index-cap.

Fiore, M. C., Jaen, C. R., Baker, T. B., Bailey, W., Benowitz, N. L., Curry, S. J., ...Wewers, M. E. (2008). Treating tobacco use and depenence: 2008 update. Retrieved June 8, 2018 from https://bphc.hrsa.gov/ buckets/treatingtobacco.pdf.

Garvey, C., Bayles, M. P., Hannon, L. F., Hill, K., Holland, A., Linberg, T. M., & Sprint, M. A. (2016). Pulmonary rehab exercise prescription in COPD: A review of selected guidelines. Official statement for the American Association of Cardiovascular & Pulmonary Rehab. *Journal of Cardiopulmonary Rehab & Prevention, 36*(2), 75–83.

Givertz, M.M. (2017). Noncardiogenic pulmonary edema. *UptoDate.* Retrieved on January 18, 2018 from http://uptodate.com.

Global Initiative for Asthma (GINA). (2010). *Global strategy for asthma management and prevention.* Retrieved January 11, 2018 from http://www.ginasthma.org/Guidelines.

Global Initiative for Asthma. (2018). Pocket Guide for Asthma Management and Prevention. Retrieved June 7, 2018 from https:// ginasthma.org/2018-pocket-guide-for-asthma-management-and-prevention/.

Global Initiative for Chronic Obstructive Lung Disease (GOLD). (2017). *Global strategy for the diagnosis, management and prevention of COPD.* Retrieved January 17, 2018, from http://www. goldcopd.org/.

Kanabus, A. (2017). Countries with TB – High & low burden countries. Retrieved June 7, 2018 from https://www.tbfacts.org/countries-tb/.

Kapur, V. K., Auckley, D. H., Chowdhuri, S., Mehra, K., Ramari, K., & Harrod, C. G. (2017). Clinical practice guidelines for diagnosis and treatment of adults with obstructive sleep apnea. *Journal of Clinical Sleep Medicine, 13*(3), 479–504.

Knechel, N. (2009). Tuberculosis: Pathophysiology, clinical features, and diagnosis. *Critical Care Nurse, 29*(2), 34–43.

Lareau, S., Mosesen, E., & Slatore, C. G. (2014). American Thoracic Society. Patient Information Source. Exacerbation of COPD. *American Journal of Respiratory and Critical Care Medicine, 189*, 11–12.

Lewis, S. M., Dirksen, S., Heitkemper, M. M., et al. (2011). *Medical-surgical nursing: assessment and management of clinical problems* (8th ed.). St. Louis, MO: Mosby.

Lucas, C., & Martin, J. (2013). Smoking and drug interactions. *Australian Prescriber, 36*, 102–104. https://doi.org/10.18773/ austprescr.2013.037.

Malone, M. J. (2011). Lower respiratory problems. In S. M. Lewis, S. R. Dirksen, & M. M. Heitkemper, et al. (Eds.), *Medical-surgical nursing: assessment and management of clinical problems* (8th ed.). St. Louis, MO: Mosby.

Marthaler, M., Keresztes, P., & Tazbir, J. (2003). SARS: what have we learned? *RN, 66*(8), 59.

Mayo Clinic. (2014). *Pulmonary edema: treatment and drugs.* Retrieved January 2014, from http://www.mayoclinic.org/diseases-conditions/pulmonary-edema/treatments-and-drugs.

McCance, K. L., & Huether, S. E. (2014). *Pathophysiology* (7th ed.). St. Louis, MO: Elsevier.

McIntosh, K. (2017). Severe acute respiratory symdrome(SARS). *UptoDate.* Retrieved January 18, 2018 from http://uptodate.com.

Moorhead, S., Johnson, M., Maas, M., & Swanson, E. (2008). *Nursing outcomes classification (NOC)* (4th ed.). St Louis: Mosby/Elsevier.

National Cancer Institute (NCI). (2017). *Lung cancer.* Retrieved January 15, 2018 from http://www.cancer.gov.

Pinto, D.S. (2017). Pathophysiology of cardiogenic pulmonary edema. Uptodate. Retrieved January 16, 2018 from http://uptodate.com.

Polo, F., Molteni, M., Del Sorbo, D., Pasciuti, L., Crippa, M., Villa, G., … Cimminiello, C. (2015). Mortality at 30 and 90 days in elderly patients with pulmonary embolus: A retrospective cohort study. *Intern Emergency Medicine, 10*(4), 431–436. https://doi.org/10.1007/s11739-014-1179-z.

Sarna, L., & Bialous, S. (2010). Using evidence-based guidelines to help patients stop smoking. *American Nurse Today, 5*(1), 44–47.

Singanayagam, A., Chalmers, J. D., & Hill, A. T. (2009). Severity assessment in community-acquired pneumonia: a review. *The Quarterly Journal of Medicine, 102*, 379–388.

Sorenson, H.M. (2017). Arterial oxygenation in the elderly. *Advance.* Retrieved from http://respiratory-care-sleep-medicine.advanceweb.com/Article/Arterial-Oxygenation-in-the-Elderly.aspx.

Sovari, A.A. (2017). Cardiogenic pulmonary edema treatment and management. Retrieved January 16, 2018 from http://emedicine.medscape.com.

Stupka, E., & deShazo, R. (2009). Asthma in seniors: part 1. Evidence for underdiagnosis, undertreatment and increasing morbidity and mortality. *The American Journal of Medicine, 122*(1), 6–11.

Surgeon General. (2014). Current status of tobacco control. Surgeon General's report. Retrieved from http://www.surgeongeneral.gov/library/reports.

Thompson, T. Kabrhel, C., & Pena, C. (2017). Clinical presentation, evaluation and diagnosis of the nonpregnant adult with acute PE. *Uptodate.* Retrieved January 11, 2018, from http://uptodate.com.

Vaz Fragoso, C. A., & Gill, T. M. (2011). Respiratory impairment and the aging lung: A novel paradigm for assessing pulmonary function. *The Journals of Gerontology: Series A, 67A*(3), 264–275. https://doi.org/10.1093/gerona/glr198.

Vallerand, A. H., & Sanoski, C. A. (2017). *Davis' Drug Guide for Nurses* (15th ed.). Philadelphia, PA: F.A. Davis Company.

Weaver, T. (2017). Adherence with continuous positive airway pressure. *UptoDate.* Retrieved on January 16, 2018 from www.uptodate.com.

Woo, T. M., & Robinson, M. V. (2016). *Pharmacotherapeutics for advanced practice nurse prescribers* (4th ed.). Philadelphia, PA: F.A. Davis Company.

Workman, M. L. (2013). *Care of patients with noninfectious lower respiratory problems.* In D. Ignatavicius, M. L. Workman, & C. R. Rebar (Eds.), *Medical-surgical nursing: Concepts for interprofessional collaborative care* (9th ed.). St. Louis, MO: Elsevier.

World Health Organization (WHO). (2018a). Obesity. Retrieved January 11, 2018, from http://www.who.int/topics/obesity/en.

World Health Organization (WHO). (2018b). World Health Guide on TB. Retrieved January 2018, from http://www.who.int./publications/guidelines/tuberculosis/en.

21

Gastrointestinal Function

Jennifer J. Yeager, PhD, RN, APRN

ⓔ http://evolve.elsevier.com/Meiner/gerontologic

LEARNING OBJECTIVES

On completion of this chapter, the reader will be able to:

1. Describe the age-related physiologic and functional changes in the gastrointestinal system.
2. Explain primary and secondary preventive care related to the gastrointestinal tract for older patients and the rationalizations for such care.
3. Discuss the alterations of normal structure and function accompanying common gastrointestinal diseases of older adults.
4. Describe appropriate evaluation of older patients with symptoms related to a gastrointestinal disorder.
5. Describe the cause, incidence, and pathophysiology of the various types of gastrointestinal disorders, including cancer and liver disease.
6. Discuss the nursing management of gastrointestinal disorders in older adults.
7. Write an appropriate care plan for an older patient with a gastrointestinal disorder.

WHAT WOULD YOU DO?

What would you do if you were faced with the following situations?

- While rounding on your patient, she asks you for "something for constipation." You note her records indicate a bowel movement yesterday. What should you do?
- Your patient reports nausea, trouble eating and lack of appetite, vague abdominal pain, decreased peripheral sensation, and edema. What additional assessment data should you gather? What interventions should you plan?

The gastrointestinal (GI) system functions in the ingestion, digestion, and absorption of nutrients as well as in the excretion of solid wastes from the body. The accessory organs of digestion—salivary glands, liver, pancreas, and gallbladder—aid in the absorption of nutrients by secreting enzymes involved in the digestive process. GI system–related symptoms and complaints are common with advancing age, and the nurse is often the first health care provider to identify and acknowledge them. Therefore knowledge of normal and age-related changes in the GI system is essential in providing appropriate nursing care.

AGE-RELATED CHANGES IN STRUCTURE AND FUNCTION

Although many health-related complaints from older adults pertain to the GI system, these complaints are rarely responsible for death. Older adults are usually aware of alterations in GI function, and many of these changes can be alleviated through

appropriate self-care practices. Normal aging causes some changes in the GI tract (Table 21.1); however, multiple factors such as polypharmacy, stress, poor nutrition, multiple comorbidities, and poor hygiene may all contribute to alterations in GI function. Misinformation about changes in GI function may lead to more complex problems because of failure to seek health care or engage in appropriate preventive and treatment measures. The nurse has the responsibility for teaching health promotion and disease prevention strategies to these patients.

Many of the systemic changes in the digestion and absorption of nutrients from the GI tract result from changes in older adults' cardiovascular and neurologic systems, rather than their GI systems. For example, atherosclerosis and other cardiovascular problems may cause a decrease in mesenteric blood flow, leading to a decrease in absorption in the small intestine. Additionally, the central and peripheral nervous systems affect the motility of the entire GI system, and any change may alter peristalsis, thereby altering transit time. A decrease in mobility, often seen in the older adult, may also affect GI function.

Oral Cavity and Pharynx

Changes in the oral cavity have an effect not only on an older person's well-being, comfort, and health, but also on overall nutrition and digestion. The most obvious change in the mouth is the loss of teeth. One-fourth of adults 65 or older are edentulous (without teeth). Periodontal gum disease, caused by bacterial infection and inflammation under the gum line, damages bone and connective tissue. Teeth become loose, chewing becomes more difficult, and often the teeth must be extracted (Centers for Disease Control and Prevention [CDC], 2009a).

TABLE 21.1 Alterations in Assessment Findings: Gastrointestinal System

Expected Aging Changes	Alterations in Assessment Findings
Gingival retraction	Loss of teeth, presence of dentures, difficulty chewing
Decreased taste buds, decreased sense of smell	Diminished sense of taste (especially salty and sweet)
Decreased volume of saliva	Dry oral mucosa
Atrophy of gingival tissue	Poor-fitting dentures
Esophagus	
Lower esophageal sphincter pressure decreased, motility decreased	Epigastric distress, dysphagia, potential for hiatal hernia and aspiration
Abdominal Wall	
Thinner and less taut	More visible peristalsis, easier palpation of organs
Decrease in number and sensitivity of sensory receptors	Less sensitivity to surface pain
Stomach	
Atrophy of gastric mucosa, decrease in blood flow	Food intolerances, signs of anemia as result of cobalamin malabsorption, decreased gastric emptying
Small Intestines	
Slight decreases in secretion of most digestive enzymes and motility	Complaints of indigestion, slowed intestinal transit, delayed absorption of fat-soluble vitamins
Liver	
Decreased size and lower in position	Easier palpation because of lower border extending past costal margin
Decrease in protein synthesis, ability to regenerate decreased	Decrease in drug metabolism
Large Intestine, Anus, Rectum	
Decreased anal sphincter tone and nerve supply to rectal area	Fecal incontinence
Decreased muscular tone, decreased motility	Flatulence, abdominal distention, relaxed perineal musculature
Increase in transit time, sensation to defecation decreased	Constipation, fecal impaction
Pancreas	
Pancreatic ducts distended, lipase production decreased, pancreatic reserve impaired	Impaired fat absorption, decreased glucose tolerance

From Lewis, S. L., Bucher, L., Heitkemper, M. M., & Harding, M. M. (2017). *Medical-surgical nursing: Assessment and management of clinical problems* (10th ed.). St. Louis, MO: Elsevier.

Taste buds both decrease in number and atrophy beginning at age 60, resulting in decreased ability to discriminate among salty and sweet followed by bitter and sour. This may contribute to decreased enjoyment of food, resulting in poor eating habits and nutritional deficiencies. Drugs such as diuretics, anticholinergics, certain antidepressants, and antipsychotics reduce saliva production, leading to xerostomia (dry mouth). A reduction in saliva increases the risk for tooth decay and gum disease. Saliva normally protects the oral tissues by cleaning teeth and neutralizing acids (Lewis, Bucher, Heitkemper, & Harding, 2017).

Healthy People 2020 reflects on the importance of oral health as an integral component of health and well-being. Poor oral health and periodontal disease lead to pain and disability. One of the goals of *Healthy People 2020* is to improve access to preventive oral care and early treatment efforts for older adults (Healthy People 2020 website, 2013).

Esophagus

Age-related changes in the smooth muscle lining the esophagus contribute to a decrease in the strength of esophageal contractions and lower esophageal sphincter weakness, leading to decreased food transit time. Esophageal sphincter weakness causes older adults to be more prone to reflux of acid from the stomach or gastroesophageal reflux (LeMone & Burke, 2008). Neurogenic, hormonal, and vascular changes secondary to comorbidities may also contribute to a decrease in esophageal motility. These changes may lead to complaints of dysphagia, heartburn, or vomiting of undigested foods. Subsequently, poor nutrition, dehydration, and decreased food intake result.

Stomach

Age-related changes in the stomach include decreased production of gastric acid, pepsin, bicarbonate, prostaglandins, and mucus. By the age of 60, gastric secretions decrease to 70% to 80% of those of the average adult. A decrease in pepsin may hinder protein digestion, whereas a decrease in hydrochloric acid and intrinsic factor may lead to malabsorption of iron, vitamin B_{12}, calcium, and folic acid. Altered absorption and decreased gastric acid production, combined with altered gastric defense mechanisms, increase the incidence of pernicious anemia, peptic ulcer disease (PUD), and stomach cancer. Gastric emptying time is increased secondary to decreased elasticity of the stomach wall (Lewis et al., 2017). The stomach of an older adult is not able to accommodate large amounts of food, resulting in a feeling of fullness or early satiation.

Small Intestine

Age-related changes in the small intestine include atrophy and broadening of the villi, leading to a decrease in absorptive surface. This results in a decrease in the absorption of lipids. Aging may also lead to a decrease in the production of lactase, resulting in intolerance to dairy products. As individuals age, they may also experience an increase in the overpopulation of certain intestinal bacteria, leading to bloating, pain, and weight loss. The increase in intestinal bacteria may also lead to a decrease in the absorption of calcium, folic acid, and iron (Shaheen, 2006).

Large Intestine

The main function of the large intestine is storage, propulsion, and evacuation of feces. Age-related changes in the large intestine include atrophy of the muscle layers and mucosa. These normal changes with aging may lead to a decrease in contraction of the muscle wall when the rectum is filled with feces, resulting in constipation. In addition, the incidence of diverticuli is increased in older adults. Diverticuli are prevalent in nearly half of people older than 60 years (Shaheen, 2006). Diverticuli are small outpouchings of the colon, where it bulges at weak spots in the intestinal wall.

Gallbladder

The gallbladder and bile ducts are unaffected by aging. However, the incidence of gallstones does increase with age. Bile may become more lithogenic with advancing age, possibly because of an increase in biliary cholesterol related to diet and hormonal changes that affect cholesterol metabolism. The bile salt pool also decreases as a result of a decrease in bile salt synthesis. These predispositions for stone development, along with a tendency for dehydration in older adults, explain the increased incidence of cholelithiasis and cholecystitis in older adults. The complications of cholelithiasis in older adults include empyema, perforation, and choledocholithiasis (calculi in the common bile duct). These complications are often seen in persons older than age 65 and those with diabetes (Lewis et al., 2017).

Pancreas

The pancreas shows some age-related changes such as fibrosis, fatty acid deposits, and atrophy; weight, but not size, is affected (Lewis et al., 2017). Evidence suggests that the volume of pancreatic secretions (chymotrypsin and pancreatic lipase) decline with age. This decrease in enzyme activity affects the digestion of fats and may account for a vague intolerance of fatty foods in older adults. The incidence of pancreatic cancer and pancreatitis increases in older adults.

Liver

The liver is a sturdy organ and retains most of its functions throughout the life span. Although the liver size decreases after age 50, liver function tests may remain within normal limits. A decline in cardiac output associated with aging contributes to a decrease in hepatic blood flow. As hepatic blood flow slows, drug metabolism is reduced, which leaves the aging liver more susceptible to drugs and toxins. Older persons have a decreased ability to compensate for infectious, immunologic, and metabolic disorders (Lewis et al., 2017). Some evidence suggests that normal aging may adversely affect liver tissue regeneration. The mechanism of this effect is not fully known, but it may be a result of a generalized slowing of repair or an inadequate response to regeneration of liver tissue.

PREVENTION

Although some changes in the GI system are associated with aging, strategies for both primary and secondary prevention of problems arising from these changes are available (Table 21.2). Nurses caring for older patients should educate their patients concerning these guidelines.

COMMON GASTROINTESTINAL SYMPTOMS

No clear-cut GI diseases can be attributed directly to the aging process. However, many conditions show a higher incidence in older adults and have a greater effect on their physical and social well-being. These complaints may be related to normal physiologic changes associated with aging but must be distinguished from pathologic problems that increase in frequency with aging.

Older adults may report GI symptoms not related to a specific diagnosis. Any symptom reported by an older patient needs thorough assessment by the nurse. What follows are the most frequently reported GI symptoms experienced by older adults. The sections include information on their definitions, assessment, nursing interventions, and self-care measures.

Nausea and Vomiting

Vomiting is controlled through a central vomiting center in the medulla. This center is close to the pain and respiratory centers; it is also near the centers that control vestibular and vasomotor function. Occasionally, stimuli from one center spill over to another, and symptoms may become mixed (Fig. 21.1).

Nausea may be difficult for patients to describe; many use the phrase "I feel sick" to convey the symptom of nausea. It is important to keep in mind that, although nausea usually precedes vomiting, it may also be an isolated symptom. In general, nausea in the absence of vomiting is of central, rather than peripheral, origin (i.e., the symptom is initiated centrally in the brain rather than peripherally in the GI tract). Central nausea is usually a response to a metabolic disorder.

It is important to obtain a detailed description of events surrounding a complaint of nausea and vomiting. Data should be elicited about precipitating factors (e.g., the relationship of nausea and vomiting to food intake, drugs, and activity). The patient should be questioned about the presence of nausea and vomiting, as well as diarrhea or constipation. It is important to obtain information about the amount and characteristics of the emesis and whether the vomitus contained food particles, bile, or blood (bright red or the color of coffee grounds). Other symptoms such as a fever, sweating, pallor, dizziness, and pain should be determined. Because older adults are at risk for dehydration and electrolyte imbalances, it is essential to establish the frequency and amount of vomiting and to examine patients for signs and symptoms of fluid and electrolyte imbalances.

Nursing interventions include establishing many self-help measures, including dietary changes such as drinking clear liquids, progressing from eating bland foods to solid foods, and small, frequent meals. If vomiting occurs, fluid replacement should be a priority. Sips of fluids every 15 minutes until more can be tolerated may decrease episodes of dehydration. Older adults are at high risk for aspiration, and they should be placed in the semi-Fowler or side-lying position when drinking liquids. It is important that older adults be made aware of the signs and symptoms of dehydration and electrolyte imbalances, as well as when to seek medical care. Any episodes of prolonged nausea or vomiting require careful evaluation by a health care provider. In addition, it should be made clear that pharmacologic therapy used to treat nausea and vomiting may cause sedation, confusion, and delirium in the older adult.

TABLE 21.2   Guidelines for Screening for the Early Detection of Colorectal Cancer and Adenomas for Average-Risk Women and Men Aged 50 Years and Older

The following options are acceptable choices for colorectal cancer screening in average-risk adults beginning at age 50 years. Since each of the following tests has inherent characteristics related to prevention potential, accuracy, costs, and potential harms, individuals should have an opportunity to make an informed decision when choosing one of the following options.

In the opinion of the guidelines development committee, *colon cancer prevention* should be the primary goal of colorectal cancer screening. Tests that are designed to detect both early cancer and adenomatous polyps should be encouraged if resources are available and patients are willing to undergo an invasive test.

Tests That Detect Adenomatous Polyps and Cancer

Test	Interval	Key Issue for Informed Decisions
FSIG with insertion to 40 cm or to splenic flexure	Every 5 years	• Complete or partial bowel prep is required • Sedation usually is not used, so there may be some discomfort during the procedure • The protective effect of sigmoidoscopy is primarily limited to the portion of the colon examined • Patients should understand that positive findings on sigmoidoscopy usually result in a referral for colonoscopy
Colonoscopy	Every 10 years	• Complete bowel prep is required • Conscious sedation is used in most centers; patients will miss a day of work and will need a chaperone for transportation from the facility • Risks include perforation and bleeding, which are rare but potentially serious; most of the risk is associated with polypectomy
DCBE	Every 5 years	• Complete bowel prep is required • If patients have one or more polyps ≥6 mm, colonoscopy will be recommended; follow-up colonoscopy will require complete bowel prep • Risks of DCBE are low; rare cases of perforation have been reported
CTC	Every 5 years	• Complete bowel prep is required • If patients have one or more polyps ≥6 mm, colonoscopy will be recommended; if same day colonoscopy is not available, a second complete bowel prep will be required before colonoscopy • Risks of CTC are low; rare cases of perforation have been reported • Extracolonic abnormalities may be identified on CTC that could require further evaluation

Tests That Primarily Detect Cancer

Test	Interval	Key Issues for Informed Decisions
gFOBT with high sensitivity for cancer	Annual	• Depending on manufacturer's recommendations, 2 to 3 stool samples collected at home are needed to complete testing; a single sample of stool gathered during a digital exam in the clinical setting is not an acceptable stool test and should not be done
FIT with high sensitivity for cancer	Annual	• Positive tests are associated with an increased risk of colon cancer and advanced neoplasia; CSPY should be recommended if the test results are positive • If the test is negative, it should be repeated annually • Patients should understand that one-time testing is likely to be ineffective
sDNA with high sensitivity for cancer	Interval uncertain	• An adequate stool sample must be obtained and packaged with appropriate preservative agents for shipping to the laboratory • The unit cost of the currently available test is significantly higher than other forms of stool testing • If the test is positive, CSPY will be recommended • If the test is negative, the appropriate interval for a repeat test is uncertain

CTC, Computed tomography colonoscopy; *DCBE,* double-contrast barium enema; *FIT,* fecal immunochemical test; *FSIG,* flexible sigmoidoscopy; *gFOBT,* guaiac-based fecal occult blood test; *sDNA,* stool DNA test.
From Levin, B., Lieberman, D.A., McFarland, B., Smith, R.A., Brooks, D., Andrews, K.S., . . . Sinawer, S.J. (2008). Screening and surveillance for the early detection of colorectal cancer and adenomatous polyps, 2008: A joint guideline from the American Cancer Society, the US Multi-Society Task Force on Colorectal Cancer, and the American College of Radiology. *CA: A Cancer Journal for Clinicians, 58*(3):130–160, Table 2.

Anorexia

Anorexia as a symptom should not be confused with anorexia nervosa, which is an eating disorder of psychiatric significance. The term *anorexia* literally means "lack of appetite." Hunger and appetite are not synonymous; hunger is related to the physiologic need for food. It is important for the nurse to ascertain whether food intake is decreased truly because of loss of appetite. Once that is determined, the nurse must ask questions regarding other symptoms, including weight loss, nausea, vomiting, abdominal pain, diarrhea, and constipation. In addition, psychosocial factors such as stress, grief, pain, and concomitant illnesses may also need to be assessed. Older adults are often faced with limited financial resources resulting in a decreased overall ability to purchase adequate food (Lewis et al., 2017).

Nursing interventions for older patients with anorexia include monitoring of intake, output, and weight. It is important

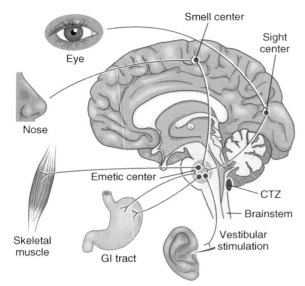

Fig. 21.1 Stimuli involved in the act of vomiting. *CTZ,* Chemoreceptor trigger zone; *GI,* gastrointestinal. (Modified from McKenry, L., Tessier, E., & Hogan, M. [2006]. *Mosby's pharmacology in nursing* [22nd ed.]. St. Louis, MO: Mosby.)

to acknowledge a patient's symptoms and provide gentle encouragement to eat for nutritional purposes. Small, frequent meals may be helpful. Encouraging older patients to seek medical attention for anorexia is also important because patients may not be aware of the problem.

Abdominal Pain

Abdominal pain as a symptom is often difficult to assess in a complete manner. With older adults, it may be even more difficult, even for a skilled clinician. The assessment of pain may be made easier by thinking in terms of the three pathways for pain impulses. The first are the *visceral pain pathways,* which are activated by receptors in the wall of the abdominal viscera and develop from stretching or distending the abdominal wall or from inflammation. This type of pain is often diffuse; is poorly localized; and has a gnawing, burning, or cramping quality. The second are *somatic* or *parietal pathways,* which are activated by receptors in the parietal peritoneum and other supporting tissues. This type of pain is usually sharp, more intense, constant, and better localized than visceral pain. The third are *referral pathways,* which account for referred pain (i.e., pain felt at a different site than the source of the pain but sharing the same dermatome). This type of pain is usually sharp and well localized; it may resemble somatic pain (Fig. 21.2).

In assessing any type of pain, the nurse should elicit information about its duration, location, mode of onset (sudden or gradual), intensity, quality, rhythm, relationship to food, alleviating and aggravating factors, and radiation (e.g., back, neck, or groin), as well as the older patient's ability to pass stool and gas. Older persons may complain of vague symptoms and wait much longer than their younger counterparts to seek medical care. Older adults are also less likely to exhibit leukocytosis (increased white blood cell [WBC] count), fevers, rebound tenderness, or local rigidity (Tazkarji, 2008).

Nursing interventions include measures to increase comfort and pain relief. The nurse should encourage older patients to see their health care provider for a complete evaluation of the abdominal pain. Abdominal pain that is severe is often referred to as an *acute abdomen.* Nursing procedures for acute abdomen

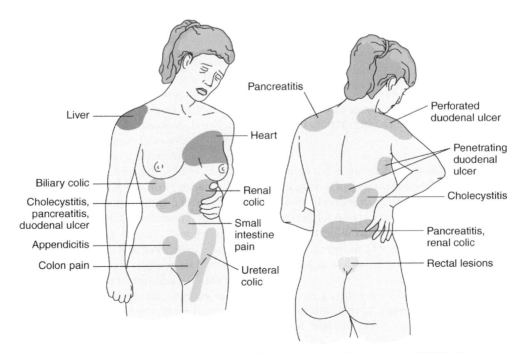

Fig. 21.2 Common sites of referred abdominal pain. (From Saxton, D., Green, J., et al. [2009]. *Mosby's comprehensive review of nursing for NCLEX-RN® Examination* [19th ed.]. St. Louis, MO: Mosby.)

include (1) starting intravenous fluids, as ordered; (2) placing a nasogastric tube for decompression of the stomach; (3) monitoring and recording vital signs and reporting abnormal findings; (4) monitoring intake and output accurately every hour; and (5) completing an assessment on the onset of pain, presence of vomiting or diarrhea, and presence of fever, and taking an accurate medical and surgical history.

Gas

Belching, bloating, fullness, and flatus are some of the complaints associated with gas. About 99% of the gas present in the GI tract of adults comprises five gases: nitrogen, oxygen, hydrogen, carbon dioxide, and methane. The percentage of each individual gas depends on the source; these sources include swallowing, diffusion of gas from the bloodstream to the intestinal lumen, and processing of food. All these gases are odorless; the unpleasant odor associated with flatus is probably a result of hydrogen sulfide metabolized from sulfur-containing foods. A frequency of 7 to 20 expulsions of gas a day is considered normal. Intestinal gas is frequently accompanied by intense abdominal pain, which may be relieved by repositioning or walking.

Although belching primarily comes from the unconscious swallowing of air, it is important to assess patients for other symptoms suggestive of gastritis or PUD. Many complaints of bloating and fullness are related to a motility disorder or malabsorption; however, in older adults, the complaints must be taken seriously. Further assessment through questioning about changes in bowel function, pain, and other GI tract symptoms is required.

Although the expulsion of flatus is a normal event, excessive flatus may have several causes. Some patients form more gas within the gut, some swallow more air, and others may have excessive flatus because of the nature of the foods consumed. Common culprits include beans, cabbage, legumes, raisins, and artificial sweeteners. In addition, patients who are lactose intolerant may produce more gas. Careful questioning may reveal one or a combination of these causes.

Nursing interventions focus on patient education about the cause and nature of intestinal gas. The keys to treatment are changes in dietary factors (e.g., focusing on eating more slowly and avoiding gas-producing foods) and a routine exercise plan.

Diarrhea

Diarrhea is an increase in the frequency of defecation, but many definitions also include a change in the consistency of feces (e.g., watery stools). Diarrhea may be caused by increased bowel motility or interference in the normal absorption of water and nutrients from the GI tract. When an older adult reports diarrhea, it is important to ascertain exactly what is meant. Keep in mind that the description of diarrhea is useless unless a patient's normal bowel habits are known.

The nurse should ask about precipitating events (e.g., travel out of the country or eating at a restaurant), timing (intermittent or continuous), associated factors (fever, weight loss, abdominal pain, vomiting, dietary or drug changes, and any systemic diseases), characteristics of the diarrhea (frequency, consistency, volume, foul smell, presence of mucus or blood, incontinence, awakening from sleep [e.g., nocturnal diarrhea usually points to an organic cause rather than a functional or infectious cause]), and whether the onset was sudden. All these questions help assess the diarrhea further to aid in determining the cause.

Nursing care focuses on maintaining adequate fluid and electrolyte balance, assessing for complications, and providing emotional support as necessary. Usual water loss accompanying bowel movements is 150 milliliters per day (mL/day); severe diarrhea can account for up to 5 to 10 liters (L) of water loss daily. Therefore assessing for signs and symptoms of dehydration and volume depletion in older patients is important. Patients and their families need to be taught to report complications such as increased thirst, weakness, dizziness, palpitations, and fatigue. If fluid and electrolyte imbalances occur, either oral or parenteral therapy may be required because diarrhea in older adults may be life-threatening. Nursing interventions should also be aimed at identifying and correcting the cause. Administration of antibiotics may be necessary for infectious diarrhea. Depending on the causative factor, antispasmodic and antidiarrheal drugs may also be used. Education of patients and their families should include instruction on dietary changes. Older patients with chronic diarrhea should avoid gas-forming foods, vegetables, spices, and milk products; patients with acute diarrhea should consume bland foods, such as the BRAT (bananas, rice, applesauce, toast) diet and clear liquids.

Constipation

Constipation is a common problem among older adults secondary to physiologic changes and is often a complication of polypharmacy. Among those older than 65, women are affected more often compared with men. Constipation is often defined according to the patient's perception of abnormal bowel function (Berman, Brooks, & Silver, 2007). Typical definitions of constipation also include hard, dry stools that are difficult to pass. Bowel movements less than three times a week are often associated with constipation. However, normal bowel patterns differ greatly among individuals. Nurses can use the Bristol Stool Chart to help communication about bowel habits (Patel, Chen, Fewel, & Stock, 2016) (Fig. 21.3).

Common causes of constipation in older adults include diet (decreased fiber intake), mechanical obstruction (fecal impaction and cancer), drug side effects (aluminum- and calcium-based antacids, iron preparations, anticholinergics, narcotics, antidepressants, antipsychotics, calcium channel blockers, and overuse of laxatives), multiple comorbidities, and mobility and functional issues (Ginsberg, Phillips, Wallace, & Josephson, 2007). Perhaps the most widespread cause of constipation in older adults is diet. It is usually a lack of certain foods, rather than the addition of certain foods, that leads to the problem. For example, many foods such as fresh fruits and vegetables contain natural laxatives, although older adults may have difficulty eating these foods because of dental problems. A second dietary cause of constipation is the lack of fiber or bulk and a decrease in fluid intake. In general, unrefined foods have more fiber than the refined foods popular in American society.

Bristol Stool Chart

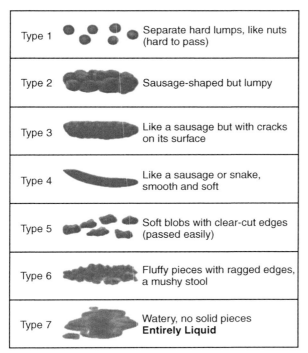

Type 1		Separate hard lumps, like nuts (hard to pass)
Type 2		Sausage-shaped but lumpy
Type 3		Like a sausage but with cracks on its surface
Type 4		Like a sausage or snake, smooth and soft
Type 5		Soft blobs with clear-cut edges (passed easily)
Type 6		Fluffy pieces with ragged edges, a mushy stool
Type 7		Watery, no solid pieces **Entirely Liquid**

Fig. 21.3 Bristol stool chart. (From Kliegman, R. M., Stanton, B. F., St. Geme, J. W., et al. [2016] *Nelson textbook of pediatrics* [20th ed.]. Philadelphia, PA: Elsevier.)

It is important to keep in mind that constipation might be a result of overuse or improper use of laxatives because of an older adult's excessive concern about the frequency of defecation. In this instance, the nurse may reinforce with a patient and family that, as long as the consistency is normal and the bowel movements occur at regular intervals, it is not necessary to take laxatives.

Limitations on mobility may greatly affect the ability of an older person to feed themselves and to reach the toilet. They may feel awkward about depending on others for these functions. Subsequently, they may ignore the urge to defecate rather than ask for help to get to the toilet. They may also decrease fluid intake to prevent urinary incontinence. These factors may greatly influence regular bowel patterns (Lewis et al., 2017).

Constipation is treated through dietary measures such as increasing fluid intake and increasing fiber, combined with light exercise and development of a regular toileting routine that includes responding to the urge to defecate. In teaching older adults about dietary changes, the nurse should educate them about fiber being a "food" rather than a "medicine."

Multiple drugs are available to treat constipation, and many of them are available over the counter (OTC). Laxatives are defined as drugs used to facilitate or stimulate the passage of feces and are classified as bulking agents (bran, psyllium), surfactants (stool softeners), emollients (mineral oil), contact stimulants (cascara, castor oil, bisacodyl), saline cathartics (magnesium hydroxide [Milk of Magnesia], citrate, sodium or potassium phosphate), and osmotic agents (lactulose, sorbitol). Laxatives may also be categorized by speed of action: (1) group I

drugs (castor oil, saline laxatives in high doses) act in 2 to 6 hours and produce watery stool; (2) group II drugs (other contact stimulants, low-dose saline laxatives) act in 6 to 12 hours and produce a semiformed stool; and (3) group III drugs (bulking agents, surfactants, lactulose) produce soft stools in 1 to 3 days.

In addition to oral laxatives, several rectal agents are available. Enemas provide immediate relief but should be limited in their use for long-term treatment. Soapsud enemas should never be used because they lead to mucosal irritation. Small-volume enemas such as Fleets are the easiest to use. Rectal suppositories (bisacodyl, glycerin) may also be used, but they must be retained for 20 to 30 minutes for optimal results and so may be more difficult for older patients to use.

EVIDENCE-BASED PRACTICE
Using Probiotics as Treatment of Constipation

Background
Chronic constipation is a problem among older adults. Some studies report the incidence of constipation as high as 50% in long-term care residents. Studies have reported probiotics can reduce the incidence of constipation by increasing colonic transit, defecation frequency, and feces stiffening.

Sample/Setting
Following full-text screening and analysis of identified studies, nine articles were identified as meeting all inclusion criteria for the review.

Methods
Articles in this review came from Medline, Embase, Scopus, Lilacs, and Cochrane databases. They were analyzed using Preferred Reporting Items for Systematic reviews and Meta-Analysis (PRISMA) guidelines. Search terms were *constipation* and *probiotics*.

Findings
Among the nine articles meeting criteria for the review, five were observational studies and four were randomized, placebo-controlled trials. Analysis of study findings indicates administration of probiotics significantly improved constipation in the elderly by 10% to 40%. The strain of bacteria most commonly used was *Bifidobacterium longum*.

Implications
Caution should be taken in the interpretation of these findings as there was much heterogeneity between studies (e.g., evaluation tools, different probiotic strains, and reporting of side effects). Further placebo-controlled studies should be conducted to determine the most appropriate strain of probiotic, dosing, and duration of treatment.

From Martinez-Martinez, M. I., Calabuig-Tolsa, R., & Cauli, O. (2017). The effect of probiotics as a treatment for constipation in elderly people: A systematic review. *Archives of Gerontology and Geriatrics, 71*, 142-149. doi: 10.1016/j.archger.2017.04.004.

Fecal Incontinence

Fecal incontinence, the involuntary passing of feces, may be acute or chronic, and it demands evaluation. For older adults, the loss of bowel control is devastating and may significantly alter their quality of life. Fecal incontinence may be a result of colorectal lesions (perianal disease, proctitis, and tumors), neurologic problems (dementia, stroke, and spinal cord lesions), laxative abuse, unrecognized lactose intolerance, diabetic neuropathy, poor dietary habits, or immobility (Kane, Ouslander, Abrass, & Resnick, 2009).

Nursing interventions focus on education concerning the prevention and treatment of incontinence in older adults. Examining the cause of the incontinence is important for the nurse, patient, and family. Laxative abuse is completely preventable and treatable with education and reassurance to the patient that being "regular" does not necessarily mean one or two bowel movements a day.

Regardless of the cause, a program of bowel control (see Patient/Family Teaching box) may usually help an older patient who is aware of and distressed by incontinence. It is important to reassure older patients that control and retraining are achievable because many older adults believe that fecal incontinence is the first step on the road to permanent institutionalization. Other nursing interventions include methods to deal with the embarrassment caused by the incontinence, ways to decrease fecal odor, use of adult diapers, and skin care.

🧍 PATIENT/FAMILY TEACHING

Bowel Training for the Patient With Incontinence

Overview
Bowel incontinence refers to the inability to voluntarily control defecation. It may result from decreased anal muscle tone, disturbances in the neural innervations of the rectum, loss of cortical control, rectal prolapse, diarrhea, constipation with overflow related to impaction, or altered cognition.

Goal
Control of bowel elimination

Actions
- Record and evaluate patient's fecal elimination pattern.
- Establish consistent time to toilet based on pattern.
- Position patient in best physiologic position for defecation: sitting with normal posture.
- Have patient lean forward or prop feet on stool to increase intraabdominal pressure.
- Instruct patient to bear down and attempt to defecate.
- Record results; ensure patient does not develop fecal impaction.
- If necessary, stimulate anorectal reflex with glycerin suppository 30 to 45 minutes before scheduled fecal elimination.
- Supplement toilet activities with exercise and good fluid (minimally 1,500 milliliters per day [mL/day]) and fiber intake, unless contraindicated.

From Eliopoulos, C. (2005). *Gerontological nursing* (6th ed.). Philadelphia, PA: Lippincott Williams & Wilkins.

COMMON DISEASES OF THE GASTROINTESTINAL TRACT

The following is an overview of common GI disorders seen in older patients, including the related nursing care.

Gingivitis and Periodontitis

The gingivae, or gums, are subject to localized and systemic diseases, problems caused by drug therapy, poor oral hygiene, and poor nutrition. *Gingivitis,* an inflammation of the gums surrounding the teeth, may result in pain and bleeding; it may lead to *periodontitis,* a spreading of the inflammation to the underlying tissues, bones, or roots of teeth. This is the most common reason for tooth loss with advancing age. Gingivitis resulting from overgrowth of the gingivae may occur in people taking phenytoin on a long-term basis.

Candida albicans, or thrush, is an infection causing white lesions on the oral mucosa. It is often seen in persons with compromised immune systems and in those with suppressed immunity such as individuals taking immunosuppressant drugs and antibiotics. The condition is most common in denture-bearing tissues of the mouth. The patient may complain of an unpleasant taste, burning, or itching, or may be asymptotic (Duthie, Katz, & Malone, 2007).

NURSING MANAGEMENT

Assessment

Assessment begins with a good history of dental care and dental hygiene practices. A complete health history focusing on other illnesses and concomitant drugs, as well as a physical assessment of the mouth, is necessary.

Diagnosis

The most common nursing diagnoses for an older patient with gingivitis or periodontitis include the following:
- Inadequate oral mucous membrane
- Inadequate dentition
- Inadequate health maintenance
- Inadequate nutrition, resulting from pain

Planning and Expected Outcomes

An older adult must understand the relationship between oral health and overall health and well-being. The nurse must determine a patient's feelings and attitude about performing the self-care necessary to achieve the desired goals.

Expected outcomes for an older patient with gingivitis or periodontitis include the following:
1. The patient will maintain a comfortable and functional oral cavity.
2. The patient will establish and maintain a mouth care routine, including regular professional dental care.
3. The patient will maintain normal body weight and nutritional status.

Intervention

Nursing management of an older patient with gingivitis or periodontitis includes promotion of regular oral hygiene, regular preventive dental care, and maintenance of nutritional status. In addition, assessing the patient's knowledge of the importance of oral hygiene and frequently reinforcing oral hygiene practices are important roles for the nurse. Oral hygiene includes flossing regularly, brushing teeth or dentures, and using saline mouth rinses, as needed. Professional dental care should be sought routinely every 6 months or more often, as needed. Proper fit of dentures initially and at all subsequent visits to both the dentist and the primary health care provider is also encouraged. Pain relief, which will facilitate adequate nutrition, may be managed with nonnarcotics (e.g., acetaminophen), frequent mouth rinses, and a liquid or soft diet.

The key to treatment of gingivitis and periodontitis is prevention. Although good oral hygiene needs to begin early in life, it is never too late for an older patient to begin routine dental care and oral hygiene. The nurse should discuss with the patient the use of nutritional foods that are nonirritating, for example, soft foods such as pudding or custard, and the use of nutritional supplements such as Ensure.

Evaluation

Evaluation includes documentation of achievement of the expected outcomes, establishment and maintenance of regular dental care and oral hygiene practices, and prevention of infection. Evaluation focuses on an older adult's ability to carry out the recommendations and whether any changes in self-care have occurred as a result. Findings of an oral cavity inspection should be noted, as should any instructions or explanations provided to the patient. The patient's response to recommended treatment measures should also be documented.

Dysphagia

Dysphagia (difficult swallowing) is a common problem in the older adult population. Weakened esophageal smooth muscle and incompetent sphincter function are contributory in the older adult who develops dysphagia. Dysphagia is a symptom with many underlying causes, including stroke, neurologic disease (e.g., Alzheimer's disease and Parkinson's disease), local trauma or tissue damage, and tumors that may obstruct the flow of food and liquids in the esophagus. Symptoms may range from mild to severe to a complete inability to swallow (Lewis et al., 2017). Dysphagia may compromise the nutritional status in the older adult, increase the risk of aspiration pneumonia, and lead to a decreased quality of life (Box 21.1).

Nursing care is aimed at ensuring the patient receives adequate evaluation, nutrition, hydration, and safe positioning during meals to prevent aspiration. Dietary modification may be recommended following speech–language pathologist evaluation and modified barium swallow.

NURSING MANAGEMENT

Assessment

Assessment begins with an accurate and precise history that focuses on whether the dysphagia occurs with liquids, solids, or both, as well as the time frame for the progression of the dysphagia. A thorough physical examination includes (1) neurologic assessment; (2) assessment of oral cavity and salivary glands; (3) observation of swallowing capability, both liquid and solid substances; and (4) examination of neck and thyroid glands.

Diagnosis

Nursing diagnoses for an older patient with dysphagia include the following:

- Inadequate nutrition
- Potential for aspiration resulting from abnormal swallowing
- Acute pain resulting from odynophagia (painful swallowing in the mouth or esophagus)
- Fear resulting from the diagnosis and prognosis

BOX 21.1 Feeding Tubes in Advanced Dementia

The American Geriatrics Society has stated that feeding tubes are not recommended in persons with advanced dementia. Instead, they recommend careful hand feeding in a quiet and calm environment, stating "hand feeding has been shown to be as good as tube feeding for the outcomes of death, aspiration pneumonia, functional status, and comfort" (American Geriatrics Society Ethics Committee and Clinical Practice and Models of Care Committee, 2014, p. 1590). Additionally, they note patients with tube feedings have an increased risk of agitation, use of chemical restraints, and development of new pressure injuries. Studies have indicated as many as 34% of nursing home residents with cognitive impairment have feeding tubes. These were placed to reduce weight loss and aspiration pneumonia, and improve survival. However, the evidence shows 22.9% of residents with feeding tubes continue to aspirate. Additionally, the use of feeding tubes increases the risk of future hospitalizations and increases mortality (Rhodes, 2014). Patient-centered approaches to feeding (e.g., choice of food, tempo of feeding, and pleasant environment) should be part of usual care for older adults with advanced dementia. The health care team should assist caregivers in making an informed decision about how best to meet their loved one's nutritional needs. In doing so, options other than feeding tube placement may be available and should be discussed.

From Rhodes, R. (2014). When evidence clashes with emotion: Feeding tubes in advanced dementia. *Annals of Long-Term Care: Clinical Care and Aging, 22*(9), 24-26. https://www.managedhealthcareconnect.com/article/when-evidence-clashes-emotion-feeding-tubes-advanced-dementia; and American Geriatrics Society Ethics Committee and Clinical Practice and Models of Care Committee. (2014). American Geriatrics Society feeding tubes in advanced dementia position statement. *Journal of the American Geriatrics Society, 62*(8), 1590-3. doi: 10.1111/jgs.12924.

Planning and Expected Outcomes

It is essential to determine whether an older patient is ready and able to learn the self-care measures necessary to reduce the symptoms associated with dysphagia. Determining the extent of a patient's specific fears created by learning of the nature of interventions is important because the type and degree of fear affects the nurse's specificity in intervention strategies.

Expected outcomes for an older patient with dysphagia include the following:

1. The patient will maintain weight within 10% of ideal body weight.
2. The patient will remain free from aspiration.
3. The patient will learn techniques to swallow that minimize aspiration and pain.
4. The patient will be free from epigastric discomfort.
5. The patient will be able to verbalize fears related to the diagnosis and prognosis.

Intervention

Nursing management of an older patient with dysphagia includes maintenance of hydration and nutritional status, prevention of aspiration, and provision of emotional support and information regarding the diagnosis and prognosis. Additionally, the nurse provides support and reassurance directed at a patient's fear of eating related to pain, difficulty swallowing, and frequent regurgitation. Optimizing nutritional status and preventing weight loss are important because fear of eating may lead to chronic weight loss. Instruction regarding eating habits and swallowing techniques, and maintaining weight and nutrition are important. For example, eating small, frequent meals consisting of pureed or soft high-protein, high-calorie foods; taking only small sips of fluid or using thickened liquids; and turning head to the side are helpful. The nurse should instruct the patient to elevate the head of the bed to prevent nocturnal aspiration.

Evaluation

Evaluation includes documentation of achievement of the expected outcomes, prevention of aspiration, and maintenance of nutrition. Evaluation of how the patient is coping with the diagnosis may be assessed through a patient's resumption of activities and ability to verbalize feelings. Additionally, evaluation focuses on a patient's ability to satisfactorily incorporate and adhere to the dietary recommendations and modify behaviors and lifestyle to reduce symptoms.

Gastroesophageal Reflux and Esophagitis

Gastroesophageal reflux disease (GERD) is a prevalent condition found in 20% to 25% of the older adult population. Causes are lower esophageal sphincter dysfunction, delayed gastric emptying, hiatal hernia, and increased intraabdominal pressure. Older adults also take drugs that increase the symptoms of GERD. Examples of such drugs include tetracycline, alendronate, potassium chloride, quinidine, aspirin, ascorbic acid, nonsteroidal antiinflammatory drugs (NSAIDs), clindamycin, and theophylline. Older adults often take drugs in the supine position and with inadequate fluids, which may worsen symptoms (Wolfe, 2006).

Esophagitis refers to inflammation of the esophagus. Most often this results from gastroesophageal reflux caused by either prolonged vomiting or an incompetent lower esophageal sphincter. The amount of mucosal damage is related to the contact time between the esophageal mucosa and the gastric contents, as well as the acidity and quantity of gastric secretions. Additional causes of esophagitis include viral, fungal, or bacterial infections.

Symptoms of GERD and esophagitis include heartburn, retrosternal discomfort, and the regurgitation of sour, bitter material. Symptoms are often precipitated by the ingestion of a large amount of fatty or spicy foods or alcohol. Strictures, caused by esophageal scarring, may develop and make food passage difficult. Dysphagia for both liquids and solids occurs as scar tissue builds and the esophageal lining stiffens, leading to esophageal narrowing. If regurgitation occurs often, substernal pain may result, occasionally mimicking a heart attack. Reflux may be aggravated by postural changes such as sleeping in the supine position but may occur in any position. Pulmonary aspiration because of reflux is common; when severe, it may lead to pneumonia.

Hiatal Hernia

In hiatal hernia (diaphragmatic or esophageal hernia), a major cause of reflux and esophagitis, part of the stomach protrudes through an opening of the diaphragm (Fig. 21.4). The condition may be intermittent or continuous. The continuous type is least common, accounting for only about 10% of cases. Either part or all the stomach, and even the intestines, may herniate, causing dyspepsia, severe pain, and often a gastric ulceration. The

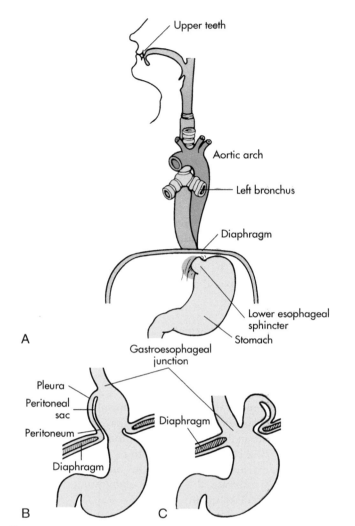

Fig. 21.4 Hiatal hernias. **A,** Normal esophagus. **B,** Sliding hiatal hernia. **C,** Rolling or paraesophageal hernia. (From Salvo, S. G. [2009]. *Mosby's pathology for massage therapists* [2nd ed.]. St. Louis, MO: Mosby Elsevier.)

intermittent type, or sliding hernia, occurs with changes in position or with increased peristalsis. The stomach is forced through the opening of the diaphragm when the person is prone and moves back to its normal position when the person stands up. Most hiatal hernias are asymptomatic and require no treatment. Symptoms, when they arise, include heartburn, gastric regurgitation, dysphagia, and indigestion. These symptoms are accentuated (1) when assuming the supine position after meals, (2) after overeating, (3) after physical exertion, or (4) with a sudden change in posture (Lewis et al., 2017).

NURSING MANAGEMENT

Assessment

Assessment begins with a history of symptoms and possible aggravating factors. Older patients may use terms such as *indigestion* or *heartburn*, rather than *pain*, and these terms need to be clearly defined. Patients also may not understand what *regurgitation* means, especially in relationship to vomiting. Older persons may have atypical symptoms, including hoarseness, chest pain, postprandial fullness, respiratory symptoms, and belching. Alcohol and drug use must also be determined, as these are contributing factors. Drug and diet histories are also important components of the assessment.

Diagnosis

Nursing diagnoses for an older patient with gastroesophageal reflux include the following:

- Potential for aspiration resulting from regurgitation
- Inadequate nutrition resulting from pain or dysphagia
- Need for health teaching resulting from lack of exposure to disease process and treatment modalities

Planning and Expected Outcomes

It is essential to determine whether a patient is ready to learn the preventive measures necessary for reducing symptoms. The presence of additional health problems may affect an older patient's ability to participate in an educational plan or carry out the interventions.

Expected outcomes for an older patient with gastroesophageal reflux include the following:

1. The patient will remain free from aspiration.
2. The patient will maintain weight within 10% of ideal body weight.
3. The patient will verbalize an understanding of the disease process and treatment approaches.

Intervention

Nursing management of older patients with GERD includes maintenance of adequate nutrition, prevention of aspiration, and instruction to patients and their families about the disease process and treatment approach. Nonpharmacologic treatment includes avoiding foods that increase symptoms, maintenance of health, and smoking cessation. Support from caregivers, spouses, or significant others is key to success.

Evaluation

Evaluation includes documentation of achievement of expected outcomes, prevention of complications, and appropriate dietary and lifestyle changes. Because most patients improve after 1 month of conservative management with antacids and lifestyle changes, it is important for the nurse to ascertain whether symptoms have subsided. If they have not, referral for further medical management is warranted.

Vitamin B_{12} Deficiency

Vitamin B_{12} deficiency is a condition present in more than 20% of older adults. Malabsorption causes the majority of cases; however, pernicious anemia accounts for about one-fifth of known cases. Causes of malabsorption include gastritis, alcoholism, gastric surgery, inflammatory bowel disease, autoimmune disorders, and long-term use of proton-pump inhibitors (PPIs) or histamine-2 (H_2) blockers (Chaparro & Mauricio, 2013). In pernicious anemia, degeneration of the parietal cells in the gastric mucosa leads to a decrease in production of the intrinsic factor, resulting in reduced absorption of vitamin B_{12}. Vitamin B_{12} deficiency impairs the production of red blood cells (RBCs). This results in large, oval, fragile cells that have a short lifetime.

Persons with pernicious anemia are typically treated with injections of vitamin B_{12} as oral vitamin B_{12} is not well absorbed (Lewis et al., 2017). However, supplementation with 1,000 micrograms (mcg) cyanocobalamin orally has been shown to elevate B_{12} levels, even in those with pernicious anemia. Oral supplementation is preferred for older adults with malabsorption or other causes of B_{12} deficiency (Nettina, 2009).

Gastritis

Gastritis refers to inflammation of the gastric mucosa and occurs in acute or chronic forms. The amount of gastric acid secretion might not be excessive in cases of gastritis.

Acute gastritis causes transient inflammation, hemorrhages, and erosion into the gastric mucosal lining. Although the cause may be undetermined, it is frequently associated with alcoholism, aspirin or NSAID ingestion, smoking, and severely stressful conditions such as burns, trauma, central nervous system (CNS) damage, chemotherapy, and radiotherapy.

Chronic gastritis involves inflammation of the stomach lining that may occur repeatedly or continue over time. Among its possible causes are ulcers, hiatal hernias, vitamin deficiencies, chronic alcohol use, gastric mucosal atrophy, achlorhydria, and peptic ulceration. The continual loss of gastric mucosa eventually decreases gastric secretion and may lead to pernicious anemia, PUD, or gastric cancer.

The major symptom of gastritis is abdominal pain. Other symptoms include indigestion, distention, decreased appetite, nausea, and vomiting. Many patients with chronic gastritis are asymptomatic.

Stress-Induced Gastritis

Stress-induced gastritis or erosion may occur in critically ill patients such as those with burns, sepsis, multiorgan failure, major surgery, or head injury. These erosions are superficial defects of the stomach mucosa that usually do not penetrate the muscularis layer; however, they may result in significant blood loss.

Two mechanisms are thought to produce stress ulcers: (1) mucosal ischemia resulting from a lack of blood supply to the gastric mucosa during the poststress period and (2) a decrease in mucosal bicarbonate concentration leading to increased sensitivity of the gastric mucosa to hydrochloric acid and pepsin.

The major clinical manifestation of stress ulcers is painless, gastric bleeding. Because of the danger of bleeding after acute stress and the difficulty of stopping it once it has started, preventive measures are routinely used to decrease hydrogen ion secretion and neutralize gastric acid. These include administration of antacids, as well as histamine blockers, sucralfate, or both.

NURSING MANAGEMENT

Assessment

Assessment begins with a history and review of systems, which may include complaints of indigestion, abdominal or epigastric discomfort, nausea, vomiting, or anorexia. Questioning patients about possible GI blood loss (e.g., hematemesis or melena) is also important. With acute gastritis, signs of dehydration may be present.

Diagnosis

Nursing diagnoses for an older patient with gastritis include the following:

- Acute pain resulting from epigastric discomfort, cramping secondary to acidity, or both
- Dehydration resulting from decreased intake, vomiting and blood loss, or both
- Need for health teaching resulting from the disease process

Planning and Expected Outcomes

Because most patients receive treatment on an outpatient basis, the nurse must determine an older patient's ability to adhere to the recommended treatment strategies. Expected outcomes for an older patient with gastritis include the following:

1. The patient will experience relief of epigastric symptoms.
2. The patient will maintain adequate fluid and electrolyte balance.
3. The patient will verbalize understanding of the disease and factors that contribute to the disease.

Intervention

Nursing management of an older patient with gastritis includes acid-suppressant drugs, as ordered; small, frequent, easily digested meals; maintenance of a calm environment to decrease the effects of stress; monitoring of fluid and electrolyte status; and teaching the older patient about precipitating and contributory factors. GI bleeding is a possible complication of gastritis, and prevention and early diagnosis are important. An older patient must understand the necessity of limiting or eliminating alcohol and tobacco use, avoiding aspirin and other NSAIDs, and seeking prompt medical attention for symptoms of indigestion and epigastric pain.

Evaluation

Evaluation includes documentation of achieved expected outcomes, a decrease in symptoms, and no evidence of GI hemorrhaging or other complications. The nurse should note an older patient's adherence to necessary lifestyle changes.

Peptic Ulcer Disease

PUD is an ulcerative condition caused by the erosion of the GI mucosa resulting from the digestive action of hydrochloric acid and pepsin. Although PUD refers to injury anywhere in the GI tract, the most common occurrence is in the stomach and duodenum (Fig. 21.5).

The exact cause of peptic ulcers is unclear, but research has identified conditions that predispose individuals to their development. *Helicobacter pylori* infection plays a central role in the development of PUD in nearly 70% of cases in older adults (Pilotto, Franceschi, Maggi et al., 2010). The infection leads to bacterial gastritis and subsequent gastric atrophy. Long-term effects of gastric mucosal atrophy include decreased gastric acid production, intestinal metaplasia, and gastric carcinoma. The organism secretes urease, which generates free ammonia, and a protease that breaks down the gastric mucus. These substances mediate inflammation in the gastric mucosa, which makes it more vulnerable (Lewis et al., 2017). Gastric ulcers and duodenal ulcers (DUs) are typically associated with NSAID use. Other drugs associated with PUD include

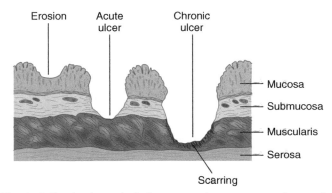

Fig. 21.5 Peptic ulcers, including an erosion, an acute ulcer, and a chronic ulcer. (From Lewis, S. L., Bucher, L., Heitkemper, M. M., & Harding, M. M. [2017]. *Medical-surgical nursing: Assessment and management of clinical problems* [10th ed.]. St. Louis, MO: Elsevier.)

warfarin, selective serotonin reuptake inhibitors (SSRIs), and bisphosphonates (Pilotto et al., 2010).

Both genetic and environmental factors have been proposed as the cause of peptic ulcers because both gastric ulcers and DUs tend to occur in families. At present, no direct evidence exists that indicates dietary or occupational factors as causes of ulcer disease. In addition, although psychological factors such as anxiety or stress play a role in the response of peptic ulcers to treatment, little evidence supports the common belief that only a person with the type A personality, who is constantly striving for perfection, develops ulcers. However, prolonged stress may produce a stress ulcer in anyone.

Gastric Ulcers

In gastric ulcers, the level of hydrochloric acid secretion is usually normal or reduced. The problem lies in the increased rate of diffusion of gastric acid back into the tissue. Patients with benign gastric ulcers should be encouraged to receive frequent follow-up and monitoring because these ulcers can become malignant. Risk factors for the formation of gastric ulcers include *H. pylori* infection, NSAID use, cigarette smoking, and alcohol use disorder. Caffeine and excessive stress may aggravate symptoms.

The most common symptom with gastric ulcers is gnawing or burning pain in the epigastric region that comes and goes; eating may lead to pain relief. Pain may be worse on an empty stomach. If the ulcer has eroded through the mucosa, food aggravates symptoms rather than alleviating them (Lewis et al., 2017). Nausea, vomiting, and weight loss are common. Perforation may lead to hemorrhage and peritonitis. Healing and recurrences are common. A lack of healing or failure to decrease in size suggests malignancy.

Duodenal Ulcers

In contrast to gastric ulcers, people with DUs have a normal back diffusion of gastric acid but an increased rate of gastric acid secretion. They also have an increased emptying rate of acid from the stomach to the duodenum. If the increase in acid is not buffered in the stomach, the acid is propelled into the duodenum, which leads to irritation of the duodenal mucosa. Most of these ulcerations occur in the first part of the duodenum, close to the pylorus. It is believed that the bacterium *H. pylori* migrates from the stomach to the duodenum in the presence of dysplastic changes in the duodenal mucosa.

Typically, the symptoms of DUs are patterned by periods of exacerbation and remission and follow a pain–food–relief pattern. The pain begins 2 to 4 hours after meals and is immediately relieved by food or antacids. The pain is in the midepigastrium and may be described as a burning or cramplike pain (Lewis et al., 2017). The pain may manifest as back pain. Other GI symptoms include heartburn and regurgitation of sour acidic juice into the back of the throat. Anorexia and weight loss are rare because the patient usually seeks food to relieve the pain. A DU may rupture because of erosion through the duodenal wall, and this leads to contamination of the peritoneal cavity (peritonitis). A slowly bleeding ulcer may reveal guaiac-positive stools. On physical examination, the only abnormality observed is possibly a tender epigastrium.

NURSING MANAGEMENT

Assessment

Assessment begins with evaluation of a patient's complaint of abdominal or epigastric pain, the most common symptom of peptic ulcers. The pain should be assessed for presence, location, character, and especially alleviating and precipitating factors. Peptic ulcer pain is usually described as gnawing, burning, or aching, usually in the epigastric area, and may radiate around to the back. The pain usually begins when the stomach is empty and may disappear with the ingestion of food or an antacid. Because of this, the pain often occurs at night when the stomach is empty, especially with DUs. A patient may also exhibit signs of complications of the peptic ulcer. Hemorrhaging may be manifested as either melena or hematemesis. Older adults typically have a blunted presentation.

Diagnosis

The most frequently used nursing diagnoses for an older patient with PUD include the following:
- Acute pain resulting from mucosal lesions
- Need for health teaching resulting from lack of exposure to disease process and treatment
- Inadequate family therapeutic management resulting from complexity of health care regimen

Planning and Expected Outcomes

Because not all older patients with PUD have the same set of symptoms, the nurse must determine individual patient needs with regard to education and other interventions. Expected outcomes for an older patient with PUD include the following:
1. The patient will report a decrease in abdominal or epigastric pain.
2. The patient will adhere to the prescribed dietary, activity, and drug regimen.
3. The patient will acknowledge aggravating factors such as smoking, alcohol use, stress, or frequent use of aspirin or NSAIDs.

Intervention

Nursing management for an older patient with PUD includes education of the patient on lifestyle changes, dietary modifications, and drugs that may be used in the treatment plan. Lifestyle changes include cessation of smoking, cessation of alcohol consumption, and avoidance of other irritants such as aspirin-containing products and NSAIDs. In addition, stress reduction techniques such as exercise, relaxation training, biofeedback, and other appropriate outlets should be explored and individualized, depending on patient needs and wishes. Dietary changes include avoiding foods that irritate the mucosa of the stomach, for example, caffeine and foods that cause pain.

Drugs need to be taken as prescribed. An older patient needs to be instructed that antacids work quickly to neutralize acid in the stomach and are only to be used intermittently for heartburn and acid indigestion. Drugs to reduce or prevent acid production (H_2 receptor antagonists and PPIs) should be taken exactly as ordered, but these agents take longer to provide relief. The patient should also understand that antacids last only 20 to 30 minutes, whereas drugs to reduce or prevent acid production have a long-term effect. Another important point to discuss with the older patient is the effect of the ulcer drug on other drugs. For example, cimetidine, an H_2 receptor antagonist, interferes with the metabolism of warfarin, theophylline, and phenytoin.

If surgery is performed, more dietary modifications may be necessary because of a reduction in the size of the stomach. A response known as *dumping syndrome* is common after gastric resection; it is manifested by dizziness, nausea, and diaphoresis after meals. The institution of small, frequent meals that are low in carbohydrates will diminish the incidence of these symptoms. Resting after eating and drinking fluids between (rather than during) meals will also help alleviate these symptoms. Maintaining adequate nutrition and fluid and electrolyte balance is especially important for older patients and may be achieved by making these dietary modifications.

Evaluation

Evaluation includes documentation of achievement of the expected outcomes, prevention of complications, elimination of symptoms, and an increased knowledge base regarding PUD. Any complications from recommended medical treatments should be noted.

Enteritis

Enteritis, or *gastroenteritis,* refers to an inflammatory process of the stomach or small intestine. Bacteria, viruses, drugs, radiation, ingestion of foods that irritate the gastric mucosa, or allergic reactions may cause it. Bacterial enteritis, commonly known as "food poisoning," is often caused by ingestion of food contaminated by bacteria containing toxins. Examples of these bacteria include *Staphylococcus aureus, Salmonella,* and *Clostridium botulinum.*

In addition, enteritis may result from parasitic infections such as amebiasis and trichinosis. Amebiasis is caused by a protozoal parasite that primarily invades the large intestine. The inactive form, a cyst, is ingested through food or water contaminated by feces and passes into the intestines. There, the active form is released and enters the intestinal wall, causing ulceration of the intestinal mucosa. Amebiasis is prevalent primarily in tropical countries and in places with poor sanitation.

Trichinosis is transmitted through improperly cooked pork and is caused by the larvae of a roundworm that became imbedded in the striated muscles. When the contaminated pork is eaten, gastric acid releases the larvae from cysts; they develop into adults in the host's intestine. The adult females release larvae which move toward the host's muscles, where they may remain for many years. Acute enteritis is a result of direct bacterial or viral infection, or the effect of the toxins produced by bacteria. This results in either an increased secretion of water into the intestinal lumen or an increase in motility, causing large amounts of food and fluid to be excreted. In general, enteritis causes inflammatory changes in the intestinal mucosa, which return to normal when the offending agent is removed.

The pathologic process has varying manifestations resulting in symptoms of abdominal cramping, profuse diarrhea, and vomiting. With profuse diarrhea, large amounts of fluid and electrolytes may be lost, which leads to dehydration and electrolyte imbalances of hyponatremia and hypokalemia. Older adults are particularly at risk for dehydration and electrolyte imbalance. Prompt treatment is required.

NURSING MANAGEMENT

Assessment

Assessment begins with a history of recent food intake, nausea, vomiting, and diarrhea including amount, duration, frequency, and stool characteristics. The nurse should inquire about recent drug use, especially antibiotics, and recent travel. If food poisoning is suspected, the nurse should also question the patient regarding possible sources of contamination. Physical examination includes inspection of mucous membranes and assessment of orthostatic blood pressure, temperature, and abdominal tenderness. A urine specimen for specific gravity may be helpful in assessing hydration.

Diagnosis

The most common nursing diagnoses for an older patient with enteritis include the following:
- Dehydration resulting from vomiting and diarrhea
- Diarrhea resulting from intestinal inflammation

Planning and Expected Outcomes

Expected outcomes for an older patient with enteritis include the following:
1. The patient will maintain adequate fluid volume and electrolyte balance.
2. The patient will have a continual decline in the number of liquid, nonformed stools until baseline is achieved.

Intervention

Nursing management of an older patient with enteritis includes maintenance of hydration and monitoring of fluid and electrolyte status. With severe vomiting and diarrhea, intravenous hydration and hospitalization are required. With milder forms of enteritis, clear liquids may be offered at home. In all cases, monitoring for signs and symptoms of dehydration is imperative. In addition, it is important for the nurse to determine whether an older patient has someone nearby to assist him or her or summon for help if the condition worsens. Older patients need to be educated about the signs and symptoms of dehydration and when to seek further medical care. Prevention of bacterial and parasitic enteritis should also be discussed, and the need for thorough hand washing, especially before meals and food preparation, should be stressed.

Evaluation

Evaluation includes documentation of achievement of the expected outcomes, prevention of complications, and return to baseline status. The nurse should monitor the older patient for reduction of symptoms as the problem resolves. Careful monitoring of oral intake and tolerance of advancing diet is also documented.

Intestinal Obstruction

Intestinal obstruction occurs whenever partial or complete blockage of the GI tract occurs in either the small intestine or the large intestine. This may be the result of several conditions, which are usually classified as mechanical or paralytic ileus.

Mechanical obstructions are the most common and are primarily caused by tumors, adhesions, or hernias (Fig. 21.6). Another mechanical cause of intestinal obstruction is volvulus or the twisting of a part of the intestine. Although this is a rare cause of obstruction overall, it is more common in older adults because the mesenteric ligaments weaken over time.

Paralytic ileus involves decreased or absent peristalsis resulting from neurologic or vascular disorders. Peristalsis becomes diminished or absent because of a triggering of the inhibitory reflex by noxious stimuli such as anesthesia, peritoneal injury, interruption of the nerve supply, abdominal injury or surgical manipulation, intestinal ischemia, electrolyte imbalances, or side effects of certain drugs such as antidepressants or drugs to control pain. Neurologic causes, which may be overlooked, include diabetes-related neuropathy, multiple sclerosis, stroke, or Parkinson's disease. It is a common postoperative problem, especially after abdominal surgery.

Vascular disorders may cause intestinal or mesenteric ischemia resulting in obstruction. Prolonged ischemia results in death of the surface of the villi and epithelial cells, which, in turn, impairs the absorption of nutrients. In addition, the mucosal layer becomes necrotic, and peristalsis diminishes. Although intestinal or mesenteric ischemia is relatively rare, its high mortality rate and predominance in older adults make it important for nurses caring for older adults. Some degree of intestinal ischemia is present in all patients who have a history of other forms of ischemia, thrombosis, or infarction or in patients who have chronic ischemia, for example, those with atherosclerosis. Most of these patients have a history of cerebrovascular disease, peripheral vascular disease, coronary heart disease, or all of these conditions. Ischemic bowel disease comprises a spectrum of acute and chronic syndromes that usually affect older adults. The major syndromes of ischemic intestinal disease include acute embolic ischemia, acute thrombotic occlusion (ischemic colitis), nonocclusive ischemia, chronic intestinal ischemia (abdominal angina), and venous occlusive disease.

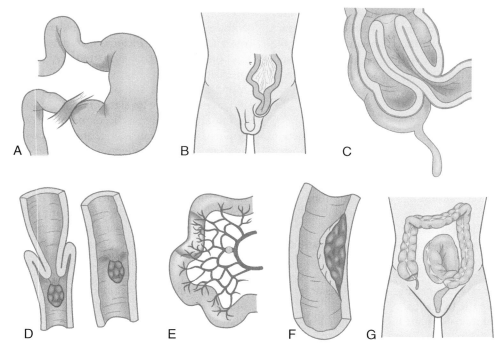

Fig. 21.6 Bowel obstructions. **A,** Adhesions. **B,** Strangulated inguinal hernia. **C,** Ileocecal intussusception. **D,** Intussusception from polyps. **E,** Mesenteric occlusion. **F,** Neoplasm. **G,** Volvulus of the sigmoid colon. (From Lewis, S. L., Bucher, L., Heitkemper, M. M., & Harding, M. M. [2017]. *Medical-surgical nursing: Assessment and management of clinical problems* [10th ed.]. St. Louis, MO: Elsevier.)

Whatever the cause of intestinal obstruction, after the blockage occurs, the bowel becomes distended by gas and air proximal to the area of blockage. If the process continues, gastric, biliary, and pancreatic secretions, along with water, electrolytes, and serum proteins, begin to accumulate in the area, causing an increase in intraluminal pressure. A third space shift may occur when the circulating blood volume decreases because of the movement of water into the intestinal lumen, which may lead to dehydration, electrolyte imbalances, and hypovolemia.

Clinical findings with an obstruction include the acute onset of severe cramping pain that correlates roughly to the area or level of obstruction. The pain may decrease in severity as the distention of the bowel increases. In mesenteric ischemia, the clinical presentation is initially nonspecific and may mimic other, more common abdominal problems such as diverticulitis, appendicitis, and cholecystitis. Although the major symptom is abdominal pain, the clue to mesenteric ischemia is that the pain is out of proportion to what is found on physical examination. Atherosclerotic ischemia may create an angina-like cramping abdominal pain that becomes worse after meals and then dissipates. In colonic ischemia, the pain is worse in the left lower quadrant. Vasospasm and emboli produce an acute, severe abdominal pain with associated vomiting and diarrhea.

Abdominal distention will be present, especially if the obstruction is in the lower small intestine or colon. Percussion will elicit a tympanic sound because of the accumulation of gas and air in the bowel. Hyperactive bowel sounds are present above the site of a mechanical obstruction as the intestine attempts to push the contents downward. The increase in the rate and force of peristalsis may cause *borborygmi* (loud and high-pitched bowel sounds); these may progress to an absence of bowel sounds as the condition persists. Bowel sounds below the obstruction will be absent. Vomiting is almost always present and may (rarely) be bilious or feculent, depending on the level of the obstruction. Diarrhea may occur if the obstruction is not complete, allowing watery contents to pass. The patient may develop signs of dehydration and shock.

Complications of intestinal obstruction include perforation of the bowel, chemical or bacterial peritonitis, hypovolemic shock, and septic shock. The increased pressure on the mucosa of the affected bowel segment may lead to bowel necrosis, resulting in changes in the permeability of the bowel wall. Normal bacteria of the intestine may then escape into the peritoneal cavity, causing peritonitis that may escalate to bacteremia. Perforation of the thinned intestinal wall results in the loss of fluid into the abdominal space, chemical peritonitis, and possible abscess formation. Infection and loss of fluid and electrolytes are major problems. Hypovolemic shock may result when there is a shift of fluid greater than 10% of body weight. Septic shock may also occur because of the contamination of the bloodstream when the bowel ruptures or becomes gangrenous. Sepsis and hypovolemic shock are life-threatening and must be treated aggressively.

NURSING MANAGEMENT

Assessment

Assessment begins with a thorough history of the precipitating event; the nurse should focus on the type and frequency of vomiting and diarrhea (e.g., profuse or fecal) and the location and character of pain (e.g., cramping, constant, or diffuse). A sudden change in a patient's description of abdominal pain from generalized and dull to localized and sharp must be taken seriously; this is a characteristic presentation of peritonitis. Physical examination should focus on the presence and character of bowel sounds (e.g., loud, frequent, absent, or weak), the presence of abdominal distention, vital signs, and urinary output. A sudden elevation of temperature is another classic sign of peritonitis.

Diagnosis

Nursing diagnoses for an older patient with bowel obstruction or ileus include the following:

- Dehydration resulting from loss of body fluids and inadequate fluid volume intake
- Inadequate nutrition resulting from vomiting and obstruction
- Nausea resulting from GI irritation
- Constipation resulting from decreased motility or obstruction

Planning and Expected Outcomes

Expected outcomes for an older patient with an ileus or intestinal obstruction include the following:

1. The patient will maintain adequate fluid volume and electrolyte balance.
2. The patient will verbalize a tolerable level of discomfort.
3. The patient will regain and maintain adequate nutrition, as evidenced by achievement of preillness body weight.
4. The patient will state relief from nausea.
5. The patient will maintain passage of soft, formed stool.

The older adult with bowel obstruction requires careful and close observation because the classic signs of pain and fluid loss may be blunted.

Intervention

Nursing management of an older patient with intestinal obstruction or ileus includes maintenance of hydration and promotion of comfort. Dehydration may be prevented through the provision of intravenous fluids and electrolytes, as ordered. Monitoring intake and output and specific gravity of urine, as well as monitoring for signs of fluid overloading or dehydration, is important. Nasogastric or nasointestinal tubes are usually required for decompression, and maintenance of their patency and placement is imperative. Pain relief measures may include drug therapy; however, narcotics are sometimes not allowed because of their effects on the bowel and their masking of important symptoms. Other comfort measures include repositioning, mouth care, skin care, and music or meditation. If surgery is required, preparation of the patient and family concerning what should be expected is also important.

Evaluation

Evaluation includes documentation of achievement of expected outcomes and prevention of complications (see Nursing Care Plan: Ileus). Vital signs, intake and output, bowel sounds, and bowel elimination patterns should also be recorded. If surgery was performed, monitoring of the incision site and wound healing status is necessary.

Diverticula

Diverticula are saclike protrusions of the mucosa along the GI tract. These small sacs are formed by herniation of the mucous membrane outward through a separation in circular muscle fibers of the intestine where blood vessels penetrate the muscle

---

◎ NURSING CARE PLAN

Ileus: Obstruction Resulting From Diverticulitis

Clinical Situation

Mrs. M is a 78-year-old retired seamstress who was recently admitted to the emergency department with abdominal pain. Her son and daughter-in-law, with whom she lives, brought her in. Her son reported that his mother had been complaining of abdominal pain for the past 24 hours, and because it did not subside, he encouraged her to seek medical attention. Over the past 24 hours, Mrs. M reported left-sided lower abdominal pain, nausea, and, more recently, vomiting. She was unsure whether she had a fever. Her daughter-in-law added that her mother-in-law had had a lot of constipation recently, for which Mrs. M had taken various types of laxatives.

Her medical history included hypertension (for which she takes nifedipine extended release and hydrochlorothiazide) and hypercholesterolemia (for which she takes lovastatin daily). Her son also remembered the doctor telling his mother a few years ago that she had diverticulosis, which was diagnosed from an incidental finding on radiography. Her only past surgery was an uncomplicated cholecystectomy about 20 years ago for cholecystitis. Mrs. M stated that she ate a regular diet, without restrictions, and did not have much weight fluctuation over the past few years.

Physical examination revealed a thin woman, weighing 128 pounds (lb), with a temperature of 100.9° F (38.3° C) (orally), pulse of 98 beats per minute (beats/min), respiratory rate of 24 breaths/min, and blood pressure of 140/84 mm Hg. She was lying on the stretcher curled in a semifetal position. Her abdomen was not obviously distended, and her only scar was a midline incisional scar from her previous cholecystectomy. She had loud, high-pitched bowel sounds, but no

audible bruits. Her abdomen was tender, and a firm mass was palpable in the lower left quadrant. She had no elicitable rebound tenderness. She had tenderness on rectal examination and was thought to have stools high up in her rectal vault. Her stool occult test was guaiac-negative.

Laboratory tests revealed a WBC count of 90,000 microliters (μL) and a normal hemoglobin count. Urinalysis was normal, as were serum electrolyte levels. Serum amylase was 500 units per deciliter (units/dL). Plain abdominal radiography revealed air–fluid levels but no free air on the abdomen. She was given the diagnosis of ileus or obstruction resulting from diverticulitis.

Mrs. M was admitted to a general medical unit and had a surgical consultation. She was started on intravenous fluids, restricted to NPO (nothing by mouth) status, and had a nasogastric tube placed on high intermittent suction. Intravenous antibiotic therapy was begun and continued for the remainder of her hospitalization. She was monitored closely and managed medically. She was found to have an ileus only and never required surgery for a small bowel obstruction or perforation. She was discharged to home on the eighth day after admission. She resumed her previous drugs.

Nursing Diagnoses

Dehydration resulting from active loss of body fluid secondary to nasogastric tube output

Inadequate nutrition resulting from prolonged NPO status

Constipation resulting from decreased mobility, daily ingestion of constipating drugs, and lack of dietary fiber

Need for health teaching resulting from lack of exposure to knowledge about prevention and complications of diverticular disease

Pain (abdominal) resulting from reluctance to take drugs to control pain

Outcomes

The patient will maintain adequate fluid volume and electrolyte balance.

The patient will maintain preadmission weight.

The patient will establish a regular pattern of fecal elimination.

The patient and family will be able to verbalize dietary changes and be able to prevent constipation and further complications.

The patient will obtain pain relief.

Interventions

Monitor vital signs every 4 hours or as ordered.

Maintain intravenous therapy, as ordered.

Monitor intake and output (hourly); skin moisture, color, and turgor; specific gravity of urine (every 4 hours); serum electrolyte levels; and level of consciousness.

Weigh the patient every day or as ordered.

Monitor serum albumin and protein levels.

Administer intravenous total perineal nutrition, as ordered.

When the patient is no longer NPO, encourage high-protein, high-calorie foods.

Administer stool-softening drugs, if ordered.

When the patient is no longer NPO, encourage a daily fluid intake of 2 liters (L) and consumption of high-fiber foods. Teach the patient about fiber-rich foods to be included in the diet.

When the patient is able, encourage her to increase her activity level.

Teach about constipating side effects of drugs.

Provide the patient and family with written and verbal information concerning the importance of a high-fiber diet, the need to maintain an adequate fluid intake, and the need for light exercise.

Provide the patient and family with written and verbal information concerning complications of diverticulosis, such as diverticulitis.

Assess and monitor the degree of pain every 4 hours.

Provide the patient with verbal and written instruction about analgesics.

Provide other measures of pain relief, such as guided imagery, repositioning, and diversional activities.

Provide encouragement by informing the patient that the pain will decrease as the ileus improves.

---

layer. Diverticula are a result of increased intraluminal pressure and can develop in any part of the digestive tract. They occur most often in the descending and sigmoid colon. Colonic diverticula are usually multiple.

The exact cause of diverticula is unknown. Because of the frequency of diverticula in older adults, it is thought that they are related to the blood supply or nutrition of the bowel. Lack of dietary fiber or roughage and decreased fecal bulk have also been correlated with this process. With an increase in food bulk (as with consumption of dietary fiber), the pressure in the colon decreases. In contrast, when little waste is present in the colon, stronger muscle contractions are necessary to excrete it, and the pressure increases. This increase in pressure leads to muscle hypertrophy and the development of diverticula. In this manner, diverticula have also been linked to chronic constipation and obesity in older adults. Atrophy of the musculature of the bowel wall may weaken the intestine and be another factor in the development of diverticula in older adults. The presence of multiple diverticula that are not inflamed is termed *diverticulosis*. This is a disease of middle age and old age. The incidence of diverticulosis increases with age and represents the fifth most important GI disease in Western countries in terms of direct and indirect health care costs. It is the most common disease of the colon in industrialized countries, and the highest rates are reported in the United States, Europe, and Australia (Petruzziello et al., 2006). Diverticulosis may be symptom-free and is often diagnosed as an incidental finding on radiography or sigmoidoscopy. When symptoms are present, it may be associated with vague abdominal discomfort, constipation, or diarrhea.

Diverticulitis is an inflammation of or around a diverticular sac usually caused by the retention of undigested food, stool, and bacteria. In diverticulitis, stasis leads to inflammation, infection, or both. The mucous membranes may erode or perforate blood vessels, causing bleeding. Obstruction of the large intestine, fistulae, and abscesses may result. Rupture of the infected material into the peritoneal cavity may result in

peritonitis. Approximately 25% of those with diverticulosis develop diverticulitis (Chapman, Davies, Wolff et al., 2005).

Clinical manifestations of symptomatic diverticular disease include constipation or diarrhea, left-sided lower abdominal pain, and fever. More than half of patients with diverticulitis experience some change in bowel habits; most complain of constipation. Other symptoms include flatulence, nausea, and vomiting. Older adults with diverticulitis may be afebrile and have little abdominal discomfort. Complications include perforation and peritonitis, ureteral obstruction, and significant lower GI bleeding. Surgery may be necessary if an obstruction or perforation is suspected.

NURSING MANAGEMENT

Assessment

Assessment begins with an older patient's history of elimination patterns and changes in these patterns such as frequency of defecation, stool characteristics (e.g., color, size, and consistency), toileting habits, and course (e.g., improving or worsening and recurrent or chronic changes in bowel habits). Exercise patterns, pain, bloating, nausea, vomiting, medical history (e.g., hemorrhoids or bowel surgery), and family history of bowel problems such as polyps or colon cancer are also important. With diverticulitis, the patient may have fever and chills. A physical examination may be unremarkable, but it may also reveal left lower quadrant tenderness or a guaiac-positive stool.

Diagnosis

The most common nursing diagnoses for an older patient with diverticulosis or diverticulitis include the following:
- Potential for constipation, resulting from decreased fluid, bulk in the diet, or both
- Acute pain, resulting from bowel obstruction
- Need for health teaching, resulting from lack of exposure to disease process, prevention, and treatment

Planning and Expected Outcomes

Expected outcomes for an older patient with diverticulosis or diverticulitis include the following:

1. The patient will experience fewer episodes of constipation, as evidenced by establishment of a regular pattern of bowel activity.
2. The patient will verbalize pain relief and remain free from abdominal pain.
3. The patient will verbalize self-care practices to minimize symptoms of diverticulosis and prevent complications of diverticulitis.

Intervention

Nursing management of an older patient with diverticulosis or diverticulitis includes the prevention and elimination of constipation and the initiation of dietary changes. This includes teaching the patient and family about the development of diverticula and the escalation to diverticulitis. In addition, teaching should include the importance of eating high-fiber foods, which include beans, whole grains, brown rice, fruits (e.g., apples, bananas, and pears) and vegetables (e.g., broccoli, carrots, corn, and squash). Patients should be encouraged to drink eight cups of fluids each day, unless contraindicated by cardiac status.

An older patient with diverticulitis needs pain management (with antispasmodics, analgesics, or other measures such as a heating pad), bowel rest (intravenous fluids if given NPO [nothing by mouth] status), and hospitalization if acutely ill. The nurse should teach self-care practices that promote bowel regularity and administration of stool softeners (such as docusate), as necessary. Preventing constipation is of the utmost importance.

Evaluation

Evaluation includes documentation of achievement of the expected outcomes, prevention of complications, and maintenance of regular bowel patterns and habits. Asking an older adult to verbalize how he or she has incorporated the self-care practices into daily life is an effective way to ascertain whether the patient understands the disease and is able to take measures to prevent complications.

Colon Polyps

Colon polyps are growths on the mucous membranes of the GI tract. A polyp may be sessile (flat, broad, and attached directly to the intestinal wall) or pedunculated (attached to the wall by a thin stem). The most common type of polyp is termed *adenomatous polyp* or *adenoma*. Adenomatous polyps may become cancerous. The larger the polyp, the more likely it is to be malignant (greater than 1 millimeter [mm]). Having numerous polyps increases the likelihood of developing cancer.

The most common nonmalignant polyps are of the hyperplastic type. These rarely grow large and never cause clinical symptoms. Many patients with polyps are asymptomatic. These growths are often discovered incidentally by sigmoidoscopy, colonoscopy, or barium enema. Occasionally, they may bleed, causing bright red blood in feces.

NURSING MANAGEMENT

Assessment

Assessment begins with a thorough history of any changes in an older adult's routine pattern of elimination and any symptoms such as blood in the stools or on the toilet paper. A detailed family history should be taken, and specific questions should be asked regarding polyps in family members. A physical examination may be unremarkable; however, guaiac-positive stools may be found on rectal examination.

Diagnosis

The most common nursing diagnoses for an older patient with polyps include the following:

- Need for health teaching, resulting from lack of exposure to disease process, importance of treatment, and follow-up
- Anxiety, resulting from threat to health status

Planning and Expected Outcomes

Expected outcomes for an older patient with polyps include the following:

1. The patient will verbalize knowledge of the disease process and potential outcomes.
2. The patient will obtain medical follow-up as suggested by the American Cancer Society (ACS) or a health care provider.

Intervention

Nursing management of an older patient with polyps includes education and reinforcement of the guidelines suggested by the ACS for prevention and early detection of colorectal cancer. Teaching of a patient who is to undergo colonoscopy may need to include reinforcement of the importance of having the polyps removed. Reminders should be given to older patients regarding the time for a repeated screening sigmoidoscopy (according to their health care provider or ACS guidelines). Patients may also need to be reminded that, although polyps are often asymptomatic, they may bleed. The presence of any blood in the stool may indicate the need for a repeated sigmoidoscopy or colonoscopy.

Evaluation

Evaluation includes documentation of achievement of the expected outcomes and prevention of complications such as invasive colorectal cancer.

Hemorrhoids

Hemorrhoids are dilations of the veins in the mucous membrane inside the rectum or near the anal opening. These dilations are common and develop in susceptible people as a result of increase in pressure on the veins in the pelvic and rectal areas. Patients may be predisposed because of diarrhea or constipation, obesity, pregnancy, liver disease, prolonged sitting, pelvic tumors, and anal intercourse.

Internal hemorrhoids may cause bleeding with defecation. The dilated venous sacs may protrude into the anal canal, where they become exposed and result in pain; thrombus, ulcerations, and bleeding then develop. External hemorrhoids produce varying degrees of pain, as well as pressure, itching, irritation, and a palpable mass. Bleeding occurs only if the external hemorrhoid is injured or ulcerated. Usually, blood loss is insignificant; however, with persistent bleeding, anemia of chronic disease may develop.

NURSING MANAGEMENT

Assessment

Assessment begins with an older patient's history of constipation and symptoms of rectal pain or blood in the stools or on toilet paper. The physical examination may be unremarkable except for a painful anus and rectum—painful to the point where thorough examination may be difficult. However, a prolapsed hemorrhoid may be detected and should be assessed for swelling, thrombosis, and ischemia. Guaiac-positive stools may be found.

Diagnosis

The most common nursing diagnoses for an older patient with hemorrhoids include the following:
- Potential for constipation resulting from pain on defecation
- Acute pain in the anal and rectal area resulting from swelling and inflammation
- Need for health teaching resulting from lack of previous exposure to treatment and prevention

Planning and Expected Outcomes

Expected outcomes for an older patient with hemorrhoids include the following:
1. The patient will experience fewer episodes of constipation.
2. The patient will establish a regular pattern of fecal elimination.
3. The patient will report a decrease in anal and rectal pain.
4. The patient will verbalize knowledge of self-care practices to minimize the occurrence of hemorrhoids.

Intervention

Nursing management of an older patient with hemorrhoids includes the prevention and elimination of constipation. This includes a review of high-fiber, high-roughage foods including indigestible fiber such as whole grains, legumes, and fresh fruits and vegetables (Berman et al., 2007). Adequate intake of fluids is also important. Older patients should be encouraged to consume up to 2000 milliliters (mL) of fluids each day unless contraindicated. The nurse should encourage light exercise on a regular basis and review the importance of a regular toileting routine. OTC anesthetic ointments and creams and sitz baths may be used for pain relief. Patients should be encouraged not to strain when defecating; this may worsen the hemorrhoids. The nurse should emphasize that it is important to report any rectal bleeding to rule out the possibility of a more serious disorder.

Evaluation

Evaluation includes documentation of achievement of the expected outcomes, prevention of complications, and maintenance of regular bowel patterns and habits.

DISORDERS OF THE ACCESSORY ORGANS

Cholelithiasis and Cholecystitis

Cholelithiasis is the presence or formation of gallstones in the gallbladder. When the gallbladder empties slowly or incorrectly, stasis occurs and encourages the aggregation of cholesterol crystals, eventually leading to stone formation. Gallstones are primarily composed of two main substances: cholesterol and calcium bilirubinate. The incidence of gallstones varies among racial groups (i.e., higher incidence in Hispanic and Native Americans) and countries; however, it is not known whether this is a result of environmental or genetic factors. Risk factors include obesity, female sex, multiparity, sedentary lifestyle, diabetes, drugs (e.g., cholesterol lowering agents, estrogen, and antibiotics), and advancing age (Lewis et al., 2017). Additionally, persons who have undergone bariatric surgery are at increased risk of developing gallstones.

Gallstones may be present for many years without signs and symptoms. The classic symptom is right upper quadrant pain, which may radiate to the right scapular area. The pain may be sharp, crampy, or dull and begins suddenly, often directly after a meal. The pain may last from 15 minutes to 6 hours, and nausea and vomiting may occur. These attacks of pain may occur as infrequently as once every few years or as often as every few days. Often, these episodes are precipitated by the ingestion of fatty foods. The symptoms of biliary pain are caused by an obstruction of the cystic or common bile duct, causing increased pressure and distention of the gallbladder. Often, the pain is so severe that it is mistaken for a heart attack. When the stones lodge along the biliary tract, they obstruct the flow of bile. This may result in jaundice because of the blockage of the flow of bilirubin. When the common bile duct becomes blocked, the bile cannot enter the duodenum, and the stool is clay-colored because the fecal matter lacks pigment. In addition, obstruction of the common bile duct may cause biliary pain, jaundice, pancreatitis, or cholangitis (inflammation of the bile ducts).

Cholecystitis may be acute or chronic and is usually associated with gallstones or other obstructions of the biliary system. The inflammation in cholecystitis results in a thickening of the wall of the gallbladder. This can lead to ischemia, necrosis, gangrene, and possible perforation of the gallbladder itself, leading to peritonitis. In chronic cholecystitis, the walls become thickened and inefficient at emptying. This is a result of chronic chemical or mechanical irritation from stones exerting pressure on the mucosa or from biliary stasis.

NURSING MANAGEMENT

Assessment

Assessment begins with a history of episodes of pain; the nurse should identify its location, quality, and duration. Associated symptoms include nausea and vomiting. Precipitating factors (e.g., large, fatty meals) and alleviating factors (e.g., pain relievers or changes of position) need to be documented. Physical examination may reveal a tender right upper quadrant and possibly jaundice.

Diagnosis

The most common nursing diagnoses for an older patient with cholelithiasis or cholecystitis include the following:

- Acute pain resulting from gallbladder inflammation
- Need for health teaching resulting from lack of previous exposure to the condition and treatment options
- Altered sleep pattern resulting from pain

Planning and Expected Outcomes

Expected outcomes for an older patient with cholelithiasis or cholecystitis include the following:

1. The patient will experience pain relief.
2. The patient will verbalize knowledge of the disease process, prevention of complications, and treatment options available.
3. The patient will verbalize feeling rested after nighttime sleeping.

Intervention

Nursing management of an older patient with cholelithiasis or cholecystitis includes providing pain relief and instructing the patient and family about the disease process, treatment options, and potential complications. Older patients with cholelithiasis need to know that foods high in fat may precipitate an attack of pain. They need to be aware of treatment options, including types of surgery, medical dissolution, and lithotripsy, as well as the advantages and disadvantages of each. The patient with cholecystitis may require hospitalization and may receive intravenous fluids and antibiotics. If managed at home, patients need to be on a clear liquid diet until pain is resolved and then slowly advance to a regular diet, avoiding fatty foods. Signs and symptoms of complications need to be reviewed with both patients and their families. Additional nursing care is based on an older patient's response to the initial treatment.

Evaluation

Evaluation includes documentation of achievement of expected outcomes, prevention of complications, prevention of infection, and assessment of a patient's knowledge of the disease process. The nurse also evaluates the patient's response to food intake and monitors the patient's food choices to ensure dietary compliance.

Pancreatitis

Pancreatitis is an inflammation of the pancreas and often has no known cause. The disorder may be acute or chronic. In acute pancreatitis, the organ returns to normal after treatment. In chronic pancreatitis, permanent and progressive destruction of the pancreas occurs, whereby the normal tissue is replaced by fibrous tissue.

Acute pancreatitis may be alcohol-induced or related to biliary tract disease; however, in nearly a third of cases, the cause is unknown. In the older adult, acute pancreatitis is most often related to biliary tract disease. Other causes of acute pancreatitis include drugs, surgery, trauma, and metabolic disorders.

Acute pancreatitis is believed to be caused by activation of pancreatic enzymes, which may cause autodigestion of the pancreas; activation of the enzymes is thought to result from reflux of bile into the pancreatic duct, obstruction of the pancreatic duct, ischemia, anorexia, trauma, and toxins.

The etiology of chronic pancreatitis is not as well understood (Evans & Draganov, 2006); however, most cases are caused by alcohol use disorder. Additional factors in the development of chronic pancreatitis include hereditary pancreatitis, cystic fibrosis, elevated triglycerides, cholelithiasis, and drugs.

Symptoms include severe abdominal pain in the epigastric to the right upper quadrant area, occasionally radiating through to the back. Pain is usually more intense in the supine position, and the patient often remains in a flexed position to relieve pain. Nausea, vomiting, abdominal distention, and fever are common. In chronic pancreatitis, the pain may be continuous and accompanied by weakness and jaundice. In addition, in chronic pancreatitis, the stools often become bulky, fatty, and foul-smelling; weight loss may occur because of malabsorption. Glucose intolerance is a late sign of chronic pancreatitis. The development of easily identifiable chronic pancreatitis may take years. Calcification of the pancreas may take decades to develop, and diabetes (glucose intolerance) and steatorrhea may only develop after 10 to 20 years of disease progression (Forsmark, 2008).

NURSING MANAGEMENT

Assessment

Assessment begins with an older patient's history of precipitating factors such as alcohol use disorder or the presence of gallstones. Symptoms of abdominal pain, anorexia, nausea, and vomiting need to be assessed in detail. The patient may be in tremendous pain and unable to answer, so reliance on information from a family member may be necessary. Depending on the patient's pain, a physical examination may be difficult.

Diagnosis

The most common nursing diagnoses for an older patient with pancreatitis include the following:

- Dehydration resulting from nausea or vomiting; restricted oral intake
- Acute pain resulting from obstruction of the pancreatic tract
- Inadequate nutrition resulting from anorexia and vomiting

Planning and Expected Outcomes

Expected outcomes for an older patient with pancreatitis include the following

1. The patient will maintain adequate fluid volume and electrolyte balance.
2. The patient will obtain pain relief.
3. The patient will stabilize and maintain weight.
4. The patient will not experience complications.

Intervention

Nursing management of an older patient with pancreatitis includes maintenance of fluid and electrolyte balance, establishment of pain relief measures, and prevention of complications. This includes monitoring intravenous therapy, vital signs, intake and output, serum electrolyte values, and weight. Pain management may be extremely difficult, especially for patients with chronic pancreatitis. Often, the expertise of a pain consultant is necessary.

An important consideration in acute pancreatitis is the prevention of recurrence. When pancreatitis results from alcohol use disorder, teaching should focus on the need to avoid alcohol consumption to prevent future acute episodes. Referral and counseling may be needed. For the patient with pancreatitis resulting from biliary tract disease, information on maintaining a low-fat diet is important. Providing information and emotional support is important for patients who may need surgery.

Evaluation

Evaluation includes documentation of achievement of expected outcomes, prevention of complications, prevention of recurrence (for acute pancreatitis), and maintenance of adequate nutrition and hydration. Older adults addicted to alcohol may go through withdrawal, requiring the nurse to carefully monitor and record patient responses to treatment of this secondary problem.

Hepatitis

Hepatitis is a general term referring to inflammation of the liver. It may be caused by a variety of factors such as drugs, chemicals, and alcohol, but the most common cause is viral infection. Although five major viruses (and possibly a sixth), as well as mononucleosis and cytomegalovirus, may act as the causative agents for hepatitis, hepatitis A, B, and C viruses are the most common causative agents in the United States.

Hepatitis A virus (HAV), a ribonucleic acid (RNA) virus, causes hepatitis A. The primary mode of transmission of this organism is the fecal–oral route, commonly through ingestion of contaminated food or water. Risk groups for hepatitis A include institutional populations such as patients in daycare centers and travelers to endemic areas. The clinical disease tends to be mild and of short duration. No residual liver disease after recovery and no indications of a chronic state are present. The rate of hepatitis A is decreasing in the United States, as routine vaccination is now given to all children, travelers to certain countries, and persons at risk for the disease (CDC, 2009b).

Hepatitis B virus (HBV), a deoxyribonucleic acid (DNA) virus, causes hepatitis B. This virus is transmitted through blood and body fluids, and risk factors include intravenous drug use and sexual contact. It is considered a sexually transmitted disease (STD) by the CDC. Hepatitis B follows a more severe course compared with hepatitis A and has an increased risk for liver disease (e.g., cirrhosis and cancer). A 5% to 10% incidence of a chronic state, defined as continuing to test positive for the viral antigen for 6 months or longer, is present. Affected individuals may be asymptomatic or have subclinical symptoms; however, they remain contagious as long as the antigen is present. Hepatitis D virus (HDV) is an obligate virus with HBV; this virus is spread by the same mechanisms as HBV and results in severe acute illness and life-threatening chronic liver disease.

Hepatitis C is caused by a small RNA virus, hepatitis C virus (HCV), and represents 85% to 90% of transfusion-related hepatitis cases. The clinical course is usually milder than that of hepatitis B, and the affected person may even be asymptomatic. The major concern about hepatitis C is the development of a chronic condition occurring in more than 75% of individuals. In an Italian study, the time to the development of cirrhosis as a complication of hepatitis C infection was shorter if the infection was acquired at an older age. Investigators also found this to be the result in a study published in Japan. Hepatitis C acquired through blood transfusion at an advanced age progresses more rapidly to the chronic state with the associated complications (Mindikoglu & Miller, 2009).

The pathophysiologic events leading to the liver inflammation seen in hepatitis are similar for all of the viruses. Once the virus is introduced into the individual by its specific mode of transmission, it enters the circulation and seeks out hepatic tissue. The virus enters the cell and uses the host cell's DNA to reproduce itself. This may directly injure or kill the hepatocyte, which is believed to be the primary cause of cell damage in hepatitis A, or the responding immunologic cells may harm the liver cell in the process of destroying the virus, which is the probable pathologic cause in hepatitis B and C (Table 21.3).

There also are viral hepatitis types D, E, and G. Hepatitis D virus (HDV) is a small virus that requires concomitant infection with HBV to survive. HDV cannot survive on its own because it requires HBV to make a surface antigen to enable it to infect liver cells. HDV is spread by shared needles among drug abusers, contaminated blood, and by sexual contact. Individuals who already have chronic HBV infection can acquire HDV infection at the same time as they acquire the HBV infection or later. Those with chronic hepatitis due to HBV and HDV develop cirrhosis rapidly. The combination of HDV and HBV is very difficult to treat (Davis, n.d.).

Hepatitis E virus (HEV) is like HAV in terms of disease and occurs mainly in Asia where it is transmitted by contaminated water. Hepatitis G virus (HGV, also termed GBV-C) was recently discovered and resembles HCV, but, more closely, the flaviviruses; the virus and its effects are under investigation, and its role in causing disease in humans is unclear (Davis, n.d.).

The clinical picture of hepatitis is essentially the same for disease caused by all the viruses, but the overall course is shorter for hepatitis A. Typically, the illness is divided into three phases. In the *prodromal phase,* patients have generalized symptoms of malaise, fatigue, possible right upper quadrant pain, nausea and vomiting, anorexia, and a low-grade fever. Patients often think they have the flu, or the infected individuals do not recall experiencing the symptoms as they are very mild. The second phase, in which jaundice and dark urine appear, is termed the *icteric phase.* Sometimes, jaundice does not occur. Patients may start to feel better during this phase. Finally, in the *convalescent phase,* jaundice and other symptoms disappear, and patients feel fully recovered. It is important that patients understand that it will take 3 to 6 months for the liver to return to its normal functioning status. Care should be taken regarding rest and drug and alcohol consumption during this phase; a relapse is possible.

TABLE 21.3   Viral Hepatitis

	Hepatitis A Virus (HAV)	Hepatitis B Virus (HBV)	Hepatitis C Virus (HCV)
Transmission	Person-to-person through the fecal–oral route or consumption of contaminated food or water	Via blood, semen, or another body fluid; can happen through sexual contact; sharing needles, syringes, or other drug-injection equipment; or from mother to baby at birth.	Most people become infected with the Hepatitis C virus by sharing needles or other equipment to inject drugs
Incubation period	May be spread without symptoms 2–6 weeks after exposure	Spread: blood, semen, or other body fluid 6 weeks–6 months	20–90 days
Risk groups	Institutional populations, including daycare centers, and travelers to endemic areas	Intravenous drug use and sexual contact; considered by the CDC to be a sexually transmitted disease	Recipients of blood or blood product transfusions
Course of disease	Self-limited disease that does not result in chronic infection Symptomatic usually less than 2 months	Course more severe than with hepatitis A 70% of adults and children older than 5 years will develop symptoms	Milder course
Chronic state	No	Approximately 90% of infected infants become chronically infected, compared with 2%–6% of adults.	For 70%–85% of people who become infected with Hepatitis C, it becomes a long-term, chronic infection
Prevention/ vaccination	Yes 2 injections, 6 months apart	Yes 3–4 shots over a 6-month period	No
Liver cancer risk	None	Yes (also other liver diseases like cirrhosis)	Yes

NOTE: Hepatitis D virus (HDV) is uncommon in the United States. Hepatitis D occurs only among people infected with the hepatitis B virus because HDV is an incomplete virus that requires the helper function of HBV to replicate. HDV can be an acute, short-term infection or a long-term, chronic infection. Hepatitis D is transmitted through percutaneous or mucosal contact with infectious blood and can be acquired either as a coinfection with HBV or as superinfection in people with HBV infection. There is no vaccine for hepatitis D, but it can be prevented in persons who are not already HBV-infected by hepatitis B vaccination.

Hepatitis E virus (HEV) is a self-limited disease that does not result in chronic infection. Although rare in the United States, hepatitis E is common in many parts of the world. It is transmitted from ingestion of fecal matter, even in microscopic amounts, and is usually associated with contaminated water supply in countries with poor sanitation. There is currently no FDA-approved vaccine for hepatitis E.

From Centers for Disease Control and Prevention. (2017). *Viral hepatitis.* Retrieved from https://www.cdc.gov/hepatitis/index.htm.

NURSING MANAGEMENT

Assessment

Assessment begins by reviewing with the patient any possible exposure to a hepatitis virus. The nurse should ask questions about recent travel, food intake, blood transfusions, and close contact with persons who may have had hepatitis in the past. Assess for clinical manifestations such as jaundice, right-upper-quadrant tenderness, fatigue, and malaise. The nurse should question the patient about changes in functional status; for example, whether the patient's activity level and ability to perform activities of daily living (ADLs) have decreased from baseline levels. The nurse should also review nutritional intake and assess for anorexia, as well as question changes in the way clothes fit and ask if family and friends have noticed weight loss in the patient. Palpation of the abdomen may reveal an enlarged liver.

Diagnosis

Nursing diagnoses for an older patient with hepatitis include the following:
- Inadequate health maintenance resulting from deficient knowledge about hepatitis, the treatment regimen, and prevention of spreading the virus
- Reduced stamina resulting from generalized weakness and fatigue

- Inadequate nutrition resulting from anorexia, nausea, and liver dysfunction
- Inadequate family therapeutic management resulting from lack of knowledge

Planning and Expected Outcomes

Expected outcomes for an older patient with hepatitis include the following:
1. The patient will verbalize the causes of hepatitis, the treatment plan, and mechanisms to prevent spreading the virus to others.
2. The patient will participate in ADLs without experiencing fatigue.
3. The patient will consume a well-balanced, high-calorie diet, as evidenced by a food diary.
4. The patient will demonstrate self-care activities as much as possible within physical limitations.

Intervention

The nurse must teach patients and their significant others about the spread of hepatitis and mechanisms for prevention. Depending on the specific mode of transmission of the virus, the nurse should also discuss hygiene practices in the home, especially with regard to feces; instruct men and women on condom use; discuss proper disposal of needles; instruct the patient and family on purchase and preparation of certain foods such as shellfish (i.e., eating raw shellfish should be avoided); and instruct the patient to avoid alcohol and drugs containing acetaminophen.

Frequent rest periods are necessary. The nurse should explain that rest is an important treatment in hepatitis, and activities such as visiting, cooking, and housework need to be curtailed. A patient with hepatitis best tolerates a high-carbohydrate, low-fat diet. Several small feedings throughout the day will help alleviate the effect of anorexia. Fluid intake should increase to 2,000 to 3,000 mL/day unless contraindicated by cardiovascular status.

The cause of jaundice should be explained, and the patient should be warned that changes in the colors of urine, skin, and sclera may be seen; this is a temporary condition that will resolve once the acute phase of illness has run its course.

If the jaundice causes pruritus (common in chronic HCV), the nurse should discuss the use of nonalcohol-based lotions, soft clothes and linens, and tepid baths using as little mild soap as possible. The nurse should instruct patients and caregivers about keeping patients' fingernails short to avoid injury from scratching.

Evaluation

Evaluation includes documentation of achievement of the expected outcomes, coupled with the patient's successful self-management of the disease. Careful attention to an older adult's food intake, weight trends, and activity tolerance is crucial.

Cirrhosis Secondary to Alcohol Use Disorder

Cirrhosis is a general term referring to a chronic disorder of the liver in which permanent, irreversible destruction of the hepatocytes and the normal architecture of the organ occurs. The causes for this disease are many and include fatty liver, hepatitis, cystic fibrosis, and primary biliary cirrhosis; however, about 80% of cases in the United States are attributed to alcohol use disorder.

The progressive loss of functioning liver tissue is manifested by the appearance of general signs and symptoms of liver failure; over time, other manifestations of declining liver function appear (Fig. 21.7). Early signs and symptoms of liver failure from cirrhosis are like those of hepatitis. The patient experiences fatigue, malaise, anorexia, changes in fecal elimination pattern (either diarrhea or constipation), nausea and vomiting, and dull, heavy pain in the right upper quadrant. Later symptoms include jaundice and edema in peripheral sites. Ultimately, serious complications such as bleeding, portal hypertension, ascites, and encephalopathy develop. Bleeding tendencies are the result of declining clotting and coagulation factors. One of the many functions of the liver is the production of clotting factors V, VII, IX, and X, as well as the production of fibrinogen and prothrombin. Decreased amounts of these proteins result in a bleeding diathesis in any patient with advanced liver disease, regardless of cause.

Ascites is the accumulation of serous fluid in the abdominal cavity. It is the result of several factors relating to poor liver function, but the most important of these is the decreased

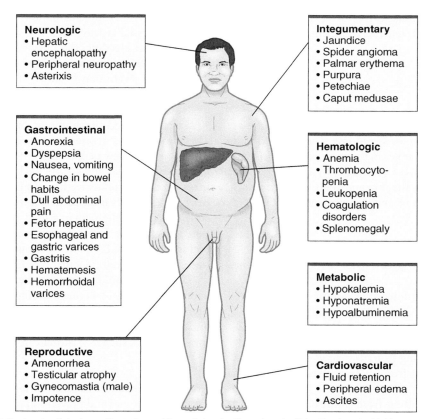

Fig. 21.7 Systemic clinical manifestations of liver cirrhosis. (From Lewis, S. L., Bucher, L., Heitkemper, M. M., & Harding, M. M. [2017]. *Medical-surgical nursing: Assessment and management of clinical problems* [10th ed.]. St. Louis, MO: Elsevier.)

production of albumin by the liver. Insufficient amounts of this major plasma protein in the blood cause the escape of plasma fluid into the abdominal space. Another factor is the increased venous pressure from portal hypertension, which forces the fluid out of the vessel. The most serious effect of ascites is respiratory compromise, which occurs when the diaphragm is pushed upward by increasing abdominal fluid, thus decreasing thoracic space for pulmonary excursion.

Portal hypertension is an increase in pressure in the portal vein and its feeders because of liver congestion or obstruction. In addition to contributing to the development of ascites, portal hypertension and the backflow of venous blood cause severe problems with hemorrhoids, splenomegaly, and esophageal varices. The effect of portal hypertension on the esophageal veins is the most dangerous because these vessels are fragile and susceptible to rupture with any increase in intraabdominal pressure. Patients who bleed from esophageal varices are gravely ill. One-third of deaths from cirrhosis are from esophageal varices.

A late-stage event in long-term liver disease is the development of *encephalopathy,* which is caused by the diseased liver's inability to carry out its function of detoxifying metabolic byproducts. One of the most critical of these is ammonia, an end-product of protein metabolism. Although it is not clear whether the ammonia is directly toxic to the brain or interferes with glucose uptake, decreasing blood ammonia levels is correlated with successful treatment. A patient with high ammonia levels will begin to exhibit changes in behavior, irrationality, agitation, combativeness, and muscle tremors (asterixis). If the condition remains untreated, hepatic coma ensues and has a mortality rate of 90%.

NURSING MANAGEMENT

Assessment

Assessment of the patient with cirrhosis involves a careful history of the onset and duration of symptoms. The nurse should question the patient about changes in the color of the stool, rectal bleeding, and bloody emesis. A thorough physical assessment of all body systems, especially the skin and abdomen, and respiratory and mental status is indicated. Assessment of nutritional status is also important.

Diagnosis

Nursing diagnoses for an older patient with cirrhosis include the following:
- Potential for reduced skin integrity resulting from pruritus, edema, and ascites
- Inadequate breathing pattern resulting from increased pressure on the diaphragm secondary to ascites
- Potential for injury resulting from decreased clotting factors
- Acute confusion resulting from increased serum ammonia levels
- Inadequate nutrition resulting from anorexia, nausea, and vomiting
- Potential for decreased self-esteem resulting from guilt about damage done to self and significant others

Planning and Expected Outcomes

Expected outcomes for an older patient with alcoholic cirrhosis include the following:
1. The patient will be free from skin breakdown.
2. The patient will demonstrate the ability to pace activity and ADLs within current ventilatory function.
3. The patient will remain free from injuries and bleeding.
4. The patient will demonstrate resolution of cerebral dysfunction, as evidenced by no injury to self or others; achieve an appropriate sleep–wake pattern; communicate meaningfully with others; and be oriented to time, person, and place.
5. The patient will maintain or gain weight to an appropriate level.
6. The patient will identify positive aspects about self and express an optimistic outlook regarding relationships.

Intervention

Interventions for an older adult with cirrhosis may be multiple and complex; a major focus is preventing complications. Skin care is a priority. The nurse should inspect the skin daily for signs of breakdown or redness. The skin should be kept clean and dry, especially after toileting. The nurse should use pressure relief devices on a patient's bed and chair. The nurse must also teach patients and caregivers the importance of changing position every 2 hours. A bed trapeze may facilitate lifting and position changes.

The nurse should position the patient in the semi-Fowler or high Fowler position to promote maximum chest expansion and maintain oxygen supplementation as indicated. Lung sounds must be assessed at least daily.

To prevent bleeding, the nurse should limit the number of venipunctures and use the smallest needle possible. A soft toothbrush or oral swabs may be used for mouth care. Male patients should use an electric razor to shave. The environment should be kept free of clutter.

Orientation and psychomotor function should be assessed. The nurse should reorient the patient on a consistent basis. The number of new people who enter the room should be limited. Mouth care should be provided before meals. The environment should be conducive to eating. Small, bland feedings may be given, especially if the patient complains of nausea. The nurse should consider the patient's food preferences and remember that a high-carbohydrate, no-protein or low-protein, low-fat diet will be ordered. The nurse should also remember that fruit juices are often well tolerated by individuals with anorexia.

The nurse should encourage the patient to discuss feelings about self-esteem while maintaining a judgment-free environment at all times. The nurse should also reinforce positive abilities and traits and help the patient identify negative automatic behaviors. Resources such as pastoral care may be used, as indicated.

Evaluation

Evaluation includes documentation of achievement of the expected outcomes and prevention or early detection of complications. Given the long-term nature of the condition, the nursing care plan should be reviewed and updated on a regular basis.

Drug-Induced Hepatitis

The older adult population has an increase in the incidence of polypharmacy and alterations in pharmacodynamics and pharmacokinetics leading to drug-induced hepatitis (Duthie et al., 2007). Because one of the major functions of the liver is the metabolism and detoxification of chemicals, including drugs, this organ is subject to potential damage from these substances. Hepatic injury may result from direct toxicity, conversion of a drug to a toxic metabolite, or immune mechanisms responding to the presence of a "foreign" invader.

Some agents cause liver cell damage in all individuals at a predictable dose level. A common example of a dose-related toxic drug is acetaminophen. With overdose of these agents, the normal metabolic pathway is exhausted and alternative means are used to clear the drug from the body. These mechanisms yield toxic byproducts.

Drugs that cause liver damage in an unpredictable manner are said to have *idiosyncratic toxicity.* These reactions are unrelated to dose and occur only in a small percentage of susceptible individuals. Idiosyncratic toxicity is manifested in a variety of ways. Massive hepatocellular injury may occur. Drugs such as isoniazid, halothane, and benoxaprofen may cause liver necrosis and possibly hepatic failure, especially in older patients. Ingestion of poisonous mushrooms causes massive cell destruction. Substances such as vinyl chloride lead to sclerosis of the portal venules and portal hypertension. Another hepatic response to toxic exposure is *cholestasis,* an arrest or cessation of normal bile flow. Drugs such as anabolic steroids, oral contraceptives, phenothiazines, and oral antidiabetes drugs cause this response. Other manifestations of liver disease from idiosyncratic toxicity include fatty changes in the liver and mass lesions such as liver cell adenoma and hyperplasia.

The clinical manifestations of drug-induced hepatitis are like those of viral hepatitis. At first, GI and influenza-like symptoms appear. Patients may be seen with jaundice, especially with the cholestatic presentation. Hepatomegaly and other signs of liver damage may also appear. The onset of symptoms may be immediate or several weeks to months after exposure to the hepatotoxic agent. In some cases, the onset of liver failure is abrupt, and the clinical course lasts only a few days, with outcomes ranging from resolution, to organ transplantation, to death.

NURSING MANAGEMENT

Assessment

In addition to the previously discussed assessments related to liver disease, it is essential that information be obtained regarding the exact name of the ingested substance, the dosage and amount taken, and the length of time since ingestion occurred. History of emesis after ingestion is also pertinent.

Diagnosis

The most common nursing diagnoses for an older patient with drug-induced hepatitis include the following:
- Need for health teaching resulting from lack of exposure to disease cause, treatment regimen, and outcome
- Potential for injury resulting from end-stage liver failure

- Need for health teaching resulting from drugs and interactions

Planning and Expected Outcomes

Expected outcomes for an older patient with drug-induced hepatitis include the following:
1. The patient will verbalize his or her understanding of the disease process and interventions.
2. The patient will not experience life-threatening complications of liver failure.
3. The patient will verbalize understanding of current drugs and their interactions.

Intervention

Nasogastric suction, if required, needs to be explained and performed in a calm manner. The nurse should also discuss the adverse effect of certain drugs with the patient and provide written material as reminders to avoid these drugs. The nurse must monitor the patient carefully for signs and symptoms of liver failure, percuss liver size, assess the skin and sclera of the eyes, and monitor the level of consciousness.

Interventions for older adults presenting with complications of liver failure are discussed in the section on Alcoholic Cirrhosis.

Evaluation

Evaluation includes documentation of achievement of the expected outcomes and prevention of complications.

GASTROINTESTINAL CANCERS

Cancers of the GI system account for more than 25% of cancer deaths in the United States each year. Cancers of the GI tract are one of the top three causes of cancer deaths in both men and women. Most tumors of the GI tract are adenocarcinomas, except for tumors of the esophagus and anus, where squamous cell malignancies predominate. Although the GI tract begins at the oral cavity and ends at the anus, oral cancer is considered along with head and neck cancers. Discussion of GI cancer will begin with cancer of the esophagus.

Esophageal Cancer

Early esophageal cancer usually remains asymptomatic. Medical evaluation is typically sought when symptoms such as dysphagia, choking when eating, hoarseness, heartburn, unintentional weight loss, and fatigue develop. Many people with esophageal cancer attribute these signs and symptoms to some of the more common disorders that affect older adults and fail to seek treatment. Because of this fact, patients with esophageal cancer have a 5-year survival rate of about 20%.

Risk factors for the development of adenocarcinoma include obesity, GERD, and a history of Barrett esophagus; for squamous cell carcinoma, risk factors include heavy alcohol consumption, cigarette smoking, diet low in fruits and vegetables, and infection with human papilloma virus (HPV). Additionally, those older than 55, men, and African Americans are at a higher risk for developing esophageal cancer.

The two main forms of esophageal cancer are adenocarcinoma and squamous cell carcinoma. Adenocarcinoma is the most prevalent form in the United States, most often affecting older white males. It typically develops at the distal portion of the esophagus. Worldwide, squamous cell carcinoma is the most common, affecting the middle of the esophagus. The tumor often metastasizes to the lungs, the liver, and the CNS.

Persons with known Barrett esophagus are urged to seek screening for esophageal cancer. The proximity of the tumor to the aorta and the trachea, in addition to the potential for metastasis, results in a generally poor prognosis. The natural history of the disease includes esophageal obstruction, coughing, hiccups, bleeding, malnutrition, cachexia, pneumonia, and death.

NURSING MANAGEMENT

Assessment

Assessment begins with an accurate history that focuses on risk factors for esophageal cancer. A review of systems may reveal symptoms of dysphagia, eating difficulties, and aspiration. A physical examination will probably reveal few findings definitive of the diagnosis. However, in advanced disease, the nurse may find palpable lymph nodes and perhaps organ enlargement resulting from metastasis. Other findings include significant and recent weight loss and substernal epigastric pain radiating to the neck, jaws, ears, and shoulder (Lewis et al., 2017).

Diagnosis

Nursing diagnoses for an older patient with esophageal cancer include the following:
- Inadequate nutrition resulting from inadequate intake of nutrients in the diet because of dysphagia
- Potential for aspiration
- Fear resulting from uncertain prognosis, possible disfigurement, and loss of ability to eat

Planning and Expected Outcomes

Expected outcomes for an older patient with esophageal cancer include the following:
1. The patient will initially stabilize weight and then achieve an individually determined weight gain.
2. The patient will remain free from aspiration.
3. The patient will verbalize fears related to the diagnosis and prognosis.

The medical treatments of radiotherapy, chemotherapy, and surgery will require additional, specific nursing interventions. The nurse should include the older adult and family in planning all aspects of nursing care related to any one or a combination of these modalities.

Intervention

Nursing management of an older patient with esophageal cancer includes maintenance of hydration and nutritional status, prevention of aspiration, maintenance of comfort, and provision of emotional support. Optimizing nutritional status and preventing further weight loss is accomplished with small, frequent feedings; high-protein, high-calorie foods; supplements such as Ensure; and tube feedings, if necessary. Nursing care to prevent aspiration focuses on assessment of respiratory status, assessment of difficulty with eating and drinking, and proper positioning during and after eating. The risk of aspiration increases in older adults when the bed is kept in the horizontal position.

The nurse's role in the prevention and early detection of esophageal cancer may lead to early identification and perhaps an improved prognosis for older patients. Persons with risk factors for esophageal cancer should be instructed on means to reduce or eliminate these factors. Counseling on the need for frequent medical follow-up, proper nutrition, and elimination of smoking and alcohol consumption is important for prevention. Older patients with frequent upper GI complaints should be advised to seek medical attention immediately.

Evaluation

Evaluation includes documentation of achievement of the expected outcomes, prevention of aspiration, and maintenance of adequate nutrition (see Nursing Care Plan: Esophageal Cancer).

Gastric Cancer

As with other forms of GI cancer, gastric cancer is insidious. Symptoms may be vague until the cancer has infiltrated and spread throughout the body, when the overt signs of cancer become evident. In addition, stomach cancer mimics other diseases such as ulcers and gastritis, so misdiagnosis and self-medication for chronic "stomach problems" are common and may delay the diagnosis and treatment of stomach cancer.

Gastric cancer is relatively uncommon in the United States; the highest incidence is currently found in Japan and China. The incidence of gastric cancer increases with age, and most individuals are diagnosed in their 70s (Rubin & Reisner, 2009). In the United States, a slight male predominance is seen. It occurs twice as often among black men and women as among whites and seems to have a familial connection. The reasons for these geographic and cultural incidences are unclear.

The cause is unknown, although the incidence is higher when gastric acid is low, as with chronic gastritis and pernicious anemia. Gastric cancer is also associated with environmental and genetic factors, including diet (e.g., diets high in salt, nitrate preserved foods and smoked foods, and diets low in fruit and vegetables), smoking, and heavy alcohol consumption. It may also be precipitated by polyps or degenerative changes in gastric ulcers, previous stomach surgery, as well as achlorhydria. Finally, occupational risks such as those faced by rubber and coal workers and those working in nickel refineries also have a role. A relationship exists between gastric cancer and infection with *H. pylori*.

Adenocarcinomas account for more than 90% of stomach cancers. Adenocarcinomas arise from the mucosal lining of the stomach. Additional types of stomach cancer are (1) lymphomas, (2) GI stromal tumors, (3) carcinoid tumors, and (4) rarely squamous cell carcinomas or small cell carcinomas. Adenocarcinomas may metastasize by extension and infiltration

◎ NURSING CARE PLAN

Esophageal Cancer

Clinical Situation

Mr. B, a 66-year-old retired salesman, has come to the outpatient clinic with a complaint of dysphagia. Within the past 4 months, he has had pain and difficulty swallowing solid food; he therefore proceeded to eating soft, then liquid foods. However, within the past month, the problem has progressed to difficulty with swallowing even liquids. He reports one episode of nocturnal regurgitation this past week. Other symptoms include a loss of 20 pounds (lb) over the past 6 months, fatigue, and a dull backache. Mr. B admits that he still smokes but has cut down from two packs to one pack a day. In addition, he admits to ingestion of beer and hard liquor, although he has cut down in amount and frequency over the past few years since his retirement.

His medical history is otherwise unremarkable. He lives alone but near his daughter, who convinced him to come to the clinic when he did not eat anything at her recent Easter dinner.

Physical examination reveals a thin, older man, with a weight of 140 lb, temperature of 98° F (36.6° C), pulse of 80 beats per minute (beats/min), respiratory rate of 18 breaths/min, and blood pressure of 120/82 mm Hg. Inspection of his oropharynx reveals no abnormalities except for poor dentition. Examination of his abdomen and rectal area is also unremarkable. Laboratory values reveal iron deficiency anemia, but initial screening is otherwise unremarkable. He is scheduled for an endoscopy the next day. He returns to the clinic 1 week later to get his results, and his diagnosis is esophageal cancer. He is scheduled for radiotherapy and possibly surgery once the tumor has shrunk in size.

Nursing Diagnoses

Inadequate nutrition resulting from inadequate intake of nutrients secondary to dysphagia

Decreased ability to swallow resulting from mechanical obstruction secondary to tumor

Fear resulting from uncertain prognosis, possible disfigurement, and loss of ability to eat

Potential for aspiration resulting from dysphagia

Outcomes

The patient will stabilize weight.

The patient will swallow safely without gagging or aspirating.

The patient will maintain adequate nutrition and hydration.

The patient and family will identify sources of fears and acquire knowledge to deal with the fears.

Interventions

Encourage small, frequent meals. Encourage the use of high-protein, high-calorie foods and the use of supplements such as Ensure. Refer to a dietitian, if necessary, for specific recommendations.

Discuss the possibility of the use of tube feedings with the patient to supplement nutrients or as the sole means of delivering necessary nutrients.

Arrange for a speech therapist consultation to provide instruction regarding swallowing.

Instruct the patient and family regarding the need for upright positioning during and after eating.

Instruct the patient and family to rotate the patient's head toward the affected side to facilitate swallowing.

Provide rest periods before, during, and after feedings.

Provide thick liquids first, adding thin liquids last; begin with cold liquids and progress to hotter ones.

Instruct the patient to begin with pureed foods, progressing to soft ones, while taking small bites.

Encourage the patient and family to verbalize fears.

Provide information to reduce distortions in perceptions.

Encourage the patient and family to attend cancer support groups.

Instruct the patient and family about impending treatments such as surgery and radiotherapy.

Assess the patient's ability to eat and drink.

Assess respiratory status before, during, and after eating.

Monitor for signs of aspiration: dyspnea, coughing, wheezing, tachycardia, and elevated temperature.

Observe and record the color and character of sputum.

Instruct the patient and family to keep the patient's head elevated during and after eating or feedings.

---

along the mucosa into the stomach wall and lymph nodes. The tumor may metastasize to the lung, bone, liver, spleen, pancreas, peritoneum, and esophagus. Once the tumor has spread outside of the stomach, cure is not possible.

Because of its elusive nature, gastric cancer is usually well advanced when symptoms begin to appear. When they do manifest, they are vague and of variable duration. Because of this, people usually delay seeking medical attention for a few months after the initial onset of symptoms. Initially, the patient may complain of a vague, uneasy sense of fullness, indigestion, and distention after meals, which may be passed off as stomach upset. As the disease progresses, anorexia, nausea, and vomiting may develop and lead to weight loss. Other symptoms include dysphagia, back pain, weakness, fatigue, hematemesis, and a change in fecal elimination patterns. Unfortunately, definitive clinical signs occur mostly with advanced disease and include weight loss, pain, vomiting, anorexia, dysphagia, and a palpable abdominal mass. Prognosis is best for tumors in the lower

stomach (antrum) and worse for tumors that occur higher in the stomach (fundus).

NURSING MANAGEMENT

Assessment

Assessment begins with a thorough history and review of symptoms pertaining to the GI system, particularly symptoms that an older patient may not report unless asked. These include indigestion, discomfort after eating, nausea, anorexia, vomiting, or any chronic "stomach problem." In addition, the nurse should question older adults regarding changes in dietary or bowel patterns and habits, use of prescription and OTC drugs, and use of home remedies. A physical examination may reveal no obvious abnormalities except that, when advanced, the tumor may be palpable, especially through the thin skin and musculature of an older patient's abdomen. In addition, lymph nodes may be palpable when metastases have occurred.

Diagnosis

The most common nursing diagnoses for an older patient with gastric cancer include the following:

- Anticipatory grieving resulting from a poor prognosis
- Inadequate nutrition resulting from gastric distress
- Acute pain resulting from gastric distress and discomfort

Planning and Expected Outcomes

Expected outcomes for an older patient with gastric cancer include the following:

1. The patient will discuss thoughts and feelings related to the diagnosis with appropriate people.
2. The patient will use appropriate resources for support counseling.
3. The patient will maintain adequate nutrition, as evidenced by stabilization and maintenance of weight and consumption of a well-balanced, high-calorie diet.
4. The patient will effectively manage pain, as evidenced by verbalization of comfort and pain relief after analgesic use.

Intervention

Nursing management of an older patient with gastric cancer includes maintenance of hydration, nutrition, and fluid and electrolyte balance, and provision of emotional support to the individual and family. Many patients and their families feel guilty and negligent about the delay in seeking medical attention for the vague symptoms of gastric cancer. The nurse may support patients and families by dispelling misconceptions and offering a realistic sense of hope.

Nursing care should also focus on the prevention and early diagnosis of gastric cancer, including encouragement for all older patients with GI symptoms, however trivial, to seek medical attention. In addition, identifying those at risk and encouraging them to seek medical care for evaluation on a regular basis is also important.

Evaluation

Evaluation includes documentation of achievement of the expected outcomes, prevention of malnutrition, maintenance of comfort, and continued family support. As the disease advances and the older patient becomes more debilitated, the focus of care will change, requiring the nurse to collaborate and coordinate with other health care team members regarding alternative care arrangements.

Colorectal Carcinoma

Cancer of the colon and rectum accounts for 14% of all cancers; it is the second cause of cancer death in the United States. Cancer of the large intestine is the third most common cause of death from a malignancy for both men and women. Colorectal cancer affects both sexes equally, and the probability of developing it increases with age. Therefore age is a significant risk factor for colorectal cancer; two-thirds of cases occur in people older than 65 years (Barker & Zieve, 2007).

Although the cause of colorectal cancer is unknown, research has indicated that diet, environment, smoking, heavy alcohol use, obesity, sedentary lifestyle, and genetics all play important parts in the development of the disease, as does a personal history of colon polyps and inflammatory disease of the bowel. Colon cancer is more prevalent in the United States, probably because the typical American diet is low in fruits and vegetables and high in red meat. A diet high in fat and refined carbohydrates and low in roughage is considered a risk factor for colorectal cancer. Genetic studies also suggest an inheritable susceptibility to colorectal cancer. Individuals with first-degree relatives diagnosed with colorectal cancer have double the risk for the development of adenomatous polyps, which are considered precursors of carcinoma.

Adenocarcinoma accounts for 95% of the carcinomas of the colon. The tumors tend to grow slowly and may remain asymptomatic for a long time. Cancer of the rectum is manifested as bright red bleeding from the rectum, along with changes in the characteristics of the stool. Carcinomas in the sigmoid and descending colon tend to grow around the bowel, encircling it and leading to an obstruction. For these patients, a change in fecal elimination pattern is a common symptom. On the right side, few symptoms are seen. If present, crampy abdominal pain may be difficult to pinpoint. Anemia may also be present.

Clinical manifestations of colorectal cancer depend on the location and extent of the tumor. Left-sided lesions often cause melena, diarrhea, constipation, and a feeling of retained stool. Right-sided tumors often cause weakness, malaise, and weight loss. Abdominal pain is rare with either type and may result from obstructions or nerve involvement. An obstruction is often the first sign of the disease. Often, if a mass is palpated on physical examination or a routine rectal examination, the stool is guaiac-positive. Although the duration of symptoms is not effective in predicting the degree of tumor advancement, the early diagnosis of cancer in asymptomatic persons has been shown to be related to improved chances of survival. Colorectal cancer in stages I, II, and III is considered curable; if the cancer does not return in 5 years after treatment, it is considered cured. Stage VI cancer is not considered curable. Should metastases occur, they are primarily to the liver and lymphatic system, although other sites include the brain, lungs, bones, and adrenal glands.

Colorectal cancers produce a wide variety of tumor antigens; the carcinoembryonic antigen (CEA) is the most well-known. The CEA level is used to gauge the effectiveness of therapy and may be useful at the time of diagnosis for prognostic value. In addition, it is used to monitor for recurrence. The current use of the CEA level in mass screening and detection is limited.

NURSING MANAGEMENT

Assessment

Assessment begins with an older patient's history of symptoms such as diarrhea, constipation, abdominal pain, blood in stools, or melena. Generalized symptoms may have been overlooked by an older patient; these include malaise, weight loss, weakness, and fatigue. Eliciting a family history of colorectal cancer, polyps, and any previous bowel surgeries is also important. Because of the potential for multiple losses with colorectal cancer, the nurse must also assess an older patient's coping skills and abilities. A physical examination may reveal a mass in the abdomen or guaiac-positive stools, or it may be unremarkable.

Diagnosis

The most common nursing diagnoses for an older patient with colorectal cancer include the following:
- Inadequate nutrition resulting from anorexia
- Acute pain resulting from GI distress
- Distorted body image resulting from a colostomy

Planning and Expected Outcomes

Expected outcomes for an older patient with colorectal cancer include the following:
1. The patient will maintain recommended weight and adequate nutrition.
2. The patient will verbalize comfort after taking an analgesic.
3. The patient will verbalize acceptance of permanent or temporary body changes resulting from a colostomy.

Intervention

Nursing management of an older patient with colorectal cancer depends on the stage of the disease and the treatment modalities necessary. In general, older patients are at risk for weight loss and malnutrition because of the cancer and symptoms of vomiting or diarrhea. Eating small, frequent, high-calorie, high-protein meals should be encouraged. Allowing patients to eat some of their favorite foods on a regular basis may help maintain the recommended weight. The use of supplements such as Ensure or nighttime tube feedings may be necessary to maintain adequate nutrition. Not every patient with colorectal cancer complains of pain, but if present, pain can be managed with both pharmacologic and nonpharmacologic relief measures. If an older patient requires a colostomy either for treatment or as a palliative measure, the patient should be encouraged to verbalize and express feelings on a regular basis. Referral to a support group or counseling may be necessary. Having an older patient speak with or visit someone with a colostomy may help reduce anxiety, concerns, and fears associated with it. If the colorectal cancer is completely resected, reminding and encouraging the older patient to have follow-up examinations and procedures to check for recurrence is of the utmost importance.

Nursing care should also focus on the prevention and early diagnosis of colorectal cancer. Nearly all colorectal cancers begin as polyps. Colonoscopy screening should begin at age 50. When caught in the early stages, colorectal cancer is nearly always curable. Older adults with identified risk factors should be taught the importance of dietary changes (e.g., low-fat, high-fiber diets) and lifestyle changes (e.g., weight loss and increased physical activity).

Evaluation

Evaluation includes documentation of achievement of the expected outcomes and prevention of complications. In addition, documentation of the patient's methods of coping with the lifestyle changes imposed by the various treatment modalities is essential.

Pancreatic Cancer

Pancreatic cancer accounts for approximately 3% of all cancer in the United States. Slightly more than 20% of affected individuals survive for 1 year after diagnosis, and the 5-year survival rate is less than 5%. Pancreatic cancer is lethal. The disease usually affects older adults; the incidence of pancreatic cancer is slightly higher in men than in women and higher in African Americans than in whites. Additional risk factors include smoking, obesity, diabetes, cirrhosis, and a family history of pancreatic cancer. An increased risk attributable to environmental factors has been suggested because the incidence is higher in those exposed to industrial pollutants or who live in urban areas.

Cancer of the pancreas is primarily an adenocarcinoma. Although the head, body, or tail of the pancreas may be involved, it is primarily a disease of the exocrine portion of the gland. It arises in the head of the organ in 60% to 70% of cases.

As tumor growth advances within the pancreas or on lymph nodes along the biliary tree, obstruction and compression of the common bile duct results. Eventually, the carcinoma may infiltrate the duodenum, stomach, transverse colon, spleen, kidney, and surrounding blood vessels. Invasion by the celiac nerve plexus accounts for the severe pain associated with cancer of the body or tail of the pancreas. Cancer of the pancreas grows rapidly, so at the time of diagnosis, the cancer has invaded locally or metastasized in 90% of individuals. Metastasis occurs through the bloodstream and by peritoneal seeding, frequently causing cancers in the lungs and bone.

Symptoms generally occur late in the course of the disease and are vague and insidious in onset. Manifestations of the disease differ according to the location of the tumor within the pancreas: pain and weight loss (tail of the pancreas), steatorrhea, weight loss, and jaundice (head of the pancreas). Nonspecific findings include anorexia, fatigue, digestive problems, blood clots, and diarrhea.

NURSING MANAGEMENT

Assessment

Assessment begins with a history of symptoms and a review of possible risk factors pancreatic cancer. An accurate assessment of the pain pattern is also important. The nurse should obtain a symptom analysis for any of the usual symptoms of nausea, vomiting, weight loss, weakness, and stool changes. A physical examination may be unremarkable.

Diagnosis

Nursing diagnoses for an older patient with pancreatic cancer include the following:
- Acute pain resulting from abdominal discomfort
- Decreased ability to cope resulting from diagnosis of terminal stage
- Decreased family's ability to cope resulting from diagnosis of terminal stage

Planning and Expected Outcomes

Expected outcomes for an older patient with pancreatic cancer include the following:

1. The patient will verbalize adequate relief of pain or ability to cope with incompletely relieved pain.
2. The patient and family will verbalize concerns and feelings related to the diagnosis and prognosis.
3. The patient and family will demonstrate improved coping strategies, as evidenced by incorporation of alternative coping behaviors and techniques in their interactions.

Intervention

Nursing management for an older patient with pancreatic cancer focuses on provision of pain relief and encouragement to verbalize feelings. Pain relief may require narcotics, and the patient and family may require teaching concerning their prolonged use. Other nonpharmacologic measures of pain relief (e.g., diversional activities, repositioning, meditation, and massage) need to be offered. The patient and family may benefit from attending a support group for cancer patients. However, because of the poor prognosis, encouraging families to spend time with the older patient is also important. Assisting the patient and family in dealing with an imminent death may also be necessary.

Evaluation

Evaluation includes documentation of achievement of expected outcomes, prevention of complications, and provision of a comfortable environment.

Liver Cancer

The incidence of primary liver cancer (hepatocellular carcinoma) is less than 5% in the United States; however, in countries where hepatitis is endemic, the incidence of primary liver cancer is as high as almost 50%. In addition to hepatitis, risk factors for the development of hepatocellular carcinoma include alcoholic cirrhosis, hemochromatosis, fatty liver disease, obesity, diabetes, anabolic steroid use, and exposure to aflatoxins (poisons produced by molds). Additionally, hepatocellular carcinoma is more common in men, Asian Americans, and Pacific Islanders.

Metastatic cancer in the liver is named after the organ in which it began (e.g., metastatic breast cancer). In the case of metastatic disease, the common original sites are the lungs, breasts, kidneys, and other organs in the GI tract. Most often, multiple masses are present in the liver and spread throughout the organ via its vascular system. The diagnosis of liver metastasis is usually an indicator that the primary cancer is incurable. Weight loss is a common early finding in cases with metastatic liver disease. Signs and symptoms of liver involvement are the late signs of organ failure (e.g., ascites and portal hypertension); by the time of the diagnosis of metastasis, the overall prognosis is poor. The 5-year survival rate is 5%; if untreated, death will occur 6 to 8 weeks after diagnosis. The cause of death is most often pneumonia, malnutrition, emboli, hepatic failure, or hemorrhage.

Nursing management of older patients with metastatic liver disease is similar to that for patients with alcoholic cirrhosis.

🏠 HOME CARE

1. Regularly monitor and assess the diagnosed GI disease or disorder for signs and symptoms indicating exacerbation or instability.
2. Weigh at regular intervals to monitor weight loss or gain; encourage homebound older adults to use nutritional supplements, if indicated.
3. Teach caregivers and homebound older adults appropriate dental hygiene practices.
4. Instruct caregivers and homebound older adults on reportable signs and symptoms related to the GI problem or disorder and when to report these symptoms to the home care nurse or health care provider.
5. Instruct caregivers and homebound older adults on the name, dose, frequency, side effects, and indications of both prescribed and OTC drugs used to treat the identified GI problem.
6. Instruct caregivers and homebound older adults about laboratory indices used to evaluate GI disturbances. Inform them of the results of any tests after the health care provider has been notified.
7. Assess and instruct older adults on the importance of maintaining hydration in the presence of GI disturbances.
8. Instruct caregivers and homebound older adults on all aspects of any treatments used to provide nutritional support in the absence of a functioning GI system (e.g., enteral nutrition, total parenteral nutrition, and formula supplements).

▌SUMMARY

Many older adults' health concerns are related to the GI system. Because these problems are often amenable to appropriate self-care practices, the nurse is responsible for teaching prevention and self-management strategies to these patients. However, the nurse must also teach older adults that GI-related symptoms should not be dismissed as part of the normal aging process; they should be reported so that an accurate determination can be made and timely interventions instituted.

▌KEY POINTS

- A decline in normal function of the GI tract may occur with aging without any effect on physiologic processes.
- A significant decrease of liver function is not an inevitable outcome of aging, but because the incidence of chronic disease increases with advancing age, liver disorders are more common in older adults.
- Any weight loss or complaint of dysphagia, indigestion, heartburn, vomiting, change in appetite, or change in stool in an older patient warrants prompt evaluation by the health care provider.

- Primary and secondary prevention of problems in the GI tract should be part of the care for all older patients (e.g., colonoscopy and dental examination).
- Smoking, alcohol, obesity, and dietary factors are important risk factors for the development of GI cancers in older patients.
- Gastric ulcers have a higher incidence of becoming malignant compared with DUs.
- Intestinal ischemia should be included in the differential diagnosis of an older patient who has a history of cardiovascular disease and complains of abdominal pain.
- Guaiac-positive stools in an older adult should be considered pathologic until proven otherwise.
- Intestinal polyps and a positive family history of polyps are the main risk factors for the development of colorectal cancer.

- Although 60% of polyps and cancers are visualized with flexible sigmoidoscopy, a colonoscopy is necessary to detect any suspected cancers in the right colon.
- Although treatment of asymptomatic gallstones is not currently recommended, the rise in new therapeutic treatment options for cholecystitis should lead to a decline in morbidity and mortality previously associated with cholecystectomies in older adults.
- GI cancers present a common concern in that the symptoms are often overlooked or self-treated until the disease has become well established.
- Although the incidence of pancreatic cancer is increasing in the United States, treatment remains palliative.
- The high correlation between polypharmacy, increased drug consumption, and age makes the older person more prone to drug-induced liver disorders.

CRITICAL-THINKING EXERCISES

1. Your patient, a 69-year-old man, has smoked at least a pack of cigarettes a day for the past 33 years. At present, he is being treated for gastric ulcers. What relationship, if any, exists between his age, smoking history, and a GI disorder?
2. Your 83-year-old neighbor confides in you that she has recently had bright red blood in her stools but thinks it is because of hemorrhoids. She is reluctant to see her doctor because she does not want to be admitted in the hospital. What advice should you give her? Why are bloody stools of particular importance in older adults? What would the plan of care be because she is older than 80 years?

3. A 65-year-old man is admitted to the hospital with a diagnosis of cirrhosis of the liver. During the shift report, his primary care nurse states that he has been agitated and anxious but has not exhibited any manifestations of alcohol withdrawal. What assumptions did the nurse make? Are these assumptions valid? Explain.
4. Discuss the nursing care measures that would be similar for an older adult patient with cirrhosis and one with hepatitis.

REFERENCES

American Geriatrics Society Ethics Committee and Clinical Practice and Models of Care Committee (2014). American Geriatrics Society feeding tubes in advanced dementia position statement. *Journal of the American Geriatrics Society, 62*(8), 1590–1593. https://doi.org/10.1111/jgs.12924.

Barker, L., & Zieve, P. (2007). *Principles of ambulatory medicine* (7th ed.). Philadelphia: Lippincott Williams & Wilkins.

Berman, H., Brooks, L., & Silver, S. (2007). A rational approach to constipation. *Geriatrics and Aging, 10*(10), 654–660.

Centers for Disease Control and Prevention. (2009a). *Oral cavity & pharynx health.* Retrieved April 10, 2009, from http://www.cdc.gov/pcd/issues/2009/jan/07_0237.htm.

Centers for Disease Control and Prevention. (2009b). *Viral hepatitis.* Retrieved April 10, 2009, from http://www.cdc.gov/hepatitis/Resources/HealthProf.htm.

Chaparro, O., & Mauricio, J. (2013). Vitamin B12 deficit and development of geriatric syndromes. *Colombia Médica, 44*(1), 43–47.

Chapman, J., Davies, M., Wolff, B., et al. (2005). Complicated diverticulitis: Is it time to rethink the rules? *Annals of Surgery, 242*(4), 576–583.

Davis, C. P. (n.d.). Hepatitis (Viral Hepatitis, A, B, C, D, E, G). Retrieved March 5, 2018 from https://www.medicinenet.com/viral_hepatitis/article.htm.

Duthie, E., Katz, P., & Malone, M. (2007). *Practice of geriatrics* (4th ed.). Philadelphia: Saunders.

Evans, W., & Draganov, P. (2006). Is empiric cholecystectomy a reasonable treatment option for idiopathic acute pancreatitis? *Nature Clinical Practice Gastroenterology & Hepatology, 3*(7), 356–357.

Forsmark, C. (2008). The early diagnosis of chronic pancreatitis. *Clinical Gastroenterology and Hepatology, 6*(12), 1291–1293.

Ginsberg, D., Phillips, S., Wallace, J., & Josephson, K. (2007). Evaluating and managing constipation in the elderly. *Urol Nurs, 27*(3), 191–200 212.

Healthy People 2020 website. (2013). http://healthypeople.gov/2020/.

Kane, R., Ouslander, J., Abrass, I., & Resnick, B. (2009). *Essentials of clinical geriatrics* (6th ed.). New York: McGraw-Hill.

LeMone, P., & Burke, K. (2008). *Medical surgical nursing: Critical thinking in patient case* (4th ed.). Upper Saddle River, NJ: Prentice Hall.

Lewis, S. L., Bucher, L., Heitkemper, M. M., & Harding, M. M. (2017). *Medical-surgical nursing: Assessment and management of clinical problems* (10th ed.). St. Louis, MO: Elsevier.

Mindikoglu, A., & Miller, R. (2009). Hepatitis C in the elderly: Epidemiology, natural history, and treatment. *Clinical Gastroenterology and Hepatology, 7*(2), 128–134.

Nettina, S. (2009). A new look at vitamin B$_{12}$ deficiency. *The Nurse Practitioner, 34*(11), 18–24. https://doi.org/10.1097/01.NPR. 0000363588.59740.6f.

Patel, J. R., Chen, A. S., Fewel, N. P., & Stock, E. M. (2016). Improving communication about constipation in a long-term care setting by using the Bristol Stool Scale. *Annals of Long-Term Care: Clinical Care and Aging, 24*(7), 25–29. https://www. managedhealthcareconnect.com/article/improving-communication-about-constipation-long-term-care-setting-using-bristol-stool-scale.

Petruzziello, L., Iacopini, F., Bulajic, M., et al. (2006). Uncomplicated diverticular disease of the colon. *Alimentary Pharmacology and Therapeutics, 23*(10), 1379–1391.

Pilotto, A., Franceschi, M., Maggi, S., Addante, F., & Sancarlo, D. (2010). Optimal management of peptic ulcer disease in the elderly. *Drugs & Aging, 27*(7), 545–558.

Rhodes, R. (2014). When evidence clashes with emotion: Feeding tubes in advanced dementia. *Annals of Long-TermCare: Clinical Care and Aging, 22*(9), 24–26. https://www.managedhealthcareconnect.com/article/when-evidence-clashes-emotion-feeding-tubes-advanceddementia.

Rubin, E., & Reisner, H. (2009). *Essentials of Rubin's pathology.* Philadelphia: Lippincott Williams & Wilkins.

Shaheen, N. J. (2006). *Effects of aging on the digestive system.* Retrieved December 2, 2013, from http://www.merckmanuals.com.

Tazkarji, M. (2008). Abdominal pain among older adults. *Geriatrics and Aging, 11*(7), 410–415.

Wolfe, M. (2006). *Therapy of digestive disorders* (2nd ed.). Philadelphia: Saunders Elsevier.

22

Urinary Function

Jennifer J. Yeager, PhD, RN, APRN

ⓔ http://evolve.elsevier.com/Meiner/gerontologic

LEARNING OBJECTIVES

On completion of this chapter, the reader will be able to:

1. Describe how aging affects normal bladder function.
2. List four possible causes of acute incontinence.
3. List the types of persistent incontinence and their clinical characteristics.
4. List the components of a continence history.
5. Discuss the role of functional and environmental assessment in the evaluation of urinary incontinence.
6. Discuss how the nurse can use tests of provocation in making a nursing diagnosis of patients with urinary incontinence.
7. Describe the behavioral interventions used to treat urinary incontinence in cognitively intact patients.
8. Develop a patient teaching plan for a patient with urge incontinence.
9. Develop a caregiver teaching plan for a patient with functional urinary incontinence resulting from dementia.
10. Describe the effects of normal aging on renal function.
11. Identify the possible causes of acute and chronic kidney disease.
12. Identify the treatment options for patients with bladder cancer.
13. List supportive services for the individual who has undergone a cystectomy.
14. Differentiate between benign prostatic hypertrophy and prostate cancer.
15. Identify the treatment options for patients with prostate cancer.
16. Apply the nursing process in the care of older adults with select urinary system conditions.

WHAT WOULD YOU DO?

What would you do if you were faced with the following situations?

- Your 72-year-old female patient denies urinary incontinence on her intake history, but you notice she brought panty liners with her to the hospital. What do you do?
- Following open reduction and internal fixation (ORIF) right femur, your patient asks if they can have a catheter inserted, as it hurts too much to get up to use the bathroom, and she is afraid she will "have an accident." How do you respond?

Urinary incontinence (UI) is one of the most common health problems affecting older adults. UI is an involuntary loss of bladder control sufficient to interfere with activities. It is a significant cause of disability and dependency. Physical health, psychological well-being, interpersonal relationships, social functioning, and health care costs are adversely affected by incontinence. Individuals with UI are at increased risk for urinary tract infection (UTI), skin problems (e.g., rashes, infections, and breakdown), and falls. Incontinence contributes to psychological distress and social isolation. It is a cause of caregiver burden and plays a significant role in the decision to place older adults in long-term care facilities. The cost of UI is staggering; the combined estimate of direct and indirect costs is upward of $65 billion per year (Ganz, Smalarz, Krupski et al., 2010).

AGE-RELATED CHANGES IN STRUCTURE AND FUNCTION

UI is not a normal part of aging. Normal age-related changes in the lower urinary tract (Fig. 22.1) increase an older adult's susceptibility to other insults in the lower urinary tract. As a result, these insults (e.g., drug side effects, UTIs, and conditions impairing mobility) are more likely to produce incontinence in older patients than in younger ones.

With age, bladder capacity decreases, the prevalence of involuntary bladder contractions increases, and more urine is produced at night. The reduction in bladder capacity and increased involuntary bladder contractions may lead to urgency and frequency. Many older adults find that they must empty their bladders more often than they did when they were younger. Increased urine formation at night leads to nocturia, defined as waking to urinate one or more times during the night (Boongird, Shah, Nolin, & Unruh, 2010). Nocturia occurs frequently in the older adult and is a major contributor to disruption in normal sleep patterns and falls.

Changes occur in the urethra because of the aging process and because of decreased levels of estrogen after menopause. Thinning and increased friability of the urethral mucosa may contribute to urgency and frequency. A decrease in muscle tone

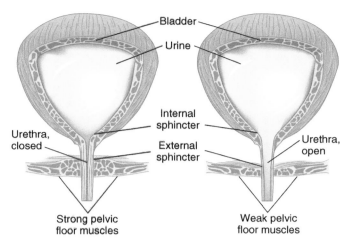

Fig. 22.1 Female urinary bladder with strong pelvic floor muscles *(left)* and weak pelvic floor muscles *(right)*. (From National Institute of Diabetes and Digestive and Kidney Diseases. [2016]. Bladder control problems in women [urinary incontinence]. Retrieved March 28, 2018, from https://www.niddk.nih.gov/health-information/urologic-diseases/bladder-control-problems-women.)

and bulk may decrease urethral resistance. In addition to the changes in the urethra, declining estrogen levels affect pelvic floor muscle tone and function.

As men age, the prevalence of benign prostatic hypertrophy (BPH) increases, with more than 50% experiencing BPH by the time they are over age 65. Enlargement of the prostate may interfere with bladder emptying and precipitate involuntary bladder contractions, resulting in incontinence or urinary retention.

PREVALENCE OF URINARY INCONTINENCE

UI is common in older adults, affecting approximately 30% of individuals (Onukwugha, Zuckerman, McNally et al., 2009). UI is more common among nursing facility residents, affecting up to 75% of all nursing facility residents (Offermans, Du Moulin, Hamers, Dassen, & Halfens, 2009). UI is an independent predictor for nursing facility admission and is associated with irritant dermatitis, pressure injuries, falls, significant sleep interruptions, and UTIs (Halter et al., 2009).

Myths and Attitudes

Despite the significant number of older adults with UI, most do not report the condition or seek medical treatment. This may be attributed to embarrassment, the belief that it is a normal consequence of aging, or the belief that it cannot be treated. Research studies have indicated that common beliefs about UI may lead older patients, particularly older women, to think that incontinence is not worth reporting to health care providers. Many health care providers do not ask patients about incontinence. And, when patients inform them about incontinence, many providers ignore the problem and do not provide adequate diagnosis and treatment.

COMMON PROBLEMS AND CONDITIONS

Acute Incontinence

UI is generally classified as either acute (transient) or chronic (persistent). Acute incontinence has a sudden onset, is generally

BOX 22.1   Causes of Acute Urinary Incontinence

- Restricted mobility
- Fecal impaction
- Atrophic vaginitis or urethritis
- Delirium
- Depression
- Psychosis
- Urinary tract infections
- Urinary calculi
- Endocrine disorders:
  - Diabetes mellitus
  - Diabetes insipidus
- Alcohol
- Caffeine
- Drugs:
  - Anticholinergics
  - Hormone therapy
  - Alpha-adrenergic blockers
  - Calcium channel blockers
  - Diuretics
  - Psychoactive drugs
  - Opioids

associated with some medical or surgical condition, and generally resolves when the underlying cause is corrected (Ouslander, 2003) (Box 22.1). Drugs are a common cause and should always be suspected in cases of new-onset incontinence. Although the exact prevalence of acute incontinence is not known, any new onset of incontinence should be considered acute and possible precipitating causes ruled out.

Chronic Incontinence

Persistent incontinence is not related to an acute illness. It continues over time, often becoming worse. Major types of persistent incontinence include urge, stress, overflow, functional, and mixed incontinence (Shenot, 2016).

Urge Incontinence

Urge incontinence is the most common type of incontinence in the older adult population. Urge incontinence may be associated with an overactive bladder. Common causes of urge incontinence include local genitourinary conditions such as UTI, drugs, bladder irritants (e.g., caffeine and carbonated drinks), bowel issues, dementia, stroke, Parkinson's disease, and cancers of the uterus and the urinary system. Individuals with urge incontinence typically give a history of involuntary urine loss after a sudden urge to void. Urgency and involuntary urine loss may be precipitated by the sound of running water, cold weather, or the sight of a toilet. Urinary accidents are sometimes large. Urge incontinence is often accompanied by nocturia and complaints of daytime frequency, with individuals often needing to void more than seven times per day (Shenot, 2016).

Stress Incontinence

Stress incontinence is the second most common form of incontinence in women. Involuntary loss of urine follows a sudden increase in intraabdominal pressure. Stress incontinence occurs as pressure in the bladder (intravesical pressure) exceeds urethral resistance. This may be caused by lack of estrogen, obesity, previous vaginal deliveries, surgeries, or all these factors. Individuals with stress incontinence often leak urine with physical exertion such as coughing, sneezing, laughing, lifting, and exercise. Older women may report leakage when they change position (e.g., get out of a chair) or lift small weights such as a small child. These activities increase intraabdominal pressure, which increases bladder pressure. If the urethra, supporting tissues, and bladder neck are abnormal, urethral resistance may be too low to withstand the increased pressure on the bladder, which results in involuntary urine loss. Stress incontinence is unusual in men, and it mainly occurs after radical prostatectomy, when the anatomic sphincters are damaged (Shenot, 2016).

Overflow Incontinence

Overflow incontinence occurs when bladder pressure in a chronically full bladder rises to a level higher than urethral resistance, causing involuntary loss of urine. Based on the history alone, overflow incontinence may be difficult to differentiate from stress or urge incontinence. It is the second most common form of incontinence in men. Typically, individuals with overflow incontinence complain of constant dribbling. They may have both daytime and nighttime accidents. Overflow incontinence may result from urethral blockage (e.g., BPH, scar tissue, stones), weakened bladder muscles, nerve injury or damage (e.g., diabetes, Parkinson's disease, and multiple sclerosis), constipation, or drugs (Shenot, 2016).

Functional Incontinence

In functional incontinence, incontinence results from physical, mental, psychological, or environmental factors interfering with the ability to make it to the toilet on time. Individuals with physical disabilities affecting their gait or their ability to undress may have difficulty reaching the bathroom on time and unbuttoning or unzipping clothes in a timely manner; individuals with cognitive impairment may not recognize their need to void or may have difficulty finding the toilet and preparing to void. Those with psychological problems such as severe depression may lack the motivation to toilet appropriately. Environmental factors may play a role in causing incontinence, especially in acute and long-term care settings. Residents confined to beds and wheelchairs, or restrained, are dependent on caregiver assistance for toileting. If that assistance is not available in a timely manner, the resident often becomes incontinent. This is especially true in the case of urgency (Shenot, 2016). Functional incontinence should be a diagnosis of exclusion.

Mixed Incontinence

Mixed incontinence is described as a combination of two or more other types: stress, urge, overflow, or functional incontinence. Among community-dwelling older adults, mixed urge incontinence and stress incontinence is common. Urge incontinence with functional incontinence is most common in residential facilities (Shenot, 2016).

Diagnosis of Urinary Incontinence

The purpose of the diagnostic evaluation for UI is threefold (Ouslander, 2003):

1. To identify potentially reversible factors that may contribute to the incontinence
2. To identify individuals who need more than a basic evaluation
3. To determine the type of incontinence so that appropriate treatment can be initiated

The basic evaluation for all persons with UI includes a history, physical examination (to include pelvic examination for women and rectal examination), postvoid residual (PVR) measurement via bladder scan, blood chemistry, and urinalysis. Urodynamic testing or cystoscopy may also be necessary (Shenot, 2016).

Incontinence can be cured, or the problem significantly alleviated, if treatable factors contributing to the incontinence are identified and appropriate medical and nursing interventions are implemented. As quality of life is significantly affected by UI, efforts to restore urinary continence should be based on an older person's satisfaction and tolerance of the interventions and strategies to achieve the outcome.

NURSING MANAGEMENT

Assessment

The purpose of the nursing assessment is to determine the type of incontinence and contributing factors so appropriate nursing interventions can be planned and implemented. In addition, nursing assessment enables the nurse to identify patients needing referral to a physician or nurse practitioner for a more complete evaluation. Assessment consists of a history assessment, functional assessment, environmental assessment, psychosocial assessment, physical examination, tests of provocation, and evaluation of bladder habits.

History

During the history assessment, information is collected about the patient's incontinence symptoms and bladder habits, general health and functional status, medical problems, current drugs, and past medical, surgical, and obstetric histories. If patients can provide the history, they are the most accurate source of data. In situations in which a patient has cognitive impairment, the nurse may need to rely on secondary sources such as family caregivers or medical records.

When taking the incontinence history, the following information should be collected:

- The onset of the incontinence
- The frequency and volume of accidents
- The circumstances that cause urine loss, including:
  - any leaking of urine when the patient coughs, sneezes, laughs, changes positions, climbs steps, exercises, has an urge to void, hears running water, is cold, or is sleeping
  - any involuntary urine loss caused by caffeine, alcohol, or any drug
  - whether the patient leaks urine and is not aware that it has occurred, has any postvoid dribbling, or leaks continuously
- Bladder habits, including the frequency and volume of daytime and nighttime urination
- Daily fluid intake, including caffeine intake

- Self-management techniques the patient has used to manage the incontinence (e.g., frequent voiding, restricting the volume or type of fluid, incontinence products, urine collection devices)
- Previous evaluation and treatment of the incontinence, including the patient's perception of the effectiveness of previous treatment measures
- Any other urinary tract symptoms, including urgency, burning, pain, hematuria, weakness of the urinary stream, intermittent stream, and difficulty emptying the bladder completely
- Bowel habits, including constipation, laxative use, and fecal incontinence

In addition to the incontinence history, the nurse should also obtain a general health history. The nurse should inquire about current medical problems, specifically problems that may affect bladder function (e.g., diabetes mellitus, congestive heart failure, bladder and kidney infections, strokes, Parkinson's disease, depression, memory problems, mobility problems, problems with coordination, and other neurologic problems or injuries). The nurse should ask about current drugs and treatments, including the use of over-the-counter (OTC) drugs or complementary and alternative medications (CAM). The nurse should inquire about previous surgeries, including past urologic or gynecologic surgery. The nurse should ask men specifically about prostate surgery and radiation; the nurse should obtain from women their obstetric history, including information about the number of pregnancies, type of delivery, any complications during delivery, and birth weights of the infants. The nurse should ask postmenopausal women about estrogen replacement therapy.

Functional Assessment

Because functional problems often contribute to UI, functional assessment is one of the most important parts of the evaluation. Information should be collected about the patient's ability to perform normal activities of daily living (ADLs), including grooming, dressing, getting in and out of bed, and walking. Patients who have difficulty performing these ADLs often have difficulty toileting. Functional status may be assessed by using unstructured questioning or by using a structured questionnaire such as the Katz Index of ADLs (Katz, Ford, Moskowitz, Jackson, & Jaffe, 1963).

Mental status should also be assessed during the functional assessment. Cognitive ability may affect the patient's ability to recognize the need to urinate, locate the toilet, and undress for toileting. In addition, knowledge of a patient's cognitive status is essential in planning nursing interventions for incontinence. The most efficient way to assess cognitive status is to use a standardized instrument such as the Montreal Cognitive Assessment (MoCA; Doerflinger, 2012).

Environmental Assessment

Environmental barriers may contribute to UI. For example, the bathroom may be too far away or inaccessible to the patient, or the toilet may be too low or difficult for the patient to get on and off. The patient may need assistance in toileting, which may not be readily available. For these reasons, environmental assessment is an important component of the evaluation of UI. It is necessary to note the following:
- Proximity of the toilet
- Any barriers between the patient's usual location and the toilet, for example, poor lighting, steps, furniture, or other objects
- The size of the bathroom: Is it large enough to accommodate the patient and any assistive devices (wheelchair or walker) that must be used?
- Toilet height: Is it adequate or too high or low?
- Presence of grab bars, if needed
- Availability of caregiver or nursing staff assistance, if needed
- Availability of a call bell, if needed

Psychosocial Assessment

Psychosocial assessment focuses on the effect of incontinence on the patient's life and on the availability and quality of caregiver assistance. The nurse should ask the patient how incontinence has affected social activities (e.g., visiting family and friends and attending social functions and church), self-esteem, mood, sexual activity, and family relationships; the nurse should also assess the patient's desire and willingness to participate in a treatment program for incontinence. Effective nursing interventions for UI require active patient involvement, so motivation is an essential component of success. If a patient does not want treatment for incontinence, the reasons should be explored. What is the reason? For example, is it knowledge deficit; depression; or an overwhelming physical, social, or psychological problem?

If the patient depends on another person's assistance in toileting, caregiver assessment is an essential component of the psychosocial assessment. Is the caregiver (1) physically able to assist the patient, (2) available on a consistent basis, and (3) willing to assist the patient? What is the caregiver's attitude toward the patient and toward incontinence? Does the caregiver have an adequate understanding of the problem and its management?

Physical Examination

The physical examination should include the following:
- Inspection of gait and balance
- Neurologic assessment of any weakness, paralysis, or sensory deficit in the lower extremities
- Abdominal examination for bladder distention, suprapubic tenderness (occurs in bladder infections), and costovertebral angle tenderness (occurs in kidney infections)
- Rectal examination for fecal impaction; rectal sensation and tone; and, in men, the size, shape, and consistency of the prostate gland
- Measurements of sitting and standing blood pressure to detect orthostatic hypotension and dizziness
- Pelvic examination, including inspection of the vagina for atrophic changes, vaginitis, cystocele, rectocele, or uterine prolapse
- Urinary stress testing: With full bladder, patient sits upright on examination table with legs spread, relaxes the perineal area, and coughs vigorously once
  - Immediate leakage that starts and stops with cough confirms stress incontinence
  - Delayed or persistent leakage suggests detrusor overactivity triggered by the cough

Bladder Habits

One of the most effective ways to assess bladder habits is to ask the patient or caregiver to keep a diary of the frequency of urination and any incontinent episodes, their relative volume, and the circumstances that precipitated their occurrence (e.g., coughing, sneezing, urgency, and changing position). Fig. 22.2 shows a sample bladder diary. Bladder diaries may be used in the home, hospital, or nursing facility and may be kept by the patient or caregiver. They provide a more objective and accurate measure of a patient's bladder habits than can be obtained by recall alone. They may be especially useful for a patient who has short-term memory problems. For bladder diaries to be accurate, patients and caregivers need careful instructions on their maintenance.

Collecting bladder diaries during assessment helps establish the type of UI and aids in planning nursing interventions.

Diagnosis

The data collected during assessment and the nurse's knowledge of UI often permit diagnosis of the type of incontinence. Sometimes, a more complex evaluation is needed to determine the cause and most appropriate treatment for UI. In any new case of incontinence, the nurse should consider acute and potentially reversible causes. If acute incontinence is ruled out or treated and involuntary urine loss persists, a diagnosis of chronic incontinence must be considered.

The following nursing diagnoses are appropriate in patients with persistent incontinence: stress UI, urge UI, overflow UI, and functional UI.

Stress Urinary Incontinence

History: The patient reports leaking urine with activities that increase intraabdominal pressure (e.g., coughing, sneezing, laughing, lifting, position changes, walking, climbing steps, or exercise).

Objective observations: Leaking urine with stress provocation; signs of pelvic floor relaxation (e.g., cystocele, rectocele, or uterine prolapse) observed on pelvic examination

Bladder records: Documentation of urine loss during physical activities that increase intraabdominal pressure

Urge Urinary Incontinence

History: The patient reports a sudden urge to void, followed by involuntary urine loss; the patient may also report that running water or cold weather precipitates involuntary urine loss.

Objective observations: Leaking urine with urge provocation

Bladder records: Documentation of urine loss associated with urgency; frequent urination and nocturia also frequently recorded

Overflow Urinary Incontinence

History: Patient histories vary, but they often show frequent involuntary urine loss of small amounts. Urine loss may be associated with physical exertion. Complaints may include decreased force of the urine stream, hesitancy, a feeling of incomplete bladder emptying, and frequent urination of small amounts of urine. Patients may also have risk factors for urinary retention such as diabetes or the use of anticholinergic drugs.

Objective observations: An elevated PVR (>100 mL) is the hallmark of overflow incontinence (Shenot, 2016). This should be part of the initial evaluation of patients with UI. On abdominal examination, a distended bladder may be detected on percussion. When overflow incontinence is associated with prostatic hypertrophy, an enlarged prostate can be detected on rectal examination. In women, a large cystocele observed during pelvic examination may suggest the cause of overflow incontinence.

Bladder records: Documentation of frequent small-volume urinary accidents

Functional Urinary Incontinence

History: The patient or caregiver reports large-volume urine loss in places other than the toilet, commode, bedpan, or urinal in the absence of symptoms of stress, urge, or overflow incontinence. The patient may be unaware of the need to void or have significant mobility impairment.

Objective observations: In pure functional incontinence, leaking is not seen with stress or urge provocation and the PVR result is normal. A mental status examination may reveal cognitive impairment. Functional assessment may reveal impaired mobility and toileting skills.

Bladder records: Documentation of involuntary urine loss (often large accidents) without symptoms of urge or stress incontinence

Planning and Expected Outcomes

For all types of UI, the nurse must determine the patient's and caregiver's desire for treatment and willingness to carry out the recommended self-care practices and interventions.

Stress Urinary Incontinence

The long-term goal is that the patient will reduce or eliminate the number of stress accidents. Short-term goals include the following:

1. The patient will master interventions (e.g., pelvic floor muscle exercises) designed to increase pelvic muscle tone.
2. The patient will recognize factors that precipitate stress accidents and use behavioral interventions to prevent accidents.

Urge Urinary Incontinence

The long-term goal is that the patient will reduce or eliminate urge accidents. Short-term goals include the following:

1. The patient will master interventions (e.g., pelvic floor muscle exercises and bladder retraining) designed to increase pelvic muscle tone and decrease urge accidents.
2. The patient will recognize factors that precipitate urge accidents and use behavioral interventions to prevent accidents.

Overflow Urinary Incontinence

The long-term goal is that the patient reduces or eliminates incontinence caused by urinary retention and overflow. Short-term goals for the patient vary, depending on the

Your Daily Bladder Diary

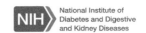

This diary will help you and your health care team figure out the causes of your bladder control trouble. The "sample" line shows you how to use the diary.

Time	Drinks		Trips to the Bathroom		Accidental Leaks	Did you feel a strong urge to go?	What were you doing at the time?
	What kind?	How much? oz, mL, cups	How many times?	How much urine?	How much urine?		Sneezing, lifting, arriving home, sleeping, etc.
Sample	Juice	8 ounces	✓✓	(sm) med lg	(sm) med lg	(Yes) No	Running
6–7 a.m.				sm med lg	sm med lg	Yes No	
7–8 a.m.				sm med lg	sm med lg	Yes No	
8–9 a.m.				sm med lg	sm med lg	Yes No	
9–10 a.m.				sm med lg	sm med lg	Yes No	
10–11 a.m.				sm med lg	sm med lg	Yes No	
11–12 noon				sm med lg	sm med lg	Yes No	
12–1 p.m.				sm med lg	sm med lg	Yes No	
1–2 p.m.				sm med lg	sm med lg	Yes No	
2–3 p.m.				sm med lg	sm med lg	Yes No	
3–4 p.m.				sm med lg	sm med lg	Yes No	
4–5 p.m.				sm med lg	sm med lg	Yes No	
5–6 p.m.				sm med lg	sm med lg	Yes No	
6–7 p.m.				sm med lg	sm med lg	Yes No	
7–8 p.m.				sm med lg	sm med lg	Yes No	
8–9 p.m.				sm med lg	sm med lg	Yes No	
9–10 p.m.				sm med lg	sm med lg	Yes No	
10–11 p.m.				sm med lg	sm med lg	Yes No	
11–12 mid.				sm med lg	sm med lg	Yes No	
12–1 a.m.				sm med lg	sm med lg	Yes No	
1–2 a.m.				sm med lg	sm med lg	Yes No	
2–3 a.m.				sm med lg	sm med lg	Yes No	
3–4 a.m.				sm med lg	sm med lg	Yes No	
4–5 a.m.				sm med lg	sm med lg	Yes No	
5–6 a.m.				sm med lg	sm med lg	Yes No	

Use this sheet as a master for making copies that you can use as a bladder diary for as many days as you need.

I used _____ pads today. I used _____ diapers today (write number).

Questions to ask my health care team: _____

_____

Fig. 22.2 Sample bladder diary. (From National Institute of Diabetes and Digestive and Kidney Diseases. [n.d.]. Your daily bladder diary. Retrieved March 28, 2018, from https://www.niddk.nih.gov/-/media/Files/Urologic-Diseases/diary_508.pdf.)

underlying mechanism responsible for the incontinence, but they might include the following:

1. The patient will seek urologic evaluation of incontinence.
2. If the patient has an atonic bladder, the patient will master in-and-out self-catheterization.

Functional Urinary Incontinence

The long-term goal is that with caregiver assistance, the patient will reduce or eliminate urinary accidents. Short-term goals for the caregiver include the following:

1. The caregiver will provide timely assistance with toileting.
2. The caregiver will remove environmental barriers to proper toileting.

Intervention

First-line nursing interventions for UI focus on lifestyle modifications and behavioral therapies. These therapies are effective for all types of UI and have limited to no side effects. Pharmacologic options are offered to patients with urge incontinence or mixed incontinence who have failed a trial lasting up to 3 months of lifestyle and behavioral therapies (Thayer et al., 2013). Despite the effectiveness of these techniques, many nurses are not skilled in their implementation. The most appropriate behavioral intervention depends on the type of incontinence and the patient's cognitive status (Du Moulin, Hamers, Paulus, Berendsen, & Halfens, 2005).

Lifestyle Modifications

Individuals with UI may decrease fluid intake to prevent accidents. This is not an effective method of managing incontinence and may lead to UTI, constipation, and dehydration. Patients and caregivers should be cautioned not to decrease fluid intake to less than six glasses a day.

Individuals with incontinence, particularly those with urge accidents, should be advised to eliminate or restrict caffeine intake. Products containing caffeine include coffee, tea, caffeinated colas, and chocolate. Caffeine has been shown to increase the occurrence of abnormal detrusor contractions, which are the cause of urge incontinence. Additionally, alcohol should be discouraged, as it is a bladder stimulant and causes increased urgency and frequency, sedation, and altered mobility.

Weight loss is another important lifestyle modification. Excessive weight increases pressure on pelvic floor muscles and the bladder. Although studies have not shown resolution of UI symptoms, significant decreases in frequency of episodes and cost of UI management have been demonstrated with decrease in weight (Cook & Sobeski, 2013).

Some older adults, even those who are continent, complain of frequent nocturia that disrupts their sleep. Getting up once at night is probably a normal effect of aging. For patients who get up more often and think that the quality of their sleep is disrupted, some measures such as restricting fluid intake in the evening may be helpful. Although it is important for patients to have adequate fluid intake, individuals with frequent nocturia should drink the bulk of this fluid before dinner. These individuals should be advised to eliminate caffeine in the evening. When an older adult goes to bed with swollen ankles and feet,

> **BOX 22.2   Suggestions for Management of Nocturia**
>
> - Restrict fluids after dinner. It is important to drink enough fluids (usually six to eight glasses a day), but the bulk of fluids should be ingested during the day.
> - Eliminate caffeine in the evening (e.g., caffeinated cola, tea, chocolate).
> - Elevate the legs in the afternoon so the feet and ankles are not swollen when going to bed.

nocturia frequently increases. Patients with such swelling should be advised to elevate their legs for several hours during the afternoon to limit the amount of edema present at bedtime (Box 22.2).

Frail older adults are at increased risk for constipation and fecal impaction, which may cause acute incontinence and exacerbate persistent incontinence. Nurses should assess bowel habits regularly and institute preventive measures such as increased fiber intake, adequate fluids, and increased activity levels.

UI increases the risk of skin rashes, infections, and skin breakdown. Frequent changes of incontinence pads and scrupulous skin care provide the best protection against these complications. For short-term use in conjunction with other treatment measures, incontinence pads or garments provide convenience and comfort. However, they are expensive for long-term use and may be associated with skin rashes and breakdown if not changed often. They should not be used as a substitute for the evaluation and treatment of incontinence.

Cognitively Intact Patients

Two behavioral interventions useful in cognitively intact individuals are bladder retraining and pelvic floor muscle exercises. These interventions may be used alone or in combination, depending on the type of incontinence.

Bladder Retraining. The patient is encouraged to adopt a gradually expanding voiding schedule with the goal of 2 to 4 hours between toileting. Retraining is useful for correcting the habit of frequent toileting and for diminishing urgency. A schedule is established for voiding times; voiding because of urgency is discouraged. This procedure is most useful for patients with urge incontinence and frequent urination.

Pelvic Floor Muscle Exercises. Kegel (1948) was the first to report pelvic floor muscle exercises as a treatment for UI. These exercises consist of alternating contraction and relaxation of the levator ani muscles, which are the muscles of the pelvic floor. These muscles, including the pubococcygeal muscle surrounding the midportion of the urethra, contract as a unit. In older adults, these muscles are often weak from disuse atrophy. Performed correctly, pelvic floor muscle exercises strengthen the muscles, increase urethral resistance, and allow the patient to use the muscles voluntarily to prevent urinary accidents (Wyman, 2003).

Clinicians often use verbal feedback during digital examination of the rectum or vagina to help patients identify their pelvic floor muscles. The nurse inserts two fingers into the vagina or one into the rectum (for men) and asks the patient to contract the pelvic floor muscles. Approximately one-third of patients can correctly identify and contract their pelvic floor muscles on digital examination and can use this exercise as a successful intervention for UI. Most older patients, however, need additional help in identifying and learning to use their pelvic floor muscles. These patients often benefit from pelvic floor muscle biofeedback. Biofeedback is not a treatment, but if appropriately used it may facilitate acquisition of the ability to contract and use the pelvic floor muscles to prevent involuntary urine loss (Burgio & Goode, 1997). During biofeedback, the patient is given immediate auditory and visual feedback of pelvic floor muscle contractions.

A variety of techniques, including vaginal probes, rectal probes, and surface electromyography, have been used to provide biofeedback. This therapy is more effective when used in conjunction with Kegel exercises.

After training with biofeedback or verbal feedback, the patient must practice the pelvic floor muscle exercises at home. The patient should be instructed to practice contracting and relaxing the pelvic floor muscles at least 45 times a day, in three or four practice sessions. The patient should exercise lying down, sitting, and standing. This facilitates the patient's ability to identify and use the muscles in any position. The nurse should remind the patient to relax the abdominal muscles when exercising, as this is essential for successful performance of exercises. The nurse may ask patients to try occasionally to slow or stop their urine stream while voiding. This allows the patients to monitor their progress in using and strengthening the correct muscles (Box 22.3).

Once patients master the exercises, they should be taught strategies to prevent involuntary urine loss (stress and urge strategies). Patients with stress accidents should be instructed to contract their pelvic floor muscles before and during activities that precipitate leaking such as coughing, sneezing, lifting, or changing position. Those with urge incontinence may be taught to contract their pelvic floor muscles to inhibit involuntary bladder contractions. A patient should respond to an urge to void by relaxing and contracting the pelvic floor muscles three or four times quickly. When the urgency subsides, the patient should walk to the toilet at a normal pace (Box 22.4).

Pessaries are an option for older women with stress or mixed UI and those with prolapse. A pessary is a stiff ring or dishlike object inserted into the vagina; it pushes against the vaginal wall and helps reposition the urethra to reduce leakage. Pessaries must be removed and cleaned monthly; if the patient is unable to perform this care, it must be done in the clinic (Thayer et al., 2013) (Fig. 22.3).

BOX 22.3 KEGEL EXERCISES

What Are Kegel Exercises?
Pelvic floor muscle exercises, also known as *Kegels* or *Kegel exercises*, are one of the best ways to improve and maintain bowel and bladder functions. They increase the strength of your pelvic floor and may improve or even eliminate bladder leakage.

There is a sling of muscles extending from the inside of the pubic bone to the anus and woven around the vagina, urethra, and rectum. This group of muscles help indirectly control the contractions of the detrusor muscle (bladder muscle) and the urethral pressures. The pelvic floor muscles relax to allow urination and tighten to stop the stream of urine. Contraction of the pelvic floor muscles closes the lower urethra, squeezing any remaining urine back up into the bladder.

Pelvic floor muscle exercises will help restore muscle function before it is permanently lost and will lessen the symptoms of incontinence.

How To Do Kegel Exercises
Like any exercise, it can be difficult at first to know that you are performing Kegels properly. But with a daily commitment, it becomes instinctive. Here are a few tips:
- **Which muscles?** If you can stop your urination flow midstream, you have identified your pelvic floor muscles. That's the most difficult part of the exercise.
- **Build up to your routine.** Performing with an empty bladder, your first goal should be to tighten your pelvic floor muscles for 5 seconds. Then relax them for 5 seconds. Try to do 5 reps on your first day. As you gain confidence from your new routine, aim for 10 seconds at a time, relaxing for 10 seconds between contractions.
- **Watch outs.** Be careful not to flex the muscles in your abdomen, thighs, or buttocks. Also, avoid holding your breath. Breathe freely during the exercises to keep from stressing the rest of your body.
- **Repeat 3 times a day.** Aim for at least 3 sets of 10 repetitions per day.
- **Give yourself encouragement.** These exercises will feel foreign in the beginning. But the longer you stay with this, the better your bladder health will become. As a bonus, Kegels have been reported to increase sexual pleasure as well.

To give your pelvic floor a full workout, there are two types of exercises you should perform. The first exercise is called a short contraction, and it works the fast twitch muscles that quickly shut off the flow of urine to prevent leakage. The muscles are quickly tightened, lifted up, and then released. You should contract as you exhale, then continue to breathe normally as you do the exercises.

The second exercise works on the supportive strength of the muscles and is referred to as a long contraction. The slow twitch muscles are gradually tightened, lifted up, and held for several seconds. At first, it may be difficult to hold the contraction for more than 1 or 2 seconds. Ultimately, the goal is to hold the contraction for 10 seconds then rest for 10 seconds between each long contraction to avoid taxing the muscles. A solid exercise plan would be to perform 3 sets of 10 short and 10 long contractions twice per day. Remember: Quality is queen here. Doing the exercises right trumps doing a bunch of them incorrectly. You should see improvements in 3 to 6 months.

As a training aid for Kegels, you can use vaginal weights, wands, or other devices that provide resistance against muscle contractions. Some of these aids are prescribed by a health professional and used under professional supervision, while others are available without prescription.

Signs of Pelvic Floor Strength Improvement
Don't be discouraged if you are not able to control your bladder as soon as you would like, but rather look for these signs as proof that your pelvic floor muscle exercises are working and that you are on your way to better bladder health:
- Longer time between bathroom visits
- Fewer "accidents"
- Ability to hold the contractions longer, or to do more repetitions
- Drier underwear, without the feeling of always being wet

Women who have difficulty performing pelvic floor muscle exercises on their own may find biofeedback therapy helpful. With professional instruction from a nurse specialist or physical therapist, many women witness significant improvement in pelvic floor muscle strength. It is crucial to remember that incontinence and pelvic floor symptoms almost always have solutions and shouldn't be shrugged off as normal. Find time each day to squeeze it into your routine.

From National Association for Continence. (2017). Kegel. Retrieved May 14, 2018, from https://www.nafc.org/kegel/.

The nurse should instruct the patient to do the following when the patient has the urge to void:
1. Stop and relax.
2. Squeeze the pelvic floor muscles three or four times quickly; do not hold.
3. Wait for the urge to pass, and then walk slowly to the bathroom during the calm period.

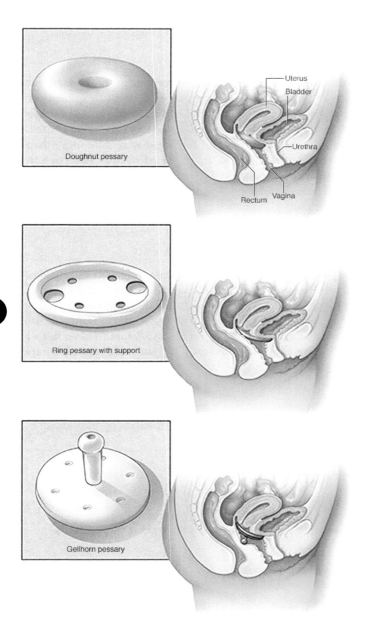

Fig. 22.3 Types of pessaries. (From Mayo Clinic Staff. [2014]. Anterior prolapse [cystocele]: Diagnosis & treatment. Retrieved March 28, 2018, from https://www.mayoclinic.org/diseases-conditions/cystocele/diagnosis-treatment/drc-20369457.)

Cognitively Impaired Patients

The techniques already described (bladder retraining, pelvic floor muscle exercises, and biofeedback) require active patient involvement. Treating UI in individuals with cognitive impairment requires the use of other behavioral techniques that depend on the caregiver rather than the patient. These include scheduled toileting, habit training, and prompted voiding. The success of these techniques in large part depends on the availability and motivation of the caregiver and the dedication of the nursing staff.

Scheduled Toileting. The patient is assisted in voiding on a regular, preset schedule. Family or professional caregivers simply take the patient to the toilet at the scheduled times, often every 2 hours.

Habit Training. Patterned urge response training (PURT) is an example of habit training. Initially, a patient's baseline voiding pattern is assessed. Once the patient's normal voiding pattern is established, the patient is assisted in voiding at the established times (Colling, Ouslander, Hadley, Eisch, & Campbell, 1992).

Prompted Voiding. Prompted voiding is most successful with patients who can recognize the need to void. It depends on active caregiver and patient involvement. The goal is to increase a patient's awareness of the need to void and increase the frequency of self-initiated toileting. Patients are approached on a regular schedule, asked if they are wet or dry, and then prompted to toilet (Box 22.5). A patient should never be forced to toilet or reprimanded for failing to toilet appropriately. Self-initiated toileting should not be discouraged. To relieve the stress that may occur because of sleep disruption for both caregiver and patient, toileting protocols may be modified for the nighttime hours.

Once contributing causes have been ruled out or treated, and if trials of scheduled toileting, habit training, and prompted voiding have failed, the use of pads and other protective garments may be the only feasible method of managing UI in the frail older adults and those with end-stage dementia (Thayer et al., 2013).

For men, external collection devices may be less expensive and less time consuming than incontinence pads or garments. However, they are associated with many complications including UTIs, skin breakdown, and ischemic disease resulting from penile constriction (U.S. Department of Health and Human Services [DHHS], 1996; Wyman, 2003). Practical external collection devices for women are not available.

The use of external collection devices requires proper preparation of the penile surface before application. The penis should be thoroughly washed and dried. It may be necessary to trim excessive hair from around the penile shaft. An adhesive-

1. Approach the patient at the scheduled times and ask if he or she is feeling wet or dry.
2. Check to see if the patient is wet or dry.
3. If the patient correctly identified his or her present continent status, give positive feedback.
4. Ask the patient if he or she prefers to use the toilet. If the response is yes, toilet the patient; if it is no, encourage the patient. *Never* force the patient to toilet.
5. Give positive feedback for appropriate toileting. Do not give any negative feedback.

enhancing skin preparation should be applied to the penile shaft and allowed to dry before condom application. Self-adhesive condom catheters, although more expensive than regular condom catheters, eliminate the need for adhesive tape. The condom catheter should be removed daily, and the penis should be inspected for irritation or skin breakdown (DHHS, 1996). The skin should be washed and dried before reapplication. If any evidence of trauma or infection is present, the condom should not be reapplied. It should be noted that treatment for genital cancer and decrease in the size of the penis associated with atherosclerosis and collagen deposition make it difficult for many older adult males to properly fit a condom catheter. A retracted penis pouch may be more appropriate in these circumstances.

Penile compression devices have been used with some success in men with mild incontinence. Issues related to comfort and decreased penile blood flow occur with improper use; penile compression devices should not be used longer than 4 hours at a time. Potential complications include edema, pain, urethral erosion, and obstruction (Moore & Lucas, 2010).

Individuals with overflow incontinence should be referred to a urologist to correct treatable causes. If the cause of incomplete bladder emptying is not correctable, measures such as the Crede method may help empty the bladder. The Crede method is performed by applying pressure over the suprapubic area to aid in the elimination of residual urine during a voiding session. If this is ineffective in emptying the bladder, the treatment of choice is often intermittent in-and-out catheterization with the use of sterile technique. Because of the high risk of associated bladder infections and urinary sepsis, indwelling catheters should be used to treat incontinence only in select circumstances (Ouslander, 2003) (Box 22.6).

BOX 22.6 Indications for Use of Indwelling Catheters

- Urinary retention that cannot be corrected medically or surgically; cannot be managed practically by intermittent catheterization; *and* is causing persistent overflow incontinence, symptomatic urinary tract infections, and/or renal dysfunction
- Pressure injury or skin lesions that are being contaminated by incontinent urine
- Provision of comfort for terminally ill or severely impaired patients

---

Evaluation

Evaluation is an integral, ongoing component of the management of UI. Patient goals are the focal point of evaluation. A patient's perception of the effectiveness of and satisfaction with his or her treatment should be assessed and documented. Many older adults with incontinence may require more than one treatment modality to achieve a satisfactory reduction in incontinence episodes. As a result, the care plan often evolves over time (see Nursing Care Plan: Mixed Incontinence and Nursing Care Plan: Functional Incontinence boxes).

AGE-RELATED RENAL CHANGES

The process of aging results in anatomic and functional changes in the renal system. Kidneys decrease in size and number of nephrons with aging. In addition, individuals with atherosclerosis experience decreased renal blood flow due to fibrous tissue and calcification-hardening renal vasculature. These factors combine, leading to a decrease in glomerular filtration rate

---

◎ NURSING CARE PLAN

Mixed Incontinence

Clinical Situation

Mrs. W is a 74-year-old retired teacher who was discharged from the hospital after amputation of a gangrenous toe. The nurse sees her three times a week to change the dressing and assess wound healing. Mrs. W's medical history includes type 2 diabetes mellitus for 26 years, complicated by peripheral neuropathy. She also has coronary artery disease (one myocardial infarction), hypertension, peptic ulcer, and rheumatoid arthritis. She has had bilateral hip replacement. She walks with a walker, and her gait is slow and sometimes unsteady. Her current drugs include insulin glargine, lansoprazole, acetaminophen, diltiazem extended release, triamterene and hydrochlorothiazide, nitroglycerin, docusate sodium, and oxybutynin. Her OTC drugs include a multivitamin, Metamucil, Citrucel, and Tums. She needs assistance with personal grooming and bathing.

She has had problems with constipation but finds that daily Metamucil and docusate sodium keep her regular. Mrs. W has been incontinent for 2 years. She describes both stress and urge symptoms, and states that she has about 14 accidents per week. She also experiences nocturia. She drinks three or four cups of regular coffee or tea a day and drinks a considerable amount of iced tea in the summer. She has seen a urologist, and he prescribed oxybutynin for her. She has been taking it for 2 years. Although it somewhat reduced the number of accidents, she does not think it is very effective. She finds the incontinence disturbing and wishes something more could be done.

Nursing Diagnosis

Inadequate urinary elimination

Outcomes

The patient will master pelvic floor muscle exercises.
The patient will experience a decrease in the number of urinary accidents.

Interventions

Ask the patient to keep a baseline bladder diary before treatment.
Teach the patient pelvic floor muscle exercises using verbal feedback of pelvic floor muscle contractions during rectal examination.
Provide written instructions for practicing the exercises.
Ask the patient to continue to keep bladder diaries during treatment.
Review the diaries and assess the patient's progress during weekly visits.
Once the patient has mastered the exercises, teach strategies to manage urge incontinence and then strategies for stress incontinence, if indicated by the diaries.
If the patient is unable to identify her pelvic floor muscles using verbal feedback or is not making adequate progress, refer her to the nurse specialist who deals with continence for biofeedback.
Advise the patient to substitute decaffeinated coffee and tea for the regular coffee and tea that she now drinks.

EVIDENCE-BASED PRACTICE

Evaluation of Function as Indicator of Urinary Incontinence

Background

UI in older adults has gained attention during the past decade as the number of older adults increase. Up to 77% of residents in long-term care are incontinent of urine. It is important to identify the risk factors for UI, so effective management strategies can be implemented.

Sample/Setting

The sample encompassed 77 older adults residing in a long-term care facility in Pingtung County, Taiwan. Participant ages ranged from 65 to 105 (mean age 76.87 ± 7.88) and included 23 women and 54 men. A total of 28 (35.9%) reported incontinence at least once a week (32.7% for men and 43.5% for women).

Methods

Face-to-face interviews were conducted that included completion of a structured sociodemographic questionnaire and the following open-ended question: "In the past 4 weeks, how often have you leaked urine?" In addition to body mass index (BMI) and waist circumference (WC), eight tests of functional status were completed: five-time chair-stand test (CST), 6-minute walk, arm curl, chair sit-and-reach (CSR), 8-foot up-and-go (UG), grip test, and back scratch.

Results

Participants with UI had poor performance on the following functional measures: five-time CST ($p = 0.017$), 8-foot UG ($p < 0.001$), CSR (right side, $p = 0.026$; left side, $p = 0.005$), and grip strength ($p = 0.017$). Just two measures were significant independent predictors for UI (8-ft UG, $p = 0.018$; CSR right $p = 0.018$, left $p = 0.010$). The 8-foot UG and CSR contribute to body strength and power and provide the ability of gait or mobility.

Implications

The study shows that "poor functional performance on the measurements of 8-foot UG and CSR are the predominant determining factors of UI for institutionalized older adults, implying that the function of the lower body has a potential role in the development of urinary incontinence" (p. 300).

From Chiu, A. F., Huang, M. H., Hsu, M. H., Liu, J. L., & Chiu, J. F. (2015). Association of urinary incontinence with impaired functional status among older people living in a long-term care setting. *Geriatrics & Gerontology International, 15*, 296-301. doi: 10.1111/ggi.12272.

◎ NURSING CARE PLAN

Functional Incontinence

Clinical Situation

Mrs. B is an 83-year-old retired housekeeper who receives visits from a nursing agency for congestive heart failure. Mrs. B was diagnosed with mild Alzheimer's disease 3 years ago. She lives with her niece, who is also her primary caregiver. Mrs. B is legally blind. She had a fall and fractured her right hip 1 year ago. She has a moderate amount of bilateral ankle and foot edema. She also suffers frequently from constipation. Her current drugs include furosemide, a calcium channel blocker, and a stool softener. She requires assistance with ambulation and ADLs. She has had UI for 3 years. Mrs. B generally feels the urge to void but has frequent accidents. Mrs. B now requires incontinence undergarments. She also has enuresis, and the pad is usually wet in the morning.

Nursing Diagnosis

Inadequate urinary elimination

Outcomes

The patient's caregiver will master a prompted voiding and toileting program with the patient.
The patient will experience a reduction in the number of episodes of incontinence.

Interventions

Collect baseline bladder diaries to establish the frequency of UI and precipitating factors.
Assess the caregiver's willingness to participate in a behavioral program to treat the patient's incontinence.
Teach the caregiver how to implement a prompted voiding program.
Assess the patient's understanding by having her conduct a return demonstration of the technique.
Visit weekly to assess implementation and success of the program.
Have the caregiver keep the bladder diaries during treatment.
Assess the patient's daily fluid intake.
If daily fluid intake is less than six to eight glasses of fluid per day, instruct the caregiver to increase the patient's fluid intake.
Instruct the caregiver to restrict the patient's fluids in the evening, providing the bulk of her fluids during the day.
Instruct the caregiver to restrict the patient's caffeine intake and eliminate caffeine in the evening.
Instruct the caregiver to have the patient elevate her legs in the afternoon to reduce the amount of edema.

(GFR). Despite the anatomic and functional changes associated with age, the kidneys remain capable of performing their functions well into the ninth decade of life unless acute illness or comorbidities result in renal dysfunction.

As persons age, renal mass decreases by 80 grams between 40 and 90 years of age. However, it has been determined that a decrease in renal mass corresponds to a decline in overall body surface area that occurs with aging. Renal blood flow decreases by 10% for every decade beyond the age of 40. With decreases in renal mass, functioning glomeruli, and blood flow, GFR is affected. GFR remains stable until about age 40, and then falls at a rate of 8 milliliters per minute (mL/min) per 1.73 square meters (m^2) per decade. Individual variances affect age-related changes in the renal system and decline in GFR; no two people age in the same way (Weinstein & Anderson, 2010).

The effect of aging on the renal system has implications for clinical management. Changes in renal function affect all aspects of pharmacokinetics. Drug dosages should be adjusted based on GFR or creatinine clearance. Older adults lack adaptive mechanisms; therefore fluid and electrolyte alterations may occur in the setting of acute illness. It is also important for nurses to recognize comorbidities likely to affect renal function in the older adult population, for example, cardiovascular disease and diabetes.

COMMON RENAL PROBLEMS AND CONDITIONS

Acute Kidney Injury

Acute kidney injury (AKI) is the sudden decline in renal function accompanied by fluid and electrolyte alterations, and acid–base disturbance. It may or may not be associated with oliguria. AKI is classified as prerenal, intrinsic, or postrenal based on causative factors (Box 22.7).

Prerenal failure occurs because of inadequate perfusion (e.g., fluid sequestration in liver failure or heart failure). It is not accompanied by parenchymal damage; therefore restoring perfusion should restore renal function.

Intrinsic failure occurs because of abnormalities within the kidney and may be caused by ischemia, sepsis, inflammation, or injury. Acute tubular necrosis (ATN) is the most common cause of intrarenal failure. The three stages of ATN are as follows:

1. **Initiation:** Blood urea nitrogen (BUN) and creatinine levels rise and urine output decreases.
2. **Maintenance:** Continued decrease in renal function lasting for 7 to 21 days during which supportive therapy (e.g., dialysis) may be necessary.
3. **Recovery:** Urine output increases accompanied by a decrease in BUN and creatinine levels. During this time, regeneration of tubular epithelial cells occurs.

Postrenal failure results from an obstructive or mechanical process in the urinary tract (e.g., renal calculi or BPH) that interferes with the outflow of urine. Removal of the obstructive process usually restores renal function.

In older adult patients who experience AKI, evaluation should begin with an attempt to determine the underlying cause. Once the cause is corrected, renal function is typically recovered. Clinical manifestations of AKI include fluid and electrolyte disturbances, metabolic acidosis, and uremic symptoms (e.g., anorexia, nausea, anemia, fatigue, edema, and crackles). The patient may also have a history of exposure to nephrotoxic substances or recent infection. Mortality from AKI exceeds 60% (Murugan & Kellulm, 2011).

The diagnosis of AKI is made based on elevated BUN level, elevation in serum creatinine, and decrease in creatinine clearance accompanied by decrease in urine output. In addition to correcting the underlying cause of AKI, treatment includes correction of acidosis and hematologic abnormalities, removal of nephrotoxic agents, and maintenance of fluid hemostasis.

Chronic Kidney Disease

Chronic kidney disease (CKD) is the presence of kidney damage for more than 3 months accompanied by decrease in GFR (Box 22.8). The symptoms manifested depend on the extent of the disease. The five stages of CKD are as follows (Arora, 2017):

- Stage 1: Kidney damage with normal or increased GFR (>90 mL/min/1.73 m^2)
- Stage 2: Mild reduction in GFR (60–89 mL/min/1.73 m^2)
- Stage 3a: Moderate reduction in GFR (45–59 mL/min/1.73 m^2)
- Stage 3b: Moderate reduction in GFR (30–44 mL/min/1.73 m^2)
- Stage 4: Severe reduction in GFR (15–29 mL/min/1.73 m^2)
- Stage 5: Kidney failure (GFR <15 mL/min/1.73 m^2 or dialysis)

BOX 22.7 Types of Acute Kidney Injury

Prerenal
- Absolute decrease in circulating volume
  - Hemorrhage
  - Dehydration
  - Burns
- Relative decrease in circulating volume
  - Distributive shock (neurogenic, anaphylactic, septic)
  - Third-spacing and edema
  - Decreased cardiac output
    - Cardiogenic shock
    - Dysrhythmias
    - Cardiac tamponade
    - Heart failure
    - Myocardial infarction
- Primary renal hemodynamic abnormalities
  - Occlusion or stenosis of renal artery*
  - Drug-induced impairment of renal autoregulation in susceptible persons†

Postrenal
- Benign prostatic hyperplasia
- Kinked or obstructed catheters
- Intraabdominal tumors
- Strictures
- Calculi

Intrarenal/Intrinsic
- Tubular (acute tubular necrosis)
  - Ischemic
    - Prolonged prerenal failure
    - Transfusion reactions
    - Rhabdomyolysis
  - Nephrotoxic
    - Prolonged postrenal failure
    - Certain antimicrobials (antibiotics; antifungal and antiviral drugs)
    - Radiographic contrast media
    - Certain cytotoxic chemotherapy agents
    - Recreational drugs (amphetamines, heroin)
    - Environmental agents (heavy metals, carbon tetrachloride, insecticides)
  - Snake and insect venom
  - Glomerular
    - Acute glomerulonephritis
  - Interstitial
    - Acute allergic interstitial nephritis
    - Acute pyelonephritis
  - Vascular
    - Vasculitis
    - Emboli
    - Nephrosclerosis (due to primary hypertension, hypertensive emergencies, and urgency)

*Use of ACE inhibitors or all receptor blockers increases the risk.
†Preexisting chronic renal insufficiency, cirrhosis, heart failure, or elderly persons (>60 years) with atherosclerotic cardiovascular disease, hypotension, diuretic use, or nephritic syndrome.
Adapted from Copstead, L., & Banasik, J. (2013). *Pathophysiology* (5th ed.). St. Louis, MO: Elsevier.

BOX 22.8 Risk Factors for Chronic Kidney Disease

- Acute tubular necrosis (not progressing beyond the oliguric stage)
- Developmental/congenital conditions
  - Renal agenesis
  - Aplastic kidneys
  - Renal hypoplasia
  - Ectopic/displaced kidneys
  - Fused kidneys
- Cystic disorders
  - Polycystic kidney disease
  - Medullary cystic disease
- Neoplasms
  - Benign tumors of the kidney
  - Malignant tumors of the kidney (including Wilms tumor)
- Infections
  - Recurrent pyelonephritis
  - Renal tuberculosis
- Glomerulonephritis

- Systemic conditions
  - Diabetes mellitus*
  - Diabetes insipidus
  - Hypertension*
  - Hyperparathyroidism
  - Liver failure/cirrhosis
  - Gout
  - Amyloidosis
  - Scleroderma
  - Goodpasture syndrome
  - Systemic lupus erythematosus (produces glomerulonephritis)
- Other
  - Genetics
  - Increasing age
  - Race (blacks)
  - Overweight/obesity
  - Dyslipidemia
  - Family history of cardiovascular disease
  - Smoking

*Most common risk factors.
Adapted from Copstead, L., & Banasik, J. (2013). *Pathophysiology* (5th ed.). St. Louis, MO: Elsevier.

PATIENT/FAMILY TEACHING

Chronic Kidney Disease

The kidneys perform crucial functions that affect all parts of the body. The kidneys, in fact, keep the rest of the body in balance and working properly. When CKD causes the kidneys to fail, the whole body stops functioning correctly, and the person can become extremely ill unless the condition is treated.

How Do the Kidneys Work?

The kidneys are the size of a person's fist and are located on either side of the spine. Each kidney has about a million working units called *nephrons*. Nephrons are the kidney's filters. Once blood is filtered, the waste products are removed from the body as urine.

The kidneys' job is to cleanse the blood of wastes, excess fluid, and drugs; release hormones and vitamins; and control red blood cell production.

The kidneys are also responsible for regulating the body's salt, potassium, and acid content.

What Causes Chronic Kidney Disease?

Several different types and causes of CKD exist. *Glomerulonephritis,* which is inflammation of the kidney, damages the nephrons. *High blood pressure,* whether a result of a kidney disorder or a cause of kidney disease, may hasten kidney failure. *Diabetes mellitus,* the leading cause of CKD, results from damage to the kidney caused by chronically high blood sugar levels. *Polycystic kidney disease* is an inherited disorder in which cysts form on kidney tissue and eventually destroy the healthy kidney tissue. *Physical abnormalities present at birth* may cause obstructions, which may lead to infection and destruction of kidney tissue. *Interstitial nephritis,* usually caused by drug use, is an inflammation of kidney tissue and leads to eventual destruction of the kidney.

What Are the Signs of Kidney Failure?

Because kidney failure sometimes gives no warning signs, it may go undiagnosed until it is well advanced. However, some warning signs may be present:

1. Decreased energy and fatigue
2. Trouble concentrating
3. Puffiness around the eyes
4. Loss of appetite
5. Nighttime muscle cramps
6. Swelling in feet and ankles
7. Dry, itchy skin
8. Urinating more frequently at night
9. Nausea and vomiting

How Is Kidney Failure Treated?

In the early stage of kidney failure, the disease may be slowed by ensuring control of high blood pressure and control of other chronic diseases such as diabetes. Additionally, the patient may be asked to take drugs to treat anemia, reduce swelling, lower cholesterol, and protect bones. The diet may be changed as well, to reduce waste products in blood. However, as the disease progresses and the kidneys no longer perform their duties of removing bodily wastes, other treatments must be used. Blood must be cleansed by using an artificial kidney (hemodialysis) three times a week at a special facility or at home or by introducing a cleansing solution into the abdomen (peritoneal dialysis), performed daily in the home. Kidney transplantation, in which healthy, donated kidneys replace the failed kidneys, may restore normal kidney function.

Outlook

No cure exists for CKD. Following the program prescribed by the health care provider is vitally important as it helps live with kidney failure. Many people with kidney disease manage to live active, productive lives.

Adapted from The National Kidney Disease Education Program. (2012). Chronic kidney disease: What does it mean for me? NIH Publication No. 12-7408. Retrieved August 30, 2014, from http://nkdep.nih.gov/resources/kidney-disease-mean-for-me-508.pdf.

Typically, patients with CKD stages 1 to 3 are asymptomatic. On entering stages 4 and 5, patients may develop weakness, edema, fatigue, hypertension, heart failure, impaired cognition and immune function, dry skin and pruritus, anorexia, nausea, malnutrition, increased bleeding, anemia, peripheral neuropathy, and an overall decreased quality of life. Management strategies include treatment of the underlying cause of CKD, aggressive control of blood pressure (systolic blood pressure [SBP] $\leq$130 mm Hg and diastolic blood pressure [DBP] $\leq$80 mm Hg), treatment of hyperlipidemia, blood sugar control in diabetics (glycated hemoglobin [Hb $_{A1c}$] <7%), avoidance of nephrotoxic drugs (e.g., nonsteroidal antiinflammatory drugs [NSAIDs]) and use of angiotensin-converting enzyme inhibitors (ACEIs) and angiotensin receptor blockers (ARBs) in individuals with proteinuria (protein >300 mg/24 hours). Additional management strategies include restricting sodium, potassium, and phosphorus in the diet; restricting protein in the diet; restricting fluid intake; weight management and promotion of exercise; and use of multivitamins and iron supplements (see Patient/Family Teaching: Chronic Kidney Disease box).

The diagnosis of CKD is usually made based on an increase in creatinine and BUN, and a decrease in creatinine clearance. Additionally, tests are performed to evaluate blood sugar levels, parathyroid hormone and calcium levels, hematocrit and hemoglobin levels, other iron studies, and reticulocyte count. Urinalysis is performed to determine the amount of protein in urine. The remainder of the evaluation is identical to that in a patient with AKI. Treatment of renal failure in an older adult is initially conservative. Older adult patients with kidney failure generally have concomitant diseases such as diabetes, cardiac disease, or cancer.

NURSING MANAGEMENT

Assessment

Assessment of an older adult with kidney disease should include thorough health history taking and physical examination; special attention should be paid to the drug history. Box 22.9 summarizes the nursing history and physical assessment data to be obtained.

Diagnosis

Appropriate nursing diagnoses for a patient with CKD include the following:
- Fluid overload resulting from compromised urinary regulatory mechanisms
- Inadequate nutrition resulting from anorexia
- Potential for infection resulting from a compromised immune system
- Need for health teaching resulting from lack of exposure to disease process, treatment regimen, and follow-up care
- Inadequate coping resulting from uncertain outcome of illness
- Reduced stamina resulting from fatigue
- Inadequate toileting self-care resulting from weakness and fatigue

---

BOX 22.9 Nursing Assessment of Renal System

History
- Personal or family history of renal disease
- Recent surgeries or illnesses (predisposing to renal dysfunction)
- Symptoms:
  - Urine (e.g., frequency, color, amount, appearance)
  - Nausea and vomiting
  - Anorexia
  - Weight loss
  - Confusion
  - Fatigue
  - Pruritus
  - Edema
- Drugs (e.g., antibiotics, antineoplastics, and nonsteroidal antiinflammatory drugs)
- Diet
- Current support systems

Physical Assessment
- Neurologic status: altered mental status and presence of asterixis
- Cardiopulmonary status: rales and pericardial rub
- Gastrointestinal status: nausea and vomiting, abdominal discomfort, and intolerance to diet
- Musculoskeletal status
- Ophthalmoscopic examination and visual inspection

- Potential for reduced skin integrity resulting from pruritus and immobility
- Reduced cardiac output resulting from fluid volume excess
- Alteration of protective mechanisms resulting from nutritional deficiencies (anemia)
- Inadequate sexuality pattern resulting from uremia and psychological effects of CKD

Planning and Expected Outcomes

The development of a care plan for an older adult with renal failure must include the patient and family or significant others because of the potential for self-care deficits. Expected outcomes include the following:
1. The patient will achieve a normal level of fluid volume use, as evidenced by reestablishment of baseline "dry" weight.
2. The patient will consume a well-balanced, appropriately restricted diet on a regular basis.
3. The patient will remain free from infection, as evidenced by an afebrile state during hospitalization.
4. The patient will demonstrate knowledge of the disease process and therapeutic regimen, as evidenced by adherence to prescribed self-care and other treatment measures.
5. The patient will demonstrate the use of effective coping strategies, as evidenced by verbalization of feelings and seeking of support.
6. The patient will demonstrate the ability to carry out ADLs without undue stress or fatigue.
7. The patient will maintain skin integrity, as evidenced by no reddened areas or broken skin.
8. The patient will have adequate cardiac output as evidenced by absence of pulmonary crackles.

BOX 22.10 Renal Diet

Managing the diet of a patient with chronic kidney disease ("renal diet") is a challenge. A balance between sufficient calories and protein must be achieved. Patients' chronic kidney disease typically have a high metabolic demand that requires a high caloric intake. Sufficient amounts of protein and calories must be provided to prevent catabolism while preserving kidney function. A renal diet is typically restricted in fluid, sodium, potassium, phosphorus, and protein. The extent of diet restriction depends on the degree of renal dysfunction. A dietitian should be involved to assist with diet modification. Following the diet prescribed by the physician will prevent further complications of renal dysfunction.

Calories

Calories are important for maintaining energy and preventing weight loss. Much of the caloric intake may come from carbohydrates and unsaturated fat. If a need to increase caloric intake exists, margarine and oils that are low in cholesterol may be considered. Jams, jellies, sugar, and honey may also be added to the diet.

Potassium

Alterations in potassium levels may cause significant illness and even life-threatening arrhythmias of the heart. It is important to maintain a low-potassium diet because in kidney failure, the kidneys are unable to rid the body of potassium in normal quantities. Foods high in potassium include dried beans, nuts, fruits, vegetables, chocolate, mushrooms, potatoes, and prune juice.

Sodium

Elevation in sodium levels causes fluid retention. This may lead to congestive heart failure and edema. It is very important to control the intake of sodium. Teaching patients to get into the habit of reading the labels on food packages is essential.

Fluid

Fluid intake consists of anything that becomes liquid at room temperature. Too much fluid may lead to weight gain, congestive heart failure, edema, shortness of breath, and high blood pressure. The amount of fluid intake is dependent on the degree of renal dysfunction.

Vitamins and Minerals

Vitamin supplementation is often necessary in patients with renal failure. Typically, supplements of folic acid, pyridoxine, and water-soluble vitamins are necessary.

Adapted from Copstead, L., & Banasik, J. (2013). *Pathophysiology* (5th ed.). St. Louis, MO: Elsevier.

BOX 22.11 What Is Peritoneal Dialysis?

Peritoneal dialysis is a type of dialysis performed when the renal system fails and can no longer adequately control the removal of waste products. It is indicated when drugs and changes in diet and fluid intake can no longer control renal dysfunction.

A membrane in the abdomen, called the *peritoneum,* lines the abdominal organs and the abdominal wall. This membrane is porous and has a rich supply of blood. Before peritoneal dialysis can begin, a catheter is inserted into the peritoneal cavity; this permits the fluid to run in. A prescribed dialysate solution is run into the peritoneum and permitted to dwell for a certain period. During the dwell period, waste products are removed from the blood through the peritoneal wall into the dialysate solution.

The patient, in conjunction with his or her health care provider, chooses one of two types of peritoneal dialysis: (1) continuous ambulatory peritoneal dialysis (CAPD) and (2) continuous cyclic peritoneal dialysis (CCPD).

CAPD is done continuously, 7 days a week. It involves the use of an indwelling catheter, connective tubing, and dialysate. If the patient needs certain electrolytes, they can be added to the dialysate solution. During the dwell period, these substances move through the peritoneal membrane and into the patient's blood supply to restore normal electrolyte concentrations. Dialysate dwells in the peritoneal cavity for 4 to 8 hours while "dialysis" occurs. The tubing is clamped, and the bag is rolled up under the patient's clothing. Normal daily activities may be performed during the dwell time. Once the dwell period ends, the dialysate is drained, and the peritoneum is filled with a new bag of dialysate.

In CCPD, an indwelling catheter, dialysate, and a cycling machine are used. Before the individual goes to sleep, he or she must be connected to the machine, which will cycle dialysate solution in and out of the peritoneum three to five times during the night, allowing for a prescribed dwell period. In the morning, the last cycle runs in and is permitted to dwell for the entire day. At the end of the day, the solution is drained, the patient is connected to the cycler, and the process is restarted.

Complications

Complications associated with peritoneal dialysis include *peritonitis,* an infection of the peritoneal wall. Infections involving the catheter tunnel and the exit site of the catheter may also occur. It is important for the patient to recognize and immediately report signs of infection (e.g., abdominal pain, fever, and dialysate solution that appears cloudy after it is drained from the abdomen).

Outlook

Peritoneal dialysis is an alternative for a failed renal system, but it does not cure the disease. Patients with chronic renal failure need to undergo some form of dialysis for the remainder of their lives or until they undergo successful transplantation. Many patients lead nearly normal lives with peritoneal dialysis and modifications in diet and fluid intake.

Data from Halter, J., Ouslander, J., Tinetti, M., Studenski, S., High, K., & Asthana, S. (2009). *Hazzard's geriatric medicine and gerontology* (6th ed). Philadelphia, PA: McGraw-Hill; Healthwise Staff. (2011). Information and resources: Peritoneal dialysis. Retrieved September 28, 2013, from http://www.webmd.com/a-to-z-guides/peritoneal-dialysis-4391.

9. The patient maintains hemoglobin above 10 g/dL.
10. The patient and partner express satisfaction with expression of intimacy.

Intervention

Interventions for an older adult with renal failure should focus on maintaining fluid and electrolyte balances; monitoring nephrotic symptoms; educating about treatment regimens, dietary management, and drug usage; and managing fatigue and low energy levels. Patients and their significant others must be educated on the interventions. The typically prescribed diet is a low-protein, low-sodium, low-potassium, and low-phosphorus diet. At times, the diet is less than palatable, so with the normal age-related changes in the sense of taste and smell, adherence to a renal diet presents a challenge. The use of spices and seasonings to enhance taste may be helpful. For those individuals with CKD who experience nausea resulting from uremic symptoms, it might be beneficial to administer a prescribed antiemetic before meals (Boxes 22.10 to 22.12, and Patient/Family Teaching: Management of Kidney Disease).

BOX 22.12 What Is Hemodialysis?

Hemodialysis is a type of dialysis performed when the renal system can no longer clear wastes effectively. It is indicated when drugs and alterations in diet and fluid intake are no longer effective in the management of kidney disease. Hemodialysis involves the use of an artificial kidney and a dialysis machine. Each hemodialysis treatment lasts 3 to 4 hours and typically is performed three times a week. Hemodialysis differs from peritoneal dialysis in that the clearance of waste products occurs outside the body and the treatments are done at an outpatient dialysis center rather than at home.

For hemodialysis, access to the bloodstream is necessary. This access could be a large intravenous tube placed in a vein in the neck or chest. If the patient has chronic kidney disease (CKD), a permanent access, termed a *fistula* or a *graft*, is surgically placed. During the hemodialysis treatment, the patient's blood and a prescribed dialysate solution circulate continuously through the artificial kidney. Waste products are cleared, and electrolytes are stabilized at this time, and cleaned blood is returned to the body. When the treatment is complete, the nurse removes the needle access to the fistula or graft. The first few hemodialysis treatments are slow and short to avoid any complications.

Complications

Complications that may occur during or after hemodialysis treatment consist of low blood pressure, rapid heart rate, and dry mouth, which could indicate that too much fluid has been removed. The patient could also experience high blood pressure, fast heart rate, and shortness of breath, which could indicate that not enough fluid has been removed from the body. If these symptoms occur during treatment, the patient should notify the nurse immediately. If they occur after treatment and the patient is at home, it is just as important to notify the physician immediately.

PATIENT/FAMILY TEACHING

Management of Kidney Disease

Patient education should include the following factors:
- Cause of the kidney disease
- Prescribed diet and fluid regimen
- Self-observation skills (e.g., measuring temperature, pulse, respiration, blood pressure, intake and output, and daily weight)
- Personal hygiene
- Exercise and rest programs
- Drug regimen (e.g., name, purpose, dosage, dosing schedule, and adverse reactions)
- Schedule of medical follow-up

Modified from National Institute of Diabetes and Digestive and Kidney Diseases. (2016). Managing chronic kidney disease. Retrieved March 5, 2018, from https://www.niddk.nih.gov/health-information/kidney-disease/chronic-kidney-disease-ckd/managing.

With the varied treatment options available to the individual with renal failure, it is important to educate patients and significant others about prescribed modalities. The National Kidney Foundation provides patient and family resources helpful to persons with CKD.

Evaluation

Evaluation is an important component in the care of older adults with CKD. Subjective data include the patient's reported symptoms and quality of life. Objective data include improved or stable renal function, as evidenced by stable levels of BUN and creatinine, hematocrit, and fluid and electrolytes.

Urinary Tract Infection

UTI and asymptomatic bacteriuria are common in the older adult population. The prevalence of bacteriuria increases dramatically in women and men older than the age of 80. The incidence of bacteriuria is higher in women than men, partly because of the proximity of the urethral meatus to the rectum. The incidence is also higher for residents of long-term care facilities compared with those living at home. Higher rates of bacteriuria in nursing facilities are likely caused by the increased incidence of soiling, incomplete bladder emptying, and bladder catheterization. Risk factors for development of UTIs include brain attack, Parkinson's disease, cognitive impairment and dementia, decreased functional status, bladder catheterization, and antibiotic use (Halter et al., 2009). *Escherichia coli* continues to be the most common infectious organism. Other common organisms are *Proteus, Klebsiella, Enterobacter, Serratia,* and *Pseudomonas.* Methicillin-resistant *Staphylococcus aureus* (MRSA), vancomycin-resistant *Enterococcus* (VRE), and fluoroquinolone-resistant gram-negative bacilli are becoming more prevalent as the causative organisms found in UTIs, especially in the long-term care setting (Phillips, Adipoju, Stone et al., 2012).

Clinical presentation of UTI in older adults includes dysuria, urgency, frequency, and hematuria secondary to damaged superficial blood vessels in the mucosa of the bladder. These symptoms are typical of lower UTIs. If the infection is in the upper urinary tract, older patients may manifest fever, chills, and flank tenderness in addition to mental status changes. If an older patient is also experiencing bacteremia, signs and symptoms of septic shock may be seen. Nurses are cautioned to remember the atypical presentation of acute illness in older adults.

Frequently, older adults present with bacteria on urinalysis (>100,000 colony-forming units per milliliter [CFU/mL] in a clean-catch specimen) without accompanying symptoms of UTI; this is referred to as *asymptomatic bacteriuria* (ASB). Research has not demonstrated any benefit to treating ASB; the use of antibiotics in this situation has the potential for harm. Despite the evidence, residents in long-term care facilities frequently receive antibiotic therapy for ASB (Phillips et al., 2012). Nurses must work collaboratively with other care providers to avoid collecting urine cultures when symptoms of UTI are absent and eliminate the inappropriate prescribing of antibiotics for ASB, which leads to multidrug resistant bacteria, increases the likelihood of adverse drug events, and increases the cost of care (Zabarsky, Sethi, & Donskey, 2008).

NURSING MANAGEMENT

Assessment

A subjective assessment of urinary elimination patterns should be completed, assessing for alterations in normal voiding patterns and symptoms such as burning, urgency, and frequency. The characteristics of the urine should also be noted. In addition, a mental status examination may be indicated, as older adults may experience altered mental status in the presence of UTI.

Diagnosis

Nursing diagnoses for an older adult patient experiencing a UTI include the following:

- Pain resulting from altered urinary elimination
- Inadequate urinary elimination resulting from the infectious process
- Need for health teaching related to unfamiliarity with treatment of UTI.

Planning and Expected Outcomes

Expected outcomes for an older patient with a UTI include the following:

1. The patient will experience adequate pain control, as evidenced by reports of no further dysuria or burning with urination.
2. The patient will resume a normal voiding pattern, free from frequency, urgency, and dysuria.
3. The patient or caregiver verbalizes knowledge of the causes and treatment of UTI.

Intervention

Nursing management should focus on education of older adults, including appropriate perihygiene measures such as showering, front-to-back wiping techniques, adequate daily fluid intake, frequent bladder emptying, adherence to the prescribed drug regimen, and reportable signs and symptoms of a recurrent infection. Sterile technique should be used with urinary catheterization; use of indwelling catheters should be minimized.

Evaluation

Evaluation includes ongoing assessment related to expected outcomes and documentation of findings. Documentation also includes routine vital signs, assessment of functional status, and other associated risk factors.

Bladder Cancer

Bladder cancer is the most common form of cancer originating in the urinary system and is most often found in persons over 70 years of age. Approximately 90% of all bladder cancers are transitional cell carcinomas originating in the epithelial lining of the urinary tract. The other 10% are typically squamous cell carcinoma, small cell carcinoma, and adenocarcinoma. Most bladder tumors are easily resected but may metastasize to the bladder wall, pelvis, liver, lungs, or bone. The biggest risk factor for developing bladder cancer is cigarette smoking. Occupational exposures to dyes, rubber, and chemicals used in processing leather, and paint are at high risk for developing bladder cancer. Chronic bladder irritation resulting from stones and chronic UTIs are risk factors for development of bladder cancer. Bladder cancer occurs more often in men than in women and more often in Caucasians than in other races. Genetics also play a role in the development of bladder cancer.

Painless hematuria is the most common symptom of bladder cancer. It may also be accompanied by dysuria, urgency, and frequency. If the tumor is large, late signs include suprapubic pain. A large tumor may also cause urinary obstruction, which, in turn, could cause low back and pelvic pain and predispose a patient to postrenal failure.

NURSING MANAGEMENT

Assessment

Nursing assessment should include a thorough history with attention to changes in urinary elimination patterns. Subjective assessment should focus on the presence of pain, hematuria, dysuria, urgency, frequency, and voiding of small volumes. Objective assessment findings include gross or microscopic hematuria.

Diagnosis

Nursing diagnoses appropriate for an older patient with bladder cancer include the following:

- Anxiety resulting from an uncertain prognosis
- Inadequate urinary elimination resulting from surgical diversion
- Distorted body image resulting from surgical diversion
- Inadequate coping resulting from uncertain outcome of treatment
- Reduced sexual expression resulting from anatomic alterations

Planning and Expected Outcomes

Developing a care plan for a patient with bladder cancer involves the patient, family, and significant others. Expected outcomes include the following:

1. The patient will experience reduced anxiety, as evidenced by a decrease in symptoms.
2. The patient will develop a routine for managing urinary diversion.
3. The patient will verbalize acceptance of urinary diversion and associated changes.
4. The patient will demonstrate the use of effective coping strategies, as evidenced by verbalization of feelings and seeking of support.
5. The patient will verbalize concerns about sexuality.
6. The patient will express satisfaction with alternative positions for intercourse.

Intervention

Nursing interventions for patients with bladder cancer focus on patient education, psychosocial support, management of pain, and maintenance of adequate fluid and nutritional intake. Surgery is performed to remove the cancer; the type of surgery depends on the stage of cancer. A transurethral resection of the bladder tumor removes noninvasive cancer. A partial or total cystectomy is used to remove invasive tumors. An ileal conduit as a means of urinary diversion is the most frequent means of managing urinary elimination following cystectomy. Social stigma associated with the excretion of body fluids into an external device compounds the patient's fears and concerns regarding the diagnosis of cancer. Because patients may have difficulty coping, it is important to encourage them to verbalize fears and concerns and to refer them to the appropriate supportive services, if necessary.

If a patient requires chemotherapy, nursing interventions include monitoring for infection, irritative voiding symptoms, allergic reactions, and bone marrow suppression. Patient education should include instructions for follow-up care and the importance of cystoscopy every 3 months for 1 year, then every 6 months to 1 year thereafter. Patients who smoke should be counseled to stop smoking.

Evaluation

Evaluation of nursing interventions is based on the achievement of expected outcomes. Documentation of ongoing biopsychosocial assessment is key in the provision of holistic nursing care.

Benign Prostatic Hypertrophy

BPH is an age-related enlargement of the prostate gland that constricts the urethra and obstructs the outflow of urine. Approximately 80% of men may be diagnosed with BPH by the age of 80. The development of BPH is the result of structural, functional, and hormonal changes.

With early prostatic enlargement, the patient may be asymptomatic because the muscles compensate for increased urethral resistance. As the prostate gland enlarges, the patient begins to manifest symptoms of an obstructive process. Symptoms include hesitancy, a decrease in the force of the urinary stream, terminal dribbling, a sensation of a full bladder after voiding, and urinary retention. Urethral obstruction may cause urinary stasis, UTIs, hydronephrosis, and renal calculi.

The purpose of the diagnostic evaluation of BPH is to determine the extent of obstruction. Diagnostic evaluation includes a history and physical examination, digital rectal examination (DRE), urinalysis, and measurement of BUN and serum creatinine levels. Although BPH is not related to prostate cancer, a prostate-specific antigen (PSA) test may be ordered in some cases to rule out prostate cancer. Although not indicated as part of the initial evaluation of BPH, abdominal ultrasonography or cystoscopy may be indicated in persons with urinary retention, renal impairment, or suspected cancer.

NURSING MANAGEMENT

Assessment

The purpose of the nursing assessment for an individual with BPH is to determine the extent of prostate enlargement and its effect on function so that appropriate nursing interventions can be planned and implemented. The assessment consists of history taking, physical examination, and evaluation of voiding patterns (Box 22.13).

Diagnosis

Nursing diagnoses appropriate for the patient experiencing BPH include the following:
- Inadequate urinary elimination resulting from bladder outlet obstruction
- Potential for infection resulting from stasis
- Reduced sexual expression resulting from erectile dysfunction
- Need for health teaching resulting from new diagnosis

Planning and Expected Outcomes

Expected outcomes for a patient with BPH include the following:
1. The patient will maintain a regular schedule of complete bladder emptying.
2. The patient will remain free from UTIs, as evidenced by using measures to prevent infection.
3. The patient will verbalize sexual concerns and describe measures to cope.

BOX 22.13 Nursing Assessment for Benign Prostatic Hypertrophy

History
- General health
- Functional status
- Medical and surgical history
- Current drugs
- Voiding habits and patterns:
  - The initiation and caliber of the urinary stream
  - Dysuria
  - Frequency
  - The presence of obstructive symptoms:
    - Diurnal frequency
    - Nocturia
    - Hesitancy
    - Urgency
    - Urge incontinence
    - Incomplete bladder emptying
    - Postvoid dribbling
    - Signs and symptoms of urinary tract infection

Physical Examination
The physical examination is usually conducted by the physician or an advanced practice nurse and includes the following:
- Digital rectal examination (DRE) to evaluate the size, shape, and consistency of the prostate gland
- Abdominal examination to determine the presence of bladder distention, suprapubic tenderness, and costovertebral angle tenderness

---

4. Patient demonstrates understanding of evaluation and treatment of BPH.

If surgery is indicated, expected outcomes might include the following:
1. The patient will have satisfactory pain control as indicated by 3 or less on a 0-to-10 scale.
2. The patient will regain urinary control like that experienced in the premorbid state.

Intervention

Nursing interventions for BPH focus on patient education regarding the diagnosis and management of the disease. Education regarding the management of alterations in urinary elimination should include establishment of frequent voiding schedules. The educational plan should also include teaching patients about the sympathomimetic actions of decongestant drugs and diet pills, as they may cause acute urinary retention.

Nursing interventions must also consider the treatment regimen. For patients treated with nonsurgical methods, interventions should focus on education about signs and symptoms of progressive BPH. As the prostate gland enlarges, the urine stream becomes weaker and hesitancy increases, and it becomes increasingly difficult to completely empty the bladder. Patient education should also focus on the drugs used to relieve symptoms, their side effects, and drug interactions. For patients undergoing surgery, nursing interventions should initially focus on immediate postoperative care. Most surgical procedures require general anesthesia and a short hospitalization. Interventions should focus on maintaining patients' levels of function and preventing postoperative complications related to immobility. Following discharge from the hospital, patients require education related to temporary activity restrictions, signs and symptoms of infection and urinary obstruction, and possible temporary incontinence. Surgical interventions may result in temporary sexual dysfunction; patients should be given the opportunity to verbalize concerns and to be referred to appropriate supportive services, such as a urologist or a certified sex therapist (see Patient/Family Teaching: Benign Prostatic Hypertrophy box).

 PATIENT/FAMILY TEACHING

Benign Prostatic Hypertrophy (BPH)

BPH may alter the flow of urine. Any of the following symptoms could indicate BPH and should be reported to the physician immediately:
* Hesitancy or difficulty beginning urination
* Frequent need to urinate during the day and at night
* Leakage of urine
* Sensation of a full bladder after having just urinated
* Weaker-than-normal flow of urine

Evaluation

Evaluation of interventions is based on the return of urinary function to the premorbid state, relief of urinary symptoms, avoidance or prompt management of UTIs, and a return to satisfactory sexual activity. Documenting the care of a patient with BPH includes noting the effectiveness of the nursing interventions, including validation the patient understands the disease process and treatment regimen and urinary elimination patterns.

Prostate Cancer

The incidence of prostate cancer increases with age; by age 90, is it estimated 70% of men have some degree of prostate cancer. Prostate cancer is the most common form of cancer in men and the second-leading cause of cancer-related death. The rate of mortality from prostate cancer is higher among black men than among white men. Risk factors include advancing age, family history of the disease, and black race.

Most prostatic cancers are adenocarcinomas; other forms include transitional cell carcinomas, small cell carcinomas, and sarcomas. Prostate cancer may metastasize through the lymphatic system and the bloodstream to the lymph nodes, bones, lungs, and liver.

Early prostate cancer is typically asymptomatic. As the tumor enlarges, it may cause symptoms of urinary obstruction. If obstruction of the urethra occurs, the patient may manifest symptoms of postrenal failure. Other symptoms may include perineal and rectal discomfort, weakness, nausea, hematuria, and lower extremity edema (with metastasis to pelvic nodes). Skeletal pain and pathologic fractures may indicate advanced disease with metastases.

It is important for men to follow the recommendations of the American Cancer Society about screening for prostate cancer. However, prostate cancer screening is not without risk:
* Finding prostate cancer may not improve your health or help you live longer.
* The results can sometimes be wrong.
* Follow-up tests, such as a biopsy, may have complications.

Men and their health care provider should discuss individual risk for prostate cancer, the pros and cons of the screening tests, and then decide if prostate screening is right for them (U.S. National Library of Medicine, 2017).

NURSING MANAGEMENT

Assessment

Assessment of a patient with prostate cancer is essentially the same as that for a patient with BPH. The nurse should assess the patient's health beliefs and fears related to a malignant process.

Diagnosis

Appropriate nursing diagnoses for a patient with prostate cancer include the following:
* Inadequate urinary elimination resulting from bladder outlet obstruction
* Anxiety resulting from uncertain prognosis
* Reduced sexual expression resulting from treatment measures
* Need for health teaching resulting from lack of previous exposure to treatment modalities and prognosis

Planning and Expected Outcomes

Expected outcomes for a patient with prostate cancer include the following:
1. The patient's urinary elimination patterns will return to the premorbid state.
2. The patient's expressions of anxiety about the diagnosis, treatment, and prognosis will be replaced with an understanding of the prognosis.
3. The patient and partner will have a mutually satisfying sexual relationship.
4. The patient will demonstrate knowledge of treatment methods and prognostic indicators.

Intervention

Nursing interventions for a patient with prostate cancer include educating the patient on diagnostic tests and treatment options. If surgery is indicated, nursing interventions should include the following:
1. Administration of analgesics for pain control
2. Suggestion of options for sexual counseling if the patient indicates a need
3. Education of the patient on the importance of a follow-up check of PSA levels and evaluation for disease progression

If hormonal therapy is indicated, the nurse should educate the patient on the administration of intramuscular or subcutaneous injections. If bone metastasis has occurred, the nurse should encourage safety measures around the home to decrease the incidence of pathologic fractures. The patient should be educated on when to report symptoms of worsening urethral obstruction, such as increased frequency, urgency, hesitancy, and urinary retention (see Nursing Care Plan: Prostate Cancer box).

Evaluation

Evaluation of interventions is based on a patient's relief of symptoms from the obstruction and his return to the premorbid

NURSING CARE PLAN

Prostate Cancer

Clinical Situation

Mr. C is a 68-year-old black male. He has no major health problems at this time. At his annual physical examination, he was found to have prostatic enlargement; serum prostate-specific antigen (PSA) testing showed a level of 30 nanograms per milliliter (ng/mL). He then underwent magnetic resonance imaging (MRI) and was found to have a grossly enlarged prostate. A needle-guided biopsy was performed, and it showed adenocarcinoma of the prostate gland. Because of the large size of the prostate mass, evaluation for metastasis, consisting of bone scintigraphy and chest radiography, was performed. The evaluation did not show any metastatic disease.

Mr. C promptly scheduled a consultation with a urologist at a major medical center for the treatment of the prostate tumor. On evaluation, he was found to have stage C prostate cancer. The decision was made to treat the prostate tumor with radical prostatectomy.

Mr. C, his wife, and children are experiencing anxiety, fear, and anticipatory grief related to the diagnosis. Mr. C lost his father 5 years ago to prostate cancer and has many bad memories of his father's illness and death.

Nursing Diagnoses

Anxiety resulting from the diagnosis of cancer

Need for health teaching resulting from lack of previous exposure to current treatment modalities and prognosis

Outcomes

Expressions of anxiety about the diagnosis and prognosis will be replaced by a realistic understanding of the disease and the likely prognosis, as evidenced by satisfactory engagement in activities.

The patient and family will verbalize understanding of the treatment regimen.

The patient and family will seek supportive services.

Interventions

Reassure the patient and family that prostate cancers are typically slow growing and treatable.

Reiterate the explanation of the diagnosis and treatment. Include the family in teaching, whenever possible.

Refer the patient and family to cancer support group services. Emphasize the importance of continuing present activities. Assist the patient in gaining awareness of anxiety.

Teach the patient relaxation techniques.

Provide written information regarding prostate disease and treatment regimens.

Encourage the patient and family members to attend educational and supportive services provided by the American Cancer Society.

---

urinary elimination pattern. The patient should verbalize an understanding of the disease process, the staging of the tumor, and the recommended treatment. The patient and his partner should regain satisfactory sexual relations. Documentation should include all ongoing assessment findings related to expected outcomes.

SUMMARY

The changes that occur in renal function with aging may be challenging. Impaired urinary elimination may cause problems that have a significant effect on day-to-day activities, self-concept, and functioning. The nurse's role includes assessment, patient advocacy, emotional support, and appropriate referral. Individualized care plans should be developed that focus on promotion of self-care and functional ability (see Health Promotion/Illness Prevention box).

HEALTH PROMOTION/ILLNESS PREVENTION

Urinary Function

Health Promotion

- Adherence to prescribed bladder training program, exercises, and techniques for UI
- Adherence to a regularly scheduled program of monitoring of conditions as appropriate (e.g., prostate-specific antigen [PSA], blood pressure, urinalysis, and laboratory tests)
- Prompt treatment of urinary tract symptoms

Disease Prevention

- Participation in a prostate cancer screening program, based on risk established by the health care provider
- Drinking at least eight glasses of water daily, unless contraindicated by other chronic conditions
- Establishment of a routine pattern of urinary elimination
- Use of appropriate hygiene measures to avoid urinary tract contamination

HOME CARE

1. Regularly monitor and assess homebound older adults for signs and symptoms of exacerbation of the diagnosed renal or urinary disease or disorder.
2. Instruct caregivers and homebound older adults on reportable signs and symptoms related to the diagnosed renal or urinary system disorder and when to report these symptoms to the home care nurse or health care provider.
3. Instruct caregivers and homebound older adults on the name, dose, frequency, and side effects of drugs prescribed to treat the diagnosed renal or urinary system disease or disorder.
4. Assess functional and environmental factors that contribute to UI in homebound older adults.
5. Instruct caregivers and homebound older adults to keep a voiding diary to help the home care nurse establish the type of UI and plan nursing interventions.
6. Instruct caregivers and homebound older adults on behavioral interventions (e.g., bladder retraining and pelvic floor exercises) to treat UI.
7. If a homebound older adult is cognitively impaired, the success of behavioral techniques (e.g., habit training, patterned urge response training [PURT], and prompted voiding) used to treat UI will depend on the caregiver's availability and motivation.
8. Instruct caregivers and homebound older adults on measures to reduce UI and maintain comfort.
9. Use indwelling catheters as a last resort to treat UI.

KEY POINTS

- UI is one of the most common health problems of older adults.
- Although the aging process does affect lower urinary tract function, aging alone does not cause UI.
- Drugs, including many OTC drugs, may cause acute UI.
- Functional and environmental assessments are important components of the evaluation of UI.
- Bladder diaries provide a more objective measure of the severity and type of incontinence than recall alone and should be part of the evaluation of UI.
- Behavioral interventions are the initial treatment of choice for many patients with UI.
- Cognitively intact patients with urge or stress incontinence often respond well to properly taught pelvic floor muscle exercises.
- Once a patient masters pelvic floor muscle exercises, the nurse may teach urge or stress strategies to prevent involuntary urine loss.
- Prompted voiding, habit training, and PURT may effectively reduce incontinence in patients with cognitive impairment, but the success of these methods depends on caregiver compliance.
- Aging affects renal function; however, impaired renal function is not a normal consequence of aging. Older adult patients must be assessed, and attention directed to adequate hydration, adjusted drug dosages, and the existence of comorbidities that may lead to renal dysfunction.
- AKI, which is classified into three types, is a reversible process. The nurse must focus on education regarding proper diet and drugs used to treat renal failure to halt the progression of AKI.
- CKD is not reversible but may be managed with drugs and diet modification unless it has progressed to end-stage renal disease; in this case, dialysis is typically required as a bridge to successful transplantation.
- Alterations in urinary elimination pattern are common in men with BPH. The nurse must be prepared to educate patients about drugs and Kegel exercises after surgery.
- PSA screening is a personal decision, made after a discussion of risks and benefits between the man and his health care provider.

CRITICAL-THINKING EXERCISES

1. Your 74-year-old female patient complains that she has leakage of urine during the day. What additional information do you need to assess her urinary function?
2. A 76-year-old man is admitted to the emergency department with complaints of nausea, fatigue, and poor appetite. The physician orders a urinalysis, BUN, and creatinine. Why does the physician suspect a urinary problem?

REFERENCES

Arora, P. (2017). *Chronic Kidney Disease*. Retrieved March 5, 2018 from https://emedicine.medscape.com/article/238798-overview.

Boongird, S., Shah, N., Nolin, T. D., & Unruh, M. L. (2010). Nocturia and aging: Diagnosis and treatment. *Advances in Chronic Kidney Disease, 17*(4), e27–e40. https://doi.org/10.1053/j.ackd.2010.04.004.

Burgio, K. L., & Goode, P. S. (1997). Behavioral interventions for incontinence in ambulatory geriatric patients. *The American Journal of the Medical Sciences, 314*, 257.

Colling, J., Ouslander, J., Hadley, B. J., Eisch, J., & Campbell, E. (1992). The effect of patterned urge-response toileting (PURT) on urinary incontinence among nursing home residents. *Journal of the American Geriatrics Society, 40*, 135–141.

Cook, K., & Sobeski, L. M. (2013). Urinary incontinence in the older adult. In G. T. Schumock, T. S. Dunsworth, D. M. Brundage, M. M. Chapman, J. W. Cheng, K. H. Chessman, & T. P. Semla (Eds.), *Geriatrics/special populations* (5th ed., pp. 3–20). Retrieved from http://www.accp.com/docs/bookstore/psap/p13b2_m1ch.pdf.

Doerflinger, D. M. (2012). *Mental Status Assessment in Older Adults: Montreal Cognitive Assessment*. Retrieved March 5, 2018 from https://consultgeri.org/try-this/general-assessment/issue-3.2.

Du Moulin, M. F., Hamers, J. P., Paulus, A., Berendsen, C., & Halfens, R. (2005). The role of the nurse in community continence care: A systematic review. *International Journal of Nursing Studies, 42*(4), 479–492.

Ganz, M. L., Smalarz, A. M., Krupski, T. L., Anger, J. T., Hu, J. C., Wittrup-Jensen, K. U., et al. (2010). Economic costs of overactive bladder in the United States. *Urology, 75*, 526–532. https://doi.org/10.1016/j.urology.2009.06.096.

Halter, J., Ouslander, J., Tinetti, M., Studenski, S., High, K., & Asthana, S. (2009). *Hazzard's geriatric medicine and gerontology* (6th ed.). Philadelphia, PA: McGraw-Hill.

Katz, S., Ford, A. B., Moskowitz, R. W., Jackson, B. A., & Jaffe, M. W. (1963). Studies of illness in the aged: The index of ADL—A standardized measure of biological and psychosocial function. *Journal of the American Medical Association, 185*, 914–919.

Kegel, A. H. (1948). Progressive resistance exercise in the functional restoration of the perineal muscles. *American Journal of Obstetrics and Gynecology, 52*, 242.

Moore, K. C., & Lucas, M. G. (2010). Management of male urinary incontinence. *Indian Journal of Urology, 26*(2), 236–244. https://doi.org/10.4103/0970-1591.65398.

Murugan, R., & Kellulm, J. A. (2011). Acute kidney injury: What's the prognosis? *National Review in Nehprology, 7*(4), 209–217. https://doi.org/10.1038/nrneph.2011.13.

Offermans, M. P., Du Moulin, M. F., Hamers, J. P., Dassen, T., & Halfens, R. J. (2009). Prevalence of urinary incontinence and associated risk factors in nursing home residents: A systematic review. *Neurourology and Urodynamics, 28*, 288–294. https://doi.org/10.1002/nau.20668.

Onukwugha, E., Zuckerman, I. H., McNally, D., Coyne, K. S., Vats, V., & Mullins, C. D. (2009). The total economic burden of overactive bladder in the United States: A disease-specific approach. *American Journal of Managed Care, 15*, S90–S97.

Ouslander, I. G. (2003). Urinary incontinence. In W. R. Hazzard, et al. (Eds.), *Principles of geriatric medicine and gerontology* (5th ed.). Philadelphia, PA: McGraw-Hill.

Phillips, C. D., Adepoju, O., Stone, N., Moudouni, D. K., Nwaiwu, O., Zhao, H., et al. (2012). Asymptomatic bacteriuria, antibiotic use, and suspected urinary tract infections in four nursing homes. *BMC Geriatrics, 12*(12). Retrieved from http://www.biomedcentral.com/1471-2318/12/73.

Shenot, P. J. (2016). *Urinary incontinence in adults.* Retrieved March 5, 2018 from http://www.merckmanuals.com/professional/SearchResults?query=urinary+incontinence.

Thayer, C., Cohen, A., Carman, L., Conn, K., Lambert, M. J., Ramos, K., et al. (2013). Urinary incontinence in women guideline. Group Health Cooperative.

U.S. Department of Health and Human Services, Agency for Healthcare Policy and Research (AHCPR). (1996). *Urinary incontinence in adults: Acute and chronic management.* Clinical Practice Guideline No. 2 Rockville, MD: AHCPR.

US National Library of Medicine. (2017). *Prostate Cancer Screening.* Retrieved March 5, 2018 from https://medlineplus.gov/prostatecancerscreening.html#cat_51.

Weinstein, J. R., & Anderson, S. (2010). The aging kidney: Physiological changes. *Advances in Chronic Kidney Disease, 17*(4), 302–307.

Wyman, J. (2003). Treatment of urinary incontinence in men and older women. *The American Journal of Nursing, 3*(Suppl), 38–45.

Zabarsky, T. F., Sethi, A. K., & Donskey, C. J. (2008). Sustained reduction in inappropriate treatment of asymptomatic bacteriuria in a long-term care facility through an educational intervention. *American Journal of Infection Control, 36*(7), 476–480. https://doi.org/10.1016/j.ajic.2007.11.007.

23

Musculoskeletal Function

Laurie Kennedy-Malone, PhD, GNP-BC, FAANP, FGSA

🌐 http://evolve.elsevier.com/Meiner/gerontologic

LEARNING OBJECTIVES

On completion of this chapter, the reader will be able to:

1. Describe the normal structure and function of the musculoskeletal system.
2. Discuss the age-related changes in the musculoskeletal system.
3. Discuss the nursing management of patients with fractures of the hip, wrist, clavicle, and vertebra.
4. Distinguish differences among osteoarthritis, rheumatoid arthritis, gout, and polymyalgia rheumatica.
5. Identify the nursing interventions associated with osteoarthritis, rheumatoid arthritis, gout, and polymyalgia rheumatica.
6. Discuss the pathophysiology, treatment, and nursing management of osteoporosis.
7. Describe the indications for amputation in older adults and the nursing management of these patients.
8. Discuss the causes and management of common foot problems in older adults.

WHAT WOULD YOU DO?

What would you do if you were faced with the following situations?

- You are taking care of a 75-year-old female who sustained a fracture of the proximal femur 3 months ago. She reports that she has completed physical therapy following the injury and is scheduled to travel overseas on a 10-day European river cruise in 6 months. She is inquiring about additional measures she can take to enhance her safety while traveling abroad. What do you advise her?
- Your patient is an 85-year-old male who has recently been diagnosed with polymyalgia rheumatica. He is currently prescribed long-term corticosteroids and has been experiencing multiple physical changes such as increased bruising, weight gain, and increased number of incidence of upper respiratory tract infections. He is requesting advice on how to maintain health while recovering from an illness yet taking the prescribed long-term corticosteroids. What do you tell him?

Musculoskeletal problems are common among older adults. Recent reports have indicated that one out of five Americans has been diagnosed with arthritis. With the aging of the population, coupled with the high incidence of obesity in this country, it is anticipated that the number of activity limitations attributable to arthritis and the number of people diagnosed with arthritis will continue to rise (Hootman, Helmick, Barbour, Theis, & Boring, 2016). Complaints in the musculoskeletal system are common because normal aging predisposes people to the development of diseases such as osteoarthritis (OA) and osteoporosis (Browne & Merrill, 2015).

Diseases of the musculoskeletal system are usually not fatal but may lead to chronic pain and disability. Chronic conditions of the musculoskeletal system may contribute to impaired function and disability in older adults in the areas of self-care and mobility. They may suffer impairments in the ability to perform activities of daily living (ADLs) such as bathing, dressing, and eating, and impairments in the ability to perform instrumental activities of daily living (IADLs) such as managing finances, preparing food, managing transportation, and keeping house. Functional impairment of ADLs and IADLs may be devastating to older adults who desire to maintain independence. When dependence occurs, it may result in loss of self-esteem, the perception of decreased quality of life, and depression (see Cultural Awareness box) (Allen et al., 2016).

AGE-RELATED CHANGES IN STRUCTURE AND FUNCTION

The musculoskeletal system is affected in numerous ways by the aging process. A pronounced decrease in muscle mass and muscle strength occurs gradually over time. The actual number of muscle cells decreases, and they are replaced by fibrous connective tissue. As a result, muscle mass, tone, and strength decrease. The elasticity of ligaments, tendons, and cartilage decreases, as does bone mass, which results in weaker bones. The intervertebral disks lose water, causing a narrowing of the vertebral space. This shrinkage may result in a loss of 1.5 to 3 inches of height. The lordotic or convex curve of the back flattens, and both flexion and extension of the lower back are decreased. Posture and gait change. Posture, as a result of the changes in the spine,

Previous author: Ramesh C. Upadhyaya, RN, CRRN, MSN, MBA, PhD-C.

CULTURAL AWARENESS

Biocultural Variations in the Musculoskeletal System

Bone	Remarks
Frontal	Thicker in black men than in white men
Parietal/occipital	Thicker in white men than in black men; occipital protuberance palpable in Eskimos

Palate	Tori (protuberances) along suture line of hard palate, which is problematic for denture wearers
	Incidence:
	  Blacks: 0%
	  Whites: 24%
	  Asian Americans: up to 50%
	  Native Americans: up to 50%

Mandible	Tori (protuberances) on lingual surface of mandible near canine and premolar teeth, which is problematic for denture wearers Most common in Asian Americans and Native Americans; exceeds 50% in some Eskimo groups
Humerus	Torsion or rotation of proximal end with muscle pull Larger in whites than in blacks Torsion in blacks is symmetric; torsion in whites usually greater on right side than on left

Radius/ulna	Length at wrist variable
	Ulna or radius may be longer
	Equal length:
	  Swedish: 61%
	  Chinese: 16%
	Ulna longer than radius:
	  Swedish: 16%
	  Chinese: 48%
	Radius longer than ulna:
	  Swedish: 23%
	  Chinese: 10%

Vertebrae	24 vertebrae found in 85%–93% of all people; racial and gender differences reveal 23 or 25 vertebrae in select groups (23 vertebrae in 11% of black women; 25 vertebrae in 12% of Eskimo and Native American men) Related to lower back pain and lordosis
Femur	Convex anterior: Native Americans Straight: blacks Intermediate: whites

Bone	Remarks
Pelvis	Hip width 1.6 centimeters (cm) (0.6 inch) smaller in black women than in white women; Asian American women have significantly smaller pelvises

Second tarsal	Second toe longer than great toe
	Incidence:
	  Whites: 8%–34%
	  Blacks: 8%–12%
	  Vietnamese: 31%
	  Melanesians: 21%–57%

Height	Clinical significance for joggers and athletes White men 1.27 cm (0.5 inch) taller than black men and 7.6 cm (2.9 inches) taller than Asian American men White women equal to black women Asian American women 4.14 cm (1.6 inches) shorter than white or black women
Composition of long bones	Longer, narrower, and denser in blacks than in whites; bone density in whites greater than in Chinese, Japanese, and Eskimos Osteoporosis lowest in black men; highest in white women

Peroneus tertius	Responsible for dorsiflexion of foot
	Muscle absent:
	  Asian Americans, Native Americans, and white: 3%–10%
	  Blacks and Berbers: 10%–15% (Sahara desert): 24%
	No clinical significance because tibialis anterior also dorsiflexes the foot

Palmaris longus	Responsible for wrist flexion
	Muscle absent:
	  Whites: 12%–20%
	  Native Americans: 2%–12%
	  Blacks: 5%
	  Asian Americans: 3%
	No clinical significance because three other muscles are also responsible for flexion

Data from Overfield, T. (1995). *Biologic variation in health and illness: Race, age, and sex differences* (2nd ed.). Boca Raton, FL: CRC Press.

assumes a position of flexion. Changes in posture result in a shift in the center of gravity. In men, the gait becomes small-stepped with a wider-based stance. Women become bowlegged (genus varus), have a narrow standing base, and walk with a waddling gait (Manini, Gundermann, & Clark, 2016). The articular cartilage erodes in older adults. It is unknown whether this is a result of the aging process or the result of wear and tear on the joints.

All the changes mentioned may cause pain, impaired mobility, self-care deficits, and increased risk of falls for older adults. Approximately one-third of those age 65 or older have falls each year. A recent report from the Centers for Disease Control and Prevention (CDC) found that, in 2016, over 2 million nonfatal falls resulted in emergency room care and more than 850,000

required hospitalization related to the injury sustained (CDC, 2018); moderate to severe injuries included hip fractures, lacerations, and traumatic brain injury (Gray-Miceli, 2017).

It has been estimated that residents have a 50% to 75% incidence of falls in nursing homes. The mean incidence is 1.5 falls per bed per year. Falls are the most common cause of accidental death in older adults. When falls result in injury and hospitalization, the risk of iatrogenic illness and immobility may lead to a downward trajectory, which may ultimately result in death. Falls may also cause a cycle of disuse. This pattern of disuse usually occurs after the individual has experienced repeated falls. The fall experience causes a fear of falling. To avoid falls, the individual decreases mobility; with decreased mobility, muscle strength decreases, joints become stiff, and pain develops, resulting in disability, loss of independence, and frailty (Gray-Miceli, 2017; Taylor-Piliae, Peterson, & Mohler, 2017). Current research has documented that some of the diseases and decline in the musculoskeletal system may be reduced or prevented through the use of regular programs of active exercise and resistive muscle strengthening (Chen, Tseng, Chang, Huang, & Li, 2013).

COMMON PROBLEMS AND CONDITIONS OF THE MUSCULOSKELETAL SYSTEM

Fractures are common problems for older adults that often result in some loss of functional ability. A *fracture* is a break or disruption in the continuity of the bone. Fractures may occur because of trauma to a bone or joint, or they may be the result of pathologic processes such as osteoporosis or neoplasms that contribute to bone fragility (Ensrud, 2013). When bones are subjected to more stress than can be withstood, a fracture occurs. Stresses on bones may be from major trauma such as automobile accidents or falls. Falls are the most common cause of fractures in older adults. The most frequently occurring fractures among older adults are hip fractures, fractures of the proximal femur, Colles (wrist) fractures, vertebral fractures, and clavicular fractures. Fractures are classified as open or closed by the location and type of fracture (Ensrud, 2013) (Fig. 23.1).

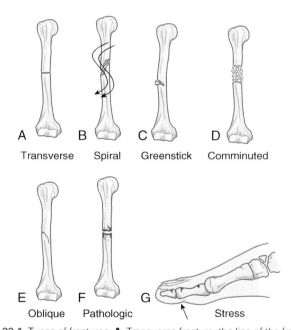

Fig. 23.1 Types of fractures. **A,** Transverse fracture: the line of the fracture extends across the bone shaft at a right angle to the longitudinal axis. **B,** Spiral fracture: the line of the fracture extends in a spiral direction along the bone shaft. **C,** Greenstick fracture: an incomplete fracture with one side splintered and the other side bent. **D,** Comminuted fracture: a fracture with more than two fragments. The smaller fragments appear to be floating. **E,** Oblique fracture: the line of the fracture extends across and down the bone. **F,** Pathologic fracture: a spontaneous fracture at the site of a diseased bone. **G,** Stress fracture: occurs in normal or abnormal bone that is subject to repeated stress, such as from jogging or running. (From Lewis, S. L., Bucher, L., Heitkemper, M. M., et al. [2017]. *Medical-surgical nursing: Assessment and management of clinical problems.* [10th ed.]. St. Louis, MO: Elsevier.)

The completed process of bone healing is termed *union.* After fractures occur, regenerative cells (fibroblasts and osteoblasts) move to the fracture site and lay down a fibrous matrix of collagen—the *callus.* This process usually occurs within 7 days of the injury. As the healing process takes place, the callus bridges the fracture site, and the distance between the bone fragments decreases. In the final stage of bone healing, remodeling (absorption of excess cells and calcification) occurs.

The history given by a patient with a fracture usually includes trauma followed by immediate local pain. Tenderness, swelling, muscle spasms, deformity, bleeding, and loss of function are also seen with fractures (Corrarino, 2015) (see Emergency Treatment box). However, it is important for the nurse to carefully evaluate vital signs and level of consciousness after a patient sustains a fall to determine what may have been the preceding factors leading up to the fall. Was the patient aware that he was falling? Did the patient know why he fell, slipped, or tripped over an object? Was the patient incontinent just before the fall? Could he move the extremities without pain (Gray-Miceli, 2017).

✚ EMERGENCY TREATMENT

Fractures

If a fracture is suspected, assess injured area for the following:
- Movement
- Pain
- Color
- Temperature
- Pulse
- Sensation

If fracture is open and bleeding is present:
- Apply pressure.
- Apply sterile dressing.
- Immobilize the fracture site.

Hip Fracture

Hip fractures are the most disabling type of fracture for older adults. They usually are caused by falls and result in direct trauma to the hip. Approximately 25% of patients with hip fractures die within 1 year after the injury (Sattui & Saag 2014). The complications of hip fractures are generally related to immobility. They include pneumonia, sepsis from urinary tract infections, and pressure ulcers. With the growing number of older adults, especially those older than 75, it is expected that the incidence of hip fractures will increase (Ensrud, 2013).

Hip fractures are classified according to their locations. *Intracapsular* fractures, or subcapital fractures, occur within the hip capsule. *Extracapsular* fractures occur outside or below the capsule and are referred to as *intertrochanteric* and *subtrochanteric* locations (Southerland, Barrie, Falk, & Menaker, 2014) (Fig. 23.2).

After the fall or injury that results in the fractured hip, the patient has an affected extremity that is usually externally rotated and shortened. Tenderness and severe pain at the fracture site may be present. Immediately after the injury, the joint should be immobilized. Buck or Russell traction (Fig. 23.3) is

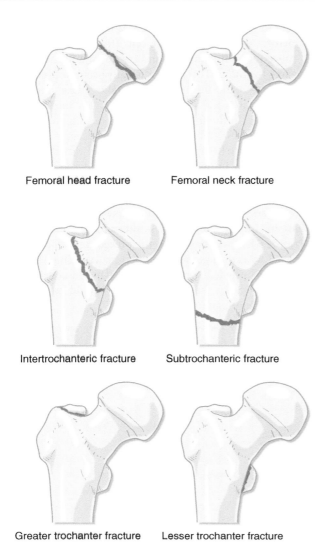

Femoral head fracture   Femoral neck fracture

Intertrochanteric fracture   Subtrochanteric fracture

Greater trochanter fracture   Lesser trochanter fracture

Fig. 23.2 Fractures of the hip. (From Adams, J. G., Barton, E. D., Collings, J. L., et al. [2013]. *Emergency medicine: Clinical essentials* [2nd ed.]. Philadelphia, PA: Saunders.)

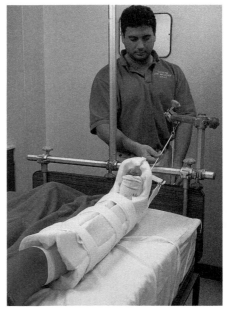

Fig. 23.3 Buck extension. Heel is supported off bed to prevent pressure on heel, weight hangs free of bed, and foot is well away from footboard of bed. The limb should lie parallel to the bed unless prevented by a slight knee flexion contracture. (From Perry, A. G., Potter, P. A., & Ostendorf, W. R. [2016]. *Nursing interventions and clinical skills* [6th ed.]. St. Louis, MO: Elsevier.)

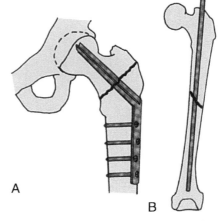

A   B

Fig. 23.4 A, Neufeld nail and screws, used in the repair of intertrochanteric fracture. **B,** Küntscher nail (intramedullary rod) used in repair of midshaft femoral fracture. (Modified from Monahan, F. D., Sands, J., Neighbors, M., et al. [2007]. *Phipps' medical-surgical nursing: Health and illness perspectives* [8th ed.]. St. Louis, MO: Mosby.)

used until the patient is stabilized. After the patient is stabilized, surgical repair, the preferred treatment, is performed. The type of surgical repair depends on the location and type of fracture, and may include internal fixation with pins, plates, and screws, or prosthetic replacement of the femoral head (Schneider et al., 2013) (Fig. 23.4).

NURSING MANAGEMENT

Assessment

Hip fractures are most often related to falls. After any fall or other injury that may cause hip trauma, the nurse assesses the hips and lower extremities for evidence of fracture. This includes inspecting the site for direct evidence of fracture, shortening of the extremity, and abnormal rotation. Also assessed is the presence of tenderness, swelling, or ecchymosis at the site of the injury (Corrarino, 2015). Note if the patient reports pain with any motion. Given that injury was severe enough to sustain

a fracture, the patient should be assessed for other injuries. A careful assessment of the patient's vital signs and level of consciousness is imperative (Eiff & Hatch, 2017).

Diagnosis

Nursing diagnoses for a patient with a hip fracture include the following:

- Pain resulting from the discomfort from the muscle and bone trauma

- Decreased mobility resulting from immobilization of the fracture and the healing process
- Potential for reduced skin integrity resulting from immobilization required for healing
- Potential for infection resulting from inadequate wound healing, compromised nutrition, and effects of immobility
- Inadequate bathing/dressing/feeding/toileting self-care resulting from discomfort and decreased mobility
- Inadequate home maintenance resulting from decreased independence and recovery period needed for fracture healing

Planning and Expected Outcomes

Nursing care of a patient with a hip fracture involves the perioperative, postoperative, and rehabilitation periods. Each of these stages of treatment and recovery requires specific nursing interventions and includes the following expected outcomes:

1. The patient will report minimum discomfort and an adequate level of pain control.
2. The patient will remain free from postoperative complications such as altered skin integrity and wound infection.
3. The patient will adhere to the prescribed physical therapy regimen to regain function of the affected joint.
4. The patient will be able to participate in physical and occupational therapies.
5. The patient will be able to safely demonstrate use of assistive devices for mobility and ADLs.
6. The patient will be able to return to the preinjury level of independence with appropriate support and assistive devices.

Intervention

On arrival in the acute care setting, the patient has his or her medical condition and hip fracture assessed and stabilized. Surgical intervention is usually recommended but is considered elective and therefore requires stability of major health conditions. During this preoperative period, the nurse's focus is on keeping the patient comfortable and hydrated, and preventing complications of immobility. Preoperatively, hip fractures may produce severe muscle spasms, causing intense pain. Pain drugs, traction, or immobilization and proper positioning are used to manage the pain. Preoperative education should include information regarding the surgical procedure, postoperative treatments, potential complications, and expected outcomes for rehabilitation and recovery.

The immediate postoperative period requires monitoring of vital signs and intake and output. Turning, deep breathing, and coughing are used to prevent respiratory complications. The operative site is monitored for signs of infection and bleeding. Movement, circulation, and sensation of the extremity are assessed to determine impaired circulation. Mental status should be assessed and any changes noted. Postoperative delirium may occur in older patients after a hip fracture; the effects of surgery, anesthesia, analgesic drugs, loss of familiar surroundings, pain, and immobility may increase the potential for delirium. Care planning should include familiarizing the patient with his or

her surroundings, providing for safety, instituting comfort measures, decreasing anxiety, and assisting with maintaining a sense of independence and identity.

EVIDENCE-BASED PRACTICE
Fall Prevention Program

Sample/Setting
This quality improvement pilot study examined the effectiveness of a fall prevention program in four assisted living facilities (ALFs) in North Carolina. All residents in the facilities were the intended population for the study. A target sample of 50 residents who met the eligibility criteria of 65 years and older, nonbed bound, nor a resident of a dementia or hospice unit were invited to participate.

Methods
The researchers collected data via observations, chart review, and conversations with the staff at baseline, and 4 months after the implementation of a fall quality improvement (QI) program. After consenting to be a subject in the study, the residents were assessed by trained researchers using the Morse Falls Scale and the Timed Get Up and Go Test. Additional data were extrapolated from the residents' Minimum Data Set scores that pertained to cognition and ADLs. The actual QI program was the Assisted Living Falls and Prevention and Monitoring Program (AL-FPMP). At each site, there was a dedicated team that that oversaw all aspects of the program.

Findings
Of the 277 residents who were eligible to participate, 175 consented to participate; after 4 months, 146 residents continued in the program. The mean age the participants was 85.7. Although there were challenges in each ALF to full implementation to the QI falls program, there was an improvement in participants' Morse Falls Scale, although results were not statistically significant.

Implications
The need for falls prevention program in ALFs remains great. To be successful, however, it was recommended that a specific falls team is established, that there is a "champion" who will lead the continued efforts of a program, that staff are trained to assess residents using the Morse Falls Scale, and finally that other programs that increase function and have been shown to reduce falls such as t'ai chi and walking be added to the AL-FPMP.

Data from Zimmerman, S., Greene, A., Sloane, P. D., Mitchell, M., Giuliani, C., Nyrop, K., & Walsh, E. (2017). Preventing falls in assisted living: Results of a quality improvement pilot study. *Geriatric Nursing, 38* (3), 185–191.

Pain is managed through careful administration of pain drugs. Because of the normal physiologic aging changes that affect pharmacokinetics and pharmacodynamics, older adults are at risk for developing changes in mental status, respiratory depression, and sedative effects with the use of narcotic analgesics. These problems are prevented with the use of lower initial doses of narcotics than those used with younger adults. The individual's response to the pain drug and the pain are closely monitored. After determining the patient's level of tolerance, the dose may be carefully increased. Keeping the affected extremity in alignment during turning also decreases pain. This is done with the use of pillows between the knees or an abduction splint.

Another common problem a patient recovering from hip surgery has is constipation and often has a fecal impaction because of the side effects of the analgesics and the hazards of immobility. Assess the patient's frequency of bowel movements and determine whether a drug is needed to relieve constipation.

Patients who have their fractures repaired with hemiarthroplasty are at risk for dislocation. The nurse should give the patient and family instructions on preventing dislocation. Dislocation may occur when the joint is adducted and internally rotated. Activities to avoid include crossing the legs and feet while seated, sitting on low seats, and adducting the legs when lying on the nonoperated side. The patient is instructed not to put on socks or shoes without the aid of assistive devices, not to cross the legs, not to lie on the affected side, to use a raised toilet seat and a shower chair, and to use a pillow between the legs while in bed. Activities that may cause dislocation should be avoided for 6 weeks until muscles surrounding the joint are healed and the joint is stabilized. Symptoms of dislocation are sudden severe pain and external rotation of the leg.

After the devastating events of hip fracture and surgery, comprehensive interdisciplinary rehabilitation focuses on returning the patient to the prior level of function and preventing disability (Della Rocca et al., 2013). Specific areas of treatment are gait and transfer training, muscle strengthening through active assistive exercises, teaching the use of adaptive techniques for dressing, and teaching the correct use of assistive devices. The patient will use walkers and canes (Fig. 23.5), and the nurse must ensure that the patient uses a safe technique with either device (see Patient/Family Teaching box: Correct Use of Walkers).

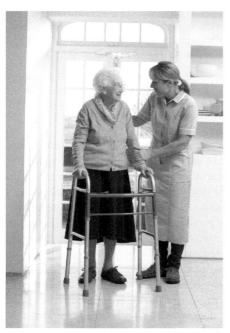

Fig. 23.5 Walking with a walker. The walker is moved about 6 inches in front of the resident. Both feet are moved up to the walker. (© monkeybusinessimages/iStock/Thinkstock.)

PATIENT/FAMILY TEACHING
Correct Use of Walkers

- A walker should always rest on all four legs, never on only two.
- Correct body position should be maintained:
  - Posture erect
  - Elbows slightly bent
  - Wrists extended
  - Shoulders relaxed
- Sturdy, comfortable, hard-soled shoes should be worn.
- Walker and affected leg should be moved together.
- Be alert for hazards such as uneven surfaces or wet floors.

The loss of independence and decreased functional ability should also be addressed during rehabilitation. These losses may lead to depression. The nurse's role is to identify the patient's strengths, give positive feedback, and reinforce the progress made in achieving goals. Discharge planning focuses on using family and social support networks and ongoing therapy programs.

Evaluation

Successful achievement of the expected outcomes after hip fracture will allow the patient to return to a preinjury level of function. Those living independently should be successful in meeting goals of therapy and should regain their self-care abilities, which will allow for returning home. Home health agencies may also be useful in successfully returning the patient to the community.

Patients who were living in other types of health care facilities before the injury should be expected to return to their previous level of activity. Complications will prolong the recovery period and may lead to long-term changes in the level of independence. Patients should report minimum pain at the fracture or surgical site and intact skin integrity. Muscle strength, joint movement, level of mobility, and degree of safety while performing ADLs should be continually evaluated throughout the recovery period. Continued physical and occupational therapies may be required to achieve goals and expected outcomes (see Nursing Care Plan: Fractured Hip).

Colles Fracture

A Colles fracture is a fracture of the distal radius that is usually a result of reaching out with an open hand to break a fall. This fracture is seen most often in perimenopausal women, and although the incidence increases following menopause, the rate of Colles fractures remains relatively stable beginning at age 65 (Ensrud, 2013). Patients with a Colles fracture have pain at the site of the fracture that begins immediately after the traumatic episode; local edema, swelling, and a visible deformity from the displacement of the distal bone fragment are also present. Treatment of a Colles fracture is usually closed reduction and immobilization with a forearm splint or cast. Nursing measures include elevating the extremity to decrease edema and neurovascular assessment to monitor for complications. The patient is instructed to actively move the thumb and fingers to improve venous return and decrease edema. Range-of-motion exercises for the elbow and shoulder prevent stiffness of the extremity.

NURSING CARE PLAN

Fractured Hip

Clinical Situation

Ms. W, an 86-year-old who still works as an executive secretary, is admitted to the skilled nursing unit of the local hospital for restorative care after surgical repair of a fractured left hip. The hip was repaired with femoral head prosthesis. Ms. W had a fall when getting on the city bus. Before this incident, Ms. W worked 3 days a week. Her general health status is good. She lives alone on the second floor of a two-story building. Her only family is a niece who lives 60 miles away.

On admission, Ms. W is a slender woman who looks younger than her stated age. She is in no acute pain. The left hip incision is clean and dry with the staples intact. Ms. W transfers with the moderate assistance of two people. During the transfer, she becomes tense and tells the nurses that she is afraid of falling and that she has to get on her feet so that she can get back to work. Because the surgical procedure has caused decreased range of motion and weakness in her left leg, Ms. W requires assistance with bathing and clothing of her lower extremities.

Nursing Diagnoses

Reduced mobility resulting from alteration in musculoskeletal function as a result of fracture and surgical repair

Inadequate bathing and dressing self-care (bathing and dressing lower extremities) resulting from alteration in musculoskeletal function secondary to fracture and surgical repair

Need for patient teaching resulting from limited exposure to home care programs

Outcomes

The patient will walk 50 feet with a pickup walker.

The patient will bathe and dress her lower extremities with the use of assistive devices.

The patient will verbalize knowledge of home care programs.

The patient will verbalize satisfaction with the discharge plans.

Interventions

Consult with a physical therapist for a program of muscle strengthening, transfer training, and gait training.

Reinforce physical therapy training.

Give positive feedback for gains made.

Instruct the patient to take deep breaths and relax before transfers.

Assist with transfers.

Give specific instructions before transfers. Instruct on hip precautions.

Teach the use of a walker.

Give a pain drug 30 to 60 minutes before physical therapy.

Consult with the occupational therapist for specific assistive devices.

Teach the use of assistive devices. Allow adequate time for bathing and dressing.

Assess support systems and the need for home services.

Instruct on wound care, home safety, and home exercise programs.

Plan for discharge with the patient and team members.

Use community services, visiting nurse, physical therapy, and niece for assistance.

Clavicular Fracture

Fractures of the clavicle, like Colles fractures, may occur after a fall on an outstretched hand or on a fall to the shoulder. The majority of these fractures occur in the middle third of the clavicle. The patient with a fractured clavicle has point tenderness, local edema, and crepitus. The shoulder is noticeably deformed, dropping downward, forward, and inward. Treatment of a clavicular fracture includes reduction of the fracture and immobilization with a sling or cast. Nursing measures include monitoring for neurovascular complications such as compartment syndrome, elevating the extremity, and instructing the patient in actively moving the hand and fingers.

Casts and Cast Care

Casts are one type of device used to immobilize an injured body part. At the same time, casts provide a means of providing pain relief and protect the injured bone from becoming contaminated (Boyd, Benjamin, & Asplund, 2009). They maintain proper positioning of the injured area, prevent further deformity, protect realigned bones, and promote healing. Used on the lower extremities, they may also allow for earlier weight bearing.

Casting materials include plaster of Paris or synthetic materials such as fiberglass. After application, plaster of Paris casts should be left uncovered to air dry. Drying time depends on the size and thickness of the cast and may take up to 48 hours. The nurse should support this type of cast with the palms of the hands rather than with the fingers to prevent indentations in the cast during the drying time. Synthetic cast materials harden quickly during and after application. The surface of this type of cast may be rough and may be covered with stockinette.

Patients are instructed to keep both types of casts dry; plastic or purchased cast protectors may be used during showering or bathing. Synthetic casts are immersed in water only with physician approval and should be dried thoroughly afterward. A hair dryer set at a low temperature may be used for this purpose.

PATIENT/FAMILY TEACHING

Cast Care

Keep casted extremity elevated for the first 24 hours.

When cast is wet, lift with palms of hands.

Observe the extremity for swelling, color changes, movement, and sensation.

If any changes occur, contact health care provider.

Do not put anything inside the cast.

Do not get plaster cast wet; cover with plastic for bathing.

Patients are instructed to keep the extremity elevated to the level of the heart to decrease edema. The patient should also be instructed to maintain movement of the extremity to prevent muscle atrophy and joint stiffness above or below the cast (see Patient/Family Teaching box: Cast Care). Nursing care includes assessment for potential areas of skin irritation or breakdown. The patient should be instructed to report any redness or discomfort along the edges of the cast and any signs of drainage or odor coming from the cast.

Neurovascular assessment of the extremity is done to determine that the cast is not constrictive. Excessive constriction caused by the cast could result in compartment syndrome, leading to ischemia and tissue destruction of the extremity. Any change in capillary refilling, skin color, skin temperature, or excessive pain not controlled with a drug should be immediately reported to the physician.

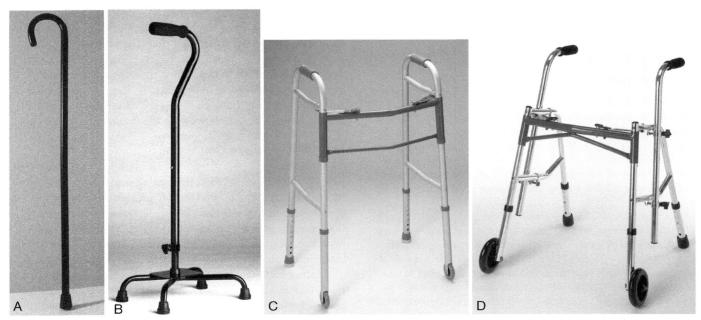

Fig. 23.6 Assistive devices. **A,** Cane. **B,** Quad cane offers more support than a single-stem walker. **C,** Walker with front wheels allows constant contact with the ground. **D,** Walker with adjustable front wheels. (From Cameron, M. H. & Monroe, L. G. [2007]. *Physical rehabilitation: Evidence-based examination, evaluation, and intervention*. St. Louis, MO: Saunders.)

Casts are generally used to immobilize fractures for 6 to 8 weeks. A variety of assistive devices may be used for patients with lower extremity casts (Fig. 23.6). The nurse prepares the patient for self-care and prevention of complications during this treatment period.

Osteoarthritis

OA, also known as *degenerative joint disease,* is a noninflammatory disease of joints characterized by progressive articular cartilage deterioration and the formation of new bone in the joint space. This is the most common type of arthritis seen in older adults and the leading cause of disability in the United States.

The exact cause of OA is not well understood. Aging alone does not cause the degeneration of the joint. Age, trauma, lifestyle, obesity, and genetics have been cited as predisposing factors in the development of OA. The underlying pain associated with OA is related to pressure of the ligaments, bone spur formation, and the stretching of the joint capsule (Ashford & Williard, 2014; Ayhan, Kesmezacar, & Akgun, 2014). In OA, the articular cartilage thins and is lost, particularly in areas of increased stress. As the cartilage deteriorates, proliferation of bone occurs at the margins of the joints. When the joint cartilage is lost, the two bone surfaces come into contact with each other. This results in joint pain. The distal interphalangeals, proximal interphalangeals, the carpometacarpal joint, first metatarsophalangeal joint, knees, hips, and spine are the joints most commonly affected by OA (Shelton, 2013; Onat, Ekiz, Biçer, & Özgirgin, 2015).

The most common symptom is a gradual onset of joint pain. The pain occurs with activity and is relieved with rest. Stiffness may occur on wakening or after periods of inactivity that resolves with movement. *Crepitus,* a grating sound and sensation, may be heard and felt with range of motion in affected joints. Affected joints also have a decreased range of motion (Onat, Ekiz, Biçer,

& Özgirgin, 2015). The degeneration of the joint structure may result in muscle spasms, gait changes, and disuse of the joint. Bony enlargements, called Heberden nodes, may be seen on the distal interphalangeals, and Bouchard nodes are the nodules of the proximal joints (Fig. 23.7) (LeBlond, Brown, Suneja, & Szot, 2015).

NURSING MANAGEMENT

Assessment

Nursing assessment of a patient with OA begins with taking a thorough history of the problem. Data gathered include information about the onset, location, quality, and duration of the joint pain. Inquire the patient about the sensation of joint locking as in the knee. Determine whether any associated muscle spasms have occurred (LeBlond, Brown, Suneja, & Szot, 2015). Questions about precipitating factors; drugs used to relieve pain, including prescription and over-the-counter (OTC) agents; nonpharmacologic interventions such as heat or cold therapy and exercise; and effect on functional abilities should be asked. Affected joints should be inspected for tenderness, swelling, redness, crepitation, and range of motion. Note the presence of muscle atrophy in surrounding muscles.

Diagnosis

Nursing diagnoses for the older adult patient with OA include the following:
- Pain resulting from inflammation and deterioration of the joint cartilage
- Reduced mobility as a result of lower extremity joint stiffness
- Inadequate self-care as a result of limitations in joint movement and strength

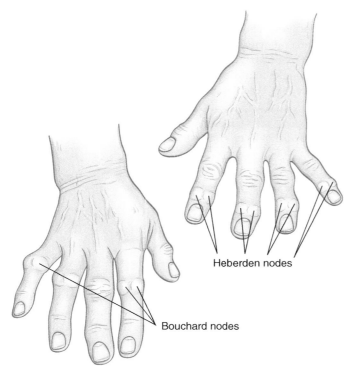

Heberden nodes

Bouchard nodes

Fig. 23.7 Nodes and arthritis. (From McCance, K. L., & Huether, S. E. [2014]. *Pathophysiology: The biologic basis for disease in adults and children* [7th ed.]. St. Louis, MO: Mosby.)

Planning and Expected Outcomes

The focus of the nursing care plan is to protect and preserve joint motion and function. Expected outcomes for the patient are individualized and specific to the joints affected. Outcomes include the following:

1. The patient will verbalize an improved level of comfort with activities.

2. The patient will be able to successfully use various adaptive devices in maintaining independence in ADLs and IADLs.
3. The patient will demonstrate safe use of assistive devices for ambulation.
4. The patient will demonstrate understanding of the use of orthotics.

Intervention

Instructions on joint protection and energy conservation are given. For patients with mild pain, a gentle exercise program that improves muscle tone and prevents joint stiffness may be used. Water therapy has been found to be effective in alleviating osteoarthritic pain and improves overall function (Bhatia, Bejarano, & Novo, 2013). Rest periods between activities are recommended. Heat or cold therapy to the joints may also be used to decrease joint pain. Simple measures such as a warm bath or shower in the morning may help reduce the early morning stiffness that may accompany the pain. Other pain relief interventions may be incorporated into the treatment plan (see Evidence-Based Practice box: Yoga Interventions for Sleep Disturbance in Older Adults with Osteoarthritis).

The physician may also prescribe various nonsteroidal antiinflammatory drugs (NSAIDs) and nonopioid analgesics to control the pain. Patients may initially be given OTC drugs then gradually advanced to a prescription antiinflammatory agent. The use of a topical antiinflammatory gel to an affected area such as the knee has been shown to reduce pain (Derry et al., 2017). Other medical treatment options for more severe pain may include directly injecting the painful joint with steroids. This may be done two or three times yearly for chronic pain. More recent developments in arthritis treatment include the injection of hyaluronic acid into a painful knee joint if more conservative measures have not been effective. The nurse should educate the patient about these conservative measures for

---

EVIDENCE-BASED PRACTICE

Osteoarthritis and Benefits of Shared Yoga Intervention for Sleep Disturbances

Background

Older adults are at cumulative risk for developing OA, with increasing age a leading risk factor. Recent studies have indicated that regular participation in yoga has reduced pain and improved function in patients with OA. This study looked at the effect of a shared yoga intervention on insomnia in older adults with OA.

Sample/Setting

Seventeen community-dwelling older adults who met the inclusion criteria of designated age range (50–85) diagnosed with OA of the hip, knee, or ankle, in pain and reported insomnia directly related to the OA were randomized to a shared yoga or individual yoga program. The age range of the participants was 50 to 72, with 53% of the sample male and 41% as female. Following telephone screenings, a baseline visit was made to obtain consent and provide participants with a sleep diary, Actigraph and yoga equipment, and an audio-guided CD to be used at home.

Methods

Before participation in the yoga classes, participants were instructed to keep a sleep diary and wear the Actigraph. The yoga programs for each group consisted

of 12 weeks of classes that consisted of a brief warm-up followed by 30 minutes of yoga. Participants were also asked to practice yoga moves at home on days when no classes were scheduled. If the participant was in the partner group, the partner also practiced yoga.

Findings

No differences were found between the two groups on attendance of classes or at home practicing yoga lessons. Participants who had a partner reported feeling motivated to go to class. Efficacy outcomes of yoga classes were found in both groups to be in perceived improvement of sleep rather than actual hours slept or on indicators of depression from the PHQ-8.

Implications

Participating in yoga, whether alone or with a partner, may improve self-reported sleep issues. Although the overall actual quality of sleep was not found to improve, nurses can recommend participation in yoga as a means of improving self-reported sleep issues, which are quite common in older adults with OA.

Data from Buchanan, T., Vitiello, & Bennett, K. (2017). Feasibility and efficacy of a shared yoga intervention for sleep disturbance in older adults with osteoarthritis. *Journal of Gerontological Nursing, 43*(8), 42-52.

treating the symptoms of arthritis. Information regarding correct dosing of oral drugs, contraindications, side effects, and adverse effects should be provided.

When conservative measures for treating chronic arthritis pain fail and the patient becomes more disabled, surgical procedures may be considered. The main indications for surgery are severe pain and increasing disability. The surgical procedure most often used is arthroplasty, a surgical replacement of the involved joint. Joint replacement surgery is currently successful for many joints that may be involved with arthritis, including the shoulders, elbows, fingers, hips, and knees. Other surgical options include arthroscopic procedures and joint fusion surgery. These procedures do not replace the joint but may result in improved function and reduced pain.

For patients undergoing joint replacement surgery for the hip or knee, the preoperative period focuses on education about the surgical procedure, its risks, any potential complications, and the postoperative course. After surgery, the goals of nursing care are to prevent complications, relieve surgical pain, and assist the patient in achieving a higher level of function and activity. Major complications after joint replacement surgery may include thromboembolism (deep venous thrombosis [DVT]), joint or wound infection, blood loss, nerve injury, joint dislocation, and surgical pain (Forster & Stewart, 2016). The risk of DVT is highest between the first and second week after surgery. Nursing interventions in the postoperative period include measures to prevent infection, control pain, and assist with daily activities. Aseptic precautions should be taken with surgical wound dressings, urinary catheters, and surgical drains to prevent infection. The patient may be given prophylactic antibiotics for a short time (24 hours) after surgery.

Infection of the site of joint replacement is a serious complication. The incidence of deep infection of joint replacement sites is 0.5% to 1%. The infection may be a result of contamination during surgery, hematoma formation, or delayed wound healing, or it may be hematogenous from a distant site, as with urinary tract infection. The most common contaminants are staphylococci and gram-positive aerobic streptococci. Because the new joint is a foreign body, pathogens may be introduced and will persist on the metal or plastic surfaces of the prosthesis, leading to chronic deep infection of the joint.

Patients with rheumatoid arthritis (RA), diabetes mellitus, or poor nutritional status and those receiving long-term corticosteroid therapies are at increased risk for developing joint infections. If infection occurs in a joint replacement, long-term intravenous antibiotic therapy is instituted for at least 6 weeks. In some cases, the infected joint may be replaced. Joint infections may lead to increased disability and prolonged rehabilitation. Various prophylactic measures should be ordered to prevent DVT. These may include various lower extremity compression devices, oral or injectable anticoagulants, and physical therapy to mobilize the patient (O'Connell et al., 2016).

Pain control during the first 24 to 48 hours may be accomplished with intravenous or epidural administration of narcotic analgesics. Patient-controlled analgesia is frequently used to provide adequate pain control. As the patient's pain decreases, oral analgesics should be ordered. Mild analgesics may be required for up to 6 weeks postoperatively as the surgical site heals.

Patients who have total hip replacement surgery are at risk for hip dislocation. The hip should be maintained in a position of abduction and neutral alignment. Some physicians may require the use of pillows or abduction splints while the patient is in bed. Nurses should reinforce hip precautions as described in the Patient/Family Teaching box: Precautions After Hip Surgery.

PATIENT/FAMILY TEACHING

Precautions After Hip Surgery

Sit with your hips at a 90-degree or greater angle.
Do *not* bend forward more than 90 degrees.
Do *not* lift the knee on the operated side higher than your hip.
Do *not* cross legs at knees or ankles.
Keep pillows between your legs when lying on your side or your back.
Do *not* bend to put on shoes; use a long shoehorn.
Do *not* bend down to reach items on the floor.
Do *not* sit in low chairs.

The goal of total knee replacement surgery is to restore at least 90 degrees of knee flexion. For patients to achieve this, active and passive physical therapy is instituted. In addition, the physician may order a continuous passive motion device, which continuously moves the knee through a preset range of flexion and extension. Rehabilitation for a patient with a joint replacement begins within 24 to 48 hours of the surgical procedure and includes muscle strengthening and range-of-motion exercises. The patient is instructed on the use of a cane, walker, or crutches. Occupational therapy provides the patient with instructions for independence in daily activities. A short stay in a rehabilitation facility may follow the acute hospital stay. However, many patients are able to quickly return to their own home with continued home therapy services.

Evaluation

The goals in caring for a patient with OA are to relieve pain and restore function. Patients should report minimum pain and improved ability to perform ADLs. Conservative measures (as outlined earlier) will improve mobility and increase comfort for many older patients. If surgical intervention is used, the patient needs to understand the expected outcomes, as well as the risks associated with the procedure. Patients with OA may benefit from support groups and group exercise programs especially designed for patients with arthritis. The patient's self-care practices should include regular exercise, the use of adaptive devices, if necessary, and adherence to prescribed drug regimens. Understanding the disease process and treatment measures will assist an older adult in maintaining function and independence.

Spinal Stenosis

Symptomatic osteoarthritic changes of the spine leading to functional limitation and pain in older adults are becoming more common. Lumbar spinal stenosis is one of the most frequently encountered, clinically important degenerative spinal disorders in the aging population (Kalff, Ewald, Waschke, Gobisch, & Hopf, 2013). Degenerative spinal stenosis is a bony overgrowth of the facet joints of the vertebrae, which leads to

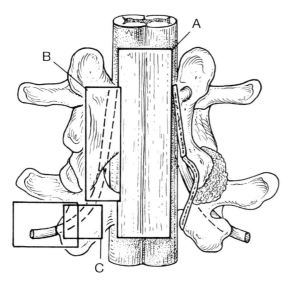

Fig. 23.8 Three-dimensional illustration of segmental stenoses. **A,** Anatomic. **B,** Segmental. **C,** Pathologic. (Redrawn from Ciric, I., Mikhael, M. A., Tarkington, J. A., & Vick, N. A. [1980]. The lateral recess syndrome: A variant of spinal stenosis. *Journal of Neurosurgery, 53,* 433–443.)

narrowing of the spinal canal and possible compression of the nerve roots. Although spinal stenosis may occur at any level of the spine, it is most frequently seen in the lumbar region at levels L3 and L4 (Fig. 23.8). Degeneration of the vertebral joints and disks of the spine, along with nerve compression, leads to progressive back pain and possible weakness of lower extremities. Patients with spinal stenosis may develop claudication-like symptoms of burning and numbness in their lower extremities (Kalff, Ewald, Waschke, Gobisch, & Hopf, 2013).

NURSING MANAGEMENT

Assessment

Goals of nursing assessment focus on the patient's symptoms. The exact location of pain or numbness, the duration of the symptoms, and successful pain relief measures should be identified. Pain caused by degenerative spinal stenosis tends to occur primarily in the back and buttocks, but it may also radiate into the thighs, calves, and feet. The pain may be unilateral or bilateral and generally worsens with prolonged standing or activity. Symptoms are generally relieved with flexion of the spine. Patients may usually report specific positions or activities that aggravate or reduce their symptoms. They may report that activities such as leaning over a grocery cart lessen their pain. Comfort levels during routine ADLs should always be assessed.

Diagnosis

Nursing diagnoses for an older patient with spinal stenosis include the following:
- Chronic pain resulting from spinal nerve root narrowing
- Reduced mobility as a result of discomfort with walking and movement
- Potential for reduced stamina as a result of chronic pain
- Potential for injury resulting from pain and difficulty with ambulation

Planning and Expected Outcomes

The focus of the nursing care plan for a patient with spinal stenosis is management of chronic pain, maintenance of strength and mobility, and promotion of independence with daily activities. The severity of symptoms and assessment of current limitations of activity will determine the individual needs of patients with degenerative spinal stenosis. Expected outcomes include the following:
1. The patient will report a minimum or tolerable level of pain.
2. The patient will demonstrate improved mobility and tolerance of activity.
3. The patient will be able to incorporate a plan for lifestyle modifications that includes activity and rest.
4. The patient will demonstrate safe use of assistive devices and make necessary environmental changes to promote safety.

Intervention

Nursing care for an older patient with spinal stenosis depends on the severity of spinal cord narrowing, the patient's state of health, and the degree of pain and immobility. For the patient being treated conservatively, the nurse should instruct him or her to allow sufficient periods of rest and to limit activities that produce pain. Physical therapy for range of motion and muscle strengthening may be ordered by the physician. Pain relief measures should be initiated and then evaluated for their effectiveness. The physician may order NSAIDs, analgesics to include injectable steroid treatments for more severe pain (Lee, Kim, Oh, Lee, Park, 2015). The use of pain assessment scales will help determine pain patterns, the severity of pain, and the effectiveness of pain relief measures. Other nursing measures to relieve pain include the use of heat or cold applications to the back, massage therapy, relaxation techniques, and position changes for the patient while in bed. Older patients with unrelieved chronic pain may be considered for pain team consultation and multidisciplinary treatment efforts. In many patients with chronic pain, depression may accompany and increase the intensity of the pain symptoms. A physician consultant may recommend the use of a mild antidepressant drug in addition to the other pain relief measures.

Evaluation

The patient's ability to perform ADLs independently with minimum discomfort should be evaluated by self-report and observation. The effectiveness of pain relief measures should be discussed with the patient, and changes should be made when drugs have lost their effectiveness. For patients undergoing epidural injections or surgical procedures, the nurse should reinforce instructions about precautions and activities. The older patient should be able to verbalize potential complications and expected outcomes of treatment. Documentation of patient interactions should include the use of an appropriate pain scale and information about current activity levels and restrictions.

Rheumatoid Arthritis

RA is a chronic, systemic, inflammatory disease that causes joint destruction and deformity, and results in disability. The onset of the disease most commonly occurs in the third or fourth decade.

However, RA may also develop in older adults, known as *elderly onset rheumatoid arthritis* (EORA). The disease is usually a chronic problem for 1% of the population, and the occurrence of the EORA has equal gender distribution compared with RA in the younger adult population (Yung, 2017).

The cause of RA is not known. The most widely accepted theory is that it is an autoimmune disease that causes inflammation, most often in the joints but sometimes also in connective tissue. Joint involvement most often starts with the proximal interphalangeals, metacarpophalangeals, and wrists; in the later stages of the disease, knees and hips are affected.

In the initial phase of RA, the synovial membrane becomes inflamed and thickens, and production of synovial fluid is increased. The change is called *pannus*. As pannus tissue develops, it causes erosion and destruction of the joint capsule and subchondral bone. These processes result in decreased joint motion, deformity, and finally ankylosis, or joint immobilization.

The course of RA is variable. Generally, the onset is gradual, and the course is one of remissions and exacerbations. The symptoms are painful, stiff joints, decreased range of motion in the joints, joint swelling, and deformity (Fig. 23.9). The joint stiffness is present in the morning and lasts from 30 minutes to 6 hours. On examination, the affected joints are warm and

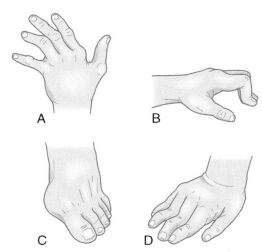

Fig. 23.10 Typical deformities of rheumatoid arthritis. **A,** Ulnar drift. **B,** Boutonnière. **C,** Hallux valgus. **D,** Swan-neck deformity. (From Lewis, S. L., Bucher, L., Heitkemper, M. M., et al. [2017]. *Medical-surgical nursing: Assessment and management of clinical problems.* [10th ed.]. St. Louis, MO: Elsevier.)

swollen. Deformities of the joints include ulnar deviation of the wrists, boutonnière deformity caused by contractures of the distal and proximal interphalangeal joints, and swan-neck deformity caused by contractures of the distal interphalangeal joint (Fig. 23.10). Patients may also develop subcutaneous nodules which feel firm and fixed, often found on the proximal side of the elbow (LeBlond, Brown, Suneja, & Szot, 2015)

Systemic symptoms may include fatigue, malaise, anorexia, weight loss, and anemia. RA in older adults may appear atypically; that is, large joints are affected more often, and the onset may be more sudden than in younger adults. Fatigue, weakness, and fever may be present (Table 23.1). Patients with long-term RA may develop comorbidities such as Sjögren syndrome, Felty syndrome, and pericarditis (Ishchenko & Lories, 2016).

NURSING MANAGEMENT

Assessment

A careful nursing history is taken. Questions are asked about family history and constitutional symptoms, including fever, anorexia, weight loss, fatigue, and duration of the joint stiffness. On physical examination, the affected joints are inspected for symmetric involvement, pain, tenderness, swelling, heat, erythema, and deformity. For patients with long-term complicated RA, assessment should also include examination of the eye for scleritis and corneal ulcers, lungs for pneumonitis, and a cardiac examination for presence of pericarditis (Ishchenko & Lories, 2016).

Diagnosis

Nursing diagnoses for a patient with RA include the following:
- Pain resulting from swollen, inflamed joint tissue
- Reduced mobility as a result of joint deformities and inflammation
- Fatigue as a result of the systemic disease process
- Inadequate nutrition as a result of loss of appetite

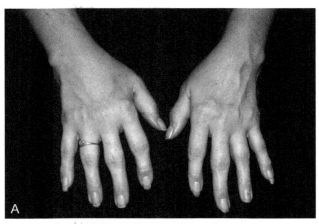

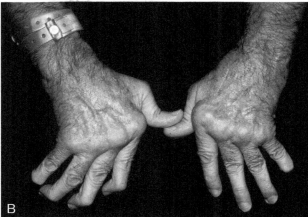

Fig. 23.9 Rheumatoid arthritis of the hand. **A,** Early stage. **B,** Advanced stage. (From Hochberg, M. C., Silman, A. J., Smolen, J. S., et al. [2009]. *Rheumatoid arthritis.* Philadelphia, PA: Mosby.)

TABLE 23.1 Differentiating Rheumatoid Arthritis From Osteoarthritis

	Rheumatoid Arthritis	Osteoarthritis
Age at onset	Fourth through sixth decades. Late onset RA peaks between 60 and 80 years of age.	Fifth and sixth decades
Onset	Gradual	Gradual
Disease course	Exacerbations and remissions	Variable, progressive
Duration of stiffness	1–24 hours	30 minutes or less
Joint pain	Worse in morning	Worse after activity
Joints involved	Proximal interphalangeal Metacarpophalangeal Metatarsophalangeal Knees, hips, wrists	Distal interphalangeal Knees, hips Lumbar, cervical Spine
Symmetric pattern	Almost always	Occasionally
Constitutional manifestations	Present	Absent
Synovial fluid	Increased cells Decreased viscosity	Few cells Normal viscosity
Radiography findings	Abnormalities present	Abnormalities present
Erythrocyte sedimentation rate	Almost always elevated	Occasionally elevated
Positive rheumatoid factor	Almost always	Never

- Inadequate bathing/dressing/feeding/toileting self-care in ADLs as a result of the loss of motion and strength in painful, swollen joints
- Distorted body image as a result of gradual onset of joint deformities

Planning and Expected Outcomes

Prevention of joint deformities, control of symptoms, and maintenance of the patient's abilities to have an active lifestyle are the focus of intervention for a patient with RA. Outcomes for the older patient include the following:

1. The patient will maintain normal joint motion in affected joints, with minimum deformities.
2. The patient's pain related to inflammation will be well controlled.
3. The patient will be able to maintain optimal functional status.

Intervention

Older patients with RA and their families require extensive education to cope effectively with the chronic nature of this disease. The nurse needs to discuss with them pain management, drug therapies, maintenance of self-care activities, promotion of safe mobility, methods of joint protection and precautions, and management of overall health.

Education on pain management includes information on appropriate drugs that have been prescribed and OTC remedies that a patient may be using. The patient should be informed that stress and anxiety may cause muscle tension that may worsen joint pain. Progressive relaxation and guided imagery are taught to decrease anxiety and stress. Application of heat and cold to the affected joints decreases cutaneous nerve stimulation. Ice packs are applied to joints during periods of acute inflammation. Moist heat is useful in relaxing muscles and increasing joint mobility.

The role of the nurse in drug management is to teach the older patient about the action, side effects, and special precautions related to the specific drugs. Table 23.2 presents multiple drugs classically used in the treatment of arthritis. In addition to those drugs listed in Table 23.2, newer pharmacologic and biologic agents are being researched and developed for use in patients with RA.

The drug management of RA is directed at disease management and at symptom control. Drugs selected for relief of the pain and inflammations include corticosteroids, analgesics, and NSAIDs. Corticosteroids along with drugs known as *disease-modifying antirheumatic drugs* (DMARDs) are prescribed to aid with disease control. Concern exists about extended corticosteroid use because of the multiple side effects of long-term use such as infection, peptic ulcer disease, and osteoporosis.

The early DMARDs, which suppress the immune response, include drugs such as methotrexate, leflunomide, hydroxychloroquine, and sulfasalazine. The newer DMARDs, which are biologic agents, are administered subcutaneously, intravenously, and orally. Drugs known as *tumor necrosis factor* (TNF) receptor antagonists are effective for the treatment of RA with methotrexate. Numerous side effects are reported to be caused by TNF receptor antagonists and include infections, potential worsening of heart failure, and demyelinating disease. Nurses need to educate patients about the numerous side effects of these drugs and stress the importance of not taking any OTC drugs without the permission of their health care provider.

Fatigue and decreased mobility of the joints of the upper extremities contribute to self-care deficits. Occupational therapists work with older patients to improve joint function and prevent disability. The modalities used include exercises, splints, methods to protect joints, and assistive devices. Splints may be used to protect joints, maintain joint function, and decrease pain. The nurse reinforces the use of these devices and monitors correct use.

Limitations of mobility because of pain and joint stiffness may lead to disuse and greater disability. To prevent excessive disability, the patient is taught body mechanics and proper body alignment, and is given recommendations for an exercise program. Using good body mechanics and keeping the body in a position of optimal alignment decrease joint stress and fatigue. Physical therapists prescribe individualized therapeutic exercise programs, which include strengthening and stretching exercises, range-of-motion exercises, and endurance training.

Fatigue is a common constitutional symptom of RA. Fatigue may interfere with the older adult's achievement of optimal functional independence. Methods used to decrease fatigue

TABLE 23.2 Drugs, Rationales, Side Effects, and Nursing Implications of Classic Drugs

Drug	Rationale for Use	Side Effects	Nursing Implications
Salicylates: aspirin	Used in early disease phase; analgesic, antipyretic, and antiinflammatory	Gastrointestinal irritation; slight elevation of liver enzyme levels; tinnitus (reversible)	Administer with milk or food. Teach use of enteric-coated tablets. Evaluate for gastrointestinal pain or bleeding, as well as tinnitus.
NSAIDs Long term: diclofenac, fenoprofen, flurbiprofen, ibuprofen, indomethacin, ketoprofen, meclofenamate, mefenamic acid, nabumetone, naproxen, oxaprozin, piroxicam, salsalate, sulindac, tolmetin	Used when salicylates are ineffective; analgesic, antipyretic, and antiinflammatory actions; generally inhibit prostaglandin synthesis	Gastrointestinal irritation; diarrhea; fluid retention, edema; interstitial nephritis; nephrotic syndrome; dizziness, tachycardia, blurred vision, headaches; cholestatic hepatitis; bone marrow depression	Must be administered for 1–2 weeks before a therapeutic response is seen. Administer with food or antacids. Assess for gastrointestinal pain and occult bleeding. Teach patient to avoid alcohol. Evaluate renal and hepatic function regularly.
Short term: phenylbutazone	Specific for adjunctive use	Same as above	Same as above; 1-week trial is suggested. Evaluate CBC. Use with caution in older adults.
Oxyphenbutazone	Effective for articular symptoms in some patients	Same as above	Same as above; use under close medical supervision.
Antimalarials: hydroxychloroquine sulfate, hydroxychloroquine phosphate	Used for severe destructive disease; 3–6 months needed to reach therapeutic levels	Gastrointestinal irritation; skin rash and changes; retinal changes; bone marrow depression	Advise ophthalmologic examination every 4–6 weeks. Allow 6–8 weeks for therapeutic effects to begin. Evaluate CBC regularly. Assess for gastrointestinal effects, headaches, dizziness, hearing effects, and hepatotoxic effects. Evaluate for water and sodium retention.
Auranofin	Effects cumulative, slow onset of effects (8–14 weeks); dosage may be gradually decreased after remission	Proteinuria; interstitial fibrosis; metallic taste	Teach skin care. Evaluate gastrointestinal discomfort. Check urine for blood and protein.
Penicillamine	As effective as gold sodium thiomalate but more toxic; unknown mechanism of action; effects seen in 2 months	Gastrointestinal irritation; taste alterations; blood dyscrasias; skin rash; stomatitis; nephrotic syndrome, glomerulonephritis; autoimmune syndrome; proteinuria	Evaluate CBC, liver, and renal function weekly for 2 months, then monthly. Teach patient to report sore throat or fever. Take between meals because food decreases absorption.
Antirheumatics: gold sodium thiomalate, aurothioglucose	Used when salicylates and NSAIDs fail; remission-inducing action suppresses inflammation	Skin rashes, pruritus; stomatitis; diarrhea; blood dyscrasias; hepatitis	Give with NSAIDs until efficacy is reached. Assess CBC and renal and liver function often.
Steroids: systemic prednisone, prednisolone, hydrocortisone	Symptom relief for months to years for certain prolonged conditions.	Multiple toxic effects, including osteoporosis, gastric ulcers, risk of infection susceptibility, hirsutism, emotional lability, edema, moon facies, hypokalemia, cataracts, glaucoma	Teach patient not to stop drug abruptly. Administer for short periods and taper dose slowly. Monitor for side effects, including hypertension and hyperglycemia.
Intraarticular	Used when only one or two joints are involved; used for pain relief, to increase function; benefits last 2 weeks to several months; joints most amenable are ankles, knees, hips, shoulders, and hands	Same as above	Teach patient that effects may be short lived. Advise that administration is limited to two to four infections per year per joint.
Immunosuppressives: azathioprine, methotrexate, cyclophosphamide	Used with advanced disease; affect immune system to decrease inflammation; teratogenic potential	Hepatitis, cirrhosis; gastrointestinal ulcers; susceptibility to infection; bone marrow suppression; alopecia; skin rash	Evaluate CBC, liver function, and renal function weekly. Assess older adults closely for signs of toxicity.
Capsaicin cream, gel, liquid, patch	Topical for pain	Irritation of skin and other mucous membranes.	Avoid contact with eyes, nares or other mucous membranes to avoid burning sensation. Avoid using with heat sources to prevent burns

CBC, Complete blood cell count; NSAIDs, nonsteroidal antiinflammatory drugs.
Modified from Roberts, D. (2013). Arthritis and connective tissue disorders. In L. Schoenly (Ed.), Core curriculum for orthopaedic nursing (7th ed.). Pitman, NJ: National Association of Orthopaedic Nurses.

include balancing rest with activity, scheduling short rest periods (1 to 2 hours), practicing relaxation techniques, and adapting the environment to simplify work. Coping with chronic illness, pain, deformity, and alterations in body image may predispose a patient to depression. If clinical depression occurs, medical evaluation and treatment are indicated.

The joint deformities and alteration in body image may negatively affect sexual function. The nurse should be aware of this and openly discuss issues of sexuality and methods of maintaining physical intimacy. Suggestions may include using analgesics before sexual activity, planning rest periods before sexual activity, assuming alternative positions, and encouraging alternative methods of maintaining physical intimacy.

Adults with RA require many types of support to cope with this chronic, disabling disease. The nurse's role is to provide the older adult with information about available resources so that optimal levels of functioning can be reached.

A good resource is the Arthritis Foundation (1330 W. Peachtree St., Atlanta, GA 30309; [800] 283–7800; http://www.arthrtitis.org), which publishes educational materials that address exercise programs, work simplification, and the disease process. Support groups and self-help classes taught in 6-week sessions are conducted by local chapters. The content of the classes includes self-efficacy, exercise, pain management, depression, stress management, and nontraditional therapies.

Evaluation

The older adult with RA should experience minimum discomfort and be able to maintain an acceptable level of function and mobility. With advances in drug therapy and active participation by the patient in activities to prevent joint deformities, the patient should experience less deformity, increased comfort levels, and understanding of the disease process.

Gouty Arthritis

Gout is a disease in which acute attacks of arthritis pain occur because of elevated levels of serum uric acid. During acute gout attacks, joint inflammation is caused by sodium urate crystals in the joint. Gout is classified as *primary* or *acquired.* Primary gout is an inborn disease of purine metabolism. Acquired gout is caused by drugs that affect excretion of uric acid. These drugs include diuretics, levodopa-carbidopa, and low-dose aspirin (Kuo, Grainge, Mallen, Zhang, & Doherty, 2015). Gout usually occurs in the middle years but also affects older adults; it is more prevalent in men than in women.

In gout, an excessive production or a decreased urinary excretion of uric acid may occur. The excess monosodium urate salts are deposited in joints and surrounding connective tissue. The deposits of the uric acid crystals are called *tophi,* often found on the helix of the ear, on the olecranon bursa, and over the Heberden nodes in patients with coexisting OA (Fig. 23.11).

Gout may manifest as an acute or a chronic condition. The onset of gout is sudden and manifested by an acute attack of pain in one or more joints. The most commonly affected area is the great toe, known as *podagra.* Other joints and periarticular structures affected by gout include the ankle, knee, wrist, and the olecranon bursa (Kuo et al., 2015). The affected joint becomes hot, reddened, and tender. The pain may be severe and interfere

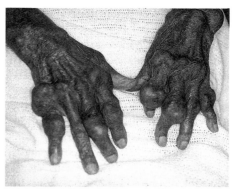

Fig. 23.11 Tophaceous gout. (Courtesy John Cook, MD. From Goldstein, B. G., & Goldstein, A. E. [1997]. *Practical dermatology* [2nd ed.]. St Louis, MO: Mosby.)

with mobility, self-care, and functional abilities. Chills and fever may also be present. Acute attacks of gout usually subside in 7 days regardless of treatment. In chronic gout, the uric acid crystals cause bone destruction and deformity. Uric acid crystals may also be deposited in the kidney and cause nephrolithiasis.

NURSING MANAGEMENT

Assessment

The onset of an acute gout attack is identified by the presence of warmth, swelling, cutaneous erythema, and severe pain in the affected joint. The initial attack is usually in one joint, and in nearly half of patients it will involve the first metatarsophalangeal joint. In older women, however, the initial presentation often begins in multiple joints (West & O'Dell, 2015). The pain is intense, and the joint is sensitive to even the slightest touch. Other symptoms may include fever, chills, and malaise. Intervals between initial attacks and subsequent acute episodes will vary, but the attacks usually become more frequent and involve more joints.

Patients with chronic gouty arthritis usually report 10 or more years of previous acute gout attacks. The involved joints are chronically uncomfortable and swollen, although the intensity of the pain is less than in the acute episodes. Tophi may or may not be detected on a physical examination (Igel et al., 2017). Nursing assessment should identify other risk factors or conditions that may predispose the patient to development of gout. These factors include obesity, hypertension, alcohol ingestion, use of diuretics, recent trauma, hyperlipidemia, diabetes mellitus, chronic kidney disease, and organ transplant.

Diagnosis

Nursing diagnoses for a patient with gouty arthritis include the following:
- Pain, acute or chronic, resulting from joint inflammation and swelling
- Reduced mobility resulting from joint deformity and discomfort secondary to the disease process
- Potential for reduced stamina resulting from pain

Planning and Expected Outcomes

The overall management plan for an older adult with gouty arthritis, either acute or chronic, is to decrease the pain and other associated symptoms. Expected outcomes for a patient with gout include the following:

1. The patient will verbalize increased comfort and pain relief with the use of appropriate analgesics and NSAIDs.
2. The patient will be able to verbalize understanding of the disease process.
3. The patient will incorporate appropriate diet modifications and lifestyle changes such as weight loss and avoidance of alcohol and food products high in purine.
4. The patient will modify his or her activity and rest pattern based on limitations imposed by the pain.
5. The patient will incorporate health practices to minimize recurrent attacks.

Intervention

In the acute phase, the goal of nursing management is to relieve pain. During an acute attack of gout, the pain may be so severe that the patient is unable to bear weight or to tolerate clothing or blankets on the affected joint. Colchicine is an effective medicine for the treatment of pain and inflammation of acute gout; severe pain subsides within 48 hours. The use of NSAIDs, especially indomethacin, provides relief comparable with that provided by colchicine. Other pain relief measures include analgesics, elevation of the affected extremity, immobilization of the joint, and heat or ice packs to the area.

Nursing interventions for chronic gout also focus on pain relief measures and prevention of recurrent attacks of gout. This is accomplished through patient education. Because obesity and diets high in protein have been linked to gout, information about the role of dietary habits should be provided. Foods high in purines, for example, shellfish and organ meats, should be avoided. Alcoholic beverages should also be avoided. Obese patients should have weight reduction diets or programs recommended. A consultation with a dietitian for diet modifications may be helpful.

A xanthine oxidase inhibitor such as allopurinol or febuxostat is the drug of choice for patients with chronic gout symptoms (Feng, Li, & Gao, 2015). Probenecid, a uricosuric agent, is another drug that may be used. Patients must be closely monitored for renal function during drug therapy. To discourage the formation of renal stones, the patient should be encouraged to have a daily intake of 2 to 3 liters (L) of fluid unless contraindicated. The patient should also be instructed to avoid salicylates, which could inhibit drug effects.

Evaluation

Patients with acute or chronic gout should be able to maintain a healthy lifestyle, incorporating the changes suggested during treatment. The patient must understand the drug therapy for acute attacks and chronic treatments. Pain management should allow a patient to participate fully in ADLs and allow for full mobility.

Osteoporosis

Osteoporosis is considered the most common metabolic bone disorder, affecting more than 10 million people in the United States (National Osteoporosis Foundation [NOF], 2014). Common among postmenopausal women, bone fractures occur every year secondary to osteoporosis (Prah, Richards, Griggs, & Simpson, 2017). The disease primarily affects women but also occurs in one of six men. Osteoporosis is commonly referred to as *porous bone disease* or *brittle bone disease* and is characterized by reduction in bone mass and loss of bone strength.

Bone is constantly remodeling itself throughout life, and the process of bone maintenance is constant. Old bone cells are removed (resorbed) by osteoclasts, and new bone cells are formed by osteoblasts. The complete process of bone remodeling takes 4 to 8 months. Bone mass is accumulated in the early part of life; bone mineral density (BMD) increases until approximately age 30, when peak bone mass is attained. Anything that interferes with the normal process of bone remodeling may lead to the development of osteoporosis. Conditions that contribute to this process include renal or hepatic failure and endocrine disorders such as hyperthyroidism, hyperparathyroidism, type 1 diabetes mellitus, RA, and chronic kidney disease. Other risk factors include heredity and genetic predisposition, lifestyle factors, and age. With osteoporosis, the bone remodeling process is altered, and the rate of bone resorption exceeds the rate of bone formation, which leads to decreased bone mass.

Osteoporosis is classified as primary osteoporosis and secondary osteoporosis. Although the cause of primary osteoporosis is not clearly understood, it is further classified into postmenopausal (type 1) osteoporosis and age-associated (type 2) osteoporosis. Type 1 osteoporosis is related to menopausal estrogen deficiency and is seen in women between ages 51 and 75. In type 1, the trabecular bone in the vertebral column, hips, and wrists is weakened. Because type I osteoporosis is related to estrogen deficiency, it is seen six times more often in women than in men. Type 2 osteoporosis occurs in both men and women older than age 70 and causes a gradual loss of cortical bone. Because this cortical bone provides support in the body, weakening of the bone is a predisposing factor in hip fractures. Age-related changes in vitamin D synthesis that result in decreased calcium absorption are thought to be the cause of type 2 osteoporosis.

Secondary osteoporosis, seen in 15% of cases, is the result of diseases such as hyperthyroidism, hyperparathyroidism, gastrointestinal disorders, neoplasms, and alcoholism. In women, early oophorectomy is a cause of secondary osteoporosis. Long-term use of corticosteroids, methotrexate, aluminum-containing antacids, phenytoin, and heparin may result in secondary osteoporosis. Prolonged immobility, which causes calcium excretion, is also a cause of secondary osteoporosis (Prah, Richards, Griggs, & Simpson, 2017).

Certain risk factors for the development of osteoporosis have been identified (Box 23.1). Risk factors that can be modified with lifestyle changes involve calcium intake, exercise, cigarette smoking, and consumption of alcoholic beverages and excessive caffeine products (Prah, Richards, Griggs, & Simpson, 2017). Age, race, gender, and body frame are risk factors that cannot be changed. The nurse may educate the older patient about these risk factors, making suggestions to modify lifestyle and nutrition. Three key essentials in preventing osteoporosis throughout life are appropriate diet, exercise, and lifestyle changes (Prah, Richards, Griggs, & Simpson, 2017).

Osteoporosis is called a "silent killer" because frequently no clinical symptoms appear until fractures occur. The initial complaint may be back pain or fatigue. The fatigue results from the increased demand on muscles to keep the body in an upright position with a decreased bone mass. Osteoporotic fractures are most commonly seen in the vertebrae of the thoracic spine, the femoral neck, and the wrist. Fractures may occur with routine activities such as bending, lifting, coughing, and straining during defecation. Osteoporosis of the spinal vertebrae causes a loss of height of 1 to 2.5 inches. Also seen is the "dowager's hump," or kyphosis, which results from the vertebrae sliding on top of each other (Fig. 23.12). Conventional radiography may provide evidence of osteoporosis, although this is often done retrospectively after a fracture. Unfortunately, at least 30% of bone mass must be lost before the disease is apparent on standard radiography. For evaluation of bone mass in individuals suspected of having osteoporosis or in those considered at risk for development of the disease, a determination of BMD appears irrefutable. Bone densitometry is commonly done with dual-energy x-ray absorptiometry (DEXA). This procedure is simple, is noninvasive, uses a low radiation dose, and is

completed in less than 30 minutes. Many physician offices are now equipped with a DEXA machine for quick and simple screening of patients. Measurement sites include the hip or lumbar spine and peripheral sites such as the wrist. Scores computed from the testing compare the older patient's score with those of normal young adults for peak bone mass and compare the older patient's score with those of gender-matched and age-matched control subjects. The T-score obtained from DEXA is a measure of how much an individual's bone mass differs (in standard deviation) from the bone mass of a healthy 20- to 29-year-old. The score obtained defines bone loss as normal, osteopenia, or osteoporosis. If a patient's T-score is 2.5 or less, it is indicative of severe osteoporosis (Mackey & Whitaker, 2015).

To more clearly establish the candidacy of patients for pharmacologic treatment of osteoporosis, the NOF recommends that clinicians use the Fracture Risk Assessment Tool (FRAX) developed by the World Health Organization (Mackey & Whitaker, 2015). FRAX can be accessed as a web-based algorithm that combines risk factors for developing osteoporosis with BMD results. The tool has been designed to be used in postmenopausal women and in men aged 40 to 90 years old. Limitations of the using the FRAX tool is that the calculated score underestimates fracture risk in patients with recent fractures, multiple osteoporosis-related fractures, and those at increased risk for falling (Cosman et al., 2014). Laboratory blood studies are obtained to differentiate osteoporosis from other diseases that may cause bone loss. Complete blood cell count (CBC) and levels of serum calcium, serum phosphorus, alkaline phosphatase, and urinary calcium are all normal in osteoporosis.

Measures to address osteoporosis should be directed at minimizing bone loss in older adults and preserving the current level of bone mass. Patient education and development of awareness of the disease are critical for prevention and risk reduction. Elimination of lifestyle risk factors, nutritional counseling, and pharmacologic management are strategies used to prevent osteoporosis (Mackey & Whitaker, 2015).

Adequate nutritional intake of calcium should be instituted in early childhood and continued throughout the life span. The current recommendation for daily calcium intake is 1000 mg for men and premenopausal women ages 25 through 49, 1,500 mg for postmenopausal women who are not taking estrogen, 1000 mg for postmenopausal women taking estrogen, and 1,500 mg for men and women older than age 65 years (Mackey & Whitaker, 2015). Milk, either low-fat or nonfat, is a good source of calcium and vitamin D. Table 23.3 identifies dietary sources of calcium. Many of these food items are also good sources of vitamin D, which is essential for the synthesis of calcium.

For individuals unable to consume adequate calcium, supplements are recommended. Various forms of calcium supplements are available. Calcium carbonate is thought to be the best supplement because it contains 40% elemental calcium, is the least expensive, and requires taking the least number of tablets. Patients, however, may find calcium citrate, which contains only 20% elemental calcium, to cause less gastrointestinal side effects, thus more tolerable for long-term therapy. Calcium supplements should be taken with meals and followed by at least 10 ounces (oz.) of water to promote absorption. No more than 600 milligrams (mg) of calcium should be taken in a single dose

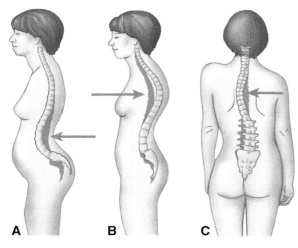

Fig. 23.12 Abnormal spinal curvatures. **A,** Lordosis. **B,** Kyphosis. **C,** Scoliosis. (From Patton, K. T., & Thibodeau, G. A. [2014]. *The human body in health & disease* [6th ed.]. St. Louis, MO: Mosby.)

TABLE 23.3	Dietary Sources of Calcium	
Food	Serving	Calcium Content (mg)
Milk		
Skim	8 oz	299
2% fat	8 oz	297
Whole	8 oz	291
Cheeses		
Swiss	1 oz	272
Processed American	1 oz	174
Mozzarella	1.5 oz	333
Cottage cheese	1 oz	135
Other Dairy Products		
Yogurt, plain low-fat	8 oz	415
Ice cream, vanilla	1 cup	168
Ice milk, vanilla	1 cup	274
Frozen Yogurt, vanilla	1 cup	206
Seafood		
Oysters	1 cup	226
Pink salmon, canned with bones	3 oz	167
Vegetables		
Collards, frozen or fresh	1 cup	357
Broccoli, fresh	1 cup	42
Turnip greens	1 cup	198
Mustard greens	1 cup	104
Kale, cooked	1 cup	94
Dried Beans (cooked and drained)		
Navy beans	1 cup	90
Pinto beans	1 cup	86
Red kidney beans, canned	1 cup	74
Other Foods		
Blackstrap molasses	2 tbsp	274
Tofu	4 oz	108
Orange Juice, calcium fortified	6 oz	261

oz, Ounce; *tbsp,* tablespoon.
Modified from National Institutes of Health Office of Dietary Supplements. (2017). Calcium. Retrieved June 12, 2018 from https://ods.od.nih.gov/factsheets/Calcium-HealthProfessional/#h3.

because absorption is compromised with higher doses. The NOF currently recommends that patients at risk take vitamin D replacement 800 to 1000 international units per day in addition to calcium (Mackey & Whitaker, 2015; NOF, 2014).

Exercise programs that include weight bearing and resistance have been shown to prevent bone loss. Exercises should be done three times a week for 30 to 60 minutes for the best results. Postural exercises to prevent or minimize kyphotic deformity are also of benefit to older adults. Moderation in any exercise program is always recommended.

According to the NOF's *Clinician's Guide to Prevention and Treatment of Osteoporosis,* pharmacologic treatment for osteoporosis is recommended for patients who have had a vertebral or hip fracture, a T-score of 2.5 or less, and a 10-year high probability of hip fracture (>3%) or a 10-year probability of any osteoporosis-related fracture from occurring (>20%), as indicated by the score on the U.S.-adapted FRAX score (NOF, 2014). Initial treatment for osteoporosis generally begins with the bisphosphonates (alendronate, risedronate, and zoledronic acid) or denosumab, a RANK ligand (RANKL) inhibitor (Buckley, Guyatt, Fink, & McAlindon, 2018). The bisphosphonates, which are classified as antiresorptive drugs, are known for their ability to slow bone breakdown by inhibiting the osteoclasts, thereby preventing bone resorption. The U.S. Food and Drug Administration (FDA) recommend bisphosphonates for the prevention and treatment of osteoporosis. Nurses need to instruct patients on the importance of following drug guidelines when taking oral bisphosphonates. Special instructions include taking the drug daily, 1 hour before any food or drug. It must be taken with 6 to 8 ounces of water, and the patient must remain upright for at least 30 minutes after taking the drug. Nurses should also instruct patients about the long-term side effects of bisphosphonates, including bone, which patients may not recognize as a drug side effect but misinterpret as progression of the disease. Denosumab, also recommended for prevention and treatment of osteoporosis, is an injectable agent that needs to be administered twice a year. It is contraindicated in patients with a known history of hypocalcemia, so calcium and vitamin D deficiencies need to be corrected before a patient is started on denosumab (NOF, 2014).

Recommendations for treatment following first-line drugs include the bisphosphonate ibandronate and raloxifene, a selective estrogen receptor modulator (SERM) that has an estrogen-like effect on bone metabolis (Mackey & Whitaker, 2015). Side effects of raloxifene include hot flashes, deep vein thrombosis (DVT), and pulmonary embolism. Patients should not only be educated on the side effects of this drug; they should also be advised to notify their health care provider if they anticipate any long-term immobility while on this drug because of the risk of thromboembolic events (NOF, 2014). Teriparatide, a parathyroid hormone that helps stimulate bone formation, is indicated for the treatment of patients at high risk of fracture from osteoporosis. This drug has been shown to be effective in increasing BMD in patients with osteoporosis related to long-term glucocorticoid therapy (Mackey & Whitaker, 2015).

Another antiresorptive drug used to treat osteoporosis is calcitonin in a parenteral or nasal spray preparation. Oral administration is not appropriate because the drug is a polypeptide hormone and is destroyed in the gastrointestinal tract. The nasal spray preparation is a formulation of synthetic salmon calcitonin, and it has been approved for use in the treatment of osteoporosis in women who are at least 5 years postmenopausal, have low bone density, and are not candidates for estrogen replacement therapy (ERT). Calcitonin is generally taken daily in one puff alternatingly through the nares. Because the drug may elicit a systemic allergic reaction in certain individuals, intradermal skin testing should precede delivery of the initial dose. Systemic adverse effects of the nasal route are reported as being minimal but may include nasal discomfort, occasional rhinitis, and itching of the nasal mucosa.

Since it was first reported, it has been recommended that the use of estrogen or hormone replacement therapy in postmenopausal women with moderately severe menopausal symptoms be limited on the basis of the findings of the Women's Health Initiative, that there is an increased risk for breast cancer, myocardial infarction, stroke, invasive breast cancer, pulmonary embolism, and DVT. Nonestrogen therapies are recommended first for the treatment of osteoporosis (NOF, 2014).

NURSING MANAGEMENT

Assessment

Nursing assessment of older patients should include taking a thorough family health history and determination of the presence of risk factors, the level of exercise, alcohol and caffeine intake, and smoking. Women should be assessed for age of onset of menopause, use of ERT, date of last mammography, and history of breast or uterine cancer. All patients should be asked about their lifelong intake of calcium, history of fractures, presence of pain, and history of falls. A physical examination includes determination of the presence of kyphosis, gait impairments, muscle weakness, and cognitive impairments (Prah, Richards, Griggs, & Simpson, 2017).

Diagnosis

Nursing diagnoses for an older patient with osteoporosis include the following:
- Inadequate nutrition resulting from a decreased intake of calcium and vitamin D
- Potential for injury resulting from weakening of the bones
- Pain resulting from inadequate pain relief secondary to bone fractures
- Distorted body image resulting from spinal deformities and loss of height
- Need for patient teaching resulting from lack of previous exposure to disease process, risk factors, and measures of prevention

Planning and Expected Outcomes

Awareness of the risk factors and education about the lifetime prevention of osteoporosis and its complications such as falls and fractures are the most important aspects of planning the care of older adults with osteoporosis. Expected outcomes for a patient with osteoporosis include the following:
1. The patient will demonstrate taking precautions at home and in the community to prevent falls and activities that may result in fractures.
2. The patient will report an adequate level of pain control in the presence of bone fractures.
3. The patient will consume nutritional supplements, food products, and drugs recommended or prescribed for meeting dietary needs, as evidenced by a diet log.
4. The patient will verbalize acceptance of changes brought about by the disease and an understanding of the treatment and prevention of further deformities (see Health Promotion box).

HEALTH PROMOTION/ILLNESS PREVENTION
Musculoskeletal Function: Osteoporosis

Health Promotion
- Routine weight-bearing exercises that do not stress the joints, such as walking
- Achievement of ideal body weight
- Initiation of a weight-training program
- Smoking cessation
- Decreased intake of alcohol and caffeine

Disease Prevention
- Participation in regular program of weight-bearing exercises
- Avoidance of injury and falls
- Maintenance of adequate dietary intake of calcium and supplementation with oral calcium supplements, as indicated
- Consideration of hormone replacement therapy
- Little to no intake of alcohol and caffeine
- Avoidance of smoking

Intervention

The nurse's role focuses on patient education about the disease process, strategies to prevent further injury or deformity, and measures to promote decreased loss of bone. Education should emphasize the identification and minimization of controllable risk factors. These include cigarette smoking, excessive consumption of alcohol, and caffeine intake. Exercise programs that will place some stress on the bones and, thus, strengthen them, for example, walking and lifting light weights, are recommended. Additional information for osteoporosis education and programs can be found through the NOF (1150, 17th Street NW, Washington, D.C. 20036; [202] 223–2226; http://www.nof.org).

Compression fractures of the vertebrae may cause pain, loss of function, and disturbance in body image brought about by the gradual loss of height caused by multiple fractures. Control of pain is achieved through the use of analgesics, NSAIDs, positioning, and relaxation techniques. Other pain management modalities include transcutaneous electrical nerve stimulation (TENS), various back supports or braces, and formal pain management consultation. Positive body image may be promoted through discussions of acceptance of changes that have occurred but with a focus on prevention of further injury and deformity (Corrarino, 2015).

Nursing care of the older adult with a hip fracture or other fracture secondary to osteoporosis includes the interventions previously noted in this chapter.

Evaluation

An older patient with osteoporosis should be able to describe measures that can be taken to decrease the potential for further bone loss as well as measures that can be taken to maintain a safe living environment so that the risk of injury resulting from falls is reduced. The patient will be able to describe the benefits of appropriate diet, lifestyle modifications, and diet supplements or drugs, if needed. The older adult will also be able to participate in regular exercise programs and to identify resources available for prevention of disease (see Nursing Care Plan: Osteoporosis With Fractured Thoracic Vertebrae).

◎ NURSING CARE PLAN

Osteoporosis With Fractured Thoracic Vertebrae

Clinical Situation

Mrs. R is a 79-year-old widow who has severe osteoporosis and who recently fractured her T4 and T5 vertebrae. After the fracture, she complained of severe pain, which has limited her daily activity and caused her to spend most of the day in bed. The period of bed rest has left her weak. Before the fracture, she was independent in mobility and self-care. She drove and participated in activities with her friends on a regular basis. She is referred to the home care agency for pain management and physical therapy to upgrade her skills for performing ADLs and to promote endurance.

Mrs. R has no other health problems. She lives alone in a two-story house. The bathroom is on the second floor. Since the fracture, Mrs. R has stayed on the second floor all day except for one trip a day to the kitchen on the first floor to fix a meal. Mrs. R's major support is her daughter, who lives in another state. She has several close friends, but they are unable to help her because of their health problems.

On the admission visit, the nurse finds Mrs. R's house to be in an unsafe condition. The rooms and stairs are cluttered with papers, boxes, and other objects. Mrs. R tells the nurse that her pain is somewhat improved, but it still limits her ability to take care of herself and her home. She also tells the nurse, "I don't understand this osteoporosis; how did that cause my fractures?"

Nursing Diagnoses

Potential for injury resulting from unsafe environment

Need for patient teaching resulting from lack of exposure to osteoporosis

Reduced mobility resulting from pain and musculoskeletal impairment

Pain resulting from inadequate knowledge of pain management

Inadequate bathing and dressing self-care (bathing and dressing lower extremities) resulting from pain and prolonged immobility

Outcomes

The patient will remain free from fractures or other injuries and will verbalize unsafe features of her home and a plan to correct.

The patient will verbalize basic information about the disease process, outcomes, and treatment.

The patient will safely walk 100 feet using a pickup walker and will participate in a daily exercise program.

The patient will verbalize that pain is tolerable. Pain will not interfere with the ability to participate in daily activities.

The patient will bathe and dress her lower extremities with the use of assistive devices.

Interventions

Discuss outcomes of an unsafe environment: risks of falling and fracture as a result of cluttered environment.

Use homemaker and friends to reduce clutter and encourage use of safety aids.

Teach safe transfer and ambulation techniques, wearing of sturdy supportive footwear, avoidance of lifting heavy objects, and how to bend from the knees when lifting.

Provide information and instruction on osteoporosis, including the pathophysiology of the disease, treatment regimen, and drug schedule, doses, and side effects.

Stress the importance of dietary intake of calcium and provide information on foods that are high in calcium.

Consult with physical therapy for a program of muscle strengthening, endurance development, stair training, and regular exercise.

Reinforce physical therapy training.

Give positive feedback for gains made.

Instruct the patient to make limited trips up and down stairs until strength is improved.

Instruct the patient on taking pain drug before the exercise program and the need for regular rest periods throughout the day.

Assess pain and the effectiveness of prescribed drugs.

Instruct the patient to take pain drug before activities and on a regular basis until pain diminishes.

Instruct the patient on the use of diversional activities and relaxation techniques.

Assist the patient in setting short-term, realistic goals.

Consult with an occupational therapist for specific assistive devices.

Instruct the patient on the use of assistive devices.

Provide assistance, supervision, and teaching, as needed, to promote self-care.

Paget's Disease

Paget's disease (osteitis deformans) is an inflammatory disease of the bone, in which both osteoclasts and osteoblasts proliferate. The processes of bone formation and bone resorption do not always proceed at the same rate. The cause of Paget's disease is not known. Recent evidence supports the theory that a viral infection of the osteoclasts causes the disease. A possible familial predisposition to Paget's disease also exists. This disease occurs most often in men older than age 40; a higher incidence occurs in individuals older than 80 years. Paget's disease is predominant in people of European descent; it is a condition that is rarely found in Asians and Africans (Ralston, 2013).

Increased activity of osteoclasts leads to increased bone resorption. Bone formation is increased to compensate. This abnormal remodeling causes deformed and enlarged bones. Vascularity in the abnormal bones is increased, which results in excessive warmth over the bones involved. Bones affected by the disease are structurally weak and prone to pathologic fractures (Ralston, 2013).

The onset of Paget's disease is insidious. Bones most often involved are the pelvis, femur, skull, tibia, and spine. The first symptom is bone pain, which is not relieved with rest and

movement. The intensity of the pain varies from mild to severe; the quality may be stabbing or dull. If the bones of the skull are involved, headaches and conductive hearing loss may occur. Barreling of the chest, kyphosis, skull enlargement, and bowing of the tibia and femur are commonly seen bone deformities. The bowing of legs and kyphosis lead to reduction in height.

The prognosis for patients with Paget's disease is not favorable because of the complications that may develop. These include pathologic fractures and loss of hearing related to changes in the temporal bone. The overgrowth of the spinal vertebrae may cause cord compression and paralysis.

NURSING MANAGEMENT

Assessment

Nursing assessment should include taking a thorough health history; information about a known family history of the disease should also be elicited. The nurse should assess for warmth, deformity, pain, and erythema over the long bones; assess the range of motion in joints; and evaluate the presence of any weakness, ataxia, or hearing loss.

Diagnosis

Nursing diagnoses for an older patient with Paget's disease include the following:

- Pain resulting from bone deformity and possible joint involvement
- Reduced mobility resulting from bone deformity, fracture, or pain
- Potential for injury resulting from limitations of mobility and altered bone metabolism
- Distorted body image resulting from deformities and disturbance in function

Planning and Expected Outcomes

Nursing care of the patient should focus primarily on pain management, if necessary, and the issues of chronic disease. Addressing the alterations in body image and impaired mobility are also critical. Expected outcomes include the following:

1. The patient will achieve a satisfactory comfort level with pain management techniques and drugs.
2. The patient will modify the home environment and take precautions in the community to prevent injuries.
3. The patient will verbalize an understanding of the chronic nature of the disease and appropriate therapies.
4. The patient will make positive coping statements related to a potential altered body image.

Intervention

Nursing care of a patient with Paget's disease includes education regarding the disease and treatment. Pain management should be addressed; pain is usually the presenting symptom. The pain is usually a deep, aching type of bone pain that may worsen with activity, especially with weight-bearing activities in patients with spinal or lower extremity deformities. For symptomatic patients, first-line drugs are nitrogen-containing bisphosphonates such as alendronate, pamidronate, risedronate, and zoledronic acid (Ralston, 2013). Patients may also be prescribed vitamin D if the 25-hydroxy vitamin D level is found to be subclinical (Ralston, 2013). Various methods of pain relief may be tried, including use of NSAIDs and analgesics. Other nursing interventions include instructing an older patient on the use of heat or cold therapy, rest, and other pain relief measures.

The patient's safety and mobility issues should be assessed. Instruction on simple exercises and the use of assistive devices or consultation with physical or occupational therapists may be of benefit. Occasionally, the patient's disease may involve the hip or knee joint, resulting in chronic, severe pain and deformity. Arthroplasty may be recommended to correct the deformity and relieve pain.

Helping the patient maintain mobility and independence with daily activities may also positively affect the patient's body image and attitude toward the chronic disease. Discussions of long-term prognosis and treatment may offer encouragement.

Evaluation

Nursing evaluation of a patient with Paget's disease includes documentation of the patient's ability to perform ADLs and his or her understanding of the importance of therapy for prevention of pain, deformity, and loss of function. Nurses should specifically evaluate the patient's need for adaptive equipment such as canes, walkers, or shoe lifts when limb shortening has occurred (Ralston, 2013).

Osteomyelitis

Osteomyelitis is an infection of the bone that may be either acute or chronic. Acute osteomyelitis resolves in 4 weeks when treated with antibiotics. Chronic osteomyelitis lasts longer than 4 weeks and does not respond to initial treatment with antibiotic.

Invasion of bone by microorganisms is the cause of osteomyelitis. Microorganisms enter the body directly through an open fracture or stage IV pressure ulcer. Bloodborne bacteria from distant sources such as urinary tract infections may indirectly inoculate bone. *Staphylococcus aureus* is the most common bacterium seen in osteomyelitis (Oliphant, 2015). Other causative agents are gram-negative bacteria such as *Escherichia coli* and *Pseudomonas aeruginosa*. Osteomyelitis is seen most often in older adults as a complication of a stage IV pressure ulcer.

Bacteria infiltrate bone through the blood supply and lodge in an area of bone where circulation is sluggish. The bacteria multiply, resulting in an inflammatory response. Pus and vascular congestion develop, causing increased pressure in bone, which leads to ischemia and vascular compromise. Necrotic bone separates from living bone. The devitalized areas are called *sequestra* (Oliphant, 2015).

In an older adult with osteomyelitis associated with a bone injury, the presenting signs are localized pain, tenderness on palpation, erythema, warmth to the touch, and edema. In osteomyelitis associated with infected pressure ulcers, the symptoms may be subtle changes in mental status, low-grade fever, chills, and increased purulent wound drainage. These signs and symptoms may go unnoticed until sepsis occurs (Oliphant, 2015).

If treated early, osteomyelitis has a good prognosis. The older adult may not have the classic signs of infection. Often, the first sign of osteomyelitis may be sepsis; in these cases, the prognosis is poor.

NURSING MANAGEMENT

Assessment

The nurse caring for older adults with osteomyelitis or for those at risk of developing osteomyelitis involves being aware of the subtlety of the presenting signs and symptoms of infection. Presenting symptoms vary in older adults and range from severe, acute onset to a clinical picture of chronic, subacute illness with minimal pain. Nursing assessment should focus on identifying risk factors predisposing a patient to osteomyelitis, examining any preexisting incisions, especially those related to insertion of a prosthetic device, wounds, decubitus ulcers or ulcers related to peripheral vascular disease or infections carefully, and monitoring vital signs and diagnostic test results (Oliphant, 2015). Another potential site for the development of osteomyelitis is the oral cavity in association with poor dentition and periodontal disease (Mears & Edwards, 2016). Close inspection of the mouth to look for eroding teeth and ill-fitting dentures and partials, which may contribute to dental abscesses, is important for the prevention of mandibular osteomyelitis (Mears & Edwards, 2016).

Diagnosis

Nursing diagnoses for a patient with osteomyelitis include the following:

- Pain resulting from swelling and tenderness
- Reduced skin integrity resulting from infected wounds
- Reduced mobility resulting from lower extremity pain

Planning and Expected Outcomes

Planning care for a patient with osteomyelitis should include a multidisciplinary approach. Treatment for this condition may be prolonged and therefore may require additional emotional and physical support. The long-term treatment for this problem requires family and significant others to be involved in the planning process. Expected outcomes include the following:

1. The patient will report minimum discomfort and adequate pain control.
2. The patient will verbalize an understanding of the need for long-term therapy to eliminate infection.
3. The patient will demonstrate safe and independent mobility.
4. The patient will exhibit intact skin surfaces and no evidence of further infection.

Intervention

Prevention of osteomyelitis includes using sterile technique during dressing changes and following strict wound precautions. A patient with infected pressure ulcers will most likely be functionally impaired and return to a long-term care setting for completion of intravenous antibiotic treatment (Oliphant, 2015. Older patients with osteomyelitis as a result of other causes will be discharged while receiving oral antibiotics. Discharge planning involves teaching about the importance of completing the course of oral antibiotics, methods of preventing infection, and specific techniques of wound management. An alternative treatment is a surgically implanted drug pump to deliver continuous antibiotic to the infection site.

The long-term treatment of chronic osteomyelitis creates psychological coping issues. Lengthy hospitalizations, immobility, and dependence may lead to feelings of anger and decreased self-worth. To help patients cope more effectively, the nurse should allow them to make informed decisions about care and should consult with therapeutic recreation specialists for diversional activities. The prolonged immobility may lead to the complications of immobility and self-care deficits. To prevent these problems, physical and occupational therapists should be consulted to provide individualized exercise programs that promote optimal functioning and prevent disability.

Evaluation

Patients with osteomyelitis should participate fully in all aspects of care. Any wounds or other potential sources of infection should show progressive healing. The patient should be able to verbalize understanding of the chronic nature of treatment, and documentation should include the patient's involvement in wound care or antibiotic therapy. For older patients who may have difficulty adjusting to the extended hospitalization required for therapy, the nurse should facilitate appropriate consultations.

Amputation

Amputation of the lower extremity is a common surgical procedure in older patients. The level of amputation depends on the extent of the disease process. Peripheral vascular disease (PVD), infections, neoplasms, and traumatic injury may all lead to lower extremity amputation; however, PVD is the most common cause in older adults.

In PVD caused by atherosclerosis and diabetes, circulation is inadequate to maintain cellular function. Atherosclerosis and diabetes are predisposing factors in the development of foot or extremity ulcers. The ulcers may be chronically infected. Osteomyelitis with bone destruction results in amputation of the extremity.

In PVD, chronic obstruction of the arteries results in inadequate circulation that causes tissue hypoxia. When the tissues are inadequately perfused for prolonged periods, atrophy of the underlying tissue occurs. This decreased circulation leads to delayed healing of injured feet or lower extremities. When ischemic ulcers do not heal, infection and necrosis or gangrene develops.

Gangrene manifests as a blackened area. The temperature in the affected area is lower than that of the unaffected area, and pain may be present. With the chronically infected extremity ulcer, the ulcer persists despite treatment with antibiotics.

NURSING MANAGEMENT

Assessment

Before the surgical procedure, a complete nursing assessment is done to determine the presence of other diseases and their effect on function. The focus of this assessment is on mobility and self-care ability. How does the patient walk? Are assistive devices required? What is the extent of self-care abilities? Assessment of the affected limb includes determining peripheral pulses, temperature, sensation, and movement. The specific characteristics of the ulcer or gangrenous area are noted, including location, size, and color. The individual's perception of the surgery is ascertained. Older patients should be asked how they feel about the impending surgical procedure and how they see the amputation affecting their health and lifestyle.

Diagnosis

Nursing diagnoses for an older patient undergoing amputation include the following:

- Pain secondary to the surgical procedure and phantom limb sensation
- Distorted body image resulting from amputation, impaired mobility, and prolonged immobilization
- Potential for reduced skin integrity resulting from the disease process, surgical procedure, and immobility
- Reduced mobility resulting from loss of an extremity
- Reduced stamina resulting from immobility
- Inadequate coping resulting from loss

Planning and Expected Outcomes

Nursing care of the patient undergoing amputation includes planning for the patient's preoperative, postoperative, and rehabilitative periods. Multidisciplinary planning is critical for the patient's recovery and long-term prognosis. Expected outcomes include the following:

1. The patient will report pain relief with the administration of analgesics.
2. The patient will demonstrate acceptance of body image changes, as evidenced by positive statements regarding the body and active involvement in treatment of the stump.
3. The patient's incisional area will remain clean and without evidence of infection.
4. The patient will safely perform self-care activities within his or her activity and energy expenditure limitations.

Intervention

Patient education is an important nursing role in preventing amputation. Because the majority of amputations are a result of PVD, patients need knowledge of how to control the factors that lead to amputation. Patients with diabetes and PVD are taught how to inspect and care for their feet and lower extremities. Instructions include information on promptly notifying a health care provider if changes occur in temperature, sensation, and color. If a sore develops, prompt treatment must be sought. Methods to protect the lower extremity from injury are included in the teaching plan.

Preoperative Care

Amputation has a major negative effect on an individual's body image and has the potential to lead to ineffective coping. To assist with adjustment in the postoperative phase, the nurse provides extensive information about the surgical procedure, including the purpose of the amputation, the potential use of prosthesis, and the rehabilitation program. To assist in the rehabilitation phase, the nurse teaches exercises to strengthen the upper extremities. Postoperative care, including positioning, turning, compression bandaging, and pain control, is discussed. Patients also require information about phantom sensations and phantom limb pain. *Phantom limb sensation* is the feeling of tingling, itching, or aching in the limb that no longer exists; *phantom limb pain* is a painful sensation that occurs in the limb that no longer exists; both these conditions may become chronic.

Postoperative Care

Routine postoperative care is provided in the immediate postoperative period. Patients are monitored carefully for complications that may be a result of preoperative health problems. Complications include hemorrhages and infection. Postoperative dressing depends on the type of prosthesis that will be used. The patient has either an immediate prosthetic fitting or a delayed prosthetic fitting. Because older adults may be debilitated from multiple chronic illnesses and the chronic condition that caused the amputation, they will probably have a delayed prosthetic fitting. Dressings are either rigid or soft in delayed prosthetic fittings. The rigid dressing may be made from either plastic or plaster of Paris. The advantage of this type of dressing is that it decreases edema. Soft dressings consist of Kerlix gauze

covered with an elastic wrap that acts as a compression dressing. The compression dressing is used to support the tissues, to decrease pain and edema, and to promote shrinking of the stump. The soft dressing is changed daily using a sterile technique. The wound is assessed for signs and symptoms of infection. A dry dressing is applied directly to the suture site.

In the immediate postoperative period (48 to 72 hours), pain drug is given on a regular schedule. Because of age-related changes in pharmacokinetics and pharmacodynamics, older patients receiving narcotic analgesics should be monitored closely for response and side effects. The effect of narcotics may last longer and may also result in excessive sedation, confusion, or respiratory depression. Initial doses should be lower than those used for younger adults. However, on the basis of the individual's pain relief and tolerance, doses may be increased. Morphine sulfate is the drug used most often in this phase of care.

Rehabilitative Care

The rehabilitative phase starts immediately after surgery with the application of the dressing. The dressing is important for prosthesis fitting because it shapes the stump for the prosthesis. The compression dressing is worn continuously and removed at least two times a day. Care is taken to properly apply the dressing. It should be wrapped snugly and securely but not so tightly that it impairs circulation. A *stump shrinker,* a continuous tube of elasticized fabric closed at one end, may be used instead of the wrap.

Physical therapy begins when the patient's condition is stable. Nursing goals for this phase include preventing complications and assisting the patient in reaching an optimal level of functioning. The physical therapy program includes active range of motion, upper extremity strengthening, and gait training. In older adults, walkers are used for ambulation, rather than crutches, because crutches require greater upper extremity strength and endurance. The nurse reinforces the importance of the exercise program and assists the patient in practicing safe transfer techniques.

Prosthetic Fitting and Adaptation

Not all older adults are candidates for prostheses. Multiple chronic illnesses may result in a state of debilitation in which the patient will not have the strength and reserve to complete a program of intense prosthetic training. These patients are taught transfer techniques and wheelchair mobility.

Prosthetic fitting is delayed until the stump is healed and well shaped. The fitting is done by a prosthetist (who makes a mold of the stump). As the stump shrinks, adjustments are made in the prosthesis. The patient is instructed to assess the stump daily for signs of irritation from an ill-fitting prosthesis.

The physical therapist and prosthetist instruct the older patient in the use of the prosthesis. The physical therapist also works on gait training. The nurse reinforces the teaching and provides the older patient with reinforcement on performance.

The individual who has had an amputation experiences loss and a major threat to body image. The normal response to loss is grief. The grieving process and adjustment to the loss are an individualized response characterized by vacillations in the recognized stages of grief: denial, isolation, anger, bargaining, depression, and acceptance.

Body image is an individual's subjective perception of the body. Gradual changes in body image are easier to adapt to than those that have an abrupt onset, as in the case of change experienced by an individual who has had an amputation. The adaptation to the change in body image does not always reflect the extent of the injury, but it is related to that individual's feelings toward himself or herself as a total person. The role of the nurse is to help the amputee discover a new self. Traumatic changes in body image may be characterized by revulsion in viewing the amputation. Viewing the amputation and looking in the mirror at the total self-picture may be difficult. Accepting the body changes is a gradual process. The nurse must allow the patient time to work through this process. The nurse may ask broad, open-ended questions about the body changes, for example, "How do you see yourself?" and "How do you think others see you?" (Touhy & Jett, 2016). Talking with other amputees on a one-on-one basis and in support groups is helpful for patients in adapting to changes in body image. The nurse should give positive but realistic feedback about the older patient's progress in functional abilities (see Nursing Care Plan: Amputation).

Evaluation

Evaluation is based on achievement of expected outcomes, as evidenced by the patient exhibiting a positive outlook about the body changes, performing self-care and other activities safely and adequately, and experiencing pain relief over time, until eventually analgesic pain drug is not needed. Documentation of these activities is critical for the multidisciplinary evaluation of the older patient's progress and is used as the basis for further care planning.

Polymyalgia Rheumatica

Polymyalgia rheumatica (PMR) is a chronic inflammatory condition characterized by sudden onset of muscle stiffness and aching (myalgia) in the neck, shoulders, and pelvic girdle. The disease occurs after the age of 50 years, most often in those 65 years or older. Women are affected more compared with men (Hancock et al., 2014). The cause of PMR is not known. Infection and an altered immune response have been suggested but not proven as the cause. Likewise, a genetic predisposition is suggested but not confirmed. The pathophysiology of PMR is not clearly understood.

The clinical presentation of PMR is similar to that of RA and OA. Symptoms include muscle stiffness and aching in the neck, shoulders, and pelvic girdle (Buttgereit, Dejaco, Matteson & Dasgupta, 2016). The muscle stiffness is present in the morning and lasts more than 1 hour. Constitutional symptoms such as fatigue, fever, often with night sweating, malaise, anorexia, depression, and weight loss may be present (Saad, 2015). Initially the pain may be limited to one area, but it generally develops in a symmetric fashion. Objective signs of muscle weakness are not present on physical examination. Check for signs of carpal tunnel syndrome such as paresthesia of the thumb and index finger. Look for swelling with pitting edema in the ankles and the top of the feet (Gonzalez-Gay & Pina, 2015).

Diagnostics indicative of PMR are an elevated erythrocyte sedimentation rate (ESR) and C-reactive protein (CRP). Patients with PMR generally are found to be anemic. PMR is treated with corticosteroids that are tapered over time. Symptoms of aching, stiffness, and fatigue may begin to resolve in about 1 to 2 days, and patients will remain on long-term corticosteroids until the laboratory values return to normal. Treatment may last one to 3 years for PMR (Dejaco et al., 2015). This marked improvement so soon after initiation of treatment is not seen in RA or OA.

NURSING MANAGEMENT

Assessment

A thorough history of the patient's symptoms, physical examination, and functional assessment are important in determining the effect of the disease on functional abilities.

Diagnosis

Nursing diagnoses for a patient with PMR include the following:
- Pain resulting from muscle stiffness and aching
- Reduced mobility resulting from pain and muscle stiffness
- Fatigue resulting from systemic symptoms
- Inadequate self-care resulting from muscle stiffness
- Inadequate coping resulting from the chronic nature of the disease

Planning and Expected Outcomes

Expected outcomes for an older patient with PMR include the following:
1. The patient will report pain relief with initiation of treatment.
2. The patient will correctly describe pharmacologic therapy, including purpose, action, and side effects of prescribed drugs.
3. The patient will establish an activity and rest pattern based on limitations imposed by the disease.
4. The patient will incorporate effective coping strategies in disease management.
5. The patient will correctly state the treatment rationale and prognosis.

Intervention

The medical diagnosis of PMR is difficult to make; because symptoms are similar to those of RA and OA, it is often misdiagnosed. The older patient who has been to many physicians in an attempt to receive the correct diagnosis and proper treatment may be frustrated, angry, and worn out. The nurse should listen to the patient's concerns and give information to the patient about the disease and the treatment plan. This includes information about the treatment with corticosteroids and their side effects. The nurse monitors the patient for the development of side effects from long-term corticosteroid use, such as

◎ NURSING CARE PLAN

Amputation

Clinical Situation

Mr. C is a 78-year-old retired truck driver with a medical history of diabetes mellitus–type 2, peripheral vascular disease (PVD), and a chronic right foot ulcer. Because the foot ulcer did not respond to conservative treatment, he underwent a right below-the-knee amputation. Before this surgical procedure, Mr. C had been hospitalized for 3 weeks for treatment of the foot ulcer. During the hospitalization he became weak and deconditioned. He now requires assistance with eating and ADLs, and maximum assistance for transfers. Mr. C complains of phantom limb pain and requires a pain drug every 4 to 6 hours.

The prolonged illness, hospitalization, and amputation have caused Mr. C to feel hopeless. He has told the nurses he is tired of being in the hospital, sick, and in pain. Mr. C has also verbalized feelings about not being the man he once was. He does not initiate any self-care and needs encouragement to complete self-care. Mr. C has a supportive wife and family. His wife has RA and thinks it will be difficult for her to care for her husband unless he participates in his care and is rehabilitated with his prosthesis. Mr. C is stable 2 days postoperatively and is beginning physical therapy for preprosthetic training.

Nursing Diagnoses

Distorted body image resulting from amputation, impaired mobility, and prolonged hospitalization

Pain resulting from the surgical procedure and phantom limb sensation

Potential for reduced skin integrity resulting from disease process, surgical procedure, age-related changes, and immobility

Reduced mobility resulting from below-the-knee amputation and prolonged immobility

Reduced stamina resulting from prolonged immobility, deconditioning, and disease processes

Inadequate coping resulting from amputation

Inadequate family coping resulting from spouse's chronic illness and disability

Outcomes

The patient will verbalize feelings of acceptance of change in body image.

The patient will verbalize that pain is tolerable.

Pain will not interfere with ability to participate in ADLs.

The incision will heal without signs or symptoms of infection.

Skin will remain free from pressure ulcers.

The patient will transfer independently and walk 10 feet with a pickup walker.

Range of motion will remain within normal limits.

Flexion contracture will not develop.

The patient will attend and participate in a daily therapy program with a normal physiologic response.

The patient will use effective coping strategies and participate in a rehabilitation program.

The family will use effective coping strategies and support the patient's participation in the rehabilitation process.

Interventions

Allow verbalization of feelings; actively listen to feelings.

Give positive feedback for progress made in self-care and mobility and for aspects of general appearance.

Encourage normal activities such as dressing in street clothes.

Encourage participation in support groups.

Assess pain and effectiveness of drugs.

Administer pain drugs, as ordered.

Provide diversional activities and alternative treatments such as relaxation techniques.

Assess incision and pressure areas (use a risk assessment scale) daily for signs of infection or pressure ulcers.

Change surgical dressing using aseptic technique.

Reposition every 2 hours; position to keep pressure off bony prominences.

Teach the patient how to change positions.

Provide adequate caloric, protein, and fluid intake.

Wrap stump with compression dressing or stump shrinker.

Consult with physical therapy for a program of muscle strengthening, transfer training, and gait training.

Reinforce physical therapy training.

Give positive feedback for gains made.

Teach transfer techniques; assist with transfers.

Teach the safe use of a walker.

Give pain drugs 30 to 60 minutes before therapy.

Do not elevate stump on pillows.

Keep stump in good alignment; prevent flexion contractures.

Reinforce the use of active range-of-motion exercises.

Encourage lying on the abdomen for 30 minutes two times a day.

Encourage participation in the therapy program.

Gradually increase activity.

Allow at least 60 minutes of rest after therapy.

Monitor vital signs before, during, and after therapy.

Assist the patient in identifying previously successful coping skills.

Suggest and describe effective coping skills.

Encourage activities that enhance self-esteem.

Encourage the use of support systems.

Encourage participation in an amputation support group; include the family, especially the spouse, in the support group.

Encourage the spouse's verbalization of feelings when the patient is not present.

Suggest and describe effective coping skills to her.

Suggest taking time to care for herself.

---

infection, osteoporosis, fractures, and diabetes mellitus. The older patient should be reassured that the dose of drug will be tapered and that eventually the symptoms will subside; however, it should be emphasized that the drug needs to be continued despite the patient becoming symptom free. Patients should also be informed that it is common to have a relapse of PMR and that, now being familiar with the disease presentation, they should report any new onset of symptoms right away to their care providers (Patil & Dasgupta, 2013).

Evaluation

Patients with PMR need to understand the chronic nature of the disease and be able to maintain functional abilities. Pain management is necessary for the older patient to perform ADLs, so the patient will need to be familiar with the drugs and their side effects. Providing appropriate education about the disease and symptom management will assist in acceptance. Documentation of education, pain assessment, and functional abilities is important for ongoing planning and care of the patient.

FOOT PROBLEMS

The foot is often overlooked in the assessment and care of older adults. Foot problems, especially pain, are common in older adults. The incidence and severity of foot problems increase with age. After age 65, 75% of the population complains of foot problems. More than 80% of those older than age 55 demonstrate arthritic changes on radiography. Foot problems may cause an unsteady gait and may result in falls (Violand, 2017).

The foot is a complex structure composed of 26 bones, 33 joints, and numerous ligaments, tendons, and muscles. The foot is necessary for ambulation. During standing and ambulation, the foot provides body support and absorbs shock. Painful feet may be the result of congenital deformities, weak structure, injuries, and diseases such as diabetes, RA, and OA. Ill-fitting shoes cause foot pain by crowding the toes and impeding normal movement. With aging, feet show signs of wear and tear. The cushioning layer of fat on the soles of feet becomes thin. Years of walking cause the metatarsal bones to spread and the ligaments to stretch, which results in widening of feet.

Corns

Corns are thickened and hardened dead or hyperkeratotic tissue that develops over bony protuberances. Corns often cause localized pain. Ill-fitting or loose shoes that constantly place pressure on bony prominences cause corns. Soft corns are produced by the bony prominence of one toe rubbing against the adjacent toe in the web space between the toes. Soft corns are macerated because of moisture in the web space. Hard corns, also known as *heloma duram,* have a dry mass of keratosis with a central hard core (Fig. 23.13). Heloma duram are found on the plantar side of the foot often over the fifth metatarsal and the surrounding metatarsal head (Feldman, 2017). Warm water soaks are used to soften corns before gently rubbing with a pumice stone or callus file. Another treatment is gentle débridement by a podiatrist. To relieve pain and prevent the development of corns, moleskin or cotton pads are placed over areas subjected to rubbing and pressure (Feldman, 2017). Wider and softer shoes are recommended; older women should avoid wearing high-heeled shoes. Use of topical applications of salicylic acid should be avoided in older adults because these may cause irritation, burns, or infection, especially in those with diabetes and impaired circulation, especially in diabetics as skin damage could occur without the patient's knowledge (Romano, 2016).

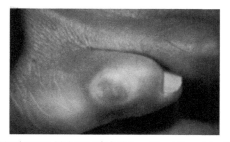

Fig. 23.13 Hard corn with keratotic buildup. (From Coughlin, M. J., Mann, R. A., & Saltzman, C. L. [2007]. *Surgery of the foot and ankle* [vol 2, 8th ed.]. Philadelphia, PA: Saunders.)

Calluses

Calluses, or plantar keratoses, are dead tissue found on the plantar surfaces of the feet. They form under the metatarsal heads, most commonly the second and third heads. Calluses are also common in people who have bunions (Hashmi, 2013). About 50% of people older than 65 years have some degree of plantar calluses. The aging changes of decreased toe function and decreased fat padding contribute to their development. Soft-soled shoes with additional cushioned insoles are recommended. Treatment is the same as for corns.

Bunions

Bunions, or *hallux valgus,* have the greatest prevalence among those older than 50 years, and women experience them four times more often compared with men because women tend to wear narrow, pointed, high-heeled shoes. Arthritis and other age-related changes such as ligament and tendon atrophy predispose older adults to bunions.

Bunions appear as bony protuberances on the side of the great toe (Fig. 23.14). With bunions, the large toe angles laterally toward the second toe. As the great toe rubs against the shoe, the bursa becomes inflamed, which results in bursitis and pain. Initial treatment of bunions involves wearing soft leather shoes that are flat, wide, and laced up. Walking or running shoes with a wide toe box prevent rubbing on the bunion. Moleskin bunion pads may be used to protect the bony protrusion. NSAIDs may be prescribed to reduce inflammation and pain. Surgical interventions are used after conservative treatment has failed. The surgical procedure includes removal of the bursa sac and correction of the bony deformity.

Hammertoe

Hammertoe is a deformity of the second toe. In this deformity, the metatarsophalangeal joint is dorsiflexed, the proximal interphalangeal joint is plantar flexed, and callus formation occurs on the dorsum of the proximal interphalangeal joint and the end of the affected toe. The result is a toe

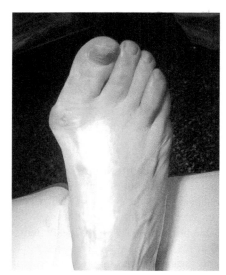

Fig. 23.14 Hallux valgus angulation of first three toes, and wide, flat metatarsus. (© Cyberprout / CC-BY-SA-1.0, via Wikimedia Commons.)

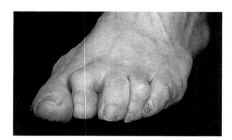

Fig. 23.15 Hammertoe associated with hallux valgus. (Courtesy Charles W. Bradley, DPM, MPA, and Caroline Harvey, DPM, California College of Podiatric Medicine; http://www.toesrus.co.uk/bunion.jpg.)

that has a clawlike appearance (Fig. 23.15). Improperly fitted shoes, muscle weakness, and arthritis are causes for hammertoe. Symptoms include pain and burning on the bottom of the foot and problems walking in shoes. Initially, pain may be relieved with the use of a moleskin toe pad. Other treatments for hammertoe include metatarsal arch support, orthotics, splints, and passive manual stretching of the proximal interphalangeal joint. Surgical correction is done if conservative treatment is ineffective.

Nail Disorders

Toenail problems are common in older adults. Older adults with problems of the nails should be referred to a podiatrist.

Onychauxis is described as hypertrophic nails whose borders curve into the soft tissue of the toes. This disorder may cause nail bed ulcers, infection, and pain.

Onychomycosis is a localized fungal infection of the toenail that is seen most frequently in older adults. Degeneration of the nail plate causes changes in the growth and appearance of the nail. Onychomycotic nails may have simple scaling or may be totally destroyed by the fungus. Initially, the nail becomes brittle and hypertrophic. The nails may be white, yellow, or brown in color. Ridges and pitting of the nail are common. Generally, the infection spreads between the nails. Predisposing factors for onychomycosis are moisture, ill-fitting footwear, recurrent trauma, and diabetes.

Treatment of onychomycosis is difficult because of the composition of the nail and the involvement of the nail matrix. Topical antifungals such as clotrimazole are generally used for several months. The oral antifungal agents such as terbinafine and itraconazole are generally not used in older adults because many older adults have a decreased pedal blood supply. The older patient with onychomycosis who does not respond to topical antifungal agents should be referred to a podiatrist. The podiatrist will débride the nail at periodic intervals.

Patient Education

The nurse should educate the older adult about the predisposing factors, prevention, and treatment of onychomycosis, and the need for ongoing foot care, including inspection of feet for signs of infection and application of the drug.

The nurse has an important role in educating patients about proper foot care and footwear. Well-fitting shoes are essential for the prevention of foot problems. The shoes should not crowd the toes and should be of the correct length and width. Shoes that are too short or narrow may force the great toe into a position of hallux valgus. Shoes should be wide enough to allow bending of the toes and movement of the foot muscles. Adequate arch support should be provided. Older women should avoid wearing high heels (Farndon, Concannon, & Stephenson, 2015).

Patients should be taught foot care that includes daily hygiene and changing of socks. Socks or stockings should be loose enough to avoid the development of pressure ulcers. Toenails should be trimmed with nail clippers; patients with impaired vision, impaired mobility, or self-care deficits may require assistance to perform this task safely. The nails should be trimmed straight across so that the development of ingrown toenails and infections is prevented. If the foot problems persist, a podiatrist should be consulted (Violand, 2017).

MUSCLE CRAMPS

Idiopathic muscle cramps without muscle weakness are common in older adults. The cramps may start during rest or after minor exercise. Muscle cramps generally affect the calf or foot muscles, producing plantar flexion of the foot or toes. They occur most frequently at night during sleep.

Stretching the affected muscles for several minutes at bedtime may prevent muscle cramps. If cramping occurs, stretching will generally relieve the discomfort. Calf muscles should be stretched, with two or three 1-minute intervals and 1-minute rest periods between stretches. Stretching exercises improve muscle flexibility and reduce the motor activity in the affected muscles.

Quinine sulfate is sometimes prescribed for muscle cramps; however, its effectiveness has been questioned. The side effects of quinine therapy for muscle cramps may increase the concentration of digoxin, and an overdose may cause confusion.

▎SUMMARY

Problems of the musculoskeletal system may have a great effect on the day-to-day life of older adults. Conditions such as OA, RA, PMR, osteoporosis, and fractures may result in functional disability, chronic pain, and a decreased quality of life. The role of the nurse working with older patients with musculoskeletal disorders is to promote safe, optimal functioning with regard to mobility and self-care. Interventions to promote comfort and to relieve pain are critical in the maintenance of function. To prevent serious disability, it is essential that patients resume activity as soon as possible after episodes of acute illness. A key nursing role is to educate patients about the importance of musculoskeletal activity in maintaining function.

🏠 HOME CARE

1. Assessment of the musculoskeletal system includes examination of bones, muscles, and joints in homebound older adults.
2. Instruct caregivers and homebound older adults about reportable signs and symptoms related to the musculoskeletal system disease or disorder being treated and when to report these changes to the home care nurse or physician.
3. Instruct caregivers and homebound older adults on the name, dose, frequency, side effects, and indications of both the prescribed and over-the-counter drugs being used to treat the identified musculoskeletal problem.
4. Musculoskeletal problems increase safety hazards (e.g., falls) in homebound older adults.
5. Assess for functional impairments such as inability to provide self-care and perform IADLs. If necessary, have social worker identify community resources for additional assistance with identified impairments, such as transportation and food preparation.
6. Assess the activity tolerance level, which may be affected by musculoskeletal problems.
7. Instruct caregivers and homebound older adults about the diagnosed musculoskeletal disease or disorder, focusing on self-care measures that maintain or promote independence.
8. Have the physical therapist and the occupational therapist evaluate and teach caregivers and homebound older adults how to adapt the environment based on the specific musculoskeletal problem (e.g., gait training, use of handheld devices to assist with eating, splints, and prostheses).
9. Encourage ambulation in a safe manner. Stretching exercises that improve posture should be part of the nursing interventions.
10. An exercise program may be suggested after consulting with the physician.
11. Instruct caregivers and homebound older adults on the necessity of calcium supplements and exercise to maintain proper skeletal function and prevent bone loss.

▎KEY POINTS

- A high incidence of musculoskeletal disorders exists among older adults.
- Musculoskeletal disorders are a major cause of functional impairments in older adults.
- Age-related changes in the musculoskeletal system may predispose older adults to falls.
- The most common sites of fractures in older adults are the hips, wrists (Colles fracture), and vertebrae.

- Demographic factors associated with osteoporosis include female gender, age, and white race.
- Lower extremity amputations in older adults are most often the result of PVD or diabetes.
- Symptoms of OA, RA, gouty arthritis, and PMR are similar, but treatments differ.
- Physical activity and exercise are key to preventing disability from musculoskeletal disorders in older adults.

▎CRITICAL-THINKING EXERCISES

1. An 83-year-old woman has suffered a musculoskeletal injury that requires a period of bed rest and limited mobility. How will age affect her ability to tolerate a period of decreased mobility? Explain.
2. You are caring for two patients: a 74-year-old man with gouty arthritis and a 68-year-old woman with RA. What aspects of their care will be similar? What aspects will be different?
3. A 72-year-old man lived a fairly sedentary lifestyle as an accountant. Now that he is retired, he recognizes the need to be active to maintain his health as long as possible. He is concerned, however, that it is too late for him to start exercising because he has never engaged in such activities. What encouragement, if any, can you give to him, and what suggestions can you make for an exercise program?

REFERENCES

Allen, K. D., Choong, P. F., Davis, A. M., Dowsey, M. M., Dziedzic, K. S., Emery, C., & Skou, S. T. (2016). Osteoarthritis: models for appropriate care across the disease continuum. *Best Practice & Research: Clinical Rheumatology, 30*(3), 503–535.

Ashford, S., & Williard, J. (2014). Osteoarthritis: A review. *The Nurse Practitioner, 39*(5), 1–8.

Ayhan, E., Kesmezacar, H., & Akgun, I. (2014). Intraarticular injections (corticosteroid, hyaluronic acid, platelet rich plasma) for the knee osteoarthritis. *World Journal of Orthopedics, 5*(3), 351.

Bhatia, D., Bejarano, T., & Novo, M. (2013). Current interventions in the management of knee osteoarthritis. *Journal of Pharmacy & Bioallied Sciences, 5*(1), 30–38. https://doi.org/10.4103/0975-7406.106561.

Boyd, A. S., Benjamin, H. J., & Asplund, C. (2009). Splints and casts: Indications and methods. *American Family Physician, 80*(5).

Browne, K. L., & Merrill, E. (2015). Musculoskeletal management matters: Principles of assessment and triage for the nurse practitioner. *The Journal for Nurse Practitioners, 11*(10), 929–939.

Buchanan, T., Vitiello, & Bennett, K. (2017). Feasibility and efficacy of a shared yoga intervention for sleep disturbance in older adults with osteoarthritis. *Journal of Gerontological Nursing, 43*(8), 42–52.

Buckley, L., Guyatt, G., Fink, H., & McAlindon, T. (2018). Reply. *Arthritis Care & Research, 70*(6), 950–951. https://doi.org/10.1002/acr.23416.

Buttgereit, F., Dejaco, C., Matteson, E. L., & Dasgupta, B. (2016). Polymyalgia rheumatica and giant cell arteritis: A systematic review.

Journal of the American Medical Association, 315(22), 2442–2458. https://doi.org/10.1001/jama.2016.5444.

Centers for Disease Control and Prevention. (2018). Nonfatal injury data. Retrieved June 12, 2018 from https://www.cdc.gov/injury/wisqars/nonfatal.html

Chen, K.-M., Tseng, W.-S., Chang, Y.-H., Huang, H.-T., & Li, C.-H. (2013). Feasibility appraisal of an elastic band exercise program for older adults in wheelchairs. *Geriatric Nursing, 34*(5), 373–376.

Corrarino, J. E. (2015). Fracture repair: Mechanisms and management. *The Journal for Nurse Practitioners, 11*(10), 960–967.

Cosman, F., de Beur, S. J., LeBoff, M. S., Lewiecki, E. M., Tanner, B., Randall, S., & Lindsay, R. (2014). Clinician's guide to prevention and treatment of osteoporosis. *Osteoporosis International, 25*(10), 2359–2381. https://doi.org/10.1007/s00198-014-2794-2.

Dejaco, C., Singh, Y. P., Perel, P., Hutchings, A., Camellino, D., Mackie, S., & Bianconi, L. (2015). 2015 Recommendations for the management of polymyalgia rheumatica: A European League Against Rheumatism/American College of Rheumatology collaborative initiative. *Arthritis & Rheumatology, 67*(10), 2569–2580.

Della Rocca, G. J., Moylan, K. C., Crist, B. D., Volgas, D. A., Stannard, J. P., & Mehr, D. A. (2013). Comanagement of geriatric patients with hip fractures: A retrospective, controlled cohort study. *Geriatric Orthopaedic Surgery & Rehabilitation, 4*(1), 10–15.

Derry, S., Wiffen, P. J., Kalso, E. A., Bell, R. F., Aldington, D., Phillips, T., ... Moore, R. A. (2017 May 12). *Cochrane Database Systematic Review, 5*. CD008609 https://doi.org/10.1002/14651858. CD008609.pub2 Review. PMID: 28497473.

Eiff, M. P., & Hatch, R. L. (2017). *Fracture Management for Primary Care Updated Edition E-Book.* Elsevier Health Sciences.

Ensrud, K. E. (2013). Epidemiology of fracture risk with advancing age. *The Journals of Gerontology: Series A, 68*(10), 1236–1242. https://doi.org/10.1093/Gerona/glt092.

Farndon, L., Concannon, M., & Stephenson, J. (2015). A survey to investigate the association of pain, foot disability and quality of life with corns. *Journal of Foot and Ankle Research, 8*, 70. https://doi.org/10.1186/s13047-015-0131-4.

Feldman, N. J. (2017). Corns and calluses. In F. J. Domingo, J. Golding, M. B. Stephens, & R. A. Baldor (Eds.), *5-Minute Clinical Consult, The 2017 – 25th Ed.* Philadelphia, PA: Lippincott Williams & Wilkins Health. Retrieved from http://online.stateref.com/Document.aspx?fxId=31&docId=430.

Feng, X., Li, Y., & Gao, W. (2015). Significance of the initiation time of urate-lowering therapy in gout patients: A retrospective research. *Joint Bone Spine, 82*(2015), 428–431.

Forster, R., & Stewart, M. (2016). Anticoagulants (extended duration) for prevention of venous thromboembolism following total hip or knee replacement or hip fracture repair. *Cochrane Database of Systematic Reviews, 2016.* Issue 3. Art. No.: CD004179 https://doi.org/10.1002/14651858.CD004179.pub2.

González-Gay, M. A., & Pina, T. (2015). Giant cell arteritis and polymyalgia rheumatica: An update. *Current Rheumatology Reports, 17*(2), 1–7.

Gray-Miceli, D. (2017). Impaired mobility and functional decline in older adults. *Nursing Clinics of North America, 52*(3), 469–487.

Hancock, A. T., Mallen, C. D., Muller, S., Belcher, J., Roddy, E., Helliwell, T., & Hider, S. L. (2014). Risk of vascular events in patients with polymyalgia rheumatica. *Canadian Medical Association Journal, 186*(13), 993. https://doi.org/10.1503/cmaj.140266.

Hashmi, F. (2013). Calluses, corns and heel fissures. *Dermatological Nursing, 12*(1). Retrieved from www.bdng.org.uk.

Hootman, J. M., Helmick, C. G., Barbour, K. E., Theis, K. A., & Boring, M. A. (2016). Updated projected prevalence of self-reported doctor-diagnosed arthritis and arthritis-attributable activity limitation among US adults, 2015–2040. *Arthritis & Rheumatology, 68*(7), 1582–1587.

Igel, T. F., Krasnokutsky, S., & Pillinger, M. H. (2017). Recent advances in understanding and managing gout. F1000 Research, Version 1, *F1000Res, 6*, 247.

Ishchenko, A., & Lories, R. J. (2016). Safety and efficacy of biological disease-modifying antirheumatic drugs in older rheumatoid arthritis patients: Staying the distance. *Drugs & Aging, 33*(6), 387–398.

Kalff, R., Ewald, C., Waschke, A., Gobisch, L., & Hopf, C. (2013). Degenerative lumbar spinal stenosis in older people: Current treatment options. *Deutsches Ärzteblatt International, 110*(37), 613–624. https://doi.org/10.3238/arztebl.2013.0613.

Kuo, C. F., Grainge, M. J., Mallen, C., Zhang, W., & Doherty, M. (2015). Rising burden of gout in the UK but continuing suboptimal management: A nationwide population study. *Annals of the Rheumatic Diseases, 74*(4), 661–667.

LeBlond, R. F., Brown, D. D., Suneja, M., & Szot, J. F. (2015). *DeGowin's diagnostic examination* (10th ed.). New York: McGraw-Hill Medical.

Lee, S. Y., Kim, T. H., Oh, J. K., Lee, S. J., & Park, M. S. (2015). Lumbar stenosis: A recent update by review of literature. *Asian Spine Journal, 9*(5), 818–828.

Mackey, P. A., & Whitaker, M. D. (2015). Osteoporosis: A therapeutic update. *The Journal for Nurse Practitioners, 11*(10), 1011–1017.

Manini, T. M., Gundermann, D. M., & Clark, B. C. (2016). Aging of the muscles and joints. In J. Halter, J. Ouslander, M. Tinetti, S. Studenski, K. High, S. Asthana, & W. Hazzard (Eds.), *Principles of geriatric medicine and gerontology* (7th ed.). New York: McGraw-Hill Medical.

Mears, S. C., & Edwards, P. K. (2016). Bone and joint infections in older adults. *Clinical Geriatric Medicine, 32*(3), 555–570. https://doi.org/10.1016/j.cger.2016.02.003.

National Osteoporosis Foundation. (2014). *Clinician's guide to prevention and treatment of osteoporosis.* http://nof.org/files/nof/public/content/resource/913/files/580.pdf. Accessed 30 October 2013.

O'Connell, S., Bashar, K., Broderick, B. J., Sheehan, J., Quondamatteo, F., Walsh, S. R., & Quinlan, L. R. (2016). The use of intermittent pneumatic compression in orthopedic and neurosurgical postoperative patients: A systematic review and meta-analysis. *Annals of Surgery, 263*(5), 888–889.

Oliphant, C. M. (2015). Management of orthopedic infections. *The Journal for Nurse Practitioners, 11*(10), 1036–1042.

Onat, Ş., Ekiz, T., Biçer, S., & Özgirgin, N. (2015). The differential diagnosis of atypical localized osteoarthritis in elderly patients: A case report. *Journal of Physical Medicine & Rehabilitation Sciences, 18*, 58–62.

Patil, P., & Dasgupta, B. (2013). Polymyalgia rheumatica in older adults. *Aging Health, 9*(5), 483–495. https://doi.org/10.2217/ahe.13.50.

Prah, A., Richards, E., Griggs, R., & Simpson, V. (2017). Enhancing osteoporosis efforts through lifestyle modifications and goal-setting techniques. *The Journal for Nurse Practitioners, 13*(8), 552–561.

Ralston, S. H. (2013). Paget's disease of bone. *New England Journal of Medicine, 368*(7), 644–650.

Romano, M. I. (2016). Corns and calluses. In T. M. Buttaro & J. Trybulski (Eds.), *Primary Care: A Collaborative Practice.* Philadelphia, PA: Elsevier. 268-269.e1.

Saad, E. R. (2015). Polymyalgia rheumatica. In H. S. Diamond (Ed.), *Medscape reference drugs, diseases & procedures.* Retrieved from http://emedicine.medscape.com/article/330815-overview.

Sattui, S. E., & Saag, K. G. (2014). Fracture mortality: Associations with epidemiology and osteoporosis treatment. *Nature Reviews Endocrinology, 10*(10), 592–602.

Schneider, A. L., Williams, E. K., Brancati, F. L., Blecker, S., Coresh, J., & Selvin, E. (2013). Diabetes and risk of fracture-related hospitalization: The atherosclerosis risk in communities study. *Diabetes Care, 36,* 1153–1158. https://doi.org/10.2337/dc12-1168.

Shelton, L. R. (2013). A closer look at osteoarthritis. *The Nurse Practitioner, 38*(7), 31–36.

Southerland, L. T., Barrie, M., Falk, J., & Menaker, J. (2014). Fractures in older adults. *Emergency Medicine Reports, 35*(11), 1–13.

Taylor-Piliae, R. E., Peterson, R., & Mohler, M. J. (2017). Clinical and community strategies to prevent falls and fall-related injuries among community-dwelling older adults. *Nursing Clinics, 52*(3), 489–497.

Touhy, T., & Jett, K. (2016). *Towards healthy aging: Human needs and nursing response* (9th ed.). St Louis, MO: Mosby.

Violand, M. (2017). Putting a healthy foot forward. *The Journal for Nurse Practitioners, 13*(7), 499–500.

West, S. G., & O'Dell, J. R. (2015). *Rheumatoid arthritis: Rheumatology secrets* (3rd ed.). Philadelphia, PA: Elsevier.

Yung, R. (2017). Rheumatoid arthritis and other autoimmune diseases. In J. B. Halter, J. G. Ouslander, S. Studenski, K. P. High, & S. Asthana (Eds.), *Hazzard's: Geriatric medicine and gerontology* (7th ed.). New York: McGraw-Hill.

Zimmerman, S., Greene, A., Sloane, P. D., Mitchell, M., Giuliani, C., Nyrop, K., & Walsh, E. (2017). Preventing falls in assisted living: Results of a quality improvement pilot study. *Geriatric Nursing, 38* (3), 185–191.

24

Cognitive and Neurologic Function

Jennifer J. Yeager, PhD, RN, APRN

http://evolve.elsevier.com/Meiner/gerontologic

LEARNING OBJECTIVES

On completion of this chapter, the reader will be able to:

1. Compare structural changes in the brain and nerve function associated with aging.
2. Describe functional changes in the neurologic system during the aging process.
3. Compare normal, age-related changes of the neurologic system with those associated with cognitive and behavioral disorders.
4. Differentiate the symptoms of depression, delirium, dementia, and other cognitive disorders.
5. Describe the symptoms and diagnostic tests and interventions related to common neurologic disorders in older adults.
6. Use the nursing process in the development of a care plan for patients with common neurologic disorders.
7. Analyze evidence-based practice that enhances management of patients with neurologic disorders.
8. Apply the nursing process to older adult patients experiencing mental health problems.
9. Identify appropriate nursing interventions when caring for older adults using psychotropic drugs.
10. Evaluate mental health resources available for older adults.

WHAT WOULD YOU DO?

What would you do if you were faced with the following situations?

- Your 72-year-old female patient, admitted yesterday for intravenous (IV) antibiotics to treat a urinary tract infection (UTI), is lethargic and has slurred speech when responding to questions. Her responses are not always appropriate to the question. What is going on?
- A 68-year-old male is brought to the emergency department (ED) via ambulance with ischemic stroke. The family states symptoms began when the evening news began (45 minutes ago). How would you determine whether the patient was appropriate for tissue plasminogen activator?

The number of older Americans (age 65 and older) continues to grow rapidly. They numbered 47.8 million in 2016, which was an increase of 11.1 million or an increase of over 30% since 2005. More than one in seven, or 14.9%, of the population in the United States is an older adult (Administration on Aging [AOA], 2017). Considering these statistics, it is imperative nurses stay abreast of the most recent findings regarding the development, manifestations, and treatment of cognitive and neurologic problems among older adults. This knowledge will assist nurses in providing safe, effective, and evidence-based nursing interventions.

The brain is a complex web of tissue and structures that allows for a series of intricate functions that continues to astonish. Understanding the brain and its function has long been an interest for health care providers. For nurses caring for older

Previous authors: Lois VonCannon, MSN, RN, and Ramesh C. Upadhyaya, RN, CRRN, MSN, MBA, PhD-C.

persons, the understanding of basic neurologic changes and common disorders is crucial.

STRUCTURAL AGE-RELATED CHANGES OF THE NEUROLOGIC SYSTEM

The nervous system is a network of complex structures that undergo many neurophysiologic changes with aging. Some changes that occur in the brain do not affect all older individuals equally, and the individual presentation of neurologic changes varies from person to person. An individual's lifestyle, nutritional intake, genetic makeup, and tissue perfusion are some of the many factors that affect the neurologic system. To appreciate the significant changes that take place with aging, one requires a brief review of the neurologic system.

The central nervous system (CNS) is divided into three major functional components: higher level brain or cerebral cortex, lower level brain (basal ganglia, thalamus, hypothalamus, brainstem, and cerebellum), and spinal cord. The brain is divided into three major areas, which include the cerebrum, brainstem, and cerebellum. The cerebrum consists of two hemispheres (right and left); each hemisphere is divided into lobes (frontal, temporal, parietal, and occipital) (Fig. 24.1). Specialized neurons located within the lobes include the hippocampus and the basal ganglia. These are the neurons that undergo structural and physiologic changes during the aging process. Another area of the CNS that undergoes significant changes in the normal aging process is the brainstem (midbrain, pons, and medulla oblongata). The reticular formation (RF) is a complex network of gray

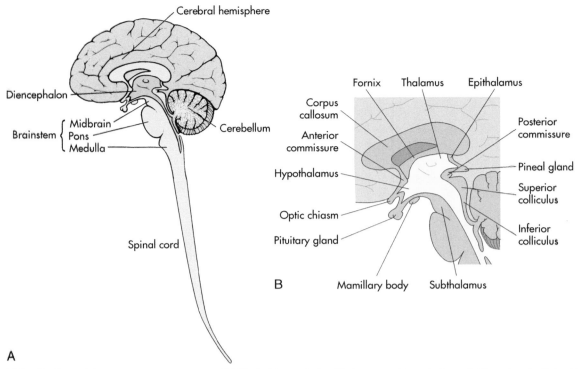

Fig. 24.1 A, Major divisions of the central nervous system (CNS). **B,** Diencephalon (thalamus and hypothalamus). (From Lewis, S. L., Dirksen, S. R., Heitkemper, M. M., et al. [2011]. *Medical surgical nursing: Assessment and management of clinical problems* [8th ed.]. St. Louis, MO: Mosby.)

matter located primarily in the brainstem area of the CNS. The RF assists and controls many functions, including skeletal muscle movement and the sleep–wake cycle, another aspect altered in aging (Black, Hawks, & Hogan, 2005; Mander et al., 2013).

Cellular and Structural Changes

Neuron

The neuron is the basic unit of the CNS and functions to transmit impulses. Some neurons are motor neurons, and some are sensory neurons. Each neuron has a cell body (soma), dendrites, and a single axon (Fig. 24.2). Synapses are structural and functional junctions between two neurons. These are the points at which the nerve impulse is transmitted from one neuron to another or from neuron to efferent organ. The two types of synapses are electrical and chemical.

Neurotransmitters

Neurotransmitters are chemical substances that enhance or inhibit nerve impulses. These substances are necessary in the synaptic transmission of information from one neuron to another. In aging, the function of these substances is altered because of the decrease of neurons. With aging, the number of neurons in various areas of the brain also decreases, and abnormal substances are deposited on the neuronal cellular structure (dendrites) (Sugarman & Huether, 2012). The loss of neurons is not as extensive in the process of aging as previously believed. Large neurons appear to shrink, and few are lost. The changes in neuron function are associated with accumulation of lipofuscin (dark fluorescent pigment) granules and neuritic plaques in the cell body of some neurons and some cellular debris in neuroglia cells (Keller, 2006) (Table 24.1).

Neuroglia and Schwann Cells

Neuroglia and Schwann cells are the supportive cells of the CNS, making up approximately half of the brain and spinal cord tissue. Their role is to protect the neurons. As individuals age, the number of these protective cells increases. Each of these cells serves a different function.

Neuroglia cells vary in size and shape and are divided into two main classes: the microglia and the macroglia (Fig. 24.3). The microglial cells are phagocytic scavenger cells related to macrophages that respond to infection or trauma to the CNS. The macroglial cells include astrocytes, oligodendrocytes, and ependymal cells. Astrocytes (astroglia) are star-shaped cells that provide the physical support for the neurons. They also regulate the chemical environment and nourish the neurons. These cells respond to brain trauma by forming scar tissue.

Oligodendrocytes and Schwann cells produce myelin within the CNS and peripheral neurons, respectively. Ependymal cells form the lining of the ventricles, CP, and central canal of the spinal cord. These cells help in the regulation of cerebrospinal fluid (CSF) and the blood-brain barrier (Sugarman & Huether, 2012).

Cerebrospinal Fluid and Ventricular System

CSF is a clear, colorless fluid. Approximately 135 milliliters (mL) of CSF circulates through the ventricles—a system of cavities within the brain—and within the subarachnoid space (80 mL in ventricles and 55 mL in the subarachnoid space). The brain and the spinal cord float in CSF, which absorbs shocks, cushions the CNS, and prevents the brain from tugging on meninges, nerve roots, and blood vessels. The choroid plexus (CP) is a group of blood vessels (capillaries) covered with a thin

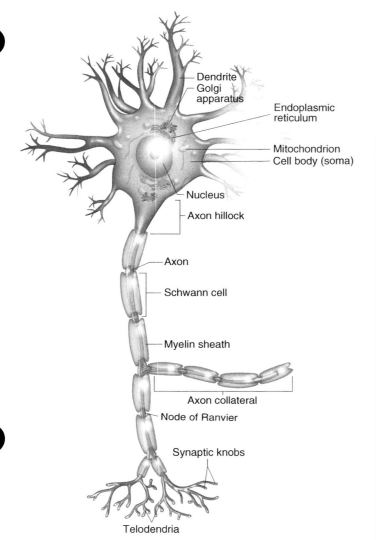

Fig. 24.2 Neuron with composite parts. (Modified from Patton, K. T., Thibodeau, G. A., & Douglas, M. M. [2012]. *Essentials of anatomy & physiology.* St. Louis, MO: Mosby.)

TABLE 24.1	**Significant Changes in the Aging Nervous System**
Neurologic Components	**Changes**
Central Nervous System	
Neurons	Shrinkage in neuron size and gradual decrease in neuron numbers
	Structural changes in dendrites
	Deposit of lipofuscin granules, neuritic plaque, and neurofibrillary bodies within cytoplasm and neurons
	Loss of myelin and decreased conduction in some nerves, especially peripheral nerves
Neurotransmitters	Changes in precursors necessary for neurotransmitter synthesis
	Change in receptor sites
	Alteration in enzymes that synthesize and degrade neurotransmitters
	Significant decreases in neurotransmitters, including ACh, glutamate, serotonin, dopamine, and gamma-aminobutyric acid
Peripheral Nervous System	
Motor	Muscular atrophy—decrease in muscle bulk
	Decrease in electrical conduction system
Sensory	Decrease in electrical conduction
	Atrophy of taste buds
	Alteration in olfactory nerve fibers
	Alteration in nerve cells of vestibular system of inner ear, cerebellum, and proprioception
Reflexes	Altered electrical conduction of the nerve caused by myelin loss
	Altered reflex responses (ankle, superficial reflexes)
Reticular formation	Physiologic changes in the RAS results in decrease in stages 3 and 4 of the sleep cycle
Autonomic Nervous System	
Basal ganglia	Slowing of autonomic nervous system response as a result of structural changes in basal ganglia

Ach, Acetylcholine; *RAS,* reticular activating system.

layer of epidermal cells. The CP is responsible for producing approximately 500 mL of CSF per day (Figs. 24.4 and 24.5).

Several physiologic changes are known to occur in the CNS of aging individuals. These may include sensory motor changes such as difficulty retrieving explicit memories and altered vision, hearing, taste, smell, vibratory sensations, and position sense. Because of neurotransmitters and hypothalamic changes in the aging process, the reticular activating system (RAS) that controls arousal and consciousness from the brainstem to the cerebral cortex is also altered. The neuroendocrine system plays a vital role in the function of the hippocampus. When any alteration occurs in this system, gradual changes in memory may be seen.

Hippocampus and the Hypothalamic–Pituitary–Adrenal Axis

The hippocampus is a part of the temporal lobe that plays an important role in memory and learning. Normal aging is associated with changes in the ability to consciously learn and retain new information easily. This occurs secondary to structural changes, synapse loss in the neurons, decreased microvascular integrity, reduction in glucose metabolism, and alterations in the neuroglia cells with aging. Because of changes in the secretory pattern of the hypothalamic–pituitary–adrenal (HPA) axis, additional alterations occur in the hippocampal area of the brain. The hippocampal area is strongly influenced by HPA hormones. The specific aspects altered by the aging process are the explicit memory (e.g., delayed recall), the ability to learn new information quickly, memory storage, and memory retrieval (Fadil, Borazanci, & Ait Ben Haddou, 2009; Keller, 2006).

Cerebrospinal Fluid

A reduction in the turnover of CSF with age decreases the distribution and efficiency with which the necessary substances are delivered from the CP to the brain target sites. These substances include the hormones necessary for metabolism and appetite, and the nutrients (e.g., transferrin, glucose, amino acids, and vitamins) necessary for nerve function. A reduction in the

CENTRAL NERVOUS SYSTEM NEUROGLIA

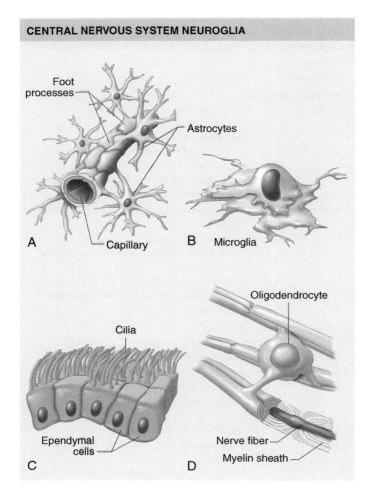

PERIPHERAL NERVOUS SYSTEM NEUROGLIA

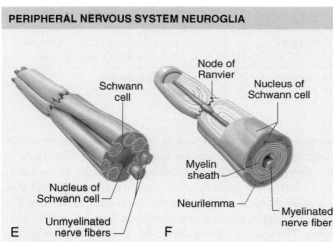

Fig. 24.3 Neuroglial cells. (From Patton, K. T., Thibodeau, G. A., & Douglas, M. M. [2012]. *Essentials of anatomy & physiology*. St. Louis, MO: Mosby.)

turnover of CSF may affect the removal of waste products, toxins (e.g., amyloid peptides and lactate), and drugs. The accumulation of these substances resulting from age-related changes may contribute to diseases causing cognitive decline. One significant factor that reduces the turnover secretion rate of CSF is the age-related increase in resistance from the vascular (sagittal venous sinus) system in the arachnoid (Redzic, Preston, Duncan et al., 2005). These changes occur in various degrees among aging individuals.

Balance and Motor Function

Age-related neurodegenerative and neurochemical changes in the cerebellum are believed to be the underlying cause of decline in motor and cognitive function. The neurodegenerative and neurochemical changes, combined with inner ear and vestibular changes, cause many older adults to experience changes in balance. These changes may further contribute to postural hypotension because of an inability to quickly respond to changes in position. The symptoms of postural hypotension are dizziness or lightheadedness when changing positions rapidly. However, compensatory processes in the cortex and subcortical areas of the brain help aging individuals maintain relatively normal motor performance (Heuninckx, Wenderoth, & Swinnen, 2008).

Reticular Formation and Sleep Patterns

The RF is a set of neurons that extends from the upper level of the spinal cord through the brainstem up to the cerebral cortex. The RF contains both motor and sensory tracts closely connected with the thalamus, basal ganglia, cerebellum, and cerebral cortex. This group of neural fibers has both excitatory and inhibitory capability. The RF contains a physiologic element, the RAS, which regulates sensory impulses transmitted to the cerebral cortex. The lower portion of the RAS in the brainstem assists in the regulation of the wake–sleep cycle and consciousness. Sleep disorders are common in aging individuals. Risk factors for sleep disturbances include physical illness, drugs, changes in social patterns (e.g., retirement or death of a spouse or loved one), and changes in circadian rhythm. Some sleep disturbances may also be part of the normal aging process resulting from neural changes in the RAS.

Normal sleep is organized into different stages that cycle throughout the night. The sleep stages are classified into the following categories (Brannon, Carroll, Vij, & Gentili, 2008; National Institute on Aging [NIA], 2012e):

- **Rapid eye movement (REM) sleep.** This is the stage of sleep during which muscle tone decreases significantly. In advanced aging, REM sleep is maintained without much decline.
- **Non-REM sleep.** This is subdivided into four stages. Stages 1 and 2 constitute light sleep, and stages 3 and 4 are deep sleep or slow-wave sleep. With aging, the duration of stage 1 sleep and the number of shifts into stage 1 sleep increase. Stages 3 and 4 decrease significantly with aging. Among the oldest-old people (older than 90 years), stages 3 and 4 may disappear completely. Some older women have normal or even increased stage 3 sleep, whereas men have normal or reduced stage 3 sleep.

As individuals age, they spend more time in bed to get the same amount of sleep they obtained when younger; however, the total sleep time is only slightly decreased, with an increase in nocturnal awakenings and daytime napping.

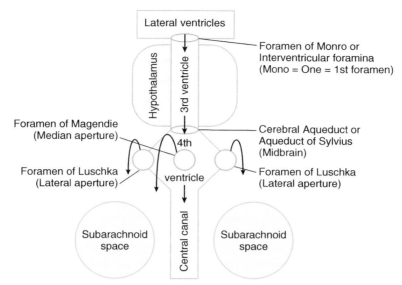

Fig. 24.4 Production, flow, and absorption of cerebrospinal fluid. (With permission from Dr. Sulabh Kumar Shrestha. Redrawn from EpoMedicine. [2016]. CSF circulation made simple. Retrieved April 17, 2018, from http://epomedicine.com/medical-students/csf-circulation-made-simple/.)

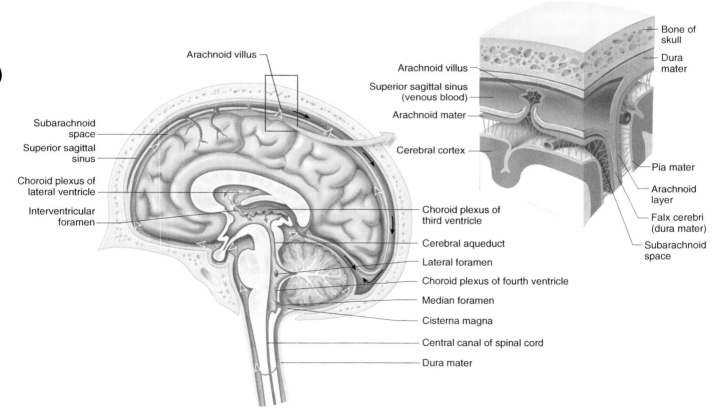

Fig. 24.5 Flow of cerebrospinal fluid. (Modified from Patton, K. T., & Thibodeau, G. A. [2013]. *Anatomy and physiology* [8th ed.]. St. Louis, MO: Mosby.)

Hence older persons often report having earlier bedtimes and increased sleep latency (time to fall asleep), with women taking longer than men, a 16% and 36% difference, respectively (NIA, 2012e).

Excessive daytime somnolence is not part of normal aging. Somnolence indicates the presence of a pathologic condition. Sleep apnea and certain movement disorders are serious sleep disorders, and older adults should be tested for these if they are having trouble with insomnia. Movement disorders, including restless leg syndrome, rapid eye movement sleep behavior disorder, and periodic limb movement disorder, are common among older adults (NIA, 2012e).

Sensorimotor Function

The nervous system depends on specialized sensory receptors to gather information about the internal and external environment. These receptors include those needed for vision, hearing, smell, touch, equilibrium, and pain sensation. Gradual changes occur in these sensory receptor sites as the aging process takes place.

Vision changes that occur with aging are significant. The lens of the eye thickens, becoming yellow, cloudy, and less elastic. The thickening of the lens reduces the amount of light passing through the lens. As the lens becomes less elastic, it loses its ability to focus on close objects. The change in elasticity also narrows the visual field and diminishes depth perception. The yellowing of the lens and changes in size and thickening of the cornea make it difficult to see at night. With aging, the fluid of the eye also becomes cloudy, reducing light sensitivity. These changes in the eyes lead to a gradual decrease in color perception, potentially affecting the ability of older individuals to distinguish between blue, green, and violet shades.

The ear consists of the outer ear, middle ear, and inner ear. Presbycusis is the hearing loss associated with the aging process. With presbycusis, older persons are unable to hear high frequencies and clearly hear consonant sounds such as *f, g, s, z, t, sh,* and *ch.* Other age-related auditory changes involve the collapse and narrowing of the auditory canal and thickening of earwax, which increase hearing difficulty.

With aging, the number of taste and smell receptors decreases and nerve transmissions are slower, although these losses are highly variable. The loss of taste and smell receptors means that food is not as appetizing to the older adult. Aging adults are also less likely to detect the bad taste or smell of spoiled food. Their reduced ability to smell also may make them unable to detect smoke, gas leaks, or other toxic fumes immediately.

The somatic receptors respond to touch, pressure, cold, pain, and body position. These receptors also become less sensitive as aging occurs. Older individuals therefore experience a decreased ability to feel pain and cope with temperature changes. These and additional age-related changes are presented in Table 24.1.

ASSESSMENT OF COGNITIVE FUNCTION

The assessment of neurocognitive function is an essential part of a comprehensive assessment in older adults. Neurocognitive function assessment includes several components and can be easily incorporated into the general assessment of older adults through history taking, physical examination, and the use of selected screening instruments. A complete mental status assessment should include attention, memory, orientation, perceptions, thought processes, thought content, insight, judgment, affect, mood, language, and higher cognitive functions.

Screening instruments are available to primary care providers for detecting mental disorders, but the actual diagnoses are based on criteria detailed in the *Diagnostic and Statistical Manual for Mental Disorders, Fifth Edition (DSM-5)* (American Psychiatric Association [APA], 2013). A multiaxial system involves assessment on several axes, each of which refers to a different domain of information that may help the clinician plan treatment and predict the outcome (APA, 2013).

Neurologic assessment includes the evaluation of cranial nerves, gait, balance, distal deep tendon reflexes, plantar responses, primary sensory modalities in the lower extremities, and cerebrovascular integrity. Complete neurocognitive examinations should be performed on all older adults to establish baseline function and to detect potentially reversible conditions causing mental and behavioral disturbances.

Few older adults recognize the symptoms of cognitive decline in themselves. It is often a friend or family member who reports these symptoms to the nurse or physician caring for the patient. An interview with the friend or family member, physical assessment, and the use of structured mental status assessments assist the nurse in identifying cognitive decline in older adults (Dick, 2013).

One of the early manifestations of cognitive decline may be observed in the functioning of older adults. It is important to include functional assessment as part of the assessment of older adults. Simple questions that may be asked in the history include their ability to perform activities of daily living (ADLs) such as bathing, dressing, toileting, and eating. Instrumental activities of daily living (IADLs) should also be addressed. These activities include the ability to clean house, shop, pay bills, and perform other functions that would allow patients to remain independent within their homes.

Selected Cognitive Function Screening Instruments
Functional Assessment

One screening tool used to identify the presence and severity of dementia symptoms based on level of function and cognition in older adults is the Dementia Severity Rating Scale (DSRS) when administered by family or caregivers. The DSRS is an 11-item instrument that can be easily and quickly administered and covers memory, orientation, judgment, community affairs, home activities, personal care, speech and language recognition, feeding, incontinence, and mobility or walking. A normal score on this instrument is four or less; the score increases as the older person's cognition decreases (Harvey, Moriarty, Kleinman et al., 2005).

Mental Status Examination

The Montreal Cognitive Assessment (MoCA) was developed in 2005 as a quick screening tool for mild cognitive impairment (MCI) and early Alzheimer's dementia. The 30-item tool assesses the domains of attention and concentration, executive functions, memory, language, visuospatial abilities, conceptual thinking, calculations, and orientation (Doerflinger, 2012). It takes about 10 minutes to administer the MoCa. Research indicates the MoCA can discriminate reliably between normal subjects, participants with MCI, and those with dementia (Maust, Cristancho, Gray, Rushing, Tjoa, & Thase, 2012). The Mini-Cog is a simple screening tool that takes about 3 minutes to administer and can be used to detect cognitive impairment quickly, during both routine visits and hospitalizations. It serves as an effective triage tool to identify patients in need of more thorough evaluation (Doerflinger, 2013).

Depression Assessment

Depression often occurs concurrently with other serious illnesses such as heart disease, stroke, diabetes, cancer, and Parkinson's disease (PD). Because many older adults face these illnesses as well as various social and economic difficulties, health care professionals may mistakenly conclude that depression is a normal consequence of these problems, an attitude often shared by patients themselves. These factors together contribute to the underdiagnoses and undertreatment of depressive disorders in older people. Depression can, and should, be treated when it occurs with other illnesses, as untreated depression may delay recovery from or worsen the outcome of the other illnesses. The relationship between depression and other illness processes in older adults is a focus of ongoing research (National Institute of Mental Health [NIMH], 2013).

The Geriatric Depression Scale (GDS) may be used with healthy older adults, as well as those who are acutely ill, and those with mild to moderate cognitive impairment. It has been used in the community and in acute and long-term care settings. The GDS short form consists of 15 items; 10 indicate the presence of depression when answered positively, whereas the rest (question numbers 1, 5, 7, 11, 13) indicate depression when answered negatively (Greenberg, 2012).

Cognitive Function and Memory in Typical Aging

Forgetfulness as an inevitable consequence of aging is a myth that has had significant influence on society's views of aging. Forgetfulness may affect both the young and old but should not be confused with true cognitive impairment. Memory and delayed recall are not substantially decreased in older persons. If allowed time to learn new material, older persons experience no more memory loss than younger persons. Cognitive impairment involves mental status changes in addition to higher level cognitive functional changes such as failure to correctly spell common words, compute simple sums, balance a checkbook, drive a car safely, plan a meal, or follow grammatical conventions. A decline in cognitive function is an effect of disease, not an effect of the normal aging process.

COGNITIVE DISORDERS ASSOCIATED WITH ALTERED THOUGHT PROCESSES

Several cognitive disorders are associated with altered thought processes in older adults. These include the three *D*s—depression, delirium, and dementia—as well as cranial tumors, subdural hematomas, and normal pressure hydrocephalus. It is often difficult to accurately diagnose the underlying cause of altered thought processes in older adults because of the similarity in their presentations. Nevertheless, accurate assessment and diagnosis are essential for ensuring appropriate treatment to improve or potentially reverse the underlying pathophysiologic condition contributing to the individual's impaired cognition.

Depression

The rate of depression increases as individuals age. The estimate is 20% to 25% of those older than 55 have evidence of a mental health disorder. These include anxiety, depression, dysthymic disorder, and severe cognitive disorders (APA, 2013; Centers for Disease Control and Prevention [CDC], 2012). The percentage of men older than the age of 85 reporting depressive symptoms is almost double that of men aged 65 to 74. Depression is associated with higher suicide rates among older adults than among younger persons with depression (CDC, 2012). Although older Americans make up nearly 15% of the U.S. population, they account for just under 19% of all suicide deaths. Older men have the highest rates of suicide of any age group, and men 85 and older have rates of suicide at 17 per 100,000. Older adults in the United States, especially those who are depressed, are more likely to commit suicide than those in any other age group, although it is difficult to estimate the true incidence of suicide among older adults (Span, 2013).

Clinical Manifestations

Depression may manifest itself through more vegetative signs such as fatigue; constipation; psychomotor retardation; depressed mood; loss of interest, energy, libido, or pleasure; changes in appetite, weight, and sleep patterns; agitation; anxiety; or crying (APA, 2013; Kyomen & Whitfield, 2008). Depression is often first seen in older adults as cognitive impairment, particularly in the areas of attention and concentration. Depressed older adults may neglect eating or caring for a chronic medical condition, predisposing them to the development of delirium.

Depression is also a common response to serious illness of any kind, particularly multiple sclerosis, hypothyroidism, lupus, hepatitis, acquired immunodeficiency syndrome (AIDS), vitamin deficiencies, and anemia. These conditions may produce depression in a more direct biologic sense. Drugs may also contribute to depression (Box 24.1). Some general medical conditions such as myocardial infarction (MI) or a hip fracture are risk factors for depression. And individuals with these conditions as well as depression have a poorer outcome compared

---

BOX 24.1 Drugs That May Contribute to Depression

- Nonnucleoside reverse transcriptase inhibitors
- Beta-blockers
- Calcium channel blockers
- Fluoroquinolones
- Opioids
- Mefloquine
- Varenicline
- Contraceptives
- Statins
- Corticosteroids
- Zovirax
- Interferon-alpha and interferon-beta
- Anticonvulsants
- Antabuse
- Benzodiazepines

with those without depression (APA, 2013). Older adults require careful medical history taking and physical examination before the diagnosis of depression can be made. The loss of physical health, employment and income, family and friends, and house and comfortable environment are difficult to accept, especially if they all occur within a relatively short period. Retirement may be difficult and depressing for many, especially those who were involved in interesting, rewarding work. *Comorbidity,* or the presence of multiple chronic health problems, may prevent older adults from enjoying life and may lead to clinical manifestations of depression.

Late-life depression is often similar in presentation to, or may be concomitant with, cognitive impairment and dementia caused by neurochemical changes and awareness of the loss of physical or intellectual functioning. Symptoms common to both depression and dementia include irritability, inability to concentrate or feel pleasure, loss of interest in life, and lack of energy and initiative. With careful assessment, it is possible to make the appropriate diagnosis. Individuals with dementia are more likely to show signs of disorientation and loss of short-term memory, and are less likely to feel sadness or guilt or to complain about pain, insomnia, and poor appetite. Table 24.2 compares selected features associated with Depression, delirium, and dementia (Sullivan, 2008).

Delirium

Delirium presents as a disturbance in attention (decreased awareness of the environment) with a reduced ability to focus, sustain, or shift attention (*DSM-5:* Neurocognitive Disorders [NCDs]). Cognitive changes (poor memory, disorientation, speech disturbance), perceptual disturbances, or both are distinct from preexisting, established, or evolving dementia. The onset of the disturbance is rapid (hours to days) and typically fluctuates over the course of the day. Delirium frequently represents a sudden and significant decline from a previous level of functioning and usually is evident after history taking, physical examination, or laboratory tests of a direct physiologic etiology of a general medical condition, substance intoxication or withdrawal, use of a drug, toxin exposure, or a combination of these factors (APA, 2013; Neufeld, Birenvenu, Rosenberg et al., 2011).

Delirium occurs in all settings, including homes, assisted living facilities, nursing facilities, and hospitals. Frequently, when an older adult becomes delirious in a community setting, it precipitates hospital admission, in part because of the underlying illness causing the delirium. It is not uncommon for hospitalized patients with cancer (25%) or AIDS (30% to 40%) to develop delirium. Approximately half of postoperative patients develop delirium, and the majority of those with terminal illness (up to 80%) develop delirium with impending death (Breitbart & Alici, 2012).

Risk Factors

The risk factors for delirium include advanced age, CNS diseases, infection, polypharmacy, hypoalbuminemia, electrolyte imbalances, trauma history, gastrointestinal or genitourinary disorders, cardiopulmonary disorders, and sensory changes. These factors may lead to physiologic imbalances increasing

TABLE 24.2 Clinical Features of Depression, Delirium, and Dementia

Clinical Feature	Depression	Delirium	Dementia
Onset	Can be abrupt or associated with life events	Sudden onset	Months to years
Duration	Weeks to months	Hours to days	Long term or lifetime
Mood	Consistent; sadness, anxiety, irritability	Labile; suspicious, mood swings	Fluctuating; depressed, apathetic, uninterested
Behavior	Variable; may have psychomotor retardation or agitation	Variable; hypokinetic or hyperkinetic	Variable with psychomotor retardation or agitation
Cognition			
Orientation	Selected disorientation	Impaired with variable severity	Slow decline over time
Alertness	Normal	Lethargic or hypervigilant	Generally normal
Memory	Selective impairment	Impairment of recent memory and attentiveness	Early recent and later remote memory impairment
Thought processes	Intact with themes of hopelessness, helplessness, and self-depreciation	Difficulty maintaining concentration; disorganized; fragmented	Impoverished; impaired abstract thinking; word-finding difficulties; impaired judgment
Perception	Normal	Possible visual, auditory, and tactile hallucinations or delusions	Misperceptions not generally present
Speech and language	Normal to slowed	Slurred, forced, or rambling	Disordered; word-finding difficulties
Mini-Mental State Examination	Performance fluctuates over time	Acute fluctuations	Moderately stable with decreasing scores over time

the risk for confusion (Fick & Mion, 2008). Specific laboratory testing should be guided by clues in the history and physical examination so that the physiologic causes of delirium can be identified.

Clinical Manifestations

Symptoms of delirium fluctuate and may include difficulty maintaining concentration or attention to external stimuli and a language disturbance, including slurred, forced, or rambling speech. Disorganized thinking demonstrated by tangential reasoning and conversation is often the presenting symptom. Other common symptoms of delirium include the following:

- Clouding of consciousness or fluctuation of awareness
- Misperceptions, illusions, or hallucinations
- Disorientation to persons, place, and time
- Memory problems
- Increased or decreased physical activity
- Impaired judgment

The Confusion Assessment Method (CAM) is a standardized evidence-based tool that enables health care personnel to identify and recognize delirium quickly and accurately in multiple settings. The CAM includes four features (onset, attention, thinking, and consciousness) found to have the greatest ability to distinguish delirium from other types of cognitive impairment (Waszynski, 2012).

Management

Many interventions are used to prevent delirium in hospitalized patients. Assessment with the use of a validated instrument such as the CAM is the first line in preventing and treating delirium. Delirium management includes rapid diagnosis and treatment of the underlying cause, management of disruptive behaviors, and supportive care. Assessment of changes in older persons' cognition is paramount. Thorough history taking and physical examination are essential for the identification of the onset, cause, direct physiologic manifestations of a general medical condition, or intoxication with or withdrawal from substances that may contribute to the onset of delirium (APA, 2013).

Nonpharmacologic Interventions. A therapeutic environment includes frequent reassurance and memory cues (calendar, clock, family photos); clear communication; caregiver consistency; decreased stimuli (noise reduction, adequate lighting, not rushing the patient); decreased stress and anxiety through frequent reassurance and providing daily routine; maintaining comfort (eyeglasses, hearing aids, personal belongings); reestablishing sleep–wake cycle by controlling nighttime noise and unnecessary disruptions; ensuring adequate food and fluid intake; ensuring elimination needs are met; providing for physical activity, ambulation, and range of motion; and avoiding chemical or physical restraint. Drugs should be used as a last resort (Tullmann, Fletcher, & Foreman, 2012).

Pharmacotherapy. Delirium that causes injury to the patient or others should be treated with drugs. Studies are equivocal on the benefit of second-generation antipsychotics in the treatment of delirium. However, risperidone, olanzapine, and quetiapine continue to be the drugs of choice in the treatment of psychotic symptoms of delirium. Doses should be kept as low as possible to minimize adverse effects. Patients should be monitored closely, as paradoxical and hypersensitivity reactions may occur. Benzodiazepines (BZs) should be avoided, except for specific indications (e.g., alcohol or gamma-hydroxybutyric acid [GHA] withdrawal delirium, delirium related to seizures) (Alagiakrishnan, 2017). Fig. 24.6 provides a sample delirium protocol.

Dementia

The number of people living with dementia worldwide is currently estimated at 46.8 million. This number is expected to

be close to 131.5 million worldwide by 2050 (Prince, Comas-Herrera, Knapp, Guerchet, & Karagiannidou, 2016). The phenomenon of potentially reversible dementia is not included in these statistics. The primary types of dementia include Alzheimer's disease (AD), vascular dementia (VaD), dementia with Lewy bodies (DLB), and frontotemporal dementia (FTD).

Dementia is a syndrome of gradual and progressive cognitive decline. It has been defined as alteration in memory, in addition to acquired persistent alteration in intellectual function (e.g., orientation, calculation, attention, and motor skills) compromising multiple cognitive domains. In dementia, individuals are unable to do the things they used to do because of the mental changes associated with this disease process. Dementia may involve language deficits, apraxia (difficulty with the manipulation of objects), agnosia (inability to recognize familiar objects), agraphia (difficulty drawing objects), and impaired executive function (Alzheimer's Association, 2013).

Although dementia is more common in older persons than in younger persons, it is not part of the normal aging process. Dementia is usually a condition occurring in later life because of changes in neurologic function caused by a disease process. Dementia has been linked to a variety of conditions. Research of the problem has been difficult because of the lack of a standard definition of mild dementia and difficulty in detecting symptoms of early dementia.

Reversible Dementia

Reversible dementia is a phenomenon that occurs when other pathologic conditions masquerade as dementia. Causes of potentially reversible dementia are presented in Box 24.2. It is important to identify and treat the underlying causes of dementia symptoms; even if these disorders are identified and treated, however, not all individuals with dementia symptoms will improve (Koedama, Pijnenburga, Deega et al., 2008).

Alzheimer Disease

Adequate, accurate diagnosis of AD is essential. Some conditions such as AD have no specific cure, but it is essential to know whether the symptoms and behavior are reversible. Even those irreversible disorders can be, and should be, treated with appropriate drugs, if useful, and with effective communication techniques and environmental strategies, as needed.

AD is the most common form of dementia in older persons and accounts for 60% to 80% of individuals with the disease (Alzheimer's Association, 2013). AD is a progressive, neurodegenerative disease characterized by the presence of neurofibrillary tangles composed of misplaced proteins within the brain, cortical amyloid plaques, and granulovascular degeneration of neurons in the pyramidal cell layer of the hippocampus. More than five million Americans have AD, and it is predicted that the number of individuals with AD could rise to 16 million by 2050. AD is the sixth leading cause of death in the United States (Alzheimer's Association, 2017).

The personal and public costs of AD are high. Medicare costs for beneficiaries with AD are expected to exceed the ability to absorb the cost (Alzheimer's Association, 2013). Costs are estimated to soar from $259 billion in 2017 to $1.1 trillion by 2050 for caring for patients with AD and other types of dementias

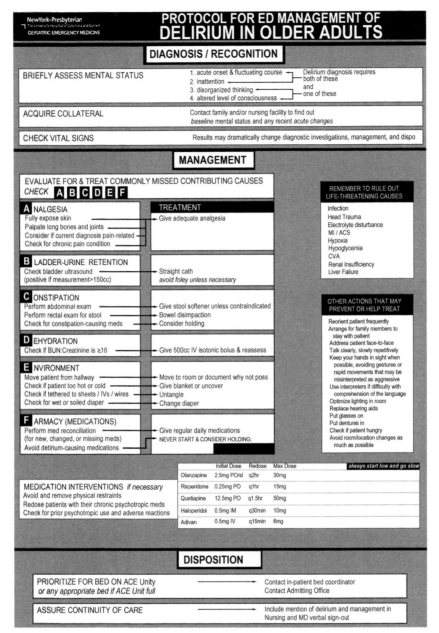

Fig. 24.6 Sample delirium protocol. (From Rosen, T., Connors, S., Clark, S., et al. [2015]. Assessment and management of delirium in older adults in the emergency department: Literature review to inform development of a novel clinical protocol. *Advanced Emergency Nursing Journal, 37*[3], 183–196.)

BOX 24.2   Causes of Potentially Reversible Dementia

- Depression
- Drug (side effects, drug interactions, drug overdose)
- Alcohol abuse
- Drug abuse
- Dietary, vitamin and mineral deficiencies (A, C, B_{12}, and folate)
- Traumas (as a result of falls, concussions, or contusions to the head)
- Hormonal dysfunction (thyroid problems)
- Metabolic disorders (dehydration, kidney failure, COPD)
- Infections
- Heart disease
- Brain disease (tumors)
- Environmental toxins

Reprinted from the Alzheimer Society of Canada. (2017). "Reversible dementias" available at http://alzheimer.ca/en/Home/About-dementia/Dementias/Reversible-dementias.

(Alzheimer's Association, 2017). Approximately 4% of people in the United States live in extended care facilities; 75% of the people with AD will be admitted to a nursing home by age 80 (Alzheimer's Association, 2013). The changing demographics of our society and the anticipated growth of the older adult population during the next few decades have created a need for health care providers to develop age-related interventions that address the mental health needs of an aging population.

Risk Factors

Research has focused on genetic, nutritional, viral, environmental, and other causes of AD. Age is the single most important risk factor for the development of AD, as the number of people with the disease doubles every 5 years beyond age 65.

EVIDENCE-BASED PRACTICE

Appropriate Antipsychotic Prescribing in Long-Term Care

Background

Approximately 25% of nursing home residents are prescribed antipsychotics despite limited efficacy and warnings against their use.

Sample/Setting

The sample encompassed the de-identified medical records of residents of a dementia special care unit. A baseline audit was conducted using American Medical Directors Association's (AMDA's) Antipsychotic Use in Dementia Assessment, which included 59 records; a second audit 2 months after in-service training included 53 records.

Methods

Roger's Diffusion of Innovations theory guided this quality improvement project. An educational in-service was designed that focused on documentation of behaviors and interventions, including Centers for Medicare & Medicaid Services (CMS) guidelines for appropriate antipsychotic use, and nonpharmacologic interventions to treat behavioral and psychiatric symptoms of dementia (BPSD).

Findings

At baseline, the antipsychotic drug prescribing rate was 20.3%. Risperidone was the most commonly prescribed antipsychotic. Documentation included the indication for use, with psychotic symptoms as the most common indication. Adverse events (33%) included falls and restlessness. Nonpharmacological interventions were documented by activities personnel (83.3%) and infrequently by nursing personnel (16.7%).

At follow-up, antipsychotic prescribing was at 15.4% (a decrease of 20.3% from baseline). There were no adverse events recorded. Nonpharmacological interventions increased to 75%, with the most common being unit-based activities, animal assisted therapy, redirection, massage, and reorientation. Physical activities increased from baseline and included walking, performing household tasks/chores, and exercise.

Implications

This quality improvement project provides evidence that staff education can positively affect the appropriate use of antipsychotic drugs and nonpharmacologic interventions for BPSD as well as improve documentation in compliance with CMS.

From Watson-Wolfe, K., Galik, E., Klinedinst, J., & Brandt, N. (2014). Application of the antipsychotic use in dementia assessment audit tool to facilitate appropriate antipsychotic use in long term care residents with dementia. *Geriatric Nursing, 35,* 71-76. doi: 10.1016/j. gerinurse.2013.09.002.

Genetic Factors

One risk factor for the development of AD is genetics, particularly in one type of early-onset AD occurring in people ages 30 to 60, but affecting less than 5% of all who have AD.

Research continues on the identification of brain abnormalities typical of AD, for example, the accumulation of amyloid in the living brain. Most cases of AD develop after age 60 and are a combination of lifestyle, genetics, and environmental factors. One genetic risk factor appears to increase the risk of developing the disease, and that is related to the apolipoprotein E (*APOE*) gene found on chromosome 19 (NIA, 2012a). Genetic testing can identify which *APOE* alleles a person has, but it cannot predict who will or will not actually develop AD.

Clinical Manifestations

Symptoms of AD that may be identified by family members and nurses include the individual repeating questions and statements, forgetting to pay bills or take drugs, increasing problems with orientation, and geographic disorientation. Other symptoms of AD include pervasive forgetfulness and memory loss, language deterioration, impaired ability to mentally manipulate visual information, poor judgment, confusion, restlessness, and mood swings. Personality changes may include apathy or loss of interest in previously enjoyed activities. Eventually, AD destroys cognition, personality, and the ability to function.

Diagnostic Studies

In 2012, both the NIA and the Alzheimer's Association proposed new guidelines to assist pathologists in describing and categorizing brain changes with AD and other dementias. One guideline is that three stages of AD exist and that, in the first stage, symptoms such as memory loss are not noticeable; it may take up to 20 years before any symptoms develop. Another guideline describes biomarkers such as beta-amyloid and tau-amyloid in CSF and blood (Alzheimer's Association, 2013). Although autopsy remains the gold standard for the definitive diagnosis of AD, clinical diagnosis has become increasingly accurate over the past several years (Alzheimer's Association, 2013). Magnetic resonance imaging (MRI) and computed tomography (CT) are used in the medical workup mainly to rule out any other brain conditions and have been used to identify the hippocampal atrophy associated with the diagnosis of AD. As with any other medical diagnosis, a complete history, physical examination, blood work, and neurologic examination and tests are essential.

Treatment

No cure exists for AD. Several pharmacologic options have been introduced to slow the progression of the disease. These drugs have transformed the care of AD patients. Cholinesterase inhibitors are prescribed for mild to moderate AD and are used to delay or prevent symptoms from becoming worse for a limited time. They may also help control some behavioral changes. These drugs include donepezil, rivastigmine, and galantamine. Tacrine was the first of the cholinesterase inhibitors, but because of the need to frequently monitor a patient's liver function, its use is limited (Dichgans, Markus, Salloway et al., 2008).

Memantine is used to treat moderate to severe AD, and its main effect is to delay the progression of some of the symptoms. The expectation with this drug is that it allows patients to maintain certain daily functions longer than they would without the drugs. Combining memantine with other AD drugs promises to be more effective than any single therapy (NIA, 2012b). Although cholinesterase inhibitors have been useful in older adults with AD, they have not been shown to have the same effects in those with other types of progressive dementia.

NURSING MANAGEMENT

Previously the management of patients with dementia consisted of helping patients and their families through progression of the disorder while allowing them as much dignity and independence as possible. This is clearly still true. However, the focus is now on maintaining cognitive and global functioning early in the disease process to postpone the need for institutional care.

Vascular Dementia

VaD is the second most frequently occurring type of dementia among older persons, causing dementia in 20% to 30% of people (Alzheimer's Association, 2013). Often referred to as *multiinfarct dementia*, depending on how it presents itself on scans, VaD is defined as a loss of cognitive function resulting from ischemic, hypoperfusive, or hemorrhagic brain lesions resulting from cerebrovascular disease or cardiovascular pathologic conditions. VaD is associated with the progressive loss of brain tissue because of a series of small infarcts caused by occlusions and blockages within the arteries to the brain. Individuals who have experienced a cerebrovascular accident (CVA) have an even greater risk of VaD (Schneck, 2008; Zekry, 2009).

Pathophysiologically, asymmetric regions of cerebral softening and hemorrhage are diffuse and irregular. If a series of infarcts occur, the rate of decline in function increases. Some recovery of function may occur over time, but full recovery never occurs. As the damage from the infarcts progresses and accumulates, more widespread evidence of diminished mental ability exists.

Risk Factors

Several medical problems place individuals at risk for the development of VaD. These include arteriosclerosis, blood dyscrasias, cardiac decompensation, hypertension, atrial fibrillation, cardiac valve replacements, systemic emboli for other reasons, diabetes mellitus, peripheral vascular disease, obesity, and smoking. Those at the highest risk are those with vasospasms in segments of the brain. Vasospasms are also referred to as transient ischemic attacks [TIAs] (Lewandowski, Rao, & Silver, 2008).

Clinical Manifestations

The onset of VaD may be gradual or abrupt. Gradual-onset VaD occurs because of small lacunar infarcts that affect a very small area of the brain, causing memory, motor, or sensory perceptual function deficits. This phenomenon may not be obvious until several small infarcts have occurred. Abrupt-onset VaD

presents with immediate neurologic symptoms such as one-sided weakness, gait abnormalities, or focal neurologic signs. Destruction of the brain tissue resulting from small emboli or brain attacks may be localized or diffuse. The usual progression of VaD follows a stepwise decline rather than the slow, steady decline associated with AD. Patients with VaD have an infarct, decline in function, and then experience a functional plateau before experiencing another insult and subsequent decline.

Symptoms of VaD depend on the location of the infarct and may include the following:
- Impaired learning and impaired retention of new information
- Impaired handling of new tasks
- Impaired reasoning ability
- Impaired spatial ability and orientation
- Impaired language

These impairments generally interfere with work and social functioning. Other symptoms may include wandering, getting lost in familiar places, moving with rapid shuffling steps, losing bladder or bowel control, inappropriately displaying emotions, and having difficulty following instructions. Not all brain attacks result in intellectual impairment; some affect movement, vision, or other functions.

Diagnostic Studies

Neuroimaging with either CT or MRI usually reveals one or more areas of cerebral infarction. VaD is most often associated with diffuse or bilateral cortical or subcortical areas of infarction or microinfarction. Other than neuroimaging and clinical examination, no other diagnostic tests or biomarkers exist for the diagnosis of VaD.

Treatment

Treatment for VaD is the same as for AD.

Lewy Body Dementia

DLB is a progressive, degenerative brain disorder causing decline in thinking, reasoning, and independent functioning caused by abnormal small deposits in the brain matter. DLB is the third most common dementia, comprising 10% to 25% of all cases. Lewy bodies may be found in persons with AD and those with PD. Individuals with PD have a sixfold increased risk for the development of DLB compared with the general population (Alzheimer's Association, 2013; Dodel et al., 2008).

Risk Factors

No risk factors or causes are known for DLB at this time.

Clinical Manifestations

The clinical manifestations of DLB are like those of AD; however, DLB is often marked by prominent fluctuations in attention and ability to communicate, and by the severity of psychiatric symptoms, particularly visual hallucinations. DLB, compared with AD, tends to have more visual–spatial processing impairments and features of subcortical dementia. These include decreased attention and deficits in verbal fluency. Extrapyramidal features are also found in DLB, including rigidity, bradykinesia, flexed posture, and shuffling gait. Other symptoms may include the following:

- Excessive daytime sleepiness and altered arousal
- Periods of reduced attention and concentration
- REM sleep disorder

Diagnostic Studies

No laboratory tests are available for the diagnosis of DLB. MRI shows less hippocampal activity than is seen in AD, but these are too minimal to be of diagnostic value. Diagnosis is based on the health care professional's best judgment after neurologic examination and tests (Alzheimer's Association, 2013; Bhasin, Rowan, Edwards, & McKeith, 2007).

Management

Management of patients with DLB focuses on symptomatic relief when psychiatric and behavioral symptoms become distressing. Treatment for PD is essential in the event of gait and balance alterations. The use of cholinesterase inhibitors has been supported in DLB, as is the use of antidepressants, especially the use of selective serotonin reuptake inhibitors (SSRIs). Antipsychotic drugs should be used with extreme caution as these may cause serious side effects in around 50% of patients (Alzheimer's Association, 2013). Because these patients also have sleep disorders involving REM sleep, clonazepam may be used.

Frontotemporal Dementia

FTD is a clinical syndrome of exclusion associated with non-AD pathologic conditions and is relatively rare in the clinical setting. This syndrome includes the spectrum of non-AD dementias and is characterized by focal atrophy of the frontal and anterior temporal regions.

Risk Factors

The risk factors for FTD are poorly understood.

Clinical Manifestations

FTDs are defined generally by the earliest symptoms: (1) progressive behavior and personality decline with a change in personality, emotions, behavior and judgment, called *behavioral variant frontotemporal dementia* or *Pick disease;* (2) progressive language decline, with early changes in language ability in speaking, reading, writing and understanding, called *primary progressive aphasia;* and (3) progressive motor decline, characterized by difficulties with physical movement, including shaking, difficulty walking, frequent falls, and poor coordination (National Institute of Neurologic Disorders and Stroke [NINDS], 2013).

Diagnostic Studies

Neuroimaging with CT or MRI may be useful in the diagnosis of FTD. Focal atrophy of the prefrontal or temporal regions confirms FTD; however, this finding is not always present. Positron emission tomography (PET) or single photon emission computed tomography (SPECT) may also assist in the confirmation of the clinical diagnosis (NINDS, 2013).

Management

In FTD, the interval between onset of symptoms and severe dementia ranges from 3 to 10 years. Currently, no treatments for FTD are available, but patients with FTD do benefit from a team approach with the use of speech therapists, physical therapists, day care, respite care, and the judicious use of drugs to control symptoms (NINDS, 2013).

Other Dementia-Related Diseases

Normal Pressure Hydrocephalus

Normal pressure hydrocephalus (NPH) is a rare but potentially reversible condition; if left untreated, it leads to permanent cognitive impairment. In NPH, CSF circulates to the cerebral subarachnoid space, enlarging the ventricles but causing no rise in the CSF pressure. It is believed that most cases of NPH are related to prior cerebral insults such as traumatic injury, viral insult, or previous surgery. NPH has a triad of symptoms that present together: (1) gait disturbance (e.g., ataxic or magnetic gait), (2) urinary incontinence, and (3) cognitive dysfunction. Patients who develop dementia before gait disturbance have poorer outcomes. Treatment involves placing a shunt to drain CSF (NINDS, 2013).

Dementia may also result from other diseases, including Huntington disease (formerly called *Huntington's chorea*), Creutzfeldt-Jakob disease, and infection with human immunodeficiency virus (HIV). These diseases are less common among the older adult population.

Subdural Hematomas

A subdural hematoma is bleeding between the cranium and the cerebral cortex. The pressure created by this bleeding may cause cognitive impairment and neurologic deficits. Older adults are at risk for the development of subdural hematomas caused by brain atrophy and corresponding vascular changes that occur with normal aging, and they are also at risk for falls and subsequent head injuries.

The two types of subdural hematomas are acute subdural hematoma and chronic subdural hematoma. Symptoms of acute subdural hematomas develop within 48 to 72 hours after a head injury but are not seen with the typical signs of increased intracranial pressure (ICP). Instead, the presentation includes insidious changes in mentation and focal neurologic signs. Chronic subdural hematomas may be caused by trauma but often are not noticed until 3 or more weeks after the initial injury because of slow bleeding into the intracranial space.

Treatments for both acute and chronic subdural hematomas include the evacuation of the hematoma, usually with the use of burr holes and a closed drainage system. Unfortunately, recurrence is not uncommon.

Intracranial Tumors

Intracranial tumors occur more frequently in older adults than in younger adults and may be either benign (meningiomas) or malignant (gliomas). Intracranial tumors in older adults rarely are seen with the typical signs of increased ICP (e.g., headaches, vomiting, and papilledema); rather, they are seen with subtly progressive changes such as withdrawal, isolation, personality changes, and slowly progressive hemiparesis. Because the symptoms are insidious and include cognitive dysfunction and withdrawal, older adults with intracranial tumors are often misdiagnosed with depression or dementia; later, when focal neurologic signs appear, brain tumors are considered.

The diagnosis of an intracranial tumor is made after cranial CT or MRI. The pathologic condition is determined through a biopsy, either by tumor extraction or stereotactic needle biopsy under CT or MRI guidance. Treatment is based on the results of the biopsy and may include surgical extraction followed by radiation if the tumor recurs (meningioma) or surgical extraction followed by radiation and concomitant chemotherapy (malignant glioma). The prognosis is generally poor; the 1-year survival rate for malignant gliomas is 23%.

The decision of whether and how to treat intracranial tumors in older adults is complex, in part because of preexisting illnesses that may complicate neurosurgery, as well as potential complications or side effects after surgery, chemotherapy, and radiation. Treatment in older patients may lead to deficits that are as serious as those resulting from no treatment or limited treatment. All treatment decisions should be made in conjunction with individuals and their families.

DIAGNOSTIC ASSESSMENT OF COGNITIVE DISORDERS

Examination

History taking, physical examination, behavioral observation, and functional and mental status examinations form the basis for a diagnosis of depression, delirium, and dementia. Medical screening alone is not sufficient for the evaluation of intellectual decline in older adults, but it does provide valuable information for ruling out treatable disorders. The only positive diagnosis for dementia-related disorders is a brain tissue biopsy or autopsy of the brain. Screening for treatable, reversible causes is essential in identifying and implementing appropriate treatment for the underlying cause of cognitive dysfunction associated with altered thought processes.

Diagnostic Studies

Laboratory tests are used to assess the nervous system or rule out medical problems causing the disorder. CT, MRI, and electroencephalography (EEG) have been used for diagnosis of delirium or dementia. CT is useful in detecting pathologic conditions such as space-occupying lesions (e.g., intracranial tumors, subdural hematomas, and hydrocephalus) that may lead to dementia. The pathologic changes seen in dementia, including ventricular enlargement, narrowing of the gyri, widening of the sulci, and brain atrophy, may be identified on CT. Images obtained by MRI have a high resolution and may be useful in detecting multiple subcortical brain attacks and white matter disease. MRI is useful in the diagnosis of VaD. The disadvantage of MRI is that the test requires the older person to lie motionless for a long time. This may be impossible for older persons with cognitive disorders. EEG may provide important information about the mental status. The background frequency of the waking EEG can be correlated with a

patient's mental state. Normal EEG results in a severely impaired patient support the diagnosis of pseudodementia. In early dementia, EEG results may demonstrate an abnormally slow response, which indicates a treatable diagnosis. PET is a noninvasive technique that allows assessment of regional glucose use, oxygen consumption, and regional cerebral blood flow. This technique may be useful in the differential diagnosis of the hippocampal atrophy seen in AD and the changes associated with FTD.

Laboratory Studies

CSF studies are useful for identifying reversible causes of dementia. Laboratory screening tests to rule out treatable medical diagnoses may include a complete blood cell count (CBC); electrolytes; chest radiography; urinalysis; liver, kidney, and thyroid function tests; serum B_{12} levels; folate; syphilis serology (with high index of suspicion of syphilis); and drug studies. Genetic testing remains controversial; however, testing for the APOE epsilon-4 allele has been considered in AD. Routine use of this test may, however, lead to overdiagnosis of AD.

Postmortem biopsy is considered the only definitive means of differentiating the type of dementia causing the symptoms. The clinical profile, obtained through history taking, physical examination, mental status examination, laboratory tests, and behavioral observations, has improved the classification of dementia.

DSM-5 Criteria

The *DSM-5* classification (APA, 2013) is the most widely accepted system of classifying abnormal behaviors and is consistent in most respects with the systems used by the World Health Organization (WHO) and the International Classification of Diseases. The *DSM-5* classification categorizes each disorder as a clinically significant behavioral or psychological syndrome or pattern that may occur in a person and is associated with present distress and disability; loss of an important freedom; or an increased risk of suffering, death, pain, or disability. It cannot be assumed that each mental disorder is a discrete entity, with sharp boundaries separating it from other disorders. The classification includes all age groups and is not specific to older adults.

The *DSM-5* disorders of delirium, dementia, and other cognitive disorders are discussed under the heading of "Neurocognitive Disorders." These disorders are further subdivided based on cause:

Delirium

- Delirium resulting from a general medical condition
- Substance-induced delirium (because of a drug or drug or toxin exposure)
- Delirium resulting from multiple causes
- Delirium not otherwise specified (if the cause is indeterminate)

Dementia

- AD
- VaD

- Dementia resulting from other general medical conditions (e.g., HIV, head trauma, PD, and Huntington disease)
- Substance-induced persisting dementia (resulting from drug abuse, drugs, or toxin exposure)
- Dementia resulting from multiple causes
- Dementia not otherwise specified (if the cause is indeterminate)

Cognitive Disorder Not Otherwise Specified

- Does not meet criteria for other disorders

TREATMENT OF BEHAVIORAL AND PSYCHOLOGICAL SYMPTOMS OF DEMENTIA

Nonpharmacological Measures

Nonpharmacological measures are first line therapy in the treatment of behavioral and psychological symptoms of dementia (BPSD). Effective interventions focus on addressing the needs a person with dementia can no longer express. This approach can be guided by the Need-driven Dementia-compromised Behavior Model, developed by a group of nurses with the purpose of elevating the standard of care for persons with dementia. The model reframes the prevailing viewpoint of BPSD. Caregivers are directed to identify triggers (such as pain or the need for toileting) leading to BPSD, instead of extinguishing these behaviors with physical or chemical restraints, thus rendering person-centered, holistic care (Algase et al., 1996).

Dementia results in the loss of the ability to communicate needs. According to Algase et al. (1996), the expressed behavior is a result of background factors and proximal factors that, when combined, result in dementia-compromised behaviors. The Need-driven Dementia-compromised Behavior Model conceptualizes behavioral issues in nursing home residents as expressions of unmet needs. Understanding the interplay between disruptive behavior and unmet needs is paramount, as individuals with significant dementia are dependent on others to meet their needs (Fig. 24.7).

Individualized Care

When initially considering the use of drugs in the treatment of altered thought processes, health care providers must remember that individual responses to drugs vary considerably. All drugs require close monitoring by health care workers and family members for action and side effects. The recommendation for pharmacotherapy in the older adult is to "start low, go slow, and titrate upward until benefits or side effects are seen" (Zwicker & Fulmer, 2012). Patient and family education is essential when a new drug is started. Education helps create realistic expectations of the drug's benefits and potential side effects. Every patient may respond differently to drug management; therefore individualized care is essential.

Pharmacotherapy

Disease Management

Drug management of each of the disorders described has been listed previously. In summary, drug management of depression requires the use of antidepressant drugs. Drug management for the treatment of delirium may include the discontinuation of drugs contributing to the older person's recent mental status changes or the addition of drugs to treat underlying conditions. The advent of cholinesterase inhibitors has revolutionized the treatment of early AD, and cholinesterase inhibitors have shown some promise in the treatment of both VaD and DLB. These drugs work to slow disease progression and decrease agitated behaviors.

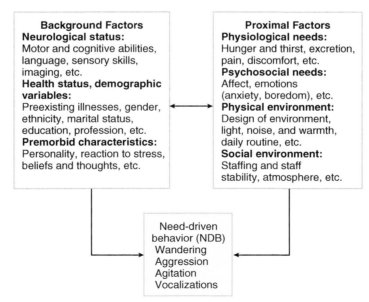

Fig. 24.7 Need-driven dementia-compromised behavior model. (Modified from Holle, D., Roes, M., Buscher, I., et al. [2014]. Process evaluation of the implementation of dementia-specific case conferences in nursing homes (FallDem): Study protocol for a randomized controlled trial. *Trials, 15*[1], 485.)

Antipsychotics

In 2012, CMS launched an initiative to reduce the off-label prescribing of antipsychotics in long-term care. At the time, CMS reported 14% of residents received antipsychotic drugs, and 83% of them were prescribed off label, many for reasons identified on boxed warnings NOT to administer them:

"Elderly patients with dementia-related psychosis treated with antipsychotic drugs are at an increased risk of death. Antipsychotics are not approved for the treatment of patients with dementia-related psychosis."

Guidelines suggest that some atypical antipsychotics can be considered but only if the resident behaviors result in "significant distress for the patient or poses a safety risk for the persons with dementia or those around them" (Kirkham et al., 2017, p. 170). Antipsychotics used in persons with dementia is associated with "increased risks of mortality, stroke, and more common side effects such as falls, sedation, and cognitive decline" (Kirkham et al., 2017, p. 170). Additionally, current evidence shows there is little benefit when prescribing antipsychotics for BPSD, and significant adverse effects. The American Psychological Association (APA) has drawn up guidelines for the appropriate use of antipsychotics in long-term care (see Box 24.3) (APA, 2016).

BOX 24.3   Guidelines for the Appropriate Prescribing of Antipsychotics in Persons With Dementia

- Nonemergency antipsychotic drug should only be used in patients with dementia when agitation and psychosis symptoms are severe, are dangerous, and/or cause significant distress to the patient.
- Response to nondrug interventions should be reviewed before use of antipsychotic drug.
- Before treatment with an antipsychotic, the potential risks and benefits should be assessed by the physician and discussed with the patient and the patient's surrogate decision maker, with input from the family.
- Treatment should be initiated at a low dose and eased up to the minimum effective dose.
- If the patient experiences significant side effects, the risks and benefits should be reviewed to determine whether the antipsychotic should be discontinued.
- If there is no significant response after a 4-week time period, the drug should be tapered and withdrawn.
- In patients who show adequate response to the drug, an attempt to taper and withdraw the antipsychotic should be made within 4 months of starting.
- In patients whose antipsychotic drugs are being tapered, symptoms should be assessed at least every month during tapering and for at least 4 months after the drug is discontinued.
- A long-acting injectable antipsychotic should not be used unless it is administered for a co-occurring chronic psychotic disorder.
- If nonemergency antipsychotic drug treatment is to be used, haloperidol should not be used first.

Reprinted with permission from American Psychiatric Association. (2016). APA releases new practice guidelines on the use of antipsychotics in patients with dementia [news release]. Retrieved from https://www.psychiatry.org/newsroom/news-releases/apa-releases-new-practice-guidelines-on-the-use-of-antipsychotics-in-patients-with-dementia.

NURSING MANAGEMENT

Nurses caring for older adults who have symptoms of an acute cognitive disorder need to support existing sensory perception until the cognitive state returns to the previous level of function. The goal of caring for older persons with dementia should be the maintenance of good health, gross and fine motor skills, and functional behaviors to maximize self-care abilities. The care provided to older adults with dementia is similar in the beginning stages, but it becomes complex and individually focused as the disease progresses. The philosophy of the care of older adults with cognitive and behavioral impairment has changed over the years. Public policy has shifted to encourage family members to care for older adults in their homes, thus decreasing health care costs and individualizing care to meet patient needs. The nurse's role has shifted from that of caregiver to one of care coordinator, that is, the nurse teaches and assists family members with home care, provides supportive care, and serves as a patient advocate.

Assessment

Performing a complete baseline physical examination, along with a neurologic examination and mental status assessment, is essential for ruling out an atypical presentation of a medical illness in an older adult. Deficits and impairments may be wrongly attributed to age or disease if accurate and complete baseline information is not available. Verbal and nonverbal responses from the patient, family members, and significant others should be used to validate assessment data. The assessment process is ongoing to ensure the accurate collection of information. The purpose of a comprehensive assessment is to determine problem areas, as well as areas of strength on which to base a care plan, including education of families and caregivers.

Assessment data gathered at the time of an acute crisis, as in a hospital setting, are critical for initial treatment. The special needs of an older adult with a cognitive disorder may require completing the assessment after treatment of the crisis to ensure discrete symptoms are not overlooked and treatment is appropriate for the disorder.

Assessment of Depression

Depression in older adults can be assessed with standardized rating scales or with a comprehensive nursing assessment that includes an evaluation of several key components of depression. Several instruments have been developed to screen older adults for depression, and other instruments provide a standardized approach to rating its severity. One of the most commonly used scales in assessing the presence or absence of depression in older adults is the Geriatric Depression Scale (GDS). Because the GDS minimizes the number of somatic depressive items, it is not necessary to upwardly adjust the cutoff score (Yesavage, 1983; Yohannes & Baldwin, 2008).

When the nursing assessment indicates the possibility of depression, the nurse may further assess the symptoms of depression previously mentioned. The comprehensive assessment includes obtaining health, nutritional, and drug histories; physical examination; mental status examination; family assessment; and assessment of performance of ADLs. Diagnostic tests that may be useful in ascertaining the presence of depression instead of another illness include certain laboratory tests (CBC, thyroid function studies, urinalysis, and dexamethasone suppression test), electrocardiography (ECG), EEG, MRI, and CT.

Level of Consciousness

Assessment of the level of consciousness provides an indication of the pathologic processes. *Consciousness* is defined as the state of awareness of the self and the environment. The most widely used and accepted tool for measuring consciousness is the Glasgow Coma Scale (GCS). The GCS measures eye opening, verbal response, and motor response. This may be the appropriate tool to use for assessment of an older person in a critical state, when the neurologic status is undetermined or rapidly changing.

Mental Status Examination

Mental status examinations for assessment of mental and cognitive function are necessary to identify impairments that may have significant and permanent effects. The choice of cognitive assessment tool varies, depending on the setting and results of the physical examination. An objective assessment may require more than obtaining orientation to person, place, and time, and should be considered before labeling a person "disoriented." It is important to thoroughly assess visual and hearing deficits and alter the environment to enhance the validity of the patient's response.

Pupil Assessment

Pupil assessment provides neurologic information and assists in the identification of the cause, responses, and location of the pathologic condition. Evaluation of an older adult's pupil size and reaction to light may be difficult because his or her pupils may appear smaller than normal, and the light reflex may be sluggish. Pupil response may also be altered by the presence of cataracts, retinal detachment, glaucoma, and sclerotic changes in the iris.

Neurologic Assessment

Neurologic disorders may cause a wide range of motor abnormalities. The extremities should be assessed for muscle strength and tone and compared for symmetry. Many older persons have normal age-related symmetric weakness and muscular fatigue. A decreased vibratory sense in the feet, a decreased Achilles tendon reflex, and decreased sensory perception may be caused by the normal loss of neurotransmitters or sensory receptors.

In the event of traumatic injury resulting in increased ICP, the classic symptoms of headache, vomiting, and papilledema may not appear in older persons or may be subtler because of normal, age-related changes caused by cerebral atrophy. These changes, including alterations in consciousness, cranial nerve deficits, and motor changes, may mimic cognitive disorders.

Behavioral Assessment

Persons with cognitive disorders commonly demonstrate problematic behaviors. These new behaviors should not be overlooked but should be viewed as symptoms requiring assessment. The type and intensity of the behavior vary, depending on the stage of disease, but each behavior exhibited requires a comprehensive, individualized assessment. Identifying the behavior

and extenuating circumstances assists in ruling out treatment causes and determining the personal meaning associated with the behavior.

Diagnosis

The selection of nursing diagnoses should be based on the assessment findings. The most commonly used nursing diagnoses for an older adult with cognitive impairment include the following:
- Reduced stamina resulting from physical illness
- Disrupted family routines resulting from cognitive impairment
- Inadequate nutrition resulting from poor oral intake
- Inadequate role performance resulting from cognitive impairment
- Anxiety resulting from misinterpretation of environmental cues
- Inadequate bathing self-care resulting from cognitive impairment
- Bowel incontinence resulting from cognitive decline and misinterpretation of physiologic needs
- Caregiver role tension resulting from older adult's cognitive decline and behavioral problems
- Confusion (acute or chronic) resulting from physiologic, emotional, or environmental processes
- Inadequate dressing self-care resulting from cognitive impairment
- Fatigue resulting from increased physical, emotional, and environmental demands
- Fear resulting from cognitive impairment
- Inadequate feeding self-care resulting from increased cognitive impairment
- Functional urinary incontinence resulting from inability to interpret physiologic and environmental cues
- Potential for injury resulting from altered ability to interpret the environment
- Decreased mobility resulting from neurologic deficits
- Reduced social interaction resulting from cognitive impairment
- Compromised family's ability to cope because of the needs of the older adult with cognitive impairment
- Disabling family's ability to cope resulting from lack of social supports
- Need for health teaching resulting from lack of previous exposure to disease process
- Decreased self-esteem resulting from awareness of cognitive deficits
- Spiritual tribulation resulting from the effect of cognitive impairment on individual and family

Planning and Expected Outcomes

Expected outcomes for older adults with cognitive changes are adapted for each diagnosis. Expected outcomes include the following:
1. The patient will exhibit no episodes of acute confusion, as evidenced by adequate hydration, nutrition, and socialization.
2. The patient will maintain continence using visual and verbal cues and regular fecal and urinary elimination routines.

3. The patient and family will demonstrate the ability to cope by accessing community agencies for support groups, Internet pages, and home health agencies for respite and support services.
4. The patient will exhibit reduced fear and anxiety by establishing a routine, keeping familiar objects, and participating individually in activities for calming down (e.g., listening to favorite music, sitting in the sun, and retreating to his or her room).
5. The patient will demonstrate fewer inappropriate behaviors such as agitation, combative behavior, and mood changes, as evidenced by identifying the triggers that cause them and decreasing or eliminating these triggers.
6. The patient will demonstrate increased socialization by voluntarily participating in activities.
7. The patient will maintain physical health.
8. Family members will participate in activities and care.
9. The spiritual health of the older adult and his or her family will be maintained, as evidenced by participation in religious services, communication with their religious organization, and participation in formal and informal spiritual practices.

Intervention

Each older adult will have a different presentation, triggers, and responses to illness; therefore the most effective interventions are based on the assessment and are individualized for each patient. When interventions are planned, it is important to consider environmental and cultural influences that affect the person's response patterns. Remaining attentive to needs as they are communicated, as well as to changes and responses in behavior, and using creativity in each situation may accomplish this. The best interventions are learned through trial and error, requiring commitment and communication with the family and the caregiver.

The efforts of health care personnel and caregivers will result in implementation of the best strategies for managing care of the patient with dementia. Identifying the stage of disease provides a baseline for management of care, but because each person's behavioral responses are based on an individual personal history and experiences, it requires persistence to determine approaches that result in desired responses. Positive responses to selected interventions may continue for a time but may decline as the disease progresses, which results in the need to reevaluate strategies. General principles of care should be individualized when caring for people with dementia.

Communication

Relaying trust, security, care, and support through simple and direct therapeutic verbal and nonverbal communication is essential when caring for older persons with dementia. In some situations, older persons are more inclined to respond to the nonverbal messages. The tone of communication should be calm and relaxed. Using eye contact and therapeutic touch when delivering a message helps the patient focus on meaning. It is important to use simple words and short sentences along with simple gestures to demonstrate meaning. At times, distraction as a form of communication may be necessary to dissuade a person with memory impairments from engaging in undesirable activities. Verbal communication may become less meaningful for the older person with altered thought processes resulting from memory loss, aphasia, apraxia, agnosia, and disorientation. Nevertheless, verbal communication on the part of the caregiver remains essential. Sounds and voices may elicit a response and provide a calming effect and an orientation to reality in these individuals.

Physical Interventions

Assessing the physical health and the ability of individuals with altered thought processes to meet their basic needs is the foundation of nursing care. Independence should be encouraged and self-esteem promoted by maintaining daily hygiene and grooming. Because a limited ability to verbally communicate may prevent an older adult from relaying a problem or symptom, nonverbal cues should be observed and considered indicative of a potential symptom requiring attention.

Nutritional Interventions

It is important to support the ongoing nutrition of individuals with dementia because they may experience decreased hunger and ability to taste food. Problems that occur during feeding may include patients' refusing to open the mouth, pocketing food in the cheeks, refusing to swallow, and coughing or choking while swallowing.

People who demonstrate symptoms of moderate to severe cognitive impairment may benefit from having meals in the same place at the same time each day. Small, frequent, nutritionally dense meals and snacks should be provided. It is important to assess the condition of the individual's teeth and ensure dentures fit well. During the later stages of dementia, the individual may need to be reminded to open the mouth and chew. Food should be soft and cut into small pieces. Thin liquids may become difficult to swallow, so serving gelatins, pudding, or ice cream may decrease problems with liquid intake. Coughing during meals is a sign of swallowing difficulties; referral to a speech therapist is recommended.

Cognitive Interventions

Reality orientation supports failing memory in early stages of dementia and preserves independent functioning for a longer duration. Although written messages and signs may become meaningless to individuals with advancing dementia, pictures often evoke a response. Persons in all stages of dementia benefit from the use of clocks, calendars, and mementos placed in their environment. As the disease progresses, daily orientation to caregivers and daily tasks improves the productivity and responses of older adults with altered thought processes.

Behavioral Interventions

Behaviors are a form of communication and may be the cognitively impaired patient's primary method of communicating needs; therefore recognizing behaviors may be the first step in ensuring that appropriate care is provided. Disruptive behaviors are a result of the disease, not deliberate actions on the part of the older person. The caregiver must realize that the patient cannot control the behaviors or be taught to change. The person displaying the symptoms may be unaware of their effect on others, whereas the family or other people involved may be more sensitive to the behaviors. It is important for care providers to learn what to expect as the older person's disease progresses. The effective management of problem behaviors should not focus on trying to change the older person but on modifying factors that may contribute to these behaviors. Careful and creative observation may identify the message in the behavior and provide opportunities for behavioral intervention (Smith, Russell, & White, 2013). Various behavior problems, possible antecedents, and strategies specific to these antecedents are listed in Table 24.3.

Because of the potential side effects of pharmacologic interventions, behavioral techniques should be the first line of treatment for older adults with altered thought processes. The use of physical or chemical restraints has demonstrated no benefit in controlling disruptive behaviors or managing disease. Unless the behaviors are upsetting or dangerous, learning how to adjust when these occur will probably result in a less stressful environment.

Social Interventions

Maintaining social interaction and human contact in a variety of ways is beneficial for older persons with cognitive decline. It provides the much-needed opportunity for participation in activities that prevent boredom and restlessness. The response from an older adult will be positive if he or she is provided the opportunity to experience success and contribute in a positive way.

TABLE 24.3	Behavioral Management Techniques	
Behavior	**Potential Causes or Antecedents**	**Management Strategies**
Wandering	Stress—noise, clutter, crowding	Reduce excessive stimulation.
	Lost—looking for someone or something familiar	Provide familiar objects, signs, pictures; offer to help find objects or place; reassure.
	Restless, bored—no stimuli	Provide meaningful activity.
	Drug side effect	Monitor, reduce, or discontinue drug.
	Lifelong pattern of being active or usual coping style	Respond to underlying mood or motivation; provide safe area to move about (e.g., secured circular path).
	Needing to use the toilet	Institute toileting schedule (such as every 2 hr); place signs or pictures on bathroom door.
	Environmental stimuli—exit signs, people leaving	Remove or camouflage environmental stimuli; provide identification or alarm bracelets.
Difficulty with personal care tasks	Task too difficult or overwhelming	Divide task into small, successive steps.
	Caregiver impatience, rushing	Be patient, allow ample time, or try again later.
	Cannot remember task	Demonstrate action or task; allow patient to perform parts of the task that can still be accomplished.
	Pain involved with movement	Treat underlying condition; consider pain medication or physiotherapy; modify or assist the movement needed.
	Cannot understand or follow caregiver instructions	Repeat request simply; state instructions one step at a time.
	Fear of task—cannot understand need for task or instructions	Reassure, comfort, distract from task with music or conversation; ask patient to help perform task.
	Inertia, apraxia; difficulty initiating and completing a task	Set up task sequence by arranging materials (such as clothing) in the order to be used; help begin the task.
Suspiciousness, paranoia	Forgot where objects were placed	Offer to help find; have more than one of same object available; have a list where objects should be placed; learn favorite hiding places.
	Misinterpreting actions or words	Do not argue or try to reason; do not take personally; distract.
	Misinterpreting who people are; suspicious of their intentions	Introduce self and role routinely; draw on old memory, connections; do not argue.
	Change in environment or routine	Reassure; familiarize; set routine.
	Misinterpreting environment	Assess vision, hearing; modify environment, as needed; explain misinterpretation simply; distract.
	Physical illness	Evaluate medically.
	Social isolation	Encourage and provide familiar social opportunities.
	Someone actually taking something from the patient	Verify the situation.
Agitation (also "sundowning," catastrophic reactions)	Discomfort, pain	Assess and manage sources of pain, constipation, infection, or full bladder; check clothing for comfort.
	Physical illness (such as urinary tract infection)	Evaluate medically; eliminate caffeine and alcohol.
	Fatigue	Schedule adequate rest; monitor activity.
	Overstimulation—noise, overhead paging, people, radio, television, activities	Reduce noise, stress; remove from situation: use television sparingly; limit crowding (e.g., dining hallways just before meals).
	Mirroring of caregiver's affect	

Continued

TABLE 24.3   Behavioral Management Techniques—cont'd

Behavior	Potential Causes or Antecedents	Management Strategies
		Control affect; model calm with low tone and slow rate; use support system and groups for outlet.
	Overextending capabilities (resulting in failure); caregiver expectations too high	Do not put in failure-oriented situations or tasks; understand losses and reduce expectations accordingly.
	Patient is being "quizzed" (multiple questions that exceed abilities)	Avoid persistent testing of memory; pose one question at a time; eliminate questions that require abstract thought, insight, or reasoning.
	Drug side effect	Assess, monitor, and reduce drug if possible; monitor health concerns.
	Patient is thwarted from desired activity (e.g., attempting to escape)	Redirect energy to similar activity; ask patient to help with meaningful activity; have diversionary tactics for outbursts; choose battles—assess whether behavior is merely irritating, rather than compromising patient safety or obstructing care.
	Lowered stress threshold	Simplify tasks, create calm; lower expectations and demands; avoid arguments and reprimands.
	Unfamiliar people or environment; change in schedule or routine	Be consistent; avoid changes, surprises; make change gradually.
	Restless	Plan calming music, massage, or meaningful activities; assign tasks that provide exercise.
Incontinence	Infection, prostate problem, chronic illness, drug side effect, stress or urge incontinence	Evaluate medically.
	Difficulty in finding bathroom	Place signs, picture on door; ensure adequate lighting.
	Lack of privacy	Provide for privacy.
	Difficulty undressing	Simplify clothing; use elastic waistbands.
	Difficulty in seeing toilet	Use contrasting colors on toilet and floor.
	Impaired mobility	Evaluate medically, treat associated pain (include physiotherapy); provide a commode; reduce diuretics when possible.
	Dependence created by socialized reinforcement	Provide increased attention for continence rather than incontinence; allow independence when possible, even if time-consuming.
	Cannot express need	Schedule toileting (such as every 2 hours while awake); reduce diuretics and bedtime liquids when possible.
	Task overwhelming	Simplify; establish step-by-step routine.
Sleep disturbance	Illness, pain, drug effect (e.g., causing daytime sleepiness or nocturnal awakening)	Evaluate medically.
	Depression	Prescribe antidepressant (consider bedtime sedative such as trazodone).
	Less need for sleep	Schedule later bedtime; allow activities or tasks safely done at night; plan more daytime exercise.
	Too hot, too cold	Adjust temperature.
	Disorientation from darkness	Use nightlights.
	Caffeine or alcohol effect	Reduce or eliminate alcohol; limit caffeine after noon.
	Hunger	Provide nighttime snack.
	Urge to void	Ensure clear, well-lit pathway to bathroom.
	Normal age- and disease-related fragmentation of sleep (like that of an infant or toddler)	Accept; plan for safety.
	Daytime sleeping	Eliminate or limit naps, provide activity and exercise instead; for naps, use recliner rather than bed.
	Fear of darkness; restless	Provide soft music, massage, nightlight.
Inappropriate or impulsive sexual behavior	Dementia-related decreased judgment and social awareness	Do not overreact or confront; respond calmly and firmly; distract and redirect.
	Misinterpreting caregivers' interaction	Do not give mixed sexual message (double entendres and innuendos—even in jest); avoid nonverbal messages; distract while performing personal care, bathing.
	Uncomfortable—too warm, clothing too tight; need to void; genital irritation	Check room temperature; assist with comfortable weather-appropriate clothing; ensure that elimination needs are met; examine for groin rash, perineal skin problems, stool impaction.
	Need for attention, affection, intimacy	Increase or meet basic need for touch and warmth; model appropriate touch; offer soothing objects (such as stuffed animals); provide hand or back massage.
	Self-stimulating, reacting to what feels good	Offer privacy; remove from inappropriate place.

From Carlson, D. L., Fleming, K. C., Smith, G. E., & Evans, J. M. (1995). Management of dementia-related behavioral disturbances: A nonpharmacologic approach. *Mayo Clinic Proceedings, 70,* 1108.

Family Interventions

Caregivers have been described as the "hidden victims" of severe dementia. It is important to provide social and emotional support to the family members caring for the individual with cognitive disorders. Day-to-day problems such as finances, legal obligations, household chores, self-care needs, troublesome behaviors, and interpersonal conflicts are just a few difficulties that must be managed by caregivers. Involving the family in care planning for a family member with dementia assists with adjustment and support.

Family members do not always understand role changes and expectations associated with caring for a loved one with a cognitive disorder. One of the most important issues faced is the loss of autonomy, not only for the older person but also for the caregiver. The encouragement and support of family members are critical to the motivation of an older person with the disability. Adjusting to the fact that dementia is irreversible and a prolonged problem places families in situations of dealing with grief over a long period. Nurses need to assist family members in understanding and accepting that each person deals with feelings differently. With this understanding, family members can serve as a strong support for the caregiver through the adjustment process.

In addition to patient assessment, the nurse must also assess the caregiver's physical health, functional status, drug regimen, nutritional status, and exercise patterns, although these may be assessed informally. The information obtained from this assessment may identify factors contributing to the caregiver's general well-being. Nurses need to encourage caregivers to take time out from their task and participate in self-care and health promotion activities. Referrals to social support groups such as dementia and AD support groups may also be beneficial for caregivers and family members.

Environmental Interventions

Individuals with dementia often have difficulty processing information, and the overloading of senses may cause confusion and anxiety. It is essential to consider the visual, auditory, olfactory, and tactile characteristics of the environment to make it more pleasant to the patient. Changes in the environment, routines, or setting may exacerbate negative behaviors in individuals with cognitive disorders. Mealtime, bath time, and activities should have a predictable pattern. Consistency is essential when the nurse identifies strategies for environmental modification. It is essential to create a feeling of security for the older adult with altered thought processes, but routines should not become so rigid that changes will not be accepted (Smith et al., 2013).

Certain routines such as sitting next to the same person during mealtime or having the same caregiver are comforting to the older adult. Changes in the routine should be introduced slowly, and a stimulus should be provided to ensure that feelings of comfort and security are not lost. Environmental modifications may be required to provide security and safety as the disease progresses. Examples of environmental modifications include decreasing stimuli by using soft colors and by limiting obstacles. Eliminating access to unsafe locations and unnecessary noises in the environment also may help with managing disruptive behaviors.

Safety and Self-Esteem Interventions

The impaired judgment, unpredictable behavior, and decreased cognitive ability in individuals diagnosed with dementia usually lead to job loss if they had been working, sometimes even before the diagnosis is made and they understand what is causing their problems. This will have a negative effect on financial status and self-esteem, and may psychologically inhibit the person from using preserved abilities. Self-esteem, independence, and autonomy are also affected when the individual with dementia must give up driving for reasons of safety. Wandering can sometimes be managed through environmental changes such as establishing fences or alarm systems and close supervision (Song & Algase, 2008).

Evaluation

Evaluation is a continual process when caring for individuals with altered thought processes related to cognitive decline. Behaviors and activities require ongoing assessment to determine variances from the baseline. Careful observation and recording of moods, behaviors, and memory provide clues to minor changes in the individual's condition. Interventions should be evaluated on an ongoing basis for efficacy. Successful and unsuccessful interventions should be communicated to other caregivers and family members to aid in the continuity of care.

CHALLENGES IN THE CARE OF OLDER ADULTS WITH COGNITIVE DISORDERS

Individuals with cognitive disorders react differently to those disorders. Because it is difficult to predict these reactions, nurses must be aware of the possible emotional, behavioral, and physical challenges they may face when caring for older persons with cognitive disorders. As a case manager and educator, the nurse also must teach family members and caregivers about potential challenges and introduce a variety of methods for facing these challenges.

Sundown Syndrome

Sundown syndrome is a commonly observed tendency in people with dementia to become more confused and agitated around late afternoon to nightfall. Sundown syndrome may resemble delirium. Along with depleted cognition, other symptoms such as reduced attention, altered sleeping and waking patterns, and disturbed psychomotor behavior are present, and these symptoms tend to be more evident in the evening. No specific cause for the occurrence of sundown syndrome has been established; however, some have hypothesized that sundowning may be the result of neurologic damage, which makes it impossible for the individual with dementia to clearly interpret environmental stimuli. Specific pathophysiologic findings that relate to sundown syndrome behaviors include disturbance in REM sleep, episodes of sleep apnea, and deterioration of the suprachiasmatic nucleus of the hypothalamus.

Sundown syndrome may also be modified through behavioral interventions, including redirection, the provision of companionship and empathy, environmental modifications in lighting, and noise reduction. Because the cause of sundowning may be different for each patient, individualized care is essential. The first step in the management of sundowning behavior includes the identification and treatment of any physiologic factors that may be contributing to those behaviors. These may include hunger, thirst, pain, and elimination needs. Nonpharmacologic management strategies for sundown syndrome include the following:

- Scheduling appointments and activities earlier in the day when the individual is rested
- Reducing environmental stimulation as the day progresses
- Providing activities that are calming in the evening, for example, playing soft music
- Increasing lighting levels: turning on room lights before dusk and providing a nightlight at bedtime
- Offering companionship and reassurance during the evening hours
- Providing 1-hour rest periods in either the late morning or the early afternoon

Drug management of these behaviors should be avoided unless the older person is a danger to self or others. If nonpharmacologic interventions are unsuccessful, low doses of specific neuroleptic agents may be indicated.

Wandering

Wandering behaviors have been described as one of the most challenging behaviors to manage in older persons with cognitive impairments. Wanderers might have experienced sleep problems, had a more active lifestyle in their younger years, and used more psychotropic drugs within their lifetime. They may wander in response to a need to use the bathroom or to combat boredom (Smith et al., 2013; Song & Algase, 2008).

Some nonpharmacologic interventions for wandering behaviors include the following:

- Ensuring an environment safe for wandering
- Informing neighbors and police of this potential problem
- Having the person wear a medical alert bracelet
- Observing potential wandering trigger behaviors
- Maintaining a regular activity and exercise program for individuals prone to wandering behavior

Paranoia or Suspiciousness

Paranoid or suspicious behaviors may reflect an individual's basic insecurity about his or her progressive memory and sensory losses. Individuals with dementia may forget where they placed certain items and then become suspicious of others and accuse them of stealing those items. Paranoia may result as a response to sensory deficits. As individuals observe others talking but are unable to hear what is being said, they may fear that others are talking about them and cling to or hoard objects, fearing they will be stolen. Nonpharmacologic interventions for suspicious or paranoid behavior include the following:

- Securing valuables in locked locations
- Avoiding the use of confrontation and the application of logic
- Looking in wastebaskets before emptying
- Not whispering or behaving in a secretive manner
- Marking all personal items with that individual's name

Hallucinations and Delusions

Hallucinations experienced by individuals with dementia are most often visual but may be auditory. Medical causes of hallucinations should be evaluated because issues such as overmedication, toxicity, fever, infection, or a combination of causes may trigger this response. If the hallucination is disturbing to the older person, offering protection and security may help calm him or her. Reasoning or logic is ineffective. Delusions occur when an individual believes something to be true when it is illogical or wrong. Depending on the stage of the disease, orientation to reality may be appropriate. If the disease has progressed, it may be best to go along with the individual's reality but attempt to change disturbing behaviors in relation to the situation. Behavior modification is the treatment of choice in the management of both hallucinations and delusions; however, if these symptoms place an individual at risk, a short course of an antipsychotic drug may be necessary.

Catastrophic Reactions

Catastrophic reactions are emotional outbursts or exaggerated reactions to minor stresses. These may be precipitated by emotional and sensory overload and aggravated by fatigue, overstimulation, inability to meet expectations, or misinterpretation of actions or words. Signs of impending reaction might include restlessness or refusals to carry out tasks. Nurses and caregivers must assess the environment for potential triggers and remove these triggers. Nonpharmacologic interventions useful in dealing with catastrophic reactions include the following:

- Removing the individual from the environment in which the reaction is occurring
- Providing a calming atmosphere to distract the individual
- Using a calm tone of voice, touch, and reassurance
- Temporarily separating the individual from the causative source

Resources

Physical and mental strain placed on caregivers can be significantly reduced if available resources are identified and used. Community resources become increasingly important as the primary caregiver grows more isolated and overextended. The nurse should identify appropriate community resources available to the patient and family and encourage family members to participate as the need becomes critical. These resources may include community mental health centers, adult day care centers, respite services, local Alzheimer's Associations and support groups, medical information and referral programs, and other family support groups specific to the disease type.

Family Support Groups

A significant increase in family support groups has created a network to help families faced with caring for a loved one with dementia. These support groups offer a variety of services ranging from assisting family members in coping with the inevitable losses faced by patients with dementia to emotional support and respite.

Respite Services

Respite service is provided to family members requiring occasional relief from the pressures of continuous caregiving. These services may prevent premature institutionalization of individuals with dementia because of caregiver stress. Respite programs offer relief services ranging from several hours to several weeks. Shared respite care is a form of respite care available in some communities, where several families join together to provide care on a rotating basis. In this setting, group members watch over several patients, which allows free time for other caregivers. Caring for loved ones in the company of others may reduce the social isolation experienced by caregivers.

Adult Day Care

Adult day care centers help keep people with dementia in the community by providing family respite, promoting activity, and encouraging the retention of previously learned skills. Some centers provide specialized social work, nursing, or physical and occupational therapy services. Adult day care centers allow family members to work during the day, do errands, rest, and yet be involved in important areas of their loved ones' lives.

Home Health Care

Home health care may provide nursing, physical and occupational therapies, services of social workers, and personal care services to patients in their homes in the later stages of dementia. Home health personnel may help with direct care needs, including meals and shopping, drugs, cleaning, laundry, transportation, appraisal of a person's condition, and companionship. However, unless the individual has an established need for skilled nursing or therapy, Medicare does not cover these services.

Legal Services

Legal services are necessary when family members must consider questions related to the person's ability to handle finances and make decisions. It is important to set up a durable power of attorney for financial matters and a health care proxy for medical matters early in the disease process while the individual can still participate in decision making. Legal guardianship is granted when the individual is no longer capable of making decisions for himself or herself. This requires that a physician or mental health professional document that the patient does not understand the ramifications of decisions or behaviors.

Community Mental Health Centers

Community mental health centers may have specialized geriatric programs, which provide a wide range of services. These services may include comprehensive assessment; psychiatric evaluations; and individual, group, and family counseling. In addition, case management services available in community mental health centers may assist in the identification of other community resources to maintain individuals in the home.

Psychiatric Hospitals

Psychiatric hospitals offer assessment and behavior stabilization. In addition, an increasing number of geriatric psychiatric units can meet the multidimensional physiologic and mental health needs of older adults with cognitive disorders. Psychiatric hospital placement usually occurs when an individual cannot be managed in the community setting, and more advanced assessment and behavior management techniques are required. Outcomes of geriatric psychiatric hospital placement may include drug management and behavior modification therapies for the individual's return to the community or may result in placement in long-term care facilities.

OTHER COMMON PROBLEMS AND CONDITIONS

Suicide

One of the leading causes of suicide among older adults is depression, often undiagnosed and untreated. The act of suicide is rarely preceded by only one cause or one reason. In older adults, common risk factors include the following:

- Recent death of a loved one
- Physical illness, uncontrollable pain, or fear of a prolonged illness
- Perceived poor health
- Social isolation and loneliness
- Major changes in social roles (e.g., retirement)

American society continues to ignore the problem of suicide in older adults. Older adults are less likely to communicate their intent to commit suicide; as a result, many health care professionals have assumed erroneously that suicide is not a significant issue among older adults. Some older adults attempt suicide to retain control by deciding on the appropriate time to die. Such acts are sometimes called *benign suicides* or *rational suicides.* These terms refer to suicides planned by individuals because they perceive their life to have no value. These types of suicide pose an ethical dilemma for nurses with regard to patient autonomy versus the value of life and often also pose a legal issue, as evidenced by the recent publicity resulting from reexamination of laws in several states. Despite the inherent uncertainty in these cases, nursing scholars have supported a nursing perspective that affirms life by enhancing the individual's quality of life rather than assuring them of their right to die (Baldessarini, 2003; Fontaine, 2008; Montross, Mohamed, Kasckow et al., 2003; Vance, Moneyham, & Farr, 2008).

Another issue that nurses deal with in caring for older adults is *passive suicide* or *subintentioned suicide.* It is a passive attempt to hasten one's death. This type of self-destructive behavior often goes unrecognized and may include nonadherence with the health care regimen (e.g., refusing safe and appropriate use of a needed drug), behaviors that harm the individual in a more active manner (e.g., continued smoking, alcohol abuse, or an eating disorder), and participating in dangerous situations (e.g., reckless driving).

Risk Factors

The risk factors for suicide in older adults are presented in Box 24.4. Evidence suggests that Protestant white men living alone in their homes are at the highest risk for suicide. They often display a neat appearance and calm behavior, and take either antianxiety or antipsychotic drugs. Many of the steps

BOX 24.4   Risk Factors for Suicide in Older Adults

- Depression
- Prior suicide attempts
- Marked feelings of hopelessness; lack of interest in future plans
- Feelings of loss of independence or sense of purpose
- Medical conditions that significantly limit functioning or life expectancy
- Impulsivity due to cognitive impairment
- Social isolation
- Family discord or losses (i.e., recent death of a loved one)
- Inflexible personality or marked difficulty adapting to change
- Access to lethal means (i.e., firearms, other weapons, etc.)
- Daring or risk-taking behavior
- Sudden personality changes
- Alcohol or drug misuse or abuse
- Verbal suicide threats such as, "You'd be better off without me" or "Maybe I won't be around"
- Giving away prized possessions

From Mental Health America in collaboration with the National Council on Aging (2015). Mental health in older adults. Retrieved from http://www.mentalhealthamerica.net/preventing-suicide-older-adults.

outlined in the nursing process of older adults with depression are also appropriate for older adults at risk for suicide.

The following steps are more specific to patients who are suicidal.

NURSING MANAGEMENT

Assessment

In assessing patients at risk for suicide, it is helpful to have on hand a series of interview questions (Box 24.5). Although not all questions are needed or appropriate for all patients, it is helpful to have a progressive series of assessment items in mind that can be adapted to the situation. The basic components of suicide risk assessment include evaluating suicidal ideation (thoughts), any prior attempts, a patient's suicide plan, the plan's lethality, the availability of the implements of the plan, coexisting substance abuse, and the pervasiveness of the despair the patient is experiencing.

BOX 24.5   Questions for Assessing the Risk for Suicide

- What has been the most difficult moment for you in the recent past?
- Have things been so bad that you have thought about escaping? If so, how?
- Are there times when death seems like an attractive option to you?
- Have you thought of harming yourself?
- Have you thought about killing yourself?
- If you were to harm yourself, how would you do it?
- Do you have access to the items you would need to carry out your plan (e.g., gun, quantities of drug, rope, enclosed garage)?
- Have you thought about harming yourself or attempted to harm yourself in the past?
- What has kept you from harming yourself thus far?
- What might keep you from harming yourself in the future?

Diagnosis

Nursing diagnoses for older adults at risk for suicide include the following:
- Decreased ability to cope resulting from multiple perceived losses
- Complex grieving resulting from multiple perceived losses
- Hopelessness resulting from deteriorating health
- Potential for self-directed violence resulting from perceived loss of control
- Spiritual tribulation resulting from hopelessness

Planning and Expected Outcomes

Planning care for an older adult patient who is suicidal requires a strong interpersonal connection with the patient. Expected outcomes include the following:
1. The patient identifies and verbalizes thoughts and feelings related to his or her emotional state.
2. The patient reports absence of suicidal ideation.
3. The patient demonstrates effective coping skills for managing stress and frustration, as evidenced by reported use of two coping strategies.
4. The patient experiences behavior control with assistance of others, as evidenced by absence of suicidal ideation.
5. The patient expresses satisfaction with spiritual well-being, as evidenced by verbalization of positive statements about self and life, including a sense of purpose in life.

Intervention

When risk of suicide is identified in an older adult patient, appropriate safety measures must be taken. These safety measures may be tailored on the basis of the patient's suicide plans, the setting in which the nurse is intervening (e.g., the patient's home, an inpatient setting), and the extent of human connection the patient has. It may be necessary for the nurse to arrange with the local mental health authorities for inpatient hospitalization (voluntary or involuntary) if patient safety cannot be ensured in an outpatient setting. The patient's significant other can often help in developing a plan for safety. It is essential for nurses to remember that no extent of environmental precautions can take the place of a strong interpersonal connection with the patient. Suicidal patients may be creative and adaptive in finding alternative methods of suicide. Without a strong therapeutic relationship to assist the patient, the nurse's best efforts to keep him or her safe may prove fruitless.

Asking patients about their suicidal thoughts does not plant the idea in their minds. If the nurse has reason to believe a patient may be suicidal, it is quite likely that he or she has already considered this option. A useful tool in working with individuals who are suicidal is a "no-suicide contract." This is an agreement (ideally written and signed) between the patient and the health care provider that the patient will not harm himself or herself. The specific wording of the agreement may differ, depending on the patient's risk factors and the setting in which the care is being provided. For example, on an inpatient unit, an agreement might state, "I commit that I will not harm myself while in the hospital, and if I have thoughts of harming myself, I will immediately inform a staff member."

Once a patient is past the immediate danger of suicidal behavior, the next step is to help him or her develop suicide prevention plans. Such plans may include alternatives other than suicide and may also include specific steps that the patient can take if he or she again experiences suicidal thoughts. These plans encourage patients to take a problem-solving (active) approach in dealing with the potential for self-harm; therefore their planning increases their sense of control. Nurses can play a significant role in the prevention of suicide among older adults. Essential components in such preventive intervention include assessing all older adults for potential self-harm issues, proactively identifying and treating depression in older adults, developing community programs focused on prevention of suicide among older adults, and informing health care professionals who work with older adults in different settings about the risk for suicide.

Evaluation

Unfortunately, despite excellent nursing assessment and intervention, older adults do continue to commit suicide at a distressingly high rate. When an older adult has committed suicide, the nurse's focus may be to assist the family and friends in coping with the resulting grief and trauma. A psychological autopsy, or the processing of events and behaviors surrounding the patient's suicide, may be useful to both the health care professionals and the patient's family and friends. Family and friends may also be encouraged to obtain assistance from support groups.

Parkinson's Disease

PD is the most common form of parkinsonism (parkinsonian syndrome). PD is a common, progressive degenerative disorder of the basal ganglia involving the dopaminergic nigrostriatal pathway (Duffy, 2010). PD is characterized by slowing in the initiation and execution of movement (bradykinesia), increased muscle tone (rigidity), tremors at rest, and impaired postural reflexes (Duffy, 2010).

Approximately 50,000 people per year are diagnosed with PD, and it affects 50% more men than women. The risk of PD increases with age, and the peak onset is in the sixth decade. Of those with PD, 5% to 50% have early onset, before age 50. In rare cases, parkinsonian symptoms occur before age 20. Although some cases have a hereditary component and others may be traced to gene mutations, most are of a sporadic nature. In fact, most researchers believe that most cases of PD result from a genetic susceptibility and that environmental factors may trigger the disease (Buter, van den Hout, Matthews, Larsen et al., 2008; NINDS, 2013).

Motor activity occurs as a result of the integrated actions originating from the cerebral cortex, basal ganglia, and cerebellum. The main area in the brain affected by PD is the basal ganglia. The basal ganglia are a group of neurons located deep within the cerebrum near the lateral ventricles. The basal ganglia control both muscle tone and the process of voluntary movement. This is accomplished through the secretion of the excitatory neurotransmitter acetylcholine (ACh) and the inhibitory neurotransmitter dopamine. Dopamine is a neurotransmitter produced in the substantia nigra and in the adrenal glands. It is then transmitted to the basal ganglia, when needed. ACh is produced in the basal ganglia and transmits excitatory messages throughout this area. Dopamine inhibits the function of ACh in the basal ganglia to control fine and voluntary movements. Therefore it is the dopamine–ACh balance that produces normal motor function (Fig. 24.8).

In PD, degeneration of the dopaminergic nigrostriatal pathway causes dopamine depletion in the basal ganglia, while the

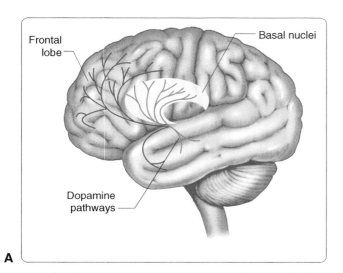

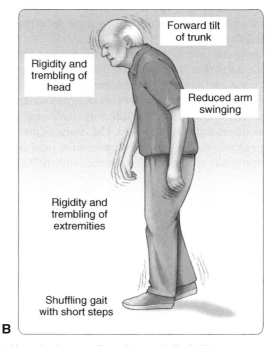

Fig. 24.8 A, Dopaminergic pathways of the brain. **B,** Signs of Parkinson's disease. (From Patton, K. T., & Thibodeau, G. A. [2010]. *Anatomy & physiology* [7th ed.]. St. Louis, MO: Mosby.)

ACh-secreting neurons remain active. This creates an imbalance between excitatory and inhibitory neural activity in neurotransmitters and is the cause of symptoms such as hypertonia (tremors and rigidity) and akinesia in PD.

Risk Factors

PD is an idiopathic syndrome. An autosomal-dominant form of parkinsonian syndrome is associated with a genetic defect of chromosome 4. Environmental factors contributing to PD include postencephalitic parkinsonism, drug-induced or toxin-induced parkinsonian syndrome, exposure to agriculture pesticides and herbicides, and trauma to the midbrain. Other related causes include hydrocephalus, hypoxia, infections, stroke, tumor, and traumas (Duffy, 2010).

Clinical Manifestations

Signs and symptoms begin subtly and include manifestations such as fatigue and a slight resting tremor. These may be the only initial symptoms. In a small portion of individuals, dementia may be the presenting symptom. The classic manifestations of PD are tremors at rest, muscle rigidity, bradykinesia, and postural abnormalities.

Balance in PD is affected by postural changes. Individuals with PD may have difficulty getting out of a chair, walking backward, or maneuvering in tight spaces. Fear of falling is a common complaint. Gait changes are caused by postural changes and a decrease in autonomic balancing reflexes. Common problems with postural and gait changes include festinating gait, freezing, propulsive gait, and retropulsion (Box 24.6).

Muscle rigidity also affects the eyes, mouth, and voice and contributes to the staring gaze. These manifestations may develop alone or in combination. As the disorder progresses, more manifestations become apparent, including uncoordinated movements; short-stepped, shuffling, and propulsive gait, which leads to increased risk of falls; postural disturbance; and trunk tilting forward.

Autonomic–neuroendocrine symptoms become noticeable and include seborrhea and excessive perspiration in the face and neck areas and absence of perspiration on the trunk and extremities. Heat intolerance, constipation, anxiety, depression, sleep disturbances, and dysphagia (difficulty swallowing) are also neuroendocrine manifestations of PD. The course of the disorder is slowly progressive. The person becomes more rigid and more disabled, eventually requiring full assistance with ADLs.

BOX 24.6   Postural and Gait Terms for Parkinson's Disease

- **Festinating gait:** occurs when the individual can only take small short steps
- **Freezing:** a phenomenon in which the individual appears to be glued to the floor, unable to move
- **Propulsive gait:** occurs when an individual begins walking, then starts running forward, unable to stop until he or she falls or runs into something
- **Retropulsion:** like propulsive gait, but the individual is walking and falling backward instead of forward

---

Diagnostic Studies

No specific studies can be used to diagnose PD. The diagnosis is based primarily on the clinical features of the disorder. Some of the diagnostic and laboratory studies used to assist in the identification of PD include CBC, which may reveal anemia. Blood chemistry profile may show low albumin and protein levels. Drug screens may be done to rule out toxic causes of the symptoms. EEG may reveal a slow pattern and disorganization of electrical activity in the brain. Upper gastrointestinal series may show delayed emptying, distention, and megacolon. Video fluoroscopy may demonstrate a slowed response of the cricopharyngeal muscles when swallowing. A diagnosis of PD is confirmed when the individual's symptoms improve with antiparkinsonian drugs (Duffy, 2010).

Management

Treatment is aimed at relieving clinical manifestations, increasing the individual's ability to perform ADLs, and decreasing the risk for injury. This is accomplished through the use of drugs, surgery, and rehabilitation aimed at optimizing the patient's functional level. A team approach is essential for high-quality care of PD patients.

Drugs

Drugs are used primarily to relieve the symptoms associated with PD. Drugs used include monoamine oxidase inhibitors (MAOIs), which are used as adjunct therapy; dopaminergics, used to provide dopamine to the basal ganglia; dopamine agonists, used to activate dopamine in the CNS; and anticholinergics, used to block the release of ACh. A new class of drug called catechol-O-methyltransferase inhibitors may be given with dopaminergics to increase the availability of dopamine in the brain (Black et al., 2005). Table 24.4 lists drugs used to treat PD. Unfortunately, the effectiveness of these drugs decreases eventually. The fluctuating response of individuals to antiparkinsonian drugs is called the *on–off response*. Antidepressants, especially amitriptyline, are used to treat depression often associated with PD. Propranolol may be used to treat tremors.

Surgical Therapy

Surgical procedures to alleviate symptoms of PD are used in patients who have not responded to drug therapy. The surgical procedures fall into three categories: (1) ablation (destruction), (2) deep brain stimulation (DBS), and (3) transplantation. Ablation and DBS work by reducing the increased neural activity produced by dopamine depletion. Transplantation of fetal neural tissue is designed to provide dopamine-producing cells in the brains of individuals with PD. This procedure is still in its experimental phase (Duffy, 2010).

NURSING MANAGEMENT

Diagnosis

Priority nursing diagnoses for a patient with PD include the following:
- Decreased mobility
- Inadequate communication

TABLE 24.4 Drugs Used to Treat Parkinson's Disease

Drug Classification and Example	Action	Indications	Common Side Effects	Nursing Implications
Anticholinergics Trihexyphenidyl Benztropine	Inhibit action of endogenous acetylcholine and muscarine agonists to block the excitatory effect of the cholinergic system	Tremors, rigidity, drooling	Dry mouth, constipation, blurred vision, confusion, hallucinations	Usually contraindicated in patients with acute-angle glaucoma and tachycardia; monitor pulse and blood pressure during periods of dosage adjustment; administer with meals; do not withdraw drug suddenly.
Dopaminergics Amantadine Carbidopa-levodopa	Cause release of dopamine in central nervous system	Rigidity, bradykinesia Tremors, rigidity, bradykinesia	Dizziness, ataxia, insomnia, leg edema Orthostatic hypotension, nausea, hallucinations, dystonia, dyskinesia	Monitor patient for postural hypotension; do not administer at bedtime. Monitor blood pressure; use elastic stockings to increase venous return; monitor patient for urinary retention.
Dopamine Agonists Bromocriptine Pergolide	Activate dopamine receptors in the central nervous system	Fluctuation of manifestations, dyskinesia, dystonia	Hallucinations, mental fogginess, orthostatic hypotension, confusion Orthostatic hypotension, nausea, insomnia	Monitor blood pressure and mental status. Monitor blood pressure; do not administer at bedtime.
COMT Tolcapone, entacapone	Enhances effect of dopamine	Adjuvant treatment	Diarrhea, elevated liver enzymes Nausea, headache	Monitor liver enzymes. Monitor for levodopa side effects.
MAOIs Selegiline*	Inhibit monoamine oxidase B, an enzyme that converts chemical by products in the brain into neurotoxins that prevent substantia nigra cell death	Adjuvant treatment	Nausea, dizziness, confusion, hallucinations, dry mouth	Monitor for levodopa side effects, as selegiline may increase effect of levodopa.

*One study showed that levodopa in combination with selegiline provided no clinical benefit over levodopa alone in treating early, mild Parkinson's disease. Moreover, the mortality rate was significantly higher when these two drugs were used together.
American Parkinson Disease Association. (2018). Medications for Parkinson's. Retrieved June 12, 2018 from https://www.apdaparkinson.org/what-is-parkinsons/treatment-medication/medication/; and, Burchum, J.R., & Rosenthal, L.D. (2019). *Lehne's pharmacology for nursing care*. St. Louis, MO: Elsevier.

- Inadequate nutrition
- Potential for injury

Planning and Expected Outcomes

Expected outcomes for a patient with PD include the following:
1. The patient will maintain an effective communication pattern.
2. The patient will maintain physical functioning and mobility and will not sustain injury.
3. The patient will maintain effective coping by demonstrating the use of coping strategies that enhance individual and family functioning.
4. The patient will maintain socialization by participation in activities.
5. The patient will verbalize satisfactory effects from drugs and safely manage the drug schedule.

The care planning and expected outcomes for a patient with PD frequently need revision because of changes in the patient's status.

Intervention

Nursing care includes teaching patients the importance of performing active range-of-motion exercises twice a day, walking at least four times a day, and using an assistive device when recommended to prevent injury associated with falls. Because PD leads to rigidity of the facial muscles, mouth, and general functioning of individuals, assessment of communication skills, speech, and writing is needed.

Consultation with a speech pathologist may be necessary if the patient develops dysphagia. Assessment of nutritional status and self-feeding abilities is crucial for preventing aspiration, respiratory complication, and nutritional imbalance. Nurses are also responsible for monitoring the intake of foods high in bulk and fluids.

Patient education includes the following:

- Teaching preventive measures for malnutrition, falls and other environmental hazards, constipation, skin breakdown from incontinence, and joint contractures
- Teaching gait training and exercises for improving ambulation, swallowing, speech, and self-care

Referral to community agencies and resources is also helpful. Some of the resources specifically available to individuals and families affected by PD include the American Parkinson Association. Recommendations of appropriate Internet sites for further information is also helpful. The nurse should encourage families and patients to communicate with their primary care provider when they have questions about PD and encourage them to keep a diary to track the symptoms, as well as the effects and side effects of drugs.

Evaluation

PD is a progressive terminal disease that has no cure. Therefore the evaluation of nursing interventions should focus on maintenance of function and engagement in activities for as long as possible. Evaluation is based on documentation of achievement of expected outcomes, as evidenced by an older adult patient exhibiting intact skin, appropriate body weight, effective communication, effective coping, and knowledge of appropriate self-care practices. Participation of family members in continued care and rehabilitation is also noted. Specific problems are documented, as is any teaching.

Cerebrovascular Accident

A disruption in the normal blood supply to the brain tissue causes a CVA (stroke or brain attack). CVAs occur suddenly and produce focal neurologic deficits lasting more than 24 hours. They are medical emergencies that should be treated immediately to prevent permanent neurologic deficits and disability. A TIA consists of the same symptoms but lasts less than 24 hours. However, about a third of those experiencing a TIA will suffer a CVA in the future.

The warning signs of a stroke are sudden numbness of face, arm, or leg, especially on one side of the body; sudden confusion; trouble speaking or understanding; sudden trouble seeing in one or both eyes; sudden trouble walking or dizziness; loss of coordination or balance; or sudden severe headache with no known cause (CDC, 2013; NINDS, 2013). Recurrence of stroke is unfortunately frequent; approximately 25% will have a recurrence within 5 years (NINDS, 2013).

Strokes are the fourth leading cause of death and the most common cause of disability in the United States; each year, they kill nearly 130,000 of the almost 800,000 who have one (American Stroke Association [ASA], 2013). The CDC reports that 60% to 75% of strokes occur in individuals older than age 65, and the risk doubles each decade after age 55. However, in 2009, 34% of those hospitalized for a stroke were under age 65 (CDC, 2013).

Approximately 30% to 50% of those who survive a CVA are left with moderate to severe disability. Blacks are more likely than whites to have a stroke, perhaps because this population has a higher incidence of hypertension and diabetes. The risk of having a stroke in their lifetime is higher among women than among men (1:5 to 1:6) (WHO, 2012). The incidence rate of stroke for Hispanic Americans is somewhere between those for African Americans and whites. American Indians and Alaska Natives are more likely to have strokes compared with other ethnic groups (not listed). Of all the groups, African Americans are more likely to die following a stroke (CDC, 2013).

In 1996, a national campaign was initiated to increase public awareness of CVA (Black et al., 2005). The NINDS conducted a study (published in 1996) that revolutionized the way we approach and treat acute ischemic stroke (AIS). The major change was the use of thrombolytic agents (recombinant tissue plasminogen activators [r-TPA]) within a 3-hour window of the onset of signs or symptoms of AIS. Findings from this study demonstrating decreased mortality and morbidity rates ignited the campaign to make the public aware of the common signs and symptoms associated with "brain attack" and to activate the emergency system for prompt diagnosis and early treatment of stroke (NINDS, 2013). Since 2004, the MERCI Retrieval System has been used for those patients beyond the 3-hour window for IV-tPA or with a response failure. It is a corkscrew-shaped device that wraps itself around the clot, which then can be removed. Approved by the Food adn Drug Administration in 2008, the Penumbra system, which uses suction to grab clots, has been used successfully as well (Fanous & Siddiqui, 2016). The NINDS continues to research and investigate new therapies to aid in the treatment and even removal of clots caused by hemorrhagic CVAs (NINDS, 2013).

Cerebral infarctions are ischemic or hemorrhagic in origin. The brain is very sensitive to any decrease in blood supply. As a result, when cerebral blood flow is reduced to a level insufficient to maintain neuronal viability, it causes a state of hypoxia. This hypoxic state leads to tissue ischemia and injury. Short-term ischemias result in TIAs. Long-term ischemia leads to permanent infarction (death of cerebral cells). Cellular events that ensue because of the ischemia alter the cell membrane. As a result, the polarization of the cell membrane changes, allowing an influx of calcium into the cell and altering cellular metabolism. Glutamate is then released, altering the cell's permeability to electrolytes. Electrolytes change the metabolic rate of the cell, leading to cellular acidosis, lactic acid production, vasodilation, and cellular hypoxia. Sustained anoxic events lead to infarct of brain tissue and irreversible neuronal injury. If an infarct occurs, the affected brain softens and liquefies.

The extent of brain infarction depends on factors such as location and size of an occluded vessel and the adequacy of the collateral circulation to the area supplied by the occluded vessel. Cell death and permanent changes may occur within 3 to 10 minutes of anoxia. The most common vessels for ischemic stroke are the middle cerebral artery and the vertebrobasilar artery. A mean arterial pressure of 50 mm Hg or less may affect brain perfusion (NINDS, 2013).

Symptoms of thrombotic stroke may be sudden but typically progress gradually over minutes to hours. The development of thrombotic strokes causes a syndrome known as *stroke-in-evolution*. The completed stroke is a CVA that has caused maximum damage with regard to neurologic deficits.

Risk Factors

The risk factors for CVAs, both genetic and lifestyle, are many. A genetic factor includes the sickle cell disease. The NINDS continues to research both the genome and biomarkers for those indicators that predispose persons to strokes over their lifetime. Lifestyle factors are high blood pressure, diabetes, cigarette smoking, and heart disease caused by atherosclerosis, obesity, and physical inactivity. Another risk factor is atrial fibrillation (NINDS, 2013).

CVAs are caused by two major pathologic events: ischemic stroke and hemorrhagic stroke. An ischemic stroke is further categorized as thrombotic, cardioembolic, and lacunar strokes. The most common cause for ischemic strokes are atherosclerosis, inflammatory disease processes, and a thrombus breaking away outside the brain or in the cardiovascular system. Hemorrhagic strokes are divided into subarachnoid and intracerebral hemorrhages, according to the site of the hemorrhage. The most common causes for hemorrhagic strokes are hypertension, a ruptured aneurysm, vascular malformations, bleeding into a tumor, hemorrhages associated with bleeding disorders or anticoagulation, head trauma, and illicit drug use (Duffy, 2010).

The incidence of deaths from stroke has gradually declined in many industrialized countries over the past 20 years. The aggressive campaign started by the NINDS in 1996 to educate the general population about the risk factors and forms of prevention has played a pivotal role in decreasing the mortality rate.

Both nonmodifiable and modifiable risk factors are associated with CVA. The nonmodifiable risk factors for CVA include gender, age, race, and heredity. Although changes cannot be made in these areas, awareness of the association of stroke could increase patients' involvement in the process of secondary prevention. Advanced age is one of the most significant risk factors for stroke. Modifiable risk factors include hypertension, diabetes mellitus, cardiovascular disease, nonvalvular atrial fibrillation, blood lipid abnormalities, smoking, substance abuse (particularly cocaine), obesity, a sedentary lifestyle, high stress levels, previous CVA or TIA, heavy alcohol use, and sudden discontinuation of antihypertensive drugs (causes hemorrhagic stroke). Modifiable risk factors may be reduced or eliminated through lifestyle changes. Hypertension is the most important modifiable risk factor for both ischemic and hemorrhagic strokes. Table 24.5 summarizes the levels of prevention for stroke.

Clinical Manifestations

Specific clinical manifestations of a TIA vary, depending on the vessel involved, the degree of obstruction of the vessel, and collateral blood supply. If the carotid system is involved, the individual may experience blurred vision, gradual visual obstruction, flashes of light, and headaches. If the posterior system is involved, symptoms may include tinnitus, vertigo (dizziness), bilateral sensory and motor symptoms, diplopia, facial weakness, and ataxia.

TABLE 24.5 Levels of Prevention for Stroke

Level	Preventive Steps
Primary prevention	Maintain ideal body weight. Manage cholesterol levels. Stop smoking. Reduce alcohol consumption. Eliminate illicit drugs.
Secondary prevention	Tightly manage blood pressure. Effectively manage diabetes mellitus. Promptly treat cardiovascular disease, transient ischemic attack, and atrial fibrillation.
Tertiary prevention	Initiate rehabilitation program early.

Early warning signs for thrombotic stroke include transient hemiparesis, loss of speech, and paresthesias (abnormal sensations) involving one side of the body and lasting a few minutes to less than 24 hours. These are considered TIAs. Common signs and symptoms that may precede cerebral hemorrhage in patients with hypertension include severe occipital or nuchal (back of the neck) headache, vertigo or syncope (fainting), paresthesias, transient paralysis, epistaxis (nose bleed), and retinal hemorrhages.

Common findings seen with strokes include headaches, vomiting, seizures, mental status changes (including coma), fevers, and ECG changes (e.g., T-wave changes, shortened P–R interval, prolonged Q–T interval, premature ventricular contractions, sinus bradycardia, ventricular tachycardia, and supraventricular tachycardia).

Clinical manifestations vary according to the cerebral vessel involved:

- **Internal carotid:** contralateral motor and sensory deficits of the arm, leg, and face. In dominant hemispheric CVA, aphasia occurs. In nondominant hemispheric CVA, apraxia, agnosia, and unilateral neglect occur, as well as homonymous hemianopia (loss of one-half of the visual field in each eye).
- **Middle cerebral artery:** drowsiness, stupor, coma, contralateral hemiplegia and sensory deficits of arm and face, aphasia, and homonymous hemianopia may be seen.
- **Anterior cerebral artery:** contralateral weakness or paralysis and sensory loss of the foot and leg, loss of ability in decision making and voluntary actions, and urinary incontinence.
- **Vertebral artery:** pain in the face, nose, or eye; numbness or weakness of the face on the ipsilateral side; problems with gait; dysphagia; and dysarthria (difficulty speaking).

Diagnostic Tests

The characteristic feature of ischemic CVA is persistent clinical manifestations that last longer than 24 hours. Therefore prompt diagnosis and treatment play a pivotal role in decreasing the progression of the injury and complications or disabilities that ensue. With the advent of improved imaging technologies, an individual experiencing any significant manifestation will receive a noncontrast CT of the head, standard MRI or diffuse-weighted MRI, or diffuse-weighted imaging (DWI).

The last procedure provides signs of the earliest changes associated with ischemia, even before injury or infarction occurs. This makes DWI a valuable tool in the early detection and treatment of CVAs. DWI performed with perfusion imaging helps improve the accuracy of the diagnosis.

Establishing an accurate diagnosis between hemorrhagic and ischemic stroke is vital. Performance of CT without contrast is the first step in trying to determine the stroke type. Because of the strong correlation between cardiovascular disease and stroke, ECG is also essential. A chest radiography and cardiac monitoring are recommended to rule out cardioembolism or any coexisting conditions such as cardiomegaly associated with valvular disease. Additional studies that may be recommended include a hematologic function laboratory test, electrolyte and glucose levels, and liver and kidney function tests. EEG is performed if the patient has seizures and a lumbar puncture if a subarachnoid hemorrhage is suspected but not seen on CT.

Management

Medical and Pharmacologic Therapy. Because of advancements in pharmacologic therapy, patients with ischemic strokes receive thrombolytic agents within 3 hours of the onset of the CVA (ASA, 2013). Confirmation of an ischemic stroke with CT without contrast is essential before r-TPA can be used. The American Heart Association/American Stroke Association have established thrombolysis guidelines for r-TPA therapy for acute ischemic strokes (Box 24.7). The desired effect of this therapy is to dissolve the clot and reperfuse the compromised brain tissue. Patients receiving r-TPA should not receive anticoagulants, antiplatelets, or any type of antithrombotic drug for at least 24 hours after treatment.

Drugs used to treat CVA patients include the following:
- Atorvastatin calcium for high cholesterol
- Baclofen for spasticity
- Onabotulinumtoxin A for upper limb spasticity and incontinence
- Dextromethorphan hydrobromide and quinidine sulfate for pseudobulbar affect
- Anticoagulants to reduce the risk of blood clots
- Antiplatelets to prevent platelets from sticking together
- Angiotensin II receptor antagonists to reduce blood pressure

Surgical management includes the following:
- Endarterectomy
- Extracranial–intracranial bypass
- Management of arteriovenous malformation
- Management of cerebral aneurysms
- Management of intracranial bleeding and evacuation of hematomas

NURSING MANAGEMENT

Diagnosis

Nursing diagnoses for an older adult with a CVA include the following:
- Potential for inadequate cerebral tissue perfusion resulting from hemorrhage, increased ICP, or both
- Inadequate breathing pattern resulting from changes in mental status
- Potential for aspiration resulting from loss of muscle tone, airway protection, and dysphagia
- Decreased mobility resulting from arm and leg weakness or paralysis (hemiparesis or hemiplegia)
- Inadequate communication resulting from aphasia and dysarthria related to alteration in the speech center
- Potential for injury resulting from seizures or hemiplegia
- Potential for reduced skin integrity resulting from prolonged immobility
- Inadequate urinary elimination resulting from immobility
- Inadequate feeding/bathing/dressing/toileting self-care resulting from impairments secondary to CVA
- Need for health teaching resulting from lack of exposure to drug use, rehabilitation, and long-term care for CVA

Planning and Expected Outcomes

Outcomes for an older adult with a CVA include the following:
1. The patient will not die.
2. The patient will have minimum residual deficits and complications.
3. The patient's increased ICP will be reduced.
4. The patient will not suffer evolution, extension, or completion of the stroke.

Intervention

Initial nursing interventions include positioning the patient at a 30- to 45-degree angle to prevent further elevation of ICP. This

---

BOX 24.7 Thrombolysis Guidelines

The American Heart Association/American Stroke Association (AHA/ASA) inclusion guidelines for the administration of rt-PA in under 3 hours are as follows:
- Diagnosis of ischemic stroke causing measurable neurologic deficit
- Neurologic signs not clearing spontaneously
- Neurologic signs not minor and isolated
- Symptoms not suggestive of subarachnoid hemorrhage
- Onset of symptoms less than 3 hours before beginning treatment
- No head trauma or prior stroke in past 3 months
- No MI in prior 3 months
- No GI/GU hemorrhage in previous 21 days
- No arterial puncture in noncompressible site during prior 7 days
- No major surgery in prior 14 days
- No history of prior intracranial bleed
- Systolic blood pressure under 185 mm Hg, diastolic blood pressure under 110 mm Hg
- No evidence of acute trauma or bleeding
- Not taking an oral anticoagulant, or if so, INR under 1.7
- If taking heparin within 48 hours, a normal activated prothrombin time (aPT)
- Platelet count of more than 100,000/μL
- Blood glucose greater than 50 mg/dL (2.7 mmol)
- No seizure with residual postictal impairments
- Computed tomography (CT) scan does not show evidence of multilobar infarction (hypodensity over one-third hemisphere)
- The patient and family understand the potential risks and benefits of therapy

position also helps manage or protect the airway of the patient with a neurologic deficit. Monitoring of vital signs assists the nurse in detecting signs of increased ICP and in effectively managing blood pressure. The nurse is responsible for continuous monitoring for signs of complications such as hydrocephalus, vasospasm, and increased neurologic changes.

Additional nursing interventions include the following:

- Encourage active range of motion on the unaffected side and passive range of motion on the affected side.
- Turn the patient every 2 hours.
- Monitor lower extremities for thrombophlebitis resulting from immobilization.
- Encourage the use of the unaffected arm for ADLs.
- Teach the patient to put clothing on the affected side first.
- Have the patient resume an oral diet only after he or she has successfully completed a swallowing evaluation. The patient may need thickened liquids or foods the consistency of oatmeal and may need to chew on the unaffected side of the mouth. This is sometimes referred to as a *dysphagia diet*.
- Collaborate with occupational and physical therapists for rehabilitation.
- Try alternative methods of communication with the patient who has aphasia.
- Teach the patient with homonymous hemianopia to adapt to the deficit by turning the head side to side to fully scan the visual field.
- The nurse also needs to educate the patient and family about:
  - CVA and CVA prevention
  - Community resources
  - Physical care and the need for psychosocial support
  - Drugs

🏠 HOME CARE

1. Assess sensorimotor function. A decline in this function is the most notable change in older adults and may be the cause of other changes such as slowed reaction time.
2. Memory impairment may compromise the teaching of homebound patients, so the nurse may have to use alternative approaches and rely on family and significant others involved in caregiving.
3. Assess for signs of impaired emotional control, diminished initiative, withdrawal, or other changes, which may be initial signs of brain dysfunction.
4. Altered thought processes occur with cognitive decline or disturbances in cognitive function, both of which occur in homebound patients with dementia, depression, delirium, or amnesic disorders.
5. The effects of aging must be considered when interpreting laboratory tests and alerting physicians about abnormal results.
6. Instruct caregivers about dosages and side effects of drugs, especially tranquilizers and antidepressants that are used in managing symptoms caused by dementia.
7. Instruct caregivers on methods to manage behavioral problems and caregiver stress.
8. Use social workers to assess community resources for caregivers and patients with dementia.
9. Assess the home environment of the older person with cognitive impairment for safety hazards and provide caregivers with tips and strategies for reducing and eliminating the identified hazards.

Evaluation

Patient progress occurs in small increments, and interventions are modified to assist patients in meeting their goals. Evaluation criteria include the following:

- Maintenance and improvement of cerebral tissue perfusion
- Avoidance of respiratory complications
- Prevention of aspiration from food, fluids, and secretions
- Prevention of contractures
- Prevention of edema in the affected extremity
- Maintenance of skin integrity
- Achievement of independence
- Pain management
- Increased ability to communicate, express feelings, and understand others
- Prevention of fecal and urinary incontinence
- Establishment of a normal voiding pattern
- Compensation for sensory deficits and physical and intellectual losses
- Participation by family members in the rehabilitation process

Anxiety

While anxiety does not decline with aging, many older adults are more focused on physical ailments and do not report feelings of anxiety. Generalized anxiety disorder (GAD) is common among older adults (Anxiety and Depression Association of America, n.d.) with a prevalence between 10% and 20% (Glasofer, 2018). Typical symptoms of GAD include chronic worry during most waking hours, restlessness, fatigue, decreased concentration, irritability, muscle tension, or disturbed sleep. Older adults may also present with physical symptoms (tachycardia, diaphoresis, and muscle tension; Glasofer, 2018).

Anxiety disorders in older adults may develop because of a specific event or a general pattern of change seen by patients as threatening. Such changes may include declines in health, illness, financial strain, an actual or potential change in living situation, the death of a significant other, or a loss of independence. Retirement is a change that often is associated with the development of an anxiety disorder in older adults.

NURSING MANAGEMENT

Assessment

Older adult patients with anxiety disorders are usually able to describe their anxiety without the nurse needing to probe extensively. They may also exhibit behavioral clues such as pacing, irritability, and fidgeting. When patients lack insight into their anxiety, the nurse may find it helpful to describe the symptoms observed as indicating anxiety. The nurse should also assess associated changes such as sleeping habits and appetite, the presence or absence of depression, and any complaints of physical pain, which may accompany the anxiety.

Somatic complaints are often seen in older adult patients experiencing anxiety. This may be attributed to the physical toll that anxiety takes on the physical systems or to a patient being more comfortable reporting a physical health concern rather than a mental health one. If the nurse believes the somatic concerns may be related to anxiety, a thorough anxiety assessment should be conducted.

Diagnosis

The nursing diagnoses for older adults with an anxiety disorder usually include the following:
- Anxiety resulting from a situational crisis
- Inadequate coping resulting from perceived vulnerability

Planning and Expected Outcomes

Expected outcomes include the following:
1. The patient identifies his or her own anxiety and coping patterns.
2. The patient reports an increase in psychological and physiologic comfort.
3. The patient demonstrates effective coping skills, as evidenced by his or her ability to solve problems and meet self-care needs.
4. The patient demonstrates the use of appropriate relaxation techniques.

Intervention

The nurse may intervene with older adults experiencing anxiety in a number of ways. It may be helpful to assist patients in examining their own "worst case scenario." By developing strategies that could be used to cope with the worst possible situation, patients may feel an increased ability to cope with their current situation. Relaxation strategies such as progressive muscle relaxation, breathing techniques, therapeutic use of music, and exercise are useful in helping patients alleviate the acute anxiety states that are most distressing to them. The nurse should help patients learn to identify increasing anxiety early in the anxiety cycle so that they can take steps to reduce it to a lower level. Family education may also be beneficial to obtain support systems for patients. Patients experiencing moderate to panic-level anxiety may need a referral for antianxiety drugs. Patients who continue to experience distress as a result of anxiety may benefit from psychotherapy. Behavior modification techniques are especially effective with phobic disorders.

Evaluation

The nurse may evaluate the care that has been provided to patients experiencing anxiety by monitoring their progress toward achievement of the expected outcomes and documenting the results. Effectiveness of any health teaching is evident in a patient's ability to use relaxation techniques and constructive problem solving.

Schizophrenia

Schizophrenia is a thought disorder characterized by altered perceptions of reality, alterations in thought processes (both form and content), and declines in patients' ADLs and occupational and social functioning. The onset of schizophrenia usually occurs between the late teens and the mid-30s. However, in rare cases, schizophrenia has an onset after age 45 (APA, 2013).

Typically, older adult patients with schizophrenia have been dealing with the disorder for a long time but may experience exacerbations of the schizophrenic symptoms with the stress of the aging process. The presentation is more likely to include delusions and hallucinations, and less likely to include disorganized and negative symptoms (Cohen, Vahia, Reyes et al., 2008; Jeste & Maglione, 2013).

NURSING MANAGEMENT

Assessment

The reader is referred to a general psychiatric nursing textbook for a complete review of the assessment process in individuals with a diagnosis of schizophrenia.

Diagnosis

Nursing diagnoses appropriate to the older adult with schizophrenia include the following:
- Social isolation resulting from altered mental status
- Anxiety resulting from unconscious conflict with reality
- Inadequate coping resulting from unrealistic perceptions
- Altered sleep pattern resulting from psychological status

Planning and Expected Outcomes

Schizophrenia is an illness that shows periods of exacerbation and remission. The goal of nursing intervention in individuals with schizophrenia is safe, effective treatment, rather than a cure. The goals for the patient that the nurse should work toward are reduction in symptoms and an improved quality of life. Other goals include reducing patient anxiety (anxiety usually exacerbates the schizophrenic symptoms), building a therapeutic relationship with the patient, providing continuity of care, and eliciting the support of family and friends to enhance the patient's function and experience. Expected outcomes include the following:
1. The patient develops a trusting relationship, as evidenced by the presence of supportive significant others.
2. The patient maintains contact with mental health caregivers, as evidenced by weekly meetings with a counselor.
3. The patient experiences a decrease in hallucinations and distress, as evidenced by verbalized reports of fewer hallucinations and feelings of distress, as well as demonstration of methods to handle hallucinations.
4. The patient gets adequate sleep, as evidenced by reports of sleeping through the night or verbalization of feeling rested after a night's sleep.

Intervention

Nursing interventions for older adults with schizophrenia should provide a comprehensive approach to the maintenance of ADLs, nutrition, hygiene, health promotion, and reality orientation. The reader is referred to a general psychiatric nursing text for a thorough review of nursing interventions for patients with schizophrenia. Interventions that may be most essential in dealing with older adults with schizophrenia include providing adequate family or social support, responding to patient symptoms, using touch appropriately, and dealing with aggressive behavior.

If patients give evidence (verbal or nonverbal) of hallucinations or delusions, the nurse should focus on responding to the feelings without arguing about the reality of their perceptual experiences. For example, if a patient states that the television is broadcasting his or her thoughts, the nurse could respond by saying, "That must be frightening," rather than saying, "Now, Mr. D, you know that the television can't do that!" Attempting to argue perception with patients only escalates their anxiety. It may, however, be helpful to reorient patients without being confrontational.

Patients with schizophrenia may easily misinterpret touch by the nurse as being harmful or threatening to them. Therefore the nurse should only touch the patient for a specific purpose and only with permission from the patient.

Older adults with schizophrenia may at times present a danger to themselves or others. The nurse should assess the level of danger that each patient presents. If the assessment shows that a patient has a potential for aggression, the nurse should take steps to deescalate the patient's anger and to provide safety for the patient and others.

Evaluation

Evaluation is based on achievement of the identified expected outcomes. The nature of the disorder may make it difficult for the nurse to establish a relationship with a patient; the nurse may therefore feel hopeless, frustrated, and inadequate while attempting to provide care. It is often helpful to establish short-term goals for patients with schizophrenia that are easily achievable and specific. The nurse is responsible for documenting progress toward achievement of the objectives, as well as the level of safety achieved.

Delusional Disorders

Delusional disorders involve nonbizarre delusions. (An example of a *nonbizarre delusion* would be a person with the false belief that he or she is under surveillance by the police. An example of a *bizarre delusion* would be that one's bodily organs have been removed and replaced by someone else's organs.) Except for the delusion, the patient's thinking is otherwise normal. Hallucinations rarely occur. These patients usually do not respond well to antipsychotic drugs (Calandra, 2003).

The following types are designated based on the predominant delusional theme (APA, 2013):
- **Erotomanic type:** delusions that another person, usually of higher status, is in love with the individual
- **Grandiose type:** delusions of inflated worth, power, knowledge, identity, or special relationship to a deity or famous person
- **Jealous type:** delusions that the individual's sexual partner is unfaithful
- **Persecutory type:** delusions that the person (or someone to whom the person is close) is being malevolently treated in some way

- **Somatic type:** delusions that the person has some physical defect or general medical condition
- **Mixed type:** delusions characteristic of more than one of those previously mentioned but with no one theme predominant
- **Unspecified type**

Intellectual Disability

Intellectual disability is characterized by below-average intellectual functioning. The onset occurs before age 18 and is accompanied by an alteration in an individual's ability to cope with life's demands and to function independently (APA, 2013). The individual's functioning, including such things as communication, self-care ability, performance of ADLs, interpersonal relationships, occupational functioning, and health and safety behaviors, may all be affected by the mental retardation. Multiple causes of intellectual disability exist. The functioning of patients with intellectual disability is affected throughout the life span, including the later years. These individuals are also more susceptible to alterations in emotional states.

NURSING MANAGEMENT

Assessment

Variables that may determine a patient's level of functioning should be assessed to determine the extent to which they enhance or detract from patient well-being.

Diagnosis

The most common nursing diagnosis seen in older adults with intellectual disability is delayed growth and development. This may be evidenced by delusions, a decreased attention span, or impaired problem solving. This diagnosis represents the ongoing challenge that older adults with intellectual disability are living with. Other common nursing diagnoses for older adults with intellectual disability include inadequate self-care and a potential for self- or outward-directed violence.

Planning and Expected Outcomes

In planning short-term and long-term goals, the nurse should customize the care plan to a patient's intellectual abilities. Adaptations to routine interventions may be needed to assist patients in comprehending their care, thereby allowing them to participate in the care. It may be useful to know a patient's intellectual functioning in terms of age level so that interventions can be adapted accordingly. Expected outcomes include the following:
1. The patient demonstrates the ability to maintain personal safety, as evidenced by the ability to communicate anger and frustration, appropriately use methods for coping with feelings, and exhibit appropriate self-control.
2. The patient demonstrates the ability to care for self independently within limitations, as evidenced by demonstration of appropriate self-care activities on a regular, consistent basis with minimum supervision.

Intervention

Nursing interventions that are specifically useful in dealing with older adults with intellectual disability primarily involve customizing the care routines to their level of intellectual functioning. When communicating with a patient, the nurse should use clear, simple instructions. Caregivers may be assigned a parental role by patients with intellectual disability. This role may represent a challenge for these patients because of their continued dependence throughout their life span; this is especially true if parents or other family members who have cared for patients throughout their life have become disabled or are now deceased. Therefore many older adults with intellectual disability as well as physical problems are admitted to nursing facilities for care.

Evaluation

In evaluating the care provided to older adult patients with intellectual disability, the nurse should also be aware of the need for an expanded nursing focus in this population. The opportunities for nursing research and service, especially in community settings, are varied and abundant. Documentation focuses on achievement of the expected outcomes and on the adaptations required because of age-related changes superimposed on the intellectual disability.

DRUG MANAGEMENT

Psychotropic Drugs

The second most common type of drug used by older adults is psychotropic agents. These drugs affect patient brain function, behavior, or experience (Reeves & Brister, 2008; Vahia, Diwan, Bankole et al., 2008). Older adults exhibit changes in the absorption, distribution, metabolism, and excretion of drugs, as well as changes in the CNS neurotransmitters and receptor sites that these drugs affect. Therefore a corresponding change occurs in the indications and contraindications for appropriate use of these drugs.

In the past, psychotropics were commonly used for residents of long-term care facilities. This use was often inappropriate or excessive. In 1987, federal regulations were developed (the Omnibus Budget Reconciliation Act) to decrease the inappropriate use of antipsychotic drugs. A corresponding decline has been seen in the frequency of use of antipsychotic agents in residents of long-term care facilities. Psychotropic drugs are appropriate when used in long-term care settings for what Drinka (1993) terms the *three Ds*: "danger to the resident or others; distress for the resident; dysfunction of the resident including interference with basic nursing care."

A primary goal in drug management for older adult patients is to find the lowest effective dose with the least adverse effects. When psychotropic drugs are used in older adults, it is also essential to remain aware of drug–drug interactions, drug–food interactions, nonadherence issues, and substance abuse and dependency issues. The nursing implications of antianxiety drugs, antidepressants, antimanic agents, antipsychotics, and other psychoactive drugs used in older adults are discussed in this section (Zagaria, 2009).

Antianxiety Agents

Antianxiety drugs are also called *anxiolytics.* In the past, barbiturates were the main types of drugs used for anxiety; however, BZs are now used because of their improved safety compared with barbiturates. Long-term use of BZs (usually defined as longer than 1 to 2 months) puts patients at risk for the development of dependence, and BZs do have potential adverse interactions, especially with sedative agents and alcohol. The two broad categories of BZs are short-acting BZs (e.g., alprazolam, lorazepam, and oxazepam) and long-acting BZs (e.g., diazepam, chlordiazepoxide, and clonazepam). The short-acting agents are preferred for older adults because of their lower potential for buildup leading to sedation and depression.

When used for anxiety, BZs should be given in the lowest possible dose for the shortest possible time. Therefore the precipitating cause of the anxiety needs to be evaluated and addressed while the BZ is being used. Although alprazolam may be used on a long-term basis for panic in older adults, most BZs should be used for less than 30 days. When BZs are used for longer periods, patients may experience withdrawal symptoms that can be as severe as seizures. When a drug is discontinued, it should be tapered slowly to prevent withdrawal symptoms or rebound anxiety symptoms. Of concern in older adults is the potential for BZs to exacerbate sleep apnea. Therefore older adults should be assessed for alterations in sleep patterns (especially snoring) before using a BZ.

Other options besides BZs are available for older adults who need an anxiolytic. Buspirone is a chemically unique antianxiety agent that does not produce dependence or interaction with BZs or alcohol. Its drawback lies in its slow onset of action (often up to 2 weeks), which tends to limit patient adherence. Nurses play an important role in educating patients about the slow onset of buspirone, thereby improving the patients' adherence to their drug regimens and giving older adults a safer option for reducing anxiety. Other drugs used to manage anxiety in older adults include antidepressants and beta-blockers such as propranolol.

Antidepressants

Antidepressant drugs include MAOIs, tricyclic antidepressants (TCAs), and SSRIs. MAOIs affect the monoamine neurotransmitter system but are rarely used because of their potential drug–food interaction with tyramine, which may precipitate a hypertensive crisis. They are used in older adults with refractory depression or cardiac arrhythmias because they do not produce the cardiovascular side effects of other antidepressants (McNamara, 2006b). Patients taking MAOIs must adhere to a tyramine-free diet and must be warned of the potential for a hypertensive crisis from drug–drug interactions with many other drugs. Their health care providers and pharmacists should monitor any new prescription or OTC drugs.

TCAs block the reuptake of norepinephrine and serotonin. The side effects include anticholinergic effects, sedation, hypotension, dry mouth, tachycardia, blurred vision, constipation, and urinary retention. These drugs are contraindicated in patients with recent MI or cardiac arrhythmias. They are rarely used since the development of the new SSRIs.

One of the most recent additions to the antidepressant category are SSRIs. SSRIs are selective and potent inhibitors of serotonin reuptake, but each differs slightly in its effect on other neurotransmitter receptors and enzymes, which may make a difference in the tolerability and efficacy of individual agents. When using SSRIs with the older population, the recommendation is to start with a low dose and go slow. Antidepressants should be withdrawn over 2 to 6 weeks to avoid withdrawal symptoms. SSRIs are considered safe in older adults because of the low risk of CNS, anticholinergic, and cardiovascular effects. However, the older population is at increased risk for impaired balance and falls with any antidepressant, especially at a higher dose. Older patients may need up to 12 weeks of these drugs for evaluation of a full response. It is important to monitor for drug–drug interactions and for excessive weight loss, especially in those who are debilitated. Improved cognitive function has been noted in the older patient with depression treated with antidepressants.

Bupropion is a norepinephrine dopamine reuptake inhibitor. The main consideration in its use is identifying patients with a history of seizures, organic brain disorder, or alcohol withdrawal. Older adults are at risk for increased accumulation of bupropion because of decreased clearance of the drug and its metabolites.

Venlafaxine and duloxetine, selective serotonin norepinephrine reuptake inhibitors (SNRIs), are considered three drugs in one. At the lower dose, an SNRI is a potent inhibitor of serotonin; at moderate doses, both serotonin and norepinephrine reuptake occurs; and at the higher doses, neuronal uptake pumps for serotonin, norepinephrine, and dopamine are inhibited. SNRIs are an excellent choice for GAD and for anxiety with comorbid depression.

Mirtazapine is a nonadrenergic-specific serotonergic antidepressant and is very sedating at 15 mg or less and less sedating at doses greater than 15 mg. It may increase appetite and cause weight gain because of its strong antihistaminic properties, but the side effects sometimes diminish over time. The nurse should monitor for sedation, hypotension, and anticholinergic effects, and taper this drug gradually, as with all antidepressants, to avoid withdrawal symptoms. Clearance of the drug is reduced in older men by up to 40% and in older women by up to 10% (Zagaria, 2009).

Additional helpful information about antidepressants includes the course of treatment. Antidepressants are commonly used until patients have been free of the symptoms of depression for 6 months to 2 years. Patients then gradually stop taking the drug to prevent the development of rebound depression. Some patients with recurrent major depression may continue to use antidepressants indefinitely. Adherence problems may be more common in older adults because of the side effects of the drug (Box 24.8). However, because of concerns about side effects, the recommendation for prescribing this drug in this age group has been to "start low, go slow, and never go high," often resulting in doses that do not achieve "a full response." Careful monitoring of drug dosage and drug interactions will aid in patient adherence, safety, and recovery. Electroconvulsive therapy (ECT) may be used in patients with life-threatening depression if antidepressants have not been effective. The usual course

of ECT would be 10 to 14 treatments every other day. ECT is now considered a humane and effective treatment for depression because of the use of anesthesia and muscle relaxants during the procedure.

Mood Stabilizers

In the older population with bipolar disorder, lithium and anticonvulsants are used as mood stabilizers. The older adult is more sensitive to lithium and is at a higher risk for neurotoxicity and cognitive impairment, even at therapeutic plasma levels. Before beginning lithium use, patients should have baseline ECG, CBC, and renal, thyroid, and liver function studies. In the older adult, lithium is started at a low dosage (e.g., 300 mg/day), and blood level is obtained in 3 or 4 days. Blood should be drawn 12 hours after the last dose of lithium. The dose is then titrated until a therapeutic blood level is reached (usually 0.4 to 1.5 milliequivalents per liter [mEq/L]). Blood levels are determined every 3 or 4 days until the therapeutic level is attained. The frequency of obtaining blood for the study may then be decreased to once a month for the first 6 months and every 2 to 3 months for an indefinite period. Renal, liver, and thyroid studies should be performed every 6 months because of the drug's potential toxicity.

Side effects seen in older adults taking lithium include gastrointestinal distress, hand tremors, ataxia, and weight gain. Cardiovascular side effects may also occur; therefore periodic ECG may be performed, as needed. Lithium toxicity may occur if blood levels are greater than 1.5 mEq/L; moderate to severe toxicity may be seen if levels are greater than 2 mEq/L; and death may occur if blood levels are greater than 2.5 mEq/L. Patients should inform all physicians and pharmacists involved in their care of any lithium use because of the potential for drug–drug interactions.

Anticonvulsants are also considered a good option for treating bipolar mood disorders, but, again, dosing should be graduated in the older population and in those with liver impairment (Lavretsky, 2008). These drugs may cause confusion, cognitive impairments, or ataxia that may lead to falls. Additional caution is warranted if anticonvulsants are combined with other drugs

---

BOX 24.8 Side Effects Associated With Antidepressants

- Nausea
- Increased appetite and weight gain
- Loss of sexual desire and other sexual problems, such as erectile dysfunction and decreased orgasm
- Fatigue and drowsiness
- Insomnia
- Dry mouth
- Blurred vision
- Constipation
- Dizziness
- Agitation
- Irritability
- Anxiety
- Headaches

that affect the CNS or have anticholinergic properties. Valproate, one of the anticonvulsants, causes an increased risk for thrombocytopenia in the older population.

Antipsychotic Drugs

Antipsychotic drugs are also called *neuroleptics.* They work by blocking the action of dopamine. Neuroleptics are used in the treatment of schizophrenia, acute psychosis, and delirium. The specific choice of a neuroleptic agent is made by both considering patients' clinical symptoms and examining the side effect profiles of the various neuroleptic agents. Older adults usually are started on lower doses (one-half to one-third of the normal dose) of high-potency neuroleptics. The high-potency neuroleptics have a lower frequency of anticholinergic, cardiovascular, and sedative side effects compared with low-potency neuroleptics. However, high-potency neuroleptics cause an increased rate of extrapyramidal symptoms (EPSs) in comparison with low-potency neuroleptics. Therefore it is essential to monitor all patients taking neuroleptics for EPSs, which are discussed later in this chapter. Haloperidol and fluphenazine are neuroleptics that are available in long-acting decanoate forms for nonadherent patients and may be administered weekly to monthly (Sangani & Saadabadi, 2017). However, the decanoates are rarely used in older adults because of their long half-life of 1 to 4 weeks. Older adults with renal or hepatic impairment, and those with decreased fluid volume are at increased risk of developing orthostatic hypotension, dizziness and falls, along with parkinsonism and tardive dyskinesia with the use of decanoates (Singh & O'Connor, 2009).

The atypical antipsychotics have a decreased incidence of side effects and EPSs. Unfortunately, clozapine carries with it the potentially dangerous side effect of agranulocytosis; therefore weekly CBCs must be obtained for all patients receiving clozapine. All antipsychotics carry a boxed warning related to use in older adults.

Side Effects

Extrapyramidal Symptoms

Nurses play a vital role in the monitoring, education, and evaluation of EPSs in patients receiving neuroleptic drugs. EPSs are described in Table 24.6.

EPSs are treated with anticholinergic or antiparkinsonian agents such as diphenhydramine, benztropine, or trihexyphenidyl. Amantadine, a dopamine agonist, may be used, especially in older

TABLE 24.6	Extrapyramidal Symptoms
Symptom	**Characteristics**
Acute dystonic reaction	Muscle rigidity; eyes fixed in deviated position; arched posture; should be treated with an anticholinergic agent such as diphenhydramine
Akathisia	Inability to sit still
Akinesia	Decreased psychomotor movements; shuffling gait
Pseudoparkinsonism	Tremor in the extremities that resembles Parkinson disease
Perioral tremor (rabbit syndrome)	Fine, rapid lip movements

patients and in those with cardiovascular dysfunction because of its reduced anticholinergic effects.

Tardive Dyskinesia

Tardive dyskinesia (TD) is a potentially permanent neurologic side effect of neuroleptic drugs. Patients and their families must be informed of the risk of TD before initiating neuroleptic therapy. Involuntary movements, especially in the face, lips, and tongue, characterize TD. The trunk and extremities may also be involved. TD is most likely to develop in patients who have used neuroleptics longer than 2 years. Patients should be evaluated for TD at each appointment. Unfortunately, no effective treatment for TD exists. The best prevention is using the lowest possible dose of a neuroleptic for the shortest time necessary.

Neuroleptic Malignant Syndrome

Neuroleptic malignant syndrome (NMS) is a rare but serious side effect that may lead to death. Its frequency increases with the use of high-potency antipsychotics. The initial symptoms include a decreased temperature, the development of EPSs, and delirium. If untreated, it then progresses to hyperthermia, stupor, severe EPSs, and coma. It is treated by immediately discontinuing any neuroleptic drug. In addition, dantrolene sodium, which may cause liver toxicity, or bromocriptine may also be used. Because of the potential for death from NMS, all patients receiving neuroleptic drugs in an inpatient or long-term care setting should have their vital signs assessed daily. Patients who take neuroleptics on an outpatient basis should be educated on the signs of NMS, particularly the cardinal sign of a temperature change.

EPSs, TD, and NMS all present significant risks for patients taking neuroleptic drugs. It is therefore essential that nurses educate patients and their caregivers of the need for routine monitoring for the development of these side effects.

Other Psychoactive Drugs Used in Older Adults

Anafranil

Clomipramine is a TCA that is specifically helpful for OCD. Its side effect profile is consistent with that of other TCAs.

Antiparkinsonian Agents

As discussed earlier, antiparkinsonian agents such as benztropine and trihexyphenidyl are used to treat the side effects of antipsychotic drugs.

Sedative-Hypnotic Agents

Sleep patterns change with age, and older adults may experience a decrease in both the quantity and quality of sleep. Delayed onset of sleep and nighttime awakenings are not uncommon in older adults. Sedative–hypnotic agents may be dangerous when used in older adults; therefore they are used only if patients are unable to function because of insomnia. Long-term use of sedative–hypnotics may produce a disturbed sleep–wake cycle and may lead to dependence and a decrease in the sense of being rested, even after an adequate amount of sleep. In older adults whose symptoms include insomnia, other causes should be ruled out first. Early night insomnia may be indicative of anxiety or pain (e.g., arthritis), and middle-of-the-night to late-night insomnia may be seen with depression.

MENTAL HEALTH CARE RESOURCES

The number and quality of resources for the care of mental health problems in older adults are minimal because geropsychiatric care is a relatively new specialty within gerontology. These resources include human resources (e.g., mental health professionals [physicians and nurses]), physical resources (e.g., hospitals, clinics, nursing facilities, and dementia units), and financial resources needed to pay for mental health care (e.g., Medicare, Medicaid, and health insurance coverage).

Human Resources

Geropsychiatric nurses and geriatric mental health nurses are trained at the master's and doctoral levels, usually in programs that offer some combination of psychiatric or mental health nursing and gerontologic nursing course work (Hoeffer, 1994). The primary major is usually psychiatric or mental health nursing with some courses in gerontologic nursing. These nurses may be certified by the American Nurses Credentialing Center as psychiatric and mental health nurse practitioners, as adult-gerontology clinical nurse specialists, or both if they have master's degree preparation in one or both specialties. These specialists should be prepared to assess and care for individuals who often have multiple, complex physical *and* mental or emotional problems. No national certification is currently offered in geropsychiatric nursing.

More geropsychiatric nurses are needed to work as staff or consultants in hospitals, nursing facilities, outpatient clinics, day treatment centers, adult day services programs, and home health agencies. Geropsychiatric advanced practice nurses, often working with geriatric psychiatrists, provide much needed care in nursing facilities. They perform assessments, manage drugs, participate in individual and group therapy on a regular schedule, and provide in-service education for the nursing staff. As previously mentioned, many older adults are never adequately diagnosed or treated for underlying psychopathologic problems. Nurses in these settings can help resolve this problem. These nurses are also greatly needed to teach technical nursing staff members, who have close contact with patients, how to communicate with and relate to older adults with mental and emotional disturbances. Patient abuse may occur when nonprofessional staff members do not know how to respond to aggressive, hostile, and combative behavior.

Because an interdisciplinary approach is important in the health care of older adults, psychiatrists, social workers, dietitians, clergy, speech pathologists, and physical and occupational therapists with some formal preparation in geriatrics and gerontology are also essential in providing high-quality care for geropsychiatric patients.

Physical Resources

Older patients with mental and emotional problems are increasingly being treated on an outpatient basis, primarily because of available methods of payment. Some of these outpatient choices are as follows:

- Community mental health centers (which may include emergency psychiatric services during the evening or night)
- The clinic or offices of a geriatric psychiatrist, geriatric mental health nurse, or advanced practice nurse specializing in geriatric mental health
- Senior partial-hospitalization programs where patients receive assessment, diagnosis, and treatment (including various types of drugs and other therapy) and return home in the late afternoon
- In-home assessments, diagnosis, treatment, care, and follow-up in patients' own residences

On the one hand, these types of programs may be more effective for older patients than residential treatment in hospitals, which may cause relocation confusion, loss of familiar environmental and sensory stimulation, and functional decline associated with the hospitalization. On the other hand, individuals without family members or an adequate support system may have problems managing difficult drug regimens alone at home. Those with major depression are at greater risk for potential suicide.

Some general hospitals have geropsychiatric units staffed and equipped to care for the mental *and* physical needs of older patients. These units provide thorough assessments and an interdisciplinary approach to total care and rehabilitation on a relatively short-term basis for older patients with primarily mental and emotional problems. Unless the general psychiatric hospital has a specific unit planned for older patients, such a facility may have difficulty meeting their needs. In fact, many general psychiatric hospitals do not even admit patients who also have physical problems and needs. Most geropsychiatric units are in psychiatric facilities associated with medical schools, where fellowships are available to psychiatrists specializing in this area. Some psychiatric hospitals have well-developed day hospitalization programs that provide treatment, care, and supervision daily. However, adequate transportation to and from the hospital each day may be a problem for older persons. Some hospitals and community agencies provide this type of medical transportation when individuals or their families cannot provide it. However, escort services from the van to the area of treatment may not be available, so the older person cannot make the trip alone for safety reasons.

Most older persons who have some type of chronic mental health problems are found in long-term care nursing facilities with some type of dementia or depression related to physical or environmental factors. In fact, Brower (1993) has stated that nursing facilities "are, in reality, minigeropsychiatric facilities, but without the trained psychiatric staff." Many of the residents in these facilities have not had the benefit of a thorough mental status assessment and diagnosis, and therefore lack proper treatment and care. In addition to ageism, a reason for this problem is the lack of adequate financial resources for the necessary assessment and treatment.

TRENDS AND NEEDS

The need to focus more on the mental and emotional health care needs of older adults will continue to increase (Box 24.9). Nurses and family members must advocate for older persons with mental health problems, who are not being adequately diagnosed and treated. State and local ombudsman programs are expanding, with plans to have at least one or two certified trained volunteer ombudsmen in all long-term care facilities, including

---

BOX 24.9 Trends and Needs in Mental Health Care of Older Adults

- Strong advocacy
- Increased outpatient care
- Expanded community resources
- Improved quality of long-term care
  - Additional legislation and regulations related to psychosocial training for staff in long-term care facilities
  - More emphasis on gerontologic, geriatric, and geropsychiatric education for health care providers
- More educational programs for family members
- Short-term respite care for family members

---

nursing facilities, hospital skilled nursing units, and assisted living facilities (sometimes called *personal care homes*).

Long periods of hospitalization in a psychiatric hospital are rare. More people are treated in the home setting and in partial hospitalization and outpatient settings. Other community organizations such as churches and congregations, senior citizens' groups, and other social organizations are developing programs to help older persons maintain their mental health by preventing loneliness and depression. Increased emphasis will be placed on improving the quality of care in long-term care facilities. The

primary need is to focus more on mental health problems, psychosocial issues, and communication skills (e.g., in-service training for all personnel). This goal may be accomplished through state legislation or the efforts of regulatory agencies. Emphasis will also be placed on increasing gerontologic, geriatric, and geropsychiatric content in the curricula of medical, nursing, and social work educational programs. Advocacy groups should work toward including more of such content in state licensing examinations.

Family members also need to learn more about the aging process, especially the normal, common changes as well as abnormal changes in behavior with aging so that they will be better able to relate to and care for their older family members in the home, if needed. Although respite care (e.g., adult day programs and nursing facilities) is available to some extent for those family members who care for older persons with mental and behavioral problems, additional short-term respite care is greatly needed. Family members caring for older persons in the home need a couple of hours of relief now and then, perhaps by a volunteer from a church, so that they may take a walk, go to a movie, or go shopping. Trained volunteers can easily provide this kind of short-term respite care to assist the caregiver and, ultimately, the older family member (Bharani & Lantz, 2009).

SUMMARY

Nurses caring for older adults face many challenges as the population of older adults continues to increase in the United States and around the world. A significant percentage of older adults suffer from some form of cognitive impairment, all of whom could benefit from nursing care focusing on the special needs of these people. Without radical changes in the way health care is allocated and delivered in this country, as well as issues of shrinking health care dollars, accessibility to care could threaten the care of older adults. Those with cognitive impairment continue to be at high risk for limited access to appropriate and cost-effective care.

Cost-effective models for care should be developed and tested along the continuum of care, from prevention of illness to management of acute illness to restoration of function and, finally, to staying in the community or home environment.

The practice of gerontologic nursing is collaborative and interdisciplinary in scope. This is necessitated by the vast complexity, diversity, and heterogeneity of older adults in terms of their physical and mental conditions, health care needs, past life experiences, current lifestyles, culture, ethnicity, and resources. The family is an extremely important aspect of gerontologic practice, not only because many older adults live within a family setting but also because the family is becoming a primary provider of care.

The most serious health problems occur in those older than 80 years old, and this group is likely to be cared for by relatives who are older than 65 years of age. The blend of medical–surgical, psychiatric, and community health nursing skills and the expertise required to care for older adults with cognitive impairments provides unique and unlimited opportunities and challenges in practice.

KEY POINTS

- The nervous system is a network of complex structures that change as an individual ages.
- Normal aging is associated with changes in the ability to consciously learn and retain new information *easily.*
- The age-related neurodegenerative and neurochemical changes in the cerebellum are believed to be the underlying cause of decline in motor and cognitive function.
- Sleep disorders are common in aging individuals. Excessive daytime somnolence is not part of normal aging.
- Vision changes that occur with aging are significant. The lens of the eye thickens, becoming yellow, cloudy, and less elastic.

- Presbycusis is hearing loss associated with the aging process.
- The loss of taste and smell receptors means that food is not as appetizing to the older adult.
- It is important to include functional assessment as part of the assessment of older adults.
- A decline in cognitive function is an effect of disease, not an effect of the normal aging process.
- Depression may manifest itself through signs such as fatigue; constipation; psychomotor retardation; depressed mood; loss of interest, energy, libido, or pleasure; changes in appetite, weight, and sleep patterns; agitation; anxiety; or crying.

- The risk factors for delirium include advanced age, CNS diseases, infection, polypharmacy, hypoalbuminemia, electrolyte imbalances, trauma history, gastrointestinal or genitourinary disorders, cardiopulmonary disorders, and sensory changes.
- The treatment of delirium is focused on the identification and treatment of the underlying cause.
- Nonpharmacologic approaches for delirium may include removing bladder catheters, improving nutritional intake, using reality orientation, decreasing sensory overstimulation or deprivation, and reassuring the older adult and their family members.
- Dementia is a syndrome of gradual and progressive cognitive decline.
- Although dementia is more common in old age, it is not part of the normal aging process.
- From the time of diagnosis, individuals with AD survive about half as long as those of similar age without dementia.
- Management of AD focuses on maintaining cognitive and global function early on in the disease process to postpone the need for institutional care.
- Individuals who have experienced a CVA have an even greater risk of VaD.
- Older adults are at risk for the development of subdural hematomas because of brain atrophy and corresponding vascular changes that occur with normal aging and are also at risk for falls and subsequent head injuries.
- The only positive way to diagnose dementia-related disorders is brain tissue biopsy or autopsy of the brain.
- Public policy has shifted to encourage family members to care for older adults in their homes, thus decreasing health care costs and individualizing care to meet patient needs.
- The nurse's role has shifted from caregiver to care coordinator; that is, the nurse teaches and assists the family members with home care, provides supportive care, and serves as a patient advocate.
- The purpose of a comprehensive assessment is to determine problem areas, as well as areas of strength on which to base a care plan, including education of families and caregivers.
- People who demonstrate symptoms of moderate to severe cognitive impairment may benefit from having meals in the same place at the same time each day.

- Persons in all stages of dementia benefit from the use of clocks, calendars, and mementos within the environment.
- The effective management of BPSD should not focus on trying to change the older person but on modifying factors that may be contributing to these behaviors.
- The use of physical or chemical restraints has demonstrated no benefit in controlling BPSD or managing disease.
- Maintaining social interaction and human contact in a variety of ways is beneficial for older persons with cognitive decline.
- Changes in the routine should be introduced slowly, and a stimulus should be provided to ensure that feelings of comfort and security are not lost.
- Wandering can sometimes be managed through environmental changes such as fences or alarm systems and close supervision.
- Sundown syndrome may also be modified through behavioral interventions, including redirection, the provision of companionship and empathy, and environmental modifications in lighting and noise reduction.
- PD, the most common form of parkinsonism, is a common progressive degenerative disorder of the basal ganglia involving the dopaminergic nigrostriatal pathway.
- A CVA is caused by a disruption in normal blood supply to the brain tissue.
- Strokes are the third leading cause of death and the most common cause of disability in the United States.
- A major change in the treatment of strokes is the use of thrombolytic agents (r-TPA) within a 3-hour window of the onset of signs or symptoms of AIS.
- Advanced age is one of the most significant risk factors for strokes.
- Modifiable risk factors for strokes include hypertension, diabetes mellitus, cardiovascular disease, nonvalvular atrial fibrillation, blood lipid abnormalities, smoking, substance abuse (particularly cocaine), obesity, a sedentary lifestyle, high stress levels, previous CVA or TIA, heavy alcohol use, and sudden discontinuation of antihypertensive drugs.
- Hypertension is the most important modifiable risk factor for both ischemic and hemorrhagic strokes.

CASE STUDY

Mr. J is 78-year-old black man who arrived in the emergency department lethargic, vomiting, unable to speak clearly, and with weakness on the right side of his body. Mr. J has a medical history of hypertension and diabetes mellitus type 2. His family (wife and daughter) reported that for the past 3 months he has been having right-sided weakness and slurred speech that resolved within an hour of onset. Mr. J also has glaucoma, gout, and a history of atrial fibrillation (managed with drugs). Mr. J's family reported that he was taking the following drugs at home: digoxin, allopurinol, furosemide, NPH (neutral protamine Hagedorn) insulin twice a day, lisinopril, baby acetylsalicylic acid, potassium chloride, and eye drops.

Mr. J's wife, 77 years old, reported that approximately 3 days ago Mr. J stopped taking his blood pressure drugs (lisinopril and furosemide) because he had spent the money on a horse race. Two nights ago, he started to experience more frequent numbness of the right arm and slurred speech, but she did not think it was important because it disappeared after several hours. Today, she had difficulty waking him up, and her daughter told her to call the ambulance.

Mr. J's blood pressure on admission was 220/120 mm Hg; his heart rate was 126 beats/min; respiratory rate was 28 breaths/min; and temperature was 98.9° F (37° C). He had right-sided hemiparesis and hemiplegia. His speech was slurred and at times incomprehensible. Mr. J was able to maintain his airway at this time.

Oxygen via nasal cannula is started at 2 liters per minute (L/min), and a peripheral intravenous line is started with normal saline intravenous fluid therapy at 80 milliliters per hour (mL/hr). A 12-lead electrocardiography (ECG) is performed, and Mr. J is sent for computed tomography (CT) of the head.

CRITICAL-THINKING QUESTIONS

1. Which one of Mr. J's symptoms supports a diagnosis of stroke?
2. What are the risk factors that Mr. J presents for the development of stroke?
3. Indicate the type of stroke Mr. J most likely had and support your answer.
4. What evidence is presented to support that Mr. J had experienced previous TIAs?
5. Why is atrial fibrillation a risk factor for embolic stroke?
6. Identify a nursing diagnosis based on Mr. J's assessment and develop an appropriate nursing care plan.

REFERENCES

Administration on Aging. (2017). *Profile of older Americans 2016.* Retrieved March 2, 2018 from https://www.acl.gov/aging-and-disability-in-america/data-and-research/profile-older-americans.

Alagiakrishnan, K. (2017). *Delirium medication.* Retrieved March 4, 2018 from https://emedicine.medscape.com/article/288890-medication#2.

Algase, D. L., Beck, C., Kolanowski, A., Whall, A., Berent, S., Richards, K., et al. (1996). Need-driven dementia-compromised behavior: An alternative view of disruptive behavior. *American Journal of Alzheimer's Disease, 11*(6), 10–19.

Alzheimer's Association. (2013). 2013 Alzheimer's disease facts and figures. Retrieved from www.alz.org/downloads/fact_figures_2013.pdf.

Alzheimer's Association. (2017). 2017 Alzheimer's disease facts and figures. Retrieved from https://www.alz.org/documents_custom/2017-facts-and-figures.pdf.

American Psychiatric Association. (2016). *APA releases new Practice Guidelines on the Use of Antipsychotics in Patients with Dementia [News Release].* Retrieved March 4, 2018 from https://www.psychiatry.org/newsroom/news-releases/apa-releases-new-practice-guidelines-on-the-use-of-antipsychotics-in-patients-with-dementia.

American Psychiatric Association. (2013). *Diagnostic and statistical manual of mental disorders: DSM-5* (5th ed.). Washington, DC: The Association.

American Stroke Association. (2013). http://strokeassociation.org/STROKEORG/AboutStroke/About-Stroke_UCM_308529_SubHomePage.jsp.

Anxiety and Depression Association of America. (n.d.). *Older adults.* Retrieved June 12, 2018 from https://adaa.org/living-with-anxiety/older-adults.

Baldessarini, R. (2003). Reducing suicide risk in psychiatric disorders. *Current Psychiatry Reports, 2*(9), 15.

Bharani, N., & Lantz, M. S. (2009). A case of late-onset psychosis. *Clinical Geriatrics, 17*(3), 12.

Bhasin, M., Rowan, E., Edwards, K., & McKeith, I. (2007). Cholinesterase inhibitors in dementia with Lewy bodies: A comparative analysis. *International Journal of Geriatric Psychiatry, 22*(9), 890–895.

Black, J. M., Hawks, J. H., & Hogan, M. A. (2005). *Medical-surgical nursing: Clinical management for positive outcome* (7th ed.). Philadelphia: Saunders.

Brannon, G. E., Carroll, K. S., Vij, S., & Gentili, A. (2008). *Sleep disorder, geriatric.* Retrieved May 11, 2009, from http://emedicine.nedscape.com/article/292498-overview.

Breitbart, W., & Alici, Y. (2012). Evidence-based treatment of delirium in patients with cancer. *Journal of Clinical Oncology, 30*(11), 1206–1214.

Brower, H. T. (1993). Special care units for dementia. *Journal of Gerontological Nursing, 19*(2), 3.

Buter, T. C., van den Hout, A., Matthews, F. E., Larsen, J. P., Brayne, C., & Aarsland, D. (2008). Dementia and survival in Parkinson disease: A 12-year population study. *Neurology, 70*(13), 1017–1022.

Calandra, J. (2003). Mental health and older adults: mental illness in later life, part 2. *Nurse Week, 4*(24), 25.

Centers for Disease Control and Prevention (CDC). (2013). *Stroke facts.* Retrieved October 30, 2013 from http://www.cdc.gov/stroke/facts.htm.

Centers for Disease Control and Prevention (CDC). (2012). Prevalence of stroke – United States, 2006-2010. *Morbidity and Mortality Weekly Report, 61*(20), 379–382.

Cohen, C. I., Vahia, I., Reyes, P., et al. (2008). Schizophrenia in later life: clinical symptoms and social well-being. *Psychiatric Services, 59*(3), 232.

Dichgans, M., Markus, H. S., Salloway, S., et al. (2008). Donepezil in patients with subcortical vascular cognitive impairment: A randomised double-blind trial in CADASIL. *Lancet Neurology, 7*(4), 310–318.

Dick, K. (2013). Dementia. In T. Buttaro, J. Trybulski, P. Bailey, & J. Sandberg-Cook (Eds.), *Primary care: A collaborative practice* (pp. 1003–1008). St. Louis, MO: Elsevier.

Dodel, R., Csoti, I., Ebersbach, G., et al. (2008). Lewy body dementia and Parkinson's disease with dementia. *Journal of Neurology, 255* (Suppl 5), 39–47.

Doerflinger, D. M. (2012). *Mental status assessment in older adults: Montreal Cognitive Assessment.* Retrieved March 4, 2018 from https://consultgeri.org/try-this/general-assessment/issue-3.2.

Doerflinger, D. M. (2013). *Mental status assessment of older adults: The Mini-Cog.* Retrieved March 4, 2018 from https://consultgeri.org/try-this/general-assessment/issue-3.1.

Drinka, D. (1993). OBRA-1987 nursing home regulations. *Journal of the American Geriatrics Society, 41*(4), 466.

Duffy, E. G. (2010). The neurologic system. In P. A. Tablowski (Ed.), *Gerontological nursing.* Upper Saddle River, NJ: Pearson Education.

Fadil, H., Borazanci, A., Ait Ben Haddou, E., et al. (2009). Early onset dementia. *International Review of Neurobiology, 84*(1), 245.

Fanous, A.A., & Siddiqui, A.H. (2016). Mechanical thrombectomy: Stent retrievers vs. aspiration catheters. *Cor et Vasa, 58*(2), e193–e203. https://doi.org/10.1016/j.crvasa.2016.01.004.

Fick, D., & Mion, L. (2008). Delirium superimposed on dementia. *The American Journal of Nursing, 108*, 52–60.

Fontaine, K. (2008). *Mental health nursing* (6th ed.). Prentice Hall, NJ: Pearson.

Glasofer, D. R. (2018). *Late Life Generalized Anxiety Disorder.* Retrieved June 12, 2018 from https://www.verywellmind.com/late-life-generalized-anxiety-disorder-1393060.

Greenberg, S. A. (2012). *The Geriatric Depression Scale (GDS).* Retrieved March 4, 2018 from https://consultgeri.org/try-this/general-assessment/issue-4.

Harvey, P. D., Moriarty, P. J., Kleinman, L., et al. (2005). The validation of a caregiver assessment of dementia: the dementia severity scale. *Alzheimer Dis & Assoc Disord, 19*(4), 186–194.

Heuninckx, S., Wenderoth, N., & Swinnen, S. P. (2008). Systems neuroplasticity in the aging brain: Recruiting additional neural resources for successful motor performance in elderly persons. *Journal of Neuroscience, 28*(1), 91–99.

Hoeffer, B. (1994). Essential curriculum content. *Journal of Psychosocial Nursing and Mental Health Services, 32*(4), 33.

Jeste, D. V., & Maglione, J. E. (2013). Treating Older Adults With Schizophrenia: Challenges and Opportunities. *Schizophrenia Bulletin, 39*(5), 966–968. https://doi.org/10.1093/schbul/sbt043.

Keller, J. N. (2006). Age-related neuropathology, cognitive decline, and Alzheimer's disease. *Ageing Research Reviews, 5*(1), 1–13.

Kirkham, J., Sherman, C., Velkers, C., Maxwell, C., Gill, S., Rochon, P., et al. (2017). Antipsychotic use in dementia. *Canadian Journal of Psychiatry, 62*(3), 170–181. https://doi.org/10.1177/0706743716673321.

Koedama, E. L., Pijnenburga, Y. A., Deegb, D. J., et al. (2008). Early-onset dementia is associated with higher mortality. *Dement Geriat Cogn Disord, 26*, 147–152.

Kyomen, H. H., & Whitfield, T. H. (2008). Agitation in older adults: Understanding its causes and treatments. *Psychiatr Times, 25*(8), 52.

Lavretsky, H. (2008). Geriatric mood disorders: A clinical update. *Psychiatr Times, 25*(8), 36.

Lewandowski, C. A., Rao, C. P., & Silver, B. (2008). Transient ischemic attack: definitions and clinical presentations. *Annals of Emergency Medicine, 52*(2), S7–S16.

Mander, B. A., Rao, V., Lu, B., Saletin, J. M., Lindquist, J. R., Ancoli-Israel, S., ... Walker, M. P. (2013). Prefrontal atrophy, disrupted NREM slow waves and impaired hippocampal-dependent memory in aging. *Nature Neuroscience, 16*(3), 357–364. https://doi.org/10.1038/nn.3324

Maust, D., Cristancho, M., Gray, L., Rushing, S., Tjoa, C., & Thase, E. (2012). Chapter 13 - Psychiatric rating scales. In *Handbook of Clinical Neurology, 106*, 227–237. https://doi.org/10.1016/B978-0-444-52002-9.00013-9.

McNamara, D. (2006b). New schizophrenia scale hailed as more objective. *Clinical Psychiatry News, 34*(8), 9.

Montross, L., Mohamed, S., Kasckow, J., et al. (2003). Preventing late-life suicide: 6 steps to detect the warning signs. *Current Psychiatry, 2*(8), 15.

National Institute of Mental Health (NIMH). (2013). *Older adults: depression and suicide facts.* Retrieved November 17, 2013 from http://www.nimh.nih.gov/publicat/elderlydepsuicide.cfm.

National Institute of Neurological Disorders and Stroke (NINDS). (2013). Retrieved November 17, 2013, from www.ninds.gov/disorders/alzheimersdisease. lewybodydisease; parkinsondisease; stroke.

National Institute on Aging [NIA]. (2012a). *Alzheimer's disease fact sheet.* Retrieved from http://www.nia.nih.gov/alzheimers/publication/alzheimers-disease-fact-sheet. Accessed on May 24, 2014.

National Institute on Aging [NIA]. (2012b). *Preventing Alzheimer's disease: What do we know.* Retrieved May 24, 2014, from http://www.nia.nih.gov/publication/preventing-alzheimers-disease.

National Institute on Aging [NIA]. (2012e). *A good night's sleep.* Retrieved November 17, 2013, from http://www.nia.nih.gov/health/publication/good-nights-sleep.

Neufeld, K. J., Joseph Bienvenu, O., Rosenberg, P. B., Mears, S. C., Lee, H. B., Kamdar, B. B., et al. (2011). The Johns Hopkins Delirium Consortium: A model for collaborating across disciplines and departments for delirium prevention and treatment. *Journal of the American Geriatrics Society, 59*(Suppl 2), S244–S248.

Prince, M., Comas-Herrera, A. C., Knapp, M., Guerchet, M., & Karagiannidou, M. (2016). *World Alzheimer's Report 2016.* London: Alzheimer's Disease International.

Redzic, Z. B., Preston, J. E., Duncan, J. A., et al. (2005). The choroid plexus–cerebrospinal fluid system: From development to aging. *Current Topics in Developmental Biology, 71*, 1–52.

Reeves, R. R., & Brister, J. C. (2008). Psychosis in late life: Emerging issues. *Journal of Psychosocial Nursing and Mental Health Services, 46*(11), 45.

Sangani, A., & Saadabadi, A. (2017). *Neuroleptic medications. StatPearls [Internet].* Retrieved June 12, 2018 from https://www.ncbi.nlm.nih.gov/books/NBK459150/.

Schneck, M. J. (2008). Vascular dementia. *Topics in Stroke Rehabilitation, 15*(1), 22–26.

Singh, D., & O'Connor, D.W. (2009). Efficacy and safety of risperidone long-acting injection in elderly people with schizophrenia. *Clinical Interventions in Aging, 4*, 351–355.

Smith, M., Russell, D., & White, M. (2013). *Alzheimer's behavior problems.* Retrieved from www.helpguide.org/elder/alzheimers_behavior_problems.htm.

Song, J., & Algase, D. (2008). Premorbid characteristics and wandering behavior in persons with dementia. *Archives of Psychiatric Nursing, 22*(6), 318–327.

Span, P. (2013). Suicide rates are high among the elderly. Retrieved March 4, 2018 from https://newoldage.blogs.nytimes.com/2013/08/07/high-suicide-rates-among-the-elderly/.

Sugarman, R. A., & Huether, S. E. (2012). Structure and function of the neurologic system. In S. E. Huether, V. L. Brashers, McCance, & N. S. Rote (Eds.), *Understanding pathophysiology* (5th ed.). St. Louis, MO: Elsevier.

Sullivan, M. G. (2008). Exams differentiate delirium from dementia. *Clinical Psychiatry News, 36*(7), 31.

Tullmann, D. F., Fletcher, K., & Foreman, M. D. (2012). Delirium. In M. Boltz, E. Capezuti, T. Fulmer, & D. Zwicker (Eds.), *Evidence-based geriatric nursing protocols for best practice* (4th ed., pp. 186–199). New York: Springer.

Vahia, I. V., Diwan, S., Bankole, A. O., et al. (2008). Adequacy of medical treatment among older persons with schizophrenia. *Psychiatric Services, 59*(8), 853.

Vance, D. E., Moneyham, L., & Farr, K. F. (2008). Suicidal ideation in adults aging with HIV: Neurological and cognitive considerations. *Journal of Psychosocial Nursing and Mental Health Services, 46*(11), 33.

Waszynski, C. M. (2012). The Confusion Assessment Method (CAM). Retrieved March 4, 2018 from https://consultgeri.org/try-this/general-assessment/issue-13.

World Health Organization (WHO). (2012). Dementia facts and figures. Retrieved October 30, 2013 from http://www.who.int/mediacentre/factsheets/fs362/en/index.html.

Yesavage, J. A., et al. (1983). Development and validation of a geriatric depression screening scale: A preliminary report. *Journal of Psychiatric Research, 17,* 37.

Yohannes, A. M., & Baldwin, R. C. (2008). Late-life depression. *Psychiatr Times, 25*(13), 50.

Zagaria, M. A. (2009). Medication-related problems in seniors: Risk factors and tips for appropriate prescribing. *American Journal for Nurse Practitioners, 13*(3), 23.

Zekry, D. (2009). Is it possible to treat vascular dementia? *Frontiers of Neurology and Neuroscience, 24,* 95–106.

Zwicker, D., & Fulmer, T. (2012). *Medication: Nursing standard of practice protocol: Reducing adverse drug events.* Retrieved October 30, 2013 from http://www.consultgerirn.org/topics/medication/want_to_know_more.

WEBSITES

Alzheimer's Association: https://www.alz.org/.

American Parkinson Disease Association: https://www.apdaparkinson.org/.

Association of Rehabilitation Nurses (ARN): http://www.rehabnurse.org/.

American Stroke Association: http://www.strokeassociation.org/STROKEORG/.

Family Caregiver Alliance: https://www.caregiver.org/.

National Stroke Association: https://www.stroke.org/.

25

Endocrine Function

Mary B. Winton, PhD, RN, ACANP-BC

http://evolve.elsevier.com/Meiner/gerontologic

LEARNING OBJECTIVES

On completion of this chapter, the reader will be able to:

1. Discuss the normal age-related physiologic changes that occur in the endocrine system.
2. Describe the major characteristics of common endocrine disorders: metabolic syndrome, type 2 diabetes mellitus,

hyperthyroidism, hypothyroidism, osteoporosis, and sexual dysfunction.
3. Apply the nursing process for endocrine disorders.

WHAT WOULD YOU DO?

What would you do if you were faced with the following situations?

- A 71-year-old woman presents to the clinic complaining of excessive urination, thirst, and hunger. She is actively involved in the community and eats foods that are easily obtained. She lives alone but has a daughter who lives nearby. What would you do?
- Your 69-year-old patient tells you that lately he has been getting tired easily, has gained some weight despite eating less, and cannot get warm. What would you do?
- One of your patients, a 73-year-old man, is interested in a lady friend and would like to see her more often but is concerned about not being able to "get it up." How would you proceed?

Previously dominated by diabetes and thyroid disease, gerontologic endocrinology has recently been redefining itself through the use of innovative insights developed from the mapping of the human genome (Bergman, Heindel, Kasten et al., 2013). Our knowledge of aging endocrine physiology and genetic influences has begun to grow at a very fast pace. New animal models (Toivonen & Partridge, 2009) and genomic endocrine-related trait studies (Walter, Atzmon, Demerath et al., 2011) have led to a robust subspecialty often referred to as the *endocrinology of aging* (Michael, 2010). Andropause, circadian dysrhythmias, dehydroepiandrosterone (DHEA) replacement, erectile dysfunction (ED), glucagon-like peptide 1 (GLP-1) replacement, male osteoporosis, menopause, metabolic syndrome, and metabolic presbycusis have joined the traditional topics of diabetes and thyroid disease in the newly emerged subspecialty.

The endocrine system is closely connected with the nervous system. When combined, they are referred to as the *neuroendocrine system*. Neuroendocrine aging is discussed in terms of

decreased estrogen production in women (menopause), decreased testosterone production in men (andropause), decreased adrenal function (adrenopause), and decreased growth hormone (GH)–insulin-like growth factor (IGF) (somatopause) (Jones & Boelaert, 2015). Endocrinologic aging involves increased molecular disorderliness of the endocrine regulatory mechanisms that results in reduced vitality of the overall person. This molecular dysregulation of neurohormones from or with the central nervous system (CNS) is one of the earliest measurable characteristics of endocrine aging.

ENDOCRINE PHYSIOLOGY IN OLDER ADULTS

The endocrine system is composed of endocrine glands (without ducts) (Fig. 25.1), which secrete hormones that control numerous processes throughout the body. Table 25.1 outlines the major endocrine glands, their functions, and possible endocrine disorders due to aging. The endocrine system uses a delicate balance of chemical messengers in the bloodstream to maintain homeostasis and regulate mood, growth, organ function, metabolism, nutrition, and sexual activity (Jones & Boelaert, 2015). Dependent on a complex interplay of factors, many hormones are secreted in a cyclic pattern of minutes, hours, days, or months. Feedback control processes (see Fig. 25.2) of these intricate gland–hormone–organ–tissue systems depend on secretion and degradation of hormones classified by chemical structure and cell receptor type (Steil, Palerm, Kurtz et al., 2011). Subtle changes to the endocrine system occur with aging (Veldhuis, 2013) because of reduced production and secretion of hormones, and decreased tissue sensitivity to the hormone's action (Fig. 25.3) (Jones & Boelaert, 2015). Morbidity of the older adult may be attributed more to hormonal imbalance (Jones & Boelaert, 2015). Four basic categories are used to classify endocrine pathology: hyporesponsiveness, hyposecretion, degradation changes, and hypersecretion. The endocrine system is elaborate and

---

Previous authors: Sue E. Meiner, EdD, APRN, BC, GNP, and Jean Benzel-Lindley, PhD, RN.

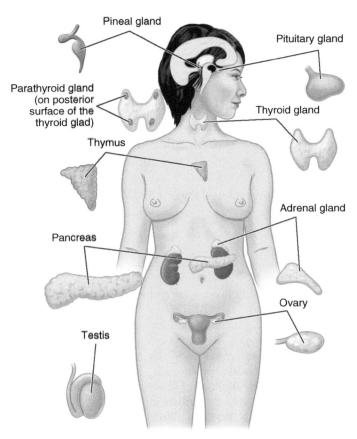

Fig. 25.1 Major endocrine glands. (From Applegate E. [2011]. *The anatomy and physiology learning system* [4th ed.]. St Louis, MO: Saunders.)

TABLE 25.1   Principal Endocrine Glands

Name	Location	Function	Aging Endocrine Disorder
Thyroid	Anterior aspect of neck	Basal metabolic rate, growth, nutrition	Obesity, hyperthyroidism, hypothyroidism, autoimmune thyroiditis, Graves' disease, euthyroid sick syndrome, thyrotoxicosis, thyroid storm, multinodular toxic goiter
Parathyroid	Back of each thyroid	Calcium and phosphorus metabolism, muscular irritability	Osteoporosis, osteomalacia, Paget disease, mineral imbalances (calcium, phosphate, magnesium)
Adrenal cortex	Above each kidney	Carbohydrate metabolism, salt–water balance, some sexual characteristics	Addison disease, Cushing syndrome, dehydration, electrolyte imbalance, acid-base imbalance, infection

Continued

TABLE 25.1   Principal Endocrine Glands—cont'd

Name	Location	Function	Aging Endocrine Disorder
Adrenal medulla	Embedded in kidney, surrounded by adrenal cortex	Sympathetic nervous system, carbohydrate metabolism	Metabolism
Anterior pituitary	Base of brain	Growth, sexual development, skin pigmentation, thyroid function, adrenocortical function (indirectly)	Hypopituitarism causing secondary dysfunction of other endocrine glands
Posterior pituitary	Attached to anterior pituitary	Uterine contraction, water balance	Dehydration, diabetes insipidus, syndrome of inappropriate antidiuretic hormone
Testes	Scrotum	Secondary sexual characteristics and function, metabolism	Andropause
Ovaries	Pelvic cavity	Secondary sexual characteristics and function, metabolism	Andropause, menopause
Pancreas	Abdomen	Sugar metabolism	Hyperglycemia, hypoglycemia, diabetes mellitus
Pineal gland	Center of brain	Daily biologic clocks	Sleep disturbance
Thymus	Chest cavity	Influences immune system response	Immune senescence: reduced response to immunization, cancer, monoclonal gammopathy, increased autoantibodies
Hypothalamus	Brain	Regulates autonomic nervous system; influences hormone production, sleep, and appetite	Kwashiorkor, obesity, hypothermia, hyperthermia, sleep disturbance

Data from Beers, M. H. & Berkow, R. (Eds.). (2014). *Merck manual of geriatrics*. Whitehouse Station, NJ: Merck. Retrieved April 30, 2014, from http://www.merckmanuals.com/professional/geriatrics.html; Copstead, L. E. & Banasik, J. K. (2013). *Pathophysiology* (5th ed.). St, Louis, MO: Elsevier; and Kronenberg, H. M., Melmed, S., Larsen, P R., & Polonsky, K. S. (2016). In S. Melmed, K. S. Polonsky, P. R. Larsen, & H. M. Kronenberg. *Williams textbook of endocrinology* (13th ed). Philadelphia, PA: Elsevier. Retrieved on December 12, 2017, from https://books.google.com/books?id=iPlACwAAQBAJ&pg=PA1237&lpg=PA1237&dq=andropause,+somatopause,+menopause,+adrenopause&source=bl&ots=UmCnwOJxKs&sig=GMPOb6BwUSY8s96DWhpjp7GoFqY&hl=en&sa=X&ved=0ahUKEwjV17Cm5lTYAhVE44MKHRq6A4cQ6AEILjAB#v=onepage&q=andropause%2C%20somatopause%2C%20menopause%2C%20adrenopause&f=false.

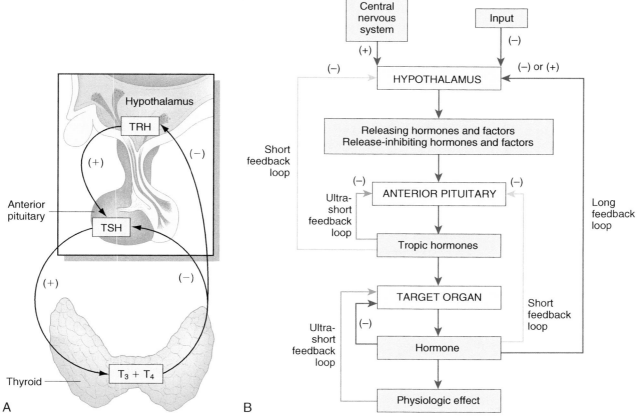

Fig. 25.2 Feedback loops. **A,** Endocrine feedback loops involving the hypothalamus-pituitary gland and end organs; in this example, the thyroid gland is illustrated (endocrine regulation). **B,** General model for control and negative feedback to hypothalamic-pituitary target organ systems. Negative-feedback regulation is possible at three levels: target organ (ultrashort feedback), anterior pituitary (short feedback), and hypothalamus (long feedback). T_3, Triiodothyronine; T_4, tetraiodothyronine (thyroxine), *TRH,* thyroid-releasing hormone; *TSH,* thyroid-stimulating hormone. (From Huether, S. E., & McCance, K. L. [2017]. *Understanding pathophysiology* [6th ed.]. St. Louis, MO: Elsevier.)

increases in complexity with the aging process (Table 25.2). The clinical manifestations due to the imbalance include decreased bone remodeling, decreased lean muscle mass, increased adipose tissue, compromised skin integrity, impaired insulin signaling, and impaired immune response (Jones & Boelarert, 2015). In addition, disease processes may alter the older person in other body systems, such as with the syndrome of inappropriate antidiuretic hormone (SIADH) secretion, which occurs with many types of tumors or infections. Therefore this chapter discusses the typical aging changes of menopause, andropause, adrenopause, and somatopause physiology without discussion of other potential superimposed pathophysiologic states.

Andropause and Menopause

Older men and women experience a decline in the biosynthesis and balance of their sex hormones (andropause) as they age (Jones & Boelaert, 2015). Women experience menopause, a complete cessation of menstruation, due to a dramatic decline in estrogen (Batrinos, 2012). In both genders, the activity of the hypothalamus–anterior pituitary–gonadal (testes and ovaries) axis declines, although the timing is gender-specific

(Lamberts & van den Beld, 2016). Both genders may experience hot flashes, night sweats, depression, and sexual dysfunction in response to age-related declines in androgen or estrogen. In contrast to the previous gender similarities in symptoms, laboratory values to determine the endocrine decline are unique to each sex: luteinizing hormone (LH) and testosterone are of primary importance in men, whereas follicle-stimulating hormone (FSH) and estrogen are of primary importance in women. Hormone replacement (HR) therapy in both genders is a hotly debated topic among health care providers because risks and benefits are unique to each patient. Ongoing debate over whether aging is a disease contributes to the controversy. Those who advocate estrogen and testosterone replacement cite the benefits of improvements in relation to bone density, libido, muscle mass, strength, visuospatial skills, depression, fatigue, hot flashes, irritability, mood, and sleep (Veldhuis, 2013). Testosterone replacement in andropause is complicated by adverse lipid effects, the risk of promoting prostate- and cardiovascular-related adverse events, and the risk of erythrocytosis (Maggio et al., 2015). Menopausal and postmenopausal HR practices continue to change on the basis of larger, more rigorous research studies. The presence

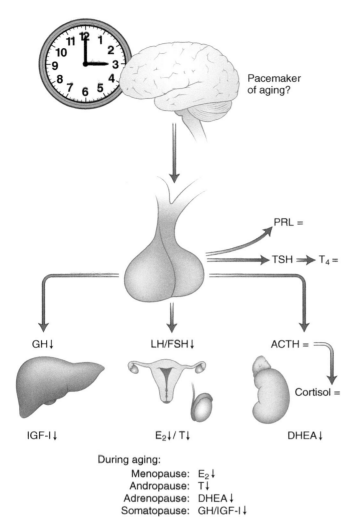

During aging:
Menopause: $E_2 \downarrow$
Andropause: $T \downarrow$
Adrenopause: DHEA $\downarrow$
Somatopause: GH/IGF-I $\downarrow$

Fig. 25.3 During aging, declines in the activities of a number of hormonal systems occur. *Left,* A decrease in growth hormone (GH) release by the pituitary gland causes a decrease in the production of insulin-like growth factor 1 (IGF-1) by the liver and other organs (somatopause). *Middle,* A decrease in release of gonadotropin luteinizing hormone (LH) and follicle-stimulating hormone (FSH) and decreased secretion at the gonadal level (from the ovaries, decreased estradiol [E_2]; from the testicle, decreased testosterone [T]) cause menopause and andropause, respectively. (Immediately after the initiation of menopause, serum LH and FSH levels increase sharply.) *Right,* The adrenocortical cells responsible for the production of dehydroepiandrosterone (DHEA) decrease in activity (adrenopause) without clinically evident changes in corticotropin (adrenocorticotropic hormone, ACTH) and cortisol secretion. A central pacemaker in the hypothalamus or higher brain areas (or both) is hypothesized, which together with changes in the peripheral organs (the ovaries, testicles, and adrenal cortex) regulates the aging process of these endocrine axes. *PRL,* Prolactin; T_4, thyroxine; *TSH,* thyrotropin. (From Melmed, S., Polonsky, K. S., Larson, P. R., & Kronenberg, H. M. [2016]. *Williams textbook of endocrinology* [13th ed.]. Philadelphia, PA: Elsevier.)

or absence of a uterus and ovaries guides clinicians on the types of hormones used in perimenopausal women (Simpson, 2012). The 2002 Women's Health Initiative findings of increased breast cancer, heart disease, stroke, and blood clots from perimenopausal HR have been confirmed (Schierbeck, Rejnmark, Tofteng et al., 2012) and joined by evidence of improved metabolic syndrome indices (Kilic, Yilmaz, Erdogan et al., 2010) and bone health with

phytoestrogen HR (Giroux, Bussières, Bureau, & Rousseau, 2012), brain health (Berent-Spillson, Persad, Love et al., 2010), and weight control. Although many clinicians continue to prescribe HRs, the benefit must outweigh the risks of developing adverse events (Maggio et al., 2015).

Adrenopause

Weighing approximately 4 grams (g), the adrenal glands sit on top of the kidneys and are composed of the adrenal medulla and cortex. The hypothalamic-pituitary-adrenal (HPA) axis regulates the body in response to stress and is important in maintaining homeostasis (Jones & Boelaert, 2015). A total loss of adrenocortical function causes death within days; however, age-related decreases in mineralocorticoids, glucocorticoids, and androgenic hormones manifest changes in body composition, skeletal mass, muscle strength, body weight, and metabolism (Jones & Boelaert, 2015). Age-related decreases in DHEA and aldosterone (Batrinos, 2012) can produce fluid and electrolyte imbalances; impair glucose, protein, and fat metabolisms; and impair immune and inflammatory responses. Other adrenal hormones either increase (epinephrine and norepinephrine) or have minimal change (cortisol) (Morley, 2016). The decline of DHEA with age parallels that of GH, so by age 65 the human body makes only 10% to 20% of what it made at age 20 (Szkrobka, Krysiak, & Okopieri, 2008). These declines closely parallel declines in the GH–IGF-1 axis, a process now referred to as *somatopause.*

Somatopause

Somatopause is often spoken of from a neuroendocrine point of view because certain neurons in the hypothalamus secrete hormones (neurosecretion). Somatopause focuses on the neuron–hypothalamus–pituitary axis and the failure of CNS integration of the endocrine and nervous systems, which causes peripheral endocrine gland insufficiency contributing to a disrupted feedback axis in aging (Di Somma, Brunelli Savanelli, Scarano et al., 2011). Somatotropin (a GH), an anabolic protein, is secreted from the hypothalamus–pituitary axis and influences many age-related changes (Batrinos, 2012). The pituitary gland secretes the GH, which in turn stimulates the liver to secrete insulin-like growth factor I (IGF-I). Current antiaging researchers who believe "you are as young as your oldest part" (Liantonio, Gramegna, Carbonara et al., 2013) have focused on various secretagogue compounds that stimulate pulsatile GH secretion and increase IGF-1 in the older adult to levels approximating those found in young adults.

COMMON ENDOCRINE PATHOPHYSIOLOGY IN OLDER ADULTS

Metabolic Syndrome–Diabetes Continuum

Pathophysiology

Metabolic syndrome is a common multifactorial syndrome of aging due to chronic low inflammation that affects the body and is characterized by central obesity, elevated triglycerides, reduced high-density lipoprotein (HDL) cholesterol, hypertension, and/or hyperglycemia (Bonomini, Rodella, & Rezzani,

TABLE 25.2 Aging Changes in the Endocrine System

Hyporesposiveness	Hyposecretion	Degradation Changes	Hypersecretion
Increased connective tissue, pigment, and structural changes in target tissue	Plasma insulin-like growth factor T_3	Thyroid hormones Cortisol Aldosterone	Norepinephrine Parathyroid hormone Atrial natriuretic peptide
Decreased receptor—ligand binding	Aldosterone Active renin Calcitonin Arginine vasopressin Growth hormone	Inactive to active renin conversion Norepinephrine clearance	Insulin Glucagon

Data from Carpenito-Moyet, L. J. (2013). *Nursing diagnosis: Application to clinical practice* (14th ed.). Philadelphia: Lippincott Williams & Wilkins.

2015). Suspected endocrine influences on the syndrome include corticosteroid axis derangement, polycystic ovary syndrome, and dysglycemia. Recent epidemiologic research has identified, defined, and measured the metabolic syndrome as a significant antecedent to illness trends in diabetes and heart disease in the United States (Chen, Lu, Pang, & Liu, 2013). Insulin resistance causes increased production of inflammatory cytokines correlating with the development of type 2 diabetes mellitus (T2DM) and atherosclerotic vascular disease. The primary risk factors for the syndrome are abdominal obesity, insulin resistance, physical inactivity, and hormonal imbalance (Look AHEAD Research Group et al., 2010). Additionally, some evidence exists for genetic influences through a variety of gene polymorphisms (Dupuis, Langenberg, Prokopenko et al., 2010).

Signs and Symptoms

Metabolic syndrome, according to the revised Adult Treatment Panel-III (ATP-III), is diagnosed when three of the following five criteria are met: obesity (waist circumference >40 inches in men or >35 inches in women), blood pressure >130/85 mm Hg, fasting plasma glucose >100 mg dL, triglyceride >150 mg dL, and HDL cholesterol >40 mg dL in men or <50 mg dL in women (Bonomini, Rodella, & Rezzani, 2015).

Medical Management

The reduction of risk factors for diabetes and atherosclerotic disease are the primary therapeutic objectives in metabolic syndrome (Pattyn, Cornelissen, Eshghi, & Vanhees, 2013). The therapeutic lifestyle changes that will improve all metabolic risk factors are detailed in Box 25.1. Nutritional management for metabolic syndrome should include meticulous attention to the amounts of low-saturated fats, trans fat, cholesterol, and simple sugars. The American Heart Association (AHA) recommends avoiding *trans* fat, reducing saturated fatty acids to 7% of daily caloric intake, reducing total daily sodium intake to be less than 2,300 mg, and increasing physical activity to 40 minutes of moderate to vigorous activity 3 to 4 days per week (Van Horn et al., 2016). A slow, modest weight loss of 7% to 10% of body weight through calorie restriction and physical activity has significant health benefits (Kaur, 2014). When the risk is high, drug therapy for hypertension, elevated low-density lipoprotein cholesterol (LDL-C), and hyperglycemia should be incorporated into the regimen.

Nursing Process Applied to Metabolic Syndrome

The nursing process is applied to the metabolic syndrome by initially focusing on the root causes of improper nutrition and inadequate physical activity, as detailed in Table 25.3.

EVIDENCE-BASED PRACTICE

Chronic Low-Calorie Sweetener Use and Risk of Abdominal Obesity Among Older Adults: A Cohort Study

Sample/Setting

Study sample includes 1454 men and women who were 20 years of age and older at the start of the study in 1958, had at least one Baltimore Longitudinal Study of Aging (BLSA) visit, lived in the community, healthy, and had complete dietary record since 1984.

Methods

An observational continuous-enrollment cohort study was established in 1958, conducted by the National Institute on Aging. Anthroprometric measures, use of low-calorie sweetener, and covariates (age, sex, race, behavioral factors that affect weight, smoking status, dietary intake of specific nutrients (e.g., fat, protein, fiber), quality of diet using Dietary Approaches to Stop Hypertension (DASH) score, and diabetes status from an oral glucose tolerance test were collected and analyzed. Statistical analysis used included marginal structural models to determine the associations of low-calorie sweetener use with body mass index, waist circumference, obesity, and abdominal obesity.

Findings

Participants who used low-calorie sweetener had higher body mass index, larger waist circumference, and higher prevalence and incidence of abdominal obesity than low-calorie sweetener nonusers.

Implications

Use of low-calorie sweeteners may not be an effective means to control weight. The brain does not sense satiety with low-calorie sweeteners. Nonsatiety encourages one to compensate by overeating, which can lead to abdominal obesity. Low-calorie sweeteners implicated in weight gain include saccharin and sucralose. Furthermore, these sweeteners worsen glucose tolerance.

From Chia, C. W., Shardell, M., Tanaka, T., Liu, D. D., Gravenstein, K. S., Simonsick, E. M., ... Ferrucci, L. (2016). Chronic low-calorie sweetener use and risk of abdominal obesity among older adults: A cohort study. *PLOS ONE 11*(11): e0167241. http://doi.dx.org/10.1371/journal.pone.0167241.

BOX 25.1 Steps Every 6 Weeks in Therapeutic Lifestyle Changes

Visit 1: Begin weight reduction, encourage physical activity, refer to dietitian.

Visit 2: Evaluate weight, waist circumference, low-density lipoprotein (LDL), high-density lipoprotein (HDL-C), triglyceride levels, blood pressure, and fasting glucose. Reinforce therapeutic lifestyle changes (TLCs). Consider meal replacements.

Visit 3: Evaluate weight, waist circumference, LDL, HDL-C, triglyceride levels, blood pressure, and fasting glucose. Reinforce TLCs. Consider meal replacements.

Visit 4: Evaluate weight, waist circumference, LDL, HDL-C, triglyceride levels, blood pressure, and fasting glucose. Reinforce TLCs. Consider meal replacements. If no improvement in parameters, consider drug therapy. Intensify weight management and physical activity.

Visit 5: Monitor adherence to TLCs and drugs, if used.

Visit 6: Reevaluate TLCs, and make adjustments to plan, as needed.

Type 2 Diabetes Mellitus

Pathophysiology

Patients with metabolic syndrome have a fivefold increased risk of developing T2DM (Garvey et al., 2014). Metabolically distinct genetic influences play a pivotal role in diabetes among older adults and require a different approach (Cigolle, Lee, Langa et al., 2011). Often starting with metabolic syndrome, the disease ultimately produces dysfunction and failure of various organs such as the heart, kidneys, nerves, eyes, and blood vessels (Grundy, 2009). Age-related changes combine with genetics and lifestyle factors to produce a hyperglycemic state. Current evidence suggests that the hyperglycemia of T2DM is caused by impaired carbohydrate metabolism, changes in pulsatile insulin release, and resistance to insulin-mediated glucose disposal (Kaur, 2014). As with metabolic syndrome, the most important variables associated with T2DM are obesity and insulin

TABLE 25.3 Metabolic Syndrome

Assessment	Diagnosis	Planning	Intervention	Evaluation
Nutrition				
1. Mini Nutritional Assessment 2. Body mass index 3. Overweight: >10% over ideal 4. Obese: >20% over ideal 5. Triceps skin fold: >15 mm in men or >25 mm in women 6. Lifetime weight trends 7. Thyroid function 8. Drugs 9. Nutrition knowledge 10. Cultural issues 11. Comorbidities 12. Drugs 13. Social support network	1. Excessive nutrition	1. Use calorie count and dietary log. 2. Use satiety and emotional scale. 3. Adjust seasonings, as needed. 4. Introduce behavior modification techniques. 5. Provide teaching on drug and dietary recommendations of National Research Council Report for older adults.	1. Review log and weight weekly. 2. Eat only at kitchen table. 3. Drink 8 ounces of water before meal. 4. Limit fat, sweets, and alcohol. Eat low-calorie snacks. 5. Control portions, eat slowly, wait 15 seconds between bites.	1. Patient is able to list dietary rules and reasons. 2. Patient demonstrates slow, steady weight loss toward goal. 3. Patient lists drug effects and dietary implications.
Activity				
1. Respiratory system 2. Cardiovascular system 3. Musculoskeletal system 4. Developmental status 5. Comorbidities 6. Drugs 7. Cultural issues 8. Social support network	1. Reduced stamina 2. Need for health teaching 3. Inadequate coping	1. Accommodate comorbidities, sensory deficits, safety concerns, financial aspects. 2. Address motivation, lifestyle, and environmental barriers. 3. Provide role models and social support. 4. Include aerobic and strength training.	1. Assess resting vital signs and 3 minutes after activity. 2. Reduce intensity or duration of activity if pulse takes longer than 3–4 minutes to return within six beats of baseline. 3. Begin with active range-of-motion exercises twice a day; add isometrics. Gradually increase tolerance from 15 minutes. 4. Provide support, safety, and fall protection. 5. Use personal incentives such as playing with grandchildren, returning to work, or going fishing. 6. Teach primary and secondary prevention related to aging and sensory deficits. 7. Teach stress-related signs and symptoms.	1. Patient will progress to specified activity level. 2. Patient is able to verbalize and engage in health maintenance behaviors. 3. Patient will make decisions and follow through with appropriate actions.

Data from McCuistion, L. E., Vuljoin-DiMaggio, K., Winton, M. B., & Yeager, J. J. (2018). *Pharmacology: A patient-centered nursing process approach* (9th ed.). St. Louis, MO: Elsevier; and Farinde, A. (2015). Oral hypoglycemia agents. *Medscape.* Retrieved on December 18, 2017, from https://emedicine.medscape.com/article/2172160-overview.

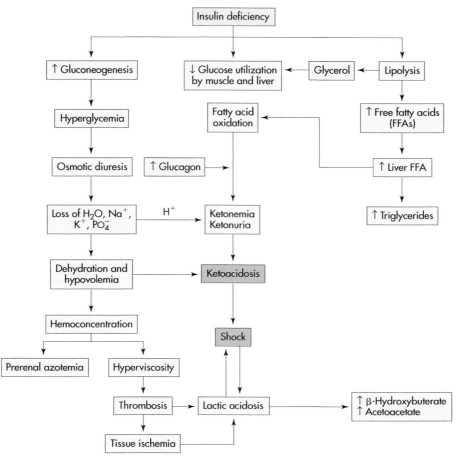

Fig. 25.4 Pathophysiology of insulin deficiency. (From Monahan, F. D., Sands J. K., Neighbors M., Marek, J. F., et al. [2007]. *Phipps' medical-surgical nursing: Health and illness perspectives* [8th ed.]. St. Louis, MO: Mosby.)

resistance. Starting with a compensatory hyperinsulinemia that affects insulin receptors on target tissues, which leads to insulin resistance that produces hyperglycemia, T2DM is a disorder of relative insulin insufficiency. The pathophysiology of T2DM in contrast to type 1 diabetes mellitus (T1DM) involves defects in the cell membrane, receptors, or intracellular pathways (Figs. 25.4 and 25.5).

Signs and Symptoms

Nearly 50% of older adults with diabetes are often undiagnosed (Lamberts & van den Beld, 2016). At the time of diagnosis, T2DM may be associated with symptoms of excessive thirst, hunger, and urination (i.e., polydipsia, polyphagia, and polyuria, respectively). However, older adults with T2DM often do not have classic symptomatology and will not complain of weight loss or fatigue along with these classic symptoms (Rejeski et al., 2012). Instead, they often describe symptoms of fatigue, blurred vision, weight change (gain or loss), and infections (McCulloch & Munshi, 2017). When questioned, older adults often attribute these changes to "aging." Individuals are often diagnosed with diabetes during a concurrent infection such as a major foot or leg wound, vaginitis, or urinary tract infection, or they may present with sexual dysfunction, numbness of the extremities, or changes in vision.

Medical Management

Diabetes management for older adults is similar as that for younger adults. Hypoglycemia should be avoided. The appropriate goal for glycated hemoglobin (A1C) is individualized with the following considerations: (1) the older adult is fit and healthy; (2) the older adult has a life expectancy of over 10 years; (3) risks of hypoglycemia; and (4) the ability for the older adult to follow the treatment regimen (McCulloch & Munshi, 2017). In general, the goal for A1C in the healthy older population should be less than 7.5%; in frail, older adults with comorbidities, the A1C should be less than or equal to 8% (McCulloch & Munshi, 2017).

The risk of hypoglycemia among the older adult is increased. Manifestations of hypoglycemia are often mistaken for other neurologic disorders, such as transient ischemic attacks (McCulloch & Munshi, 2017). A mild hypoglycemic event can lead to falls and fractures. Additionally, episodes of hypoglycemia increase an older adult's risk of cardiovascular events, dysrhythmias, and dementia.

Medical management also includes risk reduction by emphasizing cessation of smoking, controlling hypertension, managing dyslipidemia, promoting exercise, and aspirin therapy (McCulloch & Munshi, 2017). Initial drug therapy among healthy, fit older adults includes metformin along with lifestyle modification. If metformin is contraindicated or the patient is intolerant, then short-acting sulfonylurea (e.g., glipizide)

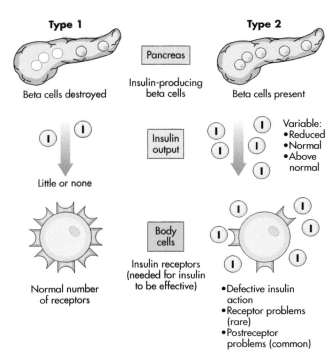

Fig. 25.5 Insulin defects in type 1 and type 2 diabetes mellitus. (From Monahan, F. D., Sands, J. K., Neighbors, M., Marek, J. F., et al. [2007]. *Phipps' medical-surgical nursing: Health and illness perspectives* [8th ed.]. St. Louis, MO: Mosby.)

TABLE 25.4	Oral Antidiabetic Agents
Classification	**Drugs**
Thiazolinediones	Rosiglitazone Pioglitazone
Biguanides	Metformin Metformin extended release
Alpha-glucosidase inhibitors	Acarbose, miglitol
Sulfonylureas	Chlorpropamide (avoid in older adults) Glipizide Glimepiride Glyburide Tolazamide Tolbutamide
Nonsulfonylurea secretagogues	Nateglinide, repaglinide
Fixed-dose combinations	Multiple combination drugs with metformin are available.

Data from McCuistion, L. E., Vuljoin-DiMaggio, K., Winton, M. B., & Yeager, J. J. (2018). *Pharmacology: A patient-centered nursing process approach* (9th ed.). St. Louis, MO: Elsevier.

is recommended. Other drugs that can be used as initial therapy include nonsulfonylurea secretagogues (e.g., repaglinide). Combination antidiabetic drugs may be more beneficial in controlling hyperglycemia than a single drug. Thiazolidinediones is not recommended for older adults due to the risk of fluid retention, weight gain, and increased risks of heart failure. Some oral antidiabetic drugs are listed in Table 25.4; dosages, drug effects, and nursing considerations are provided in Table 25.5. Insulin could be beneficial, especially if the A1C is greater than 9%, fasting plasma glucose is greater than 250 mg/dL, random glucose is consistently greater than 300 mg/dL, or ketonuria is present. Insulin is further discussed later.

NURSING MANAGEMENT

The nursing process in T2DM addresses the core defects of impaired insulin secretion and insulin action, as well as prevention of vascular and microvascular complications of the eyes, heart, kidneys, and feet (see Fig. 25.5). Lifestyle modifications are incorporated into the plan of care based on the older adult's cognitive capacity and functional limitations.

Assessment

Comprehensive nursing assessment of the older adult includes a thorough review of past medical, surgical, and family histories. The nurse should ask the patient about current drugs, particularly diuretics, beta-blockers, anticonvulsants, antihypertensives, and steroids. Patients bringing in their prescription and over-the-counter (OTC) drugs would help the nurse assess for potential problems related to drug interactions or for drugs that alter blood glucose levels.

The nurse should determine the drug's name, type, dose, and schedule; if possible, the nurse should try to observe drug administration. Self-care abilities or restrictions, self-monitoring of blood glucose levels, and any history of hypoglycemia or hyperglycemia should be assessed.

Nutritional assessment includes a current weight measurement and recent patterns of loss or gain, typical dietary patterns, changes in the sense of taste or smell, dentition, and ability to shop for and prepare foods. Because uncontrolled diabetes affects the fluid and food balance, the nurse should assess patients for signs and symptoms of nausea, vomiting, hunger, and thirst, keeping in mind that hyperglycemia may produce subtle symptoms in older adults.

Assessment of elimination in an older adult with diabetes includes obtaining a history of urinary incontinence, urinary frequency, nocturia, polyuria, sexual dysfunction, and pain during urination. The nurse should evaluate for the presence of fecal incontinence, constipation, and diarrhea. Stress incontinence, which is more common in older adults, may be intensified by hyperglycemia.

Assessment of current living conditions is essential. The nurse should ask if the individual lives alone or with others, if living arrangements afford the ability to prepare food, and if adequate financial resources are available for food and shelter. Older adults who live alone may eat little and be malnourished because of social isolation or functional impairments (Nieuwenhuizen, Weenen, Rigby, & Hetherington, 2010). The nurse should determine whether transportation to health care services is available to the older adult patient.

It is important to assess a patient's ability to learn before assessing knowledge of diabetes and its management. Cognitive function and learning styles vary, so knowing the patient's

TABLE 25.5 Common Oral Drugs for Type 2 Diabetes Mellitus

Parameter	Biguanides	Thiazolidinediones (TZDs)	Sulfonylureas	Alpha-glucosidase inhibitors
Mechanism of actions	Decreased hepatic glucose Increased skeletal muscle sensitivity, increased intestinal glucose absorption	Increased insulin sensitivity	Increased insulin secretion Decreased hepatic glucose production	Decreased carbohydrate digestion and absorption from gastrointestinal tract
Glucose effects	Fasting and postprandial	Fasting and postprandial	Fasting and postprandial	Postprandial
Hypoglycemia as monotherapy	Usually not	No	Yes	No
Weight gain	No	Yes	Yes	No
Insulin levels	Decreased	Decreased	Increased	Decreased
Side effects	Gastrointestinal (self-limiting symptoms of nausea, diarrhea, anorexia). Serious effects include lactic acidosis and hepatotoxicity	Swelling and edema; weight gain Serious side effects include heart failure	Potential allergic reaction if patient has sulfa allergy Potential drug interactions (first-generation drugs) Nervousness, tremors, weight gain, and confusion Serious side effects include aplastic anemia, thrombocytopenia, seizures, and coma	Gastrointestinal (flatulence, abdominal distention, diarrhea)
Lipid effects	Decreased	Decreased	Increased or decreased	Decreased
Starting dose for a 70-kg person	Metformin 500 mg/d with evening meal	Varies with each drug: pioglitazone 15 to 30 mg/day in monotherapy rosiglitazone 4 mg/day in monotherapy	Varies with each drug: glyburide 1.25 to 2.5 mg/day with first meal of the day; glyburide, micronized 1.5 to 3 mg/day administered with first meal of the day; glipizide 5 mg/d 30 minutes before meal; glipizide ER 5 mg/d 30 minutes before first meal of the day; glimepiride 1 mg/d	Acarbose 25 mg/tid, with first bite of each meal
Maximum dose	2550 mg/day in divided doses with meals; can be divided	Pioglitazone 45 mg/d; rosiglitazone 8 mg/d, without regard to food	Varies with each agent: glyburide 20 mg/day in single or divided doses; glyburide, micronized 12 mg/d; glipizide 40 mg/d in divided doses; glipizide extended release 20 mg/d with first meal of the day; glimepiride 8 mg/d	150–300 mg/d in divided doses based on weight Must be taken with the first bite of food at each meal
Contraindications	Type 1 diabetes Renal dysfunction Hepatic dysfunction History of alcohol abuse Chronic conditions associated with hypoxia (asthma, chronic obstructive pulmonary disease, HF) Acute conditions associated with potential for hypoxia (surgery, acute myocardial infarction, HF) Situations associated with potential renal dysfunction (e.g., intravenous contrast media) DKA	Type 1 diabetes Class III or IV Heart failure	Type 1 diabetes Hepatic dysfunction Avoid long-acting sulfonylureas to older adults DKA	Type 1 diabetes Inflammatory bowel disease DKA Bowel obstruction Cirrhosis Chronic conditions associated with maldigestion or malabsorption

d, Day; *DKA,* diabetic ketoacidosis; *HF,* heart failure; *kg,* kilogram; *mg,* milligram; *tid,* three times daily.
Data from Carpenito-Moyet, L. J. (2013). *Nursing diagnosis: Application to clinical practice* (14th ed.). Philadelphia: Lippincott Williams & Wilkins; and, McAuley, D.F. (2018). Anti-diabetic agents. Retrieved June 20, 2018 from http://www.globalrph.com/diabetes.htm#Biguanides.

preferred learning style facilitates education. Some individuals prefer to learn by visual methods, others by listening, and still others by experiencing contact in a hands-on approach.

T2DM is associated with increased depression and memory problems in older adults (McCulloch & Munshi, 2017). These problems are often aggravated by uncontrolled diabetes or hyperglycemia. It is important for the nurse to evaluate current and past blood glucose results. The nurse should assess both the older adult's ability to remember simple facts and his or her mood and level of anxiety. For example, the nurse may ask a patient to explain content that was just presented. If the patient cannot recall, the nurse needs to determine whether a learning or memory problem exists. Memory testing may be accomplished simply by asking patients to repeat number sequences or by making a short- or long-term memory assessment. The nurse should ask the older patient about neurologic symptoms such as numbness, tingling, blurred vision, headaches, and the inability to sense temperature, especially in the feet.

The nurse should assess the patient's skin condition, paying particular attention to the skin on the feet, legs, and elbows because these areas are at greatest risk for skin breakdown from pressure. The nurse should assess the skin for intactness, color, presence of swelling, discharge, odor, turgor, dryness, peeling, and lesions. Assessment of the skin in the perianal area may provide information on current skin status and general hygiene practices. Patients with hyperglycemia are prone to yeast and fungal infections in this area. Poor hygiene may predispose an individual to urinary or vaginal infections.

To assess circulation, the nurse should take an apical pulse, noting rate and rhythm; check pedal pulses bilaterally; and note the presence of hair on the lower extremities. The nurse should take blood pressure measurements with the patient in both the recumbent position and the sitting position; note any dizziness associated with a change of position; and assess the respiratory rate, depth, and chest sounds.

Diagnosis

Nursing diagnoses for an older patient with T2DM include the following:

- Inadequate or excessive nutrition resulting from decreased functional capacity, altered taste, and deficient knowledge
- Decreased tissue perfusion, peripheral, resulting from decreased or interrupted arterial flow
- Reduced sexual expression resulting from metabolic alterations
- Inadequate coping resulting from metabolic alteration or feelings of distress
- Need for health teaching resulting from diabetes self-management and skills
- Potential for reduced skin integrity resulting from impaired circulation

Planning and Expected Outcomes

The goal of nursing management for the older adult with diabetes mellitus is the achievement and maintenance of desired blood glucose control, prevention of hypoglycemia and complications, and self-care management, when feasible. Expected outcomes for the plan of care include the following:

1. The patient follows the plan of care by taking action on the basis of professional advice, as evidenced by:
   a. Reports of following the prescribed regimen.
   b. Correct modification of the regimen as directed by a health professional.
   c. Performance of self-screening currently and routinely.
2. The patient shows evidence of successful individual coping, as evidenced by:
   a. Verbalization of a sense of control.
   b. Verbalization of acceptance of the situation.
   c. Use of available social support.
3. The patient demonstrates increased knowledge of the American Diabetes Association (ADA) diet, as evidenced by:
   a. Verbalization of the rationale for a prescribed diet.
   b. Setting of goals for the diet.
   c. Selection of foods recommended in the diet.
4. The patient demonstrates understanding of drug administration, as evidenced by:
   a. Statement of correct drug name, dose, and schedule.
   b. Correct demonstration of drawing up and self-injection of insulin.
   c. Description of side effects of drug.
5. The patient maintains peripheral circulation, as evidenced by:
   a. Pink, warm extremities without lesions or ulcers.
   b. Verbalization of the need for daily skin and extremity inspections.
6. The patient correctly demonstrates foot care regimen of foot cleansing and inspection techniques.
7. The patient verbalizes satisfaction with the degree of sexual functioning and ability.

The family or significant others should be involved in the care planning because they so often provide the support and reinforcement needed for long-term management of such a chronic condition.

Interventions

The nursing care of an older adult patient with T2DM is often complex. Usually, many issues must be dealt with; therefore it is important to prioritize problems. In general, emergent issues or life-threatening crises such as severe hyperglycemia, hypoglycemia, and sepsis are top priorities. Once crises are resolved, the nurse may provide education to support diabetes management.

Education

The nurse provides or coordinates education on a variety of recommended diabetic topics such as drug, pathophysiology of diabetes, monitoring of blood glucose levels, hypoglycemia and hyperglycemia, sick day management, foot care, eye care, complications, the diabetic diet, product supplies, and instructions on when to contact the health care team. Teaching is facilitated if older patients and significant others are actively involved in learning (e.g., having patients demonstrate glucose monitoring or insulin injection techniques to the nurse). Teaching aids such as booklets and handouts may enhance learning. Resources for patient educational handouts may be obtained from the American Dietetic Association (ADA), the National Diabetes Information Clearinghouse, and commercial sources.

Diet

Although diet is the cornerstone of therapy for diabetes, it may be difficult to persuade an older adult to change his or her dietary pattern. Other factors that may affect dietary adherence include limited finances, social isolation, and lack of motivation (Wood, 2017). Dietary planning with a registered dietitian may be helpful in achieving dietary goals. Dietary goals include achieving good nutrition and reaching or maintaining ideal body weight while decreasing the risk of hyperlipidemia, atherosclerosis, and hypertension. When a diet plan is established, nursing interventions are directed at supporting the dietitian's recommendations through assessment of the patient's understanding of and adherence to the plan (see Nutritional Considerations box).

NUTRITIONAL CONSIDERATIONS

Nutritional Goals for Patients With Diabetes Mellitus

Calories
Based on achievement and maintenance of ideal body weight

Protein
Approximately 12% to 20% of total calories
Recommended daily allowance: 0.8 grams per kilogram (g/kg) of body weight for adults. (Most adults consume twice the amount of protein needed.)

Carbohydrates
Approximately 45% to 60% of total calories
Emphasis placed on total carbohydrate intake rather than eliminating simple sugars
Modest sucrose intake perhaps acceptable based on metabolic control
Consistent mealtime carbohydrate intake

Fats
No more than 30% of total calories
May need further reduction depending on lipid profile
Polyunsaturated fats: 6% to 8%
Saturated fats: 10%
Monounsaturated fats: remaining percentage

Fiber
25 g per 1000 kilocalories (kcal) for low-calorie intake
Up to 40 g/day

Sodium
3000 milligrams per day (mg/day) or less
May be reduced for medical conditions such as hypertension, congestive heart failure, and edema

Vitamins and Minerals
No specific recommendations

From Muñoz-Pareja, M., León-Muñoz, L., Guallar-Castillón, P., Graciani, A., López-García, E., Banegas, J., & Rodríguez-Artalejo, F. (2012). The diet of diabetic patients in Spain in 2008 to 2010: Accordance with the main dietary recommendations—a cross-sectional study. *PLOS One, 7*(6), e39454.

Insulin and Oral Hypoglycemic Drugs

Simple is better when treating older adults to reduce the risk of hypoglycemic events. The ability for the older adult to self-manage (e.g., cognitive function) should be considered before initiating insulin. Many older patients have difficulty in managing frequent glucose testings and insulin injections (ADA, 2018). Insulin therapy requires the older patient or their caregiver to give the insulin; therefore either the patient or the caregiver should have adequate visual, motor, and cognitive skills to properly administer the drug (ADA, 2018). Insulin doses should be individualized, and hypoglycemia should be avoided. Once-daily basal insulin is usually best and with minimal side effects (ADA, 2018). Written instructions about the drug regimen should be provided for a patient and his or her significant other.

The nurse should observe the patient and his or her significant other preparing the prescribed insulin dosages; observe the patient actually injecting insulin; and note if the patient draws up an accurate amount of insulin, injects it into an appropriate site, and discards the sharp needle in a puncture-proof container. Vision or manual dexterity problems common among older adults, which may interfere with proper insulin delivery, may be identified through observation. The patient's physician should be notified of visual concerns to obtain appropriate medical equipment for visually impaired persons.

Older patients may require two insulin injections a day to adequately control blood glucose levels. Splitting the intermediate insulin dose or adding short-acting insulin may help prevent hypoglycemia and offer flexibility for older adults with eating pattern variations or decreased renal function. Home care or visiting nurse services may be useful to older adults in the initial phases of insulin therapy (Farmer, Hardeman, Hughes et al., 2012).

Because hypoglycemia is the major complication of insulin and oral hypoglycemic therapy, patients should be instructed about this complication. Oral drugs are associated with other adverse effects such as rashes, itching, nausea, vomiting, liver damage, and increased urinary frequency and urgency. Routine medical visits that include laboratory testing for complications are important. Patients taking drugs that lower glucose levels should recognize the symptoms of mild hypoglycemia and test their blood glucose accordingly; if the result is abnormal, they should ingest a source of rapid-acting carbohydrate such as 4 ounces of orange juice. The early recognition and treatment of mild hypoglycemia prevents the more serious neuroglycopenic symptoms associated with moderate and severe hypoglycemia. Unrecognized and untreated hypoglycemia puts an individual with diabetes at risk for seizures and even death.

Emergency Identification

Patients should be advised to carry medical emergency identification. In the event that an individual who takes oral hypoglycemic experiences a major complication such as severe hypoglycemia, medical emergency identification facilitates treatment of the condition by health care workers or others (Table 25.6).

Monitoring

Monitoring the blood glucose level is recommended for older patients with T2DM because they tend to have higher renal thresholds. Blood glucose monitoring is used to achieve

TABLE 25.6   Hypoglycemia Levels, Symptoms, and Treatment

Hypoglycemia Level	Symptoms	Treatment
Mild	Hunger, diaphoresis, nervousness, shakiness, tachycardia, and pale skin	15 grams (g) of carbohydrate 4 ounces (oz) of juice (no sugar added)
Moderate	Headache, irritability, fatigue, blurred vision, and mood changes	15 g of carbohydrate; may repeat
Severe	Unresponsiveness, confusion, coma, and convulsions	Glucagon; intravenous glucose

Data from Carpenito-Moyet, L. J. (2013). *Nursing diagnosis: Application to clinical practice* (14th ed.). Philadelphia: Lippincott Williams & Wilkins.

and maintain desired glucose goals; detect complications such as hyperglycemia and hypoglycemia; and educate patients about the effects of diet, drugs, activity, and stress (Mbaezue, Mayberry, Gazmararian et al., 2010). Blood glucose monitoring is particularly important for individuals taking drugs that lower blood glucose levels (e.g., oral hypoglycemics and insulin). Glucose monitoring devices are generally easy to use and reliable; however, practicing the glucose-monitoring technique is important for ensuring the accuracy of test results.

Exercise

Exercise is a strategy for decreasing insulin resistance and hyperglycemia. It is beneficial for older adults from both physiologic and psychological perspectives. The assumption that older persons are not physically capable of or willing to exercise may result in neglect of this important aspect of care. Once the patient's capabilities and limitations are considered, an exercise program is personalized to the patient. Teaching topics should include the safety rules of exercising, which include wearing a medical alert bracelet, checking blood glucose before exercise, identifying signs and symptoms of hypoglycemia, carrying a source of carbohydrate, and avoiding dehydration. Exercise-related complications or injuries are more likely to occur in this population as a result of preexisting conditions such as cardiac, musculoskeletal, and ophthalmic diseases. Precautions and exercise modifications for older adults are therefore indicated to help prevent problems.

Lifestyle Changes

Lifestyle changes are often required for individuals with diabetes. It is difficult to manage a chronic illness that affects diet, exercise, weight, drug, sexuality, and finances. Proper management of diabetes requires knowledge, skills, and the organization of a team of experts that includes the patient as the core of the team. Avoidance of smoking and alcohol is believed to improve diabetes management. An older patient's ability to adapt to lifestyle changes needs to be evaluated frequently so that additional support can be provided, when needed.

Sick Day Management

Older adults have a high incidence of chronic illness, and those with diabetes need to take special measures for "sick days." *Sick days* are generally defined as illness days that necessitate an alteration of typical treatment strategies (e.g., increasing drugs [insulin doses], meals, and fluids) or the initiation of medical interventions (e.g., antibiotics for infections). For example, when an individual with diabetes becomes ill with "stomach flu," the stress of even this common illness may precipitate severe hyperglycemia. The individual may detect significant hyperglycemia during routine blood glucose testing and should contact the health care provider for specific instructions on how to increase the insulin dosage. Individuals with nausea and vomiting are generally instructed to take 8 ounces of fluids (nondiet beverages) hourly and increase monitoring of blood glucose levels. Instructions from the provider usually indicate the levels of blood glucose that require an immediate call to the provider or a visit to the emergency department (see Emergency Treatment box).

✚ EMERGENCY TREATMENT

Sick Day Management for the Individual With Diabetes Mellitus

The term "sick days" refers to episodes of acute illness in individuals with diabetes, involving complications such as nausea, vomiting, and diarrhea. Illnesses trigger stress hormone production and result in hyperglycemia. With the onset of gastrointestinal symptoms, individuals with diabetes become easily dehydrated. If the patient's meal plan cannot be tolerated, easily digested foods such as plain soda, soups, popsicles, and crackers are taken instead. This diet may be supplemented with noncaloric liquids such as water or diet sodas to keep up with fluids lost from vomiting or diarrhea.

Individuals with diabetes must continue taking prescribed drugs such as insulin or oral hypoglycemic agents, ensure adequate hydration, and test blood more often. Urine should be tested for ketones whenever the blood glucose level is greater than 240 milligrams per deciliter (mg/dL). Other recommendations include taking temperature and weight, and recording all values and interventions. Patients with diabetes should contact their health care provider whenever they have questions or concerns or the treatment regimen is not working, as evidenced by worsening fever, decreasing alertness or ability to think, vomiting more than once, diarrhea that persists for 6 or more hours, blood glucose values of 250 mg/dL or greater despite additional insulin, or ketones in urine.

Sick day management is important in individuals with T2DM because an untreated illness may lead to a complication called *hyperglycemic hyperosmolar nonketotic coma* (HHNC). This hyperglycemic condition is more common in older patients with T2DM, whereas patients with T1DM are more likely to experience diabetic ketoacidosis. HHNC is characterized by severe dehydration and hyperglycemia (blood glucose values ≥600 mg/dL; and hyperosmolarity of blood: ≥340 milliosmoles per liter [mOsm/L] of water]). Treatment for this condition consists of insulin, intravenous fluids, and identification and treatment of the precipitating event (e.g., infection or cardiovascular problems) in the intensive care setting of a hospital.

Skin Alterations

Lower extremity amputations are a common yet preventable problem for individuals with diabetes. About 50% to 70% of all foot amputations are performed on individuals with

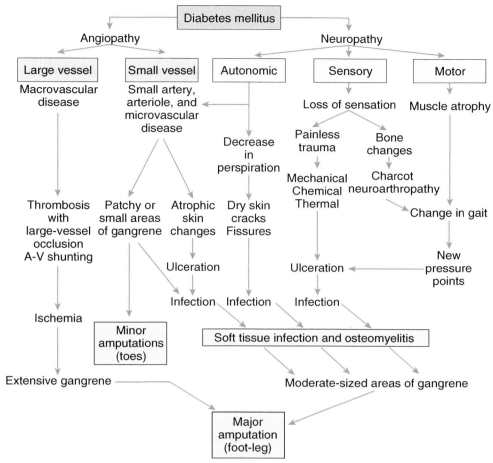

Fig. 25.6 How foot lesions of diabetes can lead to amputation. (From Levin, M. E., O'Neal, L. W., & Bowker, J. H. [1993]. *The diabetic foot* [5th ed.]. St. Louis, MO: Mosby.)

diabetes (Fig. 25.6). Prevention of foot ulcers is the key to proper foot management in older patients with diabetes. This is achieved through daily cleansing of the feet with nondrying agents, inspection of the feet, and prompt treatment of problems (see Patient/Family Teaching box). When older adult patients are unable to inspect their own feet because of mobility or vision problems, significant others should be taught how to perform thorough inspections.

👥 PATIENT/FAMILY TEACHING

Prevention of Foot Ulcers in Individuals With Diabetes Mellitus

Perform daily foot inspection.

Perform daily foot hygiene using warm (not hot) soapy water to wash feet; pat feet dry.

Gently apply mild skin cream to feet if dry or rough; do not apply between toes.

Keep toenails trimmed straight across.

Wear proper-fitting shoes, and do not go barefoot.

Break in new shoes gradually.

Do not wear tight shoes or stockings that bind.

Exercise regularly and maintain ideal body weight.

Avoid smoking because it impairs circulation to the feet.

Seek early interventions to problems (e.g., tenderness, redness, swelling, leakage of fluid).

Foot care is the same for older adults as for other persons with diabetes. Daily inspection and cleansing of feet with nondrying agents is important to eliminate potential infectious organisms. Lubrication of the feet (but not between the toes, where heat and lotions may be trapped and lead to infections) with unscented lotions is often needed to help decrease skin dryness and cracking. Appliances such as corn pads and drying agents such as alcohol should be avoided because they impair the integrity of the skin. Shoes need to be tested for good fit. Patients or caretakers should cut nails straight across to prevent complications. Individuals with diabetes who have foot neuropathy, significant hyperglycemia (blood glucose values of ≥250 mg/dL), or a history of foot infections should seek care at the first sign of a foot wound or infection.

Wound Infections

Older adults with diabetes are at a higher risk for foot complications than those without diabetes because of changes in nerves and blood vessels. Because these foot problems are common, the phrase *diabetic foot syndrome* has come into use to describe the vascular and neurologic pathology associated with diabetes. Inadequate blood flow to the feet and nerve damage contribute to the development of ulcers and infections. Hyperglycemia also plays a role in foot problems because blood glucose levels of 200 mg/dL or greater are associated with an altered immune system leukocytic response.

The clinical symptoms of foot infections vary from no symptoms to fever, erythema, warmth, discharge with ulceration, and leukocytosis (Peters, Lipsky, Berendt et al., 2012). The skin over and around the infection may appear to be white, pink, red, or shades of blue. Blood vessels may be distended and pronounced over the infection site. Nail beds may be pale and show slowed capillary refilling when pressed. The shape of the foot may be altered by infection as a result of significant soft tissue swelling. Superficial inspection of a lesion may be deceptive because the outside appearance often does not reflect the extent of the problem beneath the skin surface. Wound infections in older adults with diabetes are common and are serious events that require immediate attention. Infections may manifest symptoms such as pain, swelling, and redness, or may be symptom-free and remain undetected until they are at an advanced stage. Significant delays may occur before the health care provider is contacted and treatment is initiated, and infection may spread from the skin to fat, muscle, fascia, and bone.

Evaluation

The nurse evaluates the effectiveness of the care plan for an older patient with diabetes by frequently measuring the achievement of established specific outcomes. For example, nutritional outcomes include food selection consistent with the prescribed meal plan. Achievement of weight change goals is measured over time with weight graphs. The patient may be asked to log his or her exercise and drug compliance to enable monitoring of progress with each activity.

Insulin injection site rotations may be tracked on a chart. The patient logs blood glucose values, which are then compared with corresponding laboratory results. Patients are examined to see whether they are wearing or carrying medical alert bracelets or other emergency information. Patients may be asked to review their recent experiences with sick days and their management of fluids, nausea, vomiting, drug, and testing.

An important principle of diabetes management is having the patient "take control" of the diabetes. Self-care activities such as daily inspection of the feet and basic diabetic foot care support this self-care approach. The nurse may help a patient evaluate the effectiveness of self-care activities by direct examination and through interview techniques.

The nurse should positively reinforce effective diabetes management strategies used by an older patient. For example, when an older patient improves in foot care or the technique for insulin injections, the nurse needs to acknowledge the patient's skill. If a patient does not comply with management strategies, the situation needs to be reassessed so that adaptations can be made. An older patient may have cognitive, financial, or social support problems that are obstacles to compliance.

Documentation of assessments—including patient responses to treatment measures, patient comprehension of teaching, and patient ability to self-manage treatment measures and diet, as well as other nursing interventions—is an essential component of care for older adult patients with diabetes.

Hyperthyroidism
Pathophysiology

Primary hyperthyroidism involves hypersecretion (hyperfunctioning) of thyroid hormones, which is usually associated with an enlarged thyroid gland. Although aging causes slight decreases in thyrotropin-releasing hormone synthesis from the hypothalamus and free triiodothyronine (T_3), neither of these changes leads to thyroid-stimulating hormone (TSH) values outside the normal range (Suzuki, Nishio, Takeda, & Komatsu, 2012). Recently new data have confirmed original 1985 Framingham study estimates of hyperthyroidism incidence of 2.5% to 6% in the geriatric population, depending on the indigenous iodine supply. Hyperthyroidism in seniors is often caused by multinodular and uninodular toxic goiter rather than Graves' disease, which is the most common cause in younger adults (De Groot, 2013). Thyroid nodules are identified in 5% of people older than age 60, and 90% of nodules are benign (Fig. 25.7). Iodine-induced hyperthyroidism is another common type of hyperthyroidism among older patients using amiodarone, a cardiac drug containing iodine, which deposits in tissue and delivers iodine to the circulation over long periods.

Subclinical hyperthyroidism, a condition in which an otherwise healthy, asymptomatic patient has a suppressed serum TSH level with normal thyroxine (T_4) and T_3 levels, has been associated with an increased incidence of atrial fibrillation and decreased bone mineral density. *Thyroid storm,* or thyrotoxic crisis, is a life-threatening syndrome consisting of fever, severe tachycardia, altered mental status, dehydration, and irritability. It is most commonly seen in persons with Graves' disease, but it may result from other causes of hyperthyroidism. It may be precipitated by a concurrent illness, withdrawal from antithyroid drugs, toxic nodular hyperthyroidism, or treatment with radioactive iodine (Jones & Boelaert, 2015).

Signs and Symptoms

The classic presentation in older adults includes tachycardia, fatigue, tremors, and nervousness in contrast to tachycardia, heat intolerance, and fatigue in younger patients (Hampton, 2013). An enlarged, palpable goiter is present in 60% of older adults with hyperthyroidism. The most common complication, occurring in 27% of hyperthyroidism in older adult patients, is atrial fibrillation that does not convert back to sinus rhythm when an euthyroid state is achieved.

Medical Management

Untreated hyperthyroidism increases risks of heart failure, bone fractures, and cardiovascular events among older adults (Veldhuis, 2013). Treatment for hyperthyroidism includes antithyroid drugs and radioactive iodine (ATA, 2017). Rarely is surgical intervention required due to the risk of surgery to older adults. Adjunctive treatment, such as with beta-adrenergic blockers, can slow the heart rate of tachycardia.

NURSING MANAGEMENT

Assessment, diagnosis, planning, intervention, and evaluation for hyperthyroidism focus on the primary human response to the hypersecretion of thyroid hormone, as detailed in Table 25.7.

NURSING CARE PLAN
Diabetes Mellitus With Foot Infection

Clinical Situation

Mr. J notices that his right foot aches slightly. Taking off his shoe, he can see that his foot is red and swollen with a small amount of purulent fluid draining from a lesion on his small toe. He can even see the indentations from his shoes on the skin of his feet. He is surprised that his foot looks this bad when he had no problems earlier. He makes an appointment with his primary care provider. The appointment is 2 days after he first noticed the problem. During those 2 days, Mr. J becomes increasingly tired. Despite drinking fluids continuously, he is thirsty all the time. At the visit with his physician, Mr. J is found to have 3+ edema in the affected foot, temperature of 101° F, and blood glucose level of 250 milligrams per deciliter (mg/dL). He is diagnosed with a diabetic foot infection. Mr. J first learns of his diagnosis of diabetes mellitus at this time.

The physician sends Mr. J to the local community hospital for inpatient admission. Hospitalization is necessary to treat the foot infection and his newly diagnosed diabetes.

Nursing Diagnoses

Reduced skin integrity resulting from compromised innate defense (skin)

Pain resulting from treatments for foot ulcer (e.g., biopsy, curettage, and débridement)

Need for health teaching resulting from new experience with recently diagnosed diabetes mellitus

Need for patient teaching resulting from new experience with foot care management

Outcomes

Wound healing will occur, as demonstrated by decreasing size of wound and less purulent drainage, as well as laboratory values of complete blood cell count with differential and electrolytes within normal limits.

Circulation to affected area will be maintained, as evidenced by normal skin color and temperature, presence of pedal pulses, and no evidence of edema.

The patient will verbalize comfort after débridement procedures.

The patient will maintain stable vital signs before, during, and after the procedure.

The patient will verbalize and demonstrate understanding of diabetes and diabetes management, as evidenced by making appropriate diet selections, correctly and safely administering drugs, and accurately testing his blood glucose level.

The patient will verbalize appropriate sick day management regimen.

The patient will demonstrate daily foot care regimen of inspecting, cleansing, and using emollients.

The patient will verbalize when to contact a physician if complications occur.

The patient will achieve an optimal level of physical mobility, as evidenced by the ability to safely meet self-care needs.

The patient will protect the affected extremity, as evidenced by the ability to adhere to weight-bearing restriction.

The patient will verbalize reduced levels of anxiety with increasing knowledge and skill acquisition.

Interventions

Assess the wound at each dressing change for wound stage, epithelialization, color, edema, and discharge.

Assess vital signs.

Administer antibiotics, as prescribed.

Administer physician-ordered intravenous fluids, insulin, and drugs.

Notify the health care provider of signs and symptoms of increased pain, swelling, drainage, or fever.

Change linens, as needed, to maintain a clean wound environment.

Provide pain control during débridement by medicating before procedures.

Assess patient's vital signs and level of consciousness before administering drugs.

Assess pain level, vital signs, and level of comfort and sedation after drug.

Document the patient's tolerance of the procedure.

Assess patient understanding of the condition.

Monitor readiness and determine best methods for teaching and learning.

Provide patient information on diabetes over span of his hospitalization, including topics such as T2DM; ADA diet; exercise; drugs; sick day management; monitoring; lifestyle factors (e.g., smoking and alcohol); complications, especially of hypoglycemia and hyperglycemia; and eye, kidney, nerve, foot, and vessel problems.

Provide proper foot care teaching with demonstration, including topics such as daily inspection and cleansing, wearing shoes, avoidance of tape and drying chemicals, use of proper foot gear, applying emollients, keeping feet dry, and safe nail cutting.

Have the patient perform a return demonstration.

Instruct the patient on reportable signs and symptoms such as fever, pain, swelling, redness, and breaks in skin integrity.

Instruct the patient not to bear weight on the infected foot.

Set up the room to maximize patient independence in ADLs.

Assess the patient's mood and coping mechanisms.

Allow the patient to verbalize feelings about the diagnosis of the chronic disease of diabetes.

Support the patient in self-care and management of diabetes by (1) encouraging involvement in self-care activities, (2) providing an environment conducive to relaxation, and (3) reassuring the patient when he safely or accurately performs self-care skills and techniques.

Hypothyroidism

Pathophysiology

A common *hypofunctioning* endocrine state that results from inadequate thyroid hormone function is hypothyroidism. Diagnosis is based on sensitive, reliable assays of serum TSH and T_4 levels. The most sensitive indication of hypothyroidism caused by *primary* thyroid gland failure is an elevation of the serum TSH level. The most specific test finding is a subnormal serum-free T_4 level because it corrects for abnormalities in the T_4-binding proteins. As the thyroid gland ages, it develops moderate atrophy, fibrosis, colloid nodules, and lymphocyte infiltration (Garg & Vanderpump, 2013). The production of T_4 decreases by about 30% between young adulthood and advanced age, but serum levels are usually maintained because of the body's decreased use of T_4 as a correlate to the age-related decline in lean body mass. Hypofunctioning thyroid states may result from defects in hormone production, target tissues, or receptors. When the defect involves a hypofunctioning peripheral gland like the thyroid, it is called *primary hypothyroidism*. If the hypothyroid state is a result of a nonfunctional anterior pituitary gland, the condition is called *secondary* hypothyroidism. *Tertiary* hypothyroidism results from a defect in the hypothalamus.

Autoimmune thyroiditis is the most common cause of primary hypothyroidism in older persons. It is diagnosed in 5% of older women and in 2% of men of the same age. *Drug-induced*

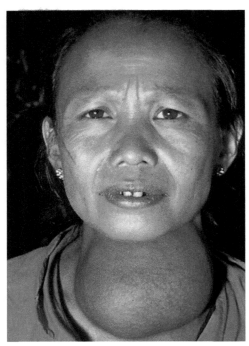

Fig. 25.7 Simple goiter. (Courtesy of Bergman, L.V. and Associates, Cold Spring, NY.)

hypothyroidism may occur with the use of lithium carbonate, amiodarone, and iodine. Other causes of hypothyroidism include ablation of the thyroid gland with radioiodine or surgery for the treatment of hyperthyroidism and postsurgical or radiation treatment of head and neck cancer. Hypothalamic or pituitary problems are rarely originating causes (Schlumberger et al., 2012).

Signs and Symptoms

The clinical symptoms of hypothyroidism in older people are atypical compared with those of younger adults. Almost all cases (99%) of hypothyroidism in older adults are subclinical, inconspicuous, and progress slowly toward thyroid failure. Because the condition is insidious, the symptoms are often attributed to old age. Older patients are seen with complaints of fatigue, cold intolerance, weight gain, muscle cramps, paresthesia, and confusion (ATA, 2017) (Table 25.8).

Medical Management

Treatment for hypothyroidism includes pure synthetic thyroxine (e.g., levothyroxine) which is instituted slowly so as not to place undue stress on the heart and the nervous system (ATA, 2017). The usual starting dose is at 25 micrograms per day. The drug is increased every 4 to 6 weeks until the serum levels of T_4 and TSH are within the normal range. For older adults without underlying cardiovascular or CNS disease, the initial dose may be higher.

NURSING MANAGEMENT

Assessment, diagnosis, planning, intervention, and evaluation for hypothyroidism focus on the human age-related response to the core defect of decreased thyroid hormone, as detailed in Table 25.8.

Primary Osteoporosis
Pathophysiology

Osteoporosis is a legitimate concern in postmenopausal women and andropausal men because of the influence of systemic sex hormones on bone (Eastell, 2013). Found six times more

---

TABLE 25.7   Hyperthyroidism

Assessment	Diagnosis	Planning	Intervention	Evaluation
1. Weight loss trends over 3 and 6 months 2. Body mass index 3. Serum albumin and thyroid-stimulating hormone 4. Mini Nutritional Assessment 5. Mini-Mental State Examination 6. Dysphagia 7. Manual dexterity 8. Financial resources 9. Dentition 10. Comorbidities 11. Drugs 12. Social support 13. Cultural influences 14. Tachycardia, defined as >90 beats per minute (beats/min) 15. Fatigue	1. Inadequate nutrition 2. Potential for reduced cardiac tissue perfusion 3. Fatigue	1. Teach disease, treatment and monitoring. 2. Teach dietary recommendations of the National Research Council Report for those older than 65 years. 3. Add 250- to 300-calorie snacks to increase body weight slowly. 4. Refer to Meals on Wheels, consultations, or other community resources as needed. 5. Monitor cardiovascular status.	1. Explain hyperthyroidism, complications, testing techniques, activity restrictions, dietary measures, drugs, radioactive iodine therapy (if needed), surgery (if needed), eye care for exophthalmos (if needed). 2. Facilitate specific meal plans, procurement, preparation, and social support. 3. Monitor for pulse rate <90 beats/min, respiratory rate <22 breaths per minute, normal blood pressure, bibasilar crackles, decreased urine output, pigmentation changes, cool or mottled skin, distended neck veins, decreased saturation of arterial oxygen (Sao_2).	1. Patient will increase intake as evidenced by gradual weight gain to normal range of body mass index. 2. Patient will maintain adequate cardiac output.

Data from Carpenito-Moyet, L. J. (2013). *Nursing diagnosis: Application to clinical practice* (14th ed.). Philadelphia: Lippincott Williams & Wilkins.

TABLE 25.8	**Hypothyroidism**			
Assessment	**Diagnosis**	**Planning**	**Intervention**	**Evaluation**
1. Fatigue on a scale of 1–10 2. Onset, pattern, and aggravating and relieving factors of fatigue 3. Effects of fatigue on activities of daily living (ADLs), instrumental ADLs (IADLs), mood, accident proneness, concentration, motivation, leisure activities, and libido 4. Depression Scale 5. Mini-Mental State Examination 6. Laboratory values of thyroid-stimulating hormone, hemoglobin, and hematocrit 7. Comorbidities 8. Drugs 9. Social support network 10. Weight as detailed in Table 25.3	1. Fatigue	1. Identify patient's energy patterns and teach energy conservation. 2. Facilitate prioritization and delegation of tasks. 3. Teach disease pathophysiology, drug management, and monitoring. 4. Facilitate appropriate community and financial resource use.	1. Explain patient's type of hypothyroidism, symptoms, complications, diagnostic tests, activity restrictions, dietary guidelines, lifelong therapy, and symptoms of accidental thyroid hormone overdose. 2. Work with patient to target ADLs and IADLs for patient performance, health care surrogate, and community services assistance.	1. Patient will achieve a balance of activity and rest. 2. Patient can verbalize pathophysiology, drug use, and monitoring required.

Data from Carpenito-Moyet, L. J. (2013). *Nursing diagnosis: Application to clinical practice* (14th ed.). Philadelphia: Lippincott Williams & Wilkins.

frequently in women, osteoporosis is a disease characterized by low bone mass leading to fragile bones that break easily. The geriatric skeleton is a metabolically active organ that experiences continuous remodeling, which provides structural integrity, support to the body, protection of vital organs, and a reservoir of calcium and other minerals (Griffith & Bao, 2013). Low bone mass may result from a failure to reach peak bone mass as a young adult, increased bone resorption, or decreased bone formation; all three of these mechanisms are believed to play a role in osteoporosis in today's older adults.

Genetic influences on osteoblast function have recently improved our understanding of osteoporosis pathogenesis. Researchers have suggested that 50% to 80% of peak bone mass is genetically determined, which supports the importance of family history in determining an individual's risk.

Hypersecretion of parathyroid hormone has also been shown to increase skeletal resorption in estrogen-deficient menopausal women; this same mechanism is believed to influence male osteoporosis (ATA, 2017). In addition, low vitamin D status in older persons contributes to bone loss mediated by the aging parathyroid gland, low daily exposure to natural sunlight, and reduced dietary intake. The primary role of calcium alone in maintaining bone mass in older persons continues to spur controversy. Osteopenia precedes osteoporosis, which is defined as bone mass less than 2.5 standard deviations below that of a young control population. Osteoporosis generally occurs in those in the sixth decade or older. Divided into primary and secondary types based on etiology, osteoporosis involves both the appendicular and axial skeleton. Other endocrine disorders such as parathyroid disease, Cushing syndrome, hypogonadism, alcohol abuse, liver disease, and amenorrhea may cause secondary osteoporosis. Osteoporosis is diagnosed by dual x-ray absorptiometry (DEXA) of the proximal femur and lumbar spine because these scans are sensitive to subtle changes in mineral density.

Signs and Symptoms

Spontaneous fractures or those caused by minimum trauma in addition to loss of height necessitate DEXA scanning in older patients because of the high incidence of occult osteoporosis. Because of its low cost and portability, ultrasonographic densitometry is frequently used on the heel; however, it is not considered as reliable as DEXA scanning. A history of fractures after age 40, family history of osteoporosis, cigarette smoking, and low body mass index have all been shown to correlate strongly with osteoporosis. Dorsal kyphosis, chronic back pain, and loss of height are common signs of primary osteoporosis in older persons (Van Meirhaeghe, Bastian, Boonen et al., 2013).

Medical Management

Calcium and vitamin D supplementation, exercise, and antiresorptive therapy are the cornerstones of medical therapy in primary osteoporosis (Bernabei, Martone, Ortolani, Landi, & Marzetti, 2014)). In the United States, the recommended intake for older adults is 500 to 1000 mg/day of elemental calcium and at least 400 international units per day (IU/day) of vitamin D in two divided doses to maximize gastrointestinal absorption. Weight-bearing and muscle-strengthening exercises add minimally to bone density, but significant benefit is seen in improved posture, balance, and reduced falls. Estrogens, bisphosphonates, selective estrogen receptor modulators, and calcitonin are used in antiresorptive therapy on the basis of the older patient's risk profile. However, patients who are at high risk for breast cancer should not take estrogen to treat osteoporosis. In addition, some physicians choose a thiazide diuretic for those with hypertension as a comorbid condition because it decreases urinary calcium excretion, which slows bone loss.

TABLE 25.9	Osteoporosis			
Assessment	**Diagnosis**	**Planning**	**Intervention**	**Evaluation**
1. Use of hormone replacement 2. Calcium and vitamin D intake 3. Exercise habits 4. Alcohol, caffeine, and protein intake 5. Current or past use of corticosteroids 6. History of thyroid, bowel, kidney, or liver disease 7. Use of excessive thyroid replacement 8. Weight as listed in Table 25.3 9. Comorbidities 10. Drugs 11. Social support 12. Cultural influences	1. Inadequate health maintenance	1. Teach disease and medical management and dietary recommendations of the National Research Council Report for those older than 65 years. 2. Teach therapeutic lifestyle changes. 3. Ensure safety and fall awareness.	1. Teach pathophysiology, testing, drugs, monitoring, complications, sources of support and information, and fall precautions. 2. Provide for supervised meal planning, encourage food label reading, and calcium and vitamin D supplementation. 3. Have patient undergo postural retraining and weight-bearing exercises.	1. Patient will have an absence of fractures, no falls, and improved bone mineral density.

Data from Carpenito-Moyet, L. J. (2013). *Nursing diagnosis: Application to clinical practice* (14th ed.). Philadelphia: Lippincott Williams & Wilkins.

NURSING MANAGEMENT

Assessment, diagnosis, planning, intervention, and evaluation for osteoporosis focus on the response to the core defect of decreased bone mass, as detailed in Table 25.9.

Sexual Dysfunction

ED and female sexual dysfunction (FSD) have garnered increased interest and research dollars in recent years as many older people strive to retain the vitality of their younger years. Previously, sexual dysfunction was discreetly minimized or overlooked in the professional literature. A recent cross-sectional study of males 40 to 88 years demonstrated the overall prevalence of ED to be 77% in men over 70 years of age (Mola, 2015). FSD remains ill-defined, even though a relatively high rate of sexual dysfunction exists among postmenopausal women because of low desire, vaginal dryness, or inability to reach orgasm (Hughes, Rostant, & Pelon, 2015) The effects of menopause appear to be incremental and additional to those characteristic of aging.

Pathophysiology

Causes of ED among males could be organic, psychological, or both; organic being vascular, hormonal, neurogenic, or anatomic in nature (Mola, 2015). Hormonal changes associated with ED begin at 40 years old in the aging man and include decreased testosterone, decreased bioavailability of testosterone, increased sex hormone–binding globulin, decreased DHEA, mildly increased estradiol-17-beta, decreased melatonin, and decreased GH and IGF-1 (Gratzke, Angulo, Chitaley et al., 2010).

The female sexual response cycle comprises a neuroendocrine-mediated vascular and nonvascular smooth muscle relaxation, which results in increased pelvic blood flow, vaginal lubrication, and clitoral engorgement. As in men, these mechanisms in women are mediated by a combination of neuromuscular and vasocongestive events. More cases of women with FSD are seen by urologists. Some researchers think that androgen deficiency or relative inactivity of the adrenal enzyme 17, 20-lyase in women is the pathophysiologic entity responsible for FSD, which is often characterized by diminished libido, diminished arousal and orgasmic capabilities, and deficient androgen levels.

Signs and Symptoms

ED is the persistent inability to achieve or sustain an erection firm enough for sexual intercourse and penetration (Wincze & Carey, 2012). ED ranges from mild to severe and occurs in 50% of 65-year-old men and 75% of men 80 years or older.

FSD is a sexual arousal disorder that may develop as women age. Menopause and declining estrogen produce a thin and dry vaginal vault. As a result, the ability to become aroused may decline because of pain during sexual intercourse. In addition, in FSD, neuroendocrine physiologic impairments interfere with the normal female sexual response and frequently bring about complaints of diminished sexual arousal, libido, genital sensation, and ability to achieve orgasm. Other physical contributors to FSD include vaginitis, cystitis, endometriosis, hypothyroidism, and diabetes mellitus. Drugs such as oral contraceptives, HR, antihypertensives, antidepressants, or sedatives can cause a sexual arousal disorder as a side effect.

Medical Management

Medical management includes pharmacologic (e.g., phosphodiesterase type 5 inhibitors and alprostadil), nonpharmacological (e.g., counseling, lifestyle modifications, vacuum constriction devices, and performing regular erection exercises), and surgery (Mola, 2015). Often, these drugs must continue to be taken, and additional medicine is added to address ED. Sildenafil, phentolamine, yohimbine, testosterone, and alprostadil are a few of the drugs prescribed to increase blood flow to the penis and thus correct ED.

Most men with ED may achieve erections by using a constriction device, with or without a vacuum device (Mola, 2015). These devices are among the least expensive treatments for ED, and they enable a man to avoid the side effects of drug treatment. Constriction bands or rings made of metal, rubber, or leather are placed at the base of the penis to slow the outflow of blood. A constriction band used alone may produce an erection in a man with mild ED, especially if the problem is maintenance of erection. If that does not work, a constriction device may also be used in combination with a vacuum device. A vacuum device consists of a hollow chamber attached to a source of suction that fits over the penis, creating an air seal. Then suction applied to the chamber draws blood into the penis, producing an erection; a binding device is then applied to

TABLE 25.10   Sexual Dysfunction

Assessment	Diagnosis	Planning	Intervention	Evaluation
1. Genital anatomy 2. Sexual identity and sexual behaviors 3. Sex drive 4. Fatigue 5. Emotional lability 6. Painful intercourse 7. Cultural influences 8. Partner availability 9. Available private time 10. Baseline function 11. Couple's connectedness 12. Erectile dysfunction, ejaculatory dysfunction, or anorgasmia 13. Depression 14. Comorbidities 15. Fears related to sexually transmitted disease 16. Medications 17. Job or financial worries 18. Values or relationship conflicts 19. Alcohol or drug use 20. Energy level 21. Laboratory abnormalities	1. Inadequate sexuality pattern	1. Explore patient's patterns of functioning. 2. Discuss relationship between sexual functioning and life stressors. 3. Reaffirm need for candid discussion between partners. 4. Intensive therapy: refer patient to appropriate therapist, counselor, or physician.	1. Permission: convey a willingness to discuss sexual matters. 2. Limited information: provide some information on likely situations and treatments. 3. Specific suggestions: offer some specific instructions based on patient's acknowledged situation. 4. Identify and problem solve acute or chronic illness and other contributing factors.	1. Patient will achieve satisfactory sexual function.

Data from Carpenito-Moyet, L. J. (2013). *Nursing diagnosis: Application to clinical practice* (14th ed.). Philadelphia: Lippincott Williams & Wilkins.

maintain the erection. Surgical implantation of firm rods or pump-operated devices is an option for men with a low risk of postoperative complications who find the 3-day hospital stay and 6-week recovery acceptable. Recently sensate focus psychotherapy has gained some popularity because of its ability to mitigate compounding psychological factors that may overlie physiologic ED.

Medical management of FSD includes watchful waiting, dose reduction of causative drugs, testosterone replacement, sensate focus psychotherapy, and prescription of bupropion, buspirone, or sildenafil. Researchers have treated women with androgen deficiency by administering 50 mg/day DHEA for 6 months; increased spontaneity, decreased time to achieve arousal, return of sexual fantasies, and an increase in desire were the significant benefits. Adverse effects were mild and limited to acne and breast tenderness (Graziottin, 2010).

NURSING MANAGEMENT

The nursing process in sexual dysfunction requires a biopsychosocial approach to the issues in ED and FSD, as detailed in Table 25.10.

SUMMARY

This chapter discussed endocrine aging as an increased molecular disorderliness of the regulatory mechanisms, which results in reduced vitality of the overall person. It described a new ensemble view in terms of decreased estrogen production in women (menopause), decreased testosterone production in men (andropause), decreased adrenal function (adrenopause), and decreased GH–IGF-1 (somatopause). This chapter included current literature on aging endocrine physiology showing current knowledge. Finally, the nursing process was applied to some of the most common endocrine diseases affecting older adults.

HOME CARE

1. Regularly assess homebound older adults diagnosed with endocrine disorders for signs and symptoms indicating exacerbation or instability.
2. Instruct caregivers and homebound older adults about reportable signs and symptoms related to the endocrine problems being monitored and about when to report these changes to the home care nurse or health care provider.
3. Instruct caregivers and homebound older adults on types, dosage, and technique of administering insulin. Have caregivers and homebound older adults do a return demonstration of this skill. Ensure that they receive written instructions to assist them in the learning process.
4. Instruct caregivers and homebound older adults about laboratory indications used to evaluate endocrine disorders. Inform them of the results of the tests after the health care provider has been notified.
5. Instruct caregivers and homebound older adults on safety tips related to insulin injection. Injecting insulin isophanne and then switching to beef or pork insulin without a physician order results in altering the times of insulin action, initiation, peak insulin action, and duration of insulin action.
6. Instruct caregivers and homebound older adults on diabetes management.
7. Instruct caregivers and homebound older adults on the proper dosage of drugs used to treat hormone imbalances associated with endocrine disorders.

KEY POINTS

- The endocrine system is regulated by feedback systems that involve a chemical connection between structures of the brain, peripheral glands, and hormones. The feedback loops regulate hormone production.
- A hypofunctioning state is one that results from inadequate endocrine secretions.
- A hyperfunctioning state is one that results from excessive secretion of hormones.
- Endocrine pathology may also be manifested in the form of hormone resistance, a condition in which the tissue response to hormones is inadequate. Resistance may be caused by a genetic defect or may be acquired, as in the case of T2DM.
- Older adults experience andropause and menopause when a decline in biosyntheses of their dominant sex hormones occurs.
- Adrenopause and somatopause are changes that occur as the result of aging.
- Metabolic syndrome is rapidly increasing in the older population. It is caused by improper nutrition, inadequate physical activity, and obesity.
- T2DM is very common in the older population.
- The most important variables associated with T2DM are obesity and insulin resistance.
- Older individuals with T2DM should strive for proper control of their blood glucose levels to reduce the risk for potential complication.

- A comprehensive nursing assessment of older patients with T2DM includes assessment of the patient's feet, the patient's knowledge of diabetes management (e.g., diet, desirable weight, exercise, drugs, and treatment of hypoglycemia and hyperglycemia), the patient's learning style, and emergency identification.
- Management of serious wounds in older patients with diabetes optimally needs to involve a multidisciplinary health team.
- Thyroid disorders are more common among older adults and more difficult to diagnose than in the younger population.
- Primary hypothyroidism in older persons may often remain unnoticed or indiscernible. Symptoms of mild depression, apathy, decreased appetite, weight loss, and weakness should be investigated.
- Thyroid HR should always be started at a low dose and increase slowly with careful monitored; follow-up appointments are essential for incremental dosing over several weeks.
- Hyperthyroidism may have an atypical presentation in older adults. Symptoms often include apathy, tiredness, weakness, anorexia, weight loss, angina, heart failure, atrial fibrillation, and absence of thyroid changes.
- Older adults need to be taught the actions and side effects of prescribed drugs and the need for lifelong monitoring of thyroid status.

CRITICAL-THINKING EXERCISES

1. Compare the endocrine gland function of a 72-year-old man with that of a 30-year-old man.
2. A 65-year-old woman was recently diagnosed with metabolic syndrome. She is sedentary, has a body mass index more than 30, and has abdominal obesity. What three issues would you prepare to teach the patient about her condition?
3. A 74-year-old man was recently diagnosed with insulin-dependent diabetes mellitus. While teaching him to administer 70/30 Humulin insulin, you note that he is unable to draw up the correct number of units into a syringe. What further information do you need about your patient before proceeding with your teaching plan?

REFERENCES

American Diabetes Association (ADA). (2018). Older adults: Standards of medical care in diabetes – 2018. *Diabetes Care, 41*(Supp. 1), S119–S125. https://doi.org/10.2337/dc18-SPPC01.

American Thyroid Association (ATA). (2017). Older patients and thyroid disease. Retrieved on December 17, 2017, from https://www.thyroid.org/thyroid-disease-older-patient/.

Batrinos, M. L. (2012). The aging of the endocrine hypothalamus and its dependent endocrine glands. *Hormones, 11*(3), 241–253.

Beers, M. H. & Berkow, R. (Eds.), (2014). *Merck manual of geriatrics.* Whitehouse Station, NJ: Merck. Retrieved April 2014, from, http://www.merckmanuals.com/professional/geriatrics/html.

Berent-Spillson, A., Persad, C., Love, T., Tkaczyk, A., Wang, H., Reame, N., et al. (2010). Early menopausal hormone use influences brain regions used for visual working memory. *Menopause, 17*(4), 692–699.

Bergman, Å., Heindel, J. J., Kasten, T., Kidd, K. A., Jobling, S., Neira, M., et al. (2013). The impact of endocrine disruption: A consensus statement on the state of the science. *Environmental Health Perspectives, 121*(4), a104.

Bernabei, R., Martone, A.M., Ortolani, E., Landi, F., & Marzetti, E. (2014). Screening, diagnosis and treatment of osteoporosis: A brief review. *Clinical Cases Mineral Bone Metabolism, 11*(13), 201-2017. Retrieved December 17, 2017, from https://www.ncbi.nlm.nih.gov/pmc/articles/PMC4269144/.

Bonomini, F., Rodella, L. F., & Rezzani, R. (2015). Metabolic syndrome, aging, and involvement of oxidative stress. *Aging and Disease, 6*(2), 109–120. https://doi.org/10.14336/AD.2014.0305.

Carpenito-Moyet, L. J. (2013). *Nursing diagnosis: Application to clinical practice* (14th ed.). Philadelphia: Lippincott Williams & Wilkins.

Chen, G., Lu, D., Pang, Z., & Liu, Q. (2013). Red and processed meat consumption and risk of stroke: A meta-analysis of prospective cohort studies. *European Journal of Clinical Nutrition, 67*(1), 91–95.

Chia, C. W., Shardell, M., Tanaka, T., Liu, D. D., Gravenstein, K. S., Simonsick, E. M., … Ferrucci, L. (2016). Chronic low-calorie sweetener use and risk of abdominal obesity among older adults: A cohort study. *PLOS ONE, 11*(11): e0167241. http://doi.dx.org/10.1371/journal.pone.0167241.

Cigolle, C. T., Lee, P. G., Langa, K. M., Lee, Y. Y., Tian, Z., & Blaum, C. S. (2011). Geriatric conditions develop in middle-aged adults with diabetes. *Journal of General Internal Medicine, 26*(3), 272–279.

Copstead, L. E., & Banasik, J. K. (2013). *Pathophysiology* (5th ed.). St.Louis: Elsevier.

De Groot, L. J. (Ed.), (2013). *THYROID MANAGER: Chapter 17-Multinodular Goiter.* Retrieved August 2013, from http://www.thyroidmanager.org/wp-content/uploads/chapters/multinodular-goiter.pdf.

Di Somma, C., Brunelli, V., Savanelli, M., Scarano, E., Savastano, S., Lombardi, G., et al. (2011). Somatopause: State of the art. *Minerva Endocrinologica, 36*(3), 243–255.

Dupuis, J., Langenberg, C., Prokopenko, I., Saxena, R., Soranzo, N., Jackson, A., et al. (2010). New genetic loci implicated in fasting glucose homeostasis and their impact on type 2 diabetes risk. *Nature Genetics, 42*(2), 105–116.

Eastell, R. (2013). Identification and management of osteoporosis in older adults. *Medicine, 41*(1), 47–52.

Farinde, A. (2015). Oral hypoglycemia agents. *Medscape.* Retrieved December 18, 2017, from https://emedicine.medscape.com/article/2172160-overview.

Farmer, A., Hardeman, W., Hughes, D., Prevost, A., Kim, Y., Craven, A., et al. (2012). An explanatory randomised controlled trial of a nurse-led, consultation-based intervention to support patients with adherence to taking glucose lowering drug for type 2 diabetes. *BMC Family Practice, 13*, 30.

Garg, A., & Vanderpump, M. (2013). Subclinical thyroid disease. *The Lancet, 379*(9821), 1142–1154.

Garvey, W. T., Ryan, D. H., Henry, R., Bohannan, N. J. V., Toplak, H., Schwiers, M., … Day, W. W. (2014). Prevention of type 2 diabetes in subjects with prediabetes and metabolic syndrome treated with phentermine and topiramate extended release. *Diabetes Care, 37*, 912–921. https://doi.org/10.2337/dc13-1518.

Giroux, S., Bussières, J., Bureau, A., & Rousseau, F. (2012). UGT2B17 gene deletion associated with an increase in bone mineral density similar to the effect of hormone replacement in postmenopausal women. *Osteoporosis International, 23*(3), 1163–1170.

Gratzke, C., Angulo, J., Chitaley, K., Dai, Y., Kim, N. N., Paick, J. S., et al. (2010). Anatomy, physiology and pathophysiology of erectile dysfunction. *The Journal of Sexual Medicine, 7*(1), 445–475.

Graziottin, A. (2010). Menopause and sexuality: Key issues in premature menopause and beyond. *Annals of the New York Academy of Science, 1205*, 254–261.

Griffith, J. F., & BAO, B. (2013). Age-related physiological changes of the bone marrow and immune system. In *Geriatric Imaging* (pp. 891–904). Berlin Heidelberg: Springer.

Grundy, S. (Ed.), (2009). *Atlas of atherosclerosis and metabolic syndrome* (5th ed.). New York: Springer.

Hampton, J. (2013). Thyroid gland disorder emergencies. *AACN Advanced Critical Care, 24*(3), 325–332.

Hughes, A. K., Rostant, O. S., & Pelon, S. (2015). Sexual problems among older women by age and race. *Journal of Women's Health, 24*(8), 663–669. http://doi.dx.org/ https://doi.org/10.1089/jwh.2014.5010.

Jones, C. M., & Boelaert, K. (2015). The endocrinology of ageing: A mini-review. *Gerontology, 61*, 291–300. https://doi.org/10.1159/000367692.

Kaur, J. (2014). A comprehensive review on metabolic syndrome. *Cardiology Research and Practice, 2014*, 1–21. https://doi.org/10.1155/2014/943162.

Kilic, S., Yilmaz, N., Erdogan, G., Aydin, M., Tasdemir, N., Doganay, M., et al. (2010). Effect of non-oral estrogen on risk markers for metabolic syndrome in early surgically menopausal women. *Climacteric: The Journal of the International Menopause Society, 13*(1), 55–62.

Kronenberg, H. M., Melmed, S., Larsen, P. R., & Polonsky, K. S. (2016). Principles of endocrinology. In S. Melmed, K. S. Polonsky, P. R. Larsen, & H. M. Kronenberg (Eds.), *Williams textbook of endocrinology* (13th ed.). Philadelphia, PA: Elsevier. Retrieved on December 12, 2017, from https://books.google.com/books?id=iPIACwAAQBAJ&pg=PA1237&lpg=PA1237&dq=andropause,+somatopause,+menopause,+adrenopause&source=bl&ots=UmCnwOJxKs&sig=GMPOb6BwUSY8s96DWhpjp7GoFqY&hl=en&sa=X&ved=0ahUKEwjV17Cm5ITYAhVE44MKHRq6A4cQ6AEILjAB#v=onepage&q=andropause%2C%20somatopause%2C%20menopause%2C%20adrenopause&f=false

Lamberts, S. W. J., & van den Beld, A. W. (2016). Endocrinology and aging. In S. Melmed, K. S. Polonsky, P. R. Larsen, & H. M. Kronenberg (Eds.), *Williams textbook of endocrinology* (13th ed.). Philadelphia, PA: Elsevier. Retrieved on December 12, 2017, from https://books.google.com/books?id=iPIACwAAQBAJ&pg=PA1237&lpg=PA1237&dq=andropause,+somatopause,+menopause,+adrenopause&source=bl&ots=UmCnwOJxKs&sig=GMPOb6BwUSY8s96DWhpjp7GoFqY&hl=en&sa=X&ved=0ahUKEwjV17Cm5ITYAhVE44MKHRq6A4cQ6AEILjAB#v=onepage&q=andropause%2C%20somatopause%2C%20menopause%2C%20adrenopause&f=false.

Liantonio, A., Gramegna, G., Carbonara, G., Sblendorio, V., Pierno, S., Fraysse, B., et al. (2013). Growth hormone secretagogues exert differential effects on skeletal muscle calcium homeostasis in male rats depending on the peptidyl/non-peptidyl structure. *Endocrinology,* en.2013-1334. Retrieved August 2013, from, http://endo.endojournals.org/content/early/2013/07/08/en.2013-1334.short.

Look AHEAD Research Group, et al. (2010). Long-term effects of a lifestyle intervention on weight and cardiovascular risk factors in individuals with type 2 diabetes mellitus: Four-year results of the Look AHEAD trial. *Archives of Internal Medicine, 170*(17), 1566–1575.

Maggio, M., De Vita, F., Fisichella, A., Lauretani, F., Ticinesi, A., Cresini, G., … Ceda, G. P. (2015). The role of the multiple hormonal dysregulation in the onset of "anemia of aging": Focus on testosterone, IGF-1, and thyroid hormones. *International Journal of Endocrinology, 2015*, 1–22. https://doi.org/10.1155/2015/292574.

Mbaezue, N., Mayberry, R., Gazmararian, J., Quarshie, A., Ivonye, C., & Heisler, M. (2010). The impact of health literacy on self-monitoring of blood glucose in patients with diabetes receiving care in an inner-city hospital. *Journal of the National Medical Association, 102*(1), 5–9.

McCance, K. L., & Huether, S. E. (2014). *Pathophysiology* (7th ed.). St. Louis, MO: Mosby.

McCuistion, L. E., Vuljoin-DiMaggio, K., Winton, M. B., & Yeager, J. J. (2018). *Pharmacology: A patient-centered nursing process approach* (9th ed.). St. Louis, MO: Elsevier.

McCulloch, D.K., & Munshi, M. (2017). Treatment of type 2 diabetes mellitus in the older adult. *UpToDate.* Retrieved on December 13, 2017, from https://www.uptodate.com/contents/treatment-of-type-2-diabetes-mellitus-in-the-older-patient.

Michael, O. T. (2010). Endocrinology of aging: The convergence of reductionist science with systems biology and integrative medicine. *Frontiers in Endocrinology, 1*(2). Retrieved August 2013, from, http://www.ncbi.nlm.nih.gov/pmc/articles/PMC3355961/.

Mola, J. R. (2015). Erectile dysfunction in the older adult male. *Urologic Nursing, 35*(2). https://doi.org/10.7257/1053-816X.2015.35.2.87.

Monahan, F. D., Sands, J. K., Neighbors, M., Marek, J. F., et al. (2007). *Phipps' medical-surgical nursing: Health and illness perspectives* (8th ed.). St. Louis, MO: Mosby.

Morley, J.E. (2016). Overview of endocrine disorders. *Merck Manual.* Retrieved December 12, 2017, from http://www.merckmanuals.com/professional/endocrine-and-metabolic-disorders/principles-of-endocrinology/overview-of-endocrine-disorders.

Muñoz-Pareja, M., León-Muñoz, L., Guallar-Castillón, P., Graciani, A., López-García, E., Banegas, J., et al. (2012). The diet of diabetic patients in Spain in 2008–2010: Accordance with the main dietary recommendations–A cross-sectional study. *PLOS One, 7*(6). e39454.

Nieuwenhuizen, W., Weenen, H., Rigby, P., & Hetherington, M. (2010). Older adults and patients in need of nutritional support: Review of current treatment options and factors influencing nutritional intake. *Clinical Nutrition, 29*(2), 160–169.

Pattyn, N., Cornelissen, V. A., Eshghi, S. R. T., & Vanhees, L. (2013). The effect of exercise on the cardiovascular risk factors constituting the metabolic syndrome. *Sports Medicine, 43*(2), 121–133.

Peters, E. J., Lipsky, B. A., Berendt, A. R., Embil, J. M., Lavery, L. A., Senneville, E., et al. (2012). A systematic review of the effectiveness of interventions in the management of infection in the diabetic foot. *Diabetes/Metabolism Research and Reviews, 28* (S1), 142–162.

Rejeski, W., Isp, E., Bertoni, A., Bray, G., Evans, G., Gregg, E., et al. (2012). Lifestyle change and mobility in obese adults with type 2 diabetes. *The New England Journal of Medicine, 366*(13), 1209–1217.

Schierbeck, L., Rejnmark, L., Tofteng, C., Stilgren, L., Eiken, P., Mosekilde, L., et al. (2012). Effect of hormone replacement therapy on cardiovascular events in recently postmenopausal women: Randomised trial. *BMJ, 345,* e6409.

Schlumberger, M., Catargi, B., Borget, I., Deandreis, D., Zerdoud, S., Bridji, B., et al. (2012). Strategies of radioiodine ablation in patients with low-risk thyroid cancer. *The New England Journal of Medicine, (36618),* 1663–1673.

Simpson, E. E. (2012). Predictors of intentions to use hormone replacement therapy in clinical postmenopausal women. *Climacteric, 15*(2), 173–180.

Steil, G., Palerm, C., Kurtz, N., Voskanyan, G., Roy, A., Paz, S., et al. (2011). The effect of insulin feedback on closed loop glucose control. *The Journal of Clinical Endocrinology and Metabolism, 96* (5), 1402–1408.

Suzuki, S., Nishio, S., Takeda, T., & Komatsu, M. (2012). Gender-specific regulation of response to thyroid hormone in aging. *Thyroid Research, 5*(1), 1.

Szkrobka, W., Krysiak, R., & Okopieri, B. (2008). Adrenopause. *Polski Merkuriusz Lekarski, 25*(145), 77–82.

Toivonen, J. M., & Partridge, L. (2009). Endocrine regulation of aging and reproduction in *Drosophilia. Molecular and Cellular Endocrinology, 299*(1), 39–50.

Van Horn, L., Appel, L. J., Burke, L. E., Economos, C., Karmally, W., … Kris-Etherton, P. (2016). Recommended dietary pattern to achieve adherence to the American Heart Association/American College of Cardiology (AHA/ACC) guidelines. *Circulation, 2016* (134), e505-e529. https://doi.org/10.1161/CIR.0000000000000462.

Van Meirhaeghe, J., Bastian, L., Boonen, S., Ranstam, J., Tillman, J. B., & Wardlaw, D. (2013). A randomized trial of balloon hypoplasty and non-surgical management for treating acute vertebral compression fractures: Outcomes and vertebral body kyphosis correction and surgical parameters. *Bone Joint Journal, 95-B* (Suppl. 17), 5–21.

Veldhuis, J. D. (2013). Changes in pituitary function with ageing and implications for patient care. *Nature Reviews Endocrinology, 9,* 205–215. https://doi.org/0.1038/nrendo.2013.38.

Walter, S., Atzmon, G., Demerath, E., Garcia, M., Kaplan, R., Kumari, M., et al. (2011). A genome-wide association study of aging. *Neurobiology of Aging, 32*(11), 2109. e15–2109. e28.

Wincze, J. P., & Carey, M. P. (2012). *Sexual dysfunction: A guide for assessment and treatment* (2nd ed.). New York: Guilford Press.

Wood, C. (2017). Ensuring good nutrition for older patients in the community. *Journal of Community Nursing, 31*(3), 50–51.

WEBSITES

American Association of Clinical Endocrinologists. http://www.aace.com.

American College of Obstetricians and Gynecologists. http://www.acog.com.

Food and Nutrition: Dietary Guidelines for Americans—USDA. http://www.health.gov/dietaryguidelines/.

North American Menopause Society. http://www.menopause.org.

National Institute of Diabetes and Digestive and Kidney Diseases of the National Institutes of Health. http://www.niddk.nih.gov.

Office of Disease Prevention and Health Promotion. http://health.gov.

Physical Activity Readiness Questionnaire (PAR-Q). http://www.d.umn.edu/student/loon/soc/phys/par-q.html.

Systematic Evidence Review: Managing Overweight and Obesity in Adults. https://www.nhlbi.nih.gov/health-topics/managing-overweight-obesity-in-adults.

PART VI

Health Care Transitions

26

Health Care Delivery Settings and Older Adults

Linda Bub, MSN, RN, GCNS-BC

ⓔ http://evolve.elsevier.com/Meiner/gerontologic

LEARNING OBJECTIVES

On completion of this chapter, the reader will be able to:

1. Describe acute care hospital use patterns in the older adult population.
2. Describe a functional model of nursing care.
3. Identify risks associated with hospitalization of older adults.
4. Identify ways to modify the physical and social environment to improve care for hospitalized older adults.
5. Identify special considerations in caring for critically ill older adults and those suffering from trauma.
6. Describe two nursing interventions for each of the three conditions that make up the geriatric triad.
7. List adaptations that can be made to facilitate learning in older adults.
8. Describe a profile of a "typical" noninstitutionalized older adult, including common diagnoses and functional limitations.
9. Distinguish the categories and types of home care organizations in existence.
10. Explain the benefits of home care.
11. Analyze the effect of the recent changes instituted by Medicare on home health agencies and home health clients.
12. Discuss the philosophy of hospice care and how it differs from traditional home health care.
13. List five common factors associated with institutionalization.
14. Identify the differences between the medical and psychosocial models of care for institutional long-term care.
15. Summarize key aspects of resident rights as they relate to the nursing facility.
16. List assessment components included in the minimum data set of the Resident Assessment Instrument.
17. Describe common clinical management programs in the nursing facility for skin problems, incontinence, nutritional problems, infection control, and mental health.
18. Differentiate types of nursing care delivery systems found in the nursing facility.
19. Describe assisted living, special care units, and subacute care units as specialty care settings of the nursing facility.

WHAT WOULD YOU DO?

What would you do if you were faced with the following situations?

• Your neighbor states her father-in-law has become forgetful and fails to take his medications at least weekly. Last week he fell; aside from bruising, there were no serious injuries. But she is concerned and does not know where to turn for help. What advice can you offer her?

• Your new admission to the general medical floor is 92 years old. He is ambulatory with the assistance of a four-point cane; he is on standby assist with ADLs. You are concerned for his safety. What do you do?

With the steady growth in the number of older adults in the United States, it is now estimated that most of a nurse's career is spent working with older adults, and almost all nurses will care for older adults in the acute care setting at some time. Older adults are a diverse, heterogeneous group in terms of age, life experiences, the aging process, health habits, attitudes, and response to illnesses. Nurses need to have specialized knowledge, skills, and abilities to care for older adults across all health care delivery settings.

CHARACTERISTICS OF OLDER ADULTS IN ACUTE CARE

The older-than-85 group is the fastest-growing segment of the U.S. population. The most common diagnosis-related groups (DRGs) in hospitalized adults over the age of 85 include heart failure, pneumonia, urinary tract infections, cerebrovascular disorders, digestive disorders, gastrointestinal hemorrhages, nutritional and metabolic disorders, rehabilitation, and renal failure (National Center for Health Statistics, 2013). The top five major causes of death in those older than 65 are heart disease, malignant neoplasms, chronic lower respiratory diseases, cerebrovascular disease, and Alzheimer's disease (National Center for Health Statistics, 2013).

Chronic conditions refer to chronic illness and impairments, and an individual's level of disability is typically categorized by the amount of assistance required in both basic activities of daily

Previous author: Marie H. Thomas, RN, PhD, FNP-C, CNE.

living (ADLs) and instrumental activities of daily living (IADLs). Arthritis, diabetes mellitus, hypertension, and heart disease are the most prevalent chronic diseases in older adults and are the leading causes of disability. The exacerbation of a chronic illness may precipitate hospitalization, and complications may profoundly affect the progress of a hospitalized patient. Because the acute event for which an older patient is hospitalized is frequently superimposed on a chronic condition or disease, this older age group is increasingly influencing the acute care environment and the professional caregiver skills required in this setting.

CHARACTERISTICS OF THE ACUTE CARE ENVIRONMENT

It is a challenge for caregivers to attend to the diverse needs of each individual admitted to the acute care setting. The older adult is not likely to be admitted to the hospital until a high level of acuity or complications exist. Reimbursement patterns can create additional complications that put stress on the care team, which, in turn, affect care. The intensity of care required for the typically emergent condition for which an older adult is admitted, compounded by the normal aging process, chronic illness, and impaired functional status, requires astute care planning and case management on the part of the health care team. The health care team's success in providing care is influenced by the philosophy of care, awareness of the risks of hospitalization, and safety features of the acute care environment.

Philosophy of Care

Rapidly rising costs and concerns over quality in acute care have fostered a climate in which the value and efficacy of hospitalization have come under increasing scrutiny. With an increasing number of hospitalized older adults, the focus on technology is being recognized as obscuring activities aimed at improving the function of those with chronic illness, physical disability, and cognitive impairment. Effective caregiving practices enable older adults to maintain or improve their independence and to return to their preferred living environment at discharge. However, in the hospital setting, health care professionals may become so involved in addressing the acute condition that they fail to appreciate the underlying problems and how these, too, influence the patient's health and recovery.

The hospital is a highly technologic system that is in a good position to address both acute and chronic problems. The focus needs to be on not only the restoration of health but also the promotion and preservation of health. The value placed on technology fosters a task orientation that may detract from the holistic focus required for the care of older adults. Acute care centers have traditionally provided care within a medical model whose focus is on diagnosis and treatment rather than providing care within a functional model, which more broadly integrates all aspects of care. With older adults, particularly those hospitalized because of an exacerbation of a chronic illness, focusing on a functional model helps address concerns related to both their medical and functional stability. The medical model practiced in the hospital needs to be expanded to include this functional model in which the main goal may not be curing the disease, but rather managing the disease, with a focus on self-care and symptom management strategies.

Risks of Hospitalization

Adverse Drug Reactions

Polypharmacy (defined as an inappropriate number of medications) is a common cause of iatrogenic illness among patients over 65 years of age and is associated with multimorbidity in older adult patients (Heppner et al., 2012). Hospitalized patients are often admitted with a large number of prescribed, over-the-counter, and homeopathic drugs that they have or have not been taking correctly or as prescribed before entering the acute care setting. Adjusting, removing, or adding to the number of medications can put the older adult at risk for adverse drug reactions.

Conversely, adverse drug reactions frequently precipitate hospitalizations and, although often unreported, are among the most common iatrogenic events in the acute care setting. Hospital staff need to obtain an accurate drug history from patients, be aware of pharmacokinetic and pharmacodynamic changes related to aging, and have a working understanding of drug–disease, drug–drug, and drug–food interactions in older adults (De Rui, Manzato, Sarti, & Sergi, 2011). Nurses should be particularly aware of drugs that may be high risk when used in older adults and carefully monitor patients taking them for signs and symptoms of toxicity (De Rui et al., 2011). Partnering with the pharmacy team to put into place pathways to identify high-risk medications, interactions, and prescribing practices is necessary to ensure safe medication prescribing for older adults in the hospital and during transitions in care.

Falls

Studies indicate that up to 79% of all adverse inpatient incidents are related to falls, and patients age 65 or older experience the most falls; approximately 10% fall more than once during their hospital stay, usually in their hospital rooms. Risk factors for hospital falls include both intrinsic and extrinsic factors. Intrinsic factors include age-related physiologic changes and diseases, as well as medications that affect cognition and balance. Extrinsic factors include environmental hazards such as the layout of older hospital rooms or cluttered hospital rooms, wheels on beds and chairs, and beds higher than what an older adult usually has at home. The hospital can be a dangerous and foreign place for older adults because of unfamiliarity and because of changes in the patient's medical condition (Rowe, 2013). The Joint Commission (2015) has emphasized the need to decrease the risk for falls, recommending the following:

- Raise awareness among staff of the need to prevent falls
- Establish an interdisciplinary falls prevention team
- Use standardized, validated tools to identify risk factors for falls
- Develop individualized plans of care based on identified risk factors for falls
- Use evidence-based practices and interventions
- Conduct postfall huddles
- Analyze contributing factors for falls on an ongoing basis to inform quality improvement efforts

Infection

Older adults are generally more vulnerable to infections because of physiologic changes in the immune system and underlying chronic disease. One in 25 patients acquire a health care–associated infection (HAI) while hospitalized (Agency for Healthcare Research and Quality [AHRQ], 2017). Of these, slightly more than 33% occur in the older patient population (Katz & Roghmann, 2016). This may be a low estimate, because older adults with infections may have an atypical presentation, making infections more difficult to diagnose. Hospital-acquired pneumonia is the most common HAI (Centers for Disease Control and Prevention [CDC], 2016); symptoms in older adults are often mental status changes or confusion, making the diagnosis more challenging (Dougdale, 2012).

Urinary tract infections (UTIs) are the second most frequent HAI (Katz & Roghmann, 2016), although bacteriuria in an older adult is often asymptomatic. Subclinical infection and inflammation may occur with presenting symptoms such as acute confusion, functional capacity deterioration and falls, anorexia, or nausea rather than the classic symptoms of fever and dysuria. Increased instrumentation and manipulation as well as decreased host immune mechanisms contribute to the increased risk of older adult patients developing sepsis originating from the urinary tract (Sollitto, 2017).

Other common sites of infection in hospitalized older adults include the gastrointestinal tract (Clostridium difficile), skin and soft tissues, and the bloodstream (CDC, 2016). Older adults are at increased risk for colonization and infection with antibiotic-resistant strains of organisms such as methicillin-resistant *Staphylococcus aureus* (MRSA), vancomycin-resistant enterococcus (VRE), and multidrug-resistant gram-negative rods (MDR-GNR; Katz & Roghmann, 2016). Control of the spread of resistant strains of organisms continues to be a problem in institutional settings. Adhering to basic principles of infection control is critical for nurses. It is essential to comply with proper hand washing, disinfection of the environment, and appropriate precautions when caring for patients infected or colonized with resistant strains.

Hazards of Immobility

Once older adults are hospitalized, immobilization through enforced bed rest or restraints often results in functional disability. Immobilized patients are vulnerable to rapid loss of muscle strength, reductions in orthostatic competence, urinary incontinence or retention, fecal impaction, atelectasis and pneumonia, acute confusion, depression, skin breakdown, and many other complications (Heppner et al., 2012). The occurrence of iatrogenic illnesses often represents a vicious cycle, referred to as the *cascade effect,* in which one problem increases the person's vulnerability to another one. Gerontologic nurses must be leaders in advocating more appropriate care and treatment of hospitalized older adults to prevent or at least reduce the occurrence of iatrogenic illness.

Safety Features

Older adults have a decreased ability to negotiate within and adapt to an unfamiliar environment. Multiple stimuli such as contact with many departments and personnel or multiple

---

BOX 26.1   Environmental Modifications

- Stabilized furnishings (e.g., removing or locking wheels)
- "Blue" fluorescent lighting
- Night-lights
- Extra lighting in bathrooms
- Consistent lighting intensity
- Light switches that glow
- Solid-color designs for floors (i.e., avoidance of patterns)
- Nonskid, nonglare floor wax
- Carpeting with uncut, low pile and padding underneath
- Contrasting color to identify boundaries between floor and wall
- Nonglossy wall surfaces
- Polarized window glass to decrease glare
- Nonglare glass over pictures; avoidance of abstract designs
- Rounded handrails for easy grasp in all areas where walking occurs; use of high-contrast colors in these areas
- Levers for doors and dressers instead of knobs
- Large-numbered, white-on-black (or black-on-white) clocks with nonglare glass
- Large-print calendars within patient's line of vision
- Telephones with large numbers
- Cases for glasses and prostheses attached to bedside and within reach
- Amplified and hearing aid-compatible phones
- Pocket talker
- Beds that lower to a height that enables patient to sit on the edge with both feet on the floor
- Use of no side rails or half-rails to deter climbing over rails
- Bed or chair exit alarms
- Chairs with armrests
- Portable elevated toilet seats
- Grab bars in shower and around toilet

Adapted from AARP. (2015). *HomeFit guide.* Retrieved December 14, 2017, from aarp.org/livable; Rein, T. (2016). *Adapting the home for grandma.* Retrieved December 14, 2017, from https://www.theseniorlist.com/2016/04/adapting-the-home-for-grandma/; and, Unwin, B. K., Andrews, C. M., Andrewes, P. M., & Hanson, J. L. (2009). Therapeutic home adaptations for older adults with disabilities. *American Family Physician, 80*(9), 963-968, 970.

---

room changes may prompt confusion and exhaustion, resulting in the loss of crucial personal items necessary for maximum functioning, such as hearing aids, prostheses, dentures, and eyeglasses. The environment may be modified in many ways for older adult patients (Box 26.1). Some modifications require additional resources, but some changes require minimum creativity on the part of the nursing staff.

NURSING IN THE ACUTE CARE SETTING

Nursing staff provides the majority of health care delivered in the hospital. Nurses are considered an integral part of the health care team and frequently provide the leadership for this team. Nurses need to be at the forefront in identifying high-quality, cost-effective interventions and transitions in care to prepare the patient and families for discharge. The quality of the nursing care provided is influenced by the philosophy of nursing, the nursing-specific competency and expertise of the nursing staff, and the various aspects of the nursing role implemented in acute care.

Nursing-Specific Competency and Expertise

Developing nursing competency helps nursing staff customize the care provided to patients age 65 or older. It enhances the nurse's job performance and the quality of care delivered. The Joint Commission (2012) requires documentation that all staff members (e.g., nurses, unlicensed assistive personnel, phlebotomists, and physical therapists) have a documented competency assessment that includes the special needs and behaviors of the specific patient age groups (e.g., geriatric, pediatric, and adolescent) that are provided cared for in the assigned area. The Joint Commission further requires that this be done on initial employment and then periodically reviewed.

A priority at the beginning of every hospitalization is the assessment of the older adult's baseline functional status so that an individual care plan can be developed (The Joint Commission, 2012). Systematic functional assessment in the acute care setting also provides a benchmark of a patient's progress as he or she moves along the continuum of care, and it promotes systematic communication of the patient's health status between health care settings (The Joint Commission, 2012). Assessment in the acute care setting includes recognition that older adults are in an unfamiliar environment, which is not conducive to optimal functioning at a time when reserves and homeostatic needs are compromised by acute illness. Many common assessment tools for ADLs and mental status assess areas of function that may not be easily evaluated at the time of admission or may not be significant at that time (i.e., assessing orientation when a calendar is not present in the room and the older adult's daily routines are disrupted). The primary goal of the acute care nurse is to maximize the older patient's independence by enhancing function. Functional strengths and weaknesses need to be identified. The care plan must provide for interventions that build on identified strengths and help the patient overcome identified weaknesses. Function integrates all aspects of the patient's condition; any change in functional status in an older adult should be interpreted as a classic sign of illness or as a complication of their illness. By knowing an older patient's baseline function, the nurse can assess new-onset signs or symptoms before they trigger a downward spiral of dependency and permanent impairment.

Nursing expertise is needed in the acute care setting to guide the staff in understanding the unique needs of older patients and enhancing their skill in managing common geriatric syndromes (Hartford Institute for Geriatric Nursing, 2008; St. Pierre & Twibell, 2012). The advanced practice nurse functions in the role of clinician, educator, consultant, and researcher. A growing number of acute care settings are recruiting and hiring advanced practice nurses to assist with the day-to-day assessment and management of patients in the acute care setting. Studies have demonstrated a significant decrease in the length of hospital stay when an advanced practice nurse is part of the care team (Kapu, Kleinpell, & Pilon, 2014; Kapu & Steaban, 2016; Moote, Krsek, Kleinpell, & Todd, 2011). The advanced practice nurse can be instrumental in developing and implementing protocols for managing common geriatric syndromes such as those defined in the geriatric triad.

The geriatric triad includes falls, changes in cognitive status, and incontinence (Chang, Tsai, Chen, & Liu, 2010). These three conditions need special attention during hospitalization. Falls may be a classic sign of illness for older adults; an older adult in the acute care setting is often at high risk for falls and consequent injuries. A strange environment, confusion, medications, immobility, urinary urgency, and age-related sensory changes all contribute to this increased risk. Falls resulting in injury may be minimized by gait training and strengthening exercises, appropriate nutrition, careful monitoring of medications, supervised toileting, environmental modifications, proper footwear, and control of orthostatic hypotension (Tinetti & Kumar, 2010). Bed and leg alarms are used in many institutions as an intervention to minimize falls but are often not successfully used as part of a comprehensive plan to reduce falls and prevent injury (see Emergency Treatment box).

✚ EMERGENCY TREATMENT
Falls

- Reassure patient and family.
- Examine for presence of injury, and call health care provider.
- Advocate for adequate assessment designed to identify covert or symptomless consequences of the fall (e.g., computed tomography, radiography, urinalysis).
- Explore the cause of the fall with the health care team by reviewing the patient's history, including any history of falls and any intrinsic or extrinsic factors that may be related to the fall.
- Document the incident and its precipitating factors, along with a plan to prevent future falls.
- Implement a fall prevention program.

Critical Care and Trauma Care

Older adults admitted to the hospital are often critically ill, and effective nursing care requires an understanding of their impaired homeostatic mechanisms, the diminished reserve capacity of their body systems, and their impaired immune response. Homeostatic mechanisms are altered with age so that the ability to generate a fever, to respond to alterations in tissue integrity, and to sense pain may be very different from those manifested by young or middle-age adults in critical care (Merck Manual of Geriatrics, 2013). The atypical and subtle nature of disease presentation becomes even more important in the intensive care unit (ICU), where the patient is often less able to articulate discomfort and new problems may arise quickly. The nurse must be aware that the most common presenting symptom of sepsis in older patients is acute mental status change (Tucker, Clark, & Abraham, 2013). Astute observation for delirium is essential in aggressively managing its underlying cause. Delirium in this setting was referred to in the past as "ICU psychosis" and was thought to be caused by sensory overload or sensory deprivation. The causes are now recognized as multifactorial and, in this environment, are often secondary to acute illness, drugs, and the environment. Critically ill individuals are at particular risk for delirium because of impaired physical and mental defenses (Monkhouse, 2013) (Table 26.1).

Two additional issues for the critical care of older adults are prevention of nutritional compromise and recognition of adverse drug reactions. Up to 65% of hospitalized older adults are malnourished on admission or acquire nutritional deficits

TABLE 26.1	**Changes in Cognitive Status**		
	Delirium	**Dementia**	**Depression**
Onset	Sudden and acute	Insidious, subtle, gradual; difficult to pinpoint	May be sudden or gradual, depending on course; may pinpoint date
Duration	Brief; often clears within 1 month or when underlying disorder is resolved	2–20 years	Weeks to years; variable
Awareness	Clouded state of consciousness; disoriented	Alert and aware	Directed inward; self-absorbed
Mood/behavior	Easily distracted; incoherent speech; difficulty with attention and concentration; hallucinations and illusions; disturbed sleep–wake cycle; increased or decreased psychomotor activity; fluctuation of symptoms: lucid at times but often worse at night	Personality changes; emotionally labile; may become easily agitated, with catastrophic reactions	Often aware of cognitive problems; apathetic, with feelings of hopelessness or worthlessness; vague somatic complaints
Task performance	Often unable to carry out tasks; difficulty following directions	Tries hard to carry out activities; gradual loss of abilities	Able but makes little effort
Mental function	Disorganized thinking; fluctuating impairments in memory, coherence, orientation, and perception	Impairments in memory, abstract thinking, judgment, and language; loss of common knowledge	Selective memory loss: "I don't know" answers on cognitive tests

while hospitalized (Monkhouse, 2013). In the critical care setting, patients are sicker and have ever-changing metabolic requirements that necessitate daily nutritional monitoring. Patients over 75 years of age admitted to the ICU after emergency surgery or for medical reasons have a mortality rate of up to 67% (Monkhouse, 2013). Clinical recognition of the pharmacokinetic and pharmacodynamic changes associated with aging is most important in the critical care setting where more drugs are used to combat more problems. Drugs given in the critical care context may be lifesaving and life-threatening at the same time (Fuchs et al., 2012).

The most common traumatic injuries experienced by those older than age 65 result from falls, automobile accidents, and burns. Older adults suffer injuries of equivalent severity to those of younger persons; however, the consequences are more severe. It is essential to obtain a thorough history of an injury from the patient and his or her family, including the circumstances surrounding the event and the events leading up to the injury. Health care professionals in the field need to realize that older adults do not tolerate hypoperfusion long and may quickly go into cardiogenic shock and multisystem organ failure. Early hemodynamic monitoring is required. The vital signs of an older adult might be restored to normal, yet the person might still be in cardiogenic shock. As much as volume depletion is a concern, so is volume overload in patients with limited cardiac and renal reserves. Insertion of a catheter does increase the risk of infection in older adults but is often justified for its monitoring value (Legome & Shockley, 2011; Fuchs et al., 2012).

Thermoregulatory mechanisms become impaired as a person ages, and older adults with trauma are particularly vulnerable. Care should be taken to reduce heat loss with the use of warm intravenous solutions, warm blankets, and proper environmental control. The degree of long-term recovery of older adults who survive injury is variable, and aggressive rehabilitation and social support are important factors in recovery. Research supports the fact that older adults are at greater risk for complications and higher mortality even when injuries are not severe (Legome & Shockley, 2011). Frailty is defined as the presence of at least three of the following criteria: decreased strength, exhaustion, slow walking speed, low physical activity and unintentional weight loss associated with increased functional impairment, falls, prolonged hospitalizations, and death (Monkhouse, 2013). Frailty is associated with female gender, chronic disease, increased chronologic age, and decreased functional status. Frailty is a measure of vulnerability and indicates those at risk for increased mortality and institutionalization. Frail individuals have a limited capacity to respond to internal and external stressors (Hubbard & Woodhouse, 2010).

HOME CARE AND HOSPICE

Community-based service providers are challenged to develop affordable and appropriate programs to assist older adults to remain in the home while maintaining their quality of life. Community-based services for older adults include home health care, community-based alternative programs, respite care, adult day care programs, senior citizen centers, homemaker programs, home-delivered meals, and transportation, among many others (Box 26.2). In some areas, churches and neighborhoods have organized volunteer programs to help meet the needs of older adults who rarely leave home. Some of these programs rely on paid nurses and volunteers from the community.

To identify the needs of the older population, nurses in the community must have sharp assessment skills and knowledge of normal aging changes, chronic illnesses, and the effects of illnesses and treatments on older adults. They must also be aware of available community resources. Home health remains one way to help the older adult who has a physical or cognitive impairment stay in the home. Because of changes in reimbursement for federal programs that provide services for older adults and limited funds for state programs, home health nurses are challenged to use interventions that are both effective and cost efficient.

BOX 26.2   Services for Older Individuals

Access Services
- Case management
- Information and referral
- Transportation

Community-Based Services
- Adult day care
- Congregate nutrition programs
- Elder abuse/protective services
- Health screening/wellness promotion services
- Housing services
- Institutional respite care
- Legal assistance
- Multipurpose senior centers
- Psychological counseling
- Retirement planning

In-Home Services
- Home-delivered meals
- Home health services
- Home hospice care
- Homemaker services
- Home maintenance and repair or chore services
- In-home respite care
- Personal emergency response systems
- Telephone monitoring and friendly visitors

FACTORS AFFECTING THE HEALTH CARE NEEDS OF NONINSTITUTIONALIZED OLDER ADULTS

Functional Status

Functional status is a term used to describe an individual's ability to perform the normal, expected, or required activities for self-care. It is a determinant of well-being and a measure of independence in older adults. Functional measures are much more useful in describing the service needs of older adults living in the community than are measures of acute and chronic illness. Because of their ability to predict service needs, functional measures are used to determine eligibility for many state-funded and federally funded, community-based, long-term care programs. Health care providers frequently order physical or occupational therapy as part of home health when a functional deficit exists (van Hout et al., 2010).

Functional status determines whether an older adult needs home health care or whether a home health client is recertified for home care services. The use of adaptive equipment as well as barriers to the client's function should be noted. While assessing the client's functional status, the home health nurse considers cognitive status, respiratory and cardiovascular status, and skin integrity. Deficits in these areas could impair the client's ability to perform ADLs and IADLs safely. The client's perception of self-care is also important because they may believe that no assistance is required when, in fact, a deficit exists (van Hout et al., 2010).

For older adults, adapting to functional limitations is crucial for maintaining independence. The outcomes of severe functional impairments are costly (e.g., institutionalization). The home health nurse must assess for functional impairments. Early detection of limitations leads to interventions that help preserve function and avoid more severe disability. *Frailty,* as previously defined, has become a predictor for older adults. Frail older adults are more likely to require assistance in the home care setting or require a supervised care setting (Monkhouse, 2013).

Cognitive Function

Cognitive impairment, which often affects an individual's functional status, is another eligibility criterion used by various community programs. Cognitive status is assessed on admission and again with every nursing visit. Other disciplines are also responsible for reporting a change in cognition to the nurse or case manager in home health. A change in cognitive status frequently signals a change in another body system. The home health nurse must establish a baseline assessment and be alert to deviations. Cognitive impairments may be reversible or irreversible, and home health personnel are in a key position to detect any changes.

Cognitive impairments are associated with functional limitations. For example, individuals with deficits in memory, language, abstract thinking, and judgment have great difficulty executing ADLs or IADLs (e.g., shopping, paying bills, preparing meals, and personal care tasks), even though they may have no *physical* impairments or disabilities. Cognitively impaired individuals often need supervision and cueing, rather than physical assistance, to perform ADLs and IADLs.

Although cognitive impairment alone does not meet the criteria for home health care services covered by Medicare, many states provide services for individuals with Alzheimer's disease and related dementias through Medicaid and Medicare waiver programs. Medicare covers skilled nursing visits when (1) the skill is necessary to maintain the client's health, (2) the cognitive impairment interferes with the client's ability to perform the skill, and (3) no caregiver is present or able to perform the skill. An older adult who requires daily insulin injections but is unable to draw up or administer the insulin because of a cognitive impairment is an example of someone who qualifies for home health care.

Housing Options for Older Adults

Although older adults prefer to live independently, it is not always possible or appropriate; financial status, functional status, frailty, and physical health may dictate consideration of alternative housing options that provide a more protective and supportive environment. Table 26.2 describes the most common housing options for older adults. Each option has its advantages and disadvantages. The decision about which option is most appropriate depends on such factors as the amount and type of assistance an older person requires, financial resources, geographic mobility, preferences for privacy and social contact, and the types of housing available. The American Association of Retired Persons (AARP) has several publications that describe each of these options in greater detail, including issues to consider when evaluating each option.

TABLE 26.2 **Housing Options for Older Adults**

Type of Housing	Description of Housing
Accessory apartment	This is a self-contained apartment unit within a house that allows an individual to live independently without living alone. It generates additional income for older homeowners and allows older renters to live near relatives or friends and remain in a familiar community.
Assisted living facility (also called *board and care home; personal care home;* or *sheltered care, residential care,* or *domiciliary care facility*)	This is a rental housing arrangement that provides room, meals, utilities, and laundry and housekeeping services for a group of residents. Such facilities offer a homelike atmosphere in which residents share meals and have opportunities to interact. What distinguishes these facilities from simple boarding homes is that they provide protective oversight and regular contact with staff members. Some facilities offer additional services such as nonmedical personal care (e.g., bathing, grooming) and social and recreational activities. In many states, these facilities operate without specific regulation or licensure; therefore the quality of service may vary greatly.
Congregate housing	Congregate housing was authorized in 1970 by the Housing and Urban Development Act. It is a group-living arrangement, usually an apartment complex, which provides tenants with private living units (including kitchen facilities), housekeeping services, and meals served in a central dining room. It is different from board and care facilities in that it provides professional staff such as social workers, nutritionists, and activity therapists who organize social services and activities.
Elder Cottage Housing Opportunity (ECHO)	This is a small, self-contained portable unit that can be placed in the backyard or at the side of a single-family dwelling. The idea was developed in Australia (where it is called a "granny flat") to allow older adults to live near family and friends but still retain privacy and independence. ECHO units are distinct from mobile homes in that they are barrier-free and energy-efficient units specifically designed for older or disabled persons.
Foster home care	Foster care for adults is similar in concept to foster care for children. It is a social service administered by the state that places an older person who needs some protective oversight or assistance with personal care in a family environment. Foster families receive a stipend to provide board and care, and older clients have a chance to participate in family and community activities. Adult foster care is appropriate for older adults who cannot live independently but do not want or need institutional care.
Home sharing	Home sharing involves two or more unrelated people living together in a house or apartment. It may involve an older person and a younger person or two or more older people living together. The participants may share all living expenses, share rent only, or exchange services for rent. For the older homeowner, renting out a bedroom generates revenue that may make it possible to afford taxes and home expenses. Many older adults view home sharing as a practical alternative to moving in with adult children. Some communities provide house-matching programs, usually sponsored by local senior centers or the Area Agency on Aging.
Life care or continuing care retirement community (CCRC)	This is a facility designed to support the concept of "aging in place." It provides a continuum of living arrangements and care—from assistance with household chores to nursing facility care—all within a single retirement community. Residents live independently in apartments or houses and contract with the community for health and social services, as needed. If a resident's need for health and nursing care prohibits independent living, the individual can move from a residential unit to the community's health care unit or nursing facility. In addition to providing shelter, meals, and health care, a CCRC provides a variety of services and activities (e.g., religious services, adult education classes, library, trips, and recreational and social programs). The key attribute of a CCRC is that it guarantees a lifetime commitment to care of an individual as long as the person remains in the retirement community. The major disadvantage of a CCRC is that it can be expensive; most CCRCs require a nonrefundable entrance fee and charge a monthly assessment, which may increase.

Modified from American Association of Retired Persons (AARP). (2013). *Housing: Independent & assisted living senior housing 2013.* Retrieved from http://www.aarp.org/home-garden/housing/.

COMMUNITY-BASED SERVICES

Use of Community- and Home-Based Services by Older Adults

Assessment of functional status aids in determining the type of services an older adult needs to remain in their home. A score on a functional status test that indicates impairment does not necessarily indicate the need for institutionalization, but it means that the older adult needs assistance with specific activities (van Hout et al., 2010). The type of services needed, the availability of the services, the cost of the services, and the requirements to qualify for the services are determined by a home health agency.

Community services are categorized into formal and informal services. Home health care is a short-term, formal service that provides assessment, observation, teaching, certain technical skills, and personal care. A client may receive home health care for a limited time and for a specific diagnosis. Homemaker services are another formal service. To qualify for most homemaker services, the older person must demonstrate a financial requirement and a specified need for service. Informal services include senior citizen centers, adult day care services, nutrition services, transportation services, and telephone monitoring services. Community resources, formal and informal, must meet the client's needs (see Cultural Awareness box).

🌐 CULTURAL AWARENESS

Community-Based Long-Term Care for Latino Older Adults

The number of Latinos older than 65 is projected to increase 500% by the year 2030. In a national survey of 2299 Latinos (of any Hispanic ancestry but predominantly Mexican Americans and Puerto Rican Americans) age 65 or older, Wallace and Lew-Ting (1992) found that Latinos have higher rates of disability than their white counterparts and a greater need for community-based long-term care (Hanlin, Delgado-Rendón, Lerner, Hargarten & Farias, 2013).

Two major factors influence the interest and ability of Latino families to seek formal long-term care: cultural influences and structural influences. *Cultural influences* include the belief systems and preferences that cause certain patterns of health care use. Because long-term care often involves nontechnical assistance that can be provided by family members, Latino older adults tend to use nursing facilities less often as family members make sacrifices to help older relatives. More acculturated families provide lower levels of care and less informal support for older adults than less acculturated ones.

Structural influences include the way the health care system and other social institutions are organized and operated. They may present both incentives and barriers to the use of health services. Given the importance of income and insurance in determining long-term care use, a major gap exists in the health insurance status of Latino older adults. In the general population, one-third of Latinos are uninsured compared with 13% of whites and 19% of blacks. This is largely because Latinos are concentrated in industries that do not offer insurance, such as personal services and construction, and because they tend to live in states such as Texas and Florida that have stringent Medicaid eligibility criteria. As a result, serious illness in the family is considered a financial problem almost twice as often among Latinos as other non-Hispanic whites (39% versus 19%).

Research reveals that the need for in-home health services for older Latinos is substantial. Mexican American older adults are less likely than the average Latino to use in-home health services despite similar levels of need. Nurses should not assume that Latino families are taking care of their disabled older members simply because of a cultural preference. Nurses should provide information and advice on the use of in-home health services when an older Latino client is physically disabled.

From Wallace, S. & Lew-Ting, C. (1992). Getting by at home: Community-based long-term care of Latino elders. *Western Journal of Medicine 157*, 337-344. Adapted and reproduced with permission from the BMJ Medical group (supported by Hanlin, E., Delgado-Rendón, A., Lerner, E, Hargarten, & S. Farías, R. [2013]. Fall risk and prevention needs assessment in an older adult Latino population: A model community global health partnership. *Progress in Community Health Partnerships: Research, Education, and Action*, 7[2], 191-199).

Because of fragmentation, noninstitutional long-term care depends on the coordination of efforts between informal and formal care providers. In some instances, families function as case managers, ensuring that resources and services are provided appropriately. In other situations, case management services are provided by formal organizations such as home health care agencies or managed care agencies. These nurses must be familiar with community resources and should assist older individuals and their families in accessing these resources. Home health nurses have a particular responsibility to assess older adults who are receiving home health services and to determine how their individual needs can best be met. The home health nurse identifies appropriate community resources, initiates the referral process, develops a care plan, coordinates services, evaluates the services, and determines whether a need exists for additional services. Home health nurse visits that target frail older adults may have a significant effect on mortality and institutionalization (van Hout et al., 2010).

Profile of Community- and Home-Based Services
Area Agencies on Aging

The major goal of the Older Americans Act (OAA) of 1965 was to remove barriers to independent living for older individuals and to ensure the availability of appropriate services for those in need. Through Title III, the Administration on Aging (AOA) and state and community programs were designed to meet the needs of older adults, especially those at risk for loss of independence. The OAA established a national network of federal, state, and Area Agencies on Aging (AAAs), which is responsible for providing a range of community services for older adults. States are divided into areas for planning and service administration. The OAA requires that each AAA designate community "focal points" as places where anyone in the community can receive information, services, and access to all of a community's resources for older adults. Multipurpose senior citizen centers often serve as these focal points, but community centers, churches, hospitals, and town halls may also be designated as focal points. The types of services provided through the OAA and the AAAs include information and referral for medical and legal advice; psychological counseling; preretirement and postretirement planning; programs to prevent abuse, neglect, and exploitation; programs to enrich life through educational and social activities; health screening and wellness promotion services; and nutrition services (AOA, 2017; Bales & Ritchie, 2009; Smith, 2010).

Multipurpose Senior Centers

Senior centers are community facilities that provide a broad range of services to older adults in the community. These services include (1) health screening; (2) health promotion and wellness programs; (3) social, educational, and recreational activities; (4) congregate meals; and (5) information and referral services for older individuals and their families. Relatively active and independent older adults primarily use senior centers because such centers do not provide nursing and custodial care services. Older adults who require these types of services would benefit from attending an adult day care program. Funding for senior centers is provided primarily through the OAA and agencies such as the United Way.

Adult Day Care Services

Adult day care services provide a variety of health and social services to older adults who live alone or with their families in the community. Most people who use adult day care services are physically frail, cognitively impaired, or both and require supervision or assistance with ADLs. Adult day care programs help delay institutionalization for older adults who require some supervision but who do not need continuous care. This allows family members to maintain their lifestyles and employment, and allows the older adult to remain in the home.

Most adult day care services operate 5 days a week during typical business hours. Charges vary with each facility, from per week to per day to per half-day. Adult day care services vary considerably in terms of eligibility criteria and the types of services provided. Key services may include transportation to and from the facility, assistance with personal care, nursing and therapeutic services, meals, and recreational activities.

Adult day care services are not federally regulated but may be licensed or certified by the state. Certification is required to receive federal funding such as Medicaid and OAA funding. Other funding sources include private pay, foundations, and long-term care insurance. Medicaid is a major funding source for most of these programs; however, participants usually pay part of the fee. Some facilities may accept only private pay or long-term care insurance. Other private sources of funding include religious organizations, businesses, and the United Way.

Some programs accept only clients with dementia. It is difficult to combine clients with dementia and clients who have no cognitive impairment. This situation requires extra staff and usually a larger facility with separate areas for the two different groups. The staff in these programs is trained to work with persons with dementia.

Respite Care

Respite care provides short-term relief or time off for persons providing home care to ill, disabled, or frail older adults. Adult day care services are a form of respite provided outside the home. Respite care is often provided at home or in institutional settings such as specially designated hospital or nursing facility units. Respite staff includes health professionals, trained volunteers, and personal care attendants (PCAs). In-home and institutional respite may be provided on a regular schedule (e.g., 4 hours a week) or for longer time intervals (e.g., 1 week, a weekend, or on an intermittent basis). Private pay and state programs that target lower-income families are the two main funding sources for respite care.

Homemaker Services

Homemaker services include such things as housecleaning, laundry, food shopping, meal preparation, and running errands. Fees vary according to the type and frequencies of services provided and are usually not covered by Medicare or Medicaid. These services are offered through home health agencies, AAAs, the Department of Health and Human Services, and private companies and organizations that provide other services to older adults. Prices vary with the type of agency offering the homemaker services. In most states, no licensing or certification is required for the individual providing the care. Background checks and letters of recommendations are often the only qualifications for the positions.

Nutrition Services

Nutrition services provide older adults with inexpensive, nutritious meals at home or in group settings. Home delivery programs such as Meals-on-Wheels deliver hot meals to the home once or twice a day, 5 days a week, and can accommodate special diets. Some Meals-on-Wheels programs sell nutritional supplements at reduced rates to older adults who cannot leave the home. Congregate meal sites provide meals in group settings such as senior centers, churches, synagogues, schools, and senior housing. The advantage of congregate meal sites is that they provide social opportunities for older adults who are otherwise socially isolated. Most nutrition programs charge a minimum fee or ask for donations. Another advantage of home-delivered meals is that the volunteer delivering the meal is able to check on the older adult daily and report any problems to the supervisor. In some instances, a Meals-on-Wheels volunteer has been the first person to discover an older adult who fell in the home and was unable to seek assistance.

Transportation Services

Many communities provide transportation services for disabled older adults through public or private agencies. The transportation may be handled by volunteer drivers in cars or by a bus, taxi, train, or a public van equipped to accommodate wheelchairs. The fee for such transportation services is usually minimal and is often based on a sliding scale. In addition, many facilities that serve older adults (e.g., adult day care services, senior centers, and health facilities) have their own transportation services.

Telephone Monitoring and Friendly Visitors

Telephone monitoring programs provide regular phone contact (usually daily) to older persons who live alone or are alone during the day. The phone calls provide social contact, as well as a check for those who are concerned about their health and safety. Friendly visitors make home visits for the purpose of companionship, assistance with correspondence, and needs assessment. Telephone monitoring staff and friendly visitors are volunteers who work through local community organizations such as churches, synagogues, senior centers, and social service agencies. Even if older adults live in areas where these formal services are not available, nurses can encourage informal telephone monitoring and visiting by family members, friends, and neighbors. Telephone services that will call individuals to remind them to take their medications are also available, usually for a monthly fee.

Personal Emergency Response Systems

Personal emergency response systems (PERSs) are home monitoring systems that allow older persons to obtain immediate assistance in emergent situations, for example, after a fall or when suffering life-threatening symptoms. A PERS consists of a small device worn on the body (encouraged to be a necklace) and, when triggered, will send an alarm to a central monitoring station. The central monitoring station then contacts predesignated persons or the police, who respond to the emergency. A PERS may be purchased or leased for a monthly fee. Because these devices are relatively expensive, they are not a practical alternative for older adults in middle-income groups. Those in the lower-income groups or dual eligibility will have it as part of a comprehensive home management plan. They are recommended with caution for persons with dementia, because resetting the device is very difficult, and the device may be triggered too often for nonemergencies. Newer devices include GPS that look like a wristwatch, so older adults with dementia or wandering tendencies can be found.

HOME HEALTH CARE

Home care consists of multiple health and social services delivered to recovering, chronically ill, or disabled individuals of all ages in their place of residence. There are three main categories of home care providers, known as *home care organizations* (National Association for Home Care and Hospice [NAHC], 2013). Medicare-certified agencies include hospice and free-standing and facility-based home health agencies.

Medicare, Medicaid, private insurance, managed care plans, and private pay cover home health services. Persons of all ages are eligible for home health services. Criteria for services vary based on the type of insurance. Most home health care recipients are 65 or older. Medicare, the primary payer source for home health services, requires the home health client to (1) have a skilled care need, (2) be homebound, (3) be unable to perform the skilled care alone and have no one in the home to provide care, and (4) require only intermittent care. If a caregiver is present, he or she must be unwilling or unable to provide the care needed. Being homebound means that the home health client has a physical reason (e.g., being bedridden) or medical condition that limits his or her ability to leave home. The use of assistive devices or a wheelchair alone does not qualify an individual for the homebound status. The home health client is allowed to leave home for medical reasons, but it must be an *effort* to do so. In other words, if the client could get to a physician's office to receive care on a regular basis, Medicare would deny the home health services. The client must also have a physician's written plan of treatment for the service specifying the frequency and duration of care provided.

Medicare establishes specific criteria for coverage by the physician, home health agency, disciplines providing care, and other entities (e.g., medical supply companies) that provide goods or services to the client. The purpose of eligibility criteria is to ensure that Medicare dollars are being spent in the most cost-effective manner (CMS, 2017). Other payer sources (e.g., health maintenance organizations [HMOs] and private insurance) use Medicare criteria as a guideline for eligibility but have the flexibility to vary the criteria with individual circumstances (Troy, 2015).

Medicaid is delivered by each state and has its own criteria for reimbursement. Other funding sources of home health include social service block grants, OAA funds, and general state revenues. The dollar amount spent on home health by sources other than Medicare and Medicaid varies with each state. The U.S. Department of Veterans Affairs; the Veterans health care program, TRICARE; and the VA Civilian Health and Medical Program (CHAMPVA) have their own coverage guidelines and payment methods for home health, and each covers different home health services (U.S. Department of Veterans Affairs, 2017).

Managed care companies have various methods for approving services related to home health care. The admission assessment is usually approved first. Then, based on the diagnosis, the functional status of the home health client, and the ability of the caregiver to provide help, the company assigns further home health visits. Other companies approve a specified number of visits based on the diagnosis and information from the referring physician. The home health agency stays in close communication with the managed care company to report progress and request any changes in the original care plan.

Home Health Agency

The predominant and most familiar provider of home care is the home health agency. Home health agencies have as their primary function the treatment or rehabilitation of clients through the intervention of skilled nurses or therapists. Clients admitted to a home health agency must be under a physician's supervision, and services must be provided in accordance with a physician's signed order. Home health agencies can provide a different combination of services. Skilled nursing and physical therapy may stand alone, that is, either the registered nurse (RN) or physical therapist may serve as the case manager. Speech therapists, occupational therapists, and medical social workers are not allowed to admit clients to home health care but must work with a nurse or physical therapist. In addition, many agencies offer nutritional services on a limited basis. Agencies may also provide disposable medical supplies as appropriate for the diagnosis and treatment plan for a client.

Proprietary Agencies

A proprietary or for-profit home care agency is designed to make money for its owners. Until 1982, proprietary home care agencies were not allowed to participate in Medicare. This was changed in response to a concern that not enough home care services were available to meet the demand. As a result, the Omnibus Budget Reconciliation Act (OBRA) of 1982 allowed proprietary home care agencies to become Medicare certified, but they were not allowed to make a profit on the Medicare portion of their business. Owners of a for-profit entity are stockholders in the corporation.

Facility-Based Agencies

A facility-based home care agency is a department or component of an organization. It may be a part of a skilled nursing facility (SNF) or rehabilitation center, or it may be hospital based. The vast majority of agencies are hospital based, that is, they function as a department of the hospital. These agencies may or may not share clinical, financial, or management services with the hospital.

The first hospital-based home care agency was established in 1947. Its programs offered nursing care and housekeeping and chore duties. In 1958, radiology services, nutritional services, and physical therapy were offered. With the enactment of Medicare and Medicaid in 1965, nurses were able to offer more home care to the sick and the disabled. Hospital-based home care agencies were few in number until the enactment of Medicare reform (OBRA, in 1987), when hospitals began to be paid for patients receiving Medicare benefits on the basis of DRGs. With shorter lengths of stay, hospitals established home care agencies or affiliated with existing home care agencies to provide options for patients who were going home with existing health care needs. The Affordable Care Act (2011) made changes to Medicare reimbursement, resulting in a 5% reduction in reimbursement for home care visits (Eck, 2010).

What determines a facility-based home care agency from CMS's point of view is whether it receives an allocation of the institution's corporate overhead. A facility-based home care agency, according to The Joint Commission (2012), shows evidence of an organizational and functional relationship between the home care agency and the facility or public representation of the home care agency as a service of the facility.

Visiting Nurse Associations

A visiting nurse association (VNA), or community nursing service, is a community-based home care agency with a governing board consisting of community representatives. Because of the commitment to provide home care services to a defined community and a not-for-profit status, VNAs are often recipients of United Way or Community Givers funds.

Benefits of Home Care

In survey after survey, older Americans choose "home" as their treatment place of choice. Because of changes in technology, equipment is smaller, easier to manage, and less expensive. As a result, individuals who at one time could be treated only in the hospital can now be managed at home. Family, friends, and even patients themselves can be taught to manage enteral and parenteral feedings, central lines, pain control, antibiotic therapy, wound care, and urinary catheters with a minimum of assistance (TJC, 2011).

Among those older adults who can benefit from home care services are individuals who:
- Have chronic medical conditions with exacerbations such as congestive heart failure, chronic obstructive pulmonary disease (COPD), unstable diabetes, kidney or liver disease with subsequent transplantation, or recent strokes;
- Have chronic mental illnesses such as depression, schizophrenia, or other psychoses;
- Need assistance with medical regimens to prevent readmission to an acute care facility;
- Need continued treatment after discharge from a hospital or nursing facility (e.g., wound care, intravenous therapy, or physical therapy); or
- Require short-term assistance at home after same-day or outpatient surgery or are terminally ill and want hospice care to die with their families and to die with dignity in the comfort of their own homes.

Home care is less expensive than hospitalization in most cases. For example, considerable savings may be achieved using home care services for infusion therapy services. Although home care services are being used because of financial considerations, sound medical and humane reasons also exist for treatment to take place in a person's home. Evidence suggests that people recover faster at home than in institutions, and hospital-acquired infections from exposure to multiple infectious processes are minimized in a person's home.

CONTINUITY OF CARE

Enhancement of the continuum of care from hospital to home is a goal shared by both hospital and home care personnel. Continuity of care involves assisting older adults to remain in the home and avoid institutionalization by having available resources that are responsive to their needs (Sharma et al., 2009; van Hout, 2010). The American Academy of Family Physicians has endorsed the establishment of the Patient-Centered Medical Home (PCMH) care model. The PCMH is a model of care led by a primary care physician (PCP) who provides continuous and coordinated care throughout a patient's lifetime to maximize health outcomes. A PCMH service includes preventive services, treatment of acute and chronic illness, and assistance with end-of-life issues. This care model promotes improved access and communication, care coordination and integration, and care quality and safety. The Patient Protection and Affordable Care Act (2010) endorsed a move toward the PCMH model with reimbursement incentives for PCMH care. The result of this change is to ensure that a continuum of care exists from hospital to home (Davis, Abrams, & Stremikis, 2011). Health care providers should follow the "Plan, Do, Check, Act Cycle" (Box 26.3).

Box 26.4 lists client characteristics that should suggest further evaluation for a home care referral. These characteristics alone do not warrant the need for home health care, but in combination with one another or with a new diagnosis that requires monitoring, they provide an excellent guideline to determine the need for services. The assessment may be done as a prehospitalization screening, at the time of admission to the hospital, after a client's condition has changed, or as a client is being discharged. What really matters is that the client be assessed for home care needs before he or she leaves the hospital.

Ideally, a client is screened for home care needs at the time of admission to a hospital to ensure adequate time to plan for continuity of care. In most instances, unless a client is already known to a home care agency, discharge planning occurs late in the hospital stay. As hospital lengths of stay become increasingly shorter, the time available to plan adequately for a client's postdischarge care is limited. Home care agencies and hospital discharge planners or case managers need to develop a good working relationship to ensure that clients going home have a plan that picks up where the hospital plan leaves off. To ensure a smooth transition, members of all disciplines who were caring for a client in the hospital—nurses, physicians, physical therapists, social workers, and others—should provide qualitative and quantitative information about the client's disposition at

---

BOX 26.3 Plan, Do, Check, Act Cycle

Plan
- Gather data on admission.
- Identify goals for discharge.
- Identify specific functional problems.
- Validate that a problem exists.
- Structure problems by delineating components.

Do
- Gather information about resources.
- Select all possible options.
- Identify measurable objectives in terms of the client's functional problems.
- Analyze each option for capacity to fulfill objectives.
- Identify advantages and disadvantages.

Check
- Compare alternatives for probability of fulfilling discharge objectives.
- Project results of alternatives.
- Explore alternatives with the client and family.
- Choose among alternatives.

Act
- Develop the discharge plan.
- Implement the plan.
- Evaluate and follow up on the plan.
- Revise the plan, as indicated.
- Update the resource file.

BOX 26.4 High-Risk Client Indicators for Home Care Services

- Unexpected readmission to the hospital within 15 to 30 days
- Frequent readmissions
- Alteration of health care problem or management
- Changes in mental status
- Nonadherent behavior before or during hospitalization
- Terminal or preterminal condition
- Seen in the hospital by physical, occupational, or speech therapist
- After amputation
- After hip or knee replacement
- New assistive devices
- Foley catheter, ileal conduit, suprapubic catheter, and/or incontinence
- Complex health management regimen
- Enteral or parenteral feedings
- Ostomies or tubes of any kind
- Draining wounds
- After wound debridement or irrigation and debridement for pressure injury
- Pain management
- Intravenous antibiotics
- Peripherally inserted central catheter
- Intravenous chemotherapy
- Multiple medications or a major medication change
- Ventilator dependence
- Low-air-loss bed or other complex medical equipment

---

discharge. The same principles apply to the discharge process from SNFs or rehabilitation facilities.

In most cases, a social worker or case manager is responsible for notifying the home health agency of a client's discharge. The home health agency requests information needed to ensure a smooth transition from the facility to home. In addition to demographics, necessary information includes the following:
- Identification of the PCP or the PCMH who will sign the home care orders
- Orders for home health care treatments (e.g., wound care, intravenous therapy, physical therapy, occupational therapy, or speech therapy)
- A description of the client's knowledge about the disease and the treatment
- A summary of the client's independence with skills
- Quantitative measures of range of motion and client response to treatment modalities
- Known social situations that could complicate or hinder the home treatment plan
- A list of supplies and medications going home with the client
- Expectations for rehospitalization or follow-up clinic visits
- Anything that would enhance a timely and efficient response from a home care agency

Role of the Home Care Agency

Admission to the home care agency begins with the referral intake. Referrals are called in to the home care agency, and the agency confirms home care benefits; schedules the admission visit consistent with the expectation of the discharge planner, physician, or client; and communicates the referral information to the nurse who will be admitting the client into service. The client must be admitted within 48 hours of discharge, according to Medicare regulations.

Nurses are assigned to clients in various ways. Some assignments are made according to geographic areas, the client's special needs, or the nurse's specialty.

IMPLEMENTING THE PLAN OF TREATMENT

The Nurse's Role

The nurse conducts the initial evaluation visit after a client is referred for home care. During the initial visit and throughout subsequent visits, the nurse assesses the client's physical, functional, emotional, socioeconomic, and environmental well-being. Nurses initiate the care plan and make revisions as appropriate throughout the length of stay in home care.

Other activities requiring the specialized skill of RNs include the following:
- Health and self-care teaching
- Coordination and case management of complex care needs
- Medication administration (e.g., intramuscular and subcutaneous) and teaching about all medications
- Wound and pressure injury care
- Urinary catheter care and teaching
- Ostomy care and teaching
- Postsurgical care
- Care of the terminally ill client

Additional activities provided by some home care nurses are as follows:
- Case management
- Intravenous therapy, enteral and parenteral nutrition, and chemotherapy
- Psychiatric nursing care

Characteristics of a Home Care Nurse

Home health nursing is a subspecialty of community health nursing. It is community-based in that the focus is the client and family, not an aggregate population. The American Nurses Association (ANA) has endorsed practice standards for home health nurses. As with other specialties, the standards address theory, research, ethics, and professional development. The ANA's statement on *The Scope of Home Health Nursing Practice* (ANA, 2013) presents the conceptual model for home health nursing. The model depicts the holistic practice of the home health nurse. Nurses who work in home care require a diverse set of skills and abilities. Most home care agencies require a nurse to have a minimum of 2 years of hospital experience before working as a home health nurse. Working in home care requires knowledge of acute and chronic disease processes and how they affect older adults. Knowledge of gerontology, pharmacokinetics in older adults, rehabilitation nursing, and principles and presentation of disease processes in older adults are areas in which home care nurses need to be competent. The home care nurse also needs to know adult learning principles and interpersonal communication techniques, and he or she must be aware of cultural differences and how they affect health and health care.

The home care nurse coordinates care with all disciplines involved with the case and reports findings, changes, and recommendations to the primary physician. The home care nurse also works cooperatively with community resources and governmental agencies if a situation warrants. The nurse, often the sole health care provider who visits a client's home, knows that observations made must be acted on immediately and that the instruction provided must last until the next visit. If emergency hospitalization is required, the nurse coordinates it with the family, the physician, the hospital, and emergency services.

Home care nurses need to be conscious of their own safety. Some neighborhoods are dangerous, and visits sometimes need to be made in the evening or night. The home health nurse should never go into a situation that might be physically threatening or dangerous. The nurse must be self-reliant, self-assured, and comfortable in providing care in the client's locale. Taking precautions at all times, not just in potentially dangerous neighborhoods, will ensure the nurse's safety. In a recent position paper, The Joint Commission endorsed the role of the home health care nurse in managing patients in noninstitutional settings, and preventing admissions and readmissions to the institutional setting (The Joint Commission, 2012).

Role of the Home Health Aide

In 2014 nearly 1 million home health aides were working in home health, with a projected increase of 38% between 2014 and 2024. HHAs are the second largest group of employees in home care (Bureau of Labor Statistics, 2017). Under the direction of an RN, HHAs assist clients with intermittent personal care services (e.g., ADLs and hygiene), take vital signs, perform simple duties (e.g., nonsterile dressing changes and Foley catheter care), assist with medications that are normally self-administered, and report changes in clients' conditions or needs. The HHA is a nonprofessional caregiver who has completed a course of study and has been certified by an appropriate agency.

In addition, an HHA is required to complete at least 12 hours of in-service training each year of employment. The HHA must demonstrate competency in certain required skills and subjects taught at in-service training at least once a year (Sengupta, Ejaz, & Harris-Kojetin, 2012).

Because the HHA sees the client more often than caregivers from other disciplines, he or she is one of the most important members of the home care team. The client feels comfortable with the aide and often shares concerns that the nurse or therapist cannot elicit. The RN supervises the HHA on a bimonthly basis (Sengupta et al., 2012).

Home health agencies also employ PCAs. PCAs are generally hired for private duty cases in which only a sitter is required (as opposed to someone who provides personal or skilled care). No formal or informal training is required, but individual agencies may provide orientation and some training. Duties performed by PCAs may include, but are not limited to, the following:

- Preparing light meals
- Helping the client to the bathroom
- Assisting with dressing and ambulation
- Light housekeeping

OASIS

Outcome and Assessment Information Set (OASIS) is an assessment tool integrated into an agency's assessment form. It is used to monitor outcomes of home care. OASIS is mandated by the Centers for Medicare and Medicaid Services (CMS) for all adult clients except maternity clients. Its purpose is to improve performance through an approach called outcome-based quality improvement (CMS, 2012a). OASIS was developed to help shape the future direction of Medicare reimbursement and the future of home health.

OASIS data are reported to regulatory bodies at least every 30 days. The completion and reporting of OASIS data are part of the conditions of participation for the Medicare program (CMS, 2012a). OASIS is intended to focus on outcomes of care such as satisfaction and improved client outcomes. OASIS data are completed on admission, discharge, interruption of services, and resumption of services. Surveyors who monitor agencies use the data for onsite reviews. They compare the data on OASIS with data from the assessment of a client when visiting the client in the home.

HOSPICE

Dying is the final phase in the trajectory of a chronic illness. Terminal illnesses, such as certain cancers and acquired immunodeficiency syndrome (AIDS), remain incurable. However, because of pharmacologic and technologic advances in treatments, many cancers and AIDS are now considered chronic illnesses. Many chronically ill persons choose to remain in their homes during the last phase of their illness to prepare for their death in familiar surroundings, together with family and friends. Hospice provides care and services to terminally ill persons and their families that can provide a choice for the terminally ill person to die in a facility or at home.

Hospice Philosophy

Hospice is a special kind of medically directed compassionate care for dying individuals and their families. It is a concept of care, not a particular place or building. The care is designed to address the physical, emotional, psychological, and spiritual needs of dying persons and to provide support services for their families during both the dying and bereavement processes. The goal of hospice is to provide comfort care, not a cure. Individuals with incurable or irreversible diseases who do not respond to treatment may choose hospice care. In addition, when a person and the family have decided to stop pursuing aggressive medical treatment, hospice is an appropriate choice.

Hospice and Palliative Care

A clarification of the terms commonly used in the end-of-life literature and clinical practice is necessary. In the United States, the terms *hospice* and *palliative care* are frequently used. *Palliative care* refers to the broader concept—it is therapy aimed at relieving or reducing the intensity of uncomfortable symptoms; it is not aimed at producing a cure. *Hospice* refers to a specific type of palliative care. Because of reimbursement policies such as the Medicare hospice benefit (discussed later in this chapter), American hospices are mandated to include specific services and are subject to the eligibility requirements that clients have a terminal diagnosis and a 6-month prognosis. Palliative and hospice care both have the goal of comfort, not cure. However, palliative care is provided in settings outside a hospice program and currently is not subject to the same regulations as are hospice programs.

In Canada, the term *palliative care* is pervasive, and *hospice* usually refers to a particular agency or program. Many of the international journals on palliative care originate from Canada, the United Kingdom, and the United States. Therefore it is critical to understand the meaning of the terms as used in the literature about end-of-life care in the respective country of origin. In addition, the health care delivery systems and the private versus governmental insurance programs also differ among the countries. Terminally ill persons, families, and health care providers in Canada and the United Kingdom do not have the constraints of the 6-month prognosis required by the U.S. system.

A widely accepted definition of palliative care, developed by the World Health Organization (WHO), reads, in part: Palliative care is the active total care of clients whose disease is not responsive to curative treatment. Control of pain, of other symptoms, and of psychological, social, and spiritual problems is paramount. The goal of palliative care is achievement of the best possible quality of life for clients and families. It affirms life and regards dying as a normal process. Palliative care neither hastens nor postpones death. It emphasizes relief of pain and other distressing symptoms, integrates the physical, psychological, and spiritual aspects of client care, and offers a support system to help the family cope during the client's illness and in their own bereavement with a team approach to care that focuses on quality of life versus quantity (WHO, n.d.).

Since the 1990s, tremendous interest in palliative care and end-of-life issues has grown throughout the world. Palliative medicine is a recognized medical specialty in the United

Kingdom and Canada. In the United States, numerous initiatives, federal funding, and financial support from private foundations are available for research and innovative programs regarding end-of-life issues. As the research-based knowledge continues to grow, interventions to achieve the outcomes of high-quality end-of-life care for all may become a reality.

Hospice Services

In 2015 approximately 4000 Medicare-certified hospices in the United States served 1.3 million Medicare enrollees with 96 million days of care (National Hospice and Palliative Care Organization [NHPCO], 2017). Services provided by a comprehensive hospice program include physician services; nursing care; medical social work; counseling services and spiritual care; certified nursing assistant (CNA) services; additional therapies, as needed (e.g., physical, occupational, and speech therapy); inpatient care related to difficulty in managing symptoms; medications; supplies; equipment; volunteers; respite services; continuous care in times of crisis; and bereavement services. These services constitute a basic level of hospice care established through the development of the NHPCO's *Standards of a Hospice Program of Care* and the federally mandated operating standards for Medicare certification for hospice programs (NHPCO, 2013).

Hospice services are provided by an interdisciplinary team consisting of the client's own physician, hospice physicians, nurses, HHAs, medical social workers, chaplains, bereavement coordinators, and volunteers. Team members use their skills and expertise to meet the needs of dying persons and their families. These needs may include teaching family and friends how to administer medications, helping dying persons maintain as much mobility and activity as possible, and listening and responding to a dying person's needs. Help from the hospice team is available 24 hours a day. One member of the team is always on call and will make home visits as needed. However, the dying person and his or her family direct the care and are directly involved in the decision-making processes.

Hospice professionals anticipate problems and concerns, including preparing a family for the loss of a dying person. After the patient' death, various types of bereavement services are available: individual and family counseling, bereavement volunteer visits, support groups, and grief classes. The bereaved family members determine their level of participation in any of the activities and services offered.

Historically, most hospice programs in the United States follow the home care model. This means that the interdisciplinary team provides routine hospice care in a terminally ill person's own home. In contrast to traditional home health care, it is not necessary for a terminally ill person to be homebound or to have a skilled nursing need. A family member or friend is usually designated as the primary family caregiver. Family members provide the 24-hour care of the dying person, and the hospice team consults and supports the family in their commitment to care for the hospice client. However, the creativity and innovation of the hospice team enables many dying individuals to remain in their homes without family caregivers.

Based on the needs of a dying person and his or her family, other levels of care are also available. Inpatient care is available when the client experiences acute or severe pain or symptom management problems. Inpatient respite care provides family caregivers with release time from the daily care of the client. This type of respite care is usually limited to 5 consecutive days. Continuous care is reserved for times of crisis. This service is provided in the client's home by nurses and HHAs. It allows up to 24-hour care.

Medicare Benefit

Hospice services are a fully covered Medicare benefit. Anyone covered by Medicare Part A is eligible for hospice care. The following three conditions must be met to qualify for the Medicare hospice benefit. First, a terminally ill person's physician and the hospice medical director must certify that the client is terminally ill and has a life expectancy of 6 months or less. Second, a client must choose to receive care from a hospice instead of receiving standard Medicare benefits. Third, care must be provided by a Medicare-certified hospice program. The Medicare benefit pays for two 90-day periods of hospice care and an unlimited number of 60-day periods if the client is reassessed and recertified as terminally ill at the beginning of each period. Hospice clients may change their minds at any time, discontinue hospice care, and return to the cure-oriented care covered by standard Medicare benefits (NHPCO, 2012).

The Medicare hospice benefit covers pain and symptom control medications for a terminal illness. Durable medical equipment needed to care for a client in the home is also covered. The Medicare hospice benefit does not pay for treatment or services unrelated to the terminal illness. Attending physician charges continue to be reimbursed in part through Medicare Part B coverage. The standard Medicare benefit program continues to pay covered costs necessary to treat unrelated conditions that the hospice client may have concurrently with the terminal diagnosis (NHPCO, 2012).

HMOs are not required by law to provide hospice services. However, most HMOs do provide these end-of-life services. In addition, HMOs that receive Medicare funding are required to inform their members who are Medicare beneficiaries of Medicare-certified hospice programs located in their geographic area. If such a person chooses hospice care, he or she does not need to leave the HMO and will continue to receive HMO benefits not covered by Medicare (NHPCO, 2012). Most private insurance companies and Medicaid also provide hospice benefits.

Location of Care

In the United States, hospice care is primarily provided in the home. However, other sites include hospital-based units, freestanding independent facilities, and long-term care facilities (nursing facilities). The use of these facilities is based on the needs of a dying client and his or her family, and on the type of services offered in the client's geographic area.

The hospice team recognizes that circumstances change. For example, a dying person and their family may initially choose to care for the dying person at home with the support of the hospice. Later, the primary caregiver may become exhausted or sick and be unable to provide that care any longer. The hospice team will assist the family in choosing an alternative to home-based hospice care. The transition between locations of care should be seamless with the assistance of the hospice team.

OVERVIEW OF LONG-TERM CARE

Definition

Long-term care has several meanings in the gerontologic nursing literature. The phrase is most accurately used to describe a collection of health, personal, and social services provided over a prolonged period. Of people over 65, 70% will use some form of long-term care in their lifetime (U.S. Department of Health and Human Services [DHHS], 2012). Recipients of long-term care services typically include older adults but may also include developmentally disabled persons, persons permanently impaired from traumatic injuries, and chronically ill younger persons. Services range from supportive care to very complex care. Long-term care settings may be categorized on a continuum according to the complexity of care provided and the amount of skilled care and services required by the residents served. Settings go from more structure to less structure as one moves from the institutional setting to community-based programs to the home setting. Table 26.3 illustrates this continuum of long-term care settings.

Persons living in nursing facilities are called *residents*. The facility is their permanent or temporary home. Some residents require nursing care until death. Other residents are admitted from an acute care hospital. They stay for a short time to recover from an acute illness, injury, or surgery, then return home. Medical, nursing, dietary, recreational, rehabilitative, social, and spiritual care is usually provided. All nursing facilities must function under the federal regulations set forth by the OBRA. Some facilities are also accredited by The Joint Commission.

Factors Associated With Institutionalization

As life expectancy and the size of the older adult population increase, the possibility of a person entering a nursing facility at some point also increases. Personal factors associated with institutionalization include advanced age, physical disability, mental impairment, white race, living without a spouse, and the presence of chronic medical conditions such as heart

TABLE 26.3 Continuum of Settings in Which Long-Term Care Is Provided

Institutional	Community	Home
Nursing facility	Adult day care center	Home health nursing
Group home	Senior center	Home health rehabilitative services
Board and care facility	Congregate meal programs	Homemaker
Assisted living	Hospice	Home-delivered meals
Continuing care retirement communities		Adaptive devices to home environment
Hospice		Hospice

disease, arthritis, hypertension, and diabetes (Luppa, Luck, Weyerer et al., 2010). Factors contributing to the need for institutionalization may be categorized according to characteristics of the person, characteristics of the person's support system, and the community resources available to the person (Box 26.5).

According to a 2010 report by the National Center for Health Statistics (U.S. DHHS, 2012), many older persons receive long-term care services in the home from relatives and friends, and in small group settings with intermediate levels of care. Despite an older person's preference to stay at home, admission to a nursing facility becomes necessary when the person's physical and mental capabilities deteriorate to a point where adequate family and community resources are no longer available. The total number of men and women older than age 65 has continued to rise (National Center for Health Statistics, 2013).

BOX 26.5   Factors Affecting the Need for Nursing Home Admission

Characteristics of the Individual
- Age, sex, and race
- Marital status
- Living arrangements
- Degree of mobility
- Ability to perform basic activities of daily living (ADLs) and instrumental ADLs (IADLs)
- Urinary or fecal incontinence
- Diabetes
- Behavior problems, wandering
- Mental status
- Memory and cognitive impairment
- Mood disturbance
- Tendency to fall
- Clinical prognosis
- Income
- Payment eligibility
- Need for special services

Characteristics of the Support System
- Family capability
- Age and health of spouse (if married)
- Presence of responsible relative (usually an adult child)
- Family structure of responsible relative
- Employment status of responsible relative
- Physician availability
- Amount of care currently received from family and others

Community Resources
- Formal community resources
- Informal support systems
- Presence of long-term care institutions
- Characteristics of long-term care institutions

Adapted from Cipariani, G., Lucetti, C., Nuti, A., & Danti, S. (2014). Wandering and dementia. *Psychogeriatrics, 14,* 135-142; Halter, J., Ouslander, J., Tinetti, M. Studenski, S. High, K. Asthana, S., & Hazzard, W. (2009). *Hazzard's Geriatric Medicine and Gerontology.* New York: McGraw-Hill; and Holup, A. A., Hyer, K., Meng, H., & Volicer, L. (2017). Profile of nursing home residents admitted directly from home. *Journal of Post-Acute and Long-Term Care Medicine, 18,* 131-137.

Medical and Psychosocial Models of Care

Nursing facilities evolved from the acute care hospital system and the medical model. Like hospitals, nursing facilities were designed around the departments and professionals rather than the consumers they served. Although the organization of nursing facilities tends to be hierarchic and bureaucratic, alternative methods of staffing are being developed and implemented (White-Chu, Graves, Godfrey et al., 2009). This emphasis is on using more licensed nursing personnel to perform primary nursing and case manager roles. Within these models, graduates with a bachelor of science in nursing will have opportunities to fill midlevel management roles and can effect positive changes in long-term care.

The medical model places residents in a sick role and in need of physician-directed help. Adherence to the medical regimen is emphasized. Residents are expected to adhere to staff and medical decisions rather than actively participate in determining them (White-Chu et al., 2009). However, one of the changes mandated by the OBRA is an emphasis on the social and psychological health of nursing facility residents, in addition to the traditional medical concerns. Residents' subjective evaluations of their quality of life need to be solicited and valued. Psychosocial models of care emphasize resident decision making and the exercise of personal choice. The ideal long-term care facility is a combination of both medical and social models, not exclusively one or the other (Box 26.6).

Sometimes, nursing facility personnel do not fully understand resident rights. Creative strategies are necessary to enhance a resident's perception of autonomy. The baccalaureate-prepared nurse is in a wonderful position to combine their knowledge of medicine, nursing, psychology, and sociology into a model that truly provides individualized care to each resident in the nursing facility.

CLINICAL ASPECTS OF THE NURSING FACILITY

Resident Rights

One of the accomplishments of the report of the Committee on Nursing Home Regulation of the Institute of Medicine (IOM)

BOX 26.6   Major Regulatory "Level A" Requirements Defined by the Omnibus Budget Reconciliation Act of 1987

- Resident rights
- Admission, transfer, and discharge rights
- Resident behavior and facility practices
- Quality of life
- Resident assessment
- Quality of care
- Nursing services
- Dietary services
- Physician services
- Specialized rehabilitative services
- Dental services
- Pharmacy services
- Infection control
- Physical environment
- Administration

was to lay the foundation for greater regulatory support of resident rights in the nursing facility (IOM, 1986). Emphasis on resident rights was directly related to a revised view that residents really did have the right to autonomy and to be active participants and decision makers in their care and life in the institutional setting.

Resident rights unique to the nursing facility are to be promoted in several ways. These include but are not limited to the following (CMS, 2015):

- Establishment and maintenance of a resident council
- Public display of posters listing resident rights
- Public display of local ombudsman program information
- Public display of annual state inspection results
- Aggressive attempts to provide opportunities for residents to exercise their right to vote during public elections
- Manage your own money as well as get information on fees and services
- Provision of opportunities for competent residents to self-administer medications
- An informed consent process for the use of side rails and chemical and physical restraints
- An informed consent process for the withdrawal or withholding of life-sustaining treatments
- A grievance process whereby residents and families can challenge the care that is given

All departments within the nursing facility, including social services, activities, nursing, dietary, and maintenance, must share responsibility for ensuring the enforcement of these resident rights. Ideally, this effort will be the operational philosophy for all nursing facilities.

Regulatory enforcement focuses strongly on resident safety without always considering a resident's individual right to be autonomous and make a conscious decision to place themselves at risk (e.g., for falling) to retain some degree of independence. Each situation must be evaluated individually, and the legalities may be complicated (NHPCO, 2012).

Resident Assessment

Interdisciplinary functional assessment of residents is the cornerstone of clinical practice in this setting. The OBRA prescribed the method of resident assessment and care plan development in an instrument known as the Resident Assessment Instrument (RAI). The RAI consists of three parts: the minimum data set (MDS), the resident assessment protocols (RAPs), and the utilization guidelines specified by the CMS's *MDS 3.0 RAI Manual* (CMS, 2012b).

The MDS is a tool that includes a comprehensive assessment of residents (Box 26.7). Categories include resident background information; cognitive, communication and hearing, and vision patterns; physical functioning and structural problems; mood, behavior, and activity pursuit patterns; psychosocial well-being; fecal and urinary continence; health conditions; disease diagnoses; oral, nutritional, and dental status; skin condition; medication use; and special treatments and procedures. This resident profile is used to develop an individualized, comprehensive care plan for each resident.

Deadlines for completion of each section and care-planning decisions emanating from the assessment process are prescribed by regulation. Box 26.8 lists the 18 problem areas that need to be addressed in the care-planning process. The outcome of the

---

EVIDENCE-BASED PRACTICE

Culture Change in Long-Term Care

Background

Long-term care facilities have been structured as institutions where each resident's routine ADLs (e.g., eating, sleeping, bathing) have been controlled by staff. Harrison and Frampton (2017) state, "one's very notion of self is given over to the logic of institutional practices" (p. 6). The culture change movement developed as a model to increase resident control over their daily life, making the environment more homelike. The purpose of this study was to describe the experience of resident-centered care from the perspective of the resident.

Methods

Qualitative, phenomenological evaluation of data was obtained from focus groups at 10 nursing homes across the United States; 227 residents participated in 20, 1-hour focus groups. In the focus groups, residents were asked:

- "This nursing home offers resident-centered care. What does that term mean to you?"
- "What changes have you seen here since resident-centered care began?"
- "In your opinion, what could this nursing home do to be more resident-centered?"

Findings

Participating residents were a mix of men and women. Ages ranged from 52 to 101 years of age. Length of time living in the nursing homes ranged from a few days to 16 years. Analysis of the data revealed the following themes:

- More homelike environment
  - "It means that we live here, and they just work here."
- Increased resident decision making
  - "I decide what I want to do."
- Direction of his or her lifestyle
  - "No one makes you do anything you don't want to. You only do what you want to do. It's your life."
- Putting the residents first
  - "To me, it means that residents come first."

Implications

The culture change movement has led to a more homelike environment for nursing home residents, increased resident decision making and personal direction, and encourages putting residents first. Despite the positive findings, residents also identified three areas still needing improvement: call light response times, access to nature and the outdoors, and transparency when it comes to hospitalization or death of fellow residents.

From Harrison, J., & Frampton, S. (2017). Resident-centered care in 10 U.S. nursing homes: Residents' perspectives. *Journal of Nursing Scholarship, 49* (1), 6-14. doi: 10.1111/jnu.12247.

BOX 26.7 MDS 3.0 Resident Assessment Categories

- Hearing, speech, and vision
- Cognitive patterns
- Mood
- Behavior
- Preferences for customary routine and activities
- Functional status/Functional abilities and goals
- Bladder & Bowel
- Active diagnosis
- Health conditions
- Swallowing/Nutritional status
- Skin conditions
- Medications
- Special treatments, procedures and programs
- Restraints
- Participation in assessment and goal setting

Centers for Medicare & Medicaid Services. (2015). MDS 3.0 for Nursing Homes and Swing Bed Providers. Retrieved May 3, 2018 from https://www.cms.gov/Medicare/Quality-Initiatives-Patient-Assessment-Instruments/NursingHomeQualityInits/NHQIMDS30.html
Note: MDS 3.0 Frequency Report (nationwide aggregate Resident Assessment Category data) can be downloaded from https://www.cms.gov/Research-Statistics-Data-and-Systems/Computer-Data-and-Systems/Minimum-Data-Set-3-0-Public-Reports/Minimum-Data-Set-3-0-frequency-report.html

BOX 26.8 Problem Areas of the Resident Assessment Protocol Summary

- Delirium
- Cognitive loss and dementia
- Visual function
- Communication
- Activities of daily living (ADLs) functional and rehabilitative potential
- Urinary incontinence and indwelling catheter
- Psychosocial well-being
- Mood state
- Behavioral symptoms
- Activities
- Falls
- Nutritional status
- Feeding tubes
- Dehydration and fluid maintenance
- Oral and dental care
- Pressure ulcers
- Psychotropic drug use
- Physical restraints

interdisciplinary team's clinical decision making related to the 18 problem areas as it feeds into care plan development is explicitly described in the RAP summary.

The specific method used to complete the RAI varies from facility to facility. Some facilities assign one nurse to complete all documentation related to the RAI; others distribute this responsibility among all the nurses. The RAI is completed for each resident on admission, annually, when a significant change of condition occurs (as defined by the CMS *MDS 3.0 RAI*

Manual), and quarterly, using an abbreviated one-page version of the RAI. For persons admitted for skilled care under Medicare Part A, the MDS and the RAI are completed at 5 or 14 days, 30 days, 60 days, and 90 days and with any significant change.

Both licensed vocational or practical nurses and RNs may contribute to the RAI. However, only an RN can sign the document and function as the RN assessment coordinator (RAC). The RAC signs and certifies the completion of the assessment, not the accuracy of the assessment data (CMS, 2012b). Contributions to the RAI are also made by the dietary supervisor, social worker, recreational therapist, medical records clerk, and physical and occupational therapists.

The overall goal of the RAI is to provide an ongoing, comprehensive assessment of a resident, emphasizing functional ability and both a physical and a psychosocial profile. It is also a key component in the development of a national database for long-term care.

Skin Care

Skin and nail care programs are important to a resident's overall health and quality of life. Skin care programs in the nursing facility are focused on prevention and treatment of skin problems. Preventive strategies include prevention of pressure injury, skin tears, and dry skin or xerosis.

Other skin-related problems commonly occurring and treated in this setting include MRSA infections, ischemic ulcers, dermatitis, eczema, herpes zoster, scabies, pediculosis, bullous pemphigoid, and skin tumors. The prevention of skin tears, pressure injury, and ischemic ulcers is an ongoing challenge for the staff in nursing facilities. The development of pressure injuries during a person's stay in a nursing facility is considered an indicator of poor quality of care, although research and current knowledge of pressure injury etiology does not support this view as totally accurate. Aggressive and appropriate preventive measures are initiated to address each resident's specific and unique risk factors.

Most nursing facilities have a structured skin care program coordinated by an RN and involves all nursing department staff plus a physical therapist, occupational therapist, and dietitian. On admission, a resident's skin is thoroughly assessed. Individual risk for developing pressure injury is established, and preventive interventions are initiated as appropriate. These may include a special mattress, positioning devices, vitamin and nutritional supplements, skin lubricants, and a schedule for repositioning the resident in beds and chairs. The CNA plays a key role in providing effective preventive skin care by assisting the resident in routine bathing, toileting, and maintenance of schedules for turning and repositioning. The individualized care plan, developed by the interdisciplinary team, provides specific instructions concerning the preventive treatment measures for each resident.

On the basis of the physical examination as well as RAI data, a care plan is initiated. Individual states have varying regulations concerning the required frequency of the nurse's clinical staging and routine assessment of pressure ulcers. Most facilities require at least weekly monitoring by an RN. The nurse measures and stages the pressure injury and evaluates the efficacy of the treatment plan. The director of nursing may also work with the medical director or individual health care providers practicing in the facility to coordinate and standardize treatments for various stages of pressure injuries. Another alternative is to intervene in skin problems on a case-by-case basis according to the preference of the resident's attending physician.

Facilities may have sustained relationships with companies that manufacture specialized beds for residents with stage III or IV pressure injuries. Often the company provides a nurse consultant as a clinical resource to the facility. The nurse functioning as the skin care program coordinator might meet routinely with the consultant. The two nurses often work collaboratively, along with the dietitian and physical therapist, to treat skin problems. Consistently following a treatment plan is essential for positive outcomes.

Incontinence

As functional dependence increases, the prevalence of incontinence increases. This common health problem has financial, physical, and psychosocial consequences, and incontinence is a common reason for placing a person in a nursing facility.

Caring for an incontinent resident is expensive; it requires more nursing time and frequent linen and clothing changes. Physical consequences of incontinence include skin breakdown, UTIs, and an increased risk of falling and consequent hip fracture. Urinary incontinence is one of the most psychologically distressing health problems faced by older adults. It may lead to depression, decreased self-esteem, and social isolation (DuBeau, Kuchel, Johnson et al., 2010). One of the features of the OBRA was the inclusion of specific standards and recommendations for the assessment and treatment of urinary incontinence. Clinical programs in nursing facilities are directed at prevention, treatment, and management of incontinence. Prevention is aimed at reducing the risk of developing urinary incontinence among at-risk residents of nursing facilities. Preventive measures include assessment of individual patterns of elimination so that anticipatory assistance with toileting may be provided, aggressive staff response to residents' requests for assistance in toileting, and arrangement of the physical environment to minimize the physical effort involved in getting to the bathroom.

Treatment programs are resident-oriented and focus on creating changes in the function of the lower urinary tract. Treatments include surgery, pharmacologic interventions, bladder training, pelvic muscle exercises, and biofeedback procedures (DuBeau et al., 2010). It is important to identify those residents who can benefit from these therapies.

Management programs for urinary incontinence are the dominant form of intervention in the nursing facility. Some residents benefit from programs that involve behavioral approaches such as scheduled toileting, habit training, and prompted voiding. These approaches focus on changing the behavior of the caregiver and the resident to minimize the incontinence. However, residents with dementia and other cognitive impairments may not benefit from these interventions; the use of incontinence pads and protective undergarments are necessary for these individuals. External condom catheters may be helpful for men.

Intermittent self-catheterization may be appropriate for residents who are cognitively intact and have adequate manual dexterity. Long-term, indwelling catheterization is indicated for residents who cannot empty their bladders and have not responded to other treatments. Residents who are terminally ill and those with pressure injury may also benefit from indwelling catheterization. Indwelling catheterization is used only after other interventions have failed.

Effective management of urinary incontinence involves a well-coordinated and sustained effort between licensed nursing staff, CNAs, and activities staff. The nurse must play a key role in managing incontinence and preventing complications; management and treatment must be directed at the cause of incontinence.

Nutrition

Nutritional deficiencies contribute to adverse clinical outcomes in nursing facility residents. Protein-calorie undernutrition results from two broad categories of factors: those causing inadequate intake and those causing increased nutritional requirements (Kaiser, Winning, Bauer et al., 2010).

The older population is the single largest demographic group at disproportionate risk of inadequate diet and malnutrition. Aging is associated with a decline in a number of physiologic functions that may affect nutritional status, including reduced lean body mass and a resultant decrease in basal metabolic rate, decreased gastric secretion of digestive juices and changes in the oral cavity, sensory function deficits, changes in fluid and electrolyte regulation, and chronic illness. Medication, hospitalization, and other social determinants also may contribute to nutritional inadequacy. The nutritional status of older people is an important determinant of quality of life, morbidity, and mortality (Brogan & Jen, 2010). Contributing factors include loss of manual dexterity, pain, dementia-related illnesses, certain medications, and chronic medical disorders. Culture, religion, and personal choice also affect how and what a person eats. A resident's appetite is affected by personal comfort and unpleasant odors, sights, and sounds. Meeting a resident's nutritional needs requires involvement of the entire health care team. The health care provider, dietitian, nurse, speech and language pathologist, occupational therapist, social worker, and nursing assistant all play roles in the assessment of individual needs, care planning, care plan implementation, and care plan evaluation. The resident is always included, and the resident's family may also provide important information.

Increased nutritional requirements may be a consequence of hyperactivity in some persons with dementia-related illnesses. Infectious illnesses, periods of recovery after surgical interventions that require tissue healing, and recovery from pressure injuries also increase nutritional requirements of nursing facility residents.

Various clinical interventions are directed at the nutritional support of residents, including programs focused on maintaining adequate caloric intake and effective identification of residents requiring supplemental nutritional support.

Enhancement of the dining experience through improved esthetics, improved dining room service, attractive food preparation, and increased sensitivity to the social nature of mealtimes is directed toward maintenance of adequate caloric intake. Other strategies related to this goal include increasing staff assistance for residents who need help with eating and improving staff techniques for providing assistance with eating. Sensitivity to dental needs and provision of the textures of foods most easily and safely consumed by each resident are additional strategies.

In nursing facilities, the most common program for prompt identification of residents requiring supplemental nutritional support consists of routine weighing. Weights are taken daily, weekly, biweekly, or monthly, depending on the severity of weight loss or gain experienced by a resident. Interdisciplinary team members, including the nurse, restorative nursing assistant (a CNA with 30 hours of formal training beyond CNA with a focus on direct restorative care and delegated formalized therapy tasks as assigned to continue an ongoing formalized therapy program), dietitian, and speech and language pathologist, may meet routinely to review weight changes and develop interventions directed at supplemental nutritional support. In addition to the strategies already described, changes in therapeutic diets and the use of nutritional products (e.g., Ensure), vitamin supplements, and enteral nutrition products may be considered. Laboratory tests are often ordered to help monitor a resident's nutritional status.

Compliance with the OBRA requires aggressive monitoring of the variables of nutritional status with attention focused on unintended weight loss. The functional implications of reduced caloric intake are to be considered. Any unintended weight loss of 5% or greater in 30 days, or 7.5% in 90 days, or 10% in 180 days (Demling & DeSanti, n.d.) is an indicator of poor quality of care. Any weight loss or weight gain must be carefully monitored. The reasons for the loss or gain and the interventions taken must be documented.

Medications

One of the basic services provided in nursing facilities is administration of medications through oral, intravenous, intramuscular, subcutaneous, and enteral routes. In the nursing facility, the licensed nurse is often responsible for the administration, documentation, storage, ordering, cart stocking, and destruction of many medications. In some states, medication aides are used to administer medications. The RN is responsible for monitoring the medication's therapeutic effects, side effects, and any allergic reactions. The RN also monitors and evaluates the skills of medication aides on an ongoing basis. Because most nursing facilities do not have an onsite pharmacy, the nursing staff is responsible for medication-related functions that would be handled by the pharmacy staff in an acute care hospital.

Monitoring for the clinical manifestations of polypharmacy, the occurrence of adverse drug reactions, and the overuse of "as required" (prn) drug orders have increasingly been emphasized since the enactment of the OBRA. The pharmacist contributes to this monitoring effort in a monthly drug review of each resident's medical record, and the nurse has numerous structured opportunities to monitor for these medication-related problems. These opportunities include routine interactions with residents while administering medications and assessment at quarterly care-planning conferences, monthly reviews of psychotropic drug regimens, and completion of the long form of the MDS (Sergi, De Rui, Sarti, & Menzato, 2011). Facilities must have policies and procedures to monitor for drug interactions and side effects.

The routine use of certain drugs, including long-acting benzodiazepines, hypnotics, sedatives, anxiolytics, and antipsychotics, has been curtailed since the enactment of the OBRA. Recommended drug dosages and indications for the use of such medications are given to federal and state survey teams to assist them in the survey and inspection process of each nursing facility (CMS, 2012a).

Residents have the right to participate in decisions about care and treatment. They must be informed of any changes in their medication regimens. Nurses must document their ongoing instruction to each resident (or the resident's legal representative) regarding the initiation of new drug therapy and changes in the dosages of medications. If a resident is cognitively intact, the opportunity to self-administer medications is to be provided (CMS, 2012a). Facilities must have and follow policies and procedures for identifying and following up on medication errors.

Rehabilitation

The provision of rehabilitation programs in nursing facilities has increased over the past 20 years. Factors contributing to this growth in rehabilitation include the OBRA regulatory mandate that facilities provide services directed at achieving the highest practicable level of physical, mental, and psychosocial well-being for residents; the growth of the subacute level of care, including nursing facility participation in managed care programs; and sustained political will to control the growth of health care expenditures (Gronstedt, Frändin, Bergland, et al., 2013).

Rehabilitation teams in nursing facilities consist of the physician, physical therapists, occupational therapists, speech and language pathologists, and facility interdisciplinary team members, including the nurse, social services representative, activity coordinator, and clinical dietitian. Ideally, a medical director with rehabilitation training and experience coordinates the rehabilitation team.

For facilities receiving funds from Medicare, managed care organizations, or private insurance groups, weekly rehabilitation meetings are held to review clinical cases. Residents and family members participate in these meetings to mutually set goals and review progress. Weekly meetings promote communication, effective discharge planning, and resident and family education.

Rehabilitation programs may be categorized into two groups:
(1) The more intensive rehabilitation programs are reimbursed through the Medicare Part A program, managed care organizations, or private insurance groups. Some of these intensive rehabilitation programs seek credentialing by The Joint Commission and the Commission for Accreditation of Rehabilitation Facilities (CARF) to be recognized as benchmark quality programs. Intensive rehabilitation includes daily or twice-daily therapy sessions involving two or more therapy specialties. These sessions are directed toward

returning a resident to a prior level of function and to residence in the community. Endurance building, strengthening, ADL training, treatment of aphasia and dysphasia, cognitive testing and retraining, new disability adaptations training (e.g., after a stroke or an amputation), and training with new adaptive equipment are therapeutic components of these programs.

(2) The less intensive rehabilitation programs that exist in nursing facilities are reimbursed through the Medicare Part B program or private payments, or they are part of the basic services offered by the nursing facility. These services include restorative nursing programs involving ambulation, ADLs, self-feeding, and range of motion. Such programs are provided by specially trained CNAs or facility nursing staff. These programs are established, revised, and supervised by the physical and occupational therapists and the speech and language pathologist. Program goals are focused on the maintenance of functional gains achieved during the more intensive rehabilitation program, regaining a level of function lost because of a short-term illness, and prevention of unnecessary loss of function.

Facilities must provide the required rehabilitation services or obtain them from an outside source. The needs of the individual resident are based on a comprehensive assessment. The goal is to help the resident maintain or regain the highest possible level of physical, mental, and psychosocial well-being.

Infection Control

The development and spread of infections are a major health and safety hazard in nursing facilities. A written program to protect residents, staff, and visitors from infection is required. Facility policies and procedures must include the use of standard precautions and transmission-based precautions, as outlined by the CDC. They must also follow the Occupational Safety and Health Administration's (OSHA) Bloodborne Pathogen Standard.

The OBRA requires nursing facilities to have an infection control program designed to provide a safe, sanitary, and comfortable environment; its purpose is to help prevent the development and transmission of disease. Facilities must have policies and procedures for investigating, controlling, and preventing infections. Records of incidents and corrective action taken related to infections must be maintained. The infection control program should quickly identify new infections. Special attention is given to residents at high risk of infection (e.g., those who are immobilized, have invasive devices or procedures, have pressure injuries, have been recently discharged from the hospital, have decreased mental status, or are nutritionally compromised). The program must also include measures to prevent outbreaks of communicable diseases, including tuberculosis (TB), influenza, hepatitis, scabies, C. difficile, and MRSA. Preventive measures involve TB testing and screening programs for residents and staff. The facility must have procedures for following up on any positive results. Programs to make annual influenza vaccinations and pneumococcal pneumonia vaccinations available as appropriate are also in place.

According to OSHA, employees at risk for exposure to bloodborne pathogens must receive free information and training on employment and annually thereafter. Employers must make the hepatitis B vaccine available to employees within 10 working days of being hired. Personal protective equipment such as gloves, goggles, face shields, gowns, shoe covers, and surgical caps must be made available free of charge to employees; they must also receive instructions on when and how to use this equipment.

An infection control committee consisting of staff members representing each department meets either monthly or quarterly to review data describing the prevalence and incidence rates of infection. This committee discusses any new or proposed revisions in policies and procedures. Typically, one nurse is designated as the infection control nurse and is responsible for coordinating surveillance, data-collecting activities, and ongoing educational sessions for the facility (Chami et al., 2011). The infection control nurse is the facility's resource for information related to the infection control program. It is this person's responsibility to obtain and use current information from the CDC, OSHA, CMS, and state department of health to ensure that the facility's infection control program is effective and meets standards. The facility's medical director and consulting pharmacist also are valuable resources.

Every department and every employee has the responsibility to know and follow the policies and procedures outlined in the infection control program. Policies and procedures include hand washing, standard precautions, respiratory protection, the Bloodborne Pathogen Standard, linen handling, housekeeping, hazardous waste disposal, and proper use of disinfectants, antiseptics, and germicides.

Mental Health

Among the aged and institutionalized population, mental health issues of particular concern include a variety of behavioral problems that may jeopardize the safety of the resident or other residents (e.g., wandering, kicking, or hitting). Because the residents live in a community setting, disruptive behaviors are not just an issue for the affected resident. The disruptive behaviors of one resident adversely affect other residents.

Residents manifesting disruptive behavior commonly have dementia-related illnesses. More than 60% of nursing facility residents have some degree of cognitive deficit. These deficits frequently precipitate behaviors that are difficult to understand and ameliorate. The use of physical and chemical restraints is restricted, and emphasis is placed on using behavioral interventions and environmental modifications (see section on Special Care Units). Doors may have alarms to deter wandering, and exercise, music, massage, low-stimulation environments, lighting, and aromatherapy may be used to decrease agitation.

Most important, nurses are learning ways to determine the causes of the disruptive behaviors by assessing for pain, hunger, infection, and inappropriate environmental stimulation. Psychotropic medications are used only as a last resort, and the side effects must be carefully monitored. It is important to know the type of dementia a resident with disruptive behaviors has been diagnosed with. All dementia is not Alzheimer's disease, and residents with other types of dementia may experience adverse responses to psychotropic medications.

End-of-Life Care

The nurse working in a nursing facility is responsible for helping the entire health care team meet the physical, spiritual, and psychosocial needs of dying residents. Ministering to the residents' families is an important part of this care. Knowledge about a resident's culture and religious beliefs helps the team provide more effective and compassionate care. Some facilities provide hospice training for staff. Hospice programs may also provide care to residents in the nursing facility.

MANAGEMENT ASPECTS OF THE NURSING FACILITY

The Nursing Department

The nursing department is the largest department in the nursing facility. The director of nursing is responsible for managing the entire nursing staff. This consists of RNs, licensed vocational or practical nurses, CNAs, and, if employed by the facility, gerontologic nurse practitioners. In some facilities, nurse managers (usually RNs) assist the director of nursing in managing and carrying out functions of the nursing department. Nurse managers may be responsible for a specified shift, a nursing unit, or specific nursing department functions such as infection control, restorative nursing, total quality management (TQM), and nursing education. Some facilities use unit charge nurses. These are usually RNs, but in some areas they are licensed vocational or practical nurses. Some facilities employ nurse practitioners to provide clinical expertise and serve as a valuable resource for the nursing staff. Nurse practitioners often work closely with the medical director and the resident's PCP to manage the resident's day-to-day care. They may write orders for medications and treatment following collaborative practice protocols.

There are 2.8 million nurses who work in long-term care facilities, with an estimated growth rate of 16% between 2014 and 2024 (Bureau of Labor Statistics, 2017). CNAs are the largest employee group in the nursing departments and facilities as a whole; nursing assistants provide as much as 80% of direct care for long-term care residents (National Network of Career Nursing Assistants, 2012).

Working in the nursing facility presents rewards, opportunities, and challenges for nurses. Rewards include the chance to establish long-term relationships with residents and family members and an opportunity to work in a setting that has a holistic orientation toward resident care. Nurses employed in nursing facilities have many opportunities to use their professional skills as clinicians, teachers, and managers. They are part of an interdisciplinary team that provides a broad spectrum of health care services. The nurse frequently takes a leadership role in developing policies and procedures, assessing resident care needs, developing and implementing care plans, and evaluating outcomes. Excellent assessment and critical thinking skills are very important. A qualified, creative nurse can advance from staff nurse to charge nurse to nurse manager. Opportunities

to chair committees on topics such as TQM, infection control, restorative nursing, and pharmacy are also available. Opportunities for professional growth continue to increase in this evolving, challenging area of health care. However, nurses who choose long-term care as a career must be willing to function in a highly regulated industry. Funding for innovative programs and services is often limited, and in some geographic areas salaries are lower than in acute care settings.

Nursing Care Delivery Systems

Several nursing care delivery systems are found in nursing facilities. There are pros and cons for each delivery system. Unfortunately the system most likely to be in place is the one that is least expensive. Federal regulations regarding staffing requirements for nursing facilities are broad and vague. They are not based on resident acuity and allow the individual facility to determine whether it can provide the care required for any given resident. Few, if any, states have required staffing ratios that are more stringent than the federal requirements.

One nursing care delivery system is functional nursing. Jobs of licensed nurses and CNAs are determined according to work tasks. For example, these may include an MDS nurse, an admission nurse, a medication nurse, a treatment nurse, a restorative nursing assistant, and possibly a dining assistant. CNAs may take groupings of rooms as an assignment for a variable period. A charge nurse functions as the first-line manager. This care delivery system is widely used because it can carry out basic care somewhat efficiently while maintaining only the minimum staffing levels required by regulations. However, if verbal communication between staff members is poor and written documentation inadequate, many resident issues and care needs go unaddressed.

Team nursing is a more integrated care delivery system than functional nursing. The licensed nurse, working with a group of residents (usually 30 to 50), provides medications and treatments to residents, functions as charge nurse or first-line supervisor to the CNAs, and maintains the required documentation for the residents. The licensed nurse may change the resident group assignments on a scheduled basis, usually weekly or monthly. CNAs may change every week or every month. The team nursing system has several advantages. Long-term continuity cannot be provided when CNAs and licensed nurses frequently change group assignments. Staff do not form attachments to residents, and residents, particularly those with memory loss, often have difficulty coping with these changes (i.e., remembering new names and faces and adjusting to the expectations of new personnel) (Duffield, Roche, Diers, et al., 2010). The other major disadvantage of this system is the burden placed on one licensed nurse to safely and efficiently provide medications and treatments to 50 residents, thoroughly assess episodic health problems, and meet documentation requirements.

A third delivery system is primary team nursing, which is also called *total client care*. This involves the combination of a licensed nurse and a CNA working together to care for approximately 10 to 15 residents (Duffield et al., 2010). This team provides all nursing care, including admissions, assistance with ADLs, and administration of medications and treatments. The main disadvantage is that too few staff members are available to meet all the residents' needs, and a risk of inadequate coverage exists when some staff are on break (Duffield et al., 2010).

Regardless of the care delivery system used, the RN practicing in the nursing facility is challenged to work effectively with licensed vocational or practical nurses and CNAs, incorporating them into a professional practice model. It is essential that the RN practicing in this setting have excellent supervisory and management skills. The leadership positions in the department of nursing are held by RNs; these positions include director of nursing services and, increasingly, director of staff development. The baccalaureate-level nurse is the best prepared to fill these positions and significantly affect the quality of care and the quality of life of many residents.

SPECIALTY CARE SETTINGS

Assisted Living Programs

Assisted living facilities are an increasingly attractive long-term care setting, placed between home care and the nursing facility in the continuum of long-term care (Assisted Living Provider Type Definitions, 2017). Regulations are minimal, so great diversity exists in the types of service delivery models used, the types of services offered, and the setting within which assisted living is provided.

Assisted living settings are homelike and offer an array of services, including meals, assistance with bathing and dressing, social and recreational programs, personal laundry and housekeeping services, transportation, 24-hour security, an emergency call system, health checks, medication administration, and minor medical treatments (Assisted Living Provider Type Definitions, 2017). Many services are purchased individually as needed by the resident.

The professional nurse can provide a broad and holistic array of services to residents in assisted living facilities. Many opportunities exist to incorporate both health promotion and illness care into the model. Resident education may delay admission to long-term care. The professional nurse may help coordinate the services provided by various departments, for example, activities, social services, physical and occupational therapy, and housekeeping. As the need for assisted living facilities continues to grow, so will the opportunity for professional nurses to define their contributions and enhance the services offered to frail older adults.

Special Care Units

Since the 1980s, the popularity of specialized units for persons with dementia has expanded. *Special care unit* (SCU) is the designation given to freestanding facilities or units within nursing facilities that specialize in the care of people with Alzheimer's disease and other types of dementia-related illnesses. Behavioral manifestations of dementia are managed in the environment without the use of chemical or physical restraints, whenever possible.

It is advisable for SCUs to have objective, measurable criteria for admission. An objective discharge policy should also be in place. These admission and discharge criteria are helpful to both nursing staff and families who are reluctant to transfer residents to another care setting when a particular resident can no longer benefit from the specialized milieu of the SCU and no longer

requires a secured unit. Admission criteria also deter SCU placement for residents without dementia who have other behavioral problems.

SCUs have physical environmental features that control stimuli and maximize safety yet minimize environmental barriers to freedom of movement (e.g., door alarms and outside fencing to facilitate safe wandering). Program features emphasize nutrition (e.g., finger foods and portable foods), structured daily activities, family involvement, and special staff training in behavioral manifestations of dementia and communication with residents who have dementia. An interdisciplinary team coordinates services and care.

Employment opportunities for the nurse in the SCU are like those in the traditional nursing facility. The SCU is a desirable work setting if the nurse has an interest in the health care needs of persons with Alzheimer's disease and other dementia-related illnesses that have behavioral manifestations. It is not a work setting that everyone can enjoy. Nurses who work with these special resident populations are able to provide valuable consultation regarding persons with Alzheimer's disease to nurses practicing in other settings, including hospitals, home care, and nursing facilities.

Subacute Care

Subacute care, with $12 billion annual spending, has become an increasingly popular level of care (HHS, 2017). The growth of subacute care has been spurred by the belief that up to 40% of clients in acute medical or rehabilitation hospital units could be treated as effectively in less costly settings. With increased political awareness of the rising costs of the Medicare and Medicaid programs, the prospect of significant savings provided by subacute care is an attractive one. Insurance companies are looking to less costly settings to provide patient care. It is estimated that subacute care could eventually replace almost 50% of current acute care hospital lengths of stay.

Subacute care is an industry category rather than a reimbursement or regulatory category. Professional organizations have developed guidelines for the clinical and business development of this level of care. Facilities with subacute care programs can obtain accreditation through The Joint Commission and CARF. These accreditations are granted to facilities with well-defined subacute care programs. Care may be reimbursed through Medicare, HMO benefits, private payment, or Medicaid.

Persons in a subacute care unit are stable and no longer acutely ill or requiring daily physician visits. They may require services such as rehabilitation, intravenous medication therapy, parenteral nutrition, complex respiratory care, and wound management.

The nursing facility has not traditionally been considered a setting in which aggressive rehabilitative services or acute care treatments such as intense rehabilitation, ventilator care, and intravenous infusion therapy are provided. Subacute care is a growing industry in which services such as these are offered to older persons, clients of managed care organizations, and clients whose private insurance company has contracted with a nursing facility to provide care. To care for such clients, the nursing staff requires a level of clinical skill beyond what is typically needed in the nursing facility. Staffing levels, particularly related to licensed nurses, are higher in response to the increased client acuity

CASE STUDY

The following situation depicts how a team of home care providers, coupled with a determined client, can accomplish more than any one discipline working independently.

Situation

Mr. G is a 75-year-old husband, father, and grandfather who suffered a hip fracture after falling at home. He was admitted to the hospital with multiple complications after open reduction internal fixation (ORIF) repair, including delirium, pressure injury, and subsequent subacute rehabilitation. He is being discharged after 3 months of care. He has been discharged home with home health care for wound management and physical therapy. His vital signs on admission to home health were stable and within normal limits. He has had increased confusion with the transition home. He is not able to manage his medications or wound care independently. His wife is frail and has difficulty with her own medications and mobility concerns. He has been discharged with the following medications:

- Docusate (Colace) 240 mg po, qd
- Bisacodyl (Dulcolax) suppository ½ to 1 rectally, every morning as needed (prn)
- Famotidine (Pepcid) 40 mg po, every hour of sleep (qhs) prn
- Enteric-coated aspirin 325 mg po, qd
- Warfarin 5 mg daily alternating with 2.5 mg

The home health nurse is charged with creating a plan of care to meet the needs of Mr. G and his family. His children and grandchildren are not available to provide hands-on care or manage his medications.

To meet the needs of Mr. G, the following services were ordered:

- Nursing—three times weekly skilled nursing visits to manage wound care, assess medication management, and coordinate labs for warfarin.
- Physical therapy—three times weekly visits to improve stamina, stability, and improve gait.
- Medical social work—three times a month to assist with community resources and possible placement in a nursing facility
- Home health aide (HHA) service—three or four times a week to assist with personal care

Because of Mrs. G's comorbidities and minimal ability to care for her husband, he will need assistance longer.

The HHA worked with physical and occupational therapists to reinforce the exercises and safe transfer techniques. Because the aide was assisting with personal care, she was able to reinforce physical and occupational therapy exercises while assisting with transfers, walking, and bathing. The aide reported that Mr. G wanted to use the bathtub and recommended that placement of the commode in the tub could allow Mr. G to transfer safely to the commode and then into the tub. This observation and recommendation from the HHA greatly enhanced Mrs. T's progression with self-care activities.

The team members worked together to identify how Mr. G and his wife could manage at home independently but are struggling. The social worker has a meeting with Mr. and Mrs. G to discuss long-term options. The family comes to a planning meeting and is able to identify ways to assist with the care of their patients. Referrals are made to the Area on Aging to plan for assistive services in the home supplemented by family care.

(Marcantonio & Yurkofsky, 2009). The involvement of the health care provider is also significantly increased.

INNOVATIONS IN THE NURSING FACILITY

Creativity in "Everyday" Nursing Facilities

All that is required to put a little life and love into any nursing facility is some creative thinking, a desire to make life better for residents, and adequate funding. As in similar endeavors, obtaining the financial resources can be the most difficult aspect of this process. However, the innovative nurse accepts this challenge and looks beyond the usual sources to obtain the necessary resources to develop and support new interventions.

Nursing facilities all over the country have acquired dogs, cats, and other animals that can live in the facility and serve as loving companions to the residents. More functionally capable residents can sometimes take primary responsibility for walking and feeding these pets. Aviaries containing tiny birds provide hours of enjoyment for many residents. Music therapy, touch therapy, and aromatherapy are among other innovative activities currently being used in nursing facilities. Indoor and outdoor gardening projects are therapeutic for many residents.

Nurse Practitioners in the Nursing Facility

Over the past two decades, many studies have been conducted to evaluate the effect of the nurse practitioner on older adult residents of nursing facilities. Long-term care facilities that use nurse practitioners can provide more timely care to acutely ill residents. The use of nurse practitioners in collaboration with physicians has been shown to reduce emergency department transfers, hospital days, and subacute days. Several HMOs are

using physician–nurse practitioner teams to provide primary care to nursing facility residents (Bakerjian, 2008).

A nurse practitioner hired by a facility must have the full support of administration to have a real effect on care. They must be free to be an educational resource for staff without being required to participate in staff evaluations. The nurse practitioner must also have the full support of the facility medical director, who serves as a resource for the practitioner and sanctions their services and expertise.

Despite studies demonstrating the cost-effectiveness of nurse practitioners in nursing facilities, few facilities currently employ them on a full-time basis. The major employment opportunities are with groups of physicians who carry a large nursing facility practice. These nurse practitioners may go on rounds with the physician or see nursing facility residents independently on alternate months, whereas the physician sees residents in the intervening months. Medicare reimburses both the physician and the nurse practitioner for this method of overseeing residents. In addition to seeing residents in the nursing facility, the practitioner may handle telephone calls from nursing facilities, triage problems, diagnose problems, and prescribe treatments and medications as needed.

THE FUTURE OF THE NURSING FACILITY

The future of the nursing facility is complicated and uncertain. Its destiny is intimately linked to public policy regarding health care reform, long-term care, and mechanisms of reimbursement. Certain aspects of this service setting are flourishing, including subacute care and SCUs for the cognitively impaired. As the number of adults reaching retirement age increases and their need for assistance grows, it is essential for the professional nurse play a dominant role in improving and transforming this practice setting. Nurses can prepare themselves to play a role in nursing facility transformation through increased education in gerontologic nursing, nursing administration, health care regulation, and public policy related to long-term care.

Nurses need to be leaders in helping shape the future of how and where long-term health care is provided. Being creative in a highly regulated industry is a significant challenge. Professional nurses who conceptualize their practice as including care for the whole person, principles of health promotion and disease prevention, and creative use of the organizational and social environment to achieve health outcomes will make valuable contributions to society. Through such efforts by nurses and other like-minded professionals committed to achieving excellence, the nursing facility will be a place where people truly can live out their days with dignity, integrity, and a sense of personal autonomy.

SUMMARY

Although nurses work in a variety of practice settings, they are working primarily with older adults. Nurses need to provide competent, evidence-based care. The growing number of gerontologic-certified basic and advanced practice nurses will help in the endeavor, as will the inclusion of more gerontologic content in nursing school curricula. New acute care models will improve the care of hospitalized older adults, as will the development and dissemination of protocols that guide the assessment and treatment of commonly encountered geriatric syndromes.

Attitudes affect care delivery, and a nurse's respect and care for the special needs of older adults are essential. The diverse roles of acute care nurses working with older patients include those of practitioner, advocate, collaborator, educator, and case manager. In addition to ensuring safe and restorative health care in the hospital, the nurse must also address the learning needs, decision making, and ethical and legal issues involved in caring for older persons.

The health care needs of a growing, noninstitutionalized older adult population, coupled with rapid changes in today's health care delivery system, demand continued exploration of alternative services and delivery mechanisms that support the care of older persons in home and community settings.

The need for programs and services aimed at supporting older persons and their caregivers in the community setting will continue to grow. Options for care must expand, and nontraditional alternatives must be developed for use by various health care personnel. The reimbursement structure is currently challenged, and will clearly continue to be, to accommodate these developments.

The entire long-term care industry is one of the greatest challenges not only to society at large but also to all health care professionals. Attempts at regulating nursing facilities for the benefit of residents' overall health and well-being are an important yet modest step toward reform. Professional nurses must combine caring with innovative leadership to continue to make positive changes within this setting.

KEY POINTS

- Adults older than age 65 account for 47% of the country's inpatient days; the average length of hospital stay is 2 days longer than that of younger patients.
- The physical and social environment in which care occurs must be modified to facilitate maintenance of function and reduce the incidence of iatrogenic complications.
- Three conditions that require special attention during the hospitalization of older adults are falls, changes in cognitive status, and incontinence.
- New models of acute nursing care have emerged that are demonstrating improvements in the quality of the nursing care provided to hospitalized patients.
- Increasing numbers of older adults are discharged from hospitals with significant needs related to medical care and functional impairments; therefore home health care for older adults is becoming more common and more complex.
- Older adults, family members, and health care providers, including nurses, must learn about hospice care in order to make timely and appropriate referrals.
- Terminally ill older adults and their families are not maximizing the benefits of hospice care because of late referrals and misunderstanding of the Medicare hospice benefit.
- The Medicare hospice benefit covers (1) services and visits by all hospice staff, (2) durable medical equipment, (3) supplies needed for the plan of care, (4) medications related to the terminal diagnosis (may involve a small copayment at the discretion of the individual hospice), and (5) dietary supplements.
- Home care is often chosen as a preferred treatment site because people want to remain in their homes, home care is usually less expensive than hospitalization, and home care minimizes exposure to multiple infectious processes. In addition, technology has evolved to support complex treatments in the home.
- Assessment for home care should be done early in a client's hospital stay. Hospital discharge planners and home care managers must work together to ensure the continuity of care necessary for a timely and effective discharge.
- The home care nurse assesses the physical, functional, emotional, socioeconomic, and environmental well-being of clients. The nurse works in collaboration with all other members of the home care team whose services are needed to address the home care plan of treatment.
- Hospice nurses perform comprehensive, holistic assessments that are similar to those of home health nurses. In addition, the spiritual dimension is an important component of hospice care. In hospice, the terminally ill person and the family are the unit of care. Therefore all assessments by members of the interdisciplinary hospice team address both as a unit.

- Residents in nursing facilities may be categorized according to their length of stay as short-term residents or long-term residents.
- Risk factors associated with institutionalization include advanced age, physical disability, mental impairment, white race, living without a spouse, frailty, depression, and the presence of chronic medical conditions.
- The MDS includes a comprehensive and interdisciplinary assessment of residents.
- The RN plays a key role in all clinical programs, including programs for skin care, management of incontinence, nutrition, infection control, and the promotion of mental health.

- Nursing care delivery systems in nursing facilities include functional nursing, team nursing, and primary team nursing.
- Assisted living programs, SCUs for dementia, and subacute care units provide unique opportunities for RNs who wish to specialize in one aspect of the care provided in institutional settings.
- Recent innovations in the nursing facility involve self-governance programs for residents, nursing education programs, and the use of nurse practitioners.

CRITICAL-THINKING EXERCISES

1. You have admitted an 85-year-old man to your acute care unit. How will you modify or adapt the environment to meet the needs of this patient? Why will you need to make these modifications?
2. Your 92-year-old patient is ready for discharge, but she is having difficulty understanding your discharge instructions. You discuss your concerns with her family and the patient. What interventions for the transition in care can you implement for this patient and family?
3. A 79-year-old woman with mild dementia is living with her 92-year-old husband in the same home of 55 years. The husband is suffering from multiple chronic conditions including diabetes and heart failure. All of their children and other family live out of state. How will you determine interventions appropriate for this couple?
4. Symptom management is a critical part of hospice nursing care. What strategies can you implement to ensure adequate pain control along with managing complications of opioid use?
5. What is OASIS and how is it used in home health care?
6. A 96-year-old woman is living in the community and is no longer able to manage her personal care, nutritional needs, and medications. What care environment is best suited to improve her safety while letting her age in place?

REFERENCES

Administration on Aging. (2017). Retrieved December 13, 2017 from https://www.acl.gov/about-acl/administration-aging.

Agency for Healthcare Research and Quality. (2017). Health care-associated infections. Retrieved December 13, 2017, from https://psnet.ahrq.gov/primers/primer/7/health-care-associated-infections.

American Nurses Association. (2013). *Home health nursing: Scope and standards of practice* (2nd ed.). Washington, DC: American Nurses Publishing.

Assisted living provider type definitions. (2017). https://www.dhs.wisconsin.gov/guide/assisted-living.htm.

Bakerjian, D. (2008). Care of nursing home residents by advanced practice nurses: a review of the literature. *Research in Gerontological Nursing, 1*, 177.

Bales, C., & Ritchie, C. (2009). *Handbook of clinical nutrition and aging.* New York: Springer.

Brogan, K., & Jen, K. (2010). Nutrition in the elderly. In P. Lichtenberg (Ed.), *The Handbook of assessment in clinical gerontology* (pp. 357–380). London: Academic Press.

Bureau of Labor Statistics, U.S. Department of Labor, Occupational Outlook Handbook, 2016–17 Edition, Home Health Aides. Retrieved October 12, 2017 from https://www.bls.gov/ooh/healthcare/home-health-aides.htm.

Centers for Disease Control and Prevention. (2016). Healthcare-associated infections (HAIs). Retrieved December 13, 2017, from https://www.cdc.gov/winnablebattles/report/docs/wb-hai.pdf.

Centers for Medicare and Medicaid Services. (2012a). http://oig.hhs.gov/oei/reports/oei-01-10-00460.pdf.

Centers for Medicare and Medicaid Services (2012b). http://www.cms.gov/Medicare/Quality-Initiatives-Patient-Assessment-Instruments/NursingHomeQualityInits/MDS30RAIManual.html.

Centers for Medicare and Medicaid Services. (2015). Medicare Coverage of Skilled Nursing Facility Care. https://www.medicare.gov/Pubs/pdf/10153.pdf.

Centers for Medicare and Medicaid Services. (2017). Medicare home health benefit. Retrieved from https://www.cms.gov/Outreach-and-Education/Medicare-Learning-Network-MLN/MLNProducts/Downloads/Home-Health-Benefit-Fact-Sheet-ICN908143.pdf.

Chami, K., Gavazzi, G., de Wazières, B., Lejeune, B., Carrat, F., Piette, F., et al. (2011). Guidelines for infection control in nursing homes: A Delphi consensus web-based survey. *Journal of Hospital Infection, 0195-670179*(1), 75–89. https://doi.org/10.1016/j.jhin.2011.04.014. http://www.sciencedirect.com/science/article/pii/S0195670111001873.

CHAMPVA. (2013). Retrieved August 12, 2013, from http://www.va.gov/hac/forbeneficiaries/champva/faqs.asp.

Chang, H., Tsai, S., Chen, C., & Liu, W. (2010). Outcomes of hospitalized elderly patients with geriatric syndrome: Report of a community hospital reform plan in Taiwan. *Archives of Gerontology and Geriatrics, 50*(Suppl. 1), S30–S33. https://doi.org.jproxy.lib.ecu.edu/10.1016/S0167-4943(10)70009-1.

Davis, K., Abrams, M., & Stremikis, K. (2011). How the affordable care act will strengthen the nation's primary care foundation. *Journal of General Internal Medicine,* 1201–1203. https://doi.org/10.1007/s11606-011-1720-y.

De Rui, M., Manzato, E., Sarti, S., & Sergi, G. (2011). Polypharmacy in the elderly: Can comprehensive geriatric assessment reduce inappropriate medication use? *Drugs & Aging, 28*(7), 509. Retrieved from http://go.galegroup.com.jproxy.lib.ecu.edu/ps/i.do?id=GALE%7CA260943957&v=2.1&u=gree96177&it=r&p=HRCA&sw=w.

Demling, R. H., & DeSanti, L. (n.d.). Involuntary weight loss and protein-energy malnutrition: Diagnosis and treatment. *Medscape.* Retrieved July 26, 2018, from https://www.medscape.org/viewarticle/416589.

Dougdale, D. (2012). *Hospital acquired pneumonia.* National Library of Medicine National Institutes of Health. www.nlm.nih.gov/medlineplus/ency/article/000146.htm.

DuBeau, C., Kuchel, G., Johnson, T., Palmer, M., & Wagg, A. (2010). Incontinence in the frail elderly: Report from the fourth international consultation on incontinence. *Neurourology and Urodynamics, 29*(1), 165–178. https://doi.org/10.1002/nau.20842.

Duffield, C., Roche, M., Diers, D., Katling-Paull, C., & Blay, N. (2010). Staffing, skill mix and the model of care. *Journal of Clinical Nursing, 19*(15–16), 2042–2051. https://doi.org/10.11/j.1365-2702.2010.03225.x.

Eck, W. (2010). Home care, hospice care, and the Affordable Care Act. *AHLA Connections.* http://publish.healthlawyers.org/Members/PracticeGroups/LTC/Documents/LTC%20from%20AC_1011.pdf.

Fuchs, L., Chronaki, C., Park, S., Novak, V., Baumfield, Y., Scott, D., … Celi, L. (2012). ICU admission characteristics and mortality rates among elderly and very elderly patients. *Intensive Care Medicine, 38*(10), 1654–1661.

Granger, C. V., Albrecht, G. L., & Hamilton, B. B. (1979 Apr). Outcome of comprehensive medical rehabilitation: Measurement by PULSES profile and the Barthel Index. *Archives of Physical Medicine and Rehabilitation, 60*(4), 145.

Grönstedt, H., Frändin, K., Bergland, A., Helbostad, J. L., Granbo, R., Puggaard, L., et al. (2013). Effects of individually tailored physical and daily activities in nursing home residents on activities of daily living, physical performance and physical activity level: A randomized controlled trial. *Gerontology, 59,* 220–229. https://doi.org/10.1159/000345416.

Hanlin, E., Delgado-Rendón, A., Lerner, E., Hargarten, S., & Farías, R. (2013). Fall risk and prevention needs assessment in an older adult Latino population: A model community global health partnership. *Progress in Community Health Partnerships: Research, Education, and Action, 7*(2).

Hartford Institute for Geriatric Nursing. (2008). *The condition of geriatric nursing organizations.* Retrieved May 2, 2009, from http://www.hartfordign.org/policy/cgno/.

Heppner, H., Christ, M., Gosch, M., Mulhlberg, W., Bahrmann, P., Berstch, T., et al. (2012). Polypharmacy in the elderly from the clinical toxicologist perspective. *Zeitschrift für Gerontologie und Geriatrie, 45,* 473–478. https://doi.org/10.1007/s00391-012-0383-6.

Hoeck, S., François, G., Geerts, J., Van der Heyden, J., Vandewoude, M., & Van Hal, G. (2012). Health-care and home-care utilization among frail elderly persons in Belgium. *European Journal of Public Health, 22*(5), 671–677. https://doi.org/10.1093/eurpub/ckr133.

Health and Human Services, Subacute Care: Policy Synthesis and Market Area Analysis. Retrieved October 16, 2017, from https://aspe.hhs.gov/report/performance-improvement-1997/subacute-care-policy-synthesis-and-market-area-analysis.

Hubbard, R., & Woodhouse, K. (2010). Frailty inflammation and the elderly. *Biogerontology, 11,* 635–641.

Institute of Medicine: Improving the quality of care in nursing homes. (1986). New York: National Academy Press.

Kaiser, R., Winning, K., Bauer, J., Lesser, S., Stehle, P., Sieber, C., et al. (2010). Nutritional status and mortality of nursing home residents. Results of a 12-month follow-up study. *Clinical Nutrition*

Supplements, 5(2), 210. https://doi.org/10.1016/S1744-1161(10)70550-0.

Kapu, A. N., Kleinpell, R., & Pilon, B. (2014). Quality and financial impact of adding nurse practitioners to inpatient care teams. *Journal of Nursing Administration, 44*(2), 87–96. https://doi.org/10.1097/NNA.0000000000000031.

Kapu, A. N., & Steaban, R. (2016). Adding nurse practitioners to inpatient teams: Making the financial case for success. *NurseLeader, 14*(3), 198–202. https://doi.org/10.1016/j.mnl.2015.10.001.

Katz, M. J., & Roghmann, M. C. (2016). Healthcare-associated infections in the elderly: What's new. *Current Opinions in Infectious Disease, 29*(4), 388–393. https://doi.org/10.1097/QCO.0000000000000283.

Legome, E., & Shockley, L. (2011). *Trauma: A comprehensive medicine approach.* Cambridge, UK: Cambridge University Press.

Luppa, M., Luck, T., Weyerer, S., Konig, H., Brahler, E., & Riedel-Heller, S. (2010). Prediction of instutionalization in the elderly: A systematic review.*Age and. Aging, 39*(1), 31–38. https://doi.org/10.1093/aging/afp202.

Marcantonio, E., & Yurkofsky, M. (2009). Subacute Care. In J. Halter, J. Ouslander, M. Tinetti, K. Studenski, S. High, S. Asthana, & W. Hazzard (Eds.), *Hazzard's Geriatric Medicine and Gerontology.* New York, NY: McGraw-Hill.

Merck manual of geriatrics. (2013). Retrieved July 1, 2013, from http://www.merckmanuals.com/professional/geriatrics.html.

Monkhouse, D. (2013). Advances in critical care for the older patient. *Reviews in Clinical Gerontology, 23*(2), 118–130.

Moote, M., Krsek, C., Kleinpell, R., & Todd, B. (2011). Physician assistant and nurse practitioner utilization in academic medical centers. *American Journal of Medical Quality, 26,* 452–460. https://doi.org/10.1177/1062860611402984.

National Association for Home Care and Hospice (NAHC). (2013). *Basic statistics about home care.* Washington, DC: NAHC.

National Center for Health Statistics (NCHS). (2013). *Health, United States, 2012.* Hyattsville, MD: NCHS.

National Center for Health Statistics (NCHS). (2017). *Health, United States, 2016.* Hyattsville, MD: With Chartbook on Long-term Trends in Health.

National Hospice and Palliative Care Organization (NHPCO). (2017). *Facts & figures: Hospice care in America.* Alexandria, VA: NHPCO.

National Network of Career Nursing Assistants. (2012). *Who we are.* http://cna-network.org/.

Rowe, J. (2013). Preventing patient falls: What are the factors in hospital settings that help reduce and prevent inpatient falls? *Home Health Care Management and Practice, 25*(3), 98–103. https://doi.org/10.1177/1084822312467533.

Sainsbury, A., Seebass, G., Bansal, A., & Young, J. (2005). Reliability of the Barthel Index when used with older people. *Age and Ageing, 34*(3), 228.

Sengupta, M., Ejaz, F., & Harris-Kojetin, L. (2012). Training of home health aides and nurse aides: Finding form national data. *Gerontology and Geriatrics Education, 33*(4), 383–401. https://doi.org/10.1080/02701960.2012.702167.

Sergi, G., De Rui, M., Sarti, S., & Menzato, E. (2011). Polypharmacy in the elderly. *Drugs and Aging, 28*(7), 509–518. https://doi.org/10.2156/11502010-000000000-00000.

Sharma, G., Fletcher, K., Zhang, D., et al. (2009). Continuity of outpatient and inpatient care by primary care physicians for hospitalized older adults. *Journal of American Medical Association, 301*(16), 1671.

Smith, J. (2010). Area agencies on aging: A community resource for patients and families. *Home Healthcare Nurse, 28*(7), 416–422.

Sollitto, M. (2017). *Urinary tract infections in the elderly*. Retrieved December 13, 2017, from https://www.agingcare.com/articles/urinary-tract-infections-elderly-146026.htm.

St. Pierre, J., & Twibell, R. (2012). Developing nurses' geriatric expertise through the geriatric resource nurse model. *Geriatric Nursing, 0197-457233*(2), 140–149. https://doi.org/10.1016/j.gerinurse.2012.01.005. http://www.sciencedirect.com/science/article/pii/S0197457212000614.

The Joint Commission (TJC). (2011). *Home—The Best Place for Health Care*. www.jointcommission.org/assets/1/18/Home_Care_position_paper_4_5_11.pdf.

The Joint Commission (TJC). (2012). *Improving patient and worker safety*. Retrieved August 18, 2013. http://www.jointcomission.org.

The Joint Commission Sentinel Event Alert Issue 55, September 28. (2015). http://www.jointcommission.org/assets/1/18/SEA_55.pdf.

Tinetti, M., & Kumar, C. (2010). The patient who falls: "It's always a tradeoff." *Journal of American Medical Association, 303*(3), 256–258. https://doi.org/10.1001/JAMA.2009.2024.

Tucker, G., Clark, N., & Abraham, I. (2013). Enhancing ED triage to accommodate the special needs of geriatric patients. *Journal of Emergency Nursing, 39*(3), 309–314.

U.S. Department of Health and Human Services (DHHS). (2012). *What is Long term care? Long term care information*. Washington, DC: DHHS.

US Department of Veterans Affairs. (2017). Health Benefits. Retrieved December 13, 2017, from https://www.va.gov/HEALTHBENEFITS/index.asp.

van Hout, H., Jansen, L., van Marwijk, H., Pronk, M., Frijters, D., & Nijpels, G. (2010). Prevention of adverse health Trajectories in a vulnerable elderly population through nurse home visits: A randomized controlled trial. *The Journals of Gerontology Series A, Biological Sciences and Medical Sciences, 7*, 734–742. https://doi.org/10.1093/gerona/glq037.

Wallace, S., & Lew-Ting, C. (1992). Getting by at home: Community-based long-term care of Latino elders. *The Western Journal of Medicine, 157*, 337.

White-Chu, E., Graves, W., Godfrey, S., Bonner, A., & Sloane, P. (2009). Beyond the medical model: The culture change revolution in long term care. *Journal of the American Medical Directors Association, 10*(6), 370–378. https://doi.org/10.1016/j.jamda.2009.04.004.

World Health Organization (n.d.). WHO definition of palliative care. Retrieved October 12, 2017, from http://www.who.int/cancer/palliative/definition/en/.

27

Chronic Illness and Rehabilitation

Beth Culross, PhD, RN, GCNS-BC, CRRN, FNGNA

http://evolve.elsevier.com/Meiner/gerontologic

LEARNING OBJECTIVES

On completion of this chapter, the reader will be able to:

1. Define chronic illness and its relationship to rehabilitation.
2. Identify potential goals for an older adult with chronic illness.
3. Plan interventions that support an older adult's adaptation to a chronic illness or disability.
4. Describe the nurse's role in assisting older adults in managing chronic conditions.
5. Identify opportunities for change in the health care system to improve care for older adults with chronic illness and disability.

WHAT WOULD YOU DO?

What would you do if you were faced with the following situations?

- You are admitting to your unit a 75-year-old man who was diagnosed with chronic obstructive pulmonary disease (COPD) 10 years ago. He presents with an exacerbation of COPD and pneumonia. He states that his energy has not returned since that last time in the hospital. He requires 2 L of oxygen at all times. What are important interventions for him?
- An 80-year-old woman with a history of coronary artery disease and new diagnosis of heart failure reports difficulty getting around. She also has osteoporosis with a history of spinal fractures and arthritis. Her family wants her to move into a long-term care facility upon hospital discharge. She wants to know your opinion. What do you tell her?

CHRONICITY

Chronic disease affects the physical, psychological, and social aspects of the lives of individuals and families. A person's lifestyle, interactions, and relationships with others may change. Many older adults with chronic illness have limitations in mobility and are unable to be out in the community, and this decreased outside contact leads to social isolation. This may lead to being homebound or moving into long-term care. Individuals with chronic illness may perceive themselves as a burden, and families often experience caregiver stress. The individual is often stigmatized or acquires a label such as "that cancer patient" or "that person with chronic pain." The disease becomes the patient's identity. Chronic disease is the leading cause of death and disability in the United States (Centers for Disease Control and Prevention [CDC], 2017a).

It is important to differentiate between the terms *chronic disease* and *chronic illness*. Often both health care providers and the general public use these terms interchangeably. *Disease* refers to a condition viewed from a pathophysiologic model such as an alteration in structure and function; it is a physical dysfunction of the body. *Illness* is what the individuals (and their families) experience, that is, how the disease is perceived, lived with, and responded to by individuals and families (Larsen, 2013a). As health care providers, we can often modify the disease process or assist the patient in achieving optimal health; however, it is often the illness experience that we can most influence.

Just as the terms *chronic disease* and *illness* are complex, so is defining them. An early national group, the Commission on Chronic Illness (1957), defined *chronic illness* as:

All impairments or deviations from normal that have one or more of the following characteristics: (a) are permanent, (b) leave residual disability, (c) are caused by nonreversible pathological alteration, (d) require special training of the client for rehabilitation, and (e) may be expected to require a long period of supervision, observation, or care.

The CDC (Bernall & Howard, 2016) defined chronic disease as follows:

Noncommunicable illnesses that are prolonged in duration, do not resolve spontaneously, and are rarely cured completely.

The World Health Organization (WHO) also recognizes that noncommunicable disease to refer to chronic disease (WHO, 2017). According to WHO, these are diseases that cannot be passed from person to person and are slow in progression with a long duration. *Chronic condition* is another term used interchangeably but may mean slightly different things (Bernall &

Previous author: Ramesh C. Upadhyaya, RN, CRRN, MSN, MBA, PhD-C.

Howard, 2016). The suggestion by Bernall and Howard (2016) is to refer to the definition of "chronic" to help us understand. Simply stated, this is a disease or condition that will reoccur time and again over a long period of time.

Both the early definition from the Commission on Chronic Illness and the CDC definition emphasize the physicality of chronic disease, in other words, the pathology. Neither definition addresses the total experience of the individual and the family. It is important for the nurse to consider the illness-related issues that the patient and family experience. Understanding the perception of and response to the disease will allow for a more individualized plan of care.

More than 133 million adults in the United States have one or more chronic conditions, which is one of every two adults (CDC, 2016). Chronic conditions continue to be the primary causes of death in individuals 65 or older. Note the number of chronic conditions in Table 27.1. As one might expect, the costs of treating individuals with chronic conditions account for more than 75% of our nation's medical care costs each year (CDC, 2016).

The continuing increase in the prevalence of chronic conditions is caused by many factors. Primary among them are life-saving and life-extending technologies not previously available, an expanding population of older adults, and as a result, increasing life expectancy. Individuals who would have succumbed to an acute illness in the past now recover, age, and live with a chronic condition. The young adult with a spinal cord injury, who years ago would not have survived, may now have a normal life span because of lifesaving technology and preventive health care. Think about the very-low-birth-weight infants of today who would not have survived in earlier years; they are now flourishing and growing into adulthood or

they survive with chronic health problems. The individual diagnosed with cancer, heart disease, or other condition can now expect to live into "old age," as formerly acute conditions have now become chronic in nature.

Even though the prevalence of chronic conditions has increased, most health care services remain oriented to acute illness. The current U.S. health care system was largely developed in the two decades after World War II. It was designed to provide acute, episodic, and curative care, and was never intended to address the needs of those with chronic conditions. Overall, the health care system does a reputable job of caring for those with acute illness or injury. However, it is a health care system that does not know how to care for the older adult with COPD, Parkinson's disease, longstanding heart disease, or cancer. The health care system applies the "acute care model" to those individuals with chronic conditions, and as a result, a mismatch exists between the needs of older adults and what the system can provide. This conflict results in fragmented care, inadequate or inappropriate care from the system, and dissatisfaction on the part of the patient.

Prevalence of Chronic Illness

Although chronic disease and disability may occur at any age, the bulk of these conditions occurs in adults 65 years or older. Julie Gerberding, former director of the CDC, stated that, "the aging of the U.S. population is one of the major public health challenges we face in the twenty-first century" (CDC & Merck Company, 2007). By 2030, older Americans will number nearly 70 million, representing 20% of the total population (CDC, 2013d). With aging, the chances of having a chronic condition increase. *The State of Aging and Health in America* (CDC, 2013d) reported that two of every three older Americans have multiple chronic diseases and account for 66% of the health care budget. With this increasing number of individuals with a chronic condition, the health care system has to do a better job of caring for them. Nursing care, in particular, needs to focus on increasing functional ability, preventing complications, promoting the highest quality of life, and, when the end stage of life occurs, providing comfort and dignity in dying. A key role for the nurse caring for an older adult with a chronic condition is to help the patient achieve optimal physical and psychosocial health.

The most frequently occurring chronic diseases in older adults include hypertension, hyperlipidemia, heart disease, arthritis, diabetes, chronic kidney disease, ischemic heart disease, dementia, depression, and COPD (NCOA, 2017).

Individuals with chronic conditions typically have repeated hospitalizations to treat exacerbations of their illness. For both men and women ages 65 to 74, the most common reasons for hospitalization are heart disease, cancer, pneumonia, and stroke (Table 27.2). As men and women reach 75 or older, these diseases continue to predominate (Table 27.2). Hospitalizations resulting from injuries, particularly in women (e.g., hip fractures), increase significantly, as does heart disease in this age category. Changes in the rates of admissions continue to be noted in the age group over the age of 85 (Table 27.2). Given these statistics, it is easy to see that older women have significantly more hospitalizations compared with men of the same age.

TABLE 27.1   Percentage of Deaths From Leading Causes Among Persons Ages 65 and Over: United States, 2014

Cause of Death	Number of Deaths in 2014 All Ages	Percent of Deaths 65 and Over in 2014
All causes	2,626,418	100
Heart disease	614,348	22.3
Cancer	591,700	21.6
Chronic lower respiratory disease	147,101	6.0
Cerebrovascular disease (stroke)	133,103	6.0
Alzheimer disease	93,541	5.0
Unintentional injury	135,928	3.9
Diabetes	76,488	2.7
Influenza and pneumonia	55,227	2.2

From Kochanek, K. D., Murphy, S. L., Xu, J., & Tejada-Vera, B. (2016). *National vital statistics report deaths: Final data for 2014*. Retrieved from https://www.cdc.gov/nchs/data/nvsr/nvsr65/nvsr65_04.pdf.

TABLE 27.2   Discharges in Nonfederal Short-Stay Hospitals, by Gender, Age, and Selected First-Listed Diagnosis, 2009 to 2010

Diagnosis	No. of Discharges (In Thousands)
Women (ages 65–74)	
Heart disease	363
Cancer (all types)	140
Chronic Obstructive Pulmonary Disease	117
Pneumonia	92
Stroke	107
Diabetes	51
Osteoarthritis	206
Injuries: Includes hip fracture	128
Men (ages 65–74)	
Heart disease	498
Cancer (all types)	171
Chronic Obstructive Pulmonary Disease	91
Pneumonia	85
Stroke	124
Diabetes	45
Osteoarthritis	133
Injuries: Includes hip fracture	75
Women (ages 75–84)	
Heart disease	510
Cancer (all types)	119
Chronic Obstructive Pulmonary Disease	83
Pneumonia	130
Stroke	144
Diabetes	51
Osteoarthritis	129
Injuries: Includes hip fracture	208
Men (ages 75–84)	
Heart disease	466
Cancer (all types)	109
Chronic Obstructive Pulmonary Disease	91
Pneumonia	107
Stroke	116
Diabetes	37
Osteoarthritis	84
Injuries: Includes hip fracture	104
Women (ages 85+)	
Heart disease	378
Cancer (all types)	44
Chronic Obstructive Pulmonary Disease	50
Pneumonia	124
Stroke	111
Diabetes	21
Osteoarthritis	30
Injuries: Includes hip fracture	222
Men (ages 85+)	
Heart disease	228
Cancer (all types)	39
Chronic Obstructive Pulmonary Disease	32
Pneumonia	80
Stroke	52
Diabetes	13
Osteoarthritis	10
Injuries: Includes hip fracture	80

From Centers for Disease Control and Prevention. (2011). Discharges in nonfederal short-stay hospitals, by sex, age, and selected first-listed diagnosis: United States, selected years 1990 through 2009-2010. Retrieved from https://www.cdc.gov/nchs/data/hus/2011/104.pdf.

The Illness Experience

The diagnosis of a chronic disease and subsequent management of that disease bring unique experiences and meanings of the process to both the patient and family (Larsen, 2013b). Just as each individual and his or her disease process are unique, so, too, are the meanings and experiences of that disease to the individual and his or her family. However, the educational background of most health care professionals is one that fits with the medical model and does not consider the different illness perceptions and behaviors of individuals. We have been taught that patients have diseases, and the degree of their pathology dictates their treatment. Health care has even developed algorithms that tell us how and what care to provide. Nonetheless, having a chronic illness is not a black and white, quantifiable concept. The course of a chronic illness varies from one individual to another. The nurse must understand the outlying variables that affect the disease, including socioeconomic factors, psychosocial factors, culture, and other contributing comorbid disease or illness.

Health Within Illness

Health care providers typically view an older person who is ill within a disease framework. This framework is an acute care framework that "fixes and cures." However, we know that chronic conditions are not cured and probably cannot be "fixed."

In caring for older adults with chronic illness, health care professionals need a paradigm shift in attitude. After learning and mastering the requirements imposed by the condition, older adults often view themselves as "well." The disease is only one component of their life and is not their identity. The physical traits of chronic illness should not determine an older adult's state of wellness. Many older adults are now more involved in their health care than ever before and accept responsibility for their wellness. They seek education about health promotion and the management of their illness. The nurse is in a position to support older adults by working with them to identify areas that may hinder progress along the wellness continuum and by teaching self-care management in these areas (Review Appendix C for resources).

Cultural Competency

Concepts of health and illness are deeply rooted in culture, race, and ethnicity, and influence an individual's (and family's) illness perceptions and health and illness behavior (Larsen & Hardin, 2013). Ethnic minorities do not necessarily subscribe to the values or tenets associated with this country's medical system. Additionally, each culture is not homogeneous, and variations and subcultures exist within each.

According to the 2000 U.S. Census, approximately 30% of the population is racially and ethnically diverse. Projections are that, by 2100, this percentage will increase to 40%, and non-Hispanic whites will make up only 60% of the U.S. population (CDC, 2013b). With the increase in the numbers of ethnically and culturally diverse older adults, health care providers need to be better attuned to their needs.

A number of nursing frameworks can assist health care providers in providing culturally competent care. The website of the

Transcultural Nursing Society (http://www.tcns.org) provides information about six different theories and models. Madeline Leininger's Culture Care Theory is based on developing nursing care with the intention of reaching positive health outcomes based on a plan that includes and considers the needs of populations and individuals with diverse cultural backgrounds (Petiprin, 2016)

Quality of Life and Health-Related Quality of Life

Advancements in health care have increased interest in the quality of life (QOL) of persons with chronic illnesses. Multiple definitions of QOL exist, but most include physical, psychological, and social components; disease and treatment-related symptoms; and spirituality. However, no consensus on the definition exists. The following definition, although somewhat older, fits well with regard to older adults. QOL is challenging to measure due to the complex nature of the concept and the generally subjective evaluation. According to the CDC (2016) QOL has meaning to a multitude of groups from every academic discipline and walk of life and may be viewed differently by each. It is made up of multiple domains that include health, jobs, housing, education, community, culture, and spirituality. The complexity of health and function in chronic illness, particularly if one believes that health can be present within illness, suggests that neither "good" health nor functional abilities are necessary for QOL. QOL is determined by the individual, not the health care provider.

Adding to the complexity of the issue, most researchers draw a distinction between QOL and health-related quality of life (HRQOL). HRQOL is a multidimensional concept that has been used along with well-being to measure the effect of chronic illness, the treatments, and the corresponding related disabilities. The domains of HRQOL include physical, emotional, mental, and social function (HealthyPeople.gov, 2017; CDC, 2016)

How QOL and HRQOL intersect is salient to the patient with chronic illness and those providing care. For example, a person who has adjusted to a wheelchair for mobility might perceive his HRQOL and his QOL as excellent, whereas the health care provider may not rate the person's HRQOL high because a wheelchair may not be that person's optimal state of function and wellness. The subjective and objective components of both of these concepts are important.

Adherence in Chronic Illness

Patient behaviors and ability or willingness to follow a treatment plan for chronic illness are important to consider. Adherence is the term used on the global stage of health care delivery for how well the patient manages the treatment plan (Berg, Evangelista, Carruthers, & Dunbar-Jacob, 2013; AlGhurair, Hughes, Simpson, & Guirguis, 2012). A number of factors influence nonadherence. These factors include (1) individual characteristics, (2) psychological factors, (3) social support, (4) prior health behaviors, (5) somatic factors, (6) regimen characteristics, (7) economic and sociocultural factors, and (8) patient–provider interactions (Berg et al., 2013).

Although adherence, formerly compliance, has been researched for a number of years, the results of that research have not effected significant changes in patient behavior. Health care providers are perhaps better able to identify the factors that influence patient behaviors toward adherence or nonadherence, but the interventions that produce positive behaviors remain elusive.

The WHO suggests adopting the use of the five A's in an effort to assist patients with the self-management aspects of their chronic disease, of which treatment adherence is just one part (AHRQ, 2012). The five A's include **a**ssess, **a**dvise, **a**gree, **a**ssist, and **a**rrange. Although these key aspects seem straightforward and easy to follow for health care providers, data suggest that adherence to treatment regimens is only 50% in individuals with chronic illness (Khanna, Pace, Mahabaleshwarkar, Basak, Datar & Banahan, 2012; AHRQ, 2012). Data in studies that examine age and adherence behaviors are mixed. A variety of factors may interfere with the ability of the older adult to adhere to a treatment plan. However, in general, developmental issues such as age have not been well addressed in the adherence literature (Khanna et al., 2012). Adherence is a complex and

---

EVIDENCE-BASED PRACTICE

Functional Status and Quality of Life Posthospitalization

Sample/Setting

This single site study was comprised of patients 60 years and older admitted to a hospital in Hamburg, Germany. Patients included had a preexisting condition that caused impairment in functional mobility. Patients were excluded if cognitive or communication impairments were present or if the patient was not expected to live past the study timeframe. Eighty-five patients consented to participate, and 47 completed all three measures.

Method

A prospective longitudinal design was used and measurements were taken at admission, 6 months, and 12 months postadmission. The WHO Quality of Life-BREF and the Barthel-Index were used to measure QOL and activities of daily living (ADLs).

Findings

The functional status of a patient posthospitalization increased during the first 6 months but then declined over the next 6 months. Differences were noted based on gender with men having a higher level of functional status over time. QOL was also found to be higher in patients with a higher self-efficacy and mental status score on admission. However overall QOL scores also increased in the first 6 months and then decreased between months 6 and 12.

Implications

Interventions to prevent decline in function in the older adult posthospital admission need to be implemented for longer periods of time and reevaluated after 6 months posthospitalization. Physical functioning and QOL are more likely to decline after the 6-month mark. Suggestions included preventative programs to be introduced after the 6-month mark to prevent further decline or rehospitalization.

From Strupeit, S., Wolf-Ostermann, K., Buss, A., & Dassen, T. (2014). Mobility and quality of life after discharge from a clinical geriatric setting focused on gender and age. *Rehabilitation Nursing, 39*(4), 198-206.

multidimensional issue that may be affected by a variety of barriers. Tools to measure adherence may not address all areas of effect, such as socioeconomic factors (AlGhuarair, Hughes, Simpson, & Guirguis, 2012)

Berg et al. (2013) suggested that, although the five A's is a good framework for health care providers to use, it is also important to (1) advise the patient of the importance of the treatment plan, (2) establish agreement with the treatment plan, and (3) arrange adequate follow-up.

Overall strategies to enhance adherence include educational, behavioral, and organizational approaches. The nurse must first assess the older adult's belief in the mutually established goals. Does the older adult have self-motivation to work toward these goals, or were these goals not mutually established but rather generated by the health care provider? The assessment should include identification of strengths such as self-motivation.

The cost of today's health care requires that nurses are aware of specific needs of older adults when structuring their therapeutic regimens. Regimens should emphasize activities that build endurance and self-reliance, and that facilitate self-care and QOL. Older adults must believe that a therapeutic regimen aids in the recovery or maintenance of their functional level.

Psychosocial Needs of Older Adults With Chronic Illness

Management of the physiologic changes caused by the disease process is the primary indicator of control of the disease. Controlling the symptoms, maintaining comfort, and preventing crisis are major tasks for the patient and the provider to work on together. For this to be met, the nurse needs to understand how the patient perceives the disease, is experiencing it as an illness, and what the current standard of practice is.

Understanding the relationship among the older adult's social, psychological, and physiologic needs is important for health care providers. Each older adult and their family are unique, and the presence of one or more chronic illnesses further illuminates their uniqueness. The end result of understanding the patient's unique situation assists the health care provider in establishing interventions that support psychosocial adaptation.

Adaptation

Adaptation implies that an event or something unusual or different that has occurred is perceived as a threat or stressor to the individual and merits a reaction, a change, or a behavior by an individual (Stanton & Revenson, 2011). Other authors have seen adaptation as good QOL, well-being, vitality, positive effect, life satisfaction, and global self-esteem (Sharpe & Curran, 2006). Adaptation is a complex, multidimensional, holistic concept. Consensus exists regarding the centrality of an individual's appraisal of their adjustment; it is *their* adjustment and their perception, not the health care professional's (Hoyt & Stanton, 2012).

Just as frameworks or models are helpful in caring for those with acute, episodic disease, they may be helpful in caring for those with chronic illness as well. Three frameworks for practice are discussed here, although more are described in the literature. These frameworks demonstrate the importance of controlling

symptoms, managing the trajectory of the disease process, and engaging the patient in self-care.

Chronic Illness and Quality of Life

Around 1975, nursing pioneers were working with dying patients and determining through research what kind of "care" those patients wanted. Their work provided a rudimentary framework that addressed the issues and concerns of patients with chronic illness. The framework was simple but was an early attempt to examine the psychosocial needs of patients versus their physical needs. Basic to patient care was an understanding of the key physical and psychosocial problems:

- The prevention of medical crises and their management if they occur
- Controlling symptoms
- Carrying out the medical regimen
- Prevention of, or living with, social isolation
- Adjustment to change in the disease
- Attempts to normalize interactions and lifestyle
- Funding
- Confronting attendant psychological, marital, and familial problems (Strauss, 1984)

Trajectory Framework

Corbin and Strauss (1992) developed the trajectory framework to assist nurses in (1) gaining insight into the chronic illness experience of the patient, (2) integrating existing literature about chronicity into their practice, and (3) providing direction for building nursing models that guide practice, teaching, research, and policy making. A *trajectory* is defined as the course of an illness over time, plus the actions that patients, families, and health care providers use to manage that course. The illness trajectory is set in motion by the pathology of the patient, but the actions taken by the health care providers, patient, and family may modify the course. Even if two older adults have the same chronic condition, the illness trajectory of each individual is different and takes into account the uniqueness of the individual (Nursing Theories, 2013).

Nine phases—pretrajectory, trajectory, stable, unstable, acute, crisis, comeback, downward, and dying—are described in the trajectory model, and although the trajectory could be conceived as a continuum, it is not linear. Patients may move through a phase, regress to a former phase, or plateau for an extended period.

Chronic Care Model

The Chronic Care Model was developed by Wagner to assist with the management of multiple chronic diseases and improve outcomes by providing a method of care coordination to improve patient self-care. There are six essential elements to the model:

1. Health System: The health system must support a culture focused on mechanisms to promote safety and quality care. The system must also be prepared to seek improvement in chronic illness management and look for improvements to reduce errors and improve communication.
2. Delivery System Design: The design of the system defines roles and tasks, is based on evidence-based care, and provides

clinical case management. Care is based on the complexity of the patient and is proactive and more preventative in nature than reactive to crisis events.

3. Decision Support: Decisions are made using evidence-based guidelines. Patients are taught the guidelines to understand the underlying principles of treatment decisions. Patients are also encouraged to learn and participate in care.

4. Clinical Information Systems: A comprehensive system of communication is important for maintaining records of information. This is also important to be able to share information among providers and patients to enhance care, provide reminders of services, summarize care, and track changes. A comprehensive system can also be used to gather information of groups or populations to add to the evidence of care and create quality improvement plans.

5. Self-Management Support: The patient is central to the management of chronic illness. This element of the model empowers the patient to take responsibility for his or her own care. This is a collaboration with the providers to set priorities, educate, establish goals, and create a plan of care that can be monitored, evaluated, and changed together.

6. Community: Developing partnerships within the community leads to more effective programs. The intent of this essential is to fill gaps that exist in services and advocate for policies to improve care. Health systems may partner with local organizations. Agencies at the state level may be able to provide material or help for managing diseases based on guidelines. National organizations can also contribute by helping to promote self-care strategies.

The Chronic Care Model brings in multiple elements of care to help the patient be educated, informed, and an active participant in the treatment plan. It also encompasses the community, the health system, and a proactive health care team (Improving Chronic Illness Care, 2006-2017).

As we look at chronic illness and the older adult, a number of phenomena that may be experienced by individuals and families need to be considered. When considering the trajectory of disease and the multiple entities that may be involved in the care of the older adult with chronic illness, more than one framework may be needed to coordinate care and improve outcomes.

Powerlessness

An older adult's self-concept may be affected if he or she feels unable to control an illness or disability or feels that self-care patterns have contributed to the present disorder. Feelings of powerlessness may be a result of normal aging changes, an altered body image, or numerous losses. Older people grieve the loss of function or the loss of their former self. How they grieve depends on the individuals, and the significance of the loss also influences the grieving process. The result of powerlessness is a loss of hope. In addition, older adults who feel powerless may lose their independence to family members or health care professionals who take over and make decisions for them. This cycle of powerlessness, loss of control, and dependence may be perpetuated by well-meaning caregivers.

Stigma

Stigma is defined as "a mark of shame or discredit or an identifying mark or characteristic" (Merriam Webster, 2013), and it may be a significant factor in many chronic illnesses and disabilities. Individuals with chronic illness present deviations from what many people expect in social exchanges (Stuenkel & Wong, 2013). American values of youth, attractiveness, and personal accomplishment provide daily examples of how those with chronic illness are different. A disease characteristic or having a disease with an unknown etiology may contribute to the stigma. Thus the individual may be stigmatized by society.

However, older adults with the chronic illnesses may inflict the stigma on themselves. They may feel ashamed of their disability, disease, physical condition, and other factors. As a result, they become reclusive and socially isolated from others.

Social Isolation

Social isolation may occur as an illness or disability becomes more severe or debilitating. This isolation may be initiated by the individual or by society. From the individual's perspective, it may become too difficult to functionally participate in activities, too complex to keep up with a medical regimen when away from home, or too difficult to manage physical symptoms such as pain or fatigue. Thus the individual initiates the isolation and withdraws or limits social contact. This may be a difficult decision for individuals and their families, or it may be a relief to stay within the "safe" confines of their homes where they may have more control.

Conversely, others may withdraw from the individual and family experiencing chronic illness. Friends may tire of hearing about the physical limitations of their friend or acquaintance. The long-term time frame or the individual with recurring cancer over a number of years, for example, may cause others to withdraw. Stigma might also be involved, and others may pull away from individuals with "unpleasant" diagnoses such as HIV and AIDS. Regardless of how or why social isolation occurs, the result is that basic needs for intimacy may be unmet (Biordi & Nicholson, 2013).

Nursing Interventions to Assist Psychosocial Adaptation

The ability of older adults to cope with the issues and problems encountered in the course of living with and managing a chronic illness determines the nurse's role and the type of interventions needed. It is the role of the nurse to collaborate with the patient to develop an individualized plan that meets the needs, expectations, and perceptions of the patient. The Chronic Care Model is a consideration here. The Chronic Care Model is based on educating and providing a treatment plan that allows the patient to be in charge of the management of the chronic illness and have open communication with health care providers (Boltz, 2016). Independence is a major concern, especially for older persons in the American culture, where it is highly valued. The older adult who can have increased independence in the management of their care will be more knowledgeable and be able to prevent complications.

Adaptation is an individual process and depends on the circumstances of the disability. Developmental changes, life transitions, and meaning placed on the disability or illness influence this ongoing process. Interventions may include supporting existing relationships or referring older adults who have lost significant relationships to a senior center where they can establish new relationships. The nurse may also explore interventions that meet spiritual needs. The nurse may refer and encourage older adults to participate in formal or informal learning opportunities available in the community.

The group process is one way to assist patients in their psychosocial adaptation. Self-help groups provide a support system in which older adults redefine themselves, focus on issues, adjust to new roles, or learn about their disease processes and how others manage (Touhy & Jett, 2011).

Changes in positions within the family affect family duties and responsibilities. Successful coping requires a positive attitude toward new roles and the ability to obtain a feeling of independence and security. Traditional roles are often masked in the hospital, and patients may think that everything will be fine on returning home. However, the transition from hospital to home is often difficult for patients and their families. They discover how much has changed and begin to face their losses. Roles may need to be renegotiated, and those that are no longer applicable must be acknowledged and mourned (Hibbard, Neufeld, & Harrison, 1996).

The nurse should guide, educate, and support older adults and their families in developing positive coping strategies. Understanding the illness and what to expect is directly related to the ability to cope. In providing support to older adults and their families, the nurse assists them in identifying their feelings. A reduction in the distress that accompanies chronic illness or disability may be achieved with nursing interventions that encourage an active problem-solving and coping orientation that interrupts avoidant, passive coping patterns (Aikens, Fischer, Namey, & Rudnick, 1997). Direct questions such as "How are you dealing with this illness? What helps you deal with this change in your family? What interferes with your ability to deal with this illness?" will provide an indication of a patient's coping strategies and their effectiveness (Twibell, 1998). The nurse should also observe older adults and family members for signs of stress that may result from ineffective coping.

One of the most difficult tasks in adaptation is balancing hope and realism. A patient and his or her family may need to express frustration and anger with the course of the illness and rehabilitation. By setting mutually agreed upon goals, divided into small increments, the nurse and the older adult may succeed in achieving them. Sharing goals with family members may elicit their support or assist them in accepting the need to avoid active involvement (Twibell, 1998). Personal coping also involves problem solving. The nurse serves as a resource for older adults and their families in solving care management problems.

A supportive social network also has been found to have a significant effect on stress (Tremethick, 1997). The roles of the home, neighborhood, friends, and family need to be considered in assessing the adequacy of social support. Referrals for day care, home health nursing, temporary long-term care, or respite care may be needed.

Another obstacle is understanding and coping with role reversals. The nurse should guide older adults in finding tasks and responsibilities within their new roles and assist in conflict resolution as old roles are redefined. Chronic illness requires long-term adaptation on the part of older adults and their families. Ongoing support by health care professionals is crucial for the older adults and their families to find enough strength to continue coping.

Physiologic Needs of Chronically Ill Older Adults

A thorough nursing health history includes a comprehensive review of body systems as well as a medication and treatment review. The medication review should include both prescription drugs and over-the-counter medications. An older adult may have more than one physician prescribing drugs and additionally may be using nonprescription remedies.

Pain

A major issue with chronic disorders is the management of pain. In evaluating pain, the nurse should note its characteristics, location, and intensity (on a scale of 1 to 10). The nurse should make an assessment of causes of possible discomfort other than the chronic illness. In addition to pharmacologic therapy, the nurse may teach the patient relaxation techniques, deep breathing exercises, guided imagery, and visualization. These techniques may relieve muscular and emotional tension, enhance the sense of control, and possibly improve coping abilities.

Fatigue

Older adults living with a chronic disorder often experience fatigue. Fatigue may be unpredictable, making it difficult to manage or alleviate. The nurse should help older adults identify causes and patterns of fatigue. Older persons may need to be taught how to conserve energy to enjoy meaningful activities. Emphasizing the benefits of periodic rest, a slower pace of activity, and more time to complete tasks may help older patients cope and feel in control. The nurse should encourage older adults to choose where to expend energy and should respect the priorities established.

Immobility and Activity Intolerance

Activity may be the most important factor in maintaining or recovering health and wellness in the older adult. Physical activity and psychosocial interaction are important in maintaining chronically ill older adults on the continuum of wellness. Inactivity may result from functional loss, and as activity levels decline, even more function may be lost. Problems as a result of inactivity are compounded when patients, families, and health care professionals display reduced expectations of activity. One possible nursing goal may be to prevent complications of prolonged inactivity during an acute exacerbation of illness.

Sexual Activity

Aging, in and of itself, causes changes to the reproductive system in both men and women. Chronic disease may further affect the sexual activity and functioning of the older adult. These changes in a patient's sexual life may cause psychological distress. Effects of the condition, medications, treatments, fatigue, changes in body image, and the feeling that one is no longer attractive may present difficult emotional barriers. Open communication between partners, including frank discussions of needs and feelings, may result in helpful adjustments in sexual practices and a deeper commitment to the relationship. Counseling partners or individual patients may smooth over these transitions. In addition to a medication review, a sexual history provides the nurse with insight into a patient's needs. The nurse should create an open, accepting atmosphere to facilitate a discussion of sexuality and provide information in a nonjudgmental manner. Only when concerns are identified and discussed can problem solving occur.

Effect of Chronic Illness on Family and Caregivers

More and more families are faced with providing care for older family members with chronic illness because of the rapidly aging population and the present ability to manage chronic illness. Family caregivers constitute the overwhelming majority of unpaid caregivers and provide the equivalent of billions of dollars of care annually (Family Caregiver Alliance, 2017). Studies have enhanced our awareness of family caregiver stress and the difficulty of balancing caregiving with activities such as personal time or social activities. The primary family caregiver often receives little help from siblings or children and considers institutionalization only when he or she is physically or emotionally exhausted.

Situational factors related to caring for adults with chronic illnesses contribute to caregiver stress. As noted previously, chronic illnesses are present for a long period and have an uncertain course. Periods of improvement, stability, and exacerbations in the trajectory of the illness cause uncertainty. Anticipation of these phases may also produce stress. Some chronic conditions develop slowly, and planning for crisis periods is possible. Advance notice of impending stress may allow the caregiver to activate coping strategies and reduce the stress experienced. However, anticipation may also be related to fear of the worst possible outcome.

The characteristics of a chronic illness may contribute to caregivers' stress. Caregivers report stress when, for example, the patient does not recognize family members or does not remember previous relationships because of cognitive changes. Behavioral problems resulting from illness also contribute to stress. The patient's functional ability and the type and amount of care needed affect caregiver stress. Ongoing care or the perception that ongoing care is needed may be physically and psychologically draining. When a caregiver is faced with a spouse's illness, the marital relationship may be affected. The quality of the past and present relationship contributes to how a spousal caregiver copes. In questioning a spousal caregiver, the nurse should determine whether unresolved marital problems exist because these problems may affect the caregiver's reactions to the caregiving experience. Interventions that focus on resolution of issues in relationships and identification of negative coping skills may improve relationships and decrease the possibility of depression in spousal caregivers.

Role strain is a problematic feature inherent in balancing the role as primary caregiver with other roles within the family network. Most caregivers feel a strong sense of responsibility to caregiving, and although most have a family system in place, it is rarely used as a source of support. Maintaining a healthy sense of self and successfully coping with role strain requires a balance of caregiving and caring for one's self. Personal activities may include work outside the home. Many caregivers experience work conflicts that result in changes in work schedules or performance.

Caregivers may feel powerless when they seem to have no control over events and perceive the stressors in their life as irreversible. Fewer than 15% of all "helper days of care" for people needing help with ADLs are provided by paid caregivers or sources outside the family. Factors that influence coping with caregiver stress and powerlessness are personal characteristics (e.g., age, gender, marital status, health, and social roles) and include knowledge of the illness, knowledge of available resources, personal perceptions, and coping strategies. Female caregivers experience a greater sense of burden and stress than male caregivers. The caregiving burden and feelings of being overwhelmed are related to a subsequent decline in mental and physical health (Family Caregiver Alliance, 2017). Assumption of a role previously assigned to an older adult with chronic illness may significantly affect stress levels.

Nursing Implications of Caregiver Stress

Effective nursing care of a patient with a chronic illness requires providing care not only to the identified patient but also to the caregiver. The caregiver's personal characteristics, social and emotional support, financial resources, and perception of the caregiving situation should be assessed in relation to feelings of powerlessness. Personal coping strategies, including the ability to solve problems in managing care, need to be explored by the nurse. Questions such as "Many family member caregivers have trouble with [such and such]. Have you found that to be true for you?" may help the nurse determine stressors and problem-solving abilities in a nonthreatening manner.

Support may be obtained from other resources such as community social service agencies, local church members, visiting nurse organizations, and other family members. Support groups for caregivers are also becoming more prevalent. Group participation decreases the sense of isolation and may help a caregiver cope with new situations. The nurse should provide information about the illness and reassurance that feelings of frustration or helplessness are not unusual reactions. Referral to a social worker may be necessary to provide detailed information regarding Medicare coverage and Medicaid eligibility, as well as other means of obtaining assistance in the health care system. Stress may be reduced by the use of adult day care or home health nursing. Temporary placement in a nursing facility provides the caregiver much-needed respite.

Caring for older adults with chronic conditions requires long-term adaptation on the part of family members. To continue in a caregiving role, a family member caregiver needs ongoing support by all involved health care professionals.

REHABILITATION

Rehabilitation refers to services and programs designed to assist individuals who have experienced a trauma or illness that results in an impairment that creates a loss of function that may be physical, psychological, social, or vocational (Lewis, 2017). Rehabilitation is a philosophy of care that promotes an optimal QOL in those with chronic illness.

Gerontologic rehabilitation nursing is a specialty practice that focuses on restoring and maintaining optimal function while considering holistically the unique effects of aging on the person. The gerontological rehabilitation nurse acts as an advocate, educator, consultant, practitioner, and researcher (ARN, 2015). Interestingly, the specialty did not arise from gerontologic nursing but from rehabilitation nursing as a subspecialty. It was seen as a need because of the large number of older adults with more disease-related conditions rather than injury or trauma conditions. Clearly, these older patients needed a different approach to their care. The main goal of the gerontologic rehabilitation nurse is to assist the older adult in achieving their personal optimal level of health and well-being by providing holistic care in a therapeutic environment (ARN, 2015). What is unique about the role is that these nurses consider the special needs, roles, social relationships, and potential comorbidities that occur in the aging process.

Centenarians, the so-called elite-old, are the fastest growing segment of our population, followed by the age group that is 85 years or older, the oldest-old (Touhy, 2011a). Strokes occur more commonly after age 65, and the incidence of stroke doubles with every decade after age 55 (Reddy & Reddy, 1997). Hip fractures peak in the eighth decade of life and are expected to double by the year 2040 (Ethans & MacKnight, 1998). Older drivers are involved in more crashes per mile driven compared with middle-aged drivers (Foley & Mitchell, 1997). These data suggest an increasing need for rehabilitation with a gerontologic focus. Rehabilitation planning should begin at the time an older adult is first seen or hospitalized.

The growth of the older population has specific implications for disability, and it affects the nurses who provide preventive, restorative, and rehabilitation services to this population. Age-related physiologic changes may slow recovery and increase residual debilitation from an acute illness or injury. Age-related changes also increase the likelihood of physical limitations from a chronic illness. Studies agree that older adults are more likely to be functionally impaired in ADLs and mobility.

Care Environments

Rehabilitation services are offered in a variety of settings. Therapy in acute medical–surgical units may assist a patient in maintaining strength when confined to bed. However, the acute medical environment offers little opportunity to apply skills learned in therapy and often emphasizes inactivity. Rehabilitation services lasting 1 to 3 hours a day are available in intermediate rehabilitation facilities and skilled care facilities (Fig. 27.1). This environment is suitable for an older adult who has the goal of returning home, who is unable to tolerate more therapy, or who requires only one therapy discipline. Intensive rehabilitation (3 hours of therapy or more) is

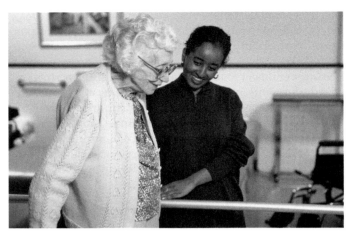

Fig. 27.1 A patient receiving therapy in a rehabilitation setting. (©KeithBrofsky/Photodisc/Thinkstock.)

available in the rehabilitation units of acute care hospitals, freestanding rehabilitation hospitals, and some geriatric assessment or rehabilitation units. Outpatient rehabilitation therapy services may be available to older adults in their homes.

Reimbursement Issues

Medicare becomes available to older adults at age 65 regardless of whether they continue to work. Part A, or basic coverage (inpatient hospital coverage), is without cost to those who qualify. Part B (more comprehensive coverage) is available for a monthly premium with deductibles. A variety of private insurance plans are available to cover the "Medigap," or the 20% of service cost not reimbursed under Medicare guidelines. Medicare is a fee-for-service delivery system. Medicare also contracts with health maintenance organizations (HMOs). HMOs provide the full range of Medicare benefits and may offer additional benefits at little or no additional charge.

Medicaid is a state-specific medical care source of funding for people with low incomes. It varies from state to state, but generally the costs of inpatient, outpatient, home health, and nursing facility rehabilitation services are partially reimbursed. Increasing fiscal constraints in local, state, and federal agencies will affect rehabilitation reimbursement and may further decrease resources available to older adults.

Public Policy and Legislation

Nurses have the power to influence public policy and legislation by advocating for the needs of older adults with disabilities and supporting and conducting relevant nursing research. The process of national public policy making started in 1951 when the first White House Conference on Aging was held. This conference made the problems of older adults visible and, since then, has been held each decade. The Older Americans Act of 1965 (last amended in 2006) introduced the concept of a focal point of services for older adults. Also in 1965, Medicare and Medicaid were established and have been revised in subsequent years. In 1982 the Tax Equity and Fiscal Responsibility Act introduced prospective reimbursement for hospitals under Medicare diagnosis-related groups.

The Americans with Disabilities Act (ADA) of 1990 outlawed discrimination on the basis of disability in employment, in programs and services provided by state and local governments, and in the provision of goods and services provided by private companies and commercial facilities (ADA, 2013). However, the ADA did not eliminate the discrimination inherent in the current system of risk-based health insurance. The Affordable Care Act of 2012 will change the issues of quality, access, and cost significantly over the next several years. This legislation and its accompanied parts provide a set of health benefits available and affordable to most citizens of the United States (Merlis, Dentzer, Haislmaier, & Turnbull, 2010).

The National Council on Disability (NCD), founded in 1978, champions the disability movement. The NCD strives to ensure full participation, equal opportunity, independent living, and economic self-sufficiency for all Americans with disabilities. Currently, 54 million Americans (of all ages) are listed as disabled (http://www.ncd.gov).

Enhancement of Fitness and Function

The goal in caring for older adults with disabilities is to maintain or improve function. Maintaining mobility, even when hospitalized, may prevent or decrease the effects of deconditioning. Referral of the older adult to physical therapy assists the nurse in developing and implementing an exercise plan. Many activities that older adults enjoy—for example, walking, swimming, cycling, rowing, and dancing—may be incorporated into exercise and endurance training. In teaching older adults that deconditioning can be reversed, the nurse should stress that activity and exercise not only increase muscle strength and endurance but also help reduce diastolic blood pressure, body fat, and the risk of coronary artery disease. Other benefits include increased bone mineral density, improved joint flexibility, and improved mental health.

Many of the nation's chronic health problems could be reduced by increases in physical activity. Finding ways to increase fitness levels, in all ages, is a national public health priority.

Older adults often think that they are too old to begin and sustain a program of exercise. However, even a small amount of time (at least 30 minutes several times a week) may improve health. In 1998, the National Institute on Aging produced their first guidelines for older adults and exercise, titled *Exercise: A Guide from the National Institute on Aging* (NIA, 1998). The updated guide, *Exercise and Physical Activity: Your Everyday Guide from the National Institute on Aging,* was published in 2009 (NIA, 2009). The guide was reprinted in 2013. The guide lists four types of exercises important in older adults. These include endurance training, which are exercises to increase breathing and heart rate; strength training, which builds muscles and increases muscle strength; balance exercises, which improve standing and gait; and flexibility exercises, which keep the body limber. Further information can be found at https://go4life.nia.nih.gov/.

Functional Assessment

Regular, comprehensive assessment of older adults is a central principle of gerontologic care. Function is a useful measure in the diagnosis of illness and self-care deficits. Functional assessment may help older adults, their families, and health care providers identify problem areas and plan appropriate interventions that assist in treatment or provision of support measures.

Similarly, in rehabilitation, progress is noted through assessments. In rehabilitation, assessment tools measure the functional status of patients. These tools provide baseline data, progress data, and outcomes of therapy. A commonly used tool is the Functional Independence Measure (FIM). This tool measures 18 abilities in six areas: (1) self-care, (2) sphincter control, (3) transfers, (4) locomotion, (5) communication, and (6) social cognition. The 18 items are all measured on an ordinal scale from 1 (dependent) to 7 (independent) (Mauk, 2013). In a rehabilitation setting, functional assessment is incorporated into the initial nursing assessment and provides information about a patient's level of functioning before any planned rehabilitation program begins. Establishing a patient's baseline level of functioning helps the nurse identify the patient's strengths and rehabilitation potential.

Keys for Completing a Functional Assessment

To successfully complete a functional assessment:
- The nurse should be aware of a patient's mental status before assessment. For example, some people with cognitive impairment deny any and all problems, whereas people with depression may just respond, "I don't know."
- The assessment approach should be adapted to the degree of potential or actual disability. Healthy older adults may not need to be to be assessed in all areas. Older adults with complex problems need specific assessments of their abilities and disabilities.
- Self-reported data and observation may be used along with data from a functional assessment tool. Some older adults may deny any functional difficulty or may minimize the amount of assistance needed. The nurse should ask the older adult what they can do rather than what they cannot do.
- The nurse should screen for safety factors that limit older adults in their self-care or in their ability to remain in their home independently: (1) confusion, (2) safety awareness, (3) toileting, (4) continence, (5) depression or poor motivation, (6) falls, and (7) transfer ability. The most important physical task for an older adult is the ability to transfer in and out of a bed or chair. A person who cannot transfer from bed to chair or chair to toilet cannot be left alone for long periods.
- A geriatric assessment must consider older adults' values and beliefs. An older patient's cultural and spiritual beliefs, feelings regarding health practices, and beliefs about quality-of-life issues should be incorporated into the care plan.

Health Promotion

Health promotion is a multidimensional concept that focuses on maintaining or improving the health of individuals, families, and communities (Huckstadt, 2013). Research over the years has demonstrated that pursuing a healthy lifestyle and making lifestyle changes prevents disease; however, health care providers and patients continue to have difficulty implementing needed changes in lifestyle. Although existing chronic disease

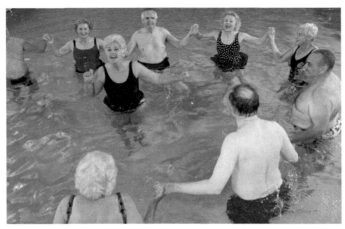

Fig. 27.2 Older adults in a water aerobics class, practicing health promotion. (©Purestock/Thinkstock.)

and disability cannot be eliminated, health promotion within rehabilitation allows older adults to achieve a maximum level of functioning and increase longevity. Health promotion in chronic illness involves behavioral change for positive lifestyle activities, accepting one's condition and making the necessary adjustments, decreasing the risk of secondary disabilities, and preventing further disease, all while striving for optimal health.

Determining reasons why an older adult participates in rehabilitation may provide the nurse with insight to further promote health in the patient. Some authors have promoted self-efficacy as a major determinant of behavior (Resnick, 2002). Other studies have found that fitness, health, independence, and socialization are important incentives to older adults (Lavie & Milani, 1997; McWilliam, Stewart, Brown, Desai, & Coderre, 1996) (Fig. 27.2). Motivational assessment tools may be used in rehabilitation programs to facilitate planning of interventions that enhance participation and compliance.

As Calloway stated, "nurses have been leaders in health promotion since the time of Florence Nightingale, whose pioneering work with the use of statistics demonstrated the positive effect of improved sanitation on the health of injured soldiers" (Calloway, 2006).

Management of Disabling Disorders

It is important for the nurse to understand the normal physiologic effects of aging and their effect on rehabilitation. For example, a cardiac rehabilitation program should focus on exercise training, education, secondary prevention, and vocational counseling. Modifications in exercise training may be needed for older adults with other physical impairments.

Peripheral vascular disease frequently limits activities of endurance. A graded reconditioning program to increase endurance is most successful. If amputation is required, rehabilitation goals and candidacy for prosthetics should be determined by premorbid function, the condition of the residual limb, and the goals of the amputee.

An older adult incapacitated by COPD can improve QOL and ease functional tasks through pulmonary rehabilitation. Success depends on the patient's motivation because improvement

may occur in symptom management but not in pulmonary function testing.

Acute presentation of neurologic disorders in older patients is confounded by comorbid conditions. Risk of stroke increases with age. With increased incidence of hypertension, atrial fibrillation, and heart disease, an older adult with a stroke is at greater risk for compromised cerebral perfusion. Functionally, an older adult who survives a brain injury needs more personal assistance. Discharge to a long-term care facility, rather than home, is more likely as a person ages (Saposnik & Black, 2009).

Life Issues

For those with lifelong conditions, complications and continued deterioration of function may go unrecognized as a result of inadequate transition from pediatric to adult health services. People with disabilities treated by rehabilitation are usually not "sick" but have a narrower margin of health. Many persons with disabilities state that they must constantly educate health professionals about the idiosyncrasies of their condition and their unique needs when treatment is prescribed.

A wide range of responses to disability exists. An individual who has had arthritis for many years may attach little significance to the condition. An individual faced with a long rehabilitation after a stroke may respond with shock, fear, and disbelief. The human spirit is remarkably resilient, adjusting to seemingly unbearable circumstances. In time, most people (in their own ways) come to accept the reality of their condition.

A person with a chronic illness or disability finds that taking health or ability for granted is no longer possible. Symptoms may spoil plans for the day, week, or month. Side effects from medication may present a variety of problems from dry mouth to ataxia. A short trip to the store may be impossible if the day is windy or the sidewalks are wet or icy. As discussed previously, fatigue is a constant companion for many older adults with chronic disabilities.

Older adults must also reorganize their lives to enhance their functional ability and rehabilitation. The nurse may assist older adults with organization. For example, calendars, schedules, and lists may assist with organizing self-care activities. Home blood glucose and blood pressure monitoring, weight measurement, self-assessments of physical condition based on the specific illness, and records of findings are examples. Organizing medications and treatments might include establishing a schedule for medications or treatments such as catheterization, toileting, or home dialysis. Organizing for working with health care professionals might include establishing a means to make and keep appointments, preparing for a visit, and obtaining the information needed to improve self-care.

The nurse should help older adult patients maximize financial resources by interpreting insurance coverage and making referrals to community agencies. Most assistive devices, handrails, canes, walkers, and hearing aids are paid for out of pocket. The nurse should encourage patients to shop around, ask questions, try the equipment, and inquire about service and cost of repairs. Used equipment may be purchased at medical supply stores or privately from individuals. Nurses need to influence legislators regarding the insurance industry's coverage of monitoring equipment, adaptive equipment, and supplies needed to maintain health. The NCD periodically reviews Medicare and Medicaid benefits packages to ensure inclusion of assistive technologies that accurately reflect contemporary health and medical practices. The NCD also recommends that the insurance term *medical necessity* be clarified to include the concept of maintaining and improving the functional capacity of individuals.

Nursing Strategies

In addition to helping older adults with rehabilitation, the nurse may assist the patient in setting and achieving goals that facilitate reintegration to former environments. As with all patients, old or young, the patient should be in agreement regarding all goals. The goals cannot be imposed by the health care providers. Potential goals for older adults in rehabilitation include the following:
- Improving range of motion
- Improving endurance and tolerance for activity
- Restoring functional ability to an acceptable level
- Improving ambulation (if appropriate)
- Maintaining safety

An important tenet of rehabilitation is setting goals; however, the goals must be the patient's goals, not the health care provider's goals of care. Often, health care providers make assumptions as to what is most important for patients (often what is most important for themselves) as opposed to listening to the patient and identifying his or her priorities. Drawing up a contract with a patient may clarify expectations. The strategy of providing homelike routines is consistent with teaching patients how to live with their illnesses and disabilities. Incorporating a patient's normal routine into teaching content can provide a sense of security that facilitates learning. Showing interest by listening to older adult patients and involving them in all decision making increases their confidence in their ability to achieve care outcomes.

Case Study

Mrs. W is a 75-year-old woman admitted to a skilled nursing facility for rehabilitation after a cerebrovascular accident (CVA) resulting in right hemiparesis. She has a history of hypertension. In addition to the hemiparesis, she displays fatigue and emotional lability. She receives physical and occupational therapy twice a day. Her goal is to return home to be with her husband. The priorities in her care are to (1) prevent complications and permanent disabilities, (2) help her achieve independence in ADLs, (3) support the coping process and integration of changes into her self-concept, and (4) provide information about the CVA, prognosis, and treatment.

The nursing staff assists Mrs. W in turning and repositioning until she masters bed mobility in physical therapy. Mrs. W becomes tearful and frustrated with her attempts at self-care. She is upset with the length of time and effort needed to complete tasks. The nurse supports Mrs. W by anticipating the time required for the self-care and getting her started. The nurse provides assistance only as necessary, maintaining a supportive but firm attitude. The nurse praises Mrs. W's efforts, and slowly Mrs. W gains a sense of self-worth that encourages her continued endeavors. She loudly expresses her feelings about her body. She refers to the affected side as "it." The nurse acknowledges Mrs. W's feeling about the betrayal of her body but retains a matter-of-fact attitude that Mrs. W can still use the unaffected side and learn to control the affected side. The staff uses words such as *weak, affected, right,* and *left* to treat that side as a part of her body. Small gains in function are celebrated. Mrs. W is also referred to social services for additional support.

After 60 days, Mrs. W is independent in ambulation with a quad cane and independent in self-care. She is able to assist in meal preparation in the sitting position. She is discharged home with her husband. Follow-up home care includes an assessment of the home environment by the occupational therapist and additional physical therapy in the home. Homemaker assistance is not necessary because of family support.

SUMMARY

Our health care system is based on acute and episodic care, and does not fit with long-term chronic disease and disability. The aging of the population and increasing prevalence of chronic disease will continue to challenge the health care system. In an ever-changing health care environment (from technology and medications to changes in payer sources), it is important to consider the chronic illness, the functional status of the older adult, and the perception of the older adult. Considering the potential trajectory of the disease and the components of the Chronic Care Model to help increase knowledge and independence, nurses can improve the QOL for patients with chronic illness.

KEY POINTS

- Health care providers need to understand the unique illness experience of each older adult and his or her chronic condition.
- It is important to recognize that health may exist within illness.
- Regular, comprehensive assessment, both physical and psychosocial, is a central principle of the care of older adults.
- Assessing what is meaningful to older adults helps the nurse plan interventions to support psychosocial adjustment to a chronic condition or illness.
- Rehabilitation of older adults focuses on improving functional ability.
- Health promotion incentives that are important to older adults are fitness, health, independence, and socialization.

CRITICAL-THINKING EXERCISE

1. An 83-year-old woman, independent and in relatively good health, has had a nagging cough for the past several months. She is concerned that the cough may indicate a serious illness. She is reluctant to seek help because she does not want to prolong her life if it means a loss of quality. Make a judgment about where she fits within the illness trajectory, and explain how a nurse can be of assistance.

REFERENCES

Administration on Aging (AOA). (2013). *Aging Statistics.* Retrieved October 10, 201, from http://www.aoa.gov/AoARoot/Aging_Statistics/future_growth/aging21/demography.aspx.

Administration on Aging (AOA). (2008). *A profile of older Americans: 2008.* Washington, DC: Department of Health and Human Services.

Agency for Healthcare Research and Quality. (2012). *Five Major Steps to Intervention (The "5 A's").* Retrieved from http://www.ahrq.gov/professionals/clinicians-providers/guidelines-recommendations/tobacco/5steps.html.

AlGhurair, S. A., Hughes, C. A., Simpson, S. H., & Guirguis, L. M. (2012). A systematic review of patient self-reported barriers of adherence to antihypertensive medication using the World Health Organization Multidimensional Adherence Model. *The Journal of Clinical Hypertension, 14*(12), 877–886.

Americans with Disabilities Act. (2013). Retrieved October 2013, from http://www.ada.gov.

Association of Rehabilitation Nurses. (2015). *The Gerontological Rehabilitation Nurse.* Retrieved from www.rehabnurse.org.

Berg, J., Evangelista, L., Carruthers, D., & Dunbar-Jacob, J. (2013). Adherence. In I. Lubkin & P. Larsen (Eds.), *Chronic illness: impact and interventions* (8th ed.). Sudbury, Mass: Jones & Bartlett.

Bernell, S., & Howard, S. W. (2016). Use your words carefully: What is a chronic disease? *Frontiers in Public Health, 4,* 159. Retrieved from ncbi.nlm.nih.gov.

Biordi, D., & Nicholson, N. (2013). Social isolation. In I. Lubkin & P. Larsen (Eds.), *Chronic illness: impact and interventions* (8th ed.). Sudbury, Mass: Jones & Bartlett.

Boltz, M., Capezuti, E., Fulmer, T., & Zwicker, D. (Eds.), (2016). *Evidenced-based geriatric nursing protocols for best practice* (5th ed.). New York: Springer Publishing.

Brown, I., Renwick, R., & Nagler, M. (1996). The centrality of quality of life in health promotion and rehabilitation. In R. Renwick, I. Brown, & M. Nagler (Eds.), *Quality of life in health promotion and rehabilitation* (pp. 3–13). Thousand Oaks, Calif: Sage.

Calloway, S. (2006). Mental health promotion: Is nursing dropping the ball? *Journal of Professional Nursing, 23*(2), 105–109.

Centers for Disease Control and Prevention. (2013a). *Minority health.* Retrieved September 11, 2013, from http://www.cdc.gov/omhd/Topic/MinorityHealth.html.

Centers for Disease Control and Prevention. (2013b). *Stroke facts and statistics.* Retrieved September 20, 2013, from http://www.cdc.gov/stroke/stroke_facts.htm.

Centers for Disease Control and Prevention (CDC). (2013c). *Chronic disease: the power to prevent, the power to control, Atlanta.* Retrieved September 21, 2013, from http://www.cdc.gov/nccdphp/publications/AAG/chronic.htm.

Centers for Disease Control and Prevention. (2013d). *State of Aging in America.* US Department of Health and Human Services. Retrieved from www.cdc.gov/aging: CDC.

Centers for Disease control and Prevention (CDC). (2016). *Health, United States, 2016 with chartbook on long-term trends in health.* Retrieved November 20, 2017 from www.cdc.gov.

Centers for Disease Control and Prevention. (2017a). *HRQOL concepts.* Retrieved from www.cdc.gov.

Centers for Disease Control and Prevention. (2017b). *Chronic Disease Overview.* Retrieved from www.cdc.gov.

Clark, G. S., Kortebein, P., & Siebens, H. C. (2012). Aging and rehabilitation. In B. Gans, N. Walsh, & L. Robinson (Eds.), *Physical medicine and rehabilitation: Principles and practice* (5th ed.). Philadelphia: Lippincott Williams & Wilkins.

Commission on Chronic Illness. (1957). *Chronic illness in the United States, prevention of chronic illness.* Cambridge, Mass: Harvard University Press.

Corbin, J. (1998). The Corbin and Strauss chronic illness trajectory model: an update. *Scholarly Inquiry for Nursing Practice, 12*(1), 33.

Curtin, M., & Lubkin, I. (1995). What is chronicity? In I. Lubkin (Ed.), *Chronic illness: impact and interventions* (3rd ed.). Sudbury, MA: Jones & Bartlett.

Easton, K. (1999). *Gerontological rehabilitation nursing.* Philadelphia: WB Saunders.

Ethans, K., & MacKnight, C. (1998). Hip fracture in the elderly. *Postgraduate Medicine, 103*(1), 157.

Federal Interagency Forum on Aging-Related Statistics (Forum). (2016). Older Americans 2016: Key indicators of well-being. Retrieved November 20, 2017 from https://agingstats.gov/docs/LatestReport/Older-Americans-2016-Key-Indicators-of-WellBeing.pdf.

Family Caregiver Alliance. (2017). Caregiving issues and strategies. Retrieved December 15, 2017 from https://www.caregiver.org/caregiving-issues-and-strategies.

Ferrans, C., & Powers, M. (1985). Quality of life index: development and psychometric properties. *Advances in Nursing Science, 8,* 15.

Foley, K., & Mitchell, S. (1997). The elderly driver: what physicians need to know. *Cleveland Clinic Journal of Medicine, 64*(8), 423.

Frankl, V. (1962). *Man's search for meaning.* New York: Simon & Schuster.

Gorina, Y., Pratt, L. A., Kramarow, E. A., & Elgaddal, N. (2015). Hospitalization, readmission, and death experience of noninstitutionalized Medicare fee-for service beneficiaries aged 65 and over. *In National Health Statistics Reports # 84.* retrieved from cdc.gov/nchs/data/nhsr/nhsr084.pdf.

Hibbard, J., Neufeld, A., & Harrison, M. J. (1996). Gender differences in the support networks of caregivers. *Journal of Gerontological Nursing, 22*(9), 15.

Holkup, P. (1998). A therapy group to facilitate understanding of intergenerational behavior patterns and to promote family healing. *Journal of Psychosocial Nursing and Mental Health Services, 36*(2), 20–26.

Holroyd, K., & Creer, T. (1986). *Self-management of chronic disease.* New York: Academic Press.

Hoyt, M., & Stanton, A. L. (2012). Adjustment to chronic illness: theory and research. In A. Baum, T. A. Revenson, & J. E. Singer (Eds.), *Handbook of health psychology* (2nd ed.). New York: Taylor & Francis.

Huckstadt, A. (2013). Health Promotion. In P. Larsen & I. Lubkin (Eds.), *Chronic illness: impact and intervention* (8th ed.). Jones & Bartlett: Sudbury, Mass.

Improving Chronic Illness Care (2017). The Chronic Care Model retrieved from www.improvingchroniccare.org.

Jablonski, A. (2004). The illness trajectory of end-stage renal disease dialysis patients. *Research and Theory for Nursing Practice, 18,* 51–72.

Khanna, R., Pace, P. F., Mahabaleshwarkar, R., Basak, R. S., Datar, M., & Banahan, B. F. (2012). Medication adherence among recipients with chronic diseases enrolled in a state Medicaid program. *Population Health Management, 15*(5), 253–260. https://doi.org/10.1089/pop.2011.0069.

Kleinmann, A. (1985). Illness meanings and illness behavior. In S. McHugh & M. Vallis (Eds.), *Illness behavior: a multidisciplinary model.* New York: Plenum.

Larsen, P. (2013a). Chronicity. In I. Lubkin & P. Larsen (Eds.), *Chronic illness: impact and intervention* (8th ed.). Sudbury, Mass: Jones & Bartlett.

Larsen, P. (2013b). The illness experience. In I. Lubkin & P. Larsen (Eds.), *Chronic illness: impact and intervention* (8th ed.). Sudbury, Mass: Jones & Bartlett.

Larsen, P., & Hardin, S. (2013). Culture and cultural competence. In I. Lubkin & P. Larsen (Eds.), *Chronic illness: impact and intervention* (8th ed.). Sudbury, Mass: Jones & Bartlett.

Lavie, C., & Milani, R. (1997). Benefits of cardiac rehabilitation and exercise training in elderly women. *The American Journal of Cardiology, 79*(5), 664.

Lee, L., Lee, D., & Woo, J. (2009). Tai Chi and health related quality of life in nursing home residents. *Journal of Nursing Scholarship, 41*(1), 35–43.

Lewis, S. M., Bucher, L., & Heitkemper, M. M. (2017). In M.M. Harding (Ed.), *Medical-surgical nursing: assessment and management of clinical problems* (10th ed.). St. Louis (MO): Elsevier.

Mauk, K. (2013). Rehabilitation. In I. Lubkin & P. Larsen (Eds.), *Chronic illness: Impact and intervention* (8th ed.). Sudbury, MA: Jones & Bartlett.

McWilliam, C., Stewart, M., Brown, J. B., Desai, K., & Coderre, P. (1996). Creating health with chronic illness. *Advances in Nursing Science, 18*(3), 1–15.

Merlis, M., Dentzer, S., Haislmaier, E., & Turnbull, N. (2010). *Health policy brief: Individual mandate. Health Affairs.* Retrieved from www.healthaffairs.org/healthpolicybriefs/brief.php/brief-id=14. Accessed November 7, 2013.

Merriam Webster Dictionary, & On-Line, Thesaurus. (2013). Retrieved October 21, 2013, from www.m-w.com.

National Center for Health Statistics (NCHS). *Health 2008 with chartbook on trends in the health of Americans.* Hyattsville, MD. The Center.

National Institute on Aging. (1998). *Exercise: a guide from the National Institute on Aging.* Washington, DC: National Institute on Aging.

National Institute on Aging. (2009). *Exercise and physical activity: your everyday guide from the National Institute on Aging.* Washington, DC: National Institute on Aging.

Office of Disease Prevention and Health Promotion (ODPHP). (2017). *Health-related quality of life and well-being.* Retrieved December 1, 2017 from www.healthypeople.gov.

Park, D. C., & Skurnik, I. (2004). Aging, cognition and patient errors in following medical instructions. In M. S. Bogner (Ed.), *Misadventures in health care: inside stories.* Mahwah, NJ: Lawrence Erlbaum.

Paterson, B. (2001). The shifting perspectives model of chronic illness. *Journal of Nursing Scholarship, 33*(1), 21–26.

Patrick, D., & Erickson, P. (1993). *Health status and health policy: quality of life in healthcare evaluation and resource allocation.* New York: Oxford.

Pinto, J. M., Kern, D. W., Wroblewski, K. E., Chen, R. C., Schumm, P., & McClintock, M. K. (2014). Sensory function: Insights from wave 2 of the national social life, health, and aging project. *Journals of Gerontology, Series B: Psychological Sciences and Social Sciences, 69*(8), S144–S153.

Reddy, M., & Reddy, V. (1997). After a stroke: strategies to restore function and prevent complications. *Geriatrics, 52*(9), 59.

Remsburg, R., & Carson, B. (2006). Rehabilitation. In I. Lubkin & P. Larsen (Eds.), *Chronic illness: impact and intervention* (6th ed.). Sudbury, MA: Jones & Bartlett.

Resnick, B. (2002). Geriatric rehabilitation: the influence of efficacy beliefs and motivation. *Rehabilitation Nursing, 27*(4), 152.

Saposnik, G., & Black, S. (2009). Stroke in the very elderly: Hospital care, case fatality and disposition. *Cerebrovascular Diseases, 27*(6), 537–543. https://doi.org/10.1159/000214216.

Sharpe, L., & Curran, L. (2006). Understanding the process of adjustment to illness. *Social Science and Medicine, 62,* 1153–1166.

Shirey, L., & Summer, L. (2000). *Caregiving: helping the elderly with activity limitations.* Washington, DC: National Academy on an Aging Society.

Skinner, B. F. (1951). How to teach animals. *Scientific American, 185,* 26–29.

Stanton, A. L., & Revenson, T. A. (2011). Adjustment to chronic disease: progress and promise in research. In H. S. Friedman (Ed.), *The Oxford handbook of health psychology.* New York: Oxford.

Strauss, A. L. (1984). *Chronic illness and the quality of life* (2nd ed.). St. Louis: Mosby.

Strauss, A., & Corbin, J. (1988). *Shaping a new health care system.* San Francisco: Jossey-Bass.

Stuenkel, D., & Wong, V. (2016). Stigma. In I. Lubkin & P. Larsen (Eds.), *Chronic illness: impact and intervention* (9th ed.). Sudbury, Mass: Jones & Bartlett.

Strupeit, Wolf-Ostermann, Buss, and Dassen (2014). Mobility and quality of life after discharge from a clinical geriatric setting focused on gender and age. *Rehabilitation Nursing, 39,* 198–206.

Thorne, S., & Paterson, B. (1998). Shifting images of chronic illness. *Image - The Journal of Nursing Scholarship, 30*(2), 173.

Touhy, T., & Jett, K. F. (2018). *Ebersole and Hess' toward healthy aging: Human needs and nursing response* (9th ed.). St Louis: Mosby.

Touhy, T. A., & Jett, K. F. (2015a). Gerontological nursing and an aging society. In T. Touhy, K. F. Jett, P. Ebersole & P. A. Hess (Eds.), *Ebersole and Hess' toward healthy aging: Human needs and nursing response* (9th ed.). St Louis: Mosby Elsevier.

Touhy, T. A., & Jett, K. F. (2015b). Health and wellness. In T. Touhy & K. F. Jett (Eds.), *Ebersole and Hess' toward healthy aging: Human needs and nursing response* (9th ed.). St Louis: Mosby Elsevier.

Tremethick, M. (1997). Thriving, not just surviving: the importance of social support among the elderly. *Journal of Psychosocial Nursing and Mental Health Services, 35*(9), 27.

Twibell, R. (1998). Family coping during critical illness. *Dimensions of Critical Care Nursing, 17*(2), 100.

World Health Organization. (2003). *Adherence in long-term therapies: evidence for action.* Geneva, Switzerland: World Health Organization. Retrieved October 10, 2013 from http://www.who.int/chp/knowledge/publications/adherence:report/en/.

World Health Organization. (2014). *Noncommunicable Diseases.* retrieved from www.who.int.

28

Cancer

Jennifer J. Yeager, PhD, RN, APRN

(e) http://evolve.elsevier.com/Meiner/gerontologic

LEARNING OBJECTIVES

On completion of this chapter, the reader will be able to:

1. Describe the physiologic and environmental factors that contribute to the increased risk of cancer in older adults.
2. Identify the malignancies most commonly found in older adults.
3. Discuss the nurse's role in cancer prevention and early detection.
4. Design therapeutic nursing plans of care by applying principles of cancer treatment to older adults.
5. Develop strategies to manage symptoms experienced by older adults receiving cancer treatment.
6. Discuss unique dimensions of psychosocial problems encountered by older adults with cancer.
7. Analyze ethical concerns related to the care of older adults with cancer.
8. Identify appropriate resources for older adults with cancer.

WHAT WOULD YOU DO?

What would you do if you were faced with the following situations?
* Your 82-year-old father is diagnosed with cancer. What crosses your mind?
* Your 68-year-old patient is diagnosed with breast cancer and voices the most concern over the side effects of treatment. How do you respond?

"Cancer is a group of diseases characterized by the uncontrolled growth and spread of abnormal cells" (American Cancer Society [ACS], 2018a, p. 1). The risk for developing cancer increases with age. Adults over the age of 65 account for 60% of all new cancer diagnoses (Cancer.net Editorial Board, 2016). Although cancer is the second leading cause of death in older adults (Centers for Disease Control and Prevention [CDC], 2017), overall cancer deaths have declined by 13% for all cancer types since 2004 (National Cancer Institute [NCI], 2017). The most common cancers in older adults are (1) lung cancer, (2) prostate and breast cancers, and (3) colon and rectal cancers (ACS, 2018a).

In the United States, the population of those 65 years or older has grown to 47.8 million people, accounting for 14.9% of the total population. By the year 2040, the number of persons older than age 65 is expected to surpass 82 million. The oldest-old population (those ages 85 or older) has grown to 6.3 million and is expected to reach 14.6 million by 2040 (Administration on Aging [AOA], 2017). As the number of older adults increases, so does the prevalence of cancer; the number of new cancer diagnoses is expected to increase by 42% by the year 2050 (Meniscus Educational Institute, 2010).

INCIDENCE

Cancer incidence refers to the number of new cases in a specified period, usually a year, in the general population. The leading types of cancer in men are lung, prostate, and colorectal cancers. The leading types of cancer in women are lung, breast, and colorectal cancers (Table 28.1). Mortality is the rate of deaths per number of incidences. Many persons survive cancer; some cancers have relatively high incidence rates and relatively low death rates.

The ACS (2018a) estimates that approximately 15.5 million Americans alive today have a history of cancer. This has increased from 7.4 million Americans in 2003. Of the survivors, some may be completely cured, whereas others still have some evidence of disease. Cancer deaths have declined over the past decade: an average of 1.6% per year (Thompson, 2013). The likelihood of developing any type of invasive cancer during one's lifetime is approximately 39.66% for men and 37.65% for women (American Cancer Society, 2018a). The 5-year survival rate for all cancers is 70% for whites and 63% for blacks (ACS, 2018a). The improvement in survival reflects progress in diagnosing certain cancers at an earlier stage and improvements in treatment. However, nearly a third of adults over 65 years have comorbidities affecting survival, including diabetes, chronic obstructive pulmonary disease (COPD), and cardiovascular and cerebrovascular diseases (Thompson, 2013).

Lung cancer remains the leading cause of cancer-related death for both men and women, accounting for 27% of cancer deaths in 2016. Lung cancer–related deaths have declined across all races and genders; however, black men and women are more

TABLE 28.1   Leading Sites of New Cancer Cases and Deaths (2018 Estimates)

Male			Female		
Estimated New Cases					
Prostate	164,690	19%	Breast	266,120	30%
Lung and bronchus	121,680	14%	Lung and bronchus	112,350	13%
Colon and rectum	75,610	9%	Colon and rectum	64,640	7%
Urinary bladder	62,380	7%	Uterine corpus	63,230	7%
Melanoma of the skin	55,150	6%	Thyroid	40,900	5%
Kidney and renal pelvis	42,680	5%	Melanoma of the skin	36,120	4%
Non-Hodgkin's lymphoma	41,730	5%	Non-Hodgkin's lymphoma	32,950	4%
Oral cavity and pharynx	37,160	4%	Pancreas	26,240	3%
Leukemia	35,030	4%	Leukemia	25,270	3%
Liver and intrahepatic bile duct	30,610	4%	Kidney and renal pelvis	22,660	3%
All sites	**856,370**	**100%**	**All sites**	**878,980**	**100%**
Estimated Deaths					
Lung and bronchus	83,550	26%	Lung and bronchus	70,500	25%
Prostate	29,430	9%	Breast	40,920	14%
Colon and rectum	27,390	8%	Colon and rectum	23,240	8%
Pancreas	23,020	7%	Pancreas	21,310	7%
Liver and intrahepatic bile duct	20,540	6%	Ovary	14,070	5%
Leukemia	14,270	4%	Uterine corpus	11,350	4%
Esophagus	12,850	4%	Leukemia	10,100	4%
Urinary bladder	12,520	4%	Liver and intrahepatic bile duct	9,660	3%
Non-Hodgkin's lymphoma	11,510	4%	Non-Hodgkin's lymphoma	8,400	3%
Kidney and renal pelvis	10,010	3%	Brain and other nervous system	7,340	3%
All sites	**323,630**	**100%**	**All sites**	**286,010**	**100%**

Note: Estimates are rounded to the nearest 10, and cases exclude basal cell and squamous cell skin cancers and in situ carcinoma except urinary bladder. Ranking is based on modeled projections and may differ from the most recent observed data.
From American Cancer Society. (2018). *Cancer facts & figures 2018.* Atlanta, GA: American Cancer Society.

likely to develop and die of lung cancer than persons of any other racial or ethnic group, despite the fact that they smoke fewer cigarettes (American Lung Association, 2016).

Racial and Ethnic Patterns

Cancer affects Americans of all racial and ethnic groups; however, the incidence of cancer does demonstrate patterns according to racial and ethnic origins. African Americans have higher overall incidence rates than Caucasians, whereas Hispanic Americans and Native Americans have lower incidence rates overall.

Racial and ethnic group age cohorts demonstrate different patterns of cancer incidence. Older Japanese immigrant women demonstrate a lower incidence of breast cancer compared with second- and third-generation Japanese women born in America. Age is an important factor, especially when environmental influences are evaluated in cases in which persons of the same race and ethnicity had different exposures as children; any examination of patterns of cancer among racial or ethnic groups should include age and environmental considerations.

Because the incidence of cancer has demonstrated patterns by race and ethnicity, both of these factors are important in determining which groups are at risk. Race and ethnicity are highly correlated with socioeconomic status. Persons living in poverty tend to lack education, employment, adequate housing, good nutrition, preventive health practices, and access to health care. Within any one race or cultural group, economic status is the major determinant for cancer risk and outcome. Economic status as a risk factor for cancer is demonstrated globally. For most cancers, notable geographic variations in incidence rates exist and reflect socioeconomic differences, particularly differences between developing and developed countries. Addressing issues of poverty among groups of people, regardless of their race or ethnic origin, will lead to decreased cancer incidence and increased survival rates (ACS, 2018a).

The leading cancers among Caucasian men are prostate, lung, colorectal, and urinary bladder cancers; melanoma; and non–Hodgkin's lymphoma. Caucasian men have a higher urinary bladder cancer incidence rate compared with men of any other racial or ethnic group; the rate is almost two times higher than that of Hispanic men, who have the second highest rate along with African American men. The incidence rate for breast cancer among Caucasian women is higher than that for women of any other racial or ethnic group. African American men have a higher overall cancer incidence rate than any other racial or ethnic group in America. In contrast, Caucasian women have the highest cancer incidence rate among all ethnic groups. In the United States, African American men and women have shorter cancer survival times and higher cancer death rates compared with other races and ethnicities.

Cancer incidence rates vary considerably among the subgroups of Asian/Pacific Islanders. Although Asian/Pacific Islanders have lower rates overall compared with other groups, they do have higher death and incidence rates for certain cancers, especially for liver and stomach cancers in both sexes. In men, the top three cancers among Chinese, Filipinos, Hawaiians, and Japanese are prostate, lung, and colorectal cancers; among Koreans, lung, stomach, and colorectal cancers; and among Vietnamese, lung, liver, and prostate cancers. Stomach cancer rates among Korean men and liver cancer rates among Vietnamese men are higher than those among men of any other racial or ethnic group. The top three cancers among Asian/Pacific Islander women are breast, lung, and colorectal cancers, with the following exceptions: stomach cancer is the leading cancer in Japanese and Korean women, and the cervix in Vietnamese women. The incidence rate of cervical cancer for Vietnamese women is more than 2½ times higher than that for any other racial or ethnic group. Asian Americans have the highest overall incidence of liver, bile duct, and stomach cancers for both men and women (ACS, 2016).

Alaskan Natives have the highest cancer incidence rates among any racial group for kidney and pelvic cancers. Alaskan Natives have a relatively high incidence of cancers of the esophagus, stomach, liver, gallbladder, and pancreas. According to the National Cancer Institute: Surveillance, Epidemiology, and End-Results program (1975–2006), American Indians who live in New Mexico and Arizona have excessive incidence rates for stomach, cervix, uterine, liver, and gallbladder cancer. American Indians have the highest gallbladder cancer incidence rate of any racial group, including blacks, Caucasians, or Hispanics (Henley, Weir, Jim, Watson & Richardson, 2015).

The leading cancers in Hispanic men and women are the same as those in Caucasians—lung, prostate, breast, and colorectal cancers. Other cancers commonly diagnosed among Hispanics include cancers of the urinary bladder and stomach in men and cervical cancer in women (ACS, 2016). (See the Cultural Awareness box.)

AGING AND ITS RELATIONSHIP TO CANCER

Cancer is a disease of aging. There are two schools of thought related to the development of cancer. These schools of thought are not mutually exclusive. First, it is thought cancer develops from "genetic mutations that are either inherited or acquired through errors in DNA replication and environmental insults" (Vassilev & DePamaphilis, 2017, p. 33). This thought correlates well with cancer and aging. Second, "cancer results from cancer stem cells (CSCs) that retain their ability to proliferate repeatedly without losing their ability to initiate uncontrolled growth, leading to cancer" (Vassilev & DePamaphilis, 2017, p. 33). This school of thought points to leukemia as a theoretical exemplar. Regardless of the underlying mechanism of cancer, cancer cells have the following distinct characteristics (Vassiley & DePamaphilis, 2017):

- Self-sufficiency in growth signals
- Insensitivity to antigrowth signals
- Evasion of apoptosis
- Unlimited proliferation
- Sustained angiogenesis
- Invasion of local tissues and metastasis to distant sites
- Utilization of abnormal metabolic pathways to generate energy
- Evasion of the immune system
- Genome instability
- Chronic inflammation

The process of cancer growth is believed to occur in four steps: tumor initiation, tumor promotion, malignant conversion, and tumor progression (Fig. 28.1). *Tumor initiation* results from activation of a protooncogene or the inactivation of a tumor-suppressor gene from exposure to an external agent that

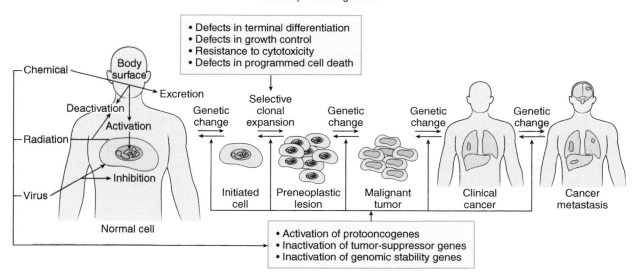

Fig. 28.1 Stages of carcinogenesis. (Redrawn from Hofseth, L. J., Weston, A., & Harris, C. C. [2017]. Chemical carcinogenesis. In R. C. Bast Jr., C. M. Croce, W. N. Hait, et al. [Eds.], *Holland-Frei cancer medicine* [9th ed.]. Hoboken, NJ: John Wiley & Sons, Inc.)

causes mutation of genetic material. The mutations are non-lethal, but they are passed on to future cell generations during replication. An initiated cell will continue to produce the mutations with each cell replication; however, the mutations alone are not enough to lead to cancer. Precancerous cell growth begins when an initiated cell encounters a promoting agent, thus the second step in cancer development is called *tumor promotion*. Tumor promotion involves selective clonal expansion of initiated cells. Promoting agents are external or environmental agents. Many substances may be considered promoters of cancer in humans; they may come from a variety of sources, including air, water, or soil, and they may be naturally occurring or chemically produced (e.g., dichlorodiphenyltrichloroethane [DDT], cigarette smoke condensate, or polychlorinated biphenyls [PCBs]). Promoting agents share the common property of inducing replication of an initiated mutant cell, thus transforming the initiated cell into a precancerous cell. Promotion is dose-dependent in its effect, and although promotion may transform a cell immediately after initiation, promotion is thought to be most successful when it involves repeated exposure to an initiated cell (Weston & Harris, 2003).

Malignant conversion is the third step in cancer growth. This step involves the transformation of preneoplastic cells to ones that express the malignant phenotype. Finally, *tumor progression* is the fourth step in cancer growth. With tumor progression, there is expression of the malignant phenotype and a tendency of malignant cells to acquire more aggressive characteristics over time. Malignant cells secrete proteases that facilitate tumor invasion of surrounding tissue. Genomic instability and uncontrolled growth are characteristics of malignant conversion (Weston & Harris, 2003).

Within normal human DNA material are genes that code cell growth–regulating substances. Oncogenes are genes that produce abnormal codes for growth-regulating substances. Oncogenes are believed to play a role in the development of cancers because, once activated, oncogenes interfere with normal physiologic regulation of cell growth. Oncogene activation is believed to result in excessive production of cell growth–regulating substances. Because oncogenes can cause improper regulation of cell growth, they can cause cancerous transformation in normal cells. The mechanism controlling oncogene activation is unclear; however, activation appears to be tightly controlled. The immune system is believed to play an important role in controlling oncogenes.

In 2003, researchers identified the sequence of the genome in the human body as part of the Human Genome Project. Each cell in the human body contains about 20,500 genes. Genes are the blueprints that direct growth and development. They are arranged in pairs and are made of genetic material called *DNA*. The totality of one's genes is known as a *genome*. Genomics is the study of what genes do and their interaction with each other.

A growing area of cancer research, cancer genome research, studies the differences in genes found in tumors to understand which ones are important in the development and proliferation of a tumor. Researchers collect thousands of samples from different types of tumors to find a tumor's genetic "fingerprint."

Different genes are involved in different tumor types, and understanding what genes are important to the development of cancer has led to improvements in detecting, diagnosing, and treating cancer.

Studying or "mapping" the cancer genome helps researchers understand the mutated genes that lead to cancer. By identifying mutated genes that cause cancer to develop or spread, researchers hope to develop drugs that target those specific genes to stop the cancer's growth. Also, identifying the genes responsible for cancer helps researchers and doctors develop tests to detect cancer earlier. The identification of many mutated genes in breast cancer, colon cancer, melanoma, and other cancers has led to the development of tests that can determine which treatment will be the most effective, as well as to the development of several new treatments that target mutated genes. For example, trastuzumab is a drug used to treat breast cancers with a specific genetic mutation that causes tumors to have too much of a protein called *HER2;* additionally, lung cancer patients with a specific gene mutation involving the ROS1 gene often respond well to treatment with crizotinib, a targeted therapy (National Cancer Institute, 2017).

One of the biggest efforts underway to map the cancer genome is The Cancer Genome Atlas (TCGA) project. The National Cancer Institute and the National Human Genome Research Institute started this project. As part of TCGA, researchers are collecting tissue samples from patients treated at cancer centers across the United States. By studying these tissue samples and comparing them with tissue samples from people who do not have cancer, researchers have identified cancer types and subtypes based on their genetics, which may lead to better tests for diagnosing cancer, as well as more effective treatments (National Cancer Institute, 2017).

Several mechanisms have been proposed to explain the way in which the aging process directly influences the cancerous transformation of cells:

- Aging increases the duration of exposure to substances that may act as promoting agents. The effects of promoters are dose-dependent; a significant dose may accumulate in older adults over decades. Also, cellular transformations and progression of cancer cells occur over time. Cancer cells grow at various rates, and in some cases significant time is needed for the small cluster of cancer cells to grow large enough to cause signs and symptoms.
- Aging cells demonstrate a tendency toward abnormal growth. Aged cells are more vulnerable to damage, thus aging likely increases the susceptibility of cells to substances that cause genetic mutations.
- Once a carcinogen damages an aged cell, it is more difficult to repair it.
- Oncogene activation might be increased in older persons, resulting in decreased regulation of cell growth and the development of cancer cells.
- Decreased immune surveillance, or immunosenescence, may contribute to increased development of cancers and their progression, although the evidence on the role of the immune system in the development of cancer is inconclusive (Crawford & Cohen, 1987; Pfeifer, 1997a).

Aging and Cancer Prevention

The risk of cancer, either increased or decreased, frequently reflects changes in the habits of a specific birth cohort. Because most cancers are the result of a lifelong exposure, the risk of developing malignant disease after age 65 is probably already determined by the time one reaches that age. Frequently, cancer risk is similar for a given birth cohort within specific environmental boundaries. Although it appears difficult to undo or reverse the cellular damage sustained in younger years, prolonged exposure to promoting agents is, nonetheless, needed for the initiated cells to be transformed. If exposure to promoters can be avoided or reduced and antipromoters can be used, cancerous transformation may not take place or may be delayed.

Interference with the promotion stage of cancer would seem to offer the best prospects for cancer prevention. Only recently has research included the search for interventions that halt the promotion phase. It is currently believed that fresh fruits and vegetables may contain antipromoters. It is possible to decrease behaviors earlier in life that promote a predisposition to certain types of cancer; for example, limiting the number of severe sunburns in youth and reducing exposure by applying sunscreen may both be ways to interfere with the promotion stage of cancer. Secondary to this, various vitamins and minerals contained in foods are being examined for their effects on the promotion phase. Older adults should be encouraged to consume the recommended daily requirements of fruits and vegetables because dietary habits may be beneficial in slowing, or halting, the cancer process. In addition, evaluation of environmental risk factors may lead to specifically targeted education and screening programs among selected high-risk cohorts.

COMMON MALIGNANCIES IN OLDER ADULTS

Lung Cancer

Lung cancer is the most common type of cancer and the leading cause of cancer death in both men and women. It occurs most often in older adults; 81% of persons with lung cancer are over the age of 60. Lung cancer accounts for 13% of all cancer diagnoses and 27% of all cancer deaths. Lung cancer–related deaths have declined across all races and genders; however, black men and women are more likely to develop lung cancer and die of it than persons of any other racial or ethnic group, despite the fact that they smoke fewer cigarettes (American Lung Association, 2016).

Risk Factors

Smoking (e.g., cigarettes, pipes, or cigars) is, by far, the most important risk factor in the development of lung cancer, both for active smokers and nonsmokers exposed to secondhand smoke. Tobacco smoke is considered a cancer promoter demonstrating a *dose–response relationship;* that is, the risk of lung cancer increases with the quantity of cigarettes smoked. The greatest lifetime cumulative exposure to cigarette smoking occurs between ages 70 and 80. It has been known for some time that the risk of lung cancer decreases over time for ex-smokers; the risk of lung cancer is increased for both current and former

smokers compared with nonsmokers (Ebbert, Yang, Vachon et al., 2003).

Other risk factors include exposure to certain industrial substances such as asbestos, chromium, nickel, arsenic, soot, tar, or radon. Radiation exposure from occupational, medical, and environmental sources is also a risk factor. Air pollution contains several substances that, with repeated exposure, may increase the risk of lung cancer (ACS, 2018a). The risk for developing lung cancer is increased for those with a family history of the disease and persons infected with the human immunodeficiency virus (HIV) (ACS, 2014). Most lung diseases are chronic and diminish the quality of life for those persons living with the disease.

Signs and Symptoms

More than a quarter of individuals diagnosed with lung cancer have no presenting symptoms. When symptoms do occur, they may be vague and attributed to other problems, especially in older adults who have underlying lung or other chronic illnesses. Others present with symptoms they develop when the tumor becomes large and the cancer metastasizes to other organs. The classic clinical presentation of lung cancer is a persistent cough, sputum streaked with blood, chest pain, fatigue and weight loss, recurring respiratory infections, shortness of breath, and hoarseness. This constellation of symptoms is also associated with cigarette smoking, and its significance as an indicator of cancer may be overlooked (ACS, 2018a).

Early Detection

Low-dose spiral computed tomography (LDCT) screening of current or former (quit within 15 years) smokers between the ages 55 to 74, who have at least a 30 pack-year smoking history has been shown to reduce lung cancer mortality by about 20%. The ACS recommends shared decision making concerning between the health care provider, the patient and their family concerning the benefits, uncertainties, and harms associated with lung cancer screening (ACS, 2018a).

Treatment

Options for treatment include surgery, radiation therapy, and chemotherapy, depending on the type and stage of disease. Lung cancer is classified into two basic types: (1) small cell lung cancer (SCLC; 13% of cases) and (2) non–small cell lung cancer (NSCLC; 84% of cases). In the case of early NSCLC, surgery is the treatment of choice, sometimes in combination with chemotherapy, other times with radiation. In advanced NSCLC, treatment is with chemotherapy and targeted drugs. In patients with SCLC, chemotherapy is used, alone or combined with radiation. Cancer stage and molecular characteristics of NSCLC and SCLC determine treatment choices (ACS, 2018a).

Breast Cancer

Breast cancer is the most common neoplasm in women, increasing in incidence with advancing age. The incidence of breast cancer decreases after age 80, although this may be attributed to a decrease in cancer screening, as opposed to an actual decrease in cancer development.

Breast cancer is the leading cause of cancer-related death in women ages 55 to 74. The primary presenting symptom is a lump in the breast (ACS, 2018a).

Although all women are at risk for developing breast cancer, the older a women is, the greater her chances are of developing breast cancer. Breast cancer is more common in Caucasian women than in other racial or ethnic groups. According to the most recent data, death rates are continuing to decline in Caucasian women; African American women of all ages have the highest mortality rates from breast cancer. Asians/Pacific Islanders have the lowest incidence of breast cancer in the United States (ACS, 2018a).

Risk Factors

The risk of breast cancer increases with age. Dominant risk factors appear to be related to duration and intensity of exposure to hormonal influences, especially estrogen, and include early menarche (before age 12), late menopause (after age 55), lengthy exposure to postmenopausal estrogen, recent use of oral contraceptives, and never having given birth or having first given live birth at a late age (after age 30). Additional risk factors for the development of breast cancer include female gender, a personal or family history of breast cancer (5% to 10% of breast cancers have a genetic predisposition), history of benign breast disease or dense breast tissue, excessive alcohol use, and smoking. Obesity and weight gain after menopause and type 2 diabetes and a sedentary lifestyle have also been shown to increase the risk of developing breast cancer (ACS, 2018a).

⊕ CULTURAL AWARENESS

Cultural Considerations in Breast Cancer Screening

Mammography screening for early detection of breast cancer has been shown to be an effective method for reducing mortality in older women.

Recent data indicate the rates of screening mammography range from 46% to 52%. Screening is lowest for Hispanics (46%) and Asians (48%). Additionally, those without insurance have less frequent mammography than those with insurance (17% versus 55%), and those with fewer than 12 years of education have less frequent mammography than those with more than 12 years of education (38% versus 53%). Finally, persons born in the United States are more likely to have screening mammography than those who have lived in the country for fewer than 10 years (52% versus 27%) (ACS, 2013a).

Barriers to early detection of breast cancer have been identified as the following: inaccurate knowledge of breast cancer and early screening, low awareness of the necessity for early detection, lack of health insurance to cover screening mammography, and lack of reimbursement to health care providers for clinical breast examinations and health teaching for early detection.

The researchers identified the following strategies to reduce barriers to early detection of breast cancer:

* Educate health care providers about the necessity of early breast cancer detection and their role in recommending it to patients.
* Conduct research to identify culturally appropriate messages and intervention strategies for each of the at-risk groups to influence their early detection behaviors.
* Use the media to increase knowledge and promote positive early detection practices among older women from culturally diverse backgrounds.

A major advance in understanding breast cancer is that the disease has a genetic basis. Approximately 5% to 10% of breast cancers are hereditary. The genes involved in most inherited breast cancers are *BRCA1* and *BRCA2*. These are tumor-suppressor genes that also serve to protect and preserve DNA. Mutation of these genes has been linked to hereditary breast and ovarian cancer. A woman's risk of developing breast cancer, ovarian cancer, or both is greatly increased if she inherits a deleterious *BRCA1* or *BRCA2* mutation. Men with these mutations also have an increased risk of breast cancer. By the age of 70, women with *BRCA1* have a 44% to 78% chance of developing breast cancer; those with *BRCA2* have a 31% to 56% chance of developing breast cancer by age 70 (ACS, 2013a; Cummings & Olopade, 1998).

Genetic tests are available to check for *BRCA1* and *BRCA2* mutations. Federal and state laws help ensure the privacy of a person's genetic information and provide protection against discrimination in health insurance and employment practices. Currently, many research studies are being conducted to discover newer and better ways of detecting, treating, and preventing cancer in carriers of *BRCA1* and *BRCA2* mutations (ACS, 2016).

Signs and Symptoms

Malignant lumps are hard and fixed, with irregular borders, and are sometimes described as "frozen peas." Nipple retraction or elevation may be caused by tumor fixation involving underlying tissues. Skin dimpling may also be present, usually because of invasion of the tumor into the ligaments and fixation on the chest wall. Localized erythema and warmth may be present and are related to inflammation. Characteristically, edema appears as "orange peel" skin. Pain is not usually a presenting symptom unless the disease is locally advanced.

Early Detection

Although the practice of breast self-examination is no longer recommended as "there is little evidence that these tests help find breast cancer early when women also get screening mammograms, … women should be familiar with how their breasts normally look and feel and report any changes to a health care provider right away" (ACS, 2017a).

Mammography can detect breast tumors before they manifest physical signs. A tumor must be about 10 millimeter (mm) in size to be palpable. A 10-mm tumor contains about 10^9, or one billion cells. Mammography screening can detect 10^7 cells. Mammography screening is more accurate for older women because breast tissue is less dense than that in younger women, making tumors easier to visualize. The ACS recommends annual mammography screening for women after age 40 until age 54; those over age 55 may change to biennial mammography if they choose. Mammography should continue "as long as overall health is good and life expectancy is 10 or more years" (ACS, 2018a).

Treatment

Breast cancer treatment should be multidisciplinary. Surgery—either breast-conserving surgery or mastectomy—is indicated for removal of the primary tumor. Radiation to the breast is recommended for most patients having breast-conserving surgery; radiation may also be recommended for women undergoing mastectomy, for large tumors, or node-involved breast cancers. Because breast cancer metastasizes early in the course of the disease, axillary lymph nodes are removed and evaluated for the presence of cancer; another alternative is sentinel node biopsy. Treatment may also involve chemotherapy (before or after surgery), hormone (antiestrogen) therapy, and/or targeted therapy (ACS, 2018a).

As with everyone, older women should be given information and support to help make treatment decisions. Breast cancer should be treated promptly, but it is not an emergency. Nurses should provide a supportive atmosphere and encourage family members to participate in treatment decisions.

Survival

The 5-year survival rate for localized breast cancer, when caught early, is 99%; for regional breast cancer, the 5-year survival rate is 90%. It is important for women to realize everyone with breast cancer is different and that survival rates are not a predictor of treatment success. Risk factors, cancer stage, and treatment choice all play into the success of any given therapy.

Prostate Cancer

Slightly more than 11% of men will develop prostate cancer during their lifetime. Prostate cancer is rare before the age of 40; the average age at diagnosis is 66. Although prostate cancer is a serious disease, most men do not die of it. The 5-year survival rate for all stages of prostate cancer is 99%; the 10-year survival rate is 98%; and the 15-year survival rate is 96%. Prostate cancer is usually adenocarcinoma that develops slowly in the gland cells of the prostate (ACS, 2017b).

Risk Factors

Prostate cancer is a disease of aging. Six out of 10 cases of prostate cancer occur in persons over the age of 65. African American men develop prostate cancer more often than Asian American and Hispanic males. Other risk factors include a family history of prostate cancer and occupational exposure to carcinogens. Smoking increases the risk of fatal prostate cancer (ACS, 2017b).

Signs and Symptoms

Prostate cancer is asymptomatic in its early stages. Signs and symptoms of cancer are related to the increased growth of the prostate that surrounds the urethra; they include weak or interrupted urine flow, difficulty or inability to begin urine flow, difficulty stopping urine flow, and urinary frequency, especially at night. Many of these symptoms are like those of infection or benign prostatic hypertrophy. As the cancer progresses, additional signs and symptoms include pain in the hips, spine, and ribs (from bony metastases); impotence; weakness or numbness in the lower extremities; and bowel and bladder incontinence (ACS, 2018a).

Early Detection

"No organizations presently endorse routine prostate cancer screening for men at average risk, because of concerns about the high rate of overdiagnosis (detecting disease that would never have caused symptoms), along with the significant potential for serious side effects associated with prostate cancer treatment" (ACS, 2018a). The ACS recommends that men, at average risk and who have a life expectancy of at least 10 years, begin discussing the risks and benefits of screening for prostate cancer with their doctor at age 50 to make an informed decision. Men at high risk of developing prostate cancer (black men, or those with a close relative diagnosed with prostate cancer before the age of 65) should have this discussion beginning at age 45 (ACS, 2018a).

Treatment

Multiple methods of treatment may be used, either alone or in combination, to manage prostate cancer: active surveillance, surgery, external beam radiation, or radioactive seed implants. Hormonal therapy may be used with surgery or radiation in advanced cases. Choice of treatment is determined by the age of the patient, comorbidities, stage and grade of the tumor, the likelihood of a cure, and the patient's inclination (ACS, 2018a).

Active surveillance involves digital rectal examination, periodic biopsy, and serial prostate specific antigen (PSA) testing. Should signs and symptoms change, treatment options may be readdressed. The primary surgery for prostate cancer is radical prostatectomy, which involves removal of the prostate and surrounding tissue. After surgery, men may develop incontinence and impotence. When the cancer has not spread beyond the prostate, radiation therapy may be effective. It may also be used in conjunction with hormone therapy, after surgery, or with advanced cancer to relieve symptoms (ACS, 2018b).

Hormone therapy is an adjunct to radiation therapy or may be used alone in patients who are not candidates for surgery or radiation. It may also be used in cases where cancer has returned or to shrink tumors so that radiation therapy is more effective. The objective of hormone therapy is to reduce circulating androgens in the body or to prevent androgens from reaching the prostate. The objective can be accomplished by using several methods: orchiectomy, luteinizing hormone (LH)–releasing hormone analogs, LH-releasing hormone antagonists, antiandrogens, and androgen-suppressing drugs. All forms of hormone therapy have similar side effects: reduced libido, impotence, shrinking of the sex organs, hot flashes, breast tenderness, osteoporosis, anemia, decreased alertness, decreased muscle mass and weight gain, elevated cholesterol, fatigue, and depression (ACS, 2018b).

Chemotherapy is not the first-line therapy for prostate cancer, although it may be used in cases of metastasis. Chemotherapy targets the rapidly dividing cancer cells. However, other cells in the body divide rapidly as well (e.g., bone marrow, mucous membranes, hair follicles), leading to side effects: hair loss, oral lesions, anorexia, nausea and vomiting, diarrhea, immunosuppression, easy bruising or bleeding, and fatigue (ACS, 2018b).

Vaccine therapy is an individualized treatment designed for advanced-stage prostate cancer. White blood cells (WBCs) from the patient are exposed to prostatic acid phosphatase (PAP) from the cancer cells; the exposed cells are then put back into the patient intravenously to stimulate the patient's immune system to attack the cancer cells (ACS, 2018b). The vaccine hasn't been shown to stop prostate cancer from growing, but it seems to help men live an average of several months longer. The cost is prohibitive ($93,000 per course of treatment).

Colorectal Cancer

Colorectal cancer is the third most common cancer, accounting for 8.6% of all cancer diagnosis. An individual's lifetime risk for developing colorectal cancer is 4.3%. Death rates are declining because of a decrease in the number of cases. Early screening with polyp removal, early diagnosis and treatment leading to cure, and improvements in treatment are the reasons for the declining rates. Five-year survival is nearly 65%. The median age at diagnosis for colorectal cancer is 67; the median age at death is 73 (National Cancer Institute, 2017b).

Risk Factors

A personal or family history of colorectal cancer, polyps, or inflammatory bowel disease has been associated with increased colorectal cancer risk, as have type 2 diabetes. Lifestyle choices linked to the development of colorectal cancer include eating a diet high in red meat and processed meats, low calcium intake, moderate to heavy alcohol consumption, and very low intake of fruits, vegetables, and whole-grain fiber. Obesity and a sedentary lifestyle have also been associated with colorectal cancer (ACS, 2018a).

Signs and Symptoms

In the early stages, colorectal cancer may not manifest any symptoms. As the disease advances, presenting signs and symptoms include a change in bowel habits or stool shape, the feeling that the bowel is not completely empty, abdominal cramping or pain, decreased appetite, and weight loss. In some cases, the cancer causes blood loss that leads to anemia, resulting in symptoms such as weakness and fatigue (ACS, 2018a).

Early Detection

According to the ACS guidelines for the early detection of colorectal cancer, starting at age 50, both men and women should have yearly guaiac-based fecal occult blood tests and flexible sigmoidoscopy every 5 years, *or* colonoscopy every 10 years, *or* double-contrast barium enema every 5 years, *or* computed tomography (CT) colonography every 5 years. Fecal occult blood testing, although inexpensive and low risk, may miss polyps, and some cancers may produce false-positive test results; however, it has been proven effective in clinical trials (ACS, 2018a). Screening is appropriate for individual older adults at high risk, but care should be taken to ensure proper testing.

Treatment

Cancer stage guides treatment, although surgery is the treatment of choice for colorectal cancer. The extent of surgery is determined by the location of the cancer and the involvement of lymph nodes. Surgical procedures include removal of the cancer and segments of the major arterial and venous blood suppliers to the affected area. Permanent colostomy is seldom needed for colon cancer. For localized cancers, surgery is frequently curative. Radiation therapy may take place before surgery to shrink the size of tumor or after surgery to reduce the chance of recurrence. Radiation has also been used in situations where patients are not surgical candidates and for palliative pain relief. Chemotherapy before surgery may help shrink the tumor; chemotherapy after surgery is beneficial for patients with cancer that has spread to the lymph nodes or cancer that has penetrated the bowel wall (ACS, 2018a).

Targeted therapies attack cancer cells directly. Unlike standard chemotherapy, which targets all rapidly dividing cells, targeted therapy interferes with specific molecules (e.g., protein enzymes, growth factor receptors) required for the cancer cells to replicate. Targeted therapies are used for treating advanced colorectal cancer. Immunotherapy is a newer option for some advanced colorectal cancers (ACS, 2018a).

SCREENING AND EARLY DETECTION: ISSUES FOR OLDER ADULTS

Primary prevention of cancer is desirable and is affected by changes in lifestyle. Older adults are likely to have had a lifetime of exposure to risk factors; although changing lifestyles is advantageous for them, the changes may not reverse the effects of exposure. Furthermore, changing habits that have developed over a lifetime is difficult, despite demonstrable benefits. Given the difficulty of cancer prevention, detection of cancer at an early stage may greatly improve survival rates. Screening asymptomatic persons at risk is feasible in many common malignancies, including breast, cervical, and colorectal cancers.

When considering a cancer screening program, the health care provider should answer two fundamental questions:
1. Is the screening test sensitive? A sensitive test will correctly identify all screened individuals who have the disease (those with true-positive results).
2. Is the screening test specific? A specific test identifies all individuals who do not have the disease (those with true-negative results).

Current efforts at advancing the science and technology of screening have resulted in greater accuracy of many screening tests. The accuracy of screening may be increased by the recognition of highly sensitive tumor-specific circulating markers (e.g., carcinoembryonic antigen [CEA] for colorectal adenocarcinoma); the development of imaging techniques capable of finding smaller lesions (e.g., 3D mammography); and the identification of early molecular changes in cancer specimens (e.g., at the cellular level using Papanicolaou [Pap] tests for cervical cancer). Given the limited effectiveness of primary prevention for older adults, screening asymptomatic persons at risk for cancer may be the most promising way to reduce the number of cancer deaths in older adults.

Yet another question to consider with a screening program is the prevalence of the disease in the population. The more prevalent the disease, the more beneficial a screening program will be. Because cancer is more common in older adults, screening is generally beneficial. The incidence of cancer increases with age; thus the positive predictive value of screening tests (i.e., the proportion of persons screened who actually have the disease) is likely to increase. In addition, screening older adults who have comorbid conditions at the time of cancer diagnosis may result in elective treatment at an early stage of disease, thus reducing the possibility of serious treatment-related morbidity and deaths.

Recommendations on planning major screening programs for older adults should be made with caution. Screening guidelines vary greatly among different national organizations. Differences among recommendations are caused by the lack of cancer screening trials that include older adults. Because more than 56% of all cancers are diagnosed in those older than 65 and 70% of all cancer deaths occur in this age group, the lack of evidence-based criteria for screening older adults makes choosing screening protocols difficult. A decision-making process that considers each older adult's personal preference and health should be used rather than relying only on age guidelines for cancer screening and detection methods. Screening should not be conducted in the absence of intent or ability to follow up on the findings with more complete evaluation and treatment. Screening is costly and useless if no follow-up occurs. Other factors that influence the decision to screen an older adult include comorbidity, functional ability, and life expectancy.

Considerable uncertainty exists concerning the use of cancer screening tests in older adults, as illustrated by the different age cutoffs recommended by various guideline panels. A framework to guide individualized cancer screening decisions in older patients may be more useful to the practicing nurse than age guidelines. Like many medical decisions, cancer screening decisions require weighing quantitative information such as risk of cancer death and likelihood of beneficial and adverse screening outcomes and qualitative factors such as individual patients' values and preferences.

Potential benefits of screening are presented as the number needed to screen to prevent one cancer-specific death based on the estimated life expectancy during which a patient will be screened. Estimates reveal substantial variability in the likelihood of benefit for patients of similar ages with varying life expectancies. In fact, patients with life expectancies of less than 5 years are unlikely to derive any survival benefit from cancer screening. The likelihood of potential harm from screening according to patient factors and test characteristics must also be considered. Some of the greatest harms of screening occur by detecting cancers that would never have become clinically significant. This becomes more likely as life expectancy decreases (Eckstrom, Feeny, Walter, Perdue, & Whitlock, 2012).

Finally, because many cancer-screening decisions in older adults cannot be made solely based on quantitative estimates of benefits and harms, considering the estimated outcomes according to the patient's own values and preferences is the final step in making informed screening decisions. As more and more cancers occur in older people, oncologists are increasingly confronted with the necessity of integrating geriatric parameters into the treatment of their patients.

The International Society of Geriatric Oncology (SIOG) created a task force to review the evidence on the use of a comprehensive geriatric assessment (CGA) in cancer patients. A systematic review of the evidence was conducted. Several biologic and clinical correlates of aging were identified. Strong evidence suggests that a CGA may detect many problems missed by a regular assessment in both general geriatric patients and older patients with cancer. Strong evidence also exists that a CGA improves function and reduces hospitalization in older adults. A CGA, with or without screening and with follow-up, should be used in older patients with cancer to detect unaddressed problems, improve functional status, and possibly improve the chances of survival (Extermann, Aapro, Bernabei et al., 2005).

Although CGA is a multidimensional tool designed to detect health problems, a barrier to its use in busy health care settings is the length of time required to complete the entire instrument. Overcash, Beckstead, Extermann, & Cobb (2005) conducted a study to determine what items contained in the instrument could be compiled to construct an abbreviated CGA (aCGA). A retrospective chart review of more than 500 patients with cancer was performed at a large southeastern cancer center. Statistical analyses revealed 15 valid and reliable items that form the aCGA. They concluded that an aCGA may be helpful in screening those seniors who would benefit from the full-length CGA.

Walter and Covinsky (2001) developed a framework for cancer screening in older adults with the following recommendations:

- Individualize the decision by conducting a CGA that includes an evaluation of comorbid conditions, polypharmacy, and the presence of dementia or depression.
- Estimate life expectancy. Reducing the risk of dying of a detectable cancer should be the main benefit of cancer screening. Although an exact determination of longevity is impossible, decisions can be made based on understanding the distribution of life expectancies at various ages. The goal of any cancer-screening program is to detect those cancers early enough for successful treatment. Therefore a patient with more than 10 years' life expectancy will benefit from a cancer-screening program (http://cancerscreening.eprognosis.org/ may provide assistance with estimating survival). Although determining life expectancy for an individual is difficult, some attempt should be made to correlate life expectancy with the potential for future development of a specific cancer. The decision to screen should consider the treatment implications, but the decisions concerning specific treatment and how aggressively to treat are separate and take place after the type and stage of cancer are diagnosed.
- Assess the risk of cancer screening. Certain clinically unimportant cancers increase as people age; therefore older patients are frequently diagnosed with these types of cancer.
- Older people have more cognitive and physical conditions that increase their fear of cancer screening. Ascertain patient preferences. Consider each older person's approach to health and discuss the risks and benefits of cancer-screening tests.
- Consult various cancer screening guidelines. The U.S. Preventive Services Task Force (USPSTF) guidelines are the

most widely used and respected; however, these guidelines are very conservative and differ significantly from those of specialty organizations such as the ACS and the AGS. A listing of all USPSTF guidelines is provided at http://www.ahrq.gov/clinic/uspstfix.htm.

Nurses working with older adults should examine the role of cancer screening and the potential benefits for the population assigned to their care. The decision to screen or not to screen should be an active one, made after thoughtful consideration within the context of a multidisciplinary health care team. Screening guidelines, individual circumstances, potential complications of aggressive evaluation workups, and associated costs are all factors to consider in deciding to screen older adults.

As a group, older persons generally require more individualized health teaching about cancer risk and detection. Older persons may lack an awareness of the risks of cancer associated with advanced age and may not know the warning signs of cancer. They may be reluctant to report physical complaints that could be indicative of cancer. In addition, many older persons are concerned about, and even fear, the diagnosis of cancer and its effect on their overall well-being and functional status. The nurse should teach older adults the following early warning signs of cancer:

- Change in bowel or bladder habits
- A sore that does not heal
- Unusual bleeding or discharge
- Thickening or lump in the breast or elsewhere
- Indigestion or difficulty swallowing
- Obvious change in a wart or mole
- Nagging cough or hoarseness

MAJOR TREATMENT MODALITIES

The five types of cancer treatment are (1) surgery, (2) radiation therapy, (3) chemotherapy, (4) targeted therapy, and (5) immunotherapy. Each form of treatment may be used alone or in combination. The type and stage of the cancer, the unique biophysiologic characteristics of the cancer cells, and an older patient's overall health status determine treatment selection at the time of diagnosis. Treatment goals also help determine the type of therapy. Cancer therapies may be directed at a *cure* or elimination of the disease; *control* or minimization of the disease; or *palliation* or relief of the symptoms.

Adjuvant therapies to the standard therapies have been developed that include angiogenesis inhibition, gene therapy, hyperthermia, laser therapy, and photodynamic therapy. Senger (1983) noted that cancerous tumors secrete chemicals, which he called *vascular permeability factors* (VPFs); these are now referred to as *vascular endothelial growth factors* (VEGFs). These substances promote the growth of new blood vessels to supply the tumor's ever-expanding need for oxygen and nutrients. In theory, blocking the secretion of these blood vessel–producing chemicals will decrease the tumor's ability to grow or survive or both.

Gene therapy involves the injection of altering substances into the cancer cells, usually in the form of viruses that make the cancer cells incapable of reproducing. Cancer cells are non-differentiated; they serve no physiologic purpose other than

reproduction. This reproduction takes place at an accelerated pace. Adding material to the cells makes replacement cells difficult to replicate. In breaking the cell replacement cycle, the tumor is rendered nonviable.

When cells in the body are heated (hyperthermia) past a specific point, usually considered to be 113° F, they are destroyed. The use of heat as an adjunct is not a new idea, but a great deal of advancement has occurred in the control and use of heat at specific sites and on the entire body.

Laser light can focus a narrow beam on specific tissues at exact locations and depths. At this time, lasers are used primarily on lesions of the skin and on endothelial lesions in the linings of cavities accessible via endoscope. Both allow for direct visualization of the process. In photodynamic therapy (PDT), photosensitizing agents, which are chemicals readily absorbed by the tumor cells, are introduced into the bloodstream and absorbed by tissues, including the tumor cells. When exposed to the light from the laser, the drugs are activated within the tumor, leading to cell death (ACS, 2013b).

Cancer is predominately a disease of older adults; however, research indicates older adults are subject to treatment bias based on age. Health care providers often fail to recommend older adults for cancer screening; older adults are subject to treatment delays and referrals, and are not offered surgical excision of tumors (Campbell, 2011). Chronologic age is not a major variable in determining a patient's ability to tolerate or respond to therapy. Functional status has been reported to be a more important pretreatment variable, influencing both the decision to treat and the type of treatment. In addition, the number of comorbid conditions is a significant predictor of the outcome of an older adult receiving cancer treatment. As with screening decisions, treatment decisions should consider the individual (ACS, 2018a). Age is but one of many factors that should be considered.

Age-related treatment bias may also occur because of the older adults or their families. Patients or family members may believe a person may be too old to tolerate treatment; thus they choose suboptimal therapies in lieu of more aggressive and curative treatments. Cancer care has changed dramatically over the years; however, many older adults remember friends or relatives who were treated with now-outdated therapies that had devastating side effects. One older woman, for instance, refused to have follow-up radiation therapy and decided to have a mastectomy when lumpectomy was an option. She remembered her mother's complications related to older methods of cobalt radiation therapy, a delivery method for external beam radiation therapy that has now been greatly improved, and declared, "No one is going to fry me like they did my poor mother." Patients and families need accurate information. Because cancer is so prevalent in older adults, many have some information about cancer, but it is often misinformation. The nurse should be sure that patients and families have accurate information and a clear understanding of the treatment options being offered.

Surgery

Surgery, the oldest method of treating cancer, is indicated for most solid tumors. Initially, with the use of sophisticated biopsy and exploratory techniques, surgery is used to diagnose the disease, by determining tumor type, and to stage the disease, by determining its extent. The primary treatment goal of surgery is to remove the tumor when localized, thus preventing regional or distant metastasis. Surgery may also be indicated for palliative care in cases where the size or location of the tumor may create such problems as compression of surrounding tissues and organs, leading to pain, necrosis, or organ failure; large primary or metastatic tumors can be reduced with surgery. Surgery may be indicated for the placement of treatment-related devices such as implanted access devices, shunts, or drains. In addition, surgery may be indicated for rehabilitation or restorative purposes such as breast reconstruction after a mastectomy. Surgery is not a treatment of choice for disseminated disease such as metastases of multiple small tumors in diffuse locations (e.g., when breast cancer metastasizes in the lungs) or for disease that is disseminated from the onset, for example, leukemia.

In the past, surgical treatment of cancer involved extensive radical procedures. Such procedures were necessary to treat large, often neglected cancers. Poor understanding of patterns of metastatic spread and little knowledge of the benefits of adjuvant therapy contributed to the focus on radical operations. Greater insight into the pathophysiology of cancer and the development of additional therapies has led to more sophisticated surgical techniques. Early detection of smaller tumors has also contributed to the decline in the number of radical procedures. Less radical procedures result in fewer complications and improved quality of life. Research has demonstrated that, in older adults with cancer, complication rates are no higher than age-matched cohorts without cancer (Audisio & Bozzett, 2004).

The curability of cancer in older adults is largely predicted by an individual's ability to tolerate major surgery. Because older adults are at risk for more complications, careful preoperative assessment is critical. In-depth evaluation of the status of the respiratory, cardiovascular, hepatic, immunologic, renal, nutritional, and central nervous systems is mandatory. The severity of underlying cancer and comorbid conditions is an important factor to consider in the decision regarding surgical therapy. In addition, a patient's rehabilitation potential should be evaluated, particularly if the intended surgery will significantly alter normal physiologic function. Some surgical procedures may produce physiologic alterations that are beyond an older adult's adaptive capabilities. Arthritic changes and diminished visual acuity are two common problems in older adults that may make the management of surgical complications and postoperative care difficult (e.g., after colostomy creation). In general, older patients have a higher surgical risk compared with younger patients; however, through careful preoperative assessment to identify risks, older patients may be offered appropriate supportive therapies that minimize complications. Although age alone is not a determinant of surgical risk, data indicate that older adults are less likely to receive surgical therapy compared with younger persons (Farrow, Hunt, & Samet, 1996).

Postoperative priorities should include preventing respiratory complications and promoting cardiac and renal function. Because of the overall reduced compensatory reserves in these systems, older adults are susceptible to many serious complications, including congestive heart failure, electrolyte imbalances, hypoxia, dehydration, and venous thromboembolism. The use of invasive lines and catheters may tax an aging immune system and predispose older patients to sepsis. The overall stress of surgery, including anesthesia and other centrally acting medications, may predispose older adults to the development of delirium. Bowel complications may include paralytic ileus and constipation. Decreased mobility and inadequate nutrition are risk factors for pressure ulcers. Careful, complete, and ongoing assessment of all body systems provides the foundation for the nurse to accurately diagnose, plan, implement, and evaluate nursing care during the postoperative period.

Radiation Therapy

Like all cancer therapies, radiation therapy is used for several different purposes. Radiation therapy may be curative for the treatment of several cancers, including skin, prostate, colorectal, lung, cervical, and Hodgkin's cancers. Radiation therapy may also be indicated as an adjuvant therapy to prevent recurrence of breast cancer after lumpectomy. In some cases, radiation therapy may be used to control cancers, adding months or years to an individual's life. Radiation therapy and chemotherapy may also be used before surgery to shrink the tumor. Often, recurrent breast and lung cancers can be controlled with radiation therapy in combination with chemotherapy, surgery, or both. Radiation therapy may also be used for palliative care. It relieves pain and prevents pathologic fractures associated with bone metastasis from breast, lung, and prostate tumors. Palliative radiation therapy is given for the relief of central nervous system symptoms caused by brain metastasis or spinal cord compression. In some cases, palliative radiation therapy may be given before a problem manifests itself, as in the treatment of vertebral lesions when spinal cord compression is imminent. According to the National Cancer Institute (2009), approximately half of all cancer patients receive radiation therapy in the course of their treatments today.

Not all cancers are sensitive to the effects of radiation therapy, but for other cancers radiation therapy may provide significant advantages over surgical procedures. Radiation encompasses wider areas around the tumor and removes tumors from regions where surgery cannot effectively excise them. The use of radiation may also result in less disability and disfigurement than some extensive surgeries. Radiation also allows simultaneous treatment to multiple metastatic sites (Davis & Lindley, 2004).

Therapeutic doses of radiation therapy are calculated to destroy or delay the growth of malignant cells without destroying normal tissue. Radiation effects at the cellular level may be either direct or indirect. Direct effects occur when key molecules within the cell—the DNA or ribonucleic acid (RNA)—are damaged. Indirect effects occur when charged particles (free radicals) are created by radiation therapy, which cause damage to cellular DNA.

The administration of radiation therapy may involve external or internal techniques. External beam therapy, which is radiation from a source at a distance from the body, is administered primarily by linear accelerators and mostly in an outpatient setting. Internal therapy involves radiation from a source placed within the body or a body cavity. Internal therapy uses various commercially available instruments or applicators that are inserted into target areas for a predetermined period. Rotation of either the target site or the radiation beam makes it possible to deliver a high dose to the tumor, yet only part of the dose reaches the surrounding noncancerous tissue.

The response of older adults to radiation therapy has not been well evaluated. Several initial reports suggest that no difference in response exists between older persons and any other age group (Host & Lunde, 1986; Nobler & Venetl, 1985). Research and clinical data suggest that the response of cancers to radiation therapy in older adults is like that in younger ones; therefore decisions to treat using radiation therapy should be based on individual factors (Greenberg & Trotti, 1992).

The associated side effects of radiation therapy are no worse in older adults than in younger ones (Larson, Lindsay, Dodd et al., 1993). However, older persons have greater difficulty compensating for temporary dysfunction in a single organ or in multiple organ systems. The challenge in treating older adults with radiation therapy is to provide appropriate supportive care to enable the patient to complete treatment without any significant alteration in functional status. Age cannot be used as a predictor for how patients will respond to radiation therapy treatment.

Chemotherapy

Because not all cancers can be cured with surgery or radiation therapy, systemic treatment with chemotherapy may be necessary. Chemotherapy is the use of drugs to destroy cancer cells. Classic chemotherapy kills cancer cells either by damaging DNA, interfering with DNA synthesis, or inhibiting cell division. In contrast to surgery and radiation therapy, which are local therapies, chemotherapy is systemic. Although single-agent chemotherapy may be successful in the treatment of certain types of cancer, most tumors show only a partial response to this type of therapy. In most cancers, specifically breast, colorectal, gastric, ovarian, and lung cancers and lymphoma, combination chemotherapy is necessary to provide a better chance of long-term, disease-free survival. Broader coverage against cells and cell lines within heterogeneous tumors is provided with combination chemotherapy (Davis & Lindley, 2004).

The objectives of chemotherapy include cure, control, and palliation. In general, the survival of older persons who receive chemotherapy is significantly longer than that of untreated older persons, even though dose adjustments may be needed to control toxicity. Table 28.2 lists commonly prescribed chemotherapeutic agents by drug classification and mechanism of action.

Pharmacokinetics

Pharmacokinetics refers to the movement of drugs throughout the body, including absorption, distribution, metabolism, and excretion. For oral chemotherapeutic agents, age-related changes in the digestive tract appear to have little effect on the absorptive capacity of the intestine. Age-related changes in body composition—decreased total body water and increased body fat—may affect drug distribution; however, no consequences for chemotherapeutic agents have been demonstrated. The liver is the main site of metabolism for many chemotherapeutic agents. A reduction in cytochrome P-450 drug metabolizing enzymes occurs with aging, which may result in reduced hepatic drug clearance in older adults. The age-related decline in kidney function has been demonstrated to have clinical consequences for drug dosing. Toxic drug levels have been demonstrated for agents primarily excreted by the kidney (Ruscin, 2014). The dosage of chemotherapeutic agents may need to be adjusted to account for age-related changes in the kidneys.

Pharmacodynamics

Pharmacodynamics refers to the interactions between the chemotherapeutic agents and their cellular targets, including the processes that modulate the activity of the agents. All agents act at the cellular level; however, their mechanisms of action vary, as do their respective administration guidelines and side effect profiles. Nurses caring for patients receiving chemotherapeutic agents should understand the specific actions and side effects of individual agents.

Targeted Therapy

Targeted cancer therapies are drugs that block the growth and spread of cancer by interfering with specific molecules (*molecular targets*) involved in the growth, progression, and spread of cancer. Targeted therapies differ from standard chemotherapy in several ways:

- They act on specific molecular targets associated with cancer, whereas most standard chemotherapies act on all rapidly dividing normal and cancerous cells.
- They are deliberately chosen or designed to interact with their target, whereas many standard chemotherapies were identified because they kill cells.
- Targeted therapies are often cytostatic (they block tumor cell proliferation), whereas standard chemotherapy agents are cytotoxic (they kill tumor cells).

Targeted therapies are the current focus of much anticancer drug development. They are a cornerstone of precision medicine, a form of medicine that uses information about a person's genes and proteins to prevent, diagnose, and treat disease (National Cancer Institute, 2018).

Immunotherapy

Immunotherapy is a type of cancer treatment designed to help the immune system fight cancer. Immunotherapy is a type of biological therapy, that is, a type of treatment that uses substances made from living organisms to treat cancer. Many different types of immunotherapy are used to treat cancer. They include (National Cancer Institute, 2017):

- Monoclonal antibodies are drugs designed to bind to specific targets in the body. They can cause an immune response that destroys cancer cells. Other types of monoclonal antibodies can "mark" cancer cells so it is easier for the immune system to find and destroy them.
- Adoptive cell transfer is a treatment that attempts to boost the natural ability of the body's T cells to fight cancer. T cells that are most active against the specific cancer are isolated from the patient's body and are then grown in large batches

TABLE 28.2 Major Chemotherapeutic Agents

Drug Classification	Major Mechanism of Action	Drugs
Alkylating agents	Alkylating agents are highly reactive compounds that act against already formed nucleic acids by cross-linking strands, thereby preventing ribonucleic acid (RNA) transcription and deoxyribonucleic acid (DNA) replication. These agents are considered cell cycle nonspecific.	Altretamine Busulfan Carboplatin Carmustine Chlorambucil Cisplatin Cyclophosphamide Dacarbazine Lomustine Melphalan Oxaliplatin Temozolomide Thiotepa
Antimetabolites	Antimetabolites are analogs of normal metabolites and act by interfering with synthesis of chromosomal nucleic acid. Some agents block an enzyme necessary for synthesis of essential factors, whereas others are incorporated into RNA or DNA, thus preventing cellular replication. Pyrimidine analogs, purine analogs, and folic acid antagonists are three major subgroups of antimetabolites, which are considered cell cycle specific.	5-fluorouracil (5-FU) 6-mercaptopurine (6-MP) Capecitabine Cytarabine Floxuridine Fludarabine Gemcitabine Hydroxyurea Methotrexate Pemetrexed
Antitumor antibiotics	Antibiotic agents are natural products of various strains of soil fungi. These agents bind to DNA, preventing RNA and DNA synthesis, and are active in all phases of the cell cycle.	Daunorubicin Doxorubicin Epirubicin Idarubicin Actinomycin-D Bleomycin Mitomycin-C Mitoxantrone

Topoisomerase inhibitors	These drugs interfere with enzymes called topoisomerases, which help separate the strands of DNA so they can be copied. Topoisomerase inhibitors are used to treat certain leukemias, as well as lung, ovarian, gastrointestinal, and other cancers. Topoisomerase inhibitors are grouped according to which type of enzyme they affect.	Topoisomerase I inhibitors:
		  Topotecan
		  Irinotecan (CPT-11)
		Topoisomerase II inhibitors:
		  Etoposide (VP-16)
		  Teniposide
		  Mitoxantrone (also acts as an antitumor antibiotic)

Mitotic inhibitors	Mitotic inhibitors are compounds derived from natural products, such as plants. They work by stopping cells from dividing to form new cells but can damage cells in all phases by keeping enzymes from making proteins needed for cell reproduction.	Docetaxel Estramustine Ixabepilone Paclitaxel Vinblastine Vincristine Vinorelbine

From American Cancer Society. (2016). How chemotherapy drugs work. Retrieved from https://www.cancer.org/treatment/treatments-and-side-effects/treatment-types/chemotherapy/how-chemotherapy-drugs-work.html.

in the laboratory. After immunosuppression, the T cells that were grown in the laboratory are given back to the patient as an intravenous (IV) infusion.

- Cytokines are proteins that are made by the body's cells. They play important roles in the body's normal immune responses and in the immune system's ability to respond to cancer. The two main types of cytokines used to treat cancer are called interferons and interleukins.

- Treatment vaccines work against cancer by boosting the body's immune system's response to cancer cells. Treatment vaccines are different from the ones that help prevent disease.
- Bacillus Calmette-Guérin (BCG) is an immunotherapy that is used to treat bladder cancer. It is a weakened form of the bacteria that causes tuberculosis. When inserted directly into the bladder with a catheter, BCG causes an immune response against cancer cells.

COMMON PHYSIOLOGIC COMPLICATIONS

Cancer treatments are aimed at destroying cancer cells. Because most treatment pharmacodynamics includes the prevention of cell division, actively dividing cell types are particularly vulnerable and may exhibit side effects. Actively dividing cell types that are most likely to exhibit side effects include those in hematopoietic tissue, the gastrointestinal tract, and hair follicles. Chemotherapy side effects are specific to the type of agent, dosage, and duration of use (see Nursing Care Plan). Radiation-related side effects depend on the location of the radiation field, intensity of the dose, and duration of the therapy. In most cases, side effects are reversible.

Bone Marrow Suppression

Chemotherapy is designed to kill rapidly growing cells, such as cancer cells, but affects all rapidly growing cells including hair follicles, the gastrointestinal tract, and bone marrow. Bone marrow suppression is a decrease in the ability of the bone marrow to manufacture hematopoietic stem cells that differentiate into the red blood cells, WBCs, and platelets that the body needs (Hughes, 2017).

- *Red blood cells* contain hemoglobin that carry oxygen to every cell in the body and return carbon dioxide to the lungs. If there are not enough red blood cells to deliver oxygen to all the tissues of the body, hypoxia occurs.
- *White blood cells* are the body's defense system, providing protection from bacteria, viruses, and other foreign substances, such as cancer cells. Neutropenia refers to a deficiency of one particular type of WBC known as a neutrophil. Without adequate neutrophils, we are predisposed to infection.
- *Platelets* are responsible for creating blood clots. A deficiency of platelets can lead to bleeding and is referred to as thrombocytopenia.

The symptoms of bone marrow suppression depend on the type of blood cells affected. In general, a deficiency of blood cells results in fatigue and weakness (Hughes, 2017).

Chemotherapy-Induced Anemia

A decreased level of red blood cells during chemotherapy is referred to as chemotherapy-induced anemia. The production of too few red blood cells to carry oxygen results in fatigue, lightheadedness or dizziness, pallor, shortness of breath, tachycardia, or palpitations.

◎ NURSING CARE PLAN

Myelosuppressive Toxicities of Chemotherapy

Clinical Situation

Mr. K is a 69-year-old man recently diagnosed with small cell cancer of the lung. He lives with his wife in a modest home. Mr. K had no functional limitations before his diagnosis of cancer. His oncologist prescribes a chemotherapy regimen of cyclophosphamide, doxorubicin, and etoposide. As with many chemotherapy regimens, a primary side effect is myelosuppression, resulting in decreased red blood cells, WBCs, and platelets. Because the therapy is given in the ambulatory care clinic, Mr. K and his wife will need to provide self-care for monitoring and managing the myelosuppressive effects of the agents.

Nursing Diagnoses

Potential for infection resulting from bone marrow depression (granulocytopenia) secondary to chemotherapy

Potential for injury bleeding caused by bone marrow depression (thrombocytopenia) secondary to chemotherapy

Inadequate peripheral tissue perfusion

Outcomes

The patient will remain free of infection.

The patient will remain free of injury and bleeding incidents.

The patient will not experience hypoxia, activity intolerance, or malaise.

Interventions

Monitor complete blood cell count and differential (absolute neutrophil count should remain above 500 cells/mm^3).

Instruct the patient and family to:
- Maintain patient defenses.
- Minimize exposure to potential pathogens.
- Assess for presence of infection:
  - Perform frequent oral hygiene using soft-bristle toothbrush and low-alcohol mouthwash.
- Lubricate dry areas using skin emollients and artificial tears.
- Maintain adequate hydration (3000 milliliters per day [mL/day] is recommended).
- Restrict visitors with colds or infections.
- Avoid large crowds.
- Perform routine bathing and perineal hygiene.
- Report temperature >100° F.

Monitor complete blood cell count and differential; platelet count should remain above 50,000 cells/mm3.

Instruct the patient and family to:
- Avoid trauma.
- Assess for the presence of bruising or bleeding:
  - Use a soft bristle toothbrush and low-alcohol mouthwash and avoid flossing and use of toothpicks.
  - Avoid tightly fitting or constrictive clothing.
  - Use a nail file or emery board; avoid clipping or pulling hangnails.
  - Use an electric razor for shaving.
  - Prevent constipation; use stool softeners and maintain adequate fluid intake.
  - Report minor bleeding such as petechiae, ecchymosis, epistaxis, and occult blood in stool, urine, or emesis.

Monitor complete blood cell count and differential:
- Hematocrit should remain above 25%.

Instruct the patient and family to:
- Increase rest and sleep periods.
- Alternate rest and activity periods.
- Incorporate foods into the diet that are high in iron, such as eggs, lean meat, green leafy vegetables, carrots, and raisins.
- Modify roles and responsibilities, as needed.

Anemia should improve after chemotherapy is completed; however, a medication to stimulate red blood cell production may be prescribed along with iron supplements. At times, blood transfusion may be necessary. Anemia is a treatable cause of fatigue; unfortunately, there are many causes of cancer fatigue, and anemia is only one of these (Hughes, 2017).

Chemotherapy-Induced Neutropenia

A low level of neutrophils during chemotherapy is referred to as chemotherapy-induced neutropenia. Suppression of the number of neutrophils is most important in raising the risk of infection. Most of the symptoms of neutropenia are related to infections and may include fever greater than 100.5° F, chills, cough, shortness of breath, and redness or drainage at the site of an injury. Persons receiving chemotherapy should be instructed to avoid situations that could result in infection, such as spending time with people who are ill or shopping in crowded malls. In the setting of neutropenia, chemotherapy treatment may be delayed or medications prescribed prevent infection or stimulate the production of WBCs (Hughes, 2017).

Chemotherapy-Induced Thrombocytopenia

A low platelet count caused by chemotherapy is referred to as chemotherapy-induced thrombocytopenia. Thrombocytopenia can result in bleeding. Signs of thrombocytopenia include easy bruising, petechiae, joint and muscle pain, blood in urine or stools, or heavy menstrual periods (if menopause has not been reached). Platelet transfusion or medications to stimulate the bone marrow to make more platelets may be prescribed if bleeding is present (Hughes, 2017).

Coping With Bone Marrow Suppression

Patients receiving chemotherapy should be taught to (Hughes, 2017):
- Wash hands properly
- Call the health care provider with any signs of infection, such as a fever greater than 100.5° F, coughing, chills, shortness of breath, or pain with urination
- Rest when feeling tired
- Stand up slowly after resting
- Avoid medications such as aspirin and ibuprofen that can increase bleeding
- Take care to avoid situations where injuries may occur

Nausea and Vomiting

Nausea is a subjectively experienced stomach distress that may be described as a heaviness, pressure, or sinking feeling in the epigastric or sternal region. It is often associated with such physical signs as pallor, sweating, and chills. Most often, patients are referring to nausea when they describe "feeling sick." *Vomiting* is the ejection of stomach contents through the mouth. Nausea and vomiting are two separate and distinct events; although they frequently occur together, it is important for the nurse to distinguish between the two when taking a patient history and planning care.

Chemotherapy-induced nausea and vomiting (CINV) are among its most distressing side effects. Not all chemotherapeutic agents cause nausea and vomiting, and those that have high emetic potential do not cause equal distress in all persons. Considerable variation exists among patients and types of agents. Some patients may expect to develop nausea and vomiting, and may begin to experience symptoms before chemotherapy starts; this is referred to as anticipatory nausea and vomiting. Because many older adults likely have friends or family members who were treated with older therapies, nurses should reassure patients that management of this side effect has changed for the better.

Nausea may lead to decreased nutritional intake, whereas vomiting may lead to severe metabolic complications, including dehydration. Older adults are less tolerant of dehydration compared with younger persons and may manifest acute confusion in response. Dehydration may create a metabolic crisis necessitating resuscitation with IV fluid administration. In addition, chemotherapeutic agents excreted by the kidney may build to toxic levels, which could lead to increased side effects and renal failure, particularly when agents with known nephrotoxic side effects are used. Electrolyte imbalances may aggravate cardiac problems and precipitate drug toxicity if a patient is taking medication to manage a cardiac condition. Episodes of severe vomiting may require the dosage of drugs to be reduced or treatment to be postponed.

Current pharmacologic management of CINV includes corticosteroids, serotonin antagonists, dopamine antagonists, neurokinin 1 (NK_1) receptor antagonists, cannabinoids, and antianxiety drugs (Fleishman, 2018).

Nursing care should begin with an in-depth emetic history and a preventive plan. Characteristics that have been linked with CINV include susceptibility to motion sickness, history of severe nausea during pregnancy, and poor emetic control during prior treatments. Nurses should evaluate the degree and duration of episodes of nausea and vomiting and monitor for signs of dehydration. Long-term nutritional compromise may result from poorly controlled nausea, and consultation with a dietitian may be helpful (see Nutritional Considerations box).

Chemotherapy-Induced Oral Mucositis

Chemotherapy-induced oral mucositis is caused by the destruction of rapidly proliferating mucosal cells in the oral cavity, which results in inflammation, ulceration, pain, and bleeding. Several chemotherapeutic agents are known to cause severe chemotherapy-induced oral mucositis. Evidence suggests that older adults are at increased risk for severe chemotherapy-induced oral mucositis. Radiation therapy that includes mucosal tissue in the radiation field may lead to dose-related oral mucositis, which generally clears when therapy is complete.

Nutritional Consequences of Cancer Treatment

The nutritional consequences of cancer treatment may be devastating, resulting in an older adult's inability to tolerate treatment and compromising his or her quality of life. Specific consequences are related to the type of treatment. Nurses should be aware of possible nutritional consequences and complete a nutritional assessment early in the course of therapy. Early assessment provides a baseline for persons at high risk. Patients should be weighed at regular intervals. Individuals at the highest risk for nutritional compromise are those experiencing weight losses of 1% to 2% in 1 week, 5% in 1 month, 7.5% in 3 months, and more than 10% in 6 months.

TREATMENT	POSSIBLE NUTRITIONAL CONSEQUENCES
Chemotherapy	Individual drugs and drug combinations produce taste alterations, notably a decreased tolerance for protein-rich foods. Drugs that cause oral mucositis and esophagitis (inflammation of the oral cavity) may lead to difficulty chewing and swallowing, resulting in decreased caloric intake and weight loss. Chemotherapy-induced nausea and vomiting may result in dehydration, decreased caloric intake, and weight loss. Drugs that cause diarrhea may lead to dehydration, electrolyte imbalance, and bleeding.
Radiation therapy of the head and neck	This may cause taste alterations, xerostomia (dry mouth), oral mucositis, and esophagitis, leading to difficulty swallowing and a decreased appetite.
Radiation therapy of the esophagus	This may cause dysphagia, sore throat, esophagitis, indigestion, and nausea, leading to difficulty swallowing and a decreased appetite.
Radiation therapy of the lung	This may lead to shortness of breath, anorexia, and nausea with generalized malaise and a decreased appetite.
Radiation therapy of the abdomen	This may cause nausea, vomiting, cramping, gas, and diarrhea, resulting in a decreased appetite.
Surgical resection of oropharynx	This surgery may cause postoperative difficulty in chewing and swallowing, changes in taste perception, and loss of appetite, leading to a dependence on tube feedings.
Esophagectomy, esophagogastrectomy, or esophageal reconstruction	This may cause gastric stasis, steatorrhea, and diarrhea, leading to a decreased appetite.
Gastrectomy (partial or complete)	This may result in dumping syndrome with symptoms of cramps, fullness, and diarrhea; malabsorption of fats, iron, vitamin B_{12}, and calcium; and early satiety secondary to decreased size of reservoir, with decreased intake of adequate nutrients and calories.
Intestinal resection	This may lead to malabsorption of nutrients, including fat, iron, vitamin B_{12}, fluids, and electrolytes, resulting in weight loss and malnutrition.
Pancreatectomy	This may result in exocrine insufficiency and malabsorption or endocrine insufficiency, leading to diabetes mellitus.

A dentist should evaluate dental and oral care needs before treatment begins, and treatment should be delayed until any dental problems are resolved. Patient should understand the importance of good oral hygiene with a soft bristle toothbrush and avoid products with alcohol, which dry the mucous membranes and increase the risk of cracking, bleeding, and infection. If toothpaste irritates the mouth, a half-teaspoon of salt in four cups of water can be used instead. Gargling with a solution made from 1 quart of water, with a half-teaspoon of salt and a half-teaspoon of baking soda may sooth mucus membranes. Prescription products are also available, and patients should be instructed to speak to their health care provider if oral mucositis persists despite conservative treatment. Nurses should routinely assess the patient's mouth, lips, and tongue for early signs of inflammation. Severe oral mucositis may result in decreased oral intake, which, in turn, may lead to dehydration and cause a metabolic crisis that may necessitate resuscitation with IV fluid administration. Also, severe oral mucositis may result in a decreased appetite, which may lead to nutritional compromise and hence decreased ability to tolerate treatment (Fleishman, 2018). In general, older persons become less tolerant of dehydration and nutritional depletion with age.

Anorexia

Many patients receiving cancer treatments complain of a general loss of appetite. Contributing factors include chemotherapeutic agents; radiation therapy, especially to the head and neck area; pain medications; and chemotherapy-induced oral mucositis. Decreased appetite leads to decreased caloric intake and weight loss. Severe weight loss has been linked to poor outcomes; patients with significant weight loss have more complications and decreased survival rates. Persons older than 80 years of age are more vulnerable to increased toxicity from radiation therapy when they are unable to maintain their weight (Zachariah, Casey, & Balducci, 1995). Anorexia may also contribute to decreased immune function, increasing the risk of infectious complications.

Dietary consultation and frequent weight monitoring are necessary to maintain optimal weight. For persons receiving chemotherapy, an increase of 4.4 calories per kilogram of body weight and 2 grams of protein per kilogram of body weight should be incorporated into an overall nutritional plan. The nurse should remember that food choices and eating patterns have strong cultural influences, and planning nutritional diets with patients and their families is critical to successful outcomes.

Diarrhea

Diarrhea results from the destruction of the actively dividing epithelial cells of the gastrointestinal tract. When these cells are destroyed, atrophy of the intestinal mucosa occurs, resulting in shortening or denuding of the intestinal villi. When the villi and microvilli become flattened, the absorptive surface area is reduced, and intestinal contents move rapidly through the gut, resulting in frequent liquid stools. Absorption of nutrients is decreased, and patients are at risk for dehydration and malnutrition. Circulatory collapse may occur, especially in older adults with cardiovascular disease. Diarrhea may aggravate perirectal problems such as hemorrhoids and may cause pain, bleeding, and infection.

Assessment of diarrhea includes the number of stools per day, their consistency, and their color. Older patients may be reluctant to discuss diarrhea, ignoring their symptoms until dehydration becomes a problem. To control diarrhea, patients should be instructed to eat small frequent meals and avoid coffee, tea, alcohol, and sweets. They should be advised to eat low-fiber foods and avoid fried, greasy, or spicy foods as well as milk and milk products. Patients should also be instructed to increase the potassium in their diet and drink plenty of room-temperature clear liquids (Fleishman, 2018). Chemotherapy is usually administered unless diarrhea is severe resulting in dehydration.

Alopecia

Alopecia is a common complication of chemotherapy. Hair loss may range from thinning of scalp hair to total body hair loss, including eyelashes, eyebrows, and pubic hair. The degree of alopecia depends on both the chemical agent and the dose. Chemotherapy-induced hair loss occurs rapidly and becomes apparent over a 2- to 3-week period after initiation of treatment. Chemotherapy-induced hair loss is temporary in most cases, and hair begins to grow back slowly after treatment has been completed. Radiation-induced hair loss occurs when the scalp is in the radiation field. Hair loss is permanent if the radiation dose causes irreversible destruction of the hair follicles; otherwise, hair loss is temporary. To date, no type of hair care product or practice has been shown to satisfactorily prevent or reduce hair loss.

Although the physiologic consequences of alopecia are minimal, the emotional distress may be enormous. Hair greatly contributes to body image and sexuality. Wigs and hairpieces should be purchased *before* total hair loss occurs. Often, patients are too embarrassed to shop for hair replacements when they are bald. Once the hair is gone, it may be difficult to match color, texture, or style (Fleishman, 2018). The nurse should not assume that hair loss is an issue only for women; men may be equally devastated by hair loss. For instance, an older, completely bald man was mortified when he lost his big bushy eyebrows, but the local university theater created a pair of high-quality eyebrows for him as a means for temporary relief.

OLDER ADULTS' EXPERIENCE OF CANCER

Cancer in older adults has been viewed as aging in the context of cancer; cancer is the prominent issue. However, cancer for older persons may be more aptly framed as "cancer in the context of aging," and aging is the predominant issue. Why do we focus on aging as the context?

Traditionally, cancer has been viewed from the perspective of younger persons. Attention has been placed on treatments that return persons to precancerous functioning and on statistics that highlight survival rates in the years after diagnosis. Successful treatment in this context means that the cancer goes away and stays away for a long time. Although a younger person's cancer experience includes looking beyond the cancer to a disease-free return to a normal lifestyle, an older person has a different experience; older adults with cancer may be close to the end of life. For a younger person, cancer may be viewed in the context of a life yet to be lived, whereas for an older person, cancer may be viewed in the context of a life mostly lived (Kagan, 1997).

A substantial body of research reveals that older adults are less likely to be offered clinical trials compared with younger adults. Older adults should be made aware that most clinical trials allow participation of older patients and do not have age limits. Older patients should ask their health care providers about available clinical trials and should use websites such as https://www.cancer.org/ and https://www.cancer.gov/ to search for clinical trials. Cancer patients may also want to seek a second opinion at a major cancer center to explore clinical trials and other treatment options.

Quality of Life

Historically, length of survival has been the most important consideration in measuring the outcome of cancer treatment. Recently, efforts have been made to address not only length of life but the circumstances of life—quality and quantity. For an older adult experiencing cancer in the context of a life mostly lived, quality is a very—if not the most—important consideration.

Determining quality of life goes beyond evaluating the severity of symptoms (such as nausea, pain, or fatigue) to considering the degree of functional status reflected in the person's ability to perform daily tasks of living. Quality of life is a multidimensional concept that includes not only functional status and the severity of symptoms but also the patient's ideas about psychological development, sociocultural issues, ethical issues, economic issues, and spirituality.

Fig. 28.2 depicts the multidimensional nature of quality of life. Attitudes in three categories—physical well-being, psychological well-being, and interpersonal well-being—have been demonstrated to be the primary determinants of overall quality of life for older adults (Padilla, Ferrell, Grant & Rhiner, 1990). Also, in older adults, quality-of-life factors are shown to be rated differently by men and women; for men, vitality and personal resources are most important, whereas for women psychosocial well-being is most important (Dibble, Padilla, Dodd & Miaskowski, 1998).

Quality-of-life evaluation is relevant to both curative and palliative care. In curative care, information obtained from a quality-of-life assessment helps guide the selection of therapeutic strategies that result in a more normal life. Older adults may need special quality-of-life consideration when choosing a

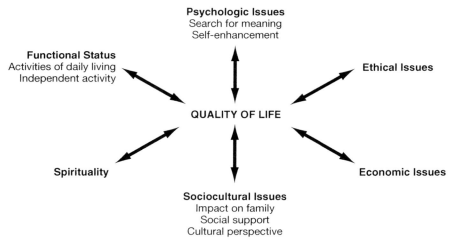

Fig. 28.2 Quality of life as a multidimensional concept.

treatment. A moderate treatment that provides relatively symptom-free disease control may be a better quality-of-life choice for an older adult than a rigorous treatment that statistically offers a prolonged disease-free period. In palliative care, quality-of-life assessment provides insight into areas that may require intervention, such as family counseling, financial planning, and management of depression.

Some measure of a person's quality of life has been included in most studies evaluating treatment modalities or chemotherapeutic agents. Historically, these studies focused on measures of functional status, primarily assessing the ability of patients to perform various activities of daily living (ADLs) using the Palliative Performance Scale (PPSv2) found at http://palliative.info/resource_material/PPSv2.pdf.

The nurse plays a central role in supporting an older patient's quality of life. Nurses manage disease-related symptoms and treatment-related side effects. Few studies have focused on the older adult's perception of health status while receiving cancer treatment. However, Steele and associates (2005) found that even patients with terminal illness can have a good quality of life when proper resources such as hospice care are initiated.

EVIDENCE-BASED PRACTICE

Symptom Management Guide for Home Health Nurses Caring for Cancer Patients

Background

Most cancer patients manage their symptoms at home with support from home health nurses. Improved support and management from nurses can facilitate improved quality of life and decreased use of health care services.

Sample/Setting

The sample encompassed six nursing agencies within a regional home care authority in Canada. The study involved 50 patient records, 14 interviews, and 150 survey responses.

Methods

This mixed methods study, guided by the Knowledge-to-Action Framework, "assessed factors influencing home care nurses' use of 15 evidence-informed symptom practice guides for providing telephone or in-home nursing services to [patients] with cancer" (p. 224). A chart audit was conducted to determine patient characteristics. Home health staff participated in semistructured interviews to determine "(1) current practice for providing symptoms support, (2) potential factors likely to influence use of 15 evidence-informed symptom practice guides, (3) need for local adaptation of the practice guises, and (4) strategies to implement the practice guides" (p. 225). Additionally, a barriers survey was administered to identify factors influencing use of the evidence-informed practice guides.

Findings

Average age of patients was 62.4 years. Of the 50 patients, 15 experienced one symptom, 11 two symptoms, and 22 three or more symptoms. Identified symptoms included nausea/vomiting, constipation, fatigue, loss of appetite, pain, diarrhea, mouth sores, anxiety, and/or depression. Nurses typically provided symptom management Monday through Friday, during normal business hours. However, patients could call 24 hours a day, 7 days a week.

Barriers to using the symptom practice guides included length and complexity of the guides; inability for a single symptom practice guide to address multiple symptoms or symptom clusters; and inadequate space for additional comments. Facilitators to using the practice guides included comprehensive and evidence-based; systematic approach, relevance to current home care nursing practice; user-friendly format with plain language; and more efficient assessment.

Implications

The nurses felt barriers to adopting the guides could be overcome through education, clear organizational mandates for using them, and integration with documentation system. Overall, the symptom guides were well received by the nurses. Implementation of these guides has the "potential to narrow the know-do gap by providing nurses with user-friendly, evidence-based tools to guide their practice" (p. 233).

From Ludwig, C., Bennis, C., Carley, M., Gifford, W., Kuziemsky, C., Lafreniere-Davis, N. ... Stacey, D. (2017). Managing symptoms during cancer treatments: Barriers and facilitators to home care nurses using symptom practice guides. *Home Health Care Management & Practice, 29*(4), 224-234. doi: 10.1177/1084822317713011.

Depression

Depressive symptoms may result from side effects of medications used to control cancer. Depressive symptoms are especially associated with hormone therapy and cortisone medications, two medication groups frequently prescribed for cancer treatment. In addition, older adults may have underlying diseases that are controlled by medications. Depressive symptoms are associated with many drugs used to manage chronic illness. In addition, depressive symptoms are known to increase with an increased number of medications taken.

Nurses should assess the older adult's risk for depression. Older adults with cancer should be educated about the psychological implications of having cancer. An understanding of how the experience of cancer may affect such things as feelings of well-being, interpersonal relationships, and self-fulfillment is needed as much as an understanding of the schedule for taking medications. Older patients and their family members should be encouraged to discuss the effects of cancer on family functioning. Individual evaluation of depressive symptoms is needed if an older person is suspected of experiencing depression. Nurses should refer older patients for further psychiatric evaluation when symptoms last longer than a week, worsen rather than improve, or interfere with the ability to carry out daily routines or cooperate with treatment plans. Management of cancer-related depression should be individualized and may include supportive interventions, cognitive intervention, psychotherapy, and psychopharmacology.

Grief and Loss

Grief is a natural and expected human reaction to loss. An older adult who is being treated for cancer may experience multiple losses, including loss of energy, loss of a body part, loss of functional ability, loss of self-esteem, and loss of control. The losses associated with cancer may overlap other losses frequently experienced by older adults, including the loss of a spouse, friends, or family; changes in living arrangements; and physical losses of vision, hearing, or mobility.

Although grief is a universal human reaction, the subject and the intensity of grief are determined by the meaning that an individual places on the loss. Grieving is a human imperative, but how people grieve varies. No one way to grieve and no one timetable for grief exist. People do not "get over" grief. They get through, reconcile with, and learn to live with the loss, but they never get over it; in some cases, a loss may be mourned forever (Bourne, 1996).

The health care literature often reports that denial is among the initial responses to loss, including losses associated with a diagnosis of cancer. Denial is believed to protect people by providing them with the time needed to assimilate the effect of the diagnosis. Unfortunately, health care providers, including nurses, often haphazardly label a person or family as being "in a state of denial." Labels reflect a judgment or conclusion, and conclusions should be supported by evidence. Most persons need some time to allow the diagnosis of cancer to reach conscious awareness. The information about the diagnosis is allowed into the awareness in increments that are tolerable to the person while that person is coming to terms with the effect of the diagnosis on his or her life. It may be more reasonable to consider that a patient is "titrating" information rather than being in a state of denial. To complicate matters, family members titrate information at different paces as they realize the effect of the diagnosis on their lives. The diagnosis of cancer often leads to a confusing and conflicting experience for the family unit.

Nurses should support older patients and families by patiently repeating information when asked, validating what the family has heard, and determining what the information means to them as individuals and as a family unit. The ongoing process of assessing a patient's and family's understanding of the information should spur nursing interventions that are often blocked when nurses judge too quickly. Although patients and families should be allowed to come to their own level of understanding of the diagnosis, the nurse should not support unrealistic ideas about the seriousness of the illness or the benefits of treatment. Interventions may be necessary when a patient and family are so threatened by the diagnosis that they are incapable of participating in decision making about the treatment choices. Nurses should validate the patient's feelings of grief and loss. Grief cannot be prevented, and nurses should give the individual permission to grieve in reaction to loss. Some older adults may have unresolved grief or complications associated with grieving. This may occur more often in older adults because they are more likely to experience multiple major losses within a short period of time: the death of spouses and friends; losses such as loss of independence, health, and decreased physical abilities, which occur as a part of the natural aging process; and the anticipation of losing someone or something special to them. In addition, some older adults need more time to adjust to change (Curtis, 2007).

Health care providers need to be alert to these signs not only to assist older adults who are grieving but also to recognize abnormal signs and symptoms so that appropriate care can be given to minimize emotional and physical complications. The following interventions adapted from Curtis (2007) may help an older adult who is grieving:

- Giving the person time. Older adults may need more time to become aware of feelings and express them. Sometimes, they also need more time to complete activities. Providing extra time shows that you are concerned and respectful of their needs.
- Pointing out signs of sadness or changes in behavior. This may help the person become aware of feelings and may help the person feel more comfortable talking with you about feelings.
- Spending time with the person. An older adult who is often alone may benefit from your company. Feelings of loneliness may last for a long time when an older adult has lost something or someone special, especially a spouse.
- Talking about the loss. Ask the person to talk about his or her loss. Older people, especially those who have experienced several losses over a short period, are often helped by sharing memories related to the losses.
- Watching for signs of prolonged grieving or depression and implementing preventive therapies.

- Older adults often have more than one loss to deal with at a time. Talking about each separate loss may help identify the person's feelings. Separating losses from one another may also help the person feel less overwhelmed and more able to cope with emotional distress.

Social Isolation

Social isolation, the sense of being cut off from people and things of importance, is an experience commonly described by older adults with cancer. Social isolation may be voluntary (i.e., a person seeks disengagement from social interaction) or involuntary (i.e., imposed by others or by circumstances). Choosing to be alone may provide important time for personal reflection, psychological rebuilding, and renewal. Involuntary social isolation, however, may have negative consequences on psychological health. Risk factors for social isolation include physical disability or illness, frailties associated with advanced age, psychological or neurologic disorders, and environmental constraints (e.g., physical surroundings, including diminished personal or material resources that are necessary to access or modify environmental factors) (Tilden & Weinert, 1987).

Voluntary social isolation may result when an older adult with cancer no longer feels comfortable in social settings because of his or her situation, including changes in body image, energy levels, or interests. Older persons with cancer may withdraw because they perceive that others are uncomfortable in their presence and because they believe, rightly or wrongly, that others are avoiding them because of the cancer diagnosis.

Involuntary social isolation may result from physical changes that prevent a person from continuing with social activities. Treatment-related side effects may interfere with the ability to drive or use public transportation, sit comfortably at a social gathering, or eat in restaurants.

Older adults experiencing cancer are particularly vulnerable to social isolation. Overall, declining physical health may limit the number or types of social activities available. The availability of social contacts may decline as family members and friends die or relocate. The recent loss of a spouse or partner may lead to social isolation, and the person may withdraw because of feelings of awkwardness or loneliness. Many older adults feel unsafe going places alone. Social isolation is not reflective of being restricted to a single place such as a home. Many older adults live a lifetime in a neighborhood only to find that the neighbors have moved, the area has changed and become less safe, and the social network that existed in the neighborhood or town has disappeared slowly over time. Older adults may perceive themselves as disconnected from the unfamiliar people in the neighborhood.

Family members may not live in geographic proximity, decreasing the ability to visit or seek assistance. It may be necessary to relocate an older adult during cancer treatment. When an older adult is relocated to live with family or in a residential care facility, he or she needs assistance with developing and maintaining social contacts.

Older adults may substitute interaction with health care personnel for meaningful social interaction. A clinic or home care visit may be an older adult's only social contact for a long time.

Nurses should evaluate the older adult's need for social interaction; assess the person's level of social activity before the cancer diagnosis, and determine whether it was satisfactory; ask what has changed in regard to social activities since the cancer diagnosis; determine what, if anything, has changed in regard to social activities as the person has gotten older; and work with the patient and family to identify strategies for maintaining social activities and contacts. Nurses should explore the importance of various activities described by the older patient. Many older adults value religious activities such as church attendance or prayer groups. In addition to meeting social needs, religious activities help meet spiritual needs.

Resources and Support

An important component to nursing care of older adults is awareness of resources and referrals to appropriate agencies or support groups. Both cancer patients and their families have found support groups sponsored by local church groups, hospitals, home health agencies, and hospices to be helpful. Nurses should have up-to-date listings for the groups in their areas.

- American Association of Retired Persons (AARP) and Grief and Loss, a national organization founded in 1973 to promote quality of life for older people, provide resources. The website on grief and loss includes community resources offering support to people grieving the death of a loved one. The website also has information on coping with the loss of a loved one and making plans such as funeral arrangements and financial decisions after a person's death: http://www.aarp.org/families/grief_loss.
- The Hospice Association of America (HAA) seeks to heighten the public visibility of hospice services. HAA offers a few helpful, practical publications for people who are considering hospice, including consumer guides, fact sheets, historical perspectives, and other background information. The website offers information from the legislative, regulatory, research, legal, and public relations departments, including "Hospice Facts and Statistics": http://hospice.nahc.org/.
- The U.S. National Hospice and Palliative Care Organization (NHPCO) offers information on local hospice and palliative care programs across America. NHPCO is committed to improving end-of-life care and expanding access to hospice care with the goal of improving quality of life for dying people and their loved ones: https://www.nhpco.org/.
- American Society of Clinical Oncology (ASCO) Resources: http://www.asco.org
- *ASCO Answers Fact Sheets:* This series of fact sheets provides a brief overview about a specific type of cancer, including a description of the cancer, how it is treated, terms to know, and questions to ask the doctor.
- *Cancer Advances:* Summaries of research advances in clinical oncology from the *Journal of Clinical Oncology,* ASCO's Annual Meetings, and ASCO's "Meet the Experts" events.
- *What to Know: ASCO's Guidelines:* Patient-friendly guides based on ASCO's Clinical Practice Guidelines for physicians.

- *Research and Meetings:* Find information on ASCO's Clinical Cancer Advances report, ASCO's Annual Meetings and Symposia, and virtual lectures: http://www.cancer.net
- *ASCO Cancer Education Slides:* Prepared cancer slide presentations, adapted from select Cancer.Net Guides to Cancer, are available for free download for oncologists, oncology nurses, and other members of the health care team.
- *Ask the ASCO Expert Series:* Read the transcripts from Cancer.Net "Ask the ASCO Expert" events, held from 2002 to 2006, in which patients, families, and the public asked ASCO experts questions about cancer and related topics, either through online chats or through month-long question-and-answer forums.

Older persons are also using web resources. Those related to cancer include the following:
- National Cancer Institute: http://www.cancer.gov
- American Cancer Society: http://www.cancer.org
- National Breast Cancer Foundation: http://www.nationalbreastcancer.org
- Prostate Cancer Foundation: https://www.pcf.org/
- American Lung Association: http://www.lungusa.org

SUMMARY

The incidence of most cancers increases with advancing age. The Oncology Nursing Society has outlined the knowledge required for nurses to provide holistic care for older adults with cancer, including the physiology of aging, geriatric assessment, symptom management, hospice and palliative care, survivorship issues, psychosocial issues, and the future of nursing care of persons with cancer (McEvoy & Cope, 2012). Cancer prevention and screening programs for older adults require special attention to ethical issues. Decisions to screen older adults should be made on an individual basis.

Older adults are more vulnerable to the development of cancer. Because the aging cell has been exposed to a lifetime of potentially carcinogenic substances, it is more susceptible to damage and is less able to repair damage. In general, older adults are capable of tolerating cancer treatment when careful attention is paid to dosage adjustments and comorbid factors. The experience of cancer for the older adult is unique. Cancer in the older adult is cancer in the context of a life mostly lived.

🏠 HOME CARE

1. Instruct homebound older adults and their caregivers to be aware of and report symptoms associated with the warning signs of cancer.
2. Educate older adults about cancer screening and self-examination.
3. Breast cancer is a disease of older women, thus breast screening is a life-long process. Instruct homebound older women on the American Cancer Society's breast self-examination (BSE) guidelines.
4. Assess nonspecific symptoms such as indigestion, loss of appetite, and weight loss in both older men and older women. These warning signs are seen in cancer of the stomach, colon, and rectum.
5. Instruct caregivers and homebound older adults with cancer about general comfort measures to promote rest and sleep, with the goal of increasing pain tolerance.
6. Assess for side effects of cancer treatment therapies (e.g., radiation therapy, chemotherapy) and report to a physician, as needed, for treatment recommendations.
7. Instruct caregivers and homebound older adults on measures to reduce the side effects of cancer treatment therapies.
8. Refer patients to hospice during the last 6 months of terminal illness.

KEY POINTS

- Three leading causes of cancer deaths in women between ages 55 and 74 are lung, breast, and colorectal cancers; in men between these same ages, the leading causes of cancer deaths are lung, colorectal, and prostate cancers.
- Aging cells show a tendency toward aberration as they replicate, probably because of the failure of growth control mechanisms. Altered growth control mechanisms make the aging cell more vulnerable to damage, leading to the development of cancer.
- Clinical manifestations of cancer in older adults may be mistakenly attributed to normal, age-related changes. Older adults should be made aware of the warning signs of cancer and report symptoms associated with them to a health care provider.
- Nurses caring for older adults have a major responsibility to recommend strategies aimed at the prevention and early detection of cancer in this age group.
- Major treatment modalities for cancer include surgery, radiation therapy, chemotherapy, targeted therapy, and immunotherapy. Therapy with any of these modalities may be used alone or in combination; therapy may be curative or palliative.
- Functional status of an older adult is the most important consideration in selecting a treatment goal and modality. Age alone is not a good predictor of treatment tolerance or response.
- Older adults generally have fewer reserves, and greater attention should be given to the status of major organs, including the kidneys, liver, heart, lungs, and gastrointestinal system. Maintenance of fluid, electrolyte balance, and caloric intake is critical to treatment outcomes for older adults.
- Older adults are especially vulnerable to the nephrologic and hematologic toxicity of some chemotherapeutic agents.
- Psychosocial care of older adults with cancer includes addressing issues related to quality of life, depression, loss and grief, and social isolation.
- The cancer experience for each older adult is unique. Cancer in an older adult is in the context of a life mostly lived.

CRITICAL-THINKING EXERCISES

1. You are asked to make a 30-minute presentation at a senior center on the benefits and risks of cancer screening in older adults. Prepare a topical outline for the presentation.

2. The director of oncology services asks you to develop a procedure for functional assessment of older adults with cancer. Develop the procedure and include any functional assessment parameters and instruments to be used.

3. The family cancer support group has asked you to facilitate a discussion on family considerations when an older family member has cancer. Prepare a list of the points that you would discuss with the group.

REFERENCES

Administration on Aging. (2017). *A profile of older Americans, 2016.* Retrieved from https://www.acl.gov/aging-and-disability-in-america/data-and-research/profile-older-americans.

American Cancer Society. (2013a). Breast cancer facts & figures: 2013-2014. Retrieved from http://www.cancer.org/acs/groups/content/@research/documents/document/acspc-040951.pdf.

American Cancer Society. (2013b). *Photodynamic therapy.* Retrieved May 1, 2014, from http://www.cancer.org/treatment/treatmentsandsideeffects/treatmenttypes/photodynamic-therapy.

American Cancer Society. (2014). How are HIV and AIDS related to cancer? Retrieved March 3, 2018, from https://www.cancer.org/cancer/cancer-causes/infectious-agents/hiv-infection-aids/hiv-aids-and-cancer.html.

American Cancer Society. (2016). Lung cancer fact sheet. Retrieved March 3, 2018, from http://www.lung.org/lung-health-and-diseases/lung-disease-lookup/lung-cancer/resource-library/lung-cancer-fact-sheet.html.

American Cancer Society. (2017a). *American Cancer Society recommendations for the early detection of breast cancer.* Retrieved March 3, 2018, from https://www.cancer.org/cancer/breast-cancer/screening-tests-and-early-detection/american-cancer-society-recommendations-for-the-early-detection-of-breast-cancer.html.

American Cancer Society. (2017b). *Survival rates for prostate cancer.* Retrieved March 3, 2018, from https://www.cancer.org/cancer/prostate-cancer/detection-diagnosis-staging/survival-rates.html.

American Cancer Society (2018a). *Cancer facts and figures, 2018.* Retrieved March 2, 2018, from https://www.cancer.org/content/dam/cancer-org/research/cancer-facts-and-statistics/annual-cancer-facts-and-figures/2018/cancer-facts-and-figures-2018.pdf.

American Cancer Society (2018b). *Hormone therapy for prostate cancer.* Retrieved March 3, 2018, from https://www.cancer.org/cancer/prostate-cancer/treating/hormone-therapy.html.

Audisio, R. A., & Bozzett, F. (2004). The surgical management of elderly cancer patients: Recommendations to the SIOG task force. *European Journal of Cancer, 40,* 926–938.

Bourne, V. (1996). Grief. In S. L. Groenwald (Ed.), *Cancer symptom management.* Boston: Jones & Bartlett.

Centers for Disease Control and Prevention. (2017). Older persons' Health. Retrieved March 2, 2018, from https://www.cdc.gov/nchs/fastats/older-american-health.htm

Crawford, J., & Cohen, H. (1987). Relationship of cancer and aging. *Clinics in Geriatric Medicine, 3*(3), 419.

Cummings, S., & Olopade, O. (1998). Predisposition testing for inherited breast cancer. *Oncology, 12*(8), 1227–1241.

Curtis, J. (2007). Grief. Retrieved June 2009, from http://www.cigna.com/healthinfo/aa122313.html.

Davis, L., & Lindley, C. (2004). Neoplastic disorders and their treatment: General principles. In M. A. Kimble, et al. (Eds.), *Applied therapeutics: The clinical use of drugs.* Philadelphia: JB Lippincott.

Dibble, S. L., Padilla, Gt. V., Dodd, M. J., & Miaskowski, C. (1998). Gender differences in the dimensions of quality of life. *Oncology Nursing Forum, 25*(3), 577–583.

Ebbert, J. O., Yang, P., Vachon, C. M., et al. (2003). Lung cancer risk reduction after smoking cessation. *Journal of Clinical Oncology, 21*(5), 921–926.

Eckstrom, E., Feeny, D. H., Walter, L. C., Perdue, L. A., & Whitlock, E. P. (2012). Individualizing cancer screening in older adults: A narrative review and framework for future research. *Journal of General Internal Medicine.*

Extermann, M., Aapro, M., Bernabei, B., et al. (2005). Use of comprehensive geriatric assessment in older cancer patients: Recommendations from the task force on CGA of the International Society of Geriatric Oncology (SIOG). *Critical Reviews in Oncology/Hematology, 55,* 241.

Farrow, D. C., Hunt, W. C., & Samet, J. M. (1996). Temporal and regional variability in the surgical treatment of cancer among older people. *Journal of the American Geriatrics Society, 44,* 559.

Fleishman, S. B. (2018). *Understanding and managing chemotherapy side effects.* Retrieved March 2, 2018, from https://www.cancercare.org/publications/24-understanding_and_managing_chemotherapy_side_effects#!introduction.

Greenberg, H. M., & Trotti, A. M. (1992). Radiation therapy of cancer in the older aged person. In L. Balducci, G. H. Lyman, & W. B. Ershler (Eds.), *Geriatric oncology.* Philadelphia: JB Lippincott.

Henley, S. J., Weir, H. K., Jim, M. A., Watson, M., & Richardson, L. C. (2015). *Gallbladder Cancer Incidence and Death Rates.* Retrieved June 12, 2018, from https://www.cdc.gov/cancer/dcpc/research/articles/gallbladder.htm.

Host, H., & Lunde, G. (1986). Age as a prognostic factor in breast cancer. *Cancer, 57,* 2217.

Hughes, G. (2017). *Bone marrow suppression during chemotherapy.* Retrieved March 4, 2018, from https://www.verywell.com/bone-marrow-suppression-during-chemotherapy-2249318.

Kagan, S. H. (1997). *Older adults coping with cancer: Integrating cancer into a life mostly lived.* New York: Garland Publishing.

Larson, P. J., Lindsay, A. M., Dodd, M. J., et al. (1993). Influence of age on problems experienced by patients with lung cancer undergoing radiation therapy. *Oncology Nursing Forum, 20,* 473.

McEvoy, L. K., & Cope, D. G. (2012). *Caring for the older adult with cancer in the ambulatory setting.* Retrieved from https://www.ons.org/sites/default/files/publication_pdfs/00_OlderAdult_AMB_Front.pdf.

Meniscus Educational Institute. (2010). *Care of the older adult with cancer.* Retrieved from http://www.managecrc.com/cefiles/cearticle-19/Care_of_the_Older_Adult_With_Cancer.pdf.

National Cancer Institute. (2017). *Cancer genomics overview.* Retrieved March 3, 2018, from https://www.cancer.gov/about-nci/organization/ccg/cancer-genomics-overview.

National Cancer Institute. (2017b). *Cancer stat facts: Colorectal cancer.* Retrieved March 3, 2018, from https://seer.cancer.gov/statfacts/html/colorect.html.

National Cancer Institute (2017). *Immunotherapy to treat cancer.* Retrieved March 4, 2018, from https://www.cancer.gov/about-cancer/treatment/types/immunotherapy.

National Cancer Institute. (2018). *Targeted cancer therapies.* Retrieved March 4, 2018, from https://www.cancer.gov/about-cancer/treatment/types/targeted-therapies/targeted-therapies-fact-sheet.

National Cancer Institute. (2009). *Cancer topics.* Washington, DC: Division of Cancer Control and Population Sciences.

Nobler, M. P., & Venetl, R. (1985). Prognostic factors in patients undergoing curative irradiation for breast cancer. *International Journal of Radiation Oncology, Biology, Physics, 11,* 1323.

Overcash, J. A., Beckstead, J., Extermann, M., & Cobb, S. (2005). The abbreviated comprehensive geriatric assessment (aCGA): A retrospective analysis. *Critical Reviews in Oncology/Hematology, 54,* 129.

Padilla, G. V., Ferrell, B., Grant, M. M., & Rhiner, M. (1990). Defining the content domain of quality of life for cancer patients with pain. *Cancer Nursing, 13*(2), 108–115.

Pfeifer, K. A. (1997a). Pathophysiology. In S. Otto (Ed.), *Oncology nursing.* St Louis: Mosby.

Ruscin, J. M. (2014). *Pharmacokinetics in the elderly.* Retrieved March 3, 2018, from http://www.merckmanuals.com/professional/geriatrics/drug-therapy-in-the-elderly/pharmacokinetics-in-the-elderly.

Senger, D. R. (1983). Tumor cells secrete a vascular permeability factor that promotes accumulation of ascites fluid. *Science, 219,* 983–985.

Steele, L. L., Mills, B., Hardin, S. R., & Hussey, L. C. (2005). The quality of life of hospice patients: patient and provider perceptions. *American Journal of Hospice and Palliative Medicine, 22*(2), 95–110.

Thompson, D. (2013, December 16). U.S. cancer death rates continue to decline: Report. U.S. News & World Report. Retrieved from http://health.usnews.com/health-news/news/articles/2013/12/16/us-cancer-death-rates-continue-to-decline-report.

Tilden, V., & Weinert, C. (1987). Social support and the chronically ill individual. *The Nursing Clinics of North America, 22,* 613.

Walter, L., & Covinsky, K. (2001). Cancer screening in elderly adults: A framework of individualized decision making. *JAMA, 285,* 2750.

Weston, A., & Harris, C. C. (2003). Multistage carcinogenesis. In D. W. Kufe, R. E. Pollock, R. R. Weichselbaum, et al. (Eds.), *Holland-Frei cancer medicine* (6th ed.). Hamilton, Ontario: BC Decker. Available from https://www.ncbi.nlm.nih.gov/books/NBK13982/.

Zachariah, B., Casey, L., & Balducci, L. (1995). Radiation therapy of the oldest old cancer patients: A study of effectiveness and toxicity. *Journal of the American Geriatrics Society, 43,* 793.

29

Loss and End-of-Life Issues

Linda Bub, MSN, RN, GCNS-BC

ⓔ http://evolve.elsevier.com/Meiner/gerontologic

LEARNING OBJECTIVES

On completion of this chapter, the reader will be able to:

1. Distinguish between loss, bereavement, grief, and mourning.
2. Discuss factors that may affect the length of time of bereavement.
3. Identify physical, psychological, social, and spiritual aspects of normal grief responses.
4. Describe four ways that complicated grief reactions may manifest themselves.
5. Discuss the tasks of mourning.
6. Describe nursing care activities for assisting bereaved older adults.
7. Discuss physical, psychological, social, and spiritual aspects of dying for older adults.
8. Explain age-related changes that affect older adults who are dying.
9. Describe nursing strategies for assisting dying older adults and their families.
10. Discuss the philosophy of palliative care.

WHAT WOULD YOU DO?

What would you do if you were faced with the following situations?

• Mr. H is an 85-year-old WWII veteran with prostate cancer with metastasis to the bones. He has been receiving chemotherapy and radiation for 2 years, but the disease has progressed. He was admitted to the acute care setting for management of postchemotherapy side effects. His oncologist is the admitting physician and has initiated his admitting orders. You are in report when you hear the code call for this patient. He is a full code and was well into being coded when his niece walked in and stated that he was a DNR, and the doctor didn't write the order! What do you do?

• Ms. K is a 90-year-old woman who is in the late stages of the dying process. Her partner of 40 years, Karen, is at her bedside in the nursing home and has been her primary caregiver since she became ill. Ms. K's family has come and demands that their wishes be followed, not her partner's. The family will not talk to Karen. What do you do?

Loss is a natural part of life and aging. The longer people live, the more losses they experience. Transitions involving loss commonly associated with aging are those such as moving from employment into retirement, from a lifelong home to a smaller home or senior apartment, from being very active to being less so, from health to chronic illness, from marriage to widowhood, and from extensive social networks to smaller circles of family and friends. These transitions are considered losses in American society and are often viewed negatively. Successful aging requires learning to deal with these losses and adapting to the changes over time. Only recently has research shown that life transitions and

crises such as the death of a loved one could act as catalysts for learning new skills and experiencing personal growth.

DEFINITIONS

The terms *loss, bereavement, grief,* and *mourning* are often used interchangeably, but these words convey different meanings (Doka, 2013). *Loss* is a broad term that connotes losing or being deprived of something such as one's health, home, or a relationship. *Bereavement* is the state or situation of having experienced a death-related loss. *Grief* is one's psychological (cognitive or affective), physical, behavioral, social, and spiritual reactions to loss. *Mourning* is often used to refer to the ritualistic behaviors in which people engage during bereavement. More recently, *mourning* is the term used for processes related to learning how to live with one's loss and grief.

LOSSES

A loss may involve a person, thing, relationship, or situation (Corless, 2010). Gradual and abrupt life transitions such as retirement, change of residence, ill health, loss of pets, and the inability to drive are losses that evoke varying responses of grief. Most of the literature and research on losses among older persons focus on the death of spouses; less attention is paid to the loss of parents, siblings, adult children, and friends. For all types of transitions—from moving to a new home to the death of a loved one—people's responses depend on their perception of the events and the meaning of the loss within the context of their lives and their physical, psychosocial, and spiritual life patterns.

Previous authors: Cindy R. Morgan, RN, MSN, CHC, CHPN, and Ramesh C. Upadhyaya, RN, CRRN, MSN, MBA, PhD-C.

Many older adults experience multiple losses with little time for grieving between the losses. The emotional crises imposed by these multiple losses can lead to disorientation, mental confusion, and withdrawal. Individual coping styles, the existence of support systems, the ability to maintain some sense of control, and the griever's health status and spiritual beliefs all influence a person's responses to multiple losses (Garrett, 1987).

Bereavement

Bereavement includes grief and mourning, both the inner emotional response and the outward response of the survivor (Corless, 2010). The time that one spends in the period of bereavement is affected by many factors. The death of one's spouse or life partner is usually the most significant loss that an older person may experience. It involves the loss of a companion who often is one's best friend, sexual partner, and partner in decision making and household management, as well as a contributing source to one's definition of self or identity. Because many older couples frequently divide the tasks of daily living to be able to remain in their home, surviving spouses must take on new responsibilities while coping with the loss of their loved ones. Perceived social support after the death of a spouse has been shown to be a factor affecting the adjustment of many surviving spouses (Balk, 2013). Other factors that may affect bereavement outcomes include ambivalent or dependent relationships, mental illness, low self-esteem, and multiple prior bereavements.

Although bereavement after the death of a spouse is a highly stressful process, the summary of studies of widowed persons by Lund (1989) concluded that many older surviving spouses are resilient. Although 72% of those studied reported that the spouse's death was the most stressful event they had ever experienced, they also reported high coping abilities. The overall effects of grief on the physical and mental health of many older adults were not as severe as expected, and both positive and negative feelings were experienced simultaneously. Loneliness and problems associated with tasks of daily living were two of the most common difficulties reported. Although bereaved older adults adjusted in many different ways to the deaths of their spouses, in general, the most difficult period was the first several months, with the process improving gradually but unsteadily over time.

The review by Lund (1989) also showed that older men and older women are more similar than dissimilar in their bereavement experiences and adjustment. Age, income, education, and anticipation or forewarning of death did not seem to have much effect on future adjustment processes. Religion-related variables also did not contribute much to adjustment. Social support was moderately helpful in the adjustment process, as were internal types of coping resources such as independence, self-efficacy, self-esteem, and competency in performing tasks of daily living.

Older adults' normal grief responses to the loss of a spouse were summarized by Lund (1989). The following conclusions, drawn from his work, speak specifically to the bereavement experiences of older persons:

- Bereavement adjustments are multidimensional in that nearly every aspect of a person's life may be affected by the loss.
- Bereavement is a highly stressful process, but many older surviving spouses are resilient.

- The overall effect of bereavement on the physical and mental health of many older spouses is not as devastating as expected.
- Older bereaved spouses commonly experience both positive and negative feelings simultaneously.
- Loneliness and problems associated with the tasks of daily living are two of the most common and difficult adjustments for older bereaved spouses.
- Spousal bereavement in later life might best be described as a process that is most difficult in the first several months but that improves gradually, if unsteadily, over time. The improvement may continue for many years, but it may never end for some.
- A great deal of diversity exists in how older bereaved adults adjust to the death of a spouse.

As indicated in the study by Lund, the time and intensity of feelings during bereavement are based on many individual factors.

Grief

Grief is the individualized and personalized emotional response that an individual makes to a real, perceived, or anticipated loss (Kissane, McKenzie, McKenzie et al., 2003). Normal grief reactions may be characterized by time: early, middle, and last phases. In the early phase, shock, disbelief, and denial are common. This phase commonly ends as people begin to accept the reality of the loss after the funeral. The middle phase is a time of intense emotional pain and separation and may be accompanied by physical symptoms and labile emotions. Lastly, reintegration and relief occur as the pain gradually subsides and a degree of physical and mental balance returns (DeSpelder & Strickland, 2010).

Human beings respond wholly to loss and manifest grief physically, psychologically, socially, and spiritually (see Patient/Family Teaching box). These are all different aspects of the whole.

PATIENT/FAMILY TEACHING

Common Symptoms of Normal Grief Responses

Grief responses have physical, psychological, social, and spiritual aspects. The duration and intensity of symptoms are highly variable. Most of the more intense symptoms subside in 6 to 12 months; however, mourning may continue for several years.

Physical symptoms commonly include crying, loss of appetite, decreased energy and fatigue, and sleep difficulties. Psychological responses commonly include feelings of sadness, guilt, anxiety, anger, depression, helplessness, and loneliness. Social changes following the loss of a loved one depend on the role of the deceased. In widowhood, a loss of social support, an adjustment to living alone, and sometimes an inability to manage tasks of daily living are frequently experienced unless new skills are learned. Spiritual responses often lead the bereaved to search for meaning in life and to reexamine his or her faith and belief system.

Physical Symptoms

Physical symptoms are commonly associated with acute grief responses. Tearfulness, crying, loss of appetite, feelings of hollowness in the stomach, decreased energy, fatigue, lethargy, and sleep difficulties are common symptoms of grief. Other physical sensations may include tension, weight loss or gain, sighing, feeling of something being stuck in the throat, tightness in the chest or throat, heart palpitations, restlessness, shortness of breath, and dry mouth (Corr & Corr, 2013).

Psychological Responses

Studies of grief responses have consistently identified common psychological responses. Feelings of sadness are the emotions most often mentioned (Worden, 2009). Other common feelings include guilt, anxiety, anger, depression, apathy, helplessness, and loneliness. Guilt and regret regarding one's relationship with the person who has died may be especially troublesome (Landman, 1993). Shock and disbelief may immediately follow the death. The bereaved person may also display diminished self-concern, a preoccupation with the deceased, and a yearning for his or her presence. Some older persons become confused and unable to concentrate after the death of someone significant to them. *Grief spasms,* periods of acute grief, may come when least expected (Rando, 1988). How the grief response manifests itself is individually determined by sociocultural factors in addition to the quality of the relationship between the deceased and the mourner. For some older persons, the grief experience may include feelings of relief and emancipation, especially after prolonged suffering or a difficult relationship,

Social Responses

The social changes that follow the loss of a loved one depend on the type of relationship and the definition of social roles within the relationship. Widowhood is the loss that generally has the greatest effect on social role change, but any loss of a person within one's household is especially difficult. In addition to deep psychological pain, the bereaved person must often learn new skills and roles to manage tasks of daily living. All these social changes occur at a time when withdrawal, a lack of interest in activities, and a lack of energy make decision making and action very difficult. Socialization and interaction patterns also change. If an older couple often socialized together with other couples, widowhood may bring dramatic changes in the type and style of interaction. For others who have strong social support and established patterns of independent interaction outside the lost relationship, the adjustment process toward creating new social roles and interactions may occur more quickly.

With the change in our society over the last 10 years, lesbian, gay, bisexual, and transgender (LGBT) individuals can have more open relationships and are now allowed to be part of the dying process with their partners. This has implications for the nurse and understanding our own biases for disenfranchised populations and how they grieve; continued discrimination in health care can create an added burden on the grieving process. It is vital that nurses understand that LGBT partners grieve differently because of previous experiences with discrimination. They often have little interaction with family due to homophobia; therefore they rely on their community or on friends for support (Patlamazoglou, Simmonds, & Snell, 2017).

Spiritual Aspects

The death of a loved one inevitably causes bereaved people to ponder the existential issues of life and to examine the meaning of not only the lost loved one's life but also their own. Spiritual issues may surface as the person searches for meaning. Anger at God, sometimes followed by a crisis of faith and meaning, may accompany bereavement. It may be important for the bereaved to view the death of their loved one as a transition to a life with God in the spirit. Meaning in life is highly individualized, but the importance of finding meaning in life is more universal. What a person finds meaningful is not as important as the ability to look back on life and see that it has been meaningful and to understand that life can continue to be meaningful even in its last stages.

Religion and spirituality can provide a stabilizing influence during grief. One's religious institution may provide the sense of belonging to a group of people who support one another in times of need. Some may experience a deep inner sense of peace that they are being cared for by a higher power. For others, however, the grief experience may precipitate a crisis in their beliefs and values. Gender, social class, ethnicity, and culture may influence one's spiritual response to grief (D'Avanzo, 2008; Doka & Davidson, 1998) (see Cultural Awareness box).

Nurses should remember that each aspect of grief is integrated within the whole person. Interventions directed at one of these areas will affect the other areas; thus an approach that separates the mind, body, and spirit is not advocated. One's responses to loss and death are characterized by (1) changes over time, (2) one's natural reaction to all kinds of losses, not just death, and (3) one's unique perception of the loss (Rando, 1988).

Types of Grief

Anticipatory grief and the responses described thus far are generally considered "normal" or uncomplicated grief reactions. When grief progresses in an unhealthy way and does not move toward resolution, it is called *complicated mourning* or *abnormal grief.* The nursing diagnosis for complicated mourning or abnormal grief is Dysfunctional Grieving, and it shares many of the defining characteristics of normal grief. Dysfunctional grieving occurs for an extended length of time and is severe in its intensity. Nurses need to be familiar with dysfunctional grieving and should refer patients to advanced practice nurses or other health professionals skilled in working with complicated grieving.

Anticipatory grief is defined as grieving that occurs before the actual loss. It includes the processes of mourning, coping, and planning, which are initiated when the impending loss of a loved one becomes apparent (Rando, 1986). These may be healthy responses to an impending death, but they also may have a negative effect on the relationship with the dying person when one's energies are predominantly focused on the future. Anticipatory grief may account for some persons' apparent lack of overt grief reactions after the death of a loved one who experienced a long terminal illness. Anticipatory grief increases as death becomes imminent and ends when the death occurs. Anticipatory grief helps reduce early shock, confusion, and depression. Survivors who resolve grief before the death of a loved one may be criticized by others or experience self-reproach for lack of a grief reaction to the actual death. These responses may lead to further problems of adjustment.

⊕ CULTURAL AWARENESS

Loss and End-of-Life Issues

Research indicates that the desire to be told of one's impending death varies according to culture: 71% of whites, 60% of blacks, 49% of Japanese Americans, and 37% of Mexican Americans want health care providers to tell them if they are dying. Each of these groups indicated that the physician is the most appropriate person to communicate the information and that a family member is the second most appropriate.

Although death is a universal human experience, culture-specific considerations exist regarding attitudes toward the loss of a loved one, including age (e.g., child versus older adult) and cause of death. In many Asian American cultures, the loss of an older adult (perceived as having accumulated years of wisdom and knowledge) may be mourned more than the loss of an infant or child (viewed as having made a lesser contribution to society because of fewer years of life experience). For many whites, the reverse may be true; relatively greater sorrow may be expressed over the loss of a younger person (perceived as having been cheated out of achieving his or her fullest potential) than is expressed over the loss of an older individual (perceived as having lived a full and productive life). It should be noted that, regardless of age, human life is valued by all cultures, and loss of life is mourned by those who knew and loved the deceased.

Among the Tohono O'odham (Papago Indians of Arizona), the concept of "good" and "bad" death is prevalent. A good death comes at the end of a full life when a person is prepared, whereas a bad death occurs unexpectedly and violently (e.g., accidents, homicides, and suicides) and leaves the victim without a chance to settle affairs or "say good-bye." Some cultural and religious groups consider suicide taboo and may impose sanctions even after death (e.g., burial in church cemeteries may be denied).

Both culture and religion influence postmortem rituals. Muslims have specific rituals for washing, dressing, and positioning the body. Jewish custom typically prohibits autopsy and embalming. Among some Asian American groups, it is customary for family and friends of the same gender to wash and prepare the body for burial or cremation. Upon death, Amish are buried in simple white garments sewn by family members. Deceased members of the Church of Jesus Christ of Latter Day Saints (Mormons) are dressed in white temple clothing before being viewed by family and friends. Some Native Americans do not say the name of the deceased out of fear the spirit will be called back to earth. Additionally, many Native Americans bury the deceased with items to help the spirit on its final journey.

Often interrelated with religious beliefs and practices, culture influences funeral and burial or cremation practices, as well as what is expected of bereaved family members (i.e., who grieves, for how long, and culturally appropriate behaviors during mourning). Among Chinese Americans, five degrees of kinship *(wu-fu)* are recognized, and these determine the degree of mourning expected according to the closeness and importance of the deceased to the mourner.

Lastly, the nurse should be aware that culture may influence the choice of a final resting place for the deceased person. For example, the bodies of older Jewish patients may be flown to Jerusalem for burial, Christians may prefer to be buried in ground blessed by a priest or minister, and those who are cremated may have expressed various preferences for the disposition of the ashes.

Disenfranchised grief is grief that is not validated or recognized by others. This complicates the grieving process both because it cannot be openly expressed and because social support is not available. Doka (in Yalom, 2010) described situations that cause disenfranchised grief: (1) when a relationship is not recognized by others (e.g., death of ex-spouse), (2) when a loss is not acknowledged (e.g., death of a pet), (3) when the griever is not felt to be capable of significant grief (e.g., very old adults or those with cognitive deficits), and (4) when the circumstances of the death are disenfranchising (e.g., deaths caused by AIDs or suicide).

Complicated grief reactions may manifest as one of four types: (1) chronic, (2) delayed, (3) exaggerated, or (4) masked. *Chronic grief reactions* are prolonged and never reach a satisfactory conclusion. Because bereaved individuals are aware of their continuing grief, this reaction is easy to recognize. A therapist can assess which tasks of grieving are not being resolved and why. The goal of intervention is to resolve these tasks (Worden, 2009). *Delayed* or *postponed grief reactions* occur when the griever's response at the time of the loss is either absent or not sufficient to deal with the loss. At some future time, the person may experience an intense grief reaction triggered by a subsequent, smaller loss or by any other event that triggers sadness. Feelings of hostility or ambivalence are usually present in this kind of reaction. *Exaggerated grief reactions* occur when normal feelings of anxiety, depression, or hopelessness grow to unmanageable proportions. People with exaggerated grief may feel an overwhelming sense of being unable to live without the deceased person. They may lose the sense that the acute grief is transient, and they may continue in this intense despair for a long time (Worden, 2009). *Masked grief reactions*

occur when bereaved persons experience feelings related to the loss but cannot express or recognize the source of these feelings. This reaction may occur as a self-protective mechanism because some people may not be able to bear the stress of mourning. Repression of grief responses usually manifests as either a physical symptom, often like one that the deceased experienced, or as some type of maladaptive behavior (Worden, 2009).

Rando (1988) outlined factors that influence how people experience and express their grief. Categories of psychological factors include the characteristics and meaning of the lost relationship, the personal characteristics of the bereaved, and the specific circumstances surrounding the death (Table 29.1). Social factors include the griever's support system, sociocultural and religious background, education and economic status, and funerary rituals. An individual's physical state also influences the grief response. Important physical factors are the use of drugs and sedatives, nutritional state, adequacy of rest and sleep, exercise, and general physical health. Nurses need to be aware of how all these factors affect dying persons and their families so that they may provide the best care possible.

MOURNING

Mourning was defined earlier as ritualistic activities such as wearing dark clothes during bereavement or lighting candles for the dead, and processes related to learning how to live with one's loss and grief. Each way is prescribed by social and cultural norms that indicate acceptable coping behaviors in a person's society (Corless, 2010). The emphasis in this section will be on the processes of learning to live with loss of a loved one

TABLE 29.1 Psychological Factors Influencing Grief Responses

Characteristics and Meaning of Lost Relationship	Personal Characteristics of Bereaved	Specific Circumstances of Death
Nature and meaning of loss Qualities of lost relationship	Coping behaviors, personality, and mental health	Immediate circumstances of death Timeliness of death
Role and function filled by deceased	Level of maturity and intelligence	Perception of preventability
Characteristics of deceased	Past experiences with loss and death	Sudden versus expected death
Amount of unfinished business between bereaved and loved one	Social, cultural, ethnic, and religious background	Length of illness before death Anticipatory grief and involvement
Perception of deceased's fulfillment in life	Gender role conditioning	
Number, type, and quality of secondary losses that accompany the death	Presence of concurrent stress or crises in life	

Modified from Rando, T. A. (Ed.) (1986). *Loss and anticipatory grief.* Lexington, MA: Lexington Books. Used with permission of Therese A. Rando, PhD.

and will include the traditional stage or phase perspectives of adjustment, tasks of mourning, and two meaning-making approaches. The complexity of the mourning process does not lend itself to a single theory.

Stage or Phase Perspectives

Most of the stage or phase theories of mourning have some aspect of the following concepts: avoidance, assimilation, and accommodation (Buglass, 2012). Avoidance is often felt when one is first confronted by the death of a loved one. The news is hard to believe; however, when the reality is viewed as a fact, strong emotions emerge. Deep emotional pain and even anger toward those seen as responsible for the death—for example, doctors, the deceased person, or God—is common. Gradually, the reality of the new situation without the loved one is assimilated. This may be a time of despair when the void left by the deceased is felt deeply. Eventually, the physical, behavioral, psychological (cognitive or affective), social, and spiritual reactions to the loss decrease, and the bereaved move into the accommodation stage or phase. This is a time when the bereaved begin to accept the loss, move on in their lives, and yet remain attached to their loved ones in a healthy way.

An example of a stage or phase approach to mourning is the early study of survivors of the 1942 Coconut Grove fire in Boston by Lindemann (1944), in which he identified physical and psychological symptoms associated with acute grief. The ages of the mourners were not known.

Although common elements in mourning seem to exist, the stage or phase models have been criticized. Much variation exists in how people respond to loss based on factors such as

the relationship the survivor had with the deceased and ways of coping with loss. Many older adults do not go through the first stage of mourning. They may have expected the death or may be beyond shock and disbelief after having experienced multiple losses in their lifetime. They may also undergo several of the stages at the same time. Regardless of whether shock or anticipation occurs, the task of accepting the reality of the loss is relevant for all.

Tasks of Mourning

The tasks of mourning defined by Worden (2009) are more active and useful descriptions of mourning among older persons. He described the following four tasks of mourning: (1) accepting the reality of the loss, (2) experiencing or working through the pain of grief, (3) adjusting to an environment in which the deceased is missing, and (4) emotionally relocating the deceased and moving on with life. The first task, accepting the reality of the loss, involves coming to the realization that the person is dead, that he or she will not return, and that reunion, at least in life as we know it, is impossible. The second task, experiencing the pain of grief, is necessary to prevent the pain from manifesting itself in some other symptom or problematic behavior. Sociocultural customs that discourage open expression of grief often contribute to unresolved grief. The third task, adjusting to an environment in which the deceased is missing, involves developing new skills and assuming the roles for which the deceased was responsible. The last task, withdrawal of emotional energy and reinvestment in another relationship, entails withdrawing emotional attachment to the lost person and loving another living person in a similar way. For many, this last task is the most difficult.

It is critical that older persons who have lost loved ones acknowledge that pain is associated with grief and loss, and that they must adjust to an environment where the loved one is absent. The expression of pain depends partly on culture and partly on the quality of the relationship with the lost loved one. Guilt may accompany the pain of grief.

Adjustment to one's environment after the loss of a loved one involves learning new roles such as those previously assumed by the deceased and new ways of interacting with others in one's social environment. This adjustment may be especially difficult if the loved one lost is the spouse and the social network consists primarily of other couples.

The final task, emotionally relocating the deceased and moving on with life, gives the bereaved person permission to invest emotionally in others without being disloyal to the lost loved one. Although Worden (2009) pointed out that, in one sense, mourning is never over, he also stated that, in losses that involve a great deal of emotional attachment, the process takes at least 1 year before the wrenching pain subsides. Some older spouses have reported that they feel as though they will never "get over" their loss but that they have learned to live with it (Lund, 1989).

In contrast to detaching or "letting go" of the deceased, Klass, Silverman, and Nickman (2006) viewed the bond between survivors and the deceased as dynamic rather than static. On the basis of their research, they suggested that bereaved persons maintain a continuing bond with the deceased. This approach is different from advocating that the mourner totally disengage or sever bonds with the deceased.

Meaning Making

Burbank (1992) found that the major source of meaning in life among older persons came from relationships with family members. When loved ones die, meaning derived from these relationships changes. Personal beliefs and attitudes, including cultural and religious ones, influence how the meanings of the losses are perceived. Some of the more common perceptions attached to illness and death are punishment by a supreme being, suffering that must be overcome or endured, a normal part of the life experience, and an opportunity for personal growth and transcendence. The meaning of a loss to a bereaved person has a significant effect on his or her responses to that loss. For this reason, it is important that caregivers explore the perceptions of the bereaved to understand and assist them as they mourn their loss.

Neimeyer (2000) proposed that reconstructing the meaning in a person's life after the death of a loved one is an important process of mourning. The bereaved are encouraged to find or create new meaning in their lives and in the deaths of the deceased. This is a cognitive process affected by one's social context as well as one's individual resources.

The multiple definitions of meaning, however, require further clarification. Holland, Currier, and Neimeyer (2006) found that the terms "sense making" and "benefit finding" were central to finding meaning. Their research indicated that better outcomes came from making sense of the death and the resulting life of the survivor than from finding benefits from the death such as reordering life priorities and becoming more empathetic.

Building on the work by Holland et al., (2006), researchers further operationalized "meaning" and "grief" to include *identity change* and *purpose in life* because they found that an important facet of meaning is the significance that some aspect of one's life experience "matters" (Hibberd, 2013).

The dual process model of coping with bereavement is another way to make meaning after the death of a loved one. In this model, Stroebe and Schut (2001) suggested that the bereaved waver between loss-oriented and restoration-oriented approaches to everyday life experiences. Regardless of whether persons are in loss-oriented or restoration-oriented states, they vacillate between positive and negative meaning (re)constructions until, over time, they become more focused on positive meaning reconstruction. For instance, persons might vacillate between positive reappraisal of the situation and negative rumination about the death, but they gradually spend more time making meaning from positive reappraisals of their situation.

Nursing Care

The goal of nursing care for older persons who are grieving and mourning is not to "make them feel better" quickly, although nurses are often tempted to try to do so. Nurses should assist and support bereaved persons through the grieving process, recognizing that pain is a normal and healthy response to loss, and allowing bereaved persons to accomplish the tasks of mourning in their own ways.

Assessment

Initial assessment of bereavement risk may be accomplished by using the Bereavement Risk Assessment Tool (BRAT) developed by the Victoria Hospice Society (2008) (Fig. 29.1). While a patient is moving through the phases of grief, progress can be measured using the 10-Mile Mourning Bridge (Huber & Gibson, 1990) (Fig. 29.2). This tool, useful for both clinical assessment and research purposes, draws on the work by Worden (2009) and is conceptualized as a journey across a 10-mile bridge. On the bridge, the 0 represents the time before grief. The 10 reflects Worden's last stage, in which patients recover the emotional energy consumed by grieving and reinvest it in their own lives. It is not suggested that people ever "get over" the death of a loved one but rather that grief could cease to be the primary focus of life. Patients may use the 10-Mile Mourning Bridge as a self-assessment tool with daily or weekly frequency, as determined by the patient. Because each person's grief experience is unique, the miles on the bridge are only defined at each end. The use of this instrument may also facilitate patient–nurse discussions about grief and progress (Huber & Bryant, 1996).

Grief Counseling

Grief counseling is used to facilitate successful progression through the grief process, whereas *grief therapy* is intended for those experiencing complicated mourning. Nurses, other health care professionals, and specially trained volunteers may provide grief counseling, whereas therapy should be conducted under the guidance of a skilled therapist (Worden, 2009). The following section discusses grief counseling.

Worden (2009) suggested four ways that grief counselors may assist grieving persons in the tasks of mourning. The aim is to (1) increase the reality of the loss, (2) help the counseled person deal with both expressed and latent effects, (3) assist the counseled person in dealing with various impediments to readjustment after the loss, and (4) encourage the counseled person to make a healthy emotional withdrawal from the deceased and to feel comfortable reinvesting that emotion in another relationship. Worden's grief counseling principles are as follows:

- *Help the survivor actualize the loss.* Nurses are often the first to initiate this process, especially after the death of a patient in a health care institution. Nurses are usually the professionals present to offer details and descriptions of the death or explanations of puzzling situations that family members may not understand. Having information about the death and the events preceding and following the death is important in helping to actualize the loss. Survivors may need to be encouraged to talk about the loss, to tell the story of events surrounding the death, and to relate memories of the deceased. This process takes time. Worden (2009) found that many survivors took up to 3 months before they began to accept the reality that their spouses were dead and not going to return.
- *Help the survivor identify and express his or her feelings.* Because they are unpleasant, some feelings accompanying bereavement may not be expressed or recognized by the

Bereavement Risk Assessment Tool
© Victoria Hospice Society 2008

Assessment Date	Assessed by	ID#	Patient / Deceased Name	Bereaved Name

Risk Indicators and Protective Factors

Comments

I. Kinship
- ☐ a) spouse/partner of patient or deceased
- ☐ b) parent/parental figure of patient or deceased

II Caregiver
- ☐ a) family member or friend who has taken primary responsibility for care

III. Mental Health
- ☐ a) significant mental illness (eg major depression, schizophrenia, anxiety disorder)
- ☐ b) significant mental disability (eg developmental, dementia, stroke, head injury)

IV. Coping
- ☐ a) substance abuse / addiction (specify)
- ☐ b) considered suicide (no plan, no previous attempt)
- ☐ c) has suicide plan and a means to carry it out OR has made previous attempt
- ☐ d) self-expressed concerns regarding own coping, now or in future
- ☐ e) heightened emotional states (anger, guilt, anxiety) as typical response to stressors
- ☐ f) yearning/pining for the deceased OR persistent disturbing thoughts/images > 3 months
- ☐ g) declines available resources or support
- ☐ h) inability to experience grief feelings or acknowledge reality of the death > 3 months

V. Spirituality / Religion
- ☐ significant challenge to fundamental beliefs / loss of meaning or faith / spiritual distress

VI. Concurrent Stressors
- ☐ a) two or more competing demands (eg single parenting, work, other caregiving)
- ☐ b) insufficient financial, practical or physical resources (eg ↓ income, no childcare, illness)
- ☐ c) recent non-death losses (eg divorce, unemployment, moving, retirement)
- ☐ d) significant other with life-threatening illness / injury (other than patient/deceased)

VII. Previous Bereavements
- ☐ a) unresolved previous bereavement(s)
- ☐ b) death of other significant person within 1 year (from time of patient's death)
- ☐ c) cumulative grief from > 2 OTHER deaths over past 3 years
- ☐ d) death or loss of parent/parental figure during own childhood (less than age 19)

VIII. Supports & Relationships
- ☐ a) lack of social support/social isolation (perceived or real - eg housebound)
- ☐ b) cultural or language barriers to support
- ☐ c) longstanding or current discordant relationship(s) within the family
- ☐ d) relationship with patient/deceased (eg abuse, dependency)

IX. Children & Youth
- ☐ a) death of parent, parental figure or sibling
- ☐ b) demonstration of extreme, ongoing behaviours/symptoms (eg sep anxiety+, nightmares)
- ☐ c) parent expresses concern regarding his/her ability to support child's grief
- ☐ d) parent/parental figure significantly compromised by his/her own grief

X. Circumstances Involving the Patient, the Care or the Death
- ☐ a) patient/deceased less than age 35
- ☐ b) lack of preparedness for the death (as perceived or demonstrated by bereaved)
- ☐ c) distress witnessing the death OR death perceived as preventable
- ☐ d) violent, traumatic OR unexplained death (eg accident, suicide, unknown cause)
- ☐ e) significant anger with OTHER health care providers (eg "my GP missed the diagnosis")
- ☐ f) significant anger with OUR hospice palliative care program (eg "you killed my wife")

XI. Protective Factors Supporting Positive Bereavement Outcome
- ☐ a) internalized belief in own ability to cope effectively
- ☐ b) perceives AND is willing to access strong social support network
- ☐ c) predisposed to high level of optimism/positive state of mind
- ☐ d) spiritual/religious beliefs that assist in coping with the death

Aug-08

Fig. 29.1 The Bereavement Risk Assessment Tool. (©Victoria Hospice Society, BRAT Manual (2008), Victoria, BC, Canada, from http://www.victoriahospice.org/health-professionals/clinical-tools.)

bereaved person. Nurses need to assess a bereaved person's feelings and ask specific questions that encourage expression. Feelings that often go unexpressed include anger, guilt, anxiety, and helplessness (Worden, 2009). Guilt and regret may be recognized and expressed through storytelling, writing in a journal, or writing a letter to the deceased. A ritual such as burying or burning the letter may assist the mourner in resolution. Sometimes, unpleasant emotions are displaced. For example, anger may be directed toward the deceased, toward God, or toward the physician or nurse who helped the family

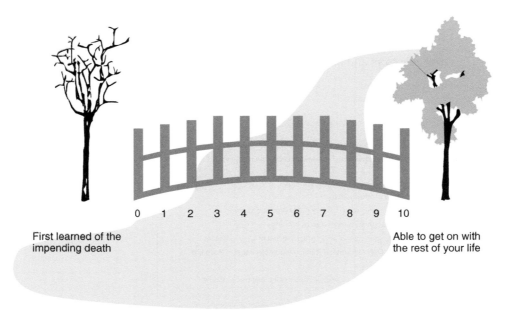

Fig. 29.2 The 10-Mile Mourning Bridge. (From Huber, R. & Gibson J. [1990]. New evidence for anticipatory grief. *The Hospice Journal, 6*[1], 49.)

care for the loved one. Such anger may be difficult to understand, but it is helpful for the targets of the anger to detach themselves and not respond defensively. Sociocultural and gender differences influence expression of emotions and need to be considered. Older persons may also express their emotions differently from how younger ones do, especially after dealing with multiple losses; for example, crying may be a less common indicator of sadness among older persons.

- *Assist the survivor in living without the deceased.* The nurse needs to assess the survivor's daily living situation and identify any existing or potential problems. The roles played by the deceased must now be assumed by the survivor (or someone else) to accomplish tasks of daily living. Knowledge of community resources and teaching of practical skills are necessary to meet this need. In general, survivors should be advised to postpone making major decisions that involve life changes such as selling property or moving. Calling on the survivor's social support system is also useful.

- *Facilitate the survivor's emotional withdrawal from the deceased.* The nurse needs to be especially sensitive to when the bereaved should emotionally withdraw from the deceased, while maintaining the bond to the deceased, and begin developing new relationships. This is especially difficult if the relationship lost was that of a spouse. Research has shown that older persons who lose a confidante are less likely than younger persons to replace the confidante. Perhaps they are unwilling to emotionally invest in another intimate relationship when the risk of repeated loss is very high. Other types of relationships such as close friendships may be encouraged to help meet an older person's needs for intimacy.

- *Give the survivor time to grieve.* It used to be believed that after the first anniversary of the death, grief should be resolved. This has been shown to be inaccurate; many factors

influence the time for adjustment, as discussed previously. Two points in time seem to be especially critical: 3 months after the death and 1 year after the death (Worden, 2009). Older persons who have experienced multiple losses may need more time. For some, the losses may never be resolved. A person may simply learn to live with the feelings of grief.

- *Interpret "normal" behavior for the survivor.* It is important that nurses, with a clear understanding of the range of normal grief responses, communicate acceptance and reassurance of the normalcy of a grieving person's responses. Grieving individuals should be reassured that they are not going crazy, that their physical and psychological responses are normal in the face of significant loss, that grief spasms may occur, and that they will feel better in time.

- *Allow for individual survivor differences.* Just as nurses must be sensitive to individual differences in styles of grieving, family and friends need to accept differences among themselves in their grief responses. Nurses may need to explain the wide range of responses and assist mourners with allowing one another to grieve in their own ways.

- *Provide continuing support for the survivor.* Although nurses' interactions with bereaved persons may be brief or intermittent, referrals may be made for outside support. This support may include community resources and support groups. Nurses should also encourage the bereaved to mobilize their own support system of family and friends.

- *Examine the survivor's defenses and coping styles.* Certain coping behaviors are healthy, whereas others are not. An older person has had a lifetime of experience coping with stressful situations and usually has well-established patterns of coping. Under normal circumstances, these defenses and coping mechanisms can often be used successfully; however, they may not be effective in dealing with monumental or accumulated losses. Unhealthy coping mechanisms may lead to destructive behaviors such as alcoholism. Nurses could help the bereaved identify their coping mechanisms, evaluate their effectiveness, and either encourage their continued use or explore other ways of coping more positively.

- *Identify pathologic conditions for the survivor and make appropriate referrals.* Assistance through grief counseling and professional guidance may not be sufficient if additional problems arise that require more intensive help. Nurses need to be particularly alert to serious depressive illness and should make referrals accordingly. Losing a spouse and living alone puts older persons at risk for depression. Older white men have the highest suicide rate of any group, which may suggest that depression is a significant problem for this age group. Discussing with older men the meaning in their lives may give the nurse clues to problems in this area.

Nurses in all settings are able to assist the bereaved at various stages of grief. Nurses are the most effective, however, when they examine their own losses, grief expectations, and patterns of coping with loss. Personal experiences with loss inevitably influence the effectiveness of the help that nurses can give to others who are mourning. A nurse who has successfully worked through a loss—big or small—and has reflected on the experience has valuable insight into the grieving process. However, a nurse who is himself of herself grieving may be unable to invest emotional energy in the care of a patient who is experiencing acute grief.

APPROACHING DEATH: OLDER PERSONS' PERSPECTIVES

The following section addresses the nature of dying among older persons, including stages of dying, attitudes toward death, and physical, psychological, social, and spiritual responses. Nursing strategies for older persons who are dying, palliative and hospice care, environmental considerations, and family and caregiver perspectives are other areas important in the optimal care of dying older adults.

In her classic work on death and dying, Kübler-Ross (1969) identified five stages widely used in practice with dying patients. This model purports that dying individuals progress through the stages of denial, anger, bargaining, depression, and, finally, acceptance of death. All people may not move through these stages in a sequential and orderly fashion, and some even move back and forth between stages; however, this stage theory has become popular in interpreting the behavior and feelings of dying persons, sometimes to their detriment. Retsinas (1988) critiqued these five stages and argued for a different model of death for older adults that takes into account the following factors: (1) that very old persons see themselves as confronting impending death, (2) that they may be accustomed to the sick role and their gradual decrease of vitality, (3) that roles have already been redefined, and (4) that death may truly be timely for older persons.

Psychological Aspects

Kastenbaum (1978) pointed to assumptions such as older persons being ready for timely deaths as evidence of our society's ageist attitudes. Although the literature demonstrates that older persons hold a wide variety of attitudes toward death, fear of their own death is relatively rare. Instead, major concerns among older persons about dying are fears of a long debilitating illness, fears of being a burden, fear of pain and suffering, concerns about quality of life, and fear of dying suddenly and not being found (Lloyd-Williams, Kennedy, Sixsmith, & Sixsmith, 2007). Cultural variations may also play a part in older peoples' attitudes toward death (Beshai, 2008; Field, 2000; Madnawat & Kachhawa, 2007; Upadhyaya & Kautz, 2009). A person who has had positive experiences of coping and is relatively well adjusted usually approaches the stress of being close to death with adaptation and acceptance. Although personal fear of death seemed generally uncommon, Field (2000) found that, even among those who accepted their nearness to death, some were not ready to die. They wished to continue living as long as possible. A "good death" for this population would be one with friends and family present (Gott, Seymour, Bellamy et al., 2004), minimal physical or mental dependency, a minimal amount of being a burden to others, being able to stay in their own homes, and having their emotional, spiritual, and financial needs met (Lloyd-Williams, Kennedy, Sixsmith & Sixsmith, 2007; Payne, Langley-Evans, & Hillierk, 1996; Steinhauser, Christakis, Clipp et al., 2000). Individual assessments of feelings about death need to be conducted, however, because older adults have widely varied experiences and attitudes.

Once people have identified themselves as nearing the end of their lives, they commonly engage in a process called *life review* (Butler, 1963), in which they try to make sense of their whole life. Erikson (1963) identified the last task of life as a psychosocial crisis of integrity versus despair. In this theory, older persons nearing death are expected to review their lives and draw some conclusions about the positive and negative aspects. If they can generally say their lives have been meaningful and worth living, a sense of ego integrity emerges. If, however, their lives are evaluated negatively, they may experience a sense of regret or meaninglessness and despair. Acceptance of death is influenced by positive memories that may help the person reach the happy conclusion that their life has been good (Young & Cullen, 1996).

Psychological issues associated with dying were found to cause the most concern to patients, families, and health care professionals (Reynolds, Henderson, Schuman, & Hanson, 2002; Wong et al., 2004). The most common unmet emotional needs of dying residents in nursing homes included sadness and depression (44%), anxiety or agitation (33%), and loneliness (21%) (Reynolds et al., 2002).

Spiritual Aspects

Religious beliefs and spiritual experiences play an important part when older persons are trying to make sense of their lives. Faith in a supreme power may give life a transcendent meaning and help people view their lives within the context of a greater purpose or meaning. Sometimes, dying or a threat of loss may trigger a crisis of faith, in which people question their previous beliefs in an effort to make sense of the present experience. Moadel et al., (1999) studied ethnically diverse patients with cancer and found that up to 51% expressed unmet spiritual or existential needs. In a study by Reynolds et al. (2002), 30% of dying nursing home residents needed more care in spiritual and emotional needs.

Three spiritual needs of dying persons have been identified by Doka (1993): (1) the need to search for the meaning of life, (2) the need to die appropriately, and (3) the need to find hope that extends beyond the grave. These three needs reflect Erikson's developmental task for the last stage of life, as well as other research findings regarding older persons' fears of dying. Religious or spiritual beliefs and experiences may be instrumental in helping older persons cope with these fears. Assessing patients' desires for religious and spiritual assistance is particularly important when they are dying. Among the many reasons for spiritual care at this time are preparing for death and the afterlife, dealing with anger over dying, seeking forgiveness for past wrongs, searching for peace, and meeting the needs of a family coping with loss (Hall, 1997). The National Consensus Project for Quality Palliative Care (NCPQPC, 2013) included assessing and treating spiritual needs in its list of nursing competencies for quality end-of-life care; however, spiritual care is not consistently provided. The Spiritual Needs Inventory (Hermann, 2006) has been validated for use in assessing the spiritual needs of patients near the end of life.

Social Aspects

Once the term *dying* is applied to an individual, role changes are often initiated or reinforced by family and friends. The adoption of the sick role may be accompanied by an acceptance of one's fate. However, some dying individuals may adopt a fighting stance, determined to do all they can to outwit or forestall death. Some move ahead with resolve to define themselves as "still living," refusing to accept the label of *dying* and thus living each day as fully as possible. The stance people take toward dying is affected by sociocultural, psychological, and life history factors. Some of these attitudes toward dying are positive and promote growth; others are negative and difficult to endure, not only for dying persons but also for those around them. For example, it is troublesome when family members want to resolve issues while the patient denies that he or she is dying and refuses to discuss matters that need resolution.

Because death and dying have been regarded as taboo topics in American society, most people are uncomfortable, at least initially, when talking about death with someone who is dying. This is partly because of having to confront one's own mortality when facing the death of others. It is fairly easy to live an illusion of stability and immortality when around young, healthy persons. However, when a loved one is dying, thoughts turn to one's own mortality and what life will be like without this person. Because these thoughts are uncomfortable for most, one way of relieving this discomfort is to avoid the dying person. Social isolation often results as friends and sometimes family seemingly abandon the dying person. A special concern for older persons results from society's attitude that they are ready to die and therefore may have less need to interact with others. It is often seen as normal and natural for them to disengage and

die quietly. This attitude also fosters social isolation. Thus social isolation, loneliness, and role changes are typical concomitants of dying for older persons. Nurses and physicians may also avoid openness in communicating with older dying patients. Costello (2001) found that nurses provided individualized physical care to dying patients, but little evidence of spiritual and emotional care was included in this practice.

Physical Aspects

An obvious and sometimes puzzling issue for those working with older persons is deciding when to consider a person to be dying. Is a diagnosis of terminal illness necessary? Are there certain physical signs that must be present? In a certain sense, all human beings are in the process of dying. Nonetheless, the probable length of time remaining before death occurs or the certainty of a fatal illness generally determines whether one is deemed to be dying. Life expectancy also enters into people's attitudes about when dying occurs. Generally, the expectation of impending death of a frail 100-year-old is greater compared with that of an energetic 75-year-old. The most commonly used definition of "terminal illness" is life expectancy of 6 months or less, which is the length of time determined by Medicare for receipt of hospice benefits. Because no clear definition of *dying* exists for older persons not diagnosed with a terminal illness, this must be explored individually.

Death for older persons usually results from complications from one or more chronic illnesses rather than from a sudden, unexpected incident or illness. The three leading causes of death, among adults older than age 65, are heart disease, cancer, and chronic lower respiratory diseases (CDC, 2016). These are expected to remain the major causes of mortality in the older adult population through the year 2020. Other major causes of death among older adults include chronic obstructive pulmonary disease (COPD), pneumonia and influenza, diabetes mellitus, injury from accidents, renal diseases, septicemia, and complications from Alzheimer's disease.

General Health Care Needs

Regardless of needs that arise from specific diseases and functional problems, dying individuals have general health care needs that must be addressed. General nursing interventions to meet these needs include (1) stabilizing and supporting vital functions and facilitating integrated functioning, (2) determining functional deviation and adjusting treatment, (3) relieving distressing symptoms and suffering, (4) assisting patient and family interaction, and (5) supporting a patient and his or her family in coping with the realities of death. Common physical problems and symptoms encountered by terminally ill patients include pain, dyspnea, constipation, delirium, altered urinary elimination patterns, altered skin integrity, loss of appetite, dry mouth, nausea and vomiting, restlessness and sleeplessness, difficulty swallowing, and nutritional problems (Derby, O'Mahoney, & Tickoo, 2010). Family coping and stress, safety needs, and self-care deficits are other important problems (Weitzner, Moody, & McMillan, 2003). Age-related changes and comorbid conditions combined with these general health care needs of dying older persons and their families make the provision of high-quality nursing care especially challenging. Skillful assessments and creative nursing strategies aimed at addressing multiple physical, psychosocial, and spiritual needs are necessary.

Effects of Age-Related Changes

Nursing care aimed at meeting the physical needs of older persons who are dying is no different from the meticulous care needed by any other patient with a debilitating condition. Age-related changes and the effects of long-term chronic illnesses predispose older persons to greater risk of problems in hygiene and skin care, nutrition, elimination, mobility and transfers, rest and sleep, pain management, respiration, and cognitive and behavioral functioning. Only the areas that pose special problems for older persons are discussed in this section.

Age-related changes in the integumentary and vascular systems, coupled with alterations in nutrition, elimination, and mobility, quickly lead to skin breakdown. Loss of the subcutaneous fat layer and a decrease in sebaceous gland activity cause the skin to become thin and dry, which makes it more susceptible to the hazards of immobility. Pressure ulcers are a problem for older, debilitated patients and are often quick to form and slow to heal. Sometimes, even the best skin care and positioning cannot prevent the formation of pressure ulcers at the end of life (Hughes, Bakos, O'Mara, & Kovner, 2005).

Rigidity of the chest wall, decreased ciliary activity, and decreased coughing and gagging reflexes all predispose older persons to respiratory problems, especially pneumonia. Aspiration pneumonia is a common problem in older patients who are unable to feed themselves and who have difficulty maintaining the upright position. The decreased effectiveness of the immune system and the often nonspecific presentation of symptoms related to pneumonia may make the diagnosis and treatment of pneumonia in older adults more complicated. Shortness of breath and altered respiratory patterns in sleep such as Cheyne-Stokes respirations or sleep apnea are more prevalent among older persons and may become problematic if these patients are seriously ill or dying.

Digestive changes associated with age include decreased amounts of saliva and digestive fluids and enzymes, decreased peristaltic activity, and decreased absorption through the intestinal wall. These changes predispose an older person who is dying to additional problems with maintaining adequate nutritional status and bowel function. They are exacerbated by immobility and often contribute to constipation, fecal impaction, and sometimes diarrhea. Although health care professionals often downplay the seriousness of constipation, this problem may cause much discomfort to the dying person and contribute to other life-threatening complications.

Changes in vision and hearing that commonly accompany advancing age reduce the stimulation that older persons receive from the environment. This is complicated by the usual practice of removing eyeglasses and hearing aids from patients who are ill and well-meaning attempts to provide a quiet, darkened, and peaceful environment. Sensory deprivation may lead to mental confusion among healthy individuals and is of even greater importance among older adults who are dying.

Environmental changes and unfamiliar people and settings also contribute to cognitive impairment among older persons. Because hospitalization or a move to a nursing facility is often a part of the dying experience for older persons, the acute confusion that may result from such a move may be permanent. Institutionalization, even if temporary, may be a rite of passage for an older person and serve as an external indicator that his or her illness is progressing, and death is becoming more imminent.

Although it is believed that the experience of superficial pain for older persons is unchanged, many older adults seem to experience less visceral pain such as organ pain (Daoust et al., 2016). Compared with younger adults, however, older people report more complaints of chronic pain and show reduced tolerance to experimentally induced pain. This may be attributed to differences in pain modulatory mechanisms associated with age (Cole, Farrell, Gibson, & Egan, 2010). All reports of pain and discomfort need to be heeded and validated by the nurse. Nonpharmacologic interventions for pain relief—for example, therapeutic touch, massage, acupressure, relaxation, and visualization—need to be used, whenever possible.

Age-related changes in pharmacokinetics and pharmacodynamics lead to atypical drug responses. Because drugs are so widely used as an essential part of medical treatment, their effectiveness, side effects, and reactions need to be closely monitored. Physiologic changes associated with dying, for example, circulatory changes, increase the difficulty in managing drug regimens. Sleep patterns are also disturbed by physiologic changes, pain, and changes in environment. Medication is the most common answer to dying persons' complaints of inability to sleep. Although medication may be appropriate in some instances, it needs to be prescribed with caution and monitored carefully. For a dying older person, sleep medications may cause new problems such as incontinence or delirium. Nonpharmacologic therapies should be used first before use of medications. Psychological causes of sleeplessness should also be explored. For example, if older persons fear dying alone in their sleep or if they have unfinished business to resolve with their families, sleep medication is not the best answer. Instead, a careful assessment of the cause of sleeplessness must be followed by appropriate treatment aimed at that cause.

Nursing Care

Excellent nursing care of dying older persons begins with examination of a nurse's own feelings about death and values regarding older people. In the youth-oriented American culture, old age is not typically highly esteemed or valued. An overworked hospital nurse must prioritize; younger patients with greater probability for survival receive more attention compared with older dying patients who bear the physician orders, "Do not resuscitate (DNR); comfort measures only." Death often comes quietly, and the nurse may not be present to care for a dying person's physical and emotional needs. Delivering high-quality nursing care to older adults may be one of the most challenging and most rewarding of all nursing experiences. It requires knowledge of the complexities of gerontologic and end-of-life nursing combined with the knowledge, skill, and compassion necessary to deliver holistic care to both dying patients and their families. Updated clinical practice guidelines for quality palliative care are available currently and will be updated again in 2018 at the following website: https://www.nationalcoalitionhpc.org/ncp-guidelines-2013/ (NCPQPC, 2013).

Assessment

As with any other nursing care, nurses must make careful and ongoing assessments of physical, psychosocial, and spiritual needs. Assessment tools for physical needs are also relevant for ill and dying older adults. Special attention, however, needs to be given to potential problem areas such as skin integrity, respiratory status, nutrition, elimination, sensory abilities, cognitive functioning, comfort, and rest. The International Association for Hospice and Palliative Care has compiled a list of assessment tools for many areas of palliative care and pain (see https://hospicecare.com/home/). Assessment tools such as the Palliative Performance Scale (Anderson, Downing, & Hill, 1996) are useful for identifying and tracking care needs of patients receiving palliative care.

The psychosocial needs of the dying person, family, and caregivers must also be carefully assessed. This may be a difficult area to approach, especially when time is limited or a patient's or family's feelings about the process of dying are unknown. Spiritual and psychosocial needs are often discussed together because they are interrelated and affect each other. Areas for careful assessment of spiritual needs include searching for meaning in life, dying appropriately, and finding hope that extends beyond the grave (Doka, 1993).

Meaning in life often emerges as a theme among those who are grieving as well as among those who are dying or nearing the end of their lives. In a study of community-living older adults by Burbank (1992), leading a meaningful life was found to be associated with both physical health and a lack of depressive symptoms. A series of questions useful in assessing the degree of meaning in life is given in Fig. 29.3.

The hierarchy of a dying person's needs, based on Maslow's hierarchy of needs framework, may assist nurses in identifying a dying older person's specific needs at each level (Touhy & Jett, 2016) (Fig. 29.4). Careful assessment of the level of a dying person's needs may indicate individualized strategies for meeting those needs.

Strategies

Little difference exists between nursing strategies for younger persons who are ill and those for dying older persons. The same actual interventions may be applied, but older adults require more frequent assessment, application, and evaluation of the effectiveness of nursing strategies. For instance, a debilitated, immobile younger person may require repositioning less often than an older person who is debilitated and immobile. Older persons may suffer from more severe xerostomia (dry mouth) compared with younger persons with the same condition. The nurse needs to ensure that care is not delivered less often because of personal biases and ageist devaluation of older persons. Pacing of care is especially important; that is, the nurse needs to exhibit patience and give the older person enough time to encourage as much independent functioning as possible.

Particularly difficult problems for older adults who are dying include pain, dyspnea, constipation, urinary incontinence, restlessness, hallucinations and delusions, and nutritional problems. Palliative care measures for these are discussed individually in this section because they often differ from strategies used with chronically ill older adults who are not close to death.

Pain is prevalent among individuals who are dying and may have a powerful, negative effect on a patient's quality of life. The pain experience is complex and its management often difficult. A stepped-care approach is recommended, with the use of aspirin or acetaminophen for mild pain, a moderate opiate such as codeine or oxycodone for more constant pain, and a strong opiate such as morphine for severe pain (World Health Organization [WHO], 2017) (Fig. 29.5). Pain medication should be given around the clock to promote stable blood pressure levels. Nursing responsibilities include careful pain assessment, education of patients and family caregivers regarding pain medication, and close communication with the prescriber for changes in medication as needed. Attention needs to be given to a patient's emotional state because psychosocial factors and emotional pain may accentuate physical pain (Wiech & Tracey, 2009).

Pain is a common complaint of older adults. The Joint Commission requires the assessment and management of pain in patients with acute illnesses and those with chronic conditions (The Joint Commission, 2016). As the number of individuals older than 65 years continues to rise, frailty and chronic diseases with associated pain are likely to increase. Therefore primary care providers will face a significant challenge in pain management in older adults. Older adults are more likely to have arthritis, bone and joint disorders, cancer, and other chronic disorders that cause pain. Between 35% and 48% of community-dwelling older adults have daily pain (Herr, 2011). Older adults residing in nursing homes have an even higher prevalence of pain, which is estimated to be between 45% and 85% (Herr, 2011; Ferrell, Ferrell, & Osterweil, 1990).

Older adults are often either untreated or undertreated for pain. Undertreatment for pain has a negative effect on the health and quality of life of older adults, resulting in depression, anxiety, social isolation, cognitive impairment, immobility, falls, malnutrition, increased health care costs, and loss of quality of life (Herr, 2011).

Dyspnea, or shortness of breath, is another common symptom feared by both patients and caregivers. Common causes include hypoxemia, poor handling of secretions, anxiety, bronchospasm, and pain. Elevation of the head of the bed, limitation of activity, a cool room with low humidity (but not completely dry), supplemental oxygen, and bronchodilators or analgesics may be sufficient to improve dyspnea. Morphine, which is often the most effective medication for decreasing dyspnea, also decreases anxiety. Constipation and a depressed respiratory rate are complications of morphine administration.

Constipation is common among older adults who require opioids for pain and whose diets and activities are restricted. Adding fiber to a patient's diet or giving bulk-forming laxatives may not be practical if the person is unable to maintain

For each of the following statements, circle the response that is most nearly true for you at this time.

1. I feel that I have found a significant meaning or meanings for leading my life.

   Strongly disagree   Disagree   Uncertain   Agree   Strongly agree

2. Even though there may be a purpose in my life, I do not try to do much about it.

   Strongly disagree   Disagree   Uncertain   Agree   Strongly agree

3. I have a belief or beliefs about life that gives my living significance.

   Strongly disagree   Disagree   Uncertain   Agree   Strongly agree

4. Something seems to stop me from doing what I really want to do.

   Strongly disagree   Disagree   Uncertain   Agree   Strongly agree

5. I do not value what I am doing in my life.

   Strongly disagree   Disagree   Uncertain   Agree   Strongly agree

6. The things that are the most important to me dominate my activities.

   Strongly disagree   Disagree   Uncertain   Agree   Strongly agree

7. In thinking of my life, it is hard for me to see a reason for my being here.

   Strongly disagree   Disagree   Uncertain   Agree   Strongly agree

8. Basically, I am living the kind of life I want to live.

   Strongly disagree   Disagree   Uncertain   Agree   Strongly agree

9. In life, I have no goals or aims at all.

   Strongly disagree   Disagree   Uncertain   Agree   Strongly agree

10. My personal existence is purposeful and meaningful.

    Strongly disagree   Disagree   Uncertain   Agree   Strongly agree

11. Life seems to be completely routine.

    Strongly disagree   Disagree   Uncertain   Agree   Strongly agree

12. Facing my daily tasks is a source of pleasure and satisfaction.

    Strongly disagree   Disagree   Uncertain   Agree   Strongly agree

Meaning Framework Question

Is there something or things so important to you in your life that they give your life meaning?

Yes   No

If no, please describe your life situation at this time. _____
_____

If yes, please list those things that are currently important to you and that give your life meaning.
_____

Fig. 29.3 Fulfillment of Meaning Scale. (From Burbank, P. M. [1992]. Assessing the meaning of life among older clients: An exploratory study. *Journal of Gerontological Nursing, 18*[9], 19-28. Reprinted with permission from SLACK Incorporated.)

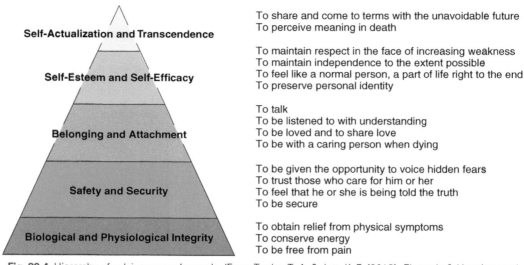

Fig. 29.4 Hierarchy of a dying person's needs. (From Touhy, T. A. & Jett, K. F. [2016]. *Ebersole & Hess' toward healthy aging: Human needs and nursing response* [9th ed.]. St. Louis, MO: Mosby.)

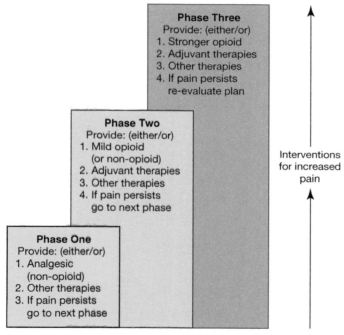

Fig. 29.5 Incorporation of analgesics in the treatment of older adults.

sufficient fluid intake and diet. Stool softeners and oral cathartics may be more effective, but suppositories, enemas, and manual disimpaction may also be necessary. Careful assessment and individualized management of constipation is essential.

A focused history, physical assessment, bladder log, and urinalysis are important for determining the cause of urinary incontinence (UI). The management of UI is based on the cause. Intermittent catheterization or an indwelling catheter may be indicated; however, the risk of infection is always a consideration with catheter placement. For the dying patient with decreased mobility and problems with skin integrity, the benefits of indwelling catheter placement may outweigh the risks.

Restlessness in a dying patient may have many causes, including constipation, urinary retention, sepsis, hypoxia, drug toxicity, increased pain, or unresolved psychosocial issues. If the cause can be identified and effective treatment implemented, restlessness can be resolved. If restlessness continues and is upsetting for the patient and family, pharmacologic management may be necessary (i.e., barbiturates, or neuroleptic drugs, such as haloperidol) (Emanuel, Ferris, von Gunten, Hauser, & Von Roenn, 2015). Nurses should keep in mind that the goal of palliative care is to maintain a level of consciousness that allows for meaningful interaction with others for as long as possible.

Dying older adults who are cognitively impaired frequently experience hallucinations and delusions. Attempts to confront and reorient the delusional person are usually unsuccessful and may cause additional agitation. A better strategy is to ignore delusional statements and divert the conversation to more neutral topics (Craun, Watkins, & Hefty, 1997). The technique of validation, based on empathic understanding of the emotion and messages behind the confusion, is effective in communicating with those experiencing delusions and hallucinations (Feil, 1993; Feil & Altman, 2004). For instance, if a person, when alone, believes that he or she is talking to his or her mother, asking the patient if he or she is feeling lonely or afraid may help the patient express underlying emotions and ease some anxiety.

Oral nutrition and hydration should be maintained if a patient is able to swallow safely. Dehydration and anorexia are often of greater concern to family members than to dying patients, who may not be experiencing any resulting discomfort. In many cases, intravenous fluids and feedings are not appropriate (see Nutritional Considerations box). Palliative care providers and nurses are aware that medically assisted nutrition and hydration rarely benefit patients at the end of life (HPNA, 2011). Adequate hydration may, in fact, increase respiratory secretions. Nasogastric tube feedings, total parenteral nutrition, and intravenous hydration increase infections and may decrease survival time (HPNA, 2011). Additional fluids may also contribute to edema caused by impaired circulation in older adults. The only documented side effect of dehydration is dry mouth, which may be relieved by administration of saliva substitutes, ice chips, and glycerin swabs, and by promotion of good oral care (HPNA, 2011). If adequate oral care is provided, it is believed that patients at the end of life do not suffer from dehydration (HPNA, 2011); however, more research is needed in this area (Dalai, Del Fabbro, & Bruera, 2009). Individual assessment and thoughtful decision making that includes the patient and family regarding hydration and nutrition are important.

🔍 NUTRITIONAL CONSIDERATIONS

Loss of appetite frequently accompanies the dying process. Families usually consider providing food as part of basic human caring and something they can do to prolong the patient's life. For the dying person, however, eating may be an unpleasant and unwanted experience. Artificial feeding with naso-gastric or gastrostomy tubes or intravenous nutrition frequently leads to further complications and earlier death. Because eating and food are often closely tied to many fond memories of loved ones, this is a difficult area and potential source of conflict between patients and their caregivers. Patients and families need to know that anorexia is a normal part of dying, and they need to have open discussion on the meaning of food and nutrition. Perhaps other meaningful and symbolic ways of providing sustenance may be achieved without artificial feeding.

Good communication skills are essential when working with persons who are dying and their families; although, a lack of effective communication by nurses and physicians about terminal diagnoses and information about death and dying have been reported (Costello, 2001). Effective communication skills such as maintaining eye contact, sensitive use of touch, and clarifying statements through reflection (i.e., restating the message as it is understood and asking for verification of its meaning) are important. Nurses' awareness of their own limitations and strengths is critical because of the level of involvement that may result from interactions with persons confronting death. Once a nurse becomes committed to working with a patient and family throughout the dying process, it is important to follow through on this commitment as much as possible.

Another important role of the nurse is to educate and support families and caregivers. Caregivers experience a multitude of problems, including decreased energy levels, health problems, deep grief, and fears about life without their loved one. Nurses need to be sensitive to caregiver needs and provide education, psychological support, and referrals for additional services.

The role of a social support system is very important during the bereavement process. As a result, it is important that the nurse assess social support networks and help mobilize support for patients and caregivers, if necessary. In addition, group therapy interventions such as forgiveness therapy for older terminally ill patients with cancer have been found to be very effective in improving quality of life (Hansen, 2009).

As caregivers, nurses are not immune to intense feelings of grief after the death of a person that they have cared for. These feelings may occur whenever close relationships develop between nurses and patients, especially in long-term care and hospice settings. A dying person may have certain characteristics that invoke memories of previous unresolved losses that the nurse has experienced. Such grief needs to be recognized, accepted, and evaluated, just as any other experience of loss and grief needs to be assessed. The first step is for the nurse to recognize unresolved grief. The next step may be to express his or her thoughts and feelings to a coworker, friend, or family member. If additional help is needed, sources such as employee assistance programs, clergy, or other counselors may be contacted.

Environment and Care Services

Fewer patients are dying in the hospital (24.6% in 2009, down from 32.6% in 2000), but they are receiving more intensive treatment at the end of life (intensive care unit admission during the last month of life increased from 24.3% in 2000 to 29.2% in 2009). Hospice care is now in place for almost one-third of Medicare beneficiaries at end of life (Teno et al., 2013). Often, an older person who is dying is moved back and forth, as their condition changes, between acute care (hospitalization) and any number of long-term care settings.

The hospital setting is particularly problematic for older persons who are dying because the primary goal in this setting is the restoration of health. Since the implementation of diagnosis-related groups, economic constraints on hospitals force patients to be discharged if they are not receiving active treatment (treatment that cannot be provided in the home or another setting) (Csordas & Kleinman, 1990). Too often, life-support technology is utilized as well as tests, treatments, and drug therapy, and the older adult experiences needless suffering.

Nursing facilities and long-term care institutions have different goals and different reimbursement systems than hospitals. The primary goal of a skilled nursing facility is to help patients regain the highest functional level possible. This may be done by using an interdisciplinary approach of nursing and rehabilitation to help patients recover from surgery or a chronic illness (Upadhyaya & Kautz, 2009). Nursing facility settings can foster a good death through their primary goal of caring; however, the reality is that care may be deficient in many nursing facilities. Thus compassionate care of the dying is often not ensured in either the hospital or the nursing facility setting.

Hospice care was founded on the philosophy of compassionate, humane care of the person who is dying and their families. Although a hospice may be an actual place where dying people go, in the United States, the term *hospice* usually refers to a philosophy of caring that can be implemented wherever the patient may be dying—at home, the hospital, or a nursing facility. The basic goal of hospice care is palliative care plus support services, that is, helping the person who is dying live as fully as possible with the highest quality of life on a day-to-day basis. During the dying process and the bereavement period, physical, emotional, social, and spiritual care are provided by an interdisciplinary team consisting of the patients, their families, health care professionals, and volunteers (Egan City & Labyak, 2010).

The term *palliative care* refers to "an approach that improves the quality of life of patients and their families facing the problems associated with life-threatening illness, through the prevention and relief of suffering by means of early identification and impeccable assessment and treatment of pain and other problems, physical, psychosocial, and spiritual" (WHO, n.d.). In the long-term end-of-life care of older adults, offering palliative care before hospice care yields many benefits. It differs from hospice care in that curative treatment can be obtained through palliative care but not through hospice care (Wittenberg-Lyles & Sanchez-Reilly, 2008). This approach has been successful in guiding the care of dying patients and their families provided by interdisciplinary health care teams.

For many older adults, home is the preferred place to die. Home care may or may not include hospice care or palliative care. Many older persons die at home, cared for only by their family or sometimes visiting nurses or home health aides. In these situations, the goals of caregivers are often like hospice goals; however, the dying person and family do not have the benefit of an interdisciplinary team and an organized approach to follow-up care.

Legislative Initiatives

Legislative initiatives regarding death and dying include the Patient Self-Determination Act, which became law in 1991; it requires all health care facilities receiving Medicare and Medicaid reimbursement to recognize advance directives. These instructions for care (living wills and durable powers-of-attorney) guide families and health care providers should the patient be incapable of decision making. Yadav et al. (2017) reviewed studies from 2011 to 2016 and found no increase in the number of patients that had advanced directives in place; despite efforts and initiatives, only 36.7% of people have completed these documents, including living wills. Confusion about the consequences of life-prolonging treatments versus the decision not to treat may undermine the older adult's ability to make informed choices about advance directives (Winter, Parker, & Schneider, 2007).

Nurses caring for very ill older adults need to understand the legal status of advance directives, living wills, and DNR orders. As natural extensions of a patient's right to self-determination, these preferences should be adhered to by the nurse (Basanta, 2002).

EVIDENCE-BASED PRACTICE

Nursing Interventions for Patients and Families at Time of Death

Background
Compassionate care at the end of life constitutes "the final act of caring." It is as important as the care given while the patient was still alive.

Sample/Setting
In this qualitative study, 13 families participated in the bathing and honoring intervention with their loved one in the Inpatient Adult Oncology Unit at Santa Barbara Cottage Hospital and follow-up semistructured telephone interview.

Method
The nurse and family participated in a step-by-step procedure "developed to bathe and honor patients with the recital of nondenominational words for those who die in the acute care setting. While the honoring words are being read, lavender oil is placed on the patient" (p. 364).

Findings
All participants felt the bathing and honoring intervention was a positive, meaningful experience that supported them in the grieving process.

Analysis of the semistructured telephone interviews revealed the following themes:

* Positive experience
* Supported grief process
* Meaningful
* Honored loved one
* Ritually or spiritually significant
* Nurses' caring
* Physicality
* New experience
* Hope that bathing and honoring becomes routine care

Implications
This study provides important information in the development of evidence-based nursing interventions that can facilitate positive, meaningful nursing care for patients and families at the end of life, which support the grieving process.

From Rodgers, D., Calmes, B., & Grotts, J. (2016). Nursing care at the time of death: A bathing and honoring practice. *Oncology Nursing Forum, 43*(3), 363-371. doi: 10.1188/16.ONF.363-371.

🏠 HOME CARE

1. Homebound older adults who have lost a spouse or significant other may manifest grief through physical symptoms.
2. Homebound older adults may develop crises of faith and express anger at God. It is important for the home care nurse to avoid being judgmental and to allow the older adult to verbalize anger and grief.
3. Refer to an advanced practice nurse or other health professional skilled in working with complicated grieving if the homebound older adult experiences dysfunctional grieving.
4. Loss of a spouse or significant other, coupled with living alone, puts homebound older adults at risk for depression.
5. Assess the terminally ill, homebound older adult's feelings toward his or her own death.
6. Provide family members and caregivers information related to the stages of dying and the physiologic changes that accompany them.
7. Use hospice care to help dying homebound older adults live as fully as possible on a day-to-day basis.
8. If hospice care is not available, home care nurses may support the homebound, terminally ill older adult through the dying process.

SUMMARY

It is important for gerontologic nurses to have a thorough understanding of the strategies related to caring for older adults who are grieving or dying. Part of understanding involves examination of the nurse's own value system and prior experience with grief and death. It is hoped that care and support for grieving or dying older persons will improve with increased knowledge and positive attitudes. This improvement should benefit both older adults and nurses, who have much knowledge and wisdom to gain from those who have the most experience in life.

KEY POINTS

- *Grief* is the acute reaction to one's perception of loss, *mourning* is the longer process of resolving acute grief reactions, and *bereavement* is the state of having experienced a significant loss.
- Grief involves many changes over time, is a natural response to all kinds of losses (not just death), and is based on one's unique perception of a loss.
- Worden (2009) views the grief process as active, involving the following four tasks of mourning: (1) accepting the reality of the loss, (2) working through the pain of grief, (3) adjusting to an environment in which the deceased is missing, and (4) emotionally relocating the deceased and moving on with life.
- Human beings respond as whole people, and their grief manifests itself in physical symptoms, psychological responses, changes in socialization patterns, and spiritual issues concerning life's meaning.
- Complicated grief reactions may manifest as one of four types of reactions: (1) chronic, (2) delayed, (3) exaggerated, or (4) masked.
- Nursing care activities that assist in the grieving process include helping the survivor express feelings, providing time to grieve, explaining "normal" grieving behaviors, examining defenses and coping styles, identifying pathologic conditions, and making appropriate referrals.
- Sociocultural and religious background, physical and functional status, social isolation and loneliness, and the meaningfulness of everyday life are all important factors in determining a person's approach to impending death.
- Age-related changes predispose older persons to greater potential problems in areas such as hygiene and skin care, nutrition, elimination, mobility, transfers, rest, sleep, pain, respiratory management, and cognitive and behavioral functioning.
- Nursing strategies for assisting dying older persons include delivering excellent physical care, using good communication skills, conducting a life review, and educating and supporting family caregivers.
- Hospice programs help dying persons live as fully as possible on a day-to-day basis by providing symptom control, addressing the psychological needs of patients, supporting family caregivers, dealing with environmental problems, and assisting patients with spiritual concerns.

CRITICAL-THINKING EXERCISES

1. An 80-year-old woman was admitted to the hospital with pneumonia and weakness. She lives alone; her children are supportive and help her around the house but do not live with her. Her husband of 51 years died within the last 6 months. She is grieving the loss, but she is relieved and feels guilty as he was an abusive spouse. How do you assist her in coping with her loss?

2. A 75-year-old man is dying from metastatic prostate cancer with bone involvement. His family has not been very close, including his children and spouse. They now want to become closer and have as much time with your patient as possible. As the hospice nurse, how do you prepare this family and spouse work through their anticipatory grieving?

REFERENCES

Anderson, F., Downing, G. M., & Hill, J. (1996). Palliative Performance Scale (PPS): a new tool. *Journal of Palliative Care, 12*(1), 5–11.

Balk, D. E. (2013). Life span issues and loss, grief, and mourning: adulthood. In D. K. Meagher & D. E. Balk (Eds.), *Handbook of Thanatology* (ed 2). Northbrook, Il: Association for Death Education and Counseling.

Basanta, W. E. (2002). Advance directives and life-sustaining treatment: a legal primer. *Hematology/Oncology Clinics of North America, 16*(6), 1381–1396.

Beshai, J. A. (2008). Are cross-cultural comparisons of norms on death anxiety valid? *Omega Journal of Death and Dying, 57*(3), 299–313.

Buglass, E. (2012). Grief and bereavement theories. *Nursing Standard, 24*(41), 44–47.

Burbank, P. M. (1992). Assessing meaning in life among older clients: an exploratory study. *Journal of Gerontological Nursing, 18*(9), 19–28.

Butler, R. (1963). The life review: an interpretation of reminiscences in the aged. *Psychiatry, 26*(1), 65.

Centers for Disease Control Fast Facts, leading cause of death in persons aged 65 and over 2016. https://www.cdc.gov/nchs/fastats/older-american-health.htm.

Cole, L. J., Farrell, M. J., Gibson, S. J., & Egan, G. F. (2010). Age-related differences in pain sensitivity and regional brain activity evoked by noxious pressure. *Neurobiology of Aging, 31*(3), 494–503.

Corless, I. (2010). Bereavement. In B. R. Ferrell & N. Coyle (Eds.), *Textbook of Palliative Nursing* (3rd ed.). New York: Oxford University Press.

Corr, C. A., & Corr, D. M. (2013). *Death and dying, life and living* (7th ed.). Belmont, CA: Wadsworth.

Costello, J. (2001). Nursing older dying patients: findings from an ethnographic study of death and dying in elderly care wards. *Journal of Advanced Nursing, 35*(1), 59–68.

Craun, M. J., Watkins, M., & Hefty, A. (1997). Hospice care of the psychotic patient. *The American Journal of Hospice & Palliative Care, 14*(4), 205.

Csordas, T. J., & Kleinman, A. (1990). The therapeutic process. In T. Johnson & C. Sargent (Eds.), *Medical anthropology: contemporary theory and method.* New York: Praeger.

D'Avanzo, C. E. (2008). *Mosby's pocket guide to cultural assessment* (4th ed.). St. Louis, MO: Mosby.

Dalai, S., Del Fabbro, E., & Bruera, E. (2009). Is there a role for hydration at the end of life? *Current Opinion in Supportive and Palliative Care, 3*(1), 72–78.

Daoust, R., Paquet, J., Piette, É., Sanogo, K., Bailey, B., & Chauny, J. M. (2016). Impact of age on pain perception for typical painful diagnoses in the emergency department. *Journal of Emergency Medicine., 50*(1), 14–20. https://doi.org/10.1016/j.jemermed.2015.06.074.

Derby, S., O'Mahoney, S., & Tickoo, R. (2010). Elderly patients. In B. R. Ferrell & N. Coyle (Eds.), *Textbook of Palliative Nursing* (3rd ed.). New York, NY: Oxford University Press.

DeSpelder, L. A., & Strickland, A. L. (2010). *The last dance: encouraging death and dying* (9th ed.). Mountain View, Calif: Mayfield.

Doka, K. J., & Davidson, J. D. (1998). *Living with grief: who we are, how we grieve.* Washington, DC: Hospice Foundation of America.

Doka, K. J. (2013). Historical and contemporary perspectives on loss, grief, and mourning. In D. K. Meagher & D. E. Balk (Eds.), *Handbook of Thanatology* (2nd ed.). Northbrook, Il: Association for Death Education and Counseling.

Doka, K. J. (1993). The spiritual needs of the dying. In K. J. Doka (Ed.), *Death and spirituality.* Amityville, NY: Baywood.

Egan City, K. A., & Labyak, M. J. (2010). Hospice palliative care for the 21st century: A model for quality end-of-life care. In B. R. Ferrell & N. Coyle (Eds.), *Textbook of Palliative Nursing* (3rd ed.). New York: Oxford University Press.

Emanuel, L. L., Ferris, F. D., von Gunten, C. F., Hauser, J. M., & Von Roenn, J. H. (2015). *The last hours of living: Practical advice for clinicians.* Retrieved January 4, 2018, from https://www.medscape.com/viewarticle/716463_4.

Erikson, E. (1963). *Childhood and society.* New York: WW Norton.

Feil, N., & Altman, R. (2004). Validation theory and the myth of the therapeutic lie. *American Journal of Alzheimer's Disease and Other Dementias, 19*(2), 77–78.

Feil, N. (1993). *The validation breakthrough.* Baltimore: Health Professions Press.

Ferrell, B. A., Ferrell, B. R., & Osterweil, D. (1990). Pain in the nursing home. *Journal of the American Geriatric Society, 38*, 409–414.

Field, D. (2000). Older people's attitudes towards death in England. *Mortality, 5*(3), 278–297.

Garrett, J. E. (1987). Multiple losses in older adults. *Journal of Gerontological Nursing, 13*(8), 8.

Gott, M., Seymour, J., Bellamy, G., et al. (2004). Older people's views about home as a place of care at the end of life. *Palliative Medicine, 18*, 460–467.

Hall, S. E. (1997). Spiritual diversity: a challenge for hospice chaplains. *The American Journal of Hospice & Palliative Care, 14*(5), 221.

Hansen, M. J. (2009). A palliative care intervention in forgiveness therapy for elderly terminally ill cancer patients. *Journal of Palliative Care, 25*(1), 51–60.

Hermann, C. P. (2006). Development and testing of the Spiritual Needs Inventory for patients near the end of life. *Oncology Nursing Forum, 33*(4), 737–744.

Herr, K. (2011). Pain assessment strategies in older patients. *The Journal of Pain, 12*(3). Supplement, S3-S13.

Hibberd, R. (2013). Meaning reconstruction in bereavement: Sense and significance. *Death Studies, 37*(7), 670–692.

Holland, J. M., Currier, J. M., & Neimeyer, R. A. (2006). Meaning reconstruction in the first two years of bereavement: the role of sense-making and benefit-finding. *Omega, 53*, 174–191.

Hospice and Palliative Nurses Association. (2011). *HPNA Position Statement Artificial Nutrition and Hydration in Advanced Illness.* Retrieved October 18, 2017 from http://hpna.advancingexpertcare.org/wp-content/uploads/2014/09/Artificial-Nutrition-and-Hydration-in-Advanced-Illness-FINAL.

Huber, R., & Bryant, J. (1996). The 10-Mile Mourning Bridge and the Brief Symptom Inventory: close relatives? *The Hospice Journal, 11*(2), 31.

Huber, R., & Gibson, J. (1990). New evidence for anticipatory grief. *The Hospice Journal, 6*(1), 49.

Hughes, R. G., Bakos, A. D., O'Mara, A., & Kovner, C. T. (2005). Palliative wound care at the end of life. *Home Health Care Management & Practice, 17*(3), 196–202.

Kastenbaum, R. (1978). Death, dying and bereavement in older age. *Aged Care & Services Review, 1*(3), 1.

Kissane, D. W., McKenzie, M., McKenzie, D. P., Forbes, A., O'Neill, I., & Bloch, S. (2003). Psychological morbidity associated with patterns of family functioning in palliative care: Baseline data from the Family Focused Grief Therapy controlled trial. *Palliative Medicine, 17*(6), 527–537.

Klass, D., Silverman, P. R., & Nickman, S. L. (2006). *Continuing bonds: new understandings of grief.* Washington, DC: Taylor & Francis.

Kübler-Ross, E. (1969). *On death and dying.* New York: Macmillan.

Landman, J. (1993). *Regret: the persistence of the possible.* New York: Oxford University Press.

Lindemann, E. (1944). Symptoms and management of acute grief. *The American Journal of Psychology, 101*, 141.

Lloyd-Williams, M., Kennedy, V., Sixsmith, A., & Sixsmith, J. (2007). The end of life: a qualitative study of the perceptions of people over the age of 80 on issues surrounding death and dying. *Journal of Pain and Symptom Management, 34*(1), 60–66.

Lund, D. A. (1989). Conclusions about bereavement in later life and implications for interventions and future research. In D. A. Lund (Ed.), *Older bereaved spouses: research with practical applications.* New York: Hemisphere.

Madnawat, A. V. S., & Kachhawa, P. S. (2007). Age, gender, and living circumstances: discriminating older adults on death anxiety. *Death Studies, 31*, 763–769.

Moadel, A., Morgan, C., Fatone, A., et al. (1999). Seeking meaning and hope: self-reported spiritual and existential needs among an ethnically diverse cancer patient population. *Psychooncology, 8,* 378–385.

National Consensus Project for Quality Palliative Care. (2013). Clinical Practice Guidelines for Quality Palliative Care (3rd ed.). Pittsburgh, PA: Author.

Neimeyer, R. A. (2000). Searching for the meaning of meaning: grief therapy and the process of reconstruction. *Death Studies, 24,* 541–558.

Patlamazoglou, L., Simmonds, J. G., Snell, T. L. (2017) Same-sex partner bereavement: non-HIV-related loss and new research directions. *OMEGA - Journal of Death and Dying.* Retrieved January 25, 2017, from https://doi-org.proxy.lib.aurora.org/10.1177/0030222817690160.

Payne, S. A., Langley-Evans, A., & Hillier, R. (1996). Perceptions of a good death: a comparative study of the views of hospice staff and patients. *Palliative Medicine, 10,* 307–312.

Rando, T. A. (Ed.), (1986). *Loss and anticipatory grief.* Lexington, Mass: Lexington Books.

Rando, T. A. (1988). *Grieving: how to go on living when someone you love dies.* Lexington, Mass: DC Heath.

Retsinas, J. (1988). The theoretical reassessment of the applicability of Kübler-Ross' stages of dying. *Death Studies, 12,* 207.

Reynolds, K., Henderson, M., Schuman, A., & Hanson, L. C. (2002). Needs of the dying in nursing homes. *Journal of Palliative Medicine,* 5(6), 895–901.

Steinhauser, K. E., Christakis, N. A., Clipp, E. C., et al. (2000). Factors considered important at the end of life by patients, family physicians, and other care providers. *JAMA, 284,* 2476–2482.

Stroebe, W., & Schut, H. (2001). Risk factors in bereavement outcome: a methodological and empirical review. In M. Stroebe, R. O. Hansson, W. Stroebe, & H. Schut (Eds.), *Handbook of bereavement research.* Washington, DC: American Psychological Association Press.

Teno, J. M., Gozalo, P. L., Bynum, J. P., Leland, N. E., Miller, S., Morden, N. E., et al. (2013). Change in end-of-life care for medicare beneficiaries site of death, place of care, and health care transitions in 2000, 2005, and 2009. *JAMA 2013, 309*(5), 470–477. https://doi.org/10.1001/jama.2012.207624.

The Joint Commission. (2016). Joint Commission statement on pain management. Retrieved January 4, 2018, from https://www.jointcommission.org/joint_commission_statement_on_pain_management/.

Touhy, T. A., & Jett, K. F. (2016). *Ebersole & Hess' Toward healthy aging: Human needs and nursing response* (9th ed.). St Louis: Mosby Elsevier.

Upadhyaya, R. C., & Kautz, D. D. (2009). Appreciating diversity and enhancing intimacy. In K. Mauk (Ed.), *Introduction to Gerontological Nursing.* Boston: Jones & Bartlett.

Victoria Hospice Society. (2008). *Bereavement risk assessment tool (BRAT).* Retrieved November 8, 2013, from http://www.victoriahospice.org/health-professionals/clinical-tools.

Weitzner, M. A., Moody, L. N., & McMillan, S. C. (2003). Symptom management issues in hospice care. *The American Journal of Hospice & Palliative Care, 14*(4), 190.

Wiech, K., & Tracey, I. (2009). The influence of negative emotions on pain: behavioral effects and neural mechanisms. *NeuroImage, 47*(3), 987–994.

Winter, L., Parker, B., & Schneider, M. (2007). Imagining the alternatives to life prolonging treatments: elders' beliefs about the dying experience. *Death Studies, 31,* 619–631.

Wittenberg-Lyles, E. M., & Sanchez-Reilly, S. (2008). Palliative care for elderly patients with advanced cancer: a long-term intervention for end-of-life care. *Patient Education and Counseling, 71,* 351–355.

Wong, F. K. Y., Liu, C. F., Szeto, Y., et al. (2004). Health problems encountered by dying patients receiving palliative home care until death. *Cancer Nursing, 27*(3), 244–250.

Worden, J. W. (2009). *Grief counseling and grief therapy: A handbook for the mental health practitioner* (4th ed.). New York: Springer.

World Health Organization. (2017). WHO's cancer pain ladder for adults. Retrieved October 18, 2017, from http://www.who.int/cancer/palliative/painladder/en/.

World Health Organization. (n.d.) WHO definition of palliative care. Retrieved November 6, 2013, from http://www.who.int/cancer/palliative/definition/en/.

Yadav K. N., et al. (2017). Approximately One In Three US Adults Completes Any Type Of Advance Directive For End-Of-Life Care. *Health Affairs (Project Hope) 36*(7), 1244–1251. https://doi.org/10.1377/hlthaff.2017.0175.

Yalom, V. (2010). Kenneth Doka on grief counseling and psychotherapy [Interview]. Retrieved January 4, 2018, from https://www.psychotherapy.net/interview/grief-counseling-doka.

Young, M., & Cullen, L. (1996). *A good death: conversations with East Londoners.* London: Routledge.

Values History Form

It is important that your medical treatment be your choice.

The purpose of this form is to assist you in thinking about and writing down what is important to you about your health. If you should at some time become unable to make health care decisions, this form may help others make a decision for you in accordance with your values.

The first section of this packet offers suggestions for using the Values History Form.

The second section, the form itself, provides an opportunity for you to discuss your values, wishes, and preferences in a number of different areas, such as your personal relationships, your overall attitude toward life, and your thoughts about illness.

The third section of this packet provides a space for indicating whether you have completed an Advance Directive (e.g., an Advance Directive for Health Care, a Living Will, Durable Power of Attorney for Health Care Decisions, or Health Care Proxy) and where such documents may be found.

Name: _____

Date: _____

If someone assisted you in completing this form, please fill in his or her name, address, and relationship to you.

Name: _____

Address: _____

Relationship: _____

From Center for Health and Law Ethics, Institute of Public Law, University of New Mexico, Albuquerque. Retrieved from http://hscethics.unm.edu/common/pdf/values-history.pdf.

OVERALL ATTITUDE TOWARD LIFE AND HEALTH

- What would you like to say to someone reading this document about your overall attitude toward life?
- What goals do you have for the future?
- How satisfied are you with what you have achieved in your life?
- What, for you, makes life worth living?
- What do you fear most? What frightens or upsets you?
- What activities do you enjoy (e.g., hobbies, watching TV, etc.)?
- How would you describe your current state of health?
- If you currently have any health problems or disabilities, how do they affect: you, your family, your work, your ability to function?
- If you have health problems or disabilities, how do you feel about them?
- What would you like others (family, friends, doctors) to know about this?
- Do you have difficulties in getting through the day and performing activities such as: eating, preparing food, sleeping, dressing, bathing, etc.?

- What would you like to say, about your general health, to someone reading this document?

PERSONAL RELATIONSHIPS

- What role do family and friends play in your life?
- How do you expect friends, family, and others to support your decisions regarding medical treatment you may need now or in the future?
- Have you made any arrangements for family or friends to make medical treatment decisions on your behalf? If so, who has agreed to make decisions for you and in what circumstances?
- What general comments would you like to make about the personal relationships in your life?

THOUGHTS ABOUT INDEPENDENCE AND SELF-SUFFICIENCY

- How does independence or dependence affect your life?
- If you were to experience decreased physical and mental abilities, how would that affect your attitude toward independence and self-sufficiency?
- If your current physical or mental health gets worse, how would you feel?

LIVING ENVIRONMENT

- Have you lived alone or with others over the last 10 years?
- How comfortable have you been in your surroundings? How might illness, disability, or age affect this?
- What general comments would you like to make about your surroundings?

RELIGIOUS BACKGROUND AND BELIEFS

- What is your spiritual/religious background?
- How do your beliefs affect your feelings toward serious, chronic, or terminal illness?
- How does your faith community, church, or synagogue support you?
- What general comments would you like to make about your beliefs?

RELATIONSHIPS WITH DOCTORS AND OTHER HEALTH CAREGIVERS

- How do you relate to your doctors? Please comment on: trust, decision making, time for satisfactory communication, and respectful treatment.
- How do you feel about other health care providers, including nurses, therapists, chaplains, social workers, etc.?
- What else would you like to say about doctors and other health care providers?

THOUGHTS ABOUT ILLNESS, DYING, AND DEATH

- What general comments would you like to make about illness, dying, and death?
- What will be important to you when you are dying (e.g., physical comfort, no pain, family members present, etc.)?
- Where would you prefer to die?
- How do you feel about the use of life-sustaining measures if you were suffering from an irreversible chronic illness (e.g., Alzheimer's disease), terminally ill, or in a permanent coma?
- What general comments would you like to make about medical treatment?

FINANCES

- What general comments would you like to make about your finances and the cost of health care?
- What are your feelings about having enough money to provide for your care?

FUNERAL PLANS

- What general comments would you like to make about your funeral and burial or cremation?

- Have you made your funeral arrangements? If so, with whom?

OPTIONAL QUESTIONS

- How would you like your obituary (announcement of your death) to read?
- Write yourself a brief eulogy (a statement about yourself to be read at your funeral).
- What would you like to say to someone reading this Values History Form?

LEGAL DOCUMENTS

- What legal documents about health care decisions have you signed? (Each state has its own special form. Feel free to add yours to the list.)
- Advance Directive for Health Care? Yes___ No___ Where and with whom can it be found?
  Name: _____
  Address: _____
  Phone: _____
- Living Will? Yes___ No___ Where and with whom can it be found?
  Name: _____
  Address: _____
  Phone: _____
- Durable Power of Attorney for Health Care Decisions? Yes___ No___ Where and with whom can it be found?
  Name: _____
  Address: _____
  Phone: _____
- Health Care Proxy? Yes___ No___ Where and with whom can it be found?
  Name: _____
  Address: _____
  Phone: _____

U.S. Advocacy Organizations for Older Adults

ORGANIZATIONS OF OLDER ADULTS

AARP
601 E Street NW
Washington, DC 20049
(888) 687-2277

Older Women's League (OWL)
666 11th Street NW
Washington, DC 20001
(202) 567-2606

ORGANIZATIONS OF PROFESSIONALS WORKING IN THE FIELD OF AGING

American Health Care Association
1201 L Street NW
Washington, DC 20005-4014
(202) 842-4444

Gerontological Society of America
1220 L Street NW, Suite 901
Washington, DC 20005
(202) 842-1275

Hispanic Council on Aging
734 15th Street NW, Suite 1050
Washington, DC 20005
(202) 347-9733

National Association of Professional Geriatric Care Managers
3275 W. Ina Road, Suite 130
Tucson, AZ 85741-2198
(520) 881-8008

National Association of Social Workers
750 First Street NE, Suite 800
Washington, DC 20002
(800) 742-4089

National Gerontological Nursing Association
121 W. State Street
Geneva, IL 60134
(630) 748-4616

ORGANIZATIONS OF BOTH PROFESSIONALS AND OLDER ADULTS

Alzheimer's Association
225 N. Michigan Avenue, Fl. 17
Chicago, IL 60601
(800) 272-3900

American Society on Aging
575 Market Street, Suite 2100
San Francisco, CA 94105-2869
(415) 974-9600

National Council on Aging (NCOA) (includes National Institute of Senior Citizens and National Institute on Adult Day Care)
251 18th Street South, Suite 500
Arlington, VA 22202
(571) 527-3900

Chronic Illness and Rehabilitation Resources

AARP
601 E Street NW
Washington, DC 20049
(888) 687-2277
http://www.aarp.org

ADA Information Line
(800) 514-0301 (voice)
(800) 514-0383 TTY
http://www.ada.gov

Administration for Community Living
330 C Street SW
Washington, DC 20201
(202) 401-4634
https://www.acl.gov

Alzheimer's Association National Office
225 N. Michigan Avenue, Fl. 17
Chicago, IL 60601
(800) 272-3900 (24/7 help line)
www.alz.org

American Academy of Physical Medicine and Rehabilitation
330 N. Wabash Avenue, Suite 2500
Chicago, IL 60611-7617
(847) 737-6000
www.aapmr.org

American Parkinson Disease Association
135 Parkinson Avenue
Staten Island, NY 10305
(800) 223-2732
www.apdaparkinson.org

Arthritis Foundation
PO Box 7669
Atlanta, GA 30357-0669
(800) 283-7800
www.arthritis.org

Association of Rehabilitation Nurses
8735 W. Higgins Road, Suite 300
Chicago, IL 60631-2738
(800) 229-7530
www.rehabnurse.org

National Council on Disability
1331 F Street NW, Suite 850
Washington, DC 20004
(202) 272-2004
(202) 272-2074 TTY
www.ncd.gov

National Institute on Aging
Building 31, Room 5C27
31 Center Drive, MSC 2292
Bethesda, MD 20892
(800) 222-2225
(800) 222-4225 TTY
www.nia.nih.gov

National Stroke Association
9707 E. Easter Lane
Centennial, CO 80112
(800) STROKES
(800) 787-6537
www.stroke.org

INDEX

Note: Page numbers followed by *f* indicate figures, *t* indicate tables, and *b* indicate boxes.

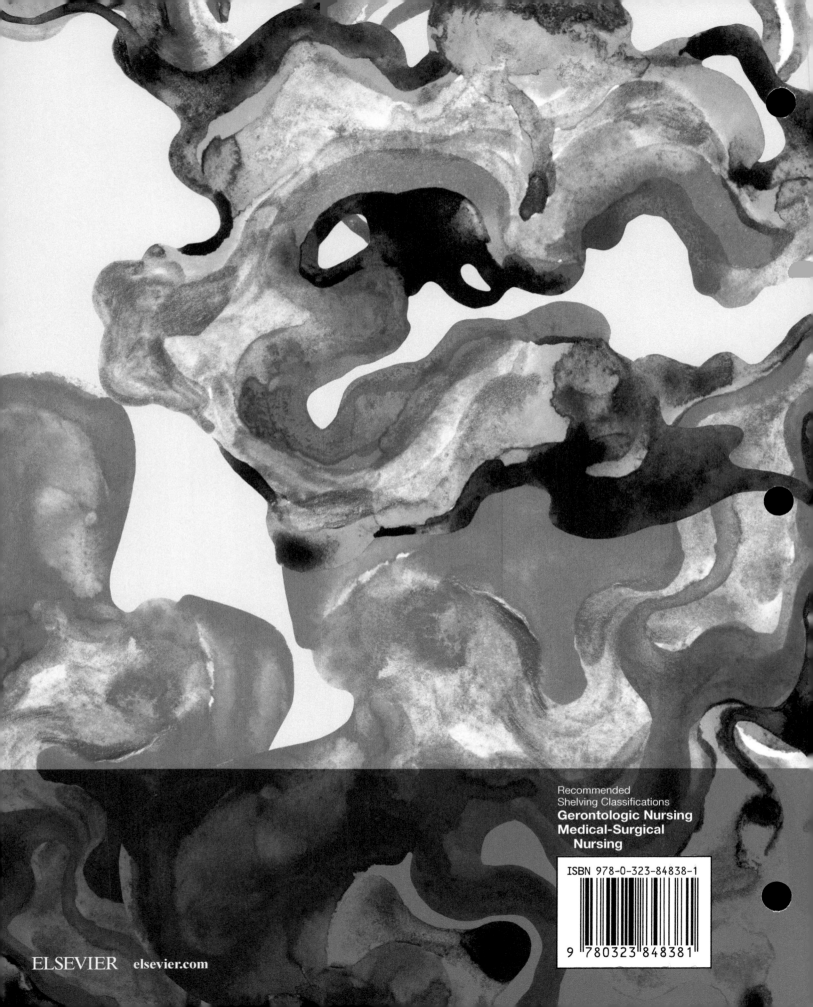

Recommended
Shelving Classifications
Gerontologic Nursing
Medical-Surgical
Nursing

ISBN 978-0-323-84838-1

9 780323 848381

ELSEVIER   elsevier.com